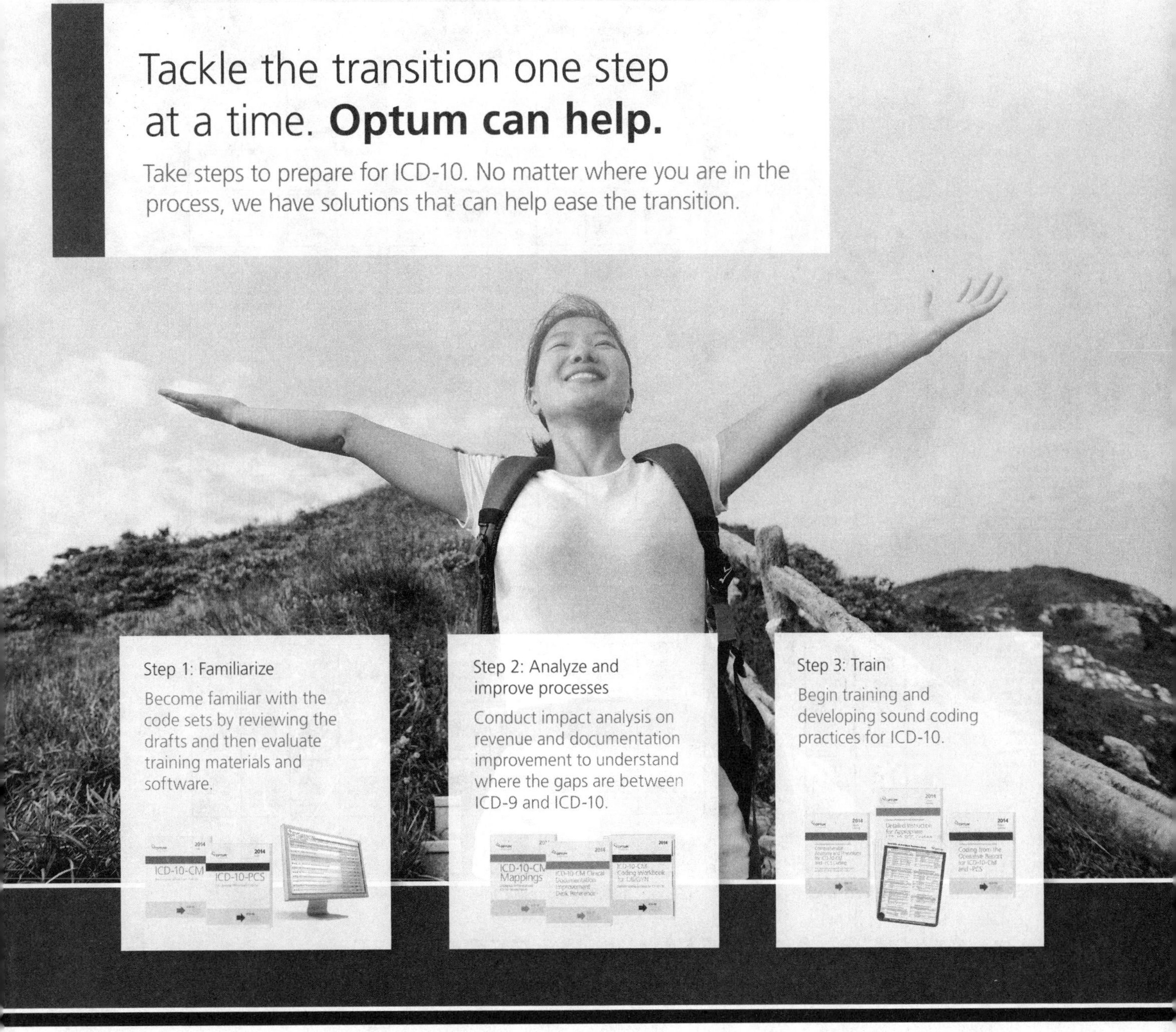

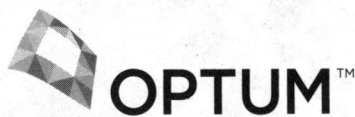

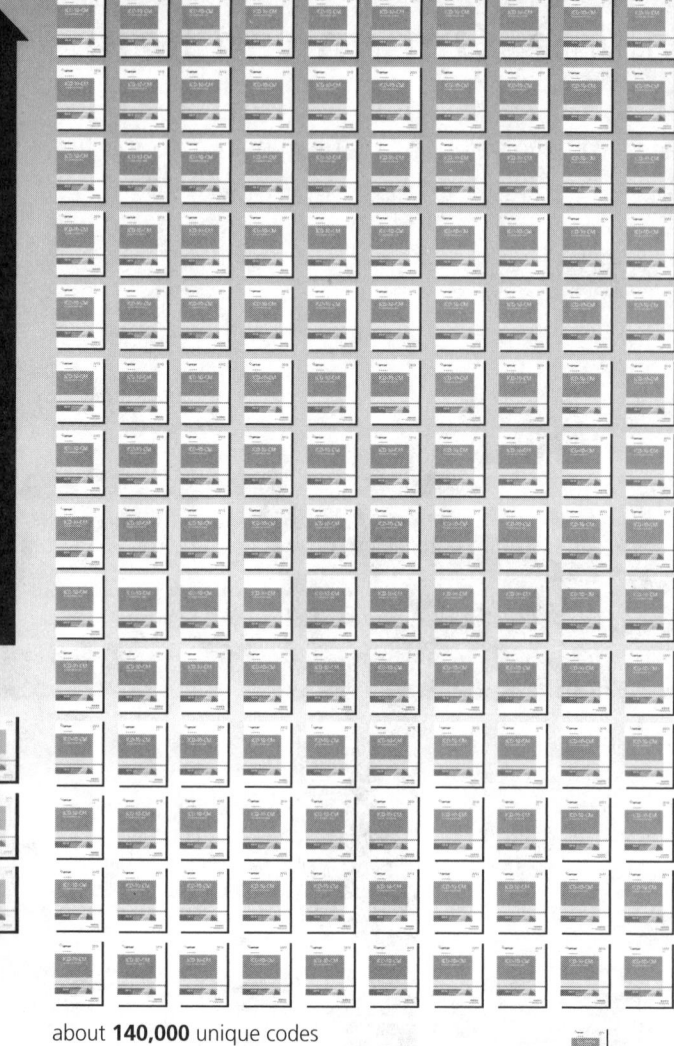
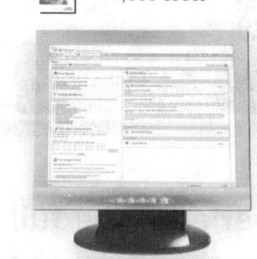

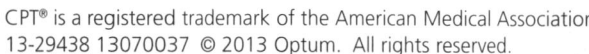
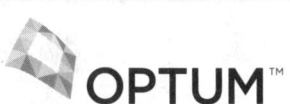

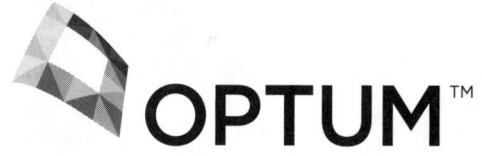

September 2013

Dear Optum Customer:

This is your FY 2014 draft of the *ICD-10-PCS: The Complete Official Draft Code Set*.

The Centers for Medicare and Medicaid Services (CMS) is the agency charged with maintaining and updating the International Procedure Coding System (ICD-10-PCS). This FY 2014 draft represents the most current changes to the ICD-10-PCS as released by CMS.

Remember, the codes in ICD-10-PCS are not currently valid for any documentation or reporting of health care services.

The Department of Health and Human Services (HHS) published the final rule regarding the adoption of both ICD-10-CM and ICD-10-PCS in the January 16, 2009, *Federal Register* (45 CFR part 162 [CMS—0013—F]). The compliance date for implementation of ICD-10-CM and ICD-10-PCS as a replacement for ICD-9-CM was October 1, 2013. On April 17, 2012, the Department of Health and Human Services (HHS) released a notice to postpone the date by which certain health care entities must comply with ICD-10 diagnosis and procedure codes. The compliance date for implementation of ICD-10-CM and ICD-10-PCS as a replacement for ICD-9-CM is now October 1, 2014.

ICD-10-PCS will replace ICD-9-CM volume 3, including the official coding guidelines, for the following procedures or other actions taken for diseases, injuries, and impairments on **hospital inpatients reported by hospitals**: prevention, diagnosis, treatment, and management.

We appreciate your choosing Optum to meet your ICD-10-PCS conversion preparation and coding training needs. If you have any questions or comments concerning your draft *ICD-10-PCS: The Complete Official Draft Code Set*, please do not hesitate to call our customer service department. The toll-free number is 1-800-464-3649, option 1.

2525 Lake Park Blvd. • Salt Lake City, UT 84120 • 800.464.3649 • Fax 801.982.4033

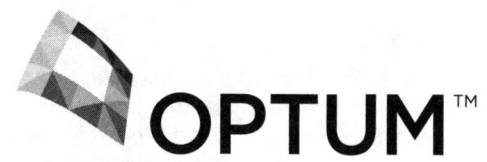

ICD-10-PCS
The Complete Official Draft
Code Set

2014

Notice

ICD-10-PCS: The Complete Official Draft Code Set is designed to be an accurate and authoritative source regarding coding and every reasonable effort has been made to ensure accuracy and completeness of the content. However, Optum makes no guarantee, warranty, or representation that this publication is accurate, complete, or without errors. It is understood that Optum is not rendering any legal or other professional services or advice in this publication and that Optum bears no liability for any results or consequences that may arise from the use of this book. Please address all correspondence to:

Optum
2525 Lake Park Blvd
Salt Lake City, UT 84120

Our Commitment to Accuracy

Optum is committed to producing accurate and reliable materials. To report corrections, please visit www.optumcoding.com/accuracy or email accuracy@optum.com. You can also reach customer service by calling 1.800.464.3649, option 1.

Copyright

Acknowledgments

Anita C. Hart, RHIA, CCS, CCS-P, *Product Manager*
Karen Schmidt, BSN, *Technical Director*
Stacy Perry, *Manager, Desktop Publishing*
Tracy Betzler, *Senior Desktop Publishing Specialist*
Hope M. Dunn, *Senior Desktop Publishing Specialist*
Katie Russell, *Desktop Publishing Specialist*
Kate Holden, *Editor*

Anita C. Hart, RHIA, CCS, CCS-P

Ms. Hart's experience includes 15 years conducting and publishing research in clinical medicine and human genetics for Yale University, Massachusetts General Hospital, and Massachusetts Institute of Technology. Her research conclusions have been published in several peer-reviewed journals. In addition, Ms. Hart has supervised medical records management, health information management, coding and reimbursement, and workers' compensation issues as the office manager for a physical therapy rehabilitation clinic. Ms. Hart is an expert in physician and facility coding, reimbursement systems, and compliance issues. She is also the author of the several Optum publications and has served as subject matter advisor on numerous other publications for hospital and physician practices. Ms. Hart is the ICD-9-CM and ICD-10-CM/PCS subject matter expert for the Optum, has served as the product manager for that product line for 15 years, and has presented at numerous national conferences. Ms. Hart is a member of the AAPC and a fully credentialed active member of the American Health Information Management Association (AHIMA). Ms Hart is a current AHIMA Approved ICD-10-CM/PCS Trainer and leads the training initiatives within Optum's Coding Solutions business unit.

Contents

Preface

This draft of the International Classification of Diseases, 10th Revision, Procedure Coding System (ICD-10-PCS) has been developed as a replacement for volume 3 of the International Classification of Diseases, Ninth Revision (ICD-9-CM). The development of ICD-10-PCS was funded by the U.S. Centers for Medicare and Medicaid Services under contract nos. 90-138, 91-22300 500-95-0005 and HHSM-550-2004-00011C to 3M Health Information Systems. ICD-10-PCS has a multi-axial, seven-character, alphanumeric code structure that provides a unique code for all substantially different procedures and allows new procedures to be easily incorporated as new codes. The initial draft was formally tested and evaluated by an independent contractor; the final version was released in 1998, with annual updates since the final release.

What's New for 2014

The Centers for Medicare and Medicaid Services is the agency charged with maintaining and updating ICD-10-PCS. CMS released the most current revisions, a summary of which may be found on the CMS website at: http://cms.hhs.gov/Medicare/Coding/ICD10/2014-ICD-10-PCS.html.

Due to the unique structure of ICD-10-PCS, a change in a character value may affect individual codes and several code tables.

Change Summary Table

2013 Total	New Codes	Revised Titles	Deleted Codes	2014 Total
71,920	7	0	3	71,924

ICD-10-PCS Code 2013 Totals, by Section

Medical and Surgical	61,898
Obstetrics	300
Placement	861
Administration	1,388
Measurement and Monitoring	339
Extracorporeal Assistance and Performance	41
Extracorporeal Therapies	42
Osteopathic	100
Other Procedures	60
Chiropractic	90
Imaging	2,934
Nuclear Medicine	463
Radiation Oncology	1,939
Rehabilitation and Diagnostic Audiology	1,380
Mental Health	30
Substance Abuse Treatment	59
Total	**71,924**

ICD-10-PCS Code Changes

- Four codes added under new technology application, valid October 1, 2013:
  — **08H005Z** Insertion of Epiretinal Visual Prosthesis into Right Eye, Open Approach
  — **08H105Z** Insertion of Epiretinal Visual Prosthesis into Left Eye, Open Approach
  — **30280B1** Transfusion of Nonautologous 4-Factor Prothrombin Complex Concentrate into Vein, Open Approach
  — **30283B1** Transfusion of Nonautologous 4-Factor Prothrombin Complex Concentrate into Vein, Percutaneous Approach

- Three new codes added and three codes deleted to correct body part value for temporary occlusion of abdominal aorta:
  — New: **04V00DJ** Restriction of Abdominal Aorta with Intraluminal Device, Temporary, Open Approach
  — New: **04V03DJ** Restriction of Abdominal Aorta with Intraluminal Device, Temporary, Percutaneous Approach
  — New: **04V04DJ** Restriction of Abdominal Aorta with Intraluminal Device, Temporary, Percutaneous Endoscopic Approach
  — Deleted: **02VW0DJ** Restriction of Thoracic Aorta with Intraluminal Device, Temporary, Open Approach
  — Deleted: **02VW3DJ** Restriction of Thoracic Aorta with Intraluminal Device, Temporary, Percutaneous Approach
  — Deleted: **02VW4DJ** Restriction of Thoracic Aorta with Intraluminal Device, Temporary, Percutaneous Endoscopic Approach

Revised Section Title

- Section title for "Radiation Oncology" revised to "Radiation Therapy" in response to public comment
  — Because the phrase "Radiation Oncology" is not used in code titles, no code titles were revised as a result of the section title change.

New Index Entries

Biopsy

Add	Bone Marrow *see* Extraction with qualifier Diagnostic

Denticulate Ligament

Revise	Denticulate Ligament *use* Spinal Cord
Revise	Denticulate Ligament *use* Spinal Meninges

Epiretinal Visual Prosthesis

Add	Epiretinal Visual Prosthesis
Add	*use* Epiretinal Visual Prosthesis in Eye
Add	Insertion of device in
Add	Left 08H105Z
Add	Right 08H005Z

Femoropatellar Joint

Add	*use* Joint, Knee, Right, Femoral Surface
Add	*use* Joint, Knee, Left, Femoral Surface

Femorotibial Joint

Add	*use* Joint, Knee, Right, Tibial Surface
Add	*use* Joint, Knee, Left, Tibial Surface

Hearing Device

Insertion of device in

Delete	Bone	
Delete		Left 0NH6[034]SZ
Delete		Right 0NH5[034]SZ
Delete	Ear	
Delete		Left 09HE[034]SZ
Delete		Right 09HD[034]SZ
Add		Right 0NH5[034]SZ
Delete	Removal of device from	
Delete		Ear
Delete		Left 09PE[078]SZ
Delete		Right 09PD[078]SZ
Delete	Skull 0NP0	
Delete	Revision of device in	
Delete		Ear
Delete		Left 09WE[078]SZ
Delete		Right 09WD[078]SZ
Delete		Skull 0NW0
Add	Removal of device from, Skull 0NP0	
Add	Revision of device in, Skull 0NW0	

Hyperthermia

Delete	Radiation Oncology
Add	Radiation Therapy

Impella®

Add	Impella® (2.5)(5.0)(LD) Cardiac Assist Device *use* Intraluminal Device

Laminotomy

Add	*see* Release, Central Nervous System 00N
Add	*see* Release, Peripheral Nervous System 01N

MicroMed HeartAssist

Add	MicroMed HeartAssist *use* Implantable Heart Assist System in Heart and Great Vessels

Patellofemoral Joint

Add	*use* Joint, Knee, Right
Add	*use* Joint, Knee, Left
Add	*use* Joint, Knee, Right, Femoral Surface
Add	*use* Joint, Knee, Left, Femoral Surface

Pneumonectomy

Revise	Pneumonectomy *see* Excision, Respiratory System 0BB

PVAD™ Ventricular Assist Device

Delete	PVAD™ Ventricular Assist Device *use* External Heart Assist System in Heart and Great Vessels

Radiation Oncology

Delete	Radiation Oncology
Delete	*see* Beam Radiation
Delete	*see* Brachytherapy

Radiation Therapy

Add	Radiation Therapy
Add	*see* Beam Radiation
Add	*see* Brachytherapy

Rectocele Repair

Revise	Rectocele Repair *see* Repair, Subcutaneous Tissue and Fascia, Pelvic Region 0JQC
Delete	*see* Repair, Subcutaneous Tissue and Fascia, Pelvic Region 0JQC

Restriction

Aorta

Revise	Thoracic 02VW[034][CDZ]Z

Spinal Nerve, Cervical

Add	Spinal Nerve, Cervical *use* Nerve, Cervical

Spinal Nerve, Lumbar

Add	Spinal Nerve, Lumbar *use* Nerve, Lumbar

Spinal Nerve, Sacral

Add	Spinal Nerve, Sacral *use* Nerve, Sacral

Spinal Nerve, Thoracic

Add	Spinal Nerve, Thoracic *use* Nerve, Thoracic

TandemHeart® System

Revise	TandemHeart® System *use* External Heart Assist System in Heart and Great Vessels

Thoratec Paracorporeal Ventricular Assist Device

Add	Thoratec Paracorporeal Ventricular Assist Device *use* External Heart Assist System in Heart and Great Vessels

Tibiofemoral Joint

Add	Tibiofemoral Joint
Add	*use* Joint, Knee, Right, Tibial Surface
Add	*use* Joint, Knee, Left, Tibial Surface
Add	*use* Joint, Knee, Right
Add	*use* Joint, Knee, Left

Transfusion

Vein

Add	4-Factor Prothrombin Complex Concentrate 3028[03]B1

New Definitions Addenda

Body Part Key

Term		Includes	
	Cervical Nerve	Add	Spinal nerve, cervical
	Knee Joint, Femoral Surface, Left	Add	Femoropatellar joint
	Knee Joint, Femoral Surface, Right	Add	Patellofemoral joint
	Knee Joint, Left	Add	Patellofemoral joint
	Knee Joint, Right	Add	Tibiofemoral joint
	Knee Joint, Tibial Surface, Left	Add	Femorotibial joint
	Knee Joint, Tibial Surface, Right	Add	Tibiofemoral joint
	Lumbar Nerve	Add	Spinal nerve, lumbar
Delete	Spinal Cord	Delete	Denticulate ligament
Add	Sacral Nerve	Add	Spinal nerve, sacral
	Spinal Meninges	Add	Denticulate ligament
	Thoracic Nerve	Add	Spinal nerve, thoracic

Device Key

Device		PCS Description	
Add	Epiretinal Visual Prosthesis in Eye	Add	Epiretinal visual prosthesis
	External Heart Assist System in Heart and Great Vessels	Delete	PVAD™ Ventricular Assist Device
		Add	TandemHeart® System
		Add	Thoratec Paracorporeal Ventricular Assist Device
	Implantable Heart Assist System in Heart and Great Vessels	Add	MicroMed HeartAssist
	Intraluminal Device	Delete	TandemHeart® System
		Add	Impella® (2.5)(5.0)(LD) cardiac assist device

Device Aggregation Table

Specific Device		For Operation		In Body System		General Device	
Add	Epiretinal Visual Prosthesis	Add	All applicable	Add	Eye	Add	Synthetic Substitute

List of Updated Files

2014 Official ICD-10-PCS Coding Guidelines
- Downloadable PDF file
- Revised in response to public comment and review by the Cooperating Parties

2014 ICD-10-PCS Code Tables and Index (Zip file)
- Downloadable PDF file, file name is PCS_2014.pdf
- Downloadable xml files for developers, file names are icd10pcs_tabular_2014.xml, icd10pcs_index_2014.xml, icd10pcs_definitions_2014.xml
- Accompanying schema for developers, file names are icd10pcs_tabular_2014.xsd, icd10pcs_index_2014.xsd, icd10pcs_definitions_2014.xsd

2014 ICD-10-PCS Code Titles, Long and Abbreviated (Zip file)
- Tabular order file defines an unambiguous order for all ICD-10-CM/PCS codes
- Text file format, file name is icd10pcs_order_2014.txt
- Provides a unique five-digit "order number" for each ICD-10-PCS table and code
- Accompanying documentation, file name is ICD10OrderFiles.pdf

2014 ICD-10-PCS Final Addenda (Zip file)
- New code titles for FY2014 shown as ICD-10-PCS table entries, file name is: PcsAddendaAdditionsNewLabels.pdf
- Deleted code titles for FY2014 shown as ICD-10-PCS table entries, file name is: PcsAddendaDeletionsOldLabels.pdf
- Downloadable xml format for developers, file names are: PcsAddendaAdditionsNewLabels.xml, PcsAddendaDeletionsOldLabels.xml
- Accompanying documentation, file name is pcs_addenda_readme2014.pdf

- Index addenda in downloadable PDF, file name is index_addenda_2014.pdf
- PCS Definitions addenda in downloadable PDF, file name is: definitions_addenda_2014.pdf
- Index and Definitions addenda in machine readable text format for developers, file names are index_addenda_2014.txt, definitions_addenda_2014.txt

2014 ICD-10-PCS Reference Manual (Zip file)
- Downloadable PDF file, file name is ICD-10-PCS Reference Manual.pdf
- Revised in response to public comment and internal review
- Addenda to 2014 version of reference manual specifies the changes, file name is pcs_ref_addenda_2014.pdf

2014 ICD-10-PCS and ICD-9-CM General Equivalence Mappings (Zip file)
- **Note: Scheduled for posting October 1, 2013**
- Downloadable text format, file names are gem_i9pcs.txt, gem_pcsi9.txt
- Contains entries for the new FY2014 ICD-9-CM and ICD-10-PCS codes and entries revised in response to public comment and internal review
- Documentation for general users and technical users, file name is: pcs_gemguide_2014.pdf
- Documentation for technical users, file name is GemsTechDoc.pdf

2014 ICD-10 Reimbursement Mappings (Zip file)
- **Note: Scheduled for posting October 1, 2013**
- Downloadable text format, file names are reimb_map_dx_2014.txt, reimb_map_pr_2014.txt
- FY2014 version uses the FY2014 GEM files
- Accompanying documentation includes rules used in the mapping, file name is: Reimb_map_guide_2014.pdf

Introduction

Volume 3 of the International Classification of Diseases Ninth Revision Clinical Modification (ICD-9-CM) has been used in the United States for reporting inpatient procedures since 1979. The structure of volume 3 of ICD-9-CM has not allowed new procedures associated with rapidly changing technology to be effectively incorporated as new codes. As a result, in 1992 the U.S. Centers for Medicare and Medicaid Services funded a project to design a replacement for volume 3 of ICD-9-CM. In 1995 CMS awarded 3M Health Information Systems a three-year contract to complete development of the replacement system. The new system is the ICD-10 Procedure Coding System (ICD-10-PCS).

History of ICD-10-PCS

The World Health Organization has maintained the International Classification of Diseases (ICD) for recording cause of death since 1893. It has updated the ICD periodically to reflect new discoveries in epidemiology and changes in medical understanding of disease.

The International Classification of Diseases Tenth Revision (ICD-10), published in 1992, is the latest revision of the ICD. The WHO authorized the National Center for Health Statistics (NCHS) to develop a clinical modification of ICD-10 for use in the United States. This version, called ICD-10-CM, is intended to replace the previous U.S. clinical modification, ICD-9-CM, that has been in use since 1979. ICD-9-CM contains a procedure classification; ICD-10-CM does not.

CMS, the agency responsible for maintaining the inpatient procedure code set in the United States, contracted with 3M Health Information Systems in 1993 to design and then develop a procedure classification system to replace volume 3 of ICD-9-CM.

The result, ICD-10-PCS, was initially completed in 1998. The code set has been updated annually since that time to ensure that ICD-10-PCS includes classifications for new procedures, devices, and technologies.

The development of ICD-10-PCS had as its goal the incorporation of the following major attributes:

- **Completeness:** There should be a unique code for all substantially different procedures. In volume 3 of ICD-9-CM, procedures on different body parts, with different approaches, or of different types are sometimes assigned to the same code.

- **Unique definitions:** Because ICD-10-PCS codes are constructed of individual values rather than lists of fixed codes and text descriptions, the unique, stable definition of a code in the system is retained. New values may be added to the system to represent a specific new approach or device or qualifier, but whole codes by design cannot be given new meanings and reused.

- **Expandability:** As new procedures are developed, the structure of ICD-10-PCS should allow them to be easily incorporated as unique codes.

- **Multi-axial codes:** ICD-10-PCS codes should consist of independent characters, with each individual component retaining its meaning across broad ranges of codes to the extent possible.

- **Standardized terminology:** ICD-10-PCS should include definitions of the terminology used. While the meaning of specific words varies in common usage, ICD-10-PCS should not include multiple meanings for the same term, and each term must be

assigned a specific meaning. There are no eponyms or common procedure terms in ICD-10-PCS.

- **Structural integrity:** ICD-10-PCS can be easily expanded without disrupting the structure of the system. ICD-10-PCS allows unique new codes to be added to the system because values for the seven characters that make up a code can be combined as needed. The system can evolve as medical technology and clinical practice evolve, without disrupting the ICD-10-PCS structure.

In the development of ICD-10-PCS, several additional general characteristics were added:

- **Diagnostic information is not included in procedure description:** When procedures are performed for specific diseases or disorders, the disease or disorder is not contained in the procedure code. The diagnosis codes, not the procedure codes, specify the disease or disorder.

- **Explicit not otherwise specified (NOS) options are restricted:** Explicit "not otherwise specified," (NOS) options are restricted in ICD-10-PCS. A minimal level of specificity is required for each component of the procedure.

- **Limited use of not elsewhere classified (NEC) option:** Because all significant components of a procedure are specified in ICD-10-PCS, there is generally no need for a "not elsewhere classified" (NEC) code option. However, limited NEC options are incorporated into ICD-10-PCS where necessary. For example, new devices are frequently developed, and therefore it is necessary to provide an "other device" option for use until the new device can be explicitly added to the coding system.

- **Level of specificity:** All procedures currently performed can be specified in ICD-10-PCS. The frequency with which a procedure is performed was not a consideration in the development of the system. A unique code is available for variations of a procedure that can be performed.

ICD-10-PCS code structure results in qualities that optimize the performance of the system in electronic applications, and maximize the usefulness of the coded healthcare data. These qualities include:

- **Optimal search capability:** ICD-10-PCS is designed for maximum versatility in the ability to aggregate coded data. Values belonging to the same character as defined in a section or sections can be easily compared, since they occupy the same position in a code. This provides a high degree of flexibility and functionality for data mining.

- **Consistent characters and values:** Stability of characters and values across vast ranges of codes provides the maximum degree of functionality and flexibility for the collection and analysis of data. Because the character definition is consistent, and only the individual values assigned to that character differ as needed, meaningful comparisons of data over time can be conducted across a virtually infinite range of procedures.

- **Code readability:** ICD-10-PCS resembles a language in the sense that it is made up of semi-independent values combined by following the rules of the system, much the way a sentence is formed by combining words and following the rules of grammar and syntax. As with words in their context, the meaning of any single value is a combination of its position in the code and any preceding values on which it may be dependent.

ICD-10-PCS Code Structure

ICD-10-PCS has a seven-character alphanumeric code structure. Each character contains up to 34 possible values. Each value represents a specific option for the general character definition. The 10 digits 0–9 and the 24 letters A–H, J–N, and P–Z may be used in each character. The letters O and I are not used so as to avoid confusion with the digits 0 and 1. An ICD-10-PCS code is the result of a process rather than as a single fixed set of digits or alphabetic characters. The process consists of combining semi-independent values from among a selection of values, according to the rules governing the construction of codes.

	Section	Body System	Root Operation	Body Part	Approach	Device	Qualifier
Characters:	1	2	3	4	5	6	7

A code is derived by choosing a specific value for each of the seven characters. Based on details about the procedure performed, values for each character specifying the section, body system, root operation, body part, approach, device, and qualifier are assigned. Because the definition of each character is also a function of its physical position in the code, the same letter or number placed in a different position in the code has different meaning.

The seven characters that make up a complete code have specific meanings that vary for each of the 16 sections of the manual. (The resource section of this manual lists character meanings for each section along with body part definitions.)

Procedures are then divided into sections that identify the general type of procedure (e.g., Medical and Surgical, Obstetrics, Imaging). The first character of the procedure code always specifies the section. The second through seventh characters have the same meaning within each section, but may mean different things in other sections. In all sections, the third character specifies the general type of procedure performed (e.g., Resection, Transfusion, Fluoroscopy), while the other characters give additional information such as the body part and approach.

In ICD-10-PCS, the term *procedure* refers to the complete specification of the seven characters.

Number of Codes in ICD-10-PCS

The table structure of ICD-10-PCS permits the specification of a large number of codes on a single page. At the time of this publication, there are 71,924 codes in the 2014 ICD-10-PCS. This is a substantial increase over the number of ICD-9-CM procedure codes. However, many codes have been eliminated from ICD-10-PCS from the Medical and Surgical section as part of a planned streamlining and refinement initiated in 2006. This code reduction has also included the deletion of certain body system values specified as "other" in order to facilitate more selective body part and system values.

For FY 2014, seven new technology codes were added to the system, and three codes were deleted, resulting in a total of 71,924 codes. The ICD-9-CM Coordination and Maintenance Committee are suspending regular updates to the ICD code sets to ease the ICD-10 transition process. These limited updates are required by section 503(a) of the Medicare Prescription Drug, Improvement, and Modernization Act of 2003.

ICD-10-PCS Manual

Index

Codes may be found in the index based on the general type of procedure (e.g., resection, transfusion, fluoroscopy), or a more commonly used term (e.g., appendectomy). For example, the code for percutaneous intraluminal dilation of the coronary arteries with an intraluminal device can be found in the Index under *Dilation*, or a synonym of *Dilation* (e.g., angioplasty). The Index then specifies the first three or four values of the code or directs the user to see another term.

Example:

> **Dilation**
> > Artery
> > > Coronary
> > > > One Site 0270

Based on the first three values of the code provided in the Index, the corresponding table can be located. In the example above, the first three values indicate table 027 is to be referenced for code completion.

The tables and characters are arranged first by number and then by letter for each character (tables for 00-, 01-, 02-, etc., are followed by those for 0B-, 0C-, 0D-, etc., followed by 0B1, 0B2, etc., followed by 0BB, 0BC, 0BD, etc.).

Note: The Tables section must be used to construct a complete and valid code by specifying the last three or four values.

Tables

The Tables section is organized differently from ICD-9-CM. Each page in the section is composed of rows that specify the valid combinations of code values. In most sections of the system, the upper portion of each table contains a description of the first three characters of the procedure code. In the Medical and Surgical section, for example, the first three characters contain the name of the section, the body system, and the root operation performed.

For instance, the values *027* specify the section *Medical and Surgical* (0), the body system *Heart and Great Vessels* (2) and the root operation *Dilation* (7). As shown in table 027, the root operation (*Dilation*) is accompanied by its definition.

The lower portion of the table specifies all the valid combinations of characters 4 through 7. The four columns in the table specify the last four characters. In the Medical and Surgical section they are labeled body part, approach, device and qualifier, respectively. Each row in the table specifies the valid combination of values for characters 4 through 7.

0   Medical and Surgical
2   Heart and Great Vessels
7   Dilation   Expanding an orifice or the lumen of a tubular body part

Body Part Character 4	Approach Character 5	Device Character 6	Qualifier Character 7
0 Coronary Artery, One Site **1** Coronary Artery, Two Sites **2** Coronary Artery, Three Sites **3** Coronary Artery, Four or More Sites	**0** Open **3** Percutaneous **4** Percutaneous Endoscopic	**4** Intraluminal Device, Drug-eluting **D** Intraluminal Device **T** Intraluminal Device, Radioactive **Z** No Device	**6** Bifurcation **Z** No Qualifier
F Aortic Valve **G** Mitral Valve **H** Pulmonary Valve **J** Tricuspid Valve **K** Ventricle, Right **P** Pulmonary Trunk **Q** Pulmonary Artery, Right **S** Pulmonary Vein, Right **T** Pulmonary Vein, Left **V** Superior Vena Cava **W** Thoracic Aorta	**0** Open **3** Percutaneous **4** Percutaneous Endoscopic	**4** Intraluminal Device, Drug-eluting **D** Intraluminal Device **Z** No Device	**Z** No Qualifier
R Pulmonary Artery, Left	**0** Open **3** Percutaneous **4** Percutaneous Endoscopic	**4** Intraluminal Device, Drug-eluting **D** Intraluminal Device **Z** No Device	**T** Ductus Arteriosus **Z** No Qualifier

The rows of this table can be used to construct 213 unique procedure codes. For example, code 02703DZ specifies the procedure for dilation of one coronary artery using an intraluminal device via percutaneous approach (i.e., percutaneous transluminal coronary angioplasty with stent).

Following are the 24 valid combinations of characters 5 through 7 for the Medical and Surgical procedure dilation of the heart and great vessels coronary artery, one site (0270):

0270046	Dilation of Coronary Artery, One Site, Bifurcation, with Drug-eluting Intraluminal Device, Open Approach
027004Z	Dilation of Coronary Artery, One Site with Drug-eluting Intraluminal Device, Open Approach
02700D6	Dilation of Coronary Artery, One Site, Bifurcation, with Intraluminal Device, Open Approach
02700DZ	Dilation of Coronary Artery, One Site with Intraluminal Device, Open Approach
02700T6	Dilation of Coronary Artery, One Site, Bifurcation, with Radioactive Intraluminal Device, Open Approach
02700TZ	Dilation of Coronary Artery, One Site with Radioactive Intraluminal Device, Open Approach
02700Z6	Dilation of Coronary Artery, One Site, Bifurcation, Open Approach
02700ZZ	Dilation of Coronary Artery, One Site, Open Approach
0270346	Dilation of Coronary Artery, One Site, Bifurcation, with Drug-eluting Intraluminal Device, Percutaneous Approach
027034Z	Dilation of Coronary Artery, One Site with Drug-eluting Intraluminal Device, Percutaneous Approach
02703D6	Dilation of Coronary Artery, One Site, Bifurcation, with Intraluminal Device, Percutaneous Approach
02703DZ	Dilation of Coronary Artery, One Site with Intraluminal Device, Percutaneous Approach
02703T6	Dilation of Coronary Artery, One Site, Bifurcation, with Radioactive Intraluminal Device, Percutaneous Approach
02703TZ	Dilation of Coronary Artery, One Site with Radioactive Intraluminal Device, Percutaneous Approach
02703Z6	Dilation of Coronary Artery, One Site, Bifurcation, Percutaneous Approach
02703ZZ	Dilation of Coronary Artery, One Site, Percutaneous Approach
0270446	Dilation of Coronary Artery, One Site, Bifurcation, with Drug-eluting Intraluminal Device, Percutaneous Endoscopic Approach
027044Z	Dilation of Coronary Artery, One Site with Drug-eluting Intraluminal Device, Percutaneous Endoscopic Approach
02704D6	Dilation of Coronary Artery, One Site, Bifurcation, with Intraluminal Device, Percutaneous Endoscopic Approach
02704DZ	Dilation of Coronary Artery, One Site with Intraluminal Device, Percutaneous Endoscopic Approach
02704T6	Dilation of Coronary Artery, One Site, Bifurcation, with Radioactive Intraluminal Device, Percutaneous Endoscopic Approach
02704TZ	Dilation of Coronary Artery, One Site with Radioactive Intraluminal Device, Percutaneous Endoscopic Approach
02704Z6	Dilation of Coronary Artery, One Site, Bifurcation, Percutaneous Endoscopic Approach
02704ZZ	Dilation of Coronary Artery, One Site, Percutaneous Endoscopic Approach

Each table contains only those combinations of values that make up a valid procedure code. In some instances, the tables are split, indicating that there is a restriction in the combination of character choices. In table 027 above, character 7, qualifier 6 Bifurcation can be used only with coronary artery body part characters 0–3. Character 7, qualifier T Ductus Arteriosus can be used only with body part character R Pulmonary Artery, Left.

The lower portion of table 001, shown below, is split into two sections; values of characters must be selected from within the same section (row) of the table.

Ø **Medical and Surgical**
Ø **Central Nervous System**
1 **Bypass**   Altering the route of passage of the contents of a tubular body part

Body Part Character 4	Approach Character 5	Device Character 6	Qualifier Character 7
6 Cerebral Ventricle	Ø Open 3 Percutaneous	7 Autologous Tissue Substitute J Synthetic Substitute K Nonautologous Tissue Substitute	Ø Nasopharynx 1 Mastoid Sinus 2 Atrium 3 Blood Vessel 4 Pleural Cavity 5 Intestine 6 Peritoneal Cavity 7 Urinary Tract 8 Bone Marrow B Cerebral Cisterns
U Spinal Canal	Ø Open 3 Percutaneous	7 Autologous Tissue Substitute J Synthetic Substitute K Nonautologous Tissue Substitute	4 Pleural Cavity 6 Peritoneal Cavity 7 Urinary Tract 9 Fallopian Tube

Body part value 6 may be in combination with device values 7, J, or K. Body part (character 4) value U may be used only in combination with qualifier (character 7) values of 4, 6, 7, and 9. In other words, code ØØ1UØ73 is invalid since the qualifier character appears above the line separating the two sections of the table.

Note: In this manual, there are instances in which some tables due to length must be continued on the next page. Each section must be used separately and value selection must be made within the same section (row) of the table.

Character Meanings

In each section each character has a specific meaning. Within a section all character meanings remain constant. The resource section of this manual lists character meanings for each section.

Sections

Procedures are divided into sections that identify the general type of procedure (e.g., Medical and Surgical, Obstetrics, Imaging). The first character of the procedure code always specifies the section.

The sections are listed below:

Medical and Surgical-related sections
Ø   Medical and Surgical

1   Obstetrics

2   Placement

3   Administration

4   Measurement and Monitoring

5   Extracorporeal Assistance and Performance

6   Extracorporeal Therapies

7   Osteopathic

8   Other Procedures

9   Chiropractic

B   Imaging

Ancillary Sections
C   Nuclear Medicine

D   Radiation Therapy

F   Physical Rehabilitation and Diagnostic Audiology

G   Mental Health

H   Substance Abuse Treatment

Medical and Surgical Section (Ø)

Character Meaning

The seven characters for Medical and Surgical procedures have the following meaning:

Character	Meaning
1	Section
2	Body System
3	Root Operation
4	Body Part
5	Approach
6	Device
7	Qualifier

The Medical and Surgical section constitutes the vast majority of procedures reported in an inpatient setting. Medical and Surgical procedure codes all have a first-character value of Ø. The second character indicates the general body system (e.g., Mouth and Throat, Gastrointestinal). The third character indicates the root operation, or specific objective, of the procedure (e.g., Excision). The fourth character indicates the specific body part on which the procedure was performed (e.g., Tonsils, Duodenum). The fifth character indicates the approach used to reach the procedure site (e.g., Open). The sixth character indicates whether a device was left in place during in the procedure (e.g., Synthetic Substitute). The seventh character is qualifier, which has a specific meaning for each root operation. For example, the qualifier can be used to identify the destination site of a *Bypass*. The first through fifth characters are always assigned a specific value, but the device (sixth character) and the qualifier (seventh character) are not applicable to all procedures. The value Z is used for the sixth and seventh characters to indicate that a specific device or qualifier does not apply to the procedure.

Section (Character 1)

Medical and Surgical procedure codes all have a first-character value of Ø.

Body Systems (Character 2)

Body systems for Medical and Surgical section codes are specified in the second character.

Body Systems

Ø	Central Nervous System
1	Peripheral Nervous System
2	Heart and Great Vessels
3	Upper Arteries
4	Lower Arteries
5	Upper Veins
6	Lower Veins
7	Lymphatic and Hemic Systems
8	Eye
9	Ear, Nose, Sinus
B	Respiratory System
C	Mouth and Throat
D	Gastrointestinal System
F	Hepatobiliary System and Pancreas
G	Endocrine System
H	Skin and Breast
J	Subcutaneous Tissue and Fascia
K	Muscles
L	Tendons
M	Bursae and Ligaments
N	Head and Facial Bones
P	Upper Bones
Q	Lower Bones
R	Upper Joints
S	Lower Joints
T	Urinary System
U	Female Reproductive System
V	Male Reproductive System
W	Anatomical Regions, General
X	Anatomical Regions, Upper Extremities
Y	Anatomical Regions, Lower Extremities

Root Operations (Character 3)

The root operation is specified in the third character. In the Medical and Surgical section there are 31 different root operations. The root operation identifies the objective of the procedure. Each root operation has a precise definition.

- *Alteration:* Modifying the natural anatomic structure of a body part without affecting the function of the body part

- *Bypass:* Altering the route of passage of the contents of a tubular body part

- *Change:* Taking out or off a device from a body part and putting back an identical or similar device in or on the same body part without cutting or puncturing the skin or a mucous membrane

- *Control:* Stopping, or attempting to stop, postprocedural bleeding

- *Creation:* Making a new genital structure that does not take over the function of a body part

- *Destruction:* Physical eradication of all or a portion of a body part by the direct use of energy, force, or a destructive agent

- *Detachment:* Cutting off all or a portion of the upper or lower extremities

- *Dilation:* Expanding an orifice or the lumen of a tubular body part

- *Division:* Cutting into a body part without draining fluids and/or gases from the body part in order to separate or transect a body part

- *Drainage:* Taking or letting out fluids and/or gases from a body part

- *Excision:* Cutting out or off, without replacement, a portion of a body part

- *Extirpation:* Taking or cutting out solid matter from a body part

- *Extraction:* Pulling or stripping out or off all or a portion of a body part by the use of force

- *Fragmentation:* Breaking solid matter in a body part into pieces

- *Fusion:* Joining together portions of an articular body part rendering the articular body part immobile

- *Insertion:* Putting in a nonbiological appliance that monitors, assists, performs, or prevents a physiological function but does not physically take the place of a body part

- *Inspection:* Visually and/or manually exploring a body part

- *Map:* Locating the route of passage of electrical impulses and/or locating functional areas in a body part

- *Occlusion:* Completely closing an orifice or lumen of a tubular body part

- *Reattachment:* Putting back in or on all or a portion of a separated body part to its normal location or other suitable location

- *Release:* Freeing a body part from an abnormal physical constraint by cutting or by use of force

- *Removal:* Taking out or off a device from a body part

- *Repair:* Restoring, to the extent possible, a body part to its normal anatomic structure and function

- *Replacement:* Putting in or on biological or synthetic material that physically takes the place and/or function of all or a portion of a body part

- *Reposition:* Moving to its normal location or other suitable location all or a portion of a body part

- *Resection:* Cutting out or off, without replacement, all of a body part

- *Restriction:* Partially closing an orifice or lumen of a tubular body part

- *Revision:* Correcting, to the extent possible, a portion of a malfunctioning device or the position of a displaced device

- *Supplement:* Putting in or on biological or synthetic material that physically reinforces and/or augments the function of a portion of a body part

- *Transfer:* Moving, without taking out, all or a portion of a body part to another location to take over the function of all or a portion of a body part

- *Transplantation:* Putting in or on all or a portion of a living body part taken from another individual or animal to physically take the place and/or function of all or a portion of a similar body part

The above definitions of root operation illustrate the precision of code values defined in the system. There is a clear distinction between each root operation.

A root operation specifies the objective of the procedure. The term *anastomosis* is not a root operation, because it is a means of joining and is always an integral part of another procedure (e.g., Bypass, Resection) with a specific objective. Similarly, *incision* is not a root operation, since it is always part of the objective of another procedure (e.g., Division, Drainage). The root operation *Repair* in the Medical and Surgical section functions as a "not elsewhere classified" option. *Repair* is used when the procedure performed is not one of the other specific root operations.

Appendix A provides additional explanation and representative examples of the Medical and Surgical root operations. Appendix B groups all root operations in the Medical and Surgical section into subcategories and provides an example of each root operation.

Body Part (Character 4)

The body part is specified in the fourth character. The body part indicates the specific anatomical site of the body system on which the procedure was performed (e.g., Duodenum). Tubular body parts are defined in ICD-10-PCS as those hollow body parts that provide a route of passage for solids, liquids, or gases. They include the cardiovascular system and body parts such as those contained in the gastrointestinal tract, genitourinary tract, biliary tract, and respiratory tract.

Approach (Character 5)

The technique used to reach the site of the procedure is specified in the fifth character. There are seven different approaches:

- *Open*: Cutting through the skin or mucous membrane and any other body layers necessary to expose the site of the procedure

- *Percutaneous*: Entry, by puncture or minor incision, of instrumentation through the skin or mucous membrane and any other body layers necessary to reach the site of the procedure

- *Percutaneous Endoscopic*: Entry, by puncture or minor incision, of instrumentation through the skin or mucous membrane and any other body layers necessary to reach and visualize the site of the procedure

- *Via Natural or Artificial Opening*: Entry of instrumentation through a natural or artificial external opening to reach the site of the procedure

- *Via Natural or Artificial Opening Endoscopic*: Entry of instrumentation through a natural or artificial external opening to reach and visualize the site of the procedure

- *Via Natural or Artificial Opening with Percutaneous Endoscopic Assistance:* Entry of instrumentation through a natural or artificial external opening and entry, by puncture or minor incision, of instrumentation through the skin or mucous membrane and any other body layers necessary to aid in the performance of the procedure

- *External*: Procedures performed directly on the skin or mucous membrane and procedures performed indirectly by the application of external force through the skin or mucous membrane

The approach comprises three components: the access location, method, and type of instrumentation.

Access location: For procedures performed on an internal body part, the access location specifies the external site through which the site of the procedure is reached. There are two general types of access locations: skin or mucous membranes, and external orifices. Every approach value except external includes one of these two access locations. The skin or mucous membrane can be cut or punctured to reach the procedure site. All open and percutaneous approach values use this access location. The site of a procedure can also be reached through an external opening. External openings can be natural (e.g., mouth) or artificial (e.g., colostomy stoma).

Method: For procedures performed on an internal body part, the method specifies how the external access location is entered. An open method specifies cutting through the skin or mucous membrane and any other intervening body layers necessary to expose the site of the procedure. An instrumentation method specifies the entry of instrumentation through the access location to the internal procedure site. Instrumentation can be introduced by puncture or minor incision, or through an external opening. The puncture or minor incision does not constitute an open approach because it does not expose the site of the procedure. An approach can define multiple methods. For example, *Via Natural or Artificial Opening with Percutaneous Endoscopic Assistance* includes both the initial entry of instrumentation to reach the site of the procedure, and the placement of additional percutaneous instrumentation into the body part to visualize and assist in the performance of the procedure.

Type of instrumentation: For procedures performed on an internal body part, instrumentation means that specialized equipment is used to perform the procedure. Instrumentation is used in all internal approaches other than the basic open approach. Instrumentation may or may not include the capacity to visualize the procedure site. For example, the instrumentation used to perform a sigmoidoscopy permits the internal site of the procedure to be visualized, while the instrumentation used to perform a needle biopsy of the liver does not. The term "endoscopic" as used in approach values refers to instrumentation that permits a site to be visualized.

Procedures performed directly on the skin or mucous membrane are identified by the external approach (e.g., skin excision). Procedures performed indirectly by the application of external force are also identified by the external approach (e.g., closed reduction of fracture).

Appendix B compares the components (access location, method, and type of instrumentation) of each approach and provides an example of each approach.

Device (Character 6)

The device is specified in the sixth character and is used only to specify devices that remain after the procedure is completed. There are four general types of devices:

- Grafts and Prostheses

- Implants

- Simple or Mechanical Appliances

- Electronic Appliances

While all devices can be removed, some cannot be removed without putting in another nonbiological appliance or body-part substitute.

When a specific device value is used to identify the device for a root operation, such as *Insertion* and that same device value is not an option for a more broad range root operation such as *Removal*, select the general device value. For example, in the body system Heart and Great Vessels, the specific device character for Cardiac Lead, Pacemaker in root operation *Insertion* is J. For the root operation *Removal*, the general device character M Cardiac Lead would be selected for the pacemaker lead.

ICD-10-PCS contains a PCS Device Aggregation Table (see appendix D) that crosswalks the *specific* device character values that have been created for specific root operations and specific body part character values to the *general* device character value that would be used for root operations that represent a broad range of procedures and general body part character values, such as Removal and Revision.

Instruments used to visualize the procedure site are specified in the approach, not the device, value.

If the objective of the procedure is to put in the device, then the root operation is *Insertion*. If the device is put in to meet an objective other than *Insertion*, then the root operation defining the underlying objective of the procedure is used, with the device specified in the device character. For example, if a procedure to replace the hip joint is performed, the root operation *Replacement* is coded, and the prosthetic device is specified in the device character. Materials that are incidental to a procedure such as clips, ligatures, and sutures are not specified in the device character. Because new devices can be developed, the value *Other Device* is provided as a temporary option for use until a specific device value is added to the system.

Qualifier (Character 7)

The qualifier is specified in the seventh character. The qualifier contains unique values for individual procedures. For example, the qualifier can be used to identify the destination site in a *Bypass*.

Medical and Surgical Section Principles

In developing the Medical and Surgical procedure codes, several specific principles were followed.

Composite Terms Are Not Root Operations

Composite terms such as colonoscopy, sigmoidectomy, or appendectomy do not describe root operations, but they do specify multiple components of a specific root operation. In ICD-10-PCS, the components of a procedure are defined separately by the characters making up the complete code. And the only component of a procedure specified in the root operation is the objective of the procedure. With each complete code the underlying objective of the procedure is specified by the root operation (third character), the precise part is specified by the body part (fourth character), and the method used to reach and visualize the procedure site is specified by the approach (fifth character). While colonoscopy, sigmoidectomy, and appendectomy are included in the Index, they do not constitute root operations in the Tables section. The objective of colonoscopy is the visualization of the colon and the root operation (character 3) is *Inspection*. Character 4 specifies the body part, which in this case is part of the colon. These composite terms, like colonoscopy or appendectomy, are included as cross-reference only. The index provides the correct root operation reference. Examples of other types of composite terms not representative of root operations are *partial* sigmoidectomy, *total* hysterectomy, and *partial* hip replacement. Always refer to the correct root operation in the Index and Tables section.

Root Operation Based on Objective of Procedure

The root operation is based on the objective of the procedure, such as *Resection* of transverse colon or *Dilation* of an artery. The assignment of the root operation is based on the procedure actually performed, which may or may not have been the intended procedure. If the intended procedure is modified or discontinued (e.g., excision instead of resection is performed), the root operation is determined by the procedure actually performed. If the desired result is not attained after completing the procedure (i.e., the artery does not remain expanded after the dilation procedure), the root operation is still determined by the procedure actually performed.

Examples:

*   Dilating the urethra is coded as *Dilation* since the objective of the procedure is to dilate the urethra. If dilation of the urethra includes putting in an intraluminal stent, the root operation remains *Dilation* and not *Insertion* of the intraluminal device because the underlying objective of the procedure is dilation of the urethra. The stent is identified by the intraluminal device value in the sixth character of the dilation procedure code.

*   If the objective is solely to put a radioactive element in the urethra, then the procedure is coded to the root operation *Insertion*, with the radioactive element identified in the sixth character of the code.

*   If the objective of the procedure is to correct a malfunctioning or displaced device, then the procedure is coded to the root operation *Revision*. In the root operation *Revision*, the original device being revised is identified in the device character. *Revision* is typically performed on mechanical appliances (e.g., pacemaker) or materials used in replacement procedures (e.g., synthetic substitute). Typical revision procedures include adjustment of pacemaker position and correction of malfunctioning knee prosthesis.

Combination Procedures Are Coded Separately

If multiple procedures as defined by distinct objectives are performed during an operative episode, then multiple codes are used. For example, obtaining the vein graft used for coronary bypass surgery is coded as a separate procedure from the bypass itself.

Redo of Procedures

The complete or partial redo of the original procedure is coded to the root operation that identifies the procedure performed rather than *Revision*.

Example:

A complete redo of a hip replacement procedure that requires putting in a new prosthesis is coded to the root operation *Replacement* rather than *Revision*.

The correction of complications arising from the original procedure, other than device complications, is coded to the procedure performed. Correction of a malfunctioning or displaced device would be coded to the root operation *Revision*.

Example:

A procedure to control hemorrhage arising from the original procedure is coded to *Control* rather than *Revision*.

Examples of Procedures Coded in the Medical Surgical Section

The following are examples of procedures from the Medical and Surgical section, coded in ICD-10-PCS.

*   Suture of skin laceration, left lower arm: 0HQEXZZ

    Medical and Surgical section (0), body system *Skin and Breast* (H), root operation *Repair* (Q), body part *Skin, Left Lower Arm* (E), *External* Approach (X) *No device* (Z), and *No qualifier* (Z).

- Laparoscopic appendectomy: ØDTJ4ZZ

  Medical and Surgical section (Ø), body system *Gastrointestinal* (D), root operation *Resection* (T), body part *Appendix* (J), *Percutaneous Endoscopic* approach (4), No Device (Z), and No qualifier (Z).

- Sigmoidoscopy with biopsy: ØDBN8ZX

  Medical and Surgical section (Ø), body system *Gastrointestinal* (D), root operation *Excision* (B), body part *Sigmoid Colon* (N), *Via Natural or Artificial Opening Endoscopic* approach (8), *No Device* (Z), and with qualifier *Diagnostic* (X).

- Tracheostomy with tracheostomy tube: ØB11ØF4

  Medical and Surgical section (Ø), body system *Respiratory* (B), root operation *Bypass* (1), body part *Trachea* (1), *Open* approach (Ø), with *Tracheostomy Device* (F), and qualifier *Cutaneous* (4).

Obstetrics Section

Character Meanings

The seven characters in the Obstetrics section have the same meaning as in the Medical and Surgical section.

Character	Meaning
1	Section
2	Body System
3	Root Operation
4	Body Part
5	Approach
6	Device
7	Qualifier

The Obstetrics section includes procedures performed on the products of conception only. Procedures on the pregnant female are coded in the Medical and Surgical section (e.g., episiotomy). The term "products of conception" refers to all physical components of a pregnancy, including the fetus, amnion, umbilical cord, and placenta. There is no differentiation of the products of conception based on gestational age. Thus, the specification of the products of conception as a zygote, embryo or fetus, or the trimester of the pregnancy is not part of the procedure code but can be found in the diagnosis code.

Section (Character 1)

Obstetrics procedure codes have a first-character value of *1*.

Body System (Character 2)

The second-character value for body system is *Pregnancy*.

Root Operation (Character 3)

The root operations *Change, Drainage, Extraction, Insertion, Inspection, Removal, Repair, Reposition, Resection,* and *Transplantation* are used in the obstetrics section and have the same meaning as in the Medical and Surgical section.

The Obstetrics section also includes two additional root operations, *Abortion* and *Delivery,* defined below:

- *Abortion*: Artificially terminating a pregnancy

- *Delivery*: Assisting the passage of the products of conception from the genital canal

A cesarean section is not a separate root operation because the underlying objective is *Extraction* (i.e., pulling out all or a portion of a body part).

Body Part (Character 4)

The body-part values in the obstetrics section are:

- *Products of conception*

- *Products of conception, retained*

- *Products of conception, ectopic*

Approach (Character 5)

The fifth character specifies approaches and is defined as are those in the Medical and Surgical section. In the case of an abortion procedure that uses a laminaria or an abortifacient, the approach is *Via Natural or Artificial Opening.*

Device (Character 6)

The sixth character is used for devices such as fetal monitoring electrodes.

Qualifier (Character 7)

Qualifier values are specific to the root operation and are used to specify the type of extraction (e.g., low forceps, high forceps, etc.), the type of cesarean section (e.g., classical, low cervical, etc.), or the type of fluid taken out during a drainage procedure (e.g., amniotic fluid, fetal blood, etc.).

Placement Section

Character Meanings

The seven characters in the Placement section have the following meaning:

Character	Meaning
1	Section
2	Anatomical Region
3	Root Operation
4	Body Region/Orifice
5	Approach
6	Device
7	Qualifier

Placement section codes represent procedures for putting a device in or on a body region for the purpose of protection, immobilization, stretching, compression, or packing.

Section (Character 1)

Placement procedure codes have a first-character value of *2*.

Body System (Character 2)

The second character contains two values specifying either *Anatomical Regions* or *Anatomical Orifices*.

Root Operation (Character 3)

The root operations in the Placement section include only those procedures that are performed without making an incision or a puncture. The root operations *Change* and *Removal* are in the

Placement section and have the same meaning as in the Medical and Surgical section.

The Placement section also includes five additional root operations, defined as follows:

- *Compression*: Putting pressure on a body region

- *Dressing*: Putting material on a body region for protection

- *Immobilization*: Limiting or preventing motion of an external body region

- *Packing*: Putting material in a body region or orifice

- *Traction*: Exerting a pulling force on a body region in a distal direction

Body Region (Character 4)
The fourth-character values are either body regions (e.g., *Upper Leg*) or natural orifices (e.g., *Ear*).

Approach (Character 5)
Since all placement procedures are performed directly on the skin or mucous membrane, or performed indirectly by applying external force through the skin or mucous membrane, the approach value is always *External*.

Device (Character 6)
The device character is always specified (except in the case of manual traction) and indicates the device placed during the procedure (e.g., cast, splint, bandage, etc.). Except for casts for fractures and dislocations, devices in the Placement section are off the shelf and do not require any extensive design, fabrication, or fitting. Placement of devices that require extensive design, fabrication, or fitting are coded in the Rehabilitation section.

Qualifier (Character 7)
The qualifier character is not specified in the Placement section; the qualifier value is always *No Qualifier*.

Administration Section

Character Meanings
The seven characters in the Administration section have the following meaning:

Character	Meaning
1	Section
2	Physiological System and Anatomical Region
3	Root Operation
4	Body System/Region
5	Approach
6	Substance
7	Qualifier

Administration section codes represent procedures for putting in or on a therapeutic, prophylactic, protective, diagnostic, nutritional, or physiological substance. The section includes transfusions, infusions, and injections, along with other similar services such as irrigation and tattooing.

Section (Character 1)
Administration procedure codes have a first-character value of *3*.

Body System (Character 2)
The body-system character contains only three values: *Indwelling Device, Physiological Systems and Anatomical Regions,* or *Circulatory System*. The *Circulatory System* is used for transfusion procedures.

Root Operation (Character 3)
There are three root operations in the Administration section.

- *Introduction*: Putting in or on a therapeutic, diagnostic, nutritional, physiological, or prophylactic substance except blood or blood products

- *Irrigation*: Putting in or on a cleansing substance

- *Transfusion*: Putting in blood or blood products

Body/System Region (Character 4)
The fourth character specifies the body system/region. The fourth character identifies the site where the substance is administered, not the site where the substance administered takes effect. Sites include *Skin and Mucous Membrane, Subcutaneous Tissue* and *Muscle*. These differentiate intradermal, subcutaneous, and intramuscular injections, respectively. Other sites include *Eye, Respiratory Tract, Peritoneal Cavity,* and *Epidural Space*.

The body systems/regions for arteries and veins are *Peripheral Artery, Central Artery, Peripheral Vein,* and *Central Vein*. The *Peripheral Artery* or *Vein* is typically used when a substance is introduced locally into an artery or vein. For example, chemotherapy is the introduction of an antineoplastic substance into a peripheral artery or vein by a percutaneous approach. In general, the substance introduced into a peripheral artery or vein has a systemic effect.

The *Central Artery* or *Vein* is typically used when the site where the substance is introduced is distant from the point of entry into the artery or vein. For example, the introduction of a substance directly at the site of a clot within an artery or vein using a catheter is coded as an introduction of a thrombolytic substance into a central artery or vein by a percutaneous approach. In general, the substance introduced into a central artery or vein has a local effect.

Approach (Character 5)
The fifth character specifies approaches as defined in the Medical and Surgical section. The approach for intradermal, subcutaneous, and intramuscular introductions (i.e., injections) is *Percutaneous*. If a catheter is placed to introduce a substance into an internal site within the circulatory system, then the approach is also *Percutaneous*. For example, if a catheter is used to introduce contrast directly into the heart for angiography, then the procedure would be coded as a percutaneous introduction of contrast into the heart.

Substance (Character 6)
The sixth character specifies the substance being introduced. Broad categories of substances are defined, such as anesthetic, contrast, dialysate, and blood products such as platelets.

Qualifier (Character 7)
The seventh character is a qualifier and is used to indicate whether the substance is *Autologous* or *Nonautologous*, or to further specify the substance.

Measurement and Monitoring Section

Character Meanings

The seven characters in the Measurement and Monitoring section have the following meaning:

Character	Meaning
1	Section
2	Physiological System
3	Root Operation
4	Body System
5	Approach
6	Function/Device
7	Qualifier

Measurement and Monitoring section codes represent procedures for determining the level of a physiological or physical function.

Section (Character 1)

Measurement and Monitoring procedure codes have a first-character value of *4*.

Body System (Character 2)

The second-character values for body system are A, *Physiological Systems* or B, *Physiological Devices*.

Root Operation (Character 3)

There are two root operations in the Measurement and Monitoring section, as defined below:

- *Measurement*: Determining the level of a physiological or physical function at a point in time

- *Monitoring*: Determining the level of a physiological or physical function repetitively over a period of time

Body System (Character 4)

The fourth character specifies the specific body system measured or monitored.

Approach (Character 5)

The fifth character specifies approaches as defined in the Medical and Surgical section.

Function/Device (Character 6)

The sixth character specifies the physiological or physical function being measured or monitored. Examples of physiological or physical functions are *Conductivity, Metabolism, Pulse, Temperature,* and *Volume*. If a device used to perform the measurement or monitoring is inserted and left in, then insertion of the device is coded as a separate Medical and Surgical procedure.

Qualifier (Character 7)

The seventh-character qualifier contains specific values as needed to further specify the body part (e.g., central, portal, pulmonary) or a variation of the procedure performed (e.g., ambulatory, stress). Examples of typical procedures coded in this section are EKG, EEG, and cardiac catheterization. An EKG is the measurement of cardiac electrical activity, while an EEG is the measurement of electrical activity of the central nervous system. A cardiac catheterization performed to measure the pressure in the heart is coded as the measurement of cardiac pressure by percutaneous approach.

Extracorporeal Assistance and Performance Section

Character Meanings

The seven characters in the Extracorporeal Assistance and Performance section have the following meaning:

Character	Meaning
1	Section
2	Physiological System
3	Root Operation
4	Body System
5	Duration
6	Function
7	Qualifier

In Extracorporeal Assistance and Performance procedures, equipment outside the body is used to assist or perform a physiological function. The section includes procedures performed in a critical care setting, such as mechanical ventilation and cardioversion; it also includes other services such as hyperbaric oxygen treatment and hemodialysis.

Section (Character 1)

Extracorporeal Assistance and Performance procedure codes have a first-character value of *5*.

Body System (Character 2)

The second-character value for body system is A, *Physiological Systems*.

Root Operation (Character 3)

There are three root operations in the Extracorporeal Assistance and Performance section, as defined below.

- *Assistance*: Taking over a portion of a physiological function by extracorporeal means

- *Performance*: Completely taking over a physiological function by extracorporeal means

- *Restoration*: Returning, or attempting to return, a physiological function to its natural state by extracorporeal means

The root operation *Restoration* contains a single procedure code that identifies extracorporeal cardioversion.

Body System (Character 4)

The fourth character specifies the body system (e.g., cardiac, respiratory) to which extracorporeal assistance or performance is applied.

Duration (Character 5)

The fifth character specifies the duration of the procedure—*Single, Intermittent,* or *Continuous*. For respiratory ventilation assistance or performance, the duration is specified in hours— *< 24 Consecutive Hours, 24–96 Consecutive Hours,* or *> 96 Consecutive Hours*. Value 6, *Multiple* identifies serial procedure treatment.

Function (Character 6)

The sixth character specifies the physiological function assisted or performed (e.g., oxygenation, ventilation) during the procedure.

Qualifier (Character 7)

The seventh-character qualifier specifies the type of equipment used, if any.

Extracorporeal Therapies Section

Character Meanings

The seven characters in the Extracorporeal Therapies section have the following meaning:

Character	Meaning
1	Section
2	Physiological Systems
3	Root Operation
4	Body System
5	Duration
6	Qualifier
7	Qualifier

In extracorporeal therapy, equipment outside the body is used for a therapeutic purpose that does not involve the assistance or performance of a physiological function.

Section (Character 1)

Extracorporeal Therapy procedure codes have a first-character value of 6.

Body System (Character 2)

The second-character value for body system is *Physiological Systems*.

Root Operation (Character 3)

There are 10 root operations in the Extracorporeal Therapy section, as defined below.

- *Atmospheric Control*: Extracorporeal control of atmospheric pressure and composition

- *Decompression*: Extracorporeal elimination of undissolved gas from body fluids

  Coding note: The root operation *Decompression* involves only one type of procedure: treatment for decompression sickness (the bends) in a hyperbaric chamber.

- *Electromagnetic Therapy*: Extracorporeal treatment by electromagnetic rays

- *Hyperthermia*: Extracorporeal raising of body temperature

  Coding note: The term hyperthermia is used to describe both a temperature imbalance treatment and also as an adjunct radiation treatment for cancer. When treating the temperature imbalance, it is coded to this section; for the cancer treatment, it is coded in section *D Radiation Therapy*.

- *Hypothermia*: Extracorporeal lowering of body temperature

- *Pheresis*: Extracorporeal separation of blood products

  Coding note: Pheresis may be used for two main purposes: to treat diseases when too much of a blood component is produced (e.g., leukemia) and to remove a blood product such as platelets from a donor, for transfusion into another patient.

- *Phototherapy*: Extracorporeal treatment by light rays

  Coding note: Phototherapy involves using a machine that exposes the blood to light rays outside the body, recirculates it, and then returns it to the body.

- *Shock Wave Therapy*: Extracorporeal treatment by shock waves

- *Ultrasound Therapy*: Extracorporeal treatment by ultrasound

- *Ultraviolet Light Therapy*: Extracorporeal treatment by ultraviolet light

Body System (Character 4)

The fourth character specifies the body system on which the extracorporeal therapy is performed (e.g., skin, circulatory).

Duration (Character 5)

The fifth character specifies the duration of the procedure (e.g., single or intermittent).

Qualifier (Character 6)

The sixth character is not specified for Extracorporeal Therapies and always has the value *No Qualifier*.

Qualifier (Character 7)

The seventh-character qualifier is used in the root operation *Pheresis* to specify the blood component on which pheresis is performed and in the root operation *Ultrasound Therapy* to specify site of treatment.

Osteopathic Section

Character Meanings

The seven characters in the Osteopathic section have the following meaning:

Character	Meaning
1	Section
2	Anatomical Region
3	Root Operation
4	Body Region
5	Approach
6	Method
7	Qualifier

Section (Character 1)

Osteopathic procedure codes have a first-character value of *7*.

Body System (Character 2)

The body-system character contains the value *Anatomical Regions*.

Root Operation (Character 3)

There is only one root operation in the Osteopathic section.

- *Treatment*: Manual treatment to eliminate or alleviate somatic dysfunction and related disorders

Body Region (Character 4)

The fourth character specifies the body region on which the osteopathic treatment is performed.

Approach (Character 5)

The approach for osteopathic treatment is always *External*.

Method (Character 6)

The sixth character specifies the method by which the treatment is accomplished.

Qualifier (Character 7)

The seventh character is not specified in the Osteopathic section and always has the value *None*.

Other Procedures Section

Character Meanings

The seven characters in the Other Procedures section have the following meaning:

Character	Meaning
1	Section
2	Body System
3	Root Operation
4	Body Region
5	Approach
6	Method
7	Qualifier

The Other Procedures section includes acupuncture, suture removal, and in vitro fertilization.

Section (Character 1)

Other Procedure section codes have a first-character value of *8*.

Body System (Character 2)

The second-character values for body systems are *Physiological Systems and Anatomical Regions* and *Indwelling Device*.

Root Operation (Character 3)

The Other Procedures section has only one root operation, defined as follows:

• *Other Procedures*: Methodologies that attempt to remediate or cure a disorder or disease.

Body Region (Character 4)

The fourth character contains specified body-region values, and also the body-region value *None* for Extracorporeal Procedures.

Approach (Character 5)

The fifth character specifies approaches as defined in the Medical and Surgical section.

Method (Character 6)

The sixth character specifies the method (e.g., *Acupuncture, Therapeutic Massage*).

Qualifier (Character 7)

The seventh character is a qualifier and contains specific values as needed.

Chiropractic Section

Character Meanings

The seven characters in the Chiropractic section have the following meaning:

Character	Meaning
1	Section
2	Anatomical Regions
3	Root Operation
4	Body Region
5	Approach
6	Method
7	Qualifier

Section (Character 1)

Chiropractic section procedure codes have a first-character value of *9*.

Body System (Character 2)

The second-character value for body system is *Anatomical Regions*.

Root Operation (Character 3)

There is only one root operation in the *Chiropractic* section.

• *Manipulation*: Manual procedure that involves a directed thrust to move a joint past the physiological range of motion, without exceeding the anatomical limit.

Body Region (Character 4)

The fourth character specifies the body region on which the chiropractic manipulation is performed.

Approach (Character 5)

The approach for chiropractic manipulation is always *External*.

Method (Character 6)

The sixth character is the method by which the manipulation is accomplished.

Qualifier (Character 7)

The seventh character is not specified in the Chiropractic section and always has the value *None*.

Imaging Section

Character Meanings

The seven characters in Imaging procedures have the following meaning:

Character	Meaning
1	Section
2	Body System
3	Root Type
4	Body Part
5	Contrast
6	Qualifier
7	Qualifier

Imaging procedures include plain radiography, fluoroscopy, CT, MRI, and ultrasound. Nuclear medicine procedures, including PET, uptakes, and scans, are in the nuclear medicine section. Therapeutic radiation procedure codes are in a separate radiation therapy section.

Section (Character 1)

Imaging procedure codes have a first-character value of *B*.

Body System (Character 2)

In the Imaging section, the second character defines the body system, such as *Heart* or *Gastrointestinal System*.

Root Type (Character 3)

The third character defines the type of imaging procedure (e.g., MRI, ultrasound). The following list includes all types in the *Imaging* section with a definition of each type:

- *Computerized Tomography (CT Scan)* : Computer-reformatted digital display of multiplanar images developed from the capture of multiple exposures of external ionizing radiation

- *Fluoroscopy*: Single plane or bi-plane real-time display of an image developed from the capture of external ionizing radiation on fluorescent screen. The image may also be stored by either digital or analog means

- *Magnetic Resonance Imaging (MRI)* : Computer reformatted digital display of multiplanar images developed from the capture of radiofrequency signals emitted by nuclei in a body site excited within a magnetic field

- *Plain Radiography*: Planar display of an image developed from the capture of external ionizing radiation on photographic or photoconductive plate

- *Ultrasonography*: Real-time display of images of anatomy or flow information developed from the capture of reflected and attenuated high-frequency sound waves

Body Part(Character 4)

The fourth character defines the body part with different values for each body system (character 2) value.

Contrast (Character 5)

The fifth character specifies whether the contrast material used in the imaging procedure is *High* or *Low Osmolar*, when applicable.

Qualifier (Character 6)

The sixth-character qualifier provides further detail regarding the nature of the substance or technologies used, such as *Unenhanced and Enhanced (contrast)*, *Laser*, or *Intravascular Optical Coherence*.

Qualifier (Character 7)

The seventh character is a qualifier that may be used to specify certain procedural circumstances, the method by which the procedure was performed, or technologies utilized, such as *Intraoperative, Intravascular*, or *Transesophageal*.

Nuclear Medicine Section

Character Meanings

The seven characters in the Nuclear Medicine section have the following meaning:

Character	Meaning
1	Section
2	Body System
3	Root Type
4	Body Part
5	Radionuclide
6	Qualifier
7	Qualifier

Nuclear Medicine is the introduction of radioactive material into the body to create an image, to diagnose and treat pathologic conditions, or to assess metabolic functions. The Nuclear Medicine section does not include the introduction of encapsulated radioactive material for the treatment of cancer. These procedures are included in the Radiation Therapy section.

Section (Character 1)

Nuclear Medicine procedure codes have a first-character value of *C*.

Body System (Character 2)

The second character specifies the body system on which the nuclear medicine procedure is performed.

Root Type (Character 3)

The third character indicates the type of nuclear medicine procedure (e.g., planar imaging or nonimaging uptake). The following list includes the types of nuclear medicine procedures with a definition of each type.

- *Nonimaging Uptake:* Introduction of radioactive materials into the body for measurements of organ function, from the detection of radioactive emissions

- *Nonimaging Probe:* Introduction of radioactive materials into the body for the study of distribution and fate of certain substances by the detection of radioactive emissions; or alternatively, measurement of absorption of radioactive emissions from an external source

- *Nonimaging Assay:* Introduction of radioactive materials into the body for the study of body fluids and blood elements, by the detection of radioactive emissions

- *Planar Imaging*: Introduction of radioactive materials into the body for single-plane display of images developed from the capture of radioactive emissions

- *Positron Emission Tomography (PET):* Introduction of radioactive materials into the body for three-dimensional display of images developed from the simultaneous capture, 180 degrees apart, of radioactive emissions

- *Systemic Therapy:* Introduction of unsealed radioactive materials into the body for treatment

- *Tomographic (Tomo) Imaging*: Introduction of radioactive materials into the body for three dimensional display of images developed from the capture of radioactive emissions

Body Part (Character 4)

The fourth character indicates the body part or body region studied. *Regional* (e.g., lower extremity veins) and *Combination* (e.g., liver and spleen) body parts are commonly used in this section.

Radionuclide (Character 5)

The fifth character specifies the radionuclide, the radiation source. The option *Other Radionuclide* is provided in the nuclear medicine section for newly approved radionuclides until they can be added to the coding system. If more than one radiopharmaceutical is given to perform the procedure, then more than one code is used.

Qualifier (Character 6 and 7)

The sixth and seventh characters are qualifiers but are not specified in the *Nuclear Medicine* section; the value is always *None*.

Radiation Therapy Section

Character Meanings

The seven characters in the Radiation Therapy section have the following meaning:

Character	Meaning
1	Section
2	Body System
3	Root Type
4	Treatment Site
5	Modality Qualifier
6	Isotope
7	Qualifier

Section (Character 1)

Radiation therapy procedure codes have a first-character value of *D*.

Body System (Character 2)

The second character specifies the body system (e.g., central nervous system, musculoskeletal) irradiated.

Root Type (Character 3)

The third character specifies the general modality used (e.g., beam radiation).

Treatment Site (Character 4)

The fourth character specifies the body part that is the focus of the radiation therapy.

Modality Qualifier (Character 5)

The fifth character further specifies the radiation modality used (e.g., photons, electrons).

Isotope (Character 6)

The sixth character specifies the isotopes introduced into the body, if applicable.

Qualifier (Character 7)

The seventh character may specify whether the procedure was performed intraoperatively.

Physical Rehabilitation and Diagnostic Audiology Section

Character Meanings

The seven characters in the Physical Rehabilitation and Diagnostic Audiology section have the following meaning:

Character	Meaning
1	Section
2	Section Qualifier
3	Root Type
4	Body System & Region
5	Type Qualifier
6	Equipment
7	Qualifier

Physical rehabilitation procedures include physical therapy, occupational therapy, and speech-language pathology. Osteopathic procedures and chiropractic procedures are in separate sections.

Section (Character 1)

Physical Rehabilitation and Diagnostic Audiology procedure codes have a first-character value of *F*.

Section Qualifier (Character 2)

The section qualifier *Rehabilitation* or *Diagnostic Audiology* is specified in the second character.

Root Type (Character 3)

The third character specifies the root type. There are 14 different root type values, which can be classified into four basic types of rehabilitation and diagnostic audiology procedures, defined as follows:

Assessment: Includes a determination of the patient's diagnosis when appropriate, need for treatment, planning for treatment, periodic assessment, and documentation related to these activities

Assessments are further classified into more than 100 different tests or methods. The majority of these focus on the faculties of hearing and speech, but others focus on various aspects of body function, and on the patient's quality of life, such as muscle performance, neuromotor development, and reintegration skills.

- *Speech Assessment*: Measurement of speech and related functions

- *Motor and/or Nerve Function Assessment*: Measurement of motor, nerve, and related functions

- *Activities of Daily Living Assessment*: Measurement of functional level for activities of daily living

- *Hearing Assessment*: Measurement of hearing and related functions

- *Hearing Aid Assessment*: Measurement of the appropriateness and/or effectiveness of a hearing device

- *Vestibular Assessment*: Measurement of the vestibular system and related functions

Caregiver Training: Educating caregiver with the skills and knowledge used to interact with and assist the patient

Caregiver Training is divided into 18 different broad subjects taught to help a caregiver provide proper patient care.

- *Caregiver Training*: Training in activities to support patient's optimal level of function

Fitting(s): Design, fabrication, modification, selection, and/or application of splint, orthosis, prosthesis, hearing aids, and/or other rehabilitation device

The fifth character used in *Device Fitting* describes the device being fitted rather than the method used to fit the device. Detailed descriptions of the devices are provided in the reference materials, the table specific to *Device Fitting*.

- *Device Fitting*: Fitting of a device designed to facilitate or support achievement of a higher level of function

Treatment: Use of specific activities or methods to develop, improve, and/or restore the performance of necessary functions, compensate for dysfunction and/or minimize debilitation

Treatment procedures include swallowing dysfunction exercises, bathing and showering techniques, wound management, gait training, and a host of activities typically associated with rehabilitation.

- *Speech Treatment*: Application of techniques to improve, augment, or compensate for speech and related functional impairment

- *Motor Treatment*: Exercise or activities to increase or facilitate motor function

- *Activities of Daily Living Treatment*: Exercise or activities to facilitate functional competence for activities of daily living

- *Hearing Treatment*: Application of techniques to improve, augment, or compensate for hearing and related functional impairment

- *Cochlear Implant Treatment*: Application of techniques to improve the communication abilities of individuals with cochlear implant

- *Vestibular Treatment*: Application of techniques to improve, augment, or compensate for vestibular and related functional impairment

The type of treatment includes training as well as activities that restore function.

Body System & Region (Character 4)

The fourth character specifies the body region and/or system on which the procedure is performed.

Type Qualifier (Character 5)

The fifth character is a type qualifier that further specifies the procedure performed. Examples include therapy to improve the range of motion and training for bathing techniques. Refer to appendix D for definitions of these types of procedures.

Equipment (Character 6)

The sixth character specifies the equipment used. Specific equipment is not defined in the equipment value. Instead, broad categories of equipment are specified (e.g., aerobic endurance and conditioning, assistive/adaptive/supportive, etc.)

Qualifier (Character 7)

The seventh character is not specified in the Physical Rehabilitation and Diagnostic Audiology section and always has the value *None*.

Mental Health Section

Character Meanings

The seven characters in the Mental Health section have the following meaning:

Character	Meaning
1	Section
2	Body System
3	Root Type
4	Type Qualifier
5	Qualifier
6	Qualifier
7	Qualifier

Section (Character 1)

Mental health procedure codes have a first-character value of *G*.

Body System (Character 2)

The second character is used to identify the body system elsewhere in ICD-10-PCS. In this section it always has the value *None*.

Root Type (Character 3)

The third character specifies the procedure type, such as crisis intervention or counseling. There are 12 types of mental health procedures, some of which are defined below.

Psychological Tests:

- Developmental: Age-normed developmental status of cognitive, social, and adaptive behavior skills

- Intellectual and Psychoeducational: Intellectual abilities, academic achievement, and learning capabilities (including behavior and emotional factors affecting learning)

- Neurobehavioral and Cognitive Status: Includes neurobehavioral status exam, interview(s), and observation for the clinical assessment of thinking, reasoning, and judgment, acquired knowledge, attention, memory, visual spatial abilities, language functions, and planning

- Neuropsychological: Thinking, reasoning and judgment, acquired knowledge, attention, memory, visual spatial abilities, language functions, planning

- Personality and Behavioral: Mood, emotion, behavior, social functioning, psychopathological conditions, personality traits, and characteristics

Crisis intervention: Includes defusing, debriefing, counseling, psychotherapy, and/or coordination of care with other providers or agencies

Individual Psychotherapy:

- Behavior: Primarily to modify behavior. Includes modeling and role playing, positive reinforcement of target behaviors, response cost, and training of self-management skills

- Cognitive/behavioral: Combining cognitive and behavioral treatment strategies to improve functioning. Maladaptive responses are examined to determine how cognitions relate to behavior patterns in response to an event. Uses learning principles and information-processing models

- Cognitive: Primarily to correct cognitive distortions and errors

- Interactive: Uses primarily physical aids and other forms of nonoral interaction with a patient who is physically, psychologically, or developmentally unable to use ordinary language for communication (e.g., the use of toys in symbolic play)

- Interpersonal: Helps an individual make changes in interpersonal behaviors to reduce psychological dysfunction. Includes exploratory techniques, encouragement of affective expression, clarification of patient statements, analysis of communication patterns, use of therapy relationship, and behavior change techniques.

- Psychoanalysis: Methods of obtaining a detailed account of past and present mental and emotional experiences to determine the source and eliminate or diminish the undesirable effects of unconscious conflicts by making the individual aware of their existence, origin, and inappropriate expression in emotions and behavior.

- Psychodynamic: Exploration of past and present emotional experiences to understand motives and drives using insight-oriented techniques (e.g., empathetic listening, clarifying self-defeating behavior patterns, and exploring adaptive alternatives) to reduce the undesirable effects of internal conflicts on emotions and behavior

- Psychophysiological: Monitoring and alternation of physiological processes to help the individual associate physiological reactions combined with cognitive and behavioral strategies to gain improved control of these processes to help the individual cope more effectively

- Supportive: Formation of therapeutic relationship primarily for providing emotional support to prevent further deterioration in functioning during periods of particular stress. Often used in conjunction with other therapeutic approaches

Counseling:

- Vocational: Exploration of vocational interest, aptitudes, and required adaptive behavior skills to develop and carry out a plan for achieving a successful vocational placement, enhancing work-related adjustment, and/or pursuing viable options in training education or preparation

Family Psychotherapy:

- Remediation of emotional or behavioral problems presented by one or more family members when psychotherapy with more than one family member is indicated

Electroconvulsive Therapy:

- Includes appropriate sedation and other preparation of the individual

Biofeedback: Includes electroencephalogram (EEG), blood pressure, skin temperature or peripheral blood flow, electrocardiogram (ECG), electrooculogram, electromyogram (EMG), respirometry or capnometry, galvanic skin response (GSR) or electrodermal response (EDR), perineometry to monitor and regulate bowel or bladder activity, and electrogastrogram to monitor and regulate gastric motility

Other Mental Health procedures include *Hypnosis, Narcosynthesis, Group Psychotherapy,* and *Light Therapy.* There are no ICD-10-PCS definitions of these procedures at this time.

Type Qualifier (Character 4)

The fourth character is a type qualifier (e.g., to indicate that counseling was educational or vocational).

Qualifier (Character 5, 6 and 7)

The fifth, sixth, and seventh characters are not specified and always have the value *None.*

Substance Abuse Treatment Section

Character Meanings

The seven characters in the Substance Abuse Treatment section have the following meaning:

Character	Meaning
1	Section
2	Body System
3	Root Type
4	Type Qualifier
5	Qualifier
6	Qualifier
7	Qualifier

Section (Character 1)

Substance Abuse Treatment codes have a first-character value of *H.*

Body System (Character 2)

The second character is used to identify the body system elsewhere in ICD-10-PCS. In this section, it always has the value *None.*

Root Type (Character 3)

The third character specifies the procedure. There are seven root type values classified in this section, as listed below:

- *Detoxification Services:* Not a treatment modality but helps the patient stabilize physically and psychologically until the body becomes free of drugs and the effects of alcohol

- *Individual Counseling:* Comprising several techniques, which apply various strategies to address drug addiction

- *Group Counseling:* Provides structured group counseling sessions and healing power through the connection with others

- *Family Counseling:* Provides support and education for family members of addicted individuals. Family member participation seen as critical to substance abuse treatment

- Other root type values in this section include *Individual Psychotherapy, Medication Management,* and *Pharmacotherapy;* there are no ICD-10-PCS definitions of these procedures at this time.

Type Qualifier (Character 4)

The fourth character further specifies the procedure type. Type Qualifier values vary dependent upon the Root Type procedure (Character 3). Root type 2, *Detoxification Services* contains only the value Z, *None* and Root type 6, *Family Counseling* contains only the value 3, *Other Family Counseling,* whereas the remainder Root Type procedures include nine to twelve total possible values.

Qualifier (Character 5, 6 and 7)

The fifth through seventh characters are designated as qualifiers but are never specified, so they always have the value *None*.

Comparison of ICD-10-PCS and ICD-9-CM

In 1993, the National Committee on Vital and Health Statistics (NCVHS) issued a report specifying recommendations for a new procedure classification system. NCVHS identified the essential characteristics that a procedure classification system should possess. Those characteristics include hierarchical structure, expandability, comprehensive, nonoverlapping, ease of use, setting and provider neutrality, multi-axial structure, and limited to classification of procedures.

ICD-10-PCS meets virtually all NCVHS characteristics, while ICD-9-CM fails to meet many NCVHS characteristics. In addition to the NCVHS characteristics, there are several other attributes of a procedure coding system that should be taken into consideration when comparing systems.

Completeness and Accuracy of Codes

The procedures coded in ICD-10-PCS provided a much more complete and accurate description of the procedure performed. The specification of the procedures performed not only affects payment, but is integral to internal management systems, external performance comparisons, and the assessment of quality of care. The detail and completeness of ICD-10-PCS is essential in today's health care environment.

General Equivalence Mappings

Due to the complexities of ICD-10-PCS and the drastic structural differences between the two coding systems, a direct code crosswalk is not possible. However, a general "mapping" of similar code choices has been developed. This network of relationships between the two code sets may be referred to as general equivalence mappings (GEMs). The purpose of these mappings, from ICD-9-CM to ICD-10-PCS, and vice versa, is to attempt to find corresponding procedure codes in lieu of a direct translation. For example:

- The ICD-9-CM to ICD-10-PCS GEM may help with analyzing or comparing data coded using the ICD-9-CM system to facilitate "forward mapping" to ICD-10-PCS.

- The ICD-10-PCS to ICD-9-CM GEM may help in comparing coded data using the ICD-10-PCS system to facilitate "backward mapping" to ICD-9-CM.

The 2014 update of the ICD-10 general equivalence mappings are posted for reference on the CMS website at the URL below: https://www.cms.gov/Medicare/Coding/ICD10/2014-ICD-10-PCS-GEMs.html.

Communications with Physicians

ICD-9-CM procedure codes often poorly describe the precise procedure performed. Physicians or others reviewing or analyzing data coded in ICD-9-CM may have difficulty developing clinical pathways, evaluating the coding for possible fraud and abuse, or conducting research. The ICD-10-PCS codes provide more clinically relevant procedure descriptions that can be more readily understood and used by physicians.

Independent evaluation of ICD-10-PCS demonstrated that there is a learning curve associated with ICD-10-PCS. Because of the additional specificity in ICD-10-PCS, it probably takes longer to attain a minimum level of coding proficiency for ICD-10-PCS than for ICD-9-CM. However, it should take less time to become *highly* proficient with ICD-10-PCS than with ICD-9-CM due to the consistency of character and value

definitions. ICD-9-CM lacks clear definitions, and many substantially different procedures are coded with the same code. Therefore, identifying the correct code required extensive knowledge of the American Hospital Association's *Coding Clinic for ICD-9-CM* and other coding guidelines.

Conclusion

ICD-10-PCS has been developed as a replacement for volume 3 of ICD-9-CM. The system has evolved during its development based on extensive input from many segments of the health care industry. The multi-axial structure of the system, combined with its detailed definition of terminology, permits a precise specification of procedures for use in health services research, epidemiology, statistical analysis, and administrative areas. ICD-10-PCS will also allow health information coders to assign accurate procedure codes with minimal effort.

Sources

All material contained in this manual is derived from the ICD-10-PCS Coding System, Reference Manual and related files revised and distributed by the Centers for Medicare and Medicaid Services, FY 2014.

ICD-10-PCS Official Conventions

The *ICD-10-PCS; The Complete Official Draft Code Set* is based on the official draft version of the International Classification of Diseases, 10th Revision, Procedure Classification System, issued by the U.S. Department of Health and Human Services, Centers for Medicare and Medicaid Services. This book is consistent with the content of the government's version of ICD-10-PCS and follows the official conventions.

Index

The user can use the Alphabetic Index to locate the appropriate table containing all the information necessary to construct a procedure code. The PCS tables should always be consulted to find the most appropriate valid code. Users may choose a valid code directly from the tables—he or she need not consult the index before proceeding to the tables to complete the code.

Main Terms

The Alphabetic Index reflects the structure of the tables. Therefore, the index is organized as an alphabetic listing. The index:

- Is based on the value of the third character

- Contains common procedure terms

- Lists anatomic sites

- Uses device terms

The main terms in the Alphabetic Index are root operations, root procedure types, or common procedure names. In addition, anatomic sites from the Body Part Key and device terms from the Device Key have been added for ease of use.

Examples:

> *Resection* (root operation)
>
> *Fluoroscopy* (root type)
>
> *Prostatectomy* (common procedure name)
>
> *Brachial artery* (body part)
>
> *Bard® Dulex™ mesh* (device)

The index provides at least the first three or four values of the code, and some entries may provide complete valid codes. However, the user should always consult the appropriate table to verify that the most appropriate valid code has been selected.

Root Operation and Procedure Type Main Terms

For the *Medical and Surgical* and related sections, the root operation values are used as main terms in the index. The subterms under the root operation main terms are body parts. For the Ancillary section of the tables, the main terms in the index are the general type of procedure performed.

Examples:

> **Destruction**
> Acetabulum
> Left 0Q55
> Right 0Q54
> Adenoids 0C5Q
> Ampulla of Vater 0F5C
> **Biofeedback** GZC9ZZZ
> **Planar Nuclear Medicine Imaging** CP1

See Reference

The second type of term in the index uses common procedure names, such as "appendectomy" or "fundoplication." These common terms are listed as main terms with a "see" reference noting the PCS root operations that are possible valid code tables based on the objective of the procedure.

Examples:

> **Tendonectomy**
> *see* Excision, Tendon 0L8
> *see* Resection, Tendon 0LT

Use Reference

The index also lists anatomic sites from the Body Part Key and device terms from the Device Key. These terms are listed with a "use" reference. The purpose of these references is to act as an additional reference to the terms located in the Appendix Keys. The term provided is the Body Part value or Device value to be selected when constructing a procedure code using the code tables. This type of index reference is not intended to direct the user to another term in the index, but to provide guidance regarding character value selection. Therefore, "use" references generally do not refer to specific valid code tables.

Examples:

> **Epitrochlear lymph node**
> *use* Lymphatic, Upper Extremity, Left
> *use* Lymphatic, Upper Extremity, Right
> **CoAxia NeuroFlo catheter**
> *use* Intraluminal Device
> **SynCardia Total Artificial Heart**
> *use* Synthetic Substitute

Code Tables

ICD-10-PCS contains 16 sections of Code Tables organized by general type of procedure. The first three characters of a procedure code define each table. The tables consist of columns providing the possible last four characters of codes and rows providing valid values for each character. Within a PCS table, valid codes include all combinations of choices in characters 4 through 7 contained in the same row of the table. All seven characters must be specified to form a valid code.

There are three main sections of tables:

- *Medical and Surgical* section:

  — *Medical and Surgical* (0)

- *Medical and Surgical*-related sections:

— *Obstetrics* (1)

— *Placement* (2)

— *Administration* (3)

— *Extracorporeal Assistance and Performance* (5)

— *Extracorporeal Therapies* (6)

— *Osteopathic* (7)

— *Other Procedures* (8)

— *Chiropractic* (9)

• Ancillary sections:

— *Imaging* (B)

— *Nuclear Medicine* (C)

— *Radiation Therapy* (D)

— *Physical Rehabilitation and Diagnostic Audiology* (F)

— *Mental Health* (G)

— *Substance Abuse Treatment* (H)

The first three character values define each table. The root operation or root type designated for each table is accompanied by its official definition.

Examples:

Table 00F provides codes for procedures on the central nervous system that involve breaking up of solid matter into pieces:

Character 1, Section	0: Medical and Surgical
Character 2, Body System	0: Central Nervous System
Character 3, Root Operation	F: Fragmentation: Breaking solid matter in a body part to pieces

Tables are arranged numerically, then alphabetically.

Examples:

Section order: Numerically ordered 0 through 9, then alphabetically ordered B through H

Table order: Tables under body system *Central Nervous System* are ordered 001 through 009, then 00B though 00X.

Character value order: As an example, table 00F in the *Central Nervous* body system, the character values for body part are arranged as follows:

3   Epidural Space

4   Subdural Space

5   Subarachnoid Space

6   Cerebral Ventricle

U   Spinal Canal

When reviewing tables, the user should keep in mind that:

• There are multiple tables for the first three characters.

• Some tables may cover multiple pages in the code book—to ensure maximum clarity about character choices, OptumInsight does not split rows of valid entries between pages. For instance, the entire table of valid characters completing a code beginning with 4A1 is split between two pages, but the split is between, not within, rows. This means that all the valid sixth and seventh characters for, say, body system *Arterial* (3) and approach *External* (X) are contained on one page.

• Individual entries may be listed in several horizontal "selection" lines.

When a table is continued onto another page, a note to this effect has been added in red.

Examples:

0   Medical and Surgical
0   Central Nervous System
F   Fragmentation   Breaking solid matter in a body part into pieces

Body Part Character 4		Approach Character 5		Device Character 6	Qualifier Character 7
3 Epidural Space	NC	0	Open	Z No Device	Z No Qualifier
4 Subdural Space	NC	3	Percutaneous		
5 Subarachnoid Space	NC	4	Percutaneous Endoscopic		
6 Cerebral Ventricle	NC	X	External		
U Spinal Canal					

NC	00F[3,4,5,6]XZZ
Non-OR	00F[3,4,5,6]XZZ

ICD-10-PCS Additional Conventions

New and Revised Text

To highlight changes to the tables with each new edition, the new and revised text is in green font.

Color-Coding and Symbol Annotations

An annotation box has been appended to every table with color-coding or symbols identifying Medicare code edits or other reimbursement edits. The box provides critical information on how the edits are applied. For example, the box may list all valid codes to which the edit applies or conditional criteria that must be met to satisfy the edits. Each table that includes a Medicare code edit or a reimbursement edit will have an annotation box. For example, see Table 00F provided on the previous page. There are two annotations one for Noncovered Procedure edit and one for Non-operating room Procedure edit. The codes to which those edits apply are listed. In some cases there will be additional criteria to satisfy the edit application, such as procedures that are noncovered except when reported with specific diagnosis codes. Because of the inherent structure of ICD-10-PCS, the edits do not always apply to all valid codes in a horizontal row of a table. The edit color-coding and symbols have been placed to the right of the fourth character for consistency and should be viewed as alerts to refer to the annotation box. It is important to *always* refer to the annotation box when applying the edits.

Bracketed Code Notation

The use of bracketed codes is an efficient convention to provide all valid character value alternatives for a specific set of circumstances. The character values in the brackets correspond to the valid values for the character in the position the bracket appears.

Examples:

In the annotation box for Table 00F provided on the previous page the Noncovered Procedure edit (NC) applies to codes represented in the bracketed code 00F[3,4,5,6]XZZ.

> 00F[3,4,5,6]XZZ Fragmentation in (Central Nervous System), External Approach

The valid fourth character values, Body Part that may be selected for this specific circumstance are as follows:

3   Epidural Space

4   Subdural Space

5   Subarachnoid Space

6   Cerebral Space

The fragmentation of matter in the spinal canal, Body Part value U, is not considered as having the noncovered edit apply under the Medicare Code Editor v30.0.

Medicare Code Edits

Medicare administrative contractors and many payers use Medicare code edits to check the coding accuracy on claims under the inpatient prospective payment system (IPPS). The Medicare code edits that apply to procedures are listed below. The coding edit information in this manual is effective from October 1, 2013, to September 30, 2014. This ICD-10 version of the Medicare Code Editor (MCE) is version 30.0. However, the MCE is not intended to be used to process claims since the

ICD-10 code set will not be mandated for use until the implementation of ICD-10 beginning on October 1, 2014.

- Invalid procedure code (tor a list of all valid ICD-10-PCS codes, see the International Classification of Diseases, Tenth Revision, Procedures Classification System)

- *Sex conflict

- *Noncovered procedure

- Nonspecific O.R. procedure (Discontinued. Effective only for claims processed using MCE version 2.0-23.0)

- *Limited coverage procedure

- Open biopsy check (Discontinued. Effective only for claims processed using MCE version (2.0-26.0)

- Bilateral procedure (Discontinued. Effective only for claims processed using MCE version 2.0-28.0)

Starred edits are identified by colors, symbols, or footnotes as described below. For a quick reference to the color codes and symbols, look at the legend/key located at the bottom of each page.

Sex Edit Symbols

The sex edit symbols below address MCE and are used to detect inconsistencies between the patient's sex and the procedure. These symbols appear in the tables to the right of the body part value (character 4):

♂   Male procedure only: this symbol appears to the right of the body part value (character 4).

♀   Female procedure only: this symbol appears to the right of the body part value (character 4).

Noncovered Procedure

Medicare does not cover all procedures. However, some noncovered procedures, due to the presence of certain diagnoses, are reimbursed. Noncovered procedures are designated by the NC symbol.

Limited Coverage

For certain procedures whose medical complexity and serious nature incur extraordinary associated costs, Medicare limits coverage to a portion of the cost. The limited coverage edit indicates the type of limited coverage. Limited procedures are designated by the LC symbol to the right of the body part value.

Other Notations in the Tabular

Under the Medicare severity diagnosis-related group (MS-DRG) system, in addition to the MCEs there are certain other circumstances that affect MS-DRG assignment. The following notations alert users to reimbursement issues related to procedure reporting.

Non-Operating Room Procedures Not Affecting MS-DRG Assignment

Some ICD-10-PCS procedure codes are valid but do not affect MS-DRG assignment when reported on a claim. These codes represent non-operating room (non-OR) procedures. A gray color bar over the body part value indicates a procedure code that does not affect

MS-DRG assignment appears **only** in the Medical/Surgical tables (ØØ1-10Y).

Non-Operating Room Procedures Affecting MS- DRG Assignment

A blue color bar over a body part value indicates a non-operating room procedure that does affect MS-DRG assignment (DRG non-OR).

Hospital-Acquired Condition Related Procedures

Procedures associated with hospital-acquired conditions (HAC) are identified with the yellow color bar over the body part value.

Combination Only

Some ICD-10-PCS procedure codes are considered "noncovered procedures" except when reported in combination with certain other procedure codes. Such codes are designated by a red color bar over the body part value.

Other Notation in the Index

▽   Subterms under main terms may continue to the next column or page. This warning statement is a reminder to always check for additional subterms and information that may continue onto the next page or column before making a final selection.

ICD-1Ø-PCS Draft Coding Guidelines

Conventions

A1. ICD-1Ø-PCS codes are composed of seven characters. Each character is an axis of classification that specifies information about the procedure performed. Within a defined code range, a character specifies the same type of information in that axis of classification.

Example: The fifth axis of classification specifies the approach in sections Ø through 4 and 7 through 9 of the system.

A2. One of 34 possible values can be assigned to each axis of classification in the seven-character code: they are the numbers Ø through 9 and the alphabet (except I and O because they are easily confused with the numbers 1 and Ø). The number of unique values used in an axis of classification differs as needed.

Example: Where the fifth axis of classification specifies the approach, seven different approach values are currently used to specify the approach.

A3. The valid values for an axis of classification can be added to as needed.

Example: If a significantly distinct type of device is used in a new procedure, a new device value can be added to the system.

A4. As with words in their context, the meaning of any single value is a combination of its axis of classification and any preceding values on which it may be dependent.

Example: The meaning of a body part value in the Medical and Surgical section is always dependent on the body system value. The body part value Ø in the Central Nervous body system specifies Brain and the body part value Ø in the Peripheral Nervous body system specifies Cervical Plexus.

A5. As the system is expanded to become increasingly detailed, over time more values will depend on preceding values for their meaning.

Example: In the Lower Joints body system, the device value 3 in the root operation Insertion specifies Infusion Device and the device value 3 in the root operation Replacement specifies Ceramic Synthetic Substitute.

A6. The purpose of the alphabetic index is to locate the appropriate table that contains all information necessary to construct a procedure code. The PCS Tables should always be consulted to find the most appropriate valid code.

A7. It is not required to consult the index first before proceeding to the tables to complete the code. A valid code may be chosen directly from the tables.

A8. All seven characters must be specified to be a valid code. If the documentation is incomplete for coding purposes, the physician should be queried for the necessary information.

A9. Within a PCS table, valid codes include all combinations of choices in characters 4 through 7 contained in the same row of the table. In the example below, ØJHT3VZ is a valid code, and ØJHW3VZ is *not* a valid code.

A10. "And," when used in a code description, means "and/or."

Example: Lower Arm and Wrist Muscle means lower arm and/or wrist muscle.

A11. Many of the terms used to construct PCS codes are defined within the system. It is the coder's responsibility to determine what the documentation in the medical record equates to in the PCS definitions. The physician is not expected to use the terms used in PCS code descriptions, nor is the coder required to query the physician when the correlation between the documentation and the defined PCS terms is clear.

Example: When the physician documents "partial resection" the coder can independently correlate "partial resection" to the root operation Excision without querying the physician for clarification.

Sample ICD-1Ø-PCS Table

Ø **Medical and Surgical**
J **Subcutaneous Tissue and Fascia**
H **Insertion**   Putting in a nonbiological appliance that monitors, assists, performs, or prevents a physiological function but does not physically take the place of a body part

Body Part Character 4	Approach Character 5	Device Character 6	Qualifier Character 7
S Subcutaneous Tissue and Fascia, Head and Neck **V** Subcutaneous Tissue and Fascia, Upper Extremity **W** Subcutaneous Tissue and Fascia, Lower Extremity	**Ø** Open **3** Percutaneous	**1** Radioactive Element **3** Infusion Device	**Z** No Qualifier
T Subcutaneous Tissue and Fascia, Trunk	**Ø** Open **3** Percutaneous	**1** Radioactive Element **3** Infusion Device **V** Infusion Pump	**Z** No Qualifier

Medical and Surgical Section Guidelines

B2. Body System

General guidelines

B2.1a. The procedure codes in the general anatomical regions body systems should only be used when the procedure is performed on an anatomical region rather than a specific body part (e.g., root operations Control and Detachment, drainage of a body cavity) or on the rare occasion when no information is available to support assignment of a code to a specific body part.

Example: Control of postoperative hemorrhage is coded to the root operation Control found in the general anatomical regions body systems.

B2.1b. Where the general body part values "upper" and "lower" are provided as an option in the Upper Arteries, Lower Arteries, Upper Veins, Lower Veins, Muscles and Tendons body systems, "upper" or "lower "specifies body parts located above or below the diaphragm respectively.

Example: Vein body parts above the diaphragm are found in the Upper Veins body system; vein body parts below the diaphragm are found in the Lower Veins body system.

B3. Root Operation

General guidelines

B3.1a. In order to determine the appropriate root operation, the full definition of the root operation as contained in the PCS Tables must be applied.

B3.1b. Components of a procedure specified in the root operation definition and explanation are not coded separately. Procedural steps necessary to reach the operative site and close the operative site are also not coded separately.

Example: Resection of a joint as part of a joint replacement procedure is included in the root operation definition of Replacement and is not coded separately. Laparotomy performed to reach the site of an open liver biopsy is not coded separately. In a resection of sigmoid colon with anastomosis of descending colon to rectum, the anastomosis is not coded separately.

Multiple procedures

B3.2. During the same operative episode, multiple procedures are coded if:

   a.   The same root operation is performed on different body parts as defined by distinct values of the body part character.

   Example: Diagnostic excision of liver and pancreas are coded separately.

   b.   The same root operation is repeated at different body sites that are included in the same body part value.

   Example: Excision of the sartorius muscle and excision of the gracilis muscle are both included in the upper leg muscle body part value, and multiple procedures are coded.

   c.   Multiple root operations with distinct objectives are performed on the same body part.

   Example: Destruction of sigmoid lesion and bypass of sigmoid colon are coded separately.

   d.   The intended root operation is attempted using one approach, but is converted to a different approach.

   Example: Laparoscopic cholecystectomy converted to an open cholecystectomy is coded as percutaneous endoscopic Inspection and open Resection.

Discontinued procedures

B3.3. If the intended procedure is discontinued, code the procedure to the root operation performed. If a procedure is discontinued before any other root operation is performed, code the root operation Inspection of the body part or anatomical region inspected.

Example: A planned aortic valve replacement procedure is discontinued after the initial thoracotomy and before any incision is made in the heart muscle, when the patient becomes hemodynamically unstable. This procedure is coded as an open Inspection of the mediastinum.

Biopsy procedures

B3.4a. Biopsy procedures are coded using the root operations , Extraction, or Drainage and the qualifier Diagnostic. The qualifier Diagnostic is used only for biopsies.

Examples: Fine needle aspiration biopsy of lung is coded to the root operation Drainage with the qualifier Diagnostic. Biopsy of bone marrow is coded to the root operation Extraction with the qualifier Diagnostic. Lymph node sampling for biopsy is coded to the root operation Excision with the qualifier Diagnostic.

Biopsy followed by more definitive treatment

B3.4b. If a diagnostic Excision, Extraction, or Drainage procedure (biopsy) is followed by a more definitive procedure, such as Destruction, Excision or Resection at the same procedure site, both the biopsy and the more definitive treatment are coded.

Example: Biopsy of breast followed by partial mastectomy at the same procedure site, both the biopsy and the partial mastectomy procedure are coded.

Overlapping body layers

B3.5. If the root operations Excision, Repair or Inspection are performed on overlapping layers of the musculoskeletal system, the body part specifying the deepest layer is coded.

Example: Excisional debridement that includes skin and subcutaneous tissue and muscle is coded to the muscle body part.

Bypass procedures

B3.6a. Bypass procedures are coded by identifying the body part bypassed "from" and the body part bypassed "to." The fourth character body part specifies the body part bypassed from, and the qualifier specifies the body part bypassed to.

Example: Bypass from stomach to jejunum, stomach is the body part and jejunum is the qualifier.

B3.6b. Coronary arteries are classified by number of distinct sites treated, rather than number of coronary arteries or anatomic name of a coronary artery (e.g., left anterior descending). Coronary artery bypass procedures are coded differently than other bypass procedures as described in the previous guideline. Rather than identifying the body part bypassed from, the body part identifies the number of coronary artery sites bypassed to, and the qualifier specifies the vessel bypassed from.

Example: Aortocoronary artery bypass of one site on the left anterior descending coronary artery and one site on the obtuse marginal coronary artery is classified in the body part axis of classification as two coronary artery sites and the qualifier specifies the aorta as the body part bypassed from.

B3.6c. If multiple coronary artery sites are bypassed, a separate procedure is coded for each coronary artery site that uses a different device and/or qualifier.

Example: Aortocoronary artery bypass and internal mammary coronary artery bypass are coded separately.

Control vs. more definitive root operations

B3.7. The root operation Control is defined as, "Stopping, or attempting to stop, postprocedural bleeding." If an attempt to stop postprocedural bleeding is initially unsuccessful, and to stop the bleeding requires performing any of the definitive root operations Bypass, Detachment, Excision, Extraction, Reposition, Replacement, or Resection, then that root operation is coded instead of Control.

Example: Resection of spleen to stop postprocedural bleeding is coded to Resection instead of Control.

Excision vs. Resection

B3.8. PCS contains specific body parts for anatomical subdivisions of a body part, such as lobes of the lungs or liver and regions of the intestine. Resection of the specific body part is coded whenever all of the body part is cut out or off, rather than coding Excision of a less specific body part.

Example: Left upper lung lobectomy is coded to Resection of Upper Lung Lobe, Left rather than Excision of Lung, Left.

Excision for graft

B3.9. If an autograft is obtained from a different body part in order to complete the objective of the procedure, a separate procedure is coded.

Example: Coronary bypass with excision of saphenous vein graft, excision of saphenous vein is coded separately.

Fusion procedures of the spine

B3.10a. The body part coded for a spinal vertebral joint(s) rendered immobile by a spinal fusion procedure is classified by the level of the spine (e.g. thoracic). There are distinct body part values for a single vertebral joint and for multiple vertebral joints at each spinal level.

Example: Body part values specify Lumbar Vertebral Joint, Lumbar Vertebral Joints, 2 or More and Lumbosacral Vertebral Joint.

B3.10b. If multiple vertebral joints are fused, a separate procedure is coded for each vertebral joint that uses a different device and/or qualifier.

Example: Fusion of lumbar vertebral joint, posterior approach, anterior column and fusion of lumbar vertebral joint, posterior approach, posterior column are coded separately.

B3.10c. Combinations of devices and materials are often used on a vertebral joint to render the joint immobile. When combinations of devices are used on the same vertebral joint, the device value coded for the procedure is as follows:

- If an interbody fusion device is used to render the joint immobile (alone or containing other material like bone graft), the procedure is coded with the device value Interbody Fusion Device

- If bone graft is the *only* device used to render the joint immobile, the procedure is coded with the device value Nonautologous Tissue Substitute or Autologous Tissue Substitute

- If a mixture of autologous and nonautologous bone graft (with or without biological or synthetic extenders or binders) is used to render the joint immobile, code the procedure with the device value Autologous Tissue Substitute

Examples: Fusion of a vertebral joint using a cage style interbody fusion device containing morsellized bone graft is coded to the device Interbody Fusion Device.

Fusion of a vertebral joint using a bone dowel interbody fusion device made of cadaver bone and packed with a mixture of local morsellized bone and demineralized bone matrix is coded to the device Interbody Fusion Device.

Fusion of a vertebral joint using both autologous bone graft and bone bank bone graft is coded to the device Autologous Tissue Substitute.

Inspection procedures

B3.11a. Inspection of a body part(s) performed in order to achieve the objective of a procedure is not coded separately.

Example: Fiberoptic bronchoscopy performed for irrigation of bronchus, only the irrigation procedure is coded.

B3.11b. If multiple tubular body parts are inspected, the most distal body part inspected is coded. If multiple non-tubular body parts in a region are inspected, the body part that specifies the entire area inspected is coded.

Examples: Cystoureteroscopy with inspection of bladder and ureters is coded to the ureter body part value.

Exploratory laparotomy with general inspection of abdominal contents is coded to the peritoneal cavity body part value.

B3.11c. When both an Inspection procedure and another procedure are performed on the same body part during the same episode, if the Inspection procedure is performed using a different approach than the other procedure, the Inspection procedure is coded separately.

Example: Endoscopic Inspection of the duodenum is coded separately when open Excision of the duodenum is performed during the same procedural episode.

Occlusion vs. Restriction for vessel embolization procedures

B3.12. If the objective of an embolization procedure is to completely close a vessel, the root operation Occlusion is coded. If the objective of an embolization procedure is to narrow the lumen of a vessel, the root operation Restriction is coded.

Examples: Tumor embolization is coded to the root operation Occlusion, because the objective of the procedure is to cut off the blood supply to the vessel.

Embolization of a cerebral aneurysm is coded to the root operation Restriction, because the objective of the procedure is not to close off the vessel entirely, but to narrow the lumen of the vessel at the site of the aneurysm where it is abnormally wide.

Release procedures

B3.13. In the root operation Release, the body part value coded is the body part being freed and not the tissue being manipulated or cut to free the body part.

Example: Lysis of intestinal adhesions is coded to the specific intestine body part value.

Release vs. Division

B3.14. If the sole objective of the procedure is freeing a body part without cutting the body part, the root operation is Release. If the sole objective of the procedure is separating or transecting a body part, the root operation is Division.

Examples: Freeing a nerve root from surrounding scar tissue to relieve pain is coded to the root operation Release. Severing a nerve root to relieve pain is coded to the root operation Division.

Reposition for fracture treatment

B3.15. Reduction of a displaced fracture is coded to the root operation Reposition and the application of a cast or splint in conjunction with the Reposition procedure is not coded separately. Treatment of a nondisplaced fracture is coded to the procedure performed.

Examples: Putting a pin in a nondisplaced fracture is coded to the root operation Insertion.

Casting of a nondisplaced fracture is coded to the root operation Immobilization in the Placement section.

Transplantation vs. Administration

B3.16. Putting in a mature and functioning living body part taken from another individual or animal is coded to the root operation Transplantation. Putting in autologous or nonautologous cells is coded to the Administration section.

Example: Putting in autologous or nonautologous bone marrow, pancreatic islet cells or stem cells is coded to the Administration section.

B4. Body Part

General guidelines

B4.1a. If a procedure is performed on a portion of a body part that does not have a separate body part value, code the body part value corresponding to the whole body part.

Example: A procedure performed on the alveolar process of the mandible is coded to the mandible body part.

B4.1b. If the prefix "peri" is combined with a body part to identify the site of the procedure, the procedure is coded to the body part named.

Example: A procedure site identified as perirenal is coded to the kidney body part.

Branches of body parts

B4.2. Where a specific branch of a body part does not have its own body part value in PCS, the body part is coded to the closest proximal branch that has a specific body part value.

Example: A procedure performed on the mandibular branch of the trigeminal nerve is coded to the trigeminal nerve body part value

Bilateral body part values

B4.3. Bilateral body part values are available for a limited number of body parts. If the identical procedure is performed on contralateral body parts, and a bilateral body part value exists for that body part, a single procedure is coded using the bilateral body part value. If no

bilateral body part value exists, each procedure is coded separately using the appropriate body part value.

Example: The identical procedure performed on both fallopian tubes is coded once using the body part value Fallopian Tube, Bilateral. The identical procedure performed on both knee joints is coded twice using the body part values Knee Joint, Right and Knee Joint, Left.

Coronary arteries

B4.4. The coronary arteries are classified as a single body part that is further specified by number of sites treated and not by name or number of arteries. Separate body part values are used to specify the number of sites treated when the same procedure is performed on multiple sites in the coronary arteries.

Examples: Angioplasty of two distinct sites in the left anterior descending coronary artery with placement of two stents is coded as Dilation of Coronary Arteries, Two Sites, with Intraluminal Device.

Angioplasty of two distinct sites in the left anterior descending coronary artery, one with stent placed and one without, is coded separately as Dilation of Coronary Artery, One Site with Intraluminal Device, and Dilation of Coronary Artery, One Site with no device.

Tendons, ligaments, bursae and fascia near a joint

B4.5. Procedures performed on tendons, ligaments, bursae and fascia supporting a joint are coded to the body part in the respective body system that is the focus of the procedure. Procedures performed on joint structures themselves are coded to the body part in the joint body systems.

Example: Repair of the anterior cruciate ligament of the knee is coded to the knee bursae and ligament body part in the bursae and ligaments body system. Knee arthroscopy with shaving of articular cartilage is coded to the knee joint body part in the Lower Joints body system.

Skin, subcutaneous tissue and fascia overlying a joint

B4.6. If a procedure is performed on the skin, subcutaneous tissue or fascia overlying a joint, the procedure is coded to the following body part:

- Shoulder is coded to Upper Arm
- Elbow is coded to Lower Arm
- Wrist is coded to Lower Arm
- Hip is coded to Upper Leg
- Knee is coded to Lower Leg
- Ankle is coded to Foot

Fingers and toes

B4.7. If a body system does not contain a separate body part value for fingers, procedures performed on the fingers are coded to the body part value for the hand. If a body system does not contain a separate body part value for toes, procedures performed on the toes are coded to the body part value for the foot.

Example: Excision of finger muscle is coded to one of the hand muscle body part values in the Muscles body system.

Upper and lower intestinal tract

B4.8 In the Gastrointestinal body system, the general body part values Upper Intestinal Tract and Lower Intestinal Tract are provided as an option for the root operations Change, Inspection, Removal and Revision. Upper Intestinal Tract includes the portion of the gastrointestinal tract from the esophagus down to and including the duodenum, and Lower Intestinal Tract includes the portion of the gastrointestinal tract from the jejunum down to and including the rectum and anus.

Example: In the root operation Change table, change of a device in the jejunum is coded using the body part Lower Intestinal Tract.

B5. Approach

Open approach with percutaneous endoscopic assistance

B5.2 Procedures performed using the open approach with percutaneous endoscopic assistance are coded to the approach Open.

Example: Laparoscopic-assisted sigmoidectomy is coded to the approach Open.

External approach

B5.3a Procedures performed within an orifice on structures that are visible without the aid of any instrumentation are coded to the approach External.

Example: Resection of tonsils is coded to the approach External.

B5.3b Procedures performed indirectly by the application of external force through the intervening body layers are coded to the approach External.

Example: Closed reduction of fracture is coded to the approach External.

Percutaneous procedure via device

B5.4 Procedures performed percutaneously via a device placed for the procedure are coded to the approach Percutaneous.

Example: Fragmentation of kidney stone performed via percutaneous nephrostomy is coded to the approach Percutaneous.

B6. Device

General guidelines

B6.1a. A device is coded only if a device remains after the procedure is completed. If no device remains, the device value No Device is coded.

B6.1b. Materials such as sutures, ligatures, radiological markers and temporary post-operative wound drains are considered integral to the performance of a procedure and are not coded as devices.

B6.1c. Procedures performed on a device only and not on a body part are specified in the root operations Change, Irrigation, Removal and Revision, and are coded to the procedure performed.

Example: Irrigation of percutaneous nephrostomy tube is coded to the root operation Irrigation of indwelling device in the Administration section.

Drainage device

B6.2. A separate procedure to put in a drainage device is coded to the root operation Drainage with the device value Drainage Device.

Obstetric Section Guidelines

C. Obstetrics Section

Products of conception

C1. Procedures performed on the products of conception are coded to the Obstetrics section. Procedures performed on the pregnant female other than the products of conception are coded to the appropriate root operation in the Medical and Surgical section.

Example: Amniocentesis is coded to the products of conception body part in the Obstetrics section. Repair of obstetric urethral laceration is coded to the urethra body part in the Medical and Surgical section.

Procedures following delivery or abortion

C2. Procedures performed following a delivery or abortion for curettage of the endometrium or evacuation of retained products of conception are all coded in the Obstetrics section, to the root operation Extraction and the body part Products of Conception, Retained. Diagnostic or therapeutic dilation and curettage performed during times other than the postpartum or post-abortion period are all coded in the Medical and Surgical section, to the root operation Extraction and the body part Endometrium.

Selection of Principal Procedure

D. Selection of Principal Procedure

The following instructions should be applied in the selection of principal procedure and clarification on the importance of the relation to the principal diagnosis when more than one procedure is performed:

1. Procedure performed for definitive treatment of both principal diagnosis and secondary diagnosis

    a. Sequence procedure performed for definitive treatment most related to principal diagnosis as principal procedure.

2. Procedure performed for definitive treatment and diagnostic procedures performed for both principal diagnosis and secondary diagnosis

    a. Sequence procedure performed for definitive treatment most related to principal diagnosis as principal procedure

3. A diagnostic procedure was performed for the principal diagnosis and a procedure is performed for definitive treatment of a secondary diagnosis.

    a. Sequence diagnostic procedure as principal procedure, since the procedure most related to the principal diagnosis takes precedence.

4. No procedures performed that are related to principal diagnosis; procedures performed for definitive treatment and diagnostic procedures were performed for secondary diagnosis

    a. Sequence procedure performed for definitive treatment of secondary diagnosis as principal procedure, since there are no procedures (definitive or nondefinitive treatment) related to principal diagnosis.

Coding Exercises

Using the ICD-10-PCS tables construct the code that accurately represents the procedure performed. Answers to these coding exercises may be found in appendix H.

Medical Surgical Section

Procedure	Code
Excision of malignant melanoma from skin of right ear	
Laparoscopy with excision of endometrial implant from left ovary	
Percutaneous needle core biopsy of right kidney	
EGD with gastric biopsy	
Open endarterectomy of left common carotid artery	
Excision of basal cell carcinoma of lower lip	
Open excision of tail of pancreas	
Percutaneous biopsy of right gastrocnemius muscle	
Sigmoidoscopy with sigmoid polypectomy	
Open excision of lesion from right Achilles tendon	
Open resection of cecum	
Total excision of pituitary gland, open	
Explantation of left failed kidney, open	
Open left axillary total lymphadenectomy	
Laparoscopic-assisted total vaginal hysterectomy	
Right total mastectomy, open	
Open resection of papillary muscle	
Radical retropubic prostatectomy, open	
Laparoscopic cholecystectomy	
Endoscopic bilateral total maxillary sinusectomy	
Amputation at right elbow level	
Right below-knee amputation, proximal tibia/fibula	
Fifth ray carpometacarpal joint amputation, left hand	
Right leg and hip amputation through ischium	
DIP joint amputation of right thumb	
Right wrist joint amputation	
Trans-metatarsal amputation of foot at left big toe	
Mid-shaft amputation, right humerus	
Left fourth toe amputation, mid-proximal phalanx	
Right above-knee amputation, distal femur	
Cryotherapy of wart on left hand	
Percutaneous radiofrequency ablation of right vocal cord lesion	

Medical Surgical Section (Continued)

Procedure	Code
Left heart catheterization with laser destruction of arrhythmogenic focus, A-V node	
Cautery of nosebleed	
Transurethral endoscopic laser ablation of prostate	
Cautery of oozing varicose vein, left calf	
Laparoscopy with destruction of endometriosis, bilateral ovaries	
Laser coagulation of right retinal vessel hemorrhage, percutaneous	
Thoracoscopic pleurodesis, left side	
Percutaneous insertion of Greenfield IVC filter	
Forceps total mouth extraction, upper and lower teeth	
Removal of left thumbnail	
Extraction of right intraocular lens without replacement, percutaneous	
Laparoscopy with needle aspiration of ova for in vitro fertilization	
Nonexcisional debridement of skin ulcer, right foot	
Open stripping of abdominal fascia, right side	
Hysteroscopy with D&C, diagnostic	
Liposuction for medical purposes, left upper arm	
Removal of tattered right ear drum fragments with tweezers	
Microincisional phlebectomy of spider veins, right lower leg	
Routine Foley catheter placement	
Incision and drainage of external perianal abscess	
Percutaneous drainage of ascites	
Laparoscopy with left ovarian cystotomy and drainage	
Laparotomy and drain placement for liver abscess, right lobe	
Right knee arthrotomy with drain placement	
Thoracentesis of left pleural effusion	
Phlebotomy of left median cubital vein for polycythemia vera	
Percutaneous chest tube placement for right pneumothorax	
Endoscopic drainage of left ethmoid sinus	
External ventricular CSF drainage catheter placement via burr hole	
Removal of foreign body, right cornea	
Percutaneous mechanical thrombectomy, left brachial artery	

Medical Surgical Section (Continued)

Procedure	Code
Esophagogastroscopy with removal of bezoar from stomach	
Foreign body removal, skin of left thumb	
Transurethral cystoscopy with removal of bladder stone	
Forceps removal of foreign body in right nostril	
Laparoscopy with excision of old suture from mesentery	
Incision and removal of right lacrimal duct stone	
Nonincisional removal of intraluminal foreign body from vagina	
Right common carotid endarterectomy, open	
Open excision of retained sliver, subcutaneous tissue of left foot	
Extracorporeal shock-wave lithotripsy (ESWL), bilateral ureters	
Endoscopic retrograde cholangiopancreatography (ERCP) with lithotripsy of common bile duct stone	
Thoracotomy with crushing of pericardial calcifications	
Transurethral cystoscopy with fragmentation of bladder calculus	
Hysteroscopy with intraluminal lithotripsy of left fallopian tube calcification	
Division of right foot tendon, percutaneous	
Left heart catheterization with division of bundle of HIS	
Open osteotomy of capitate, left hand	
EGD with esophagotomy of esophagogastric junction	
Sacral rhizotomy for pain control, percutaneous	
Laparotomy with exploration and adhesiolysis of right ureter	
Incision of scar contracture, right elbow	
Frenulotomy for treatment of tongue-tie syndrome	
Right shoulder arthroscopy with coracoacromial ligament release	
Mitral valvulotomy for release of fused leaflets, open approach	
Percutaneous left Achilles tendon release	
Laparoscopy with lysis of peritoneal adhesions	
Manual rupture of right shoulder joint adhesions under general anesthesia	
Open posterior tarsal tunnel release	
Laparoscopy with freeing of left ovary and fallopian tube	
Liver transplant with donor matched liver	
Orthotopic heart transplant using porcine heart	
Right lung transplant, open, using organ donor match	
Transplant of large intestine, organ donor match	
Left kidney/pancreas organ bank transplant	

Medical Surgical Section (Continued)

Procedure	Code
Replantation of avulsed scalp	
Reattachment of severed right ear	
Reattachment of traumatic left gastrocnemius avulsion, open	
Closed replantation of three avulsed teeth, lower jaw	
Reattachment of severed left hand	
Right hand open palmaris longus tendon transfer	
Endoscopic radial to median nerve transfer	
Fasciocutaneous flap closure of left thigh, open	
Transfer left index finger to left thumb position, open	
Percutaneous fascia transfer to fill defect, anterior neck	
Trigeminal to facial nerve transfer, percutaneous endoscopic	
Endoscopic left leg flexor hallucis longus tendon transfer	
Right scalp advancement flap to right temple	
Bilateral TRAM pedicle flap reconstruction status post mastectomy, muscle only, open	
Skin transfer flap closure of complex open wound, left lower back	
Open fracture reduction, right tibia	
Laparoscopy with gastropexy for malrotation	
Left knee arthroscopy with reposition of anterior cruciate ligament	
Open transposition of ulnar nerve	
Closed reduction with percutaneous internal fixation of right femoral neck fracture	
Trans-vaginal intraluminal cervical cerclage	
Cervical cerclage using Shirodkar technique	
Thoracotomy with banding of left pulmonary artery using extraluminal device	
Restriction of thoracic duct with intraluminal stent, percutaneous	
Craniotomy with clipping of cerebral aneurysm	
Nonincisional, transnasal placement of restrictive stent in right lacrimal duct	
Catheter-based temporary restriction of blood flow in abdominal aorta for treatment of cerebral ischemia	
Percutaneous ligation of esophageal vein	
Percutaneous embolization of left internal carotid-cavernous fistula	
Laparoscopy with bilateral occlusion of fallopian tubes using Hulka extraluminal clips	
Open suture ligation of failed A-V graft, left brachial artery	
Percutaneous embolization of vascular supply, intracranial meningioma	
Percutaneous embolization of right uterine artery, using coils	

Medical Surgical Section (Continued)

Procedure	Code
Open occlusion of left atrial appendage, using extraluminal pressure clips	
Percutaneous suture exclusion of left atrial appendage, via femoral artery access	
ERCP with balloon dilation of common bile duct	
PTCA of two coronary arteries, LAD with stent placement, RCA with no stent	
Cystoscopy with intraluminal dilation of bladder neck stricture	
Open dilation of old anastomosis, left femoral artery	
Dilation of upper esophageal stricture, direct visualization, with Bougie sound	
PTA of right brachial artery stenosis	
Transnasal dilation and stent placement in right lacrimal duct	
Hysteroscopy with balloon dilation of bilateral fallopian tubes	
Tracheoscopy with intraluminal dilation of tracheal stenosis	
Cystoscopy with dilation of left ureteral stricture, with stent placement	
Open gastric bypass with Roux-en-Y limb to jejunum	
Right temporal artery to intracranial artery bypass using Gore-Tex graft, open	
Tracheostomy formation with tracheostomy tube placement, percutaneous	
PICVA (percutaneous in situ coronary venous arterialization) of single coronary artery	
Open left femoral-popliteal artery bypass using cadaver vein graft	
Shunting of intrathecal cerebrospinal fluid to peritoneal cavity using synthetic shunt	
Colostomy formation, open, transverse colon to abdominal wall	
Open urinary diversion, left ureter, using ileal conduit to skin	
CABG of LAD using left internal mammary artery, open off-bypass	
Open pleuroperitoneal shunt, right pleural cavity, using synthetic device	
Percutaneous placement of ventriculoperitoneal shunt for treatment of hydrocephalus	
End-of-life replacement of spinal neurostimulator generator, multiple array, in lower abdomen	
Percutaneous insertion of spinal neurostimulator lead, lumbar spinal cord	
Percutaneous placement of pacemaker lead in left atrium	
Open placement of dual chamber pacemaker generator in chest wall	
Percutaneous placement of venous central line in right internal jugular	

Medical Surgical Section (Continued)

Procedure	Code
Open insertion of multiple channel cochlear implant, left ear	
Percutaneous placement of Swan-Ganz catheter in superior vena cava	
Bronchoscopy with insertion of brachytherapy seeds, right main bronchus	
Placement of intrathecal infusion pump for pain management, percutaneous	
Open insertion of interspinous process device into lumbar vertebral joint	
Open placement of bone growth stimulator, left femoral shaft	
Cystoscopy with placement of brachytherapy seeds in prostate gland	
Percutaneous insertion of Greenfield IVC filter	
Full-thickness skin graft to right lower arm, autograft (do not code graft harvest for this exercise)	
Excision of necrosed left femoral head with bone bank bone graft to fill the defect, open	
Penetrating keratoplasty of right cornea with donor matched cornea, percutaneous approach	
Bilateral mastectomy with concomitant saline breast implants, open	
Excision of abdominal aorta with Gore-Tex graft replacement, open	
Total right knee arthroplasty with insertion of total knee prosthesis	
Bilateral mastectomy with free TRAM flap reconstruction	
Tenonectomy with graft to right ankle using cadaver graft, open	
Mitral valve replacement using porcine valve, open	
Percutaneous phacoemulsification of right eye cataract with prosthetic lens insertion	
Transcatheter replacement of pulmonary valve using of bovine jugular vein valve	
Total left hip replacement using ceramic on ceramic prosthesis, without bone cement	
Aortic valve annuloplasty using ring, open	
Laparoscopic repair of left inguinal hernia with marlex plug	
Autograft nerve graft to right median nerve, percutaneous endoscopic (do not code graft harvest for this exercise)	
Exchange of liner in femoral component of previous left hip replacement, open approach	
Anterior colporrhaphy with polypropylene mesh reinforcement, open approach	
Implantation of CorCap cardiac support device, open approach	
Abdominal wall herniorrhaphy, open, using synthetic mesh	

Medical Surgical Section (Continued)

Procedure	Code
Tendon graft to strengthen injured left shoulder using autograft, open (do not code graft harvest for this exercise)	
Onlay lamellar keratoplasty of left cornea using autograft, external approach	
Resurfacing procedure on right femoral head, open approach	
Exchange of drainage tube from right hip joint	
Tracheostomy tube exchange	
Change chest tube for left pneumothorax	
Exchange of cerebral ventriculostomy drainage tube	
Foley urinary catheter exchange	
Open removal of lumbar sympathetic neurostimulator lead	
Nonincisional removal of Swan-Ganz catheter from right pulmonary artery	
Laparotomy with removal of pancreatic drain	
Extubation, endotracheal tube	
Nonincisional PEG tube removal	
Transvaginal removal of brachytherapy seeds	
Transvaginal removal of extraluminal cervical cerclage	
Incision with removal of K-wire fixation, right first metatarsal	
Cystoscopy with retrieval of left ureteral stent	
Removal of nasogastric drainage tube for decompression	
Removal of external fixator, left radial fracture	
Reposition of Swan-Ganz catheter insertion to superior vena cava	
Open revision of right hip replacement, with readjustment of prosthesis	
Adjustment of position, pacemaker lead in left ventricle, percutaneous	
External repositioning of Foley catheter to bladder	
Taking out loose screw and putting larger screw in fracture repair plate, left tibia	
Revision of VAD reservoir placement in chest wall, causing patient discomfort, open	
Thoracotomy with exploration of right pleural cavity	
Diagnostic laryngoscopy	
Exploratory arthrotomy of left knee	
Colposcopy with diagnostic hysteroscopy	
Digital rectal exam	
Diagnostic arthroscopy of right shoulder	
Endoscopy of bilateral maxillary sinus	
Laparotomy with palpation of liver	
Transurethral diagnostic cystoscopy	

Medical Surgical Section (Continued)

Procedure	Code
Colonoscopy, abandoned at sigmoid colon	
Percutaneous mapping of basal ganglia	
Heart catheterization with cardiac mapping	
Intraoperative whole brain mapping via craniotomy	
Mapping of left cerebral hemisphere, percutaneous endoscopic	
Intraoperative cardiac mapping during open heart surgery	
Hysteroscopy with cautery of post-hysterectomy oozing and evacuation of clot	
Open exploration and ligation of post-op arterial bleeder, left forearm	
Control of postoperative retroperitoneal bleeding via laparotomy	
Reopening of thoracotomy site with drainage and control of post-op hemopericardium	
Arthroscopy with drainage of hemarthrosis at previous operative site, right knee	
Radiocarpal fusion of left hand with internal fixation, open	
Posterior spinal fusion at L1–L3 level with BAK cage interbody fusion device, open	
Intercarpal fusion of right hand with bone bank bone graft, open	
Sacrococcygeal fusion with bone graft from same operative site, open	
Interphalangeal fusion of left great toe, percutaneous pin fixation	
Suture repair of left radial nerve laceration	
Laparotomy with suture repair of blunt force duodenal laceration	
Cosmetic face lift, open, no other information available	
Bilateral breast augmentation with silicone implants, open	
Cosmetic rhinoplasty with septal reduction and tip elevation using local tissue graft, open	
Abdominoplasty (tummy tuck), open	
Liposuction of bilateral thighs	
Creation of penis in female patient using tissue bank donor graft	
Creation of vagina in male patient using synthetic material	
Laparoscopic vertical sleeve gastrectomy	
Left uterine artery embolization, intraluminal biosphere injection	

Obstetrics

Procedure	Code
Abortion by dilation and evacuation following laminaria insertion	
Manually assisted spontaneous abortion	
Abortion by abortifacient insertion	
Bimanual pregnancy examination	
Extraperitoneal C-section, low transverse incision	
Fetal spinal tap, percutaneous	
Fetal kidney transplant, laparoscopic	
Open in utero repair of congenital diaphragmatic hernia	
Laparoscopy with total excision of tubal pregnancy	
Transvaginal removal of fetal monitoring electrode	

Placement

Procedure	Code
Placement of packing material, right ear	
Mechanical traction of entire left leg	
Removal of splint, right shoulder	
Placement of neck brace	
Change of vaginal packing	
Packing of wound, chest wall	
Sterile dressing placement to left groin region	
Removal of packing material from pharynx	
Placement of intermittent pneumatic compression device, covering entire right arm	
Exchange of pressure dressing to left thigh	

Administration

Procedure	Code
Peritoneal dialysis via indwelling catheter	
Transvaginal artificial insemination	
Infusion of total parenteral nutrition via central venous catheter	
Esophagogastroscopy with Botox injection into esophageal sphincter	
Percutaneous irrigation of knee joint	
Epidural injection of mixed steroid and local anesthetic for pain control	
Transfusion of antihemophilic factor, (nonautologous) via arterial central line	
Transabdominal in vitro fertilization, implantation of donor ovum	

Administration (Continued)

Procedure	Code
Autologous bone marrow transplant via central venous line	
Implantation of anti-microbial envelope with cardiac defibrillator placement, open	
Sclerotherapy of brachial plexus lesion, alcohol injection	
Percutaneous peripheral vein injection, glucarpidase	
Introduction of anti-infective envelope into subcutaneous tissue, open	

Measurement and Monitoring

Procedure	Code
Cardiac stress test, single measurement	
EGD with biliary flow measurement	
Right and left heart cardiac catheterization with bilateral sampling and pressure measurements	
Temperature monitoring, rectal	
Peripheral venous pulse, external, single measurement	
Holter monitoring	
Respiratory rate, external, single measurement	
Fetal heart rate monitoring, transvaginal	
Visual mobility test, single measurement	
Left ventricular cardiac output monitoring from pulmonary artery wedge (Swan-Ganz) catheter	
Olfactory acuity test, single measurement	

Extracorporeal Assistance and Performance

Procedure	Code
Intermittent mechanical ventilation, 16 hours	
Liver dialysis, single encounter	
Cardiac countershock with successful conversion to sinus rhythm	
IPPB (intermittent positive pressure breathing) for mobilization of secretions, 22 hours	
Renal dialysis, series of encounters	
IABP (intra-aortic balloon pump) continuous	
Intra-operative cardiac pacing, continuous	
ECMO (extracorporeal membrane oxygenation), continuous	
Controlled mechanical ventilation (CMV), 45 hours	
Pulsatile compression boot with intermittent inflation	

Extracorporeal Therapies

Procedure	Code
Donor thrombocytapheresis, single encounter	
Bili-lite UV phototherapy, series treatment	
Whole body hypothermia, single treatment	
Circulatory phototherapy, single encounter	
Shock wave therapy of plantar fascia, single treatment	
Antigen-free air conditioning, series treatment	
TMS (transcranial magnetic stimulation), series treatment	
Therapeutic ultrasound of peripheral vessels, single treatment	
Plasmapheresis, series treatment	
Extracorporeal electromagnetic stimulation (EMS) for urinary incontinence, single treatment	

Osteopathic

Procedures	Code
Isotonic muscle energy treatment of right leg	
Low velocity-high amplitude osteopathic treatment of head	
Lymphatic pump osteopathic treatment of left axilla	
Indirect osteopathic treatment of sacrum	
Articulatory osteopathic treatment of cervical region	

Other Procedures

Procedure	Code
Near infrared spectroscopy of leg vessels	
CT computer assisted sinus surgery	
Suture removal, abdominal wall	
Isolation after infectious disease exposure	
Robotic assisted open prostatectomy	
In vitro fertilization	

Chiropractic

Procedure	Code
Chiropractic treatment of lumbar region using long lever specific contact	
Chiropractic manipulation of abdominal region, indirect visceral	
Chiropractic extra-articular treatment of hip region	
Chiropractic treatment of sacrum using long and short lever specific contact	
Mechanically-assisted chiropractic manipulation of head	

Imaging

Procedure	Code
Noncontrast CT of abdomen and pelvis	
Ultrasound guidance for catheter placement, left subclavian artery	
Intravascular ultrasound, left subclavian artery	
Fluoroscopic guidance for insertion of central venous catheter in SVC, low osmolar contrast	
Chest x-ray, AP/PA and lateral views	
Endoluminal ultrasound of gallbladder and bile ducts	
MRI of thyroid gland, contrast unspecified	
Esophageal videofluoroscopy study with oral barium contrast	
Portable x-ray study of right radius/ulna shaft, standard series	
Routine fetal ultrasound, second trimester twin gestation	
CT scan of bilateral lungs, high osmolar contrast with densitometry	
Fluoroscopic guidance for percutaneous transluminal angioplasty (PTA) of left common femoral artery, low osmolar contrast	

Nuclear Medicine

Procedure	Code
Tomo scan of right and left heart, unspecified radiopharmaceutical, qualitative gated rest	
Technetium pentetate assay of kidneys, ureters, and bladder	
Uniplanar scan of spine using technetium oxidronate, with first-pass study	
Thallous chloride tomographic scan of bilateral breasts	
PET scan of myocardium using rubidium	
Gallium citrate scan of head and neck, single plane imaging	

Nuclear Medicine (Continued)

Procedure	Code
Xenon gas nonimaging probe of brain	
Upper GI scan, radiopharmaceutical unspecified, for gastric emptying	
Carbon 11 PET scan of brain with quantification	
Iodinated albumin nuclear medicine assay, blood plasma volume study	

Radiation Therapy

Procedure	Code
Plaque radiation of left eye, single port	
8 MeV photon beam radiation to brain	
IORT of colon, 3 ports	
HDR brachytherapy of prostate using palladium-103	
Electron radiation treatment of right breast, with custom device	
Hyperthermia oncology treatment of pelvic region	
Contact radiation of tongue	
Heavy particle radiation treatment of pancreas, four risk sites	
LDR brachytherapy to spinal cord using iodine	
Whole body phosphorus-32 administration with risk to hematopoetic system	

Physical Rehabilitation and Diagnostic Audiology

Procedure	Code
Bekesy assessment using audiometer	
Individual fitting of left eye prosthesis	
Physical therapy for range of motion and mobility, patient right hip, no special equipment	
Bedside swallow assessment using assessment kit	
Caregiver training in airway clearance techniques	
Application of short arm cast in rehabilitation setting	
Verbal assessment of patient's pain level	
Caregiver training in communication skills using manual communication board	
Group musculoskeletal balance training exercises, whole body, no special equipment	
Individual therapy for auditory processing using tape recorder	

Mental Health

Procedure	Code
Cognitive-behavioral psychotherapy, individual	
Narcosynthesis	
Light therapy	
ECT (electroconvulsive therapy), unilateral, multiple seizure	
Crisis intervention	
Neuropsychological testing	
Hypnosis	
Developmental testing	
Vocational counseling	
Family psychotherapy	

Substance Abuse Treatment

Procedure	Code
Naltrexone treatment for drug dependency	
Substance abuse treatment family counseling	
Medication monitoring of patient on methadone maintenance	
Individual interpersonal psychotherapy for drug abuse	
Patient in for alcohol detoxification treatment	
Group motivational counseling	
Individual 12-step psychotherapy for substance abuse	
Post-test infectious disease counseling for IV drug abuser	
Psychodynamic psychotherapy for drug-dependent patient	
Group cognitive-behavioral counseling for substance abuse	

# #

3f (Aortic) Bioprosthesis valve *use* Zooplastic Tissue in Heart and Great Vessels

A

Abdominal aortic plexus *use* Nerve, Abdominal Sympathetic
Abdominal esophagus *use* Esophagus, Lower
Abdominohysterectomy
  see Excision, Uterus ØUB9
  see Resection, Uterus ØUT9
Abdominoplasty
  see Alteration, Abdominal Wall ØWØF
  see Repair, Abdominal Wall ØWQF
  see Supplement, Abdominal Wall ØWUF
Abductor hallucis muscle
  use Muscle, Foot, Left
  use Muscle, Foot, Right
AbioCor® Total Replacement Heart *use* Synthetic Substitute
Ablation *see* Destruction
Abortion
  Abortifacient 10A07ZX
  Laminaria 10A07ZW
  Products of Conception 10AØ
  Vacuum 10A07Z6
Abrasion *see* Extraction
Accessory cephalic vein
  use Vein, Cephalic, Left
  use Vein, Cephalic, Right
Accessory obturator nerve *use* Nerve, Lumbar Plexus
Accessory phrenic nerve *use* Nerve, Phrenic
Accessory spleen *use* Spleen
Acellular Hydrated Dermis *use* Nonautologous Tissue Substitute
Acetabulectomy
  see Excision, Lower Bones ØQB
  see Resection, Lower Bones ØQT
Acetabulofemoral joint
  use Joint, Hip, Left
  use Joint, Hip, Right
Acetabuloplasty
  see Repair, Lower Bones ØQQ
  see Replacement, Lower Bones ØQR
  see Supplement, Lower Bones ØQU
Achilles tendon
  use Tendon, Lower Leg, Left
  use Tendon, Lower Leg, Right
Achillorrhaphy *see* Repair, Tendons ØLQ
Achillotenotomy, achillotomy
  see Division, Tendons ØL8
  see Drainage, Tendons ØL9
Acromioclavicular ligament
  use Bursa and Ligament, Shoulder, Left
  use Bursa and Ligament, Shoulder, Right
Acromion (process)
  use Scapula, Left
  use Scapula, Right
Acromionectomy
  see Excision, Upper Joints ØRB
  see Resection, Upper Joints ØRT
Acromioplasty
  see Repair, Upper Joints ØRQ
  see Replacement, Upper Joints ØRR
  see Supplement, Upper Joints ØRU
Activa PC neurostimulator *use* Stimulator Generator, Multiple Array in ØJH
Activa RC neurostimulator *use* Stimulator Generator, Multiple Array Rechargeable in ØJH
Activa SC neurostimulator *use* Stimulator Generator, Single Array in ØJH
Activities of Daily Living Assessment F02
Activities of Daily Living Treatment F08
ACUITY™ Steerable Lead
  use Cardiac Lead, Defibrillator in 02H
  use Cardiac Lead, Pacemaker in 02H
Acupuncture
  Breast
    Anesthesia 8EØH300
    No Qualifier 8EØH30Z

Acupuncture — *continued*
  Integumentary System
    Anesthesia 8EØH300
    No Qualifier 8EØH30Z
Adductor brevis muscle
  use Muscle, Upper Leg, Left
  use Muscle, Upper Leg, Right
Adductor hallucis muscle
  use Muscle, Foot, Left
  use Muscle, Foot, Right
Adductor longus muscle
  use Muscle, Upper Leg, Left
  use Muscle, Upper Leg, Right
Adductor magnus muscle
  use Muscle, Upper Leg, Left
  use Muscle, Upper Leg, Right
Adenohypophysis *use* Gland, Pituitary
Adenoidectomy
  see Excision, Adenoids ØCBQ
  see Resection, Adenoids ØCTQ
Adenoidotomy *see* Drainage, Adenoids ØC9Q
Adhesiolysis *see* Release
Administration
  Blood products *see* Transfusion
  Other substance *see* Introduction of substance in or on
Adrenalectomy
  see Excision, Endocrine System ØGB
  see Resection, Endocrine System ØGT
Adrenalorrhaphy *see* Repair, Endocrine System ØGQ
Adrenalotomy *see* Drainage, Endocrine System ØG9
Advancement
  see Reposition
  see Transfer
Alar ligament of axis *use* Bursa and Ligament, Head and Neck
Alimentation *see* Introduction of substance in or on
Alteration
  Abdominal Wall ØWØF
  Ankle Region
    Left ØYØL
    Right ØYØK
  Arm
    Lower
      Left ØXØF
      Right ØXØD
    Upper
      Left ØXØ9
      Right ØXØ8
  Axilla
    Left ØXØ5
    Right ØXØ4
  Back
    Lower ØWØL
    Upper ØWØK
  Breast
    Bilateral ØHØV
    Left ØHØU
    Right ØHØT
  Buttock
    Left ØYØ1
    Right ØYØØ
  Chest Wall ØWØ8
  Ear
    Bilateral Ø9Ø2
    Left Ø9Ø1
    Right Ø9ØØ
  Elbow Region
    Left ØXØC
    Right ØXØB
  Extremity
    Lower
      Left ØYØB
      Right ØYØ9
    Upper
      Left ØXØ7
      Right ØXØ6
  Eyelid
    Lower
      Left Ø8ØR
      Right Ø8ØQ
    Upper
      Left Ø8ØP
      Right Ø8ØN
  Face ØWØ2

Alteration — *continued*
  Head ØWØØ
  Jaw
    Lower ØWØ5
    Upper ØWØ4
  Knee Region
    Left ØYØG
    Right ØYØF
  Leg
    Lower
      Left ØYØJ
      Right ØYØH
    Upper
      Left ØYØD
      Right ØYØC
  Lip
    Lower ØCØ1X
    Upper ØCØØX
  Neck ØWØ6
  Nose Ø9ØK
  Perineum
    Female ØWØN
    Male ØWØM
  Shoulder Region
    Left ØXØ3
    Right ØXØ2
  Subcutaneous Tissue and Fascia
    Abdomen ØJØ8
    Back ØJØ7
    Buttock ØJØ9
    Chest ØJØ6
    Face ØJØ1
    Lower Arm
      Left ØJØH
      Right ØJØG
    Lower Leg
      Left ØJØP
      Right ØJØN
    Neck
      Anterior ØJØ4
      Posterior ØJØ5
    Upper Arm
      Left ØJØF
      Right ØJØD
    Upper Leg
      Left ØJØM
      Right ØJØL
  Wrist Region
    Left ØXØH
    Right ØXØG
Alveolar process of mandible
  use Mandible, Left
  use Mandible, Right
Alveolar process of maxilla
  use Maxilla, Left
  use Maxilla, Right
Alveolectomy
  see Excision, Head and Facial Bones ØNB
  see Resection, Head and Facial Bones ØNT
Alveoloplasty
  see Repair, Head and Facial Bones ØNQ
  see Replacement, Head and Facial Bones ØNR
  see Supplement, Head and Facial Bones ØNU
Alveolotomy
  see Division, Head and Facial Bones ØN8
  see Drainage, Head and Facial Bones ØN9
Ambulatory cardiac monitoring 4A12X45
Amniocentesis *see* Drainage, Products of Conception 10Q0
Amnioinfusion *see* Introduction of substance in or on, Products of Conception 3EØE
Amnioscopy 10J08ZZ
Amniotomy *see* Drainage, Products of Conception 10Q0
AMPLATZER® Muscular VSD Occluder *use* Synthetic Substitute
Amputation *see* Detachment
AMS 800® Urinary Control System *use* Artificial Sphincter in Urinary System
Anal orifice *use* Anus
Analog radiography *see* Plain Radiography
Analog radiology *see* Plain Radiography
Anastomosis *see* Bypass
Anatomical snuffbox
  use Muscle, Lower Arm and Wrist, Left
  use Muscle, Lower Arm and Wrist, Right

AneuRx® AAA Advantage® *use* Intraluminal Device
Angiectomy
  see Excision, Heart and Great Vessels 02B
  see Excision, Lower Arteries 04B
  see Excision, Lower Veins 06B
  see Excision, Upper Arteries 03B
  see Excision, Upper Veins 05B
Angiocardiography
  Combined right and left heart *see* Fluoroscopy, Heart, Right and Left B216
  Left Heart *see* Fluoroscopy, Heart, Left B215
  Right Heart *see* Fluoroscopy, Heart, Right B214
  SPY *see* Fluoroscopy, Heart B21
Angiography
  see Fluoroscopy, Heart B21
  see Plain Radiography, Heart B20
Angioplasty
  see Dilation, Heart and Great Vessels 027
  see Dilation, Lower Arteries 047
  see Dilation, Upper Arteries 037
  see Repair, Heart and Great Vessels 02Q
  see Repair, Lower Arteries 04Q
  see Repair, Upper Arteries 03Q
  see Replacement, Heart and Great Vessels 02R
  see Replacement, Lower Arteries 04R
  see Replacement, Upper Arteries 03R
  see Supplement, Heart and Great Vessels 02U
  see Supplement, Lower Arteries 04U
  see Supplement, Upper Arteries 03U
Angiorrhaphy
  see Repair, Heart and Great Vessels 02Q
  see Repair, Lower Arteries 04Q
  see Repair, Upper Arteries 03Q
Angioscopy 04JY4ZZ
Angiotripsy
  see Occlusion, Lower Arteries 04L
  see Occlusion, Upper Arteries 03L
Angular artery *use* Artery, Face
Angular vein
  use Vein, Face, Left
  use Vein, Face, Right
Annular ligament
  use Bursa and Ligament, Elbow, Left
  use Bursa and Ligament, Elbow, Right
Annuloplasty
  see Repair, Heart and Great Vessels 02Q
  see Supplement, Heart and Great Vessels 02U
Annuloplasty ring *use* Synthetic Substitute
Anoplasty
  see Repair, Anus 0DQQ
  see Supplement, Anus 0DUQ
Anorectal junction *use* Rectum
Anoscopy 0DJD8ZZ
Ansa cervicalis *use* Nerve, Cervical Plexus
Antabuse therapy HZ93ZZZ
Antebrachial fascia
  use Subcutaneous Tissue and Fascia, Lower Arm, Left
  use Subcutaneous Tissue and Fascia, Lower Arm, Right
Anterior cerebral artery *use* Artery, Intracranial
Anterior cerebral vein *use* Vein, Intracranial
Anterior choroidal artery *use* Artery, Intracranial
Anterior circumflex humeral artery
  use Artery, Axillary, Left
  use Artery, Axillary, Right
Anterior communicating artery *use* Artery, Intracranial
Anterior cruciate ligament (ACL)
  use Bursa and Ligament, Knee, Left
  use Bursa and Ligament, Knee, Right
Anterior crural nerve *use* Nerve, Femoral
Anterior facial vein
  use Vein, Face, Left
  use Vein, Face, Right
Anterior intercostal artery
  use Artery, Internal Mammary, Left
  use Artery, Internal Mammary, Right
Anterior interosseous nerve *use* Nerve, Median
Anterior lateral malleolar artery
  use Artery, Anterior Tibial, Left
  use Artery, Anterior Tibial, Right
Anterior lingual gland *use* Gland, Minor Salivary
Anterior (pectoral) lymph node
  use Lymphatic, Axillary, Left
  use Lymphatic, Axillary, Right

Anterior medial malleolar artery
  use Artery, Anterior Tibial, Left
  use Artery, Anterior Tibial, Right
Anterior spinal artery
  use Artery, Vertebral, Left
  use Artery, Vertebral, Right
Anterior tibial recurrent artery
  use Artery, Anterior Tibial, Left
  use Artery, Anterior Tibial, Right
Anterior ulnar recurrent artery
  use Artery, Ulnar, Left
  use Artery, Ulnar, Right
Anterior vagal trunk *use* Nerve, Vagus
Anterior vertebral muscle
  use Muscle, Neck, Left
  use Muscle, Neck, Right
Antihelix
  use Ear, External, Bilateral
  use Ear, External, Left
  use Ear, External, Right
Antitragus
  use Ear, External, Bilateral
  use Ear, External, Left
  use Ear, External, Right
Antrostomy *see* Drainage, Ear, Nose, Sinus 099
Antrotomy *see* Drainage, Ear, Nose, Sinus 099
Antrum of Highmore
  use Sinus, Maxillary, Left
  use Sinus, Maxillary, Right
Aortic annulus *use* Valve, Aortic
Aortic arch *use* Aorta, Thoracic
Aortic intercostal artery *use* Aorta, Thoracic
Aortography
  see Fluoroscopy, Lower Arteries B41
  see Fluoroscopy, Upper Arteries B31
  see Plain Radiography, Lower Arteries B40
  see Plain Radiography, Upper Arteries B30
Aortoplasty
  see Repair, Aorta, Abdominal 04Q0
  see Repair, Aorta, Thoracic 02QW
  see Replacement, Aorta, Abdominal 04R0
  see Replacement, Aorta, Thoracic 02RW
  see Supplement, Aorta, Abdominal 04U0
  see Supplement, Aorta, Thoracic 02UW
Apical (subclavicular) lymph node
  use Lymphatic, Axillary, Left
  use Lymphatic, Axillary, Right
Apneustic center *use* Pons
Appendectomy
  see Excision, Appendix 0DBJ
  see Resection, Appendix 0DTJ
Appendicolysis *see* Release, Appendix 0DNJ
Appendicotomy *see* Drainage, Appendix 0D9J
Application *see* Introduction of substance in or on
Aquapheresis 6A550Z3
Aqueduct of Sylvius *use* Cerebral Ventricle
Aqueous humour
  use Anterior Chamber, Left
  use Anterior Chamber, Right
Arachnoid mater
  use Cerebral Meninges
  use Spinal Meninges
Arcuate artery
  use Artery, Foot, Left
  use Artery, Foot, Right
Areola
  use Nipple, Left
  use Nipple, Right
AROM (artificial rupture of membranes) 10907ZC
Arterial canal (duct) *use* Artery, Pulmonary, Left
Arterial pulse tracing *see* Measurement, Arterial 4A03
Arteriectomy
  see Excision, Heart and Great Vessels 02B
  see Excision, Lower Arteries 04B
  see Excision, Upper Arteries 03B
Arteriography
  see Fluoroscopy, Heart B21
  see Fluoroscopy, Lower Arteries B41
  see Fluoroscopy, Upper Arteries B31
  see Plain Radiography, Heart B20
  see Plain Radiography, Lower Arteries B40
  see Plain Radiography, Upper Arteries B30
Arterioplasty
  see Repair, Heart and Great Vessels 02Q

Arterioplasty — continued
  see Repair, Lower Arteries 04Q
  see Repair, Upper Arteries 03Q
  see Replacement, Heart and Great Vessels 02R
  see Replacement, Lower Arteries 04R
  see Replacement, Upper Arteries 03R
  see Supplement, Heart and Great Vessels 02U
  see Supplement, Lower Arteries 04U
  see Supplement, Upper Arteries 03U
Arteriorrhaphy
  see Repair, Heart and Great Vessels 02Q
  see Repair, Lower Arteries 04Q
  see Repair, Upper Arteries 03Q
Arterioscopy 04JY4ZZ
Arthrectomy
  see Excision, Lower Joints 0SB
  see Excision, Upper Joints 0RB
  see Resection, Lower Joints 0ST
  see Resection, Upper Joints 0RT
Arthrocentesis
  see Drainage, Lower Joints 0S9
  see Drainage, Upper Joints 0R9
Arthrodesis
  see Fusion, Lower Joints 0SG
  see Fusion, Upper Joints 0RG
Arthrography
  see Plain Radiography, Non-Axial Lower Bones BQ0
  see Plain Radiography, Non-Axial Upper Bones BP0
  see Plain Radiography, Skull and Facial Bones BN0
Arthrolysis
  see Release, Lower Joints 0SN
  see Release, Upper Joints 0RN
Arthropexy
  see Repair, Lower Joints 0SQ
  see Repair, Upper Joints 0RQ
  see Reposition, Lower Joints 0SS
  see Reposition, Upper Joints 0RS
Arthroplasty
  see Repair, Lower Joints 0SQ
  see Repair, Upper Joints 0RQ
  see Replacement, Lower Joints 0SR
  see Replacement, Upper Joints 0RR
  see Supplement, Lower Joints 0SU
  see Supplement, Upper Joints 0RU
Arthroscopy
  see Inspection, Lower Joints 0SJ
  see Inspection, Upper Joints 0RJ
Arthrotomy
  see Drainage, Lower Joints 0S9
  see Drainage, Upper Joints 0R9
Artificial anal sphincter (AAS) *use* Artificial Sphincter in Gastrointestinal System
Artificial bowel sphincter (neosphincter) *use* Artificial Sphincter in Gastrointestinal System
Artificial Sphincter
  Insertion of device in
    Anus 0DHQ
    Bladder 0THB
    Bladder Neck 0THC
    Urethra 0THD
  Removal of device from
    Anus 0DPQ
    Bladder 0TPB
    Urethra 0TPD
  Revision of device in
    Anus 0DWQ
    Bladder 0TWB
    Urethra 0TWD
Artificial urinary sphincter (AUS) *use* Artificial Sphincter in Urinary System
Aryepiglottic fold *use* Larynx
Arytenoid cartilage *use* Larynx
Arytenoid muscle
  use Muscle, Neck, Left
  use Muscle, Neck, Right
Arytenoidectomy *see* Excision, Larynx 0CBS
Arytenoidopexy *see* Repair, Larynx 0CQS
Ascending aorta *use* Aorta, Thoracic
Ascending palatine artery *use* Artery, Face
Ascending pharyngeal artery
  use Artery, External Carotid, Left
  use Artery, External Carotid, Right
Aspiration *see* Drainage

▽ **Subterms under main terms may continue to next column or page**

Assessment
  Activities of daily living *see* Activities of Daily Living Assessment, Rehabilitation F02
  Hearing *see* Hearing Assessment, Diagnostic Audiology F13
  Hearing aid *see* Hearing Aid Assessment, Diagnostic Audiology F14
  Motor function *see* Motor Function Assessment, Rehabilitation F01
  Nerve function *see* Motor Function Assessment, Rehabilitation F01
  Speech *see* Speech Assessment, Rehabilitation F00
  Vestibular *see* Vestibular Assessment, Diagnostic Audiology F15
  Vocational *see* Activities of Daily Living Treatment, Rehabilitation F08
Assistance
  Cardiac
    Continuous
      Balloon Pump 5A02210
      Impeller Pump 5A0221D
      Other Pump 5A02216
      Pulsatile Compression 5A02215
    Intermittent
      Balloon Pump 5A02110
      Impeller Pump 5A0211D
      Other Pump 5A02116
      Pulsatile Compression 5A02115
  Circulatory
    Continuous
      Hyperbaric 5A05221
      Supersaturated 5A0522C
    Intermittent
      Hyperbaric 5A05121
      Supersaturated 5A0512C
  Respiratory
    24-96 Consecutive Hours
      Continuous Negative Airway Pressure 5A09459
      Continuous Positive Airway Pressure 5A09457
      Intermittent Negative Airway Pressure 5A0945B
      Intermittent Positive Airway Pressure 5A09458
      No Qualifier 5A0945Z
    Greater than 96 Consecutive Hours
      Continuous Negative Airway Pressure 5A09559
      Continuous Positive Airway Pressure 5A09557
      Intermittent Negative Airway Pressure 5A0955B
      Intermittent Positive Airway Pressure 5A09558
      No Qualifier 5A0955Z
    Less than 24 Consecutive Hours
      Continuous Negative Airway Pressure 5A09359
      Continuous Positive Airway Pressure 5A09357
      Intermittent Negative Airway Pressure 5A0935B
      Intermittent Positive Airway Pressure 5A09358
      No Qualifier 5A0935Z
Assurant (Cobalt) stent *use* Intraluminal Device
Atherectomy
  see Extirpation, Heart and Great Vessels 02C
  see Extirpation, Lower Arteries 04C
  see Extirpation, Upper Arteries 03C
Atlantoaxial joint *use* Joint, Cervical Vertebral
Atmospheric Control 6A0Z
Atrioseptoplasty
  see Repair, Heart and Great Vessels 02Q
  see Replacement, Heart and Great Vessels 02R
  see Supplement, Heart and Great Vessels 02U
Atrioventricular node *use* Conduction Mechanism
Atrium dextrum cordis *use* Atrium, Right
Atrium pulmonale *use* Atrium, Left
Attain Ability® lead
  use Cardiac Lead, Defibrillator in 02H
  use Cardiac Lead, Pacemaker in 02H
Attain Starfix® (OTW) lead
  use Cardiac Lead, Defibrillator in 02H
  use Cardiac Lead, Pacemaker in 02H
Audiology, diagnostic
  see Hearing Aid Assessment, Diagnostic Audiology F14
  see Hearing Assessment, Diagnostic Audiology F13
  see Vestibular Assessment, Diagnostic Audiology F15
Audiometry *see* Hearing Assessment, Diagnostic Audiology F13

Auditory tube
  use Eustachian Tube, Left
  use Eustachian Tube, Right
Auerbach's (myenteric) plexus *use* Nerve, Abdominal Sympathetic
Auricle
  use Ear, External, Bilateral
  use Ear, External, Left
  use Ear, External, Right
Auricularis muscle *use* Muscle, Head
Autograft *use* Autologous Tissue Substitute
Autologous artery graft
  use Autologous Arterial Tissue in Heart and Great Vessels
  use Autologous Arterial Tissue in Lower Arteries
  use Autologous Arterial Tissue in Lower Veins
  use Autologous Arterial Tissue in Upper Arteries
  use Autologous Arterial Tissue in Upper Veins
Autologous vein graft
  use Autologous Venous Tissue in Heart and Great Vessels
  use Autologous Venous Tissue in Lower Arteries
  use Autologous Venous Tissue in Lower Veins
  use Autologous Venous Tissue in Upper Arteries
  use Autologous Venous Tissue in Upper Veins
Autotransfusion *see* Transfusion
Autotransplant
  Adrenal tissue *see* Reposition, Endocrine System 0GS
  Kidney *see* Reposition, Urinary System 0TS
  Pancreatic tissue *see* Reposition, Pancreas 0FSG
  Parathyroid tissue *see* Reposition, Endocrine System 0GS
  Thyroid tissue *see* Reposition, Endocrine System 0GS
  Tooth *see* Reattachment, Mouth and Throat 0CM
Avulsion *see* Extraction
Axial Lumbar Interbody Fusion System *use* Interbody Fusion Device in Lower Joints
AxiaLIF® System *use* Interbody Fusion Device in Lower Joints
Axillary fascia
  use Subcutaneous Tissue and Fascia, Upper Arm, Left
  use Subcutaneous Tissue and Fascia, Upper Arm, Right
Axillary nerve *use* Nerve, Brachial Plexus

B

BAK/C® Interbody Cervical Fusion System *use* Interbody Fusion Device in Upper Joints
BAL (bronchial alveolar lavage), diagnostic *see* Drainage, Respiratory System 0B9
Balanoplasty
  see Repair, Penis 0VQS
  see Supplement, Penis 0VUS
Balloon Pump
  Continuous, Output 5A02210
  Intermittent, Output 5A02110
Bandage, Elastic *see* Compression
Banding *see* Restriction
Bard® Composix® Kugel® patch *use* Synthetic Substitute
Bard® Composix® (E/X)(LP) mesh *use* Synthetic Substitute
Bard® Dulex™ mesh *use* Synthetic Substitute
Bard® Ventralex™ Hernia Patch *use* Synthetic Substitute
Barium swallow *see* Fluoroscopy, Gastrointestinal System BD1
Baroreflex Activation Therapy® (BAT®)
  use Cardiac Rhythm Related Device in Subcutaneous Tissue and Fascia
  use Stimulator Lead in Upper Arteries
Bartholin's (greater vestibular) gland *use* Gland, Vestibular
Basal (internal) cerebral vein *use* Vein, Intracranial
Basal metabolic rate (BMR) *see* Measurement, Physiological Systems 4A0Z
Basal nuclei *use* Basal Ganglia
Basilar artery *use* Artery, Intracranial
Basis pontis *use* Pons
Beam Radiation
  Abdomen DW03
    Intraoperative DW033Z0
  Adrenal Gland DG02

Beam Radiation — continued
  Adrenal Gland — continued
    Intraoperative DG023Z0
  Bile Ducts DF02
    Intraoperative DF023Z0
  Bladder DT02
    Intraoperative DT023Z0
  Bone
    Intraoperative DP0C3Z0
    Other DP0C
  Bone Marrow D700
    Intraoperative D7003Z0
  Brain D000
    Intraoperative D0003Z0
  Brain Stem D001
    Intraoperative D0013Z0
  Breast
    Left DM00
      Intraoperative DM003Z0
    Right DM01
      Intraoperative DM013Z0
  Bronchus DB01
    Intraoperative DB013Z0
  Cervix DU01
    Intraoperative DU013Z0
  Chest DW02
    Intraoperative DW023Z0
  Chest Wall DB07
    Intraoperative DB073Z0
  Colon DD05
    Intraoperative DD053Z0
  Diaphragm DB08
    Intraoperative DB083Z0
  Duodenum DD02
    Intraoperative DD023Z0
  Ear D900
    Intraoperative D9003Z0
  Esophagus DD00
    Intraoperative DD003Z0
  Eye D800
    Intraoperative D8003Z0
  Femur DP09
    Intraoperative DP093Z0
  Fibula DP0B
    Intraoperative DP0B3Z0
  Gallbladder DF01
    Intraoperative DF013Z0
  Gland
    Adrenal DG02
      Intraoperative DG023Z0
    Parathyroid DG04
      Intraoperative DG043Z0
    Pituitary DG00
      Intraoperative DG003Z0
    Thyroid DG05
      Intraoperative DG053Z0
  Glands
    Intraoperative D9063Z0
    Salivary D906
  Head and Neck DW01
    Intraoperative DW013Z0
  Hemibody DW04
    Intraoperative DW043Z0
  Humerus DP06
    Intraoperative DP063Z0
  Hypopharynx D903
    Intraoperative D9033Z0
  Ileum DD04
    Intraoperative DD043Z0
  Jejunum DD03
    Intraoperative DD033Z0
  Kidney DT00
    Intraoperative DT003Z0
  Larynx D90B
    Intraoperative D90B3Z0
  Liver DF00
    Intraoperative DF003Z0
  Lung DB02
    Intraoperative DB023Z0
  Lymphatics
    Abdomen D706
      Intraoperative D7063Z0
    Axillary D704
      Intraoperative D7043Z0
    Inguinal D708
      Intraoperative D7083Z0

Beam Radiation — continued
  Lymphatics — continued
    Neck D703
      Intraoperative D7033Z0
    Pelvis D707
      Intraoperative D7073Z0
    Thorax D705
      Intraoperative D7053Z0
  Mandible DP03
    Intraoperative DP033Z0
  Maxilla DP02
    Intraoperative DP023Z0
  Mediastinum DB06
    Intraoperative DB063Z0
  Mouth D904
    Intraoperative D9043Z0
  Nasopharynx D90D
    Intraoperative D90D3Z0
  Neck and Head DW01
    Intraoperative DW013Z0
  Nerve
    Intraoperative D0073Z0
    Peripheral D007
  Nose D901
    Intraoperative D9013Z0
  Oropharynx D90F
    Intraoperative D90F3Z0
  Ovary DU00
    Intraoperative DU003Z0
  Palate
    Hard D908
      Intraoperative D9083Z0
    Soft D909
      Intraoperative D9093Z0
  Pancreas DF03
    Intraoperative DF033Z0
  Parathyroid Gland DG04
    Intraoperative DG043Z0
  Pelvic Bones DP08
    Intraoperative DP083Z0
  Pelvic Region DW06
    Intraoperative DW063Z0
  Pineal Body DG01
    Intraoperative DG013Z0
  Pituitary Gland DG00
    Intraoperative DG003Z0
  Pleura DB05
    Intraoperative DB053Z0
  Prostate DV00
    Intraoperative DV003Z0
  Radius DP07
    Intraoperative DP073Z0
  Rectum DD07
    Intraoperative DD073Z0
  Rib DP05
    Intraoperative DP053Z0
  Sinuses D907
    Intraoperative D9073Z0
  Skin
    Abdomen DH08
      Intraoperative DH083Z0
    Arm DH04
      Intraoperative DH043Z0
    Back DH07
      Intraoperative DH073Z0
    Buttock DH09
      Intraoperative DH093Z0
    Chest DH06
      Intraoperative DH063Z0
    Face DH02
      Intraoperative DH023Z0
    Leg DH0B
      Intraoperative DH0B3Z0
    Neck DH03
      Intraoperative DH033Z0
  Skull DP00
    Intraoperative DP003Z0
  Spinal Cord D006
    Intraoperative D0063Z0
  Spleen D702
    Intraoperative D7023Z0
  Sternum DP04
    Intraoperative DP043Z0
  Stomach DD01
    Intraoperative DD013Z0
  Testis DV01

Beam Radiation — continued
  Testis — continued
    Intraoperative DV013Z0
  Thymus D701
    Intraoperative D7013Z0
  Thyroid Gland DG05
    Intraoperative DG053Z0
  Tibia DP0B
    Intraoperative DP0B3Z0
  Tongue D905
    Intraoperative D9053Z0
  Trachea DB00
    Intraoperative DB003Z0
  Ulna DP07
    Intraoperative DP073Z0
  Ureter DT01
    Intraoperative DT013Z0
  Urethra DT03
    Intraoperative DT033Z0
  Uterus DU02
    Intraoperative DU023Z0
  Whole Body DW05
    Intraoperative DW053Z0
Berlin Heart Ventricular Assist Device *use* Implantable Heart Assist System in Heart and Great Vessels
Biceps brachii muscle
  use Muscle, Upper Arm, Left
  use Muscle, Upper Arm, Right
Biceps femoris muscle
  use Muscle, Upper Leg, Left
  use Muscle, Upper Leg, Right
Bicipital aponeurosis
  use Subcutaneous Tissue and Fascia, Lower Arm, Left
  use Subcutaneous Tissue and Fascia, Lower Arm, Right
Bicuspid valve *use* Valve, Mitral
Bililite therapy *see* Ultraviolet Light Therapy, Skin 6A80
Bioactive embolization coil(s) *use* Intraluminal Device, Bioactive in Upper Arteries
Biofeedback GZC9ZZZ
Biopsy
  see Drainage with qualifier Diagnostic
  see Excision with qualifier Diagnostic
  Bone Marrow *see* Extraction with qualifier Diagnostic
BiPAP *see* Assistance, Respiratory 5A09
Bisection *see* Division
Biventricular external heart assist system *use* External Heart Assist System in Heart and Great Vessels
Blepharectomy
  see Excision, Eye 08B
  see Resection, Eye 08T
Blepharoplasty
  see Repair, Eye 08Q
  see Replacement, Eye 08R
  see Reposition, Eye 08S
  see Supplement, Eye 08U
Blepharorrhaphy *see* Repair, Eye 08Q
Blepharotomy *see* Drainage, Eye 089
Block, Nerve, anesthetic injection 3E0T3CZ
Blood glucose monitoring system *use* Monitoring Device
Blood pressure *see* Measurement, Arterial 4A03
BMR (basal metabolic rate) *see* Measurement, Physiological Systems 4A0Z
Body of femur
  use Femoral Shaft, Left
  use Femoral Shaft, Right
Body of fibula
  use Fibula, Left
  use Fibula, Right
Bone anchored hearing device
  use Hearing Device, Bone Conduction in 09H
  use Hearing Device in Head and Facial Bones
Bone bank bone graft *use* Nonautologous Tissue Substitute
Bone Growth Stimulator
  Insertion of device in
    Bone
      Facial 0NHW
      Lower 0QHY
      Nasal 0NHB
      Upper 0PHY
      Skull 0NH0

Bone Growth Stimulator — continued
  Removal of device from
    Bone
      Facial 0NPW
      Lower 0QPY
      Nasal 0NPB
      Upper 0PPY
    Skull 0NP0
  Revision of device in
    Bone
      Facial 0NWW
      Lower 0QWY
      Nasal 0NWB
      Upper 0PWY
    Skull 0NW0
Bone marrow transplant *see* Transfusion
Bone screw (interlocking)(lag)(pedicle)(recessed)
  use Internal Fixation Device in Head and Facial Bones
  use Internal Fixation Device in Lower Bones
  use Internal Fixation Device in Upper Bones
Bony labyrinth
  use Ear, Inner, Left
  use Ear, Inner, Right
Bony orbit
  use Orbit, Left
  use Orbit, Right
Bony vestibule
  use Ear, Inner, Left
  use Ear, Inner, Right
Botallo's duct *use* Artery, Pulmonary, Left
Bovine pericardial valve *use* Zooplastic Tissue in Heart and Great Vessels
Bovine pericardium graft *use* Zooplastic Tissue in Heart and Great Vessels
BP (blood pressure) *see* Measurement, Arterial 4A03
Brachial (lateral) lymph node
  use Lymphatic, Axillary, Left
  use Lymphatic, Axillary, Right
Brachialis muscle
  use Muscle, Upper Arm, Left
  use Muscle, Upper Arm, Right
Brachiocephalic artery *use* Artery, Innominate
Brachiocephalic trunk *use* Artery, Innominate
Brachiocephalic vein
  use Vein, Innominate, Left
  use Vein, Innominate, Right
Brachioradialis muscle
  use Muscle, Lower Arm and Wrist, Left
  use Muscle, Lower Arm and Wrist, Right
Brachytherapy
  Abdomen DW13
  Adrenal Gland DG12
  Bile Ducts DF12
  Bladder DT12
  Bone Marrow D710
  Brain D010
  Brain Stem D011
  Breast
    Left DM10
    Right DM11
  Bronchus DB11
  Cervix DU11
  Chest DW12
  Chest Wall DB17
  Colon DD15
  Diaphragm DB18
  Duodenum DD12
  Ear D910
  Esophagus DD10
  Eye D810
  Gallbladder DF11
  Gland
    Adrenal DG12
    Parathyroid DG14
    Pituitary DG10
    Thyroid DG15
  Glands, Salivary D916
  Head and Neck DW11
  Hypopharynx D913
  Ileum DD14
  Jejunum DD13
  Kidney DT10
  Larynx D91B
  Liver DF10
  Lung DB12

Brachytherapy — continued
  Lymphatics
    Abdomen D716
    Axillary D714
    Inguinal D718
    Neck D713
    Pelvis D717
    Thorax D715
  Mediastinum DB16
  Mouth D914
  Nasopharynx D91D
  Neck and Head DW11
  Nerve, Peripheral D017
  Nose D911
  Oropharynx D91F
  Ovary DU10
  Palate
    Hard D918
    Soft D919
  Pancreas DF13
  Parathyroid Gland DG14
  Pelvic Region DW16
  Pineal Body DG11
  Pituitary Gland DG10
  Pleura DB15
  Prostate DV10
  Rectum DD17
  Sinuses D917
  Spinal Cord D016
  Spleen D712
  Stomach DD11
  Testis DV11
  Thymus D711
  Thyroid Gland DG15
  Tongue D915
  Trachea DB10
  Ureter DT11
  Urethra DT13
  Uterus DU12
Brachytherapy seeds use Radioactive Element
Broad ligament use Uterine Supporting Structure
Bronchial artery use Aorta, Thoracic
Bronchography
  see Fluoroscopy, Respiratory System BB1
  see Plain Radiography, Respiratory System BB0
Bronchoplasty
  see Repair, Respiratory System 0BQ
  see Supplement, Respiratory System 0BU
Bronchorrhaphy see Repair, Respiratory System 0BQ
Bronchoscopy 0BJ08ZZ
Bronchotomy see Drainage, Respiratory System 0B9
BRYAN® Cervical Disc System use Synthetic Substitute
Buccal gland use Buccal Mucosa
Buccinator lymph node use Lymphatic, Head
Buccinator muscle use Muscle, Facial
Buckling, scleral with implant see Supplement, Eye 08U
Bulbospongiosus muscle use Muscle, Perineum
Bulbourethral (Cowper's) gland use Urethra
Bundle of His use Conduction Mechanism
Bundle of Kent use Conduction Mechanism
Bunionectomy see Excision, Lower Bones 0QB
Bursectomy
  see Excision, Bursae and Ligaments 0MB
  see Resection, Bursae and Ligaments 0MT
Bursocentesis see Drainage, Bursae and Ligaments 0M9
Bursography
  see Plain Radiography, Non-Axial Lower Bones BQ0
  see Plain Radiography, Non-Axial Upper Bones BP0
Bursotomy
  see Division, Bursae and Ligaments 0M8
  see Drainage, Bursae and Ligaments 0M9
BVS 5000 Ventricular Assist Device use External Heart Assist System in Heart and Great Vessels
Bypass
  Anterior Chamber
    Left 08133
    Right 08123
  Aorta
    Abdominal 0410
    Thoracic 021W
  Artery
    Axillary
      Left 03160
      Right 03150

Bypass — continued
  Artery — continued
    Brachial
      Left 03180
      Right 03170
    Common Carotid
      Left 031J0
      Right 031H0
    Common Iliac
      Left 041D
      Right 041C
    Coronary
      Four or More Sites 0213
      One Site 0210
      Three Sites 0212
      Two Sites 0211
    External Carotid
      Left 031N0
      Right 031M0
    External Iliac
      Left 041J
      Right 041H
    Femoral
      Left 041L
      Right 041K
    Innominate 03120
    Internal Carotid
      Left 031L0
      Right 031K0
    Internal Iliac
      Left 041F
      Right 041E
    Intracranial 031G0
    Popliteal
      Left 041N
      Right 041M
    Radial
      Left 031C0
      Right 031B0
    Splenic 0414
    Subclavian
      Left 03140
      Right 03130
    Temporal
      Left 031T0
      Right 031S0
    Ulnar
      Left 031A0
      Right 03190
  Atrium
    Left 0217
    Right 0216
  Bladder 0T1B
  Cavity, Cranial 0W110J
  Cecum 0D1H
  Cerebral Ventricle 0016
  Colon
    Ascending 0D1K
    Descending 0D1M
    Sigmoid 0D1N
    Transverse 0D1L
  Duct
    Common Bile 0F19
    Cystic 0F18
    Hepatic
      Left 0F16
      Right 0F15
    Lacrimal
      Left 081Y
      Right 081X
    Pancreatic 0F1D
      Accessory 0F1F
  Duodenum 0D19
  Ear
    Left 091E0
    Right 091D0
  Esophagus 0D15
    Lower 0D13
    Middle 0D12
    Upper 0D11
  Fallopian Tube
    Left 0U16
    Right 0U15
  Gallbladder 0F14
  Ileum 0D1B
  Jejunum 0D1A

Bypass — continued
  Kidney Pelvis
    Left 0T14
    Right 0T13
  Pancreas 0F1G
  Pelvic Cavity 0W1J
  Peritoneal Cavity 0W1G
  Pleural Cavity
    Left 0W1B
    Right 0W19
  Spinal Canal 001U
  Stomach 0D16
  Trachea 0B11
  Ureter
    Left 0T17
    Right 0T16
  Ureters, Bilateral 0T18
  Vas Deferens
    Bilateral 0V1Q
    Left 0V1P
    Right 0V1N
  Vein
    Axillary
      Left 0518
      Right 0517
    Azygos 0510
    Basilic
      Left 051C
      Right 051B
    Brachial
      Left 051A
      Right 0519
    Cephalic
      Left 051F
      Right 051D
    Colic 0617
    Common Iliac
      Left 061D
      Right 061C
    Esophageal 0613
    External Iliac
      Left 061G
      Right 061F
    External Jugular
      Left 051Q
      Right 051P
    Face
      Left 051V
      Right 051T
    Femoral
      Left 061N
      Right 061M
    Foot
      Left 061V
      Right 061T
    Gastric 0612
    Greater Saphenous
      Left 061Q
      Right 061P
    Hand
      Left 051H
      Right 051G
    Hemiazygos 0511
    Hepatic 0614
    Hypogastric
      Left 061J
      Right 061H
    Inferior Mesenteric 0616
    Innominate
      Left 0514
      Right 0513
    Internal Jugular
      Left 051N
      Right 051M
    Intracranial 051L
    Lesser Saphenous
      Left 061S
      Right 061R
    Portal 0618
    Renal
      Left 061B
      Right 0619
    Splenic 0611
    Subclavian
      Left 0516
      Right 0515

▽ **Subterms under main terms may continue to next column or page**

Bypass — continued
 Vein — continued
  Superior Mesenteric 0615
  Vertebral
   Left 051S
   Right 051R
  Vena Cava
   Inferior 0610
   Superior 021V
  Ventricle
   Left 021L
   Right 021K
Bypass, cardiopulmonary 5A1221Z

C

Caesarean section *see* Extraction, Products of Conception 10D0
Calcaneocuboid joint
 use Joint, Tarsal, Left
 use Joint, Tarsal, Right
Calcaneocuboid ligament
 use Bursa and Ligament, Foot, Left
 use Bursa and Ligament, Foot, Right
Calcaneofibular ligament
 use Bursa and Ligament, Ankle, Left
 use Bursa and Ligament, Ankle, Right
Calcaneus
 use Tarsal, Left
 use Tarsal, Right
Cannulation
 see Bypass
 see Dilation
 see Drainage
 see Irrigation
Canthorrhaphy *see* Repair, Eye 08Q
Canthotomy *see* Release, Eye 08N
Capitate bone
 use Carpal, Left
 use Carpal, Right
Capsulectomy, lens *see* Excision, Eye 08B
Capsulorrhaphy, joint
 see Repair, Lower Joints 0SQ
 see Repair, Upper Joints 0RQ
Cardia *use* Esophagogastric Junction
Cardiac contractility modulation lead *use* Cardiac Lead in Heart and Great Vessels
Cardiac event recorder *use* Monitoring Device
Cardiac Lead
 Defibrillator
  Atrium
   Left 02H7
   Right 02H6
  Pericardium 02HN
  Vein, Coronary 02H4
  Ventricle
   Left 02HL
   Right 02HK
 Insertion of device in
  Atrium
   Left 02H7
   Right 02H6
  Pericardium 02HN
  Vein, Coronary 02H4
  Ventricle
   Left 02HL
   Right 02HK
 Pacemaker
  Atrium
   Left 02H7
   Right 02H6
  Pericardium 02HN
  Vein, Coronary 02H4
  Ventricle
   Left 02HL
   Right 02HK
 Removal of device from, Heart 02PA
 Revision of device in, Heart 02WA
Cardiac plexus *use* Nerve, Thoracic Sympathetic
Cardiac Resynchronization Defibrillator Pulse Generator
 Abdomen 0JH8
 Chest 0JH6

Cardiac Resynchronization Pacemaker Pulse Generator
 Abdomen 0JH8
 Chest 0JH6
Cardiac resynchronization therapy (CRT) lead
 use Cardiac Lead, Defibrillator in 02H
 use Cardiac Lead, Pacemaker in 02H
Cardiac Rhythm Related Device
 Insertion of device in
  Abdomen 0JH8
  Chest 0JH6
 Removal of device from, Subcutaneous Tissue and Fascia, Trunk 0JPT
 Revision of device in, Subcutaneous Tissue and Fascia, Trunk 0JWT
Cardiocentesis *see* Drainage, Pericardial Cavity 0W9D
Cardioesophageal junction *use* Esophagogastric Junction
Cardiolysis *see* Release, Heart and Great Vessels 02N
CardioMEMS® pressure sensor *use* Monitoring Device, Pressure Sensor in 02H
Cardiomyotomy *see* Division, Esophagogastric Junction 0D84
Cardioplegia *see* Introduction of substance in or on, Heart 3E08
Cardiorrhaphy *see* Repair, Heart and Great Vessels 02Q
Cardioversion 5A2204Z
Caregiver Training F0FZ
Caroticotympanic artery
 use Artery, Internal Carotid, Left
 use Artery, Internal Carotid, Right
Carotid glomus
 use Carotid Bodies, Bilateral
 use Carotid Body, Left
 use Carotid Body, Right
Carotid sinus
 use Artery, Internal Carotid, Left
 use Artery, Internal Carotid, Right
Carotid (artery) sinus (baroreceptor) lead *use* Stimulator Lead in Upper Arteries
Carotid sinus nerve *use* Nerve, Glossopharyngeal
Carotid WALLSTENT® Monorail® Endoprosthesis
 use Intraluminal Device
Carpectomy
 see Excision, Upper Bones 0PB
 see Resection, Upper Bones 0PT
Carpometacarpal (CMC) joint
 use Joint, Metacarpocarpal, Left
 use Joint, Metacarpocarpal, Right
Carpometacarpal ligament
 use Bursa and Ligament, Hand, Left
 use Bursa and Ligament, Hand, Right
Casting *see* Immobilization
CAT scan *see* Computerized Tomography (CT Scan)
Catheterization
 see Dilation
 see Drainage
 see Insertion of device in
 see Irrigation
 Heart *see* Measurement, Cardiac 4A02
 Umbilical vein, for infusion 06H033T
Cauda equina *use* Spinal Cord, Lumbar
Cauterization
 see Destruction
 see Repair
Cavernous plexus *use* Nerve, Head and Neck Sympathetic
Cecectomy
 see Excision, Cecum 0DBH
 see Resection, Cecum 0DTH
Cecocolostomy
 see Bypass, Gastrointestinal System 0D1
 see Drainage, Gastrointestinal System 0D9
Cecopexy
 see Repair, Cecum 0DQH
 see Reposition, Cecum 0DSH
Cecoplication *see* Restriction, Cecum 0DVH
Cecorrhaphy *see* Repair, Cecum 0DQH
Cecostomy
 see Bypass, Cecum 0D1H
 see Drainage, Cecum 0D9H
Cecotomy *see* Drainage, Cecum 0D9H
Celiac ganglion *use* Nerve, Abdominal Sympathetic
Celiac lymph node *use* Lymphatic, Aortic

Celiac (solar) plexus *use* Nerve, Abdominal Sympathetic
Celiac trunk *use* Artery, Celiac
Central axillary lymph node
 use Lymphatic, Axillary, Left
 use Lymphatic, Axillary, Right
Central venous pressure *see* Measurement, Venous 4A04
Centrimag® Blood Pump *use* Intraluminal Device
Cephalogram BN00ZZZ
Cerclage *see* Restriction
Cerebral aqueduct (Sylvius) *use* Cerebral Ventricle
Cerebrum *use* Brain
Cervical esophagus *use* Esophagus, Upper
Cervical facet joint
 use Joint, Cervical Vertebral
 use Joint, Cervical Vertebral, 2 or more
Cervical ganglion *use* Nerve, Head and Neck Sympathetic
Cervical interspinous ligament *use* Bursa and Ligament, Head and Neck
Cervical intertransverse ligament *use* Bursa and Ligament, Head and Neck
Cervical ligamentum flavum *use* Bursa and Ligament, Head and Neck
Cervical lymph node
 use Lymphatic, Neck, Left
 use Lymphatic, Neck, Right
Cervicectomy
 see Excision, Cervix 0UBC
 see Resection, Cervix 0UTC
Cervicothoracic facet joint *use* Joint, Cervicothoracic Vertebral
Cesarean section *see* Extraction, Products of Conception 10D0
Change device in
 Abdominal Wall 0W2FX
 Back
  Lower 0W2LX
  Upper 0W2KX
 Bladder 0T2BX
 Bone
  Facial 0N2WX
  Lower 0Q2YX
  Nasal 0N2BX
  Upper 0P2YX
 Bone Marrow 072TX
 Brain 0020X
 Breast
  Left 0H2UX
  Right 0H2TX
 Bursa and Ligament
  Lower 0M2YX
  Upper 0M2XX
 Cavity, Cranial 0W21X
 Chest Wall 0W28X
 Cisterna Chyli 072LX
 Diaphragm 0B2TX
 Duct
  Hepatobiliary 0F2BX
  Pancreatic 0F2DX
 Ear
  Left 092JX
  Right 092HX
 Epididymis and Spermatic Cord 0V2MX
 Extremity
  Lower
   Left 0Y2BX
   Right 0Y29X
  Upper
   Left 0X27X
   Right 0X26X
 Eye
  Left 0821X
  Right 0820X
 Face 0W22X
 Fallopian Tube 0U28X
 Gallbladder 0F24X
 Gland
  Adrenal 0G25X
  Endocrine 0G2SX
  Pituitary 0G20X
  Salivary 0C2AX
 Head 0W20X
 Intestinal Tract
  Lower 0D2DXUZ
  Upper 0D20XUZ

Collection from — continued
  Indwelling Device
    Circulatory System
      Blood 8C02X6K
      Other Fluid 8C02X6L
    Nervous System
      Cerebrospinal Fluid 8C01X6J
      Other Fluid 8C01X6L
  Integumentary System, Breast Milk 8E0HX62
  Reproductive System, Male, Sperm 8E0VX63
Colocentesis *see* Drainage, Gastrointestinal System 0D9
Colofixation
  see Repair, Gastrointestinal System 0DQ
  see Reposition, Gastrointestinal System 0DS
Cololysis *see* Release, Gastrointestinal System 0DN
Colonic Z-Stent® *use* Intraluminal Device
Colonoscopy 0DJD8ZZ
Colopexy
  see Repair, Gastrointestinal System 0DQ
  see Reposition, Gastrointestinal System 0DS
Coloplication *see* Restriction, Gastrointestinal System 0DV
Coloproctectomy
  see Excision, Gastrointestinal System 0DB
  see Resection, Gastrointestinal System 0DT
Coloproctostomy
  see Bypass, Gastrointestinal System 0D1
  see Drainage, Gastrointestinal System 0D9
Colopuncture *see* Drainage, Gastrointestinal System 0D9
Colorrhaphy *see* Repair, Gastrointestinal System 0DQ
Colostomy
  see Bypass, Gastrointestinal System 0D1
  see Drainage, Gastrointestinal System 0D9
Colpectomy
  see Excision, Vagina 0UBG
  see Resection, Vagina 0UTG
Colpocentesis *see* Drainage, Vagina 0U9G
Colpopexy
  see Repair, Vagina 0UQG
  see Reposition, Vagina 0USG
Colpoplasty
  see Repair, Vagina 0UQG
  see Supplement, Vagina 0UUG
Colporrhaphy *see* Repair, Vagina 0UQG
Colposcopy 0UJH8ZZ
Columella *use* Nose
Common digital vein
  use Vein, Foot, Left
  use Vein, Foot, Right
Common facial vein
  use Vein, Face, Left
  use Vein, Face, Right
Common fibular nerve *use* Nerve, Peroneal
Common hepatic artery *use* Artery, Hepatic
Common iliac (subaortic) lymph node *use* Lymphatic, Pelvis
Common interosseous artery
  use Artery, Ulnar, Left
  use Artery, Ulnar, Right
Common peroneal nerve *use* Nerve, Peroneal
Complete (SE) stent *use* Intraluminal Device
Compression
  see Restriction
  Abdominal Wall 2W13X
  Arm
    Lower
      Left 2W1DX
      Right 2W1CX
    Upper
      Left 2W1BX
      Right 2W1AX
  Back 2W15X
  Chest Wall 2W14X
  Extremity
    Lower
      Left 2W1MX
      Right 2W1LX
    Upper
      Left 2W19X
      Right 2W18X
  Face 2W11X
  Finger
    Left 2W1KX
    Right 2W1JX

Compression — continued
  Foot
    Left 2W1TX
    Right 2W1SX
  Hand
    Left 2W1FX
    Right 2W1EX
  Head 2W10X
  Inguinal Region
    Left 2W17X
    Right 2W16X
  Leg
    Lower
      Left 2W1RX
      Right 2W1QX
    Upper
      Left 2W1PX
      Right 2W1NX
  Neck 2W12X
  Thumb
    Left 2W1HX
    Right 2W1GX
  Toe
    Left 2W1VX
    Right 2W1UX
Computer Assisted Procedure
  Extremity
    Lower
      With Computerized Tomography 8E0YXBG
      With Fluoroscopy 8E0YXBF
      With Magnetic Resonance Imaging 8E0YXBH
      No Qualifier 8E0YXBZ
    Upper
      With Computerized Tomography 8E0XXBG
      With Fluoroscopy 8E0XXBF
      With Magnetic Resonance Imaging 8E0XXBH
      No Qualifier 8E0XXBZ
  Head and Neck Region
    With Computerized Tomography 8E09XBG
    With Fluoroscopy 8E09XBF
    With Magnetic Resonance Imaging 8E09XBH
    No Qualifier 8E09XBZ
  Trunk Region
    With Computerized Tomography 8E0WXBG
    With Fluoroscopy 8E0WXBF
    With Magnetic Resonance Imaging 8E0WXBH
    No Qualifier 8E0WXBZ
Computerized Tomography (CT Scan)
  Abdomen BW20
    Chest and Pelvis BW25
  Abdomen and Chest BW24
  Abdomen and Pelvis BW21
  Airway, Trachea BB2F
  Ankle
    Left BQ2H
    Right BQ2G
  Aorta
    Abdominal B420
      Intravascular Optical Coherence B420Z2Z
    Thoracic B320
      Intravascular Optical Coherence B320Z2Z
  Arm
    Left BP2F
    Right BP2E
  Artery
    Celiac B421
      Intravascular Optical Coherence B421Z2Z
    Common Carotid
      Bilateral B325
      Intravascular Optical Coherence B325Z2Z
    Coronary
      Bypass Graft
        Intravascular Optical Coherence B223Z2Z
        Multiple B223
      Multiple B221
        Intravascular Optical Coherence B221Z2Z
    Internal Carotid
      Bilateral B328
      Intravascular Optical Coherence B328Z2Z
    Intracranial B32R
      Intravascular Optical Coherence B32RZ2Z
    Lower Extremity
      Bilateral B42H
        Intravascular Optical Coherence B42HZ2Z
      Left B42G
        Intravascular Optical Coherence B42GZ2Z

Computerized Tomography (CT Scan) — continued
  Artery — continued
    Lower Extremity — continued
      Right B42F
        Intravascular Optical Coherence B42FZ2Z
    Pelvic B42C
      Intravascular Optical Coherence B42CZ2Z
    Pulmonary
      Left B32T
        Intravascular Optical Coherence B32TZ2Z
      Right B32S
        Intravascular Optical Coherence B32SZ2Z
    Renal
      Bilateral B428
        Intravascular Optical Coherence B428Z2Z
      Transplant B42M
        Intravascular Optical Coherence B42MZ2Z
    Superior Mesenteric B424
      Intravascular Optical Coherence B424Z2Z
    Vertebral
      Bilateral B32G
        Intravascular Optical Coherence B32GZ2Z
  Bladder BT20
  Bone
    Facial BN25
    Temporal BN2F
  Brain B020
  Calcaneus
    Left BQ2K
    Right BQ2J
  Cerebral Ventricle B028
  Chest, Abdomen and Pelvis BW25
  Chest and Abdomen BW24
  Cisterna B027
  Clavicle
    Left BP25
    Right BP24
  Coccyx BR2F
  Colon BD24
  Ear B920
  Elbow
    Left BP2H
    Right BP2G
  Extremity
    Lower
      Left BQ2S
      Right BQ2R
    Upper
      Bilateral BP2V
      Left BP2U
      Right BP2T
  Eye
    Bilateral B827
    Left B826
    Right B825
  Femur
    Left BQ24
    Right BQ23
  Fibula
    Left BQ2C
    Right BQ2B
  Finger
    Left BP2S
    Right BP2R
  Foot
    Left BQ2M
    Right BQ2L
  Forearm
    Left BP2K
    Right BP2J
  Gland
    Adrenal, Bilateral BG22
    Parathyroid BG23
    Parotid, Bilateral B926
    Salivary, Bilateral B92D
    Submandibular, Bilateral B929
    Thyroid BG24
  Hand
    Left BP2P
    Right BP2N
  Hands and Wrists, Bilateral BP2Q
  Head BW28
  Head and Neck BW29
  Heart
    Intravascular Optical Coherence B226Z2Z

▽ **Subterms under main terms may continue to next column or page**

Computerized Tomography (CT Scan) — continued

Heart — continued
Right and Left B226
Hepatobiliary System, All BF2C
Hip
Left BQ21
Right BQ20
Humerus
Left BP2B
Right BP2A
Intracranial Sinus B522
Intravascular Optical Coherence B522Z2Z
Joint
Acromioclavicular, Bilateral BP23
Finger
Left BP2DZZZ
Right BP2CZZZ
Foot
Left BQ2Y
Right BQ2X
Hand
Left BP2DZZZ
Right BP2CZZZ
Sacroiliac BR2D
Sternoclavicular
Bilateral BP22
Left BP21
Right BP20
Temporomandibular, Bilateral BN29
Toe
Left BQ2Y
Right BQ2X
Kidney
Bilateral BT23
Left BT22
Right BT21
Transplant BT29
Knee
Left BQ28
Right BQ27
Larynx B92J
Leg
Left BQ2F
Right BQ2D
Liver BF25
Liver and Spleen BF26
Lung, Bilateral BB24
Mandible BN26
Nasopharynx B92F
Neck BW2F
Neck and Head BW29
Orbit, Bilateral BN23
Oropharynx B92F
Pancreas BF27
Patella
Left BQ2W
Right BQ2V
Pelvic Region BW2G
Pelvis BR2C
Chest and Abdomen BW25
Pelvis and Abdomen BW21
Pituitary Gland B029
Prostate BV23
Ribs
Left BP2Y
Right BP2X
Sacrum BR2F
Scapula
Left BP27
Right BP26
Sella Turcica B029
Shoulder
Left BP29
Right BP28
Sinus
Intracranial B522
Intravascular Optical Coherence B522Z2Z
Paranasal B922
Skull BN20
Spinal Cord B02B
Spine
Cervical BR20
Lumbar BR29
Thoracic BR27
Spleen and Liver BF26

Computerized Tomography (CT Scan) — continued

Thorax BP2W
Tibia
Left BQ2C
Right BQ2B
Toe
Left BQ2Q
Right BQ2P
Trachea BB2F
Tracheobronchial Tree
Bilateral BB29
Left BB28
Right BB27
Vein
Pelvic (Iliac)
Left B52G
Intravascular Optical Coherence B52GZ2Z
Right B52F
Intravascular Optical Coherence B52FZ2Z
Pelvic (Iliac) Bilateral B52H
Intravascular Optical Coherence B52HZ2Z
Portal B52T
Intravascular Optical Coherence B52TZ2Z
Pulmonary
Bilateral B52S
Intravascular Optical Coherence B52SZ2Z
Left B52R
Intravascular Optical Coherence B52RZ2Z
Right B52Q
Intravascular Optical Coherence B52QZ2Z
Renal
Bilateral B52L
Intravascular Optical Coherence B52LZ2Z
Left B52K
Intravascular Optical Coherence B52KZ2Z
Right B52J
Intravascular Optical Coherence B52JZ2Z
Spanchnic B52T
Intravascular Optical Coherence B52TZ2Z
Vena Cava
Inferior B529
Intravascular Optical Coherence B529Z2Z
Superior B528
Intravascular Optical Coherence B528Z2Z
Ventricle, Cerebral B028
Wrist
Left BP2M
Right BP2L

Concerto II CRT-D *use* Cardiac Resynchronization Defibrillator Pulse Generator in 0JH

Condylectomy
see Excision, Head and Facial Bones 0NB
see Excision, Lower Bones 0QB
see Excision, Upper Bones 0PB

Condyloid process
use Mandible, Left
use Mandible, Right

Condylotomy
see Division, Head and Facial Bones 0N8
see Division, Lower Bones 0Q8
see Division, Upper Bones 0P8
see Drainage, Head and Facial Bones 0N9
see Drainage, Lower Bones 0Q9
see Drainage, Upper Bones 0P9

Condylysis
see Release, Head and Facial Bones 0NN
see Release, Lower Bones 0QN
see Release, Upper Bones 0PN

Conization, cervix *see* Excision, Uterus 0UB9

Conjunctivoplasty
see Repair, Eye 08Q
see Replacement, Eye 08R

CONSERVE® PLUS Total Resurfacing Hip System *use* Resurfacing Device in Lower Joints

Construction
Auricle, ear *see* Replacement, Ear, Nose, Sinus 09R
Ileal conduit *see* Bypass, Urinary System 0T1

Consulta CRT-D *use* Cardiac Resynchronization Defibrillator Pulse Generator in 0JH

Consulta CRT-P *use* Cardiac Resynchronization Pacemaker Pulse Generator in 0JH

Contact Radiation
Abdomen DWY37ZZ
Adrenal Gland DGY27ZZ
Bile Ducts DFY27ZZ

Contact Radiation — continued

Bladder DTY27ZZ
Bone, Other DPYC7ZZ
Brain D0Y07ZZ
Brain Stem D0Y17ZZ
Breast
Left DMY07ZZ
Right DMY17ZZ
Bronchus DBY17ZZ
Cervix DUY17ZZ
Chest DWY27ZZ
Chest Wall DBY77ZZ
Colon DDY57ZZ
Diaphragm DBY87ZZ
Duodenum DDY27ZZ
Ear D9Y07ZZ
Esophagus DDY07ZZ
Eye D8Y07ZZ
Femur DPY97ZZ
Fibula DPYB7ZZ
Gallbladder DFY17ZZ
Gland
Adrenal DGY27ZZ
Parathyroid DGY47ZZ
Pituitary DGY07ZZ
Thyroid DGY57ZZ
Glands, Salivary D9Y67ZZ
Head and Neck DWY17ZZ
Hemibody DWY47ZZ
Humerus DPY67ZZ
Hypopharynx D9Y37ZZ
Ileum DDY47ZZ
Jejunum DDY37ZZ
Kidney DTY07ZZ
Larynx D9YB7ZZ
Liver DFY07ZZ
Lung DBY27ZZ
Mandible DPY37ZZ
Maxilla DPY27ZZ
Mediastinum DBY67ZZ
Mouth D9Y47ZZ
Nasopharynx D9YD7ZZ
Neck and Head DWY17ZZ
Nerve, Peripheral D0Y77ZZ
Nose D9Y17ZZ
Oropharynx D9YF7ZZ
Ovary DUY07ZZ
Palate
Hard D9Y87ZZ
Soft D9Y97ZZ
Pancreas DFY37ZZ
Parathyroid Gland DGY47ZZ
Pelvic Bones DPY87ZZ
Pelvic Region DWY67ZZ
Pineal Body DGY17ZZ
Pituitary Gland DGY07ZZ
Pleura DBY57ZZ
Prostate DVY07ZZ
Radius DPY77ZZ
Rectum DDY77ZZ
Rib DPY57ZZ
Sinuses D9Y77ZZ
Skin
Abdomen DHY87ZZ
Arm DHY47ZZ
Back DHY77ZZ
Buttock DHY97ZZ
Chest DHY67ZZ
Face DHY27ZZ
Leg DHYB7ZZ
Neck DHY37ZZ
Skull DPY07ZZ
Spinal Cord D0Y67ZZ
Sternum DPY47ZZ
Stomach DDY17ZZ
Testis DVY17ZZ
Thyroid Gland DGY57ZZ
Tibia DPYB7ZZ
Tongue D9Y57ZZ
Trachea DBY07ZZ
Ulna DPY77ZZ
Ureter DTY17ZZ
Urethra DTY37ZZ
Uterus DUY27ZZ
Whole Body DWY57ZZ

CONTAK RENEWAL® 3 RF (HE) CRT-D *use* Cardiac Resynchronization Defibrillator Pulse Generator in ØJH
Continuous Glucose Monitoring (CGM) device *use* Monitoring Device
Continuous Negative Airway Pressure
24-96 Consecutive Hours, Ventilation 5A09459
Greater than 96 Consecutive Hours, Ventilation 5A09559
Less than 24 Consecutive Hours, Ventilation 5A09359
Continuous Positive Airway Pressure
24-96 Consecutive Hours, Ventilation 5A09457
Greater than 96 Consecutive Hours, Ventilation 5A09557
Less than 24 Consecutive Hours, Ventilation 5A09357
Contraceptive Device
Change device in, Uterus and Cervix ØU2DXHZ
Insertion of device in
Cervix ØUHC
Subcutaneous Tissue and Fascia
Abdomen ØJH8
Chest ØJH6
Lower Arm
Left ØJHH
Right ØJHG
Lower Leg
Left ØJHP
Right ØJHN
Upper Arm
Left ØJHF
Right ØJHD
Upper Leg
Left ØJHM
Right ØJHL
Uterus ØUH9
Removal of device from
Subcutaneous Tissue and Fascia
Lower Extremity ØJPW
Trunk ØJPT
Upper Extremity ØJPV
Uterus and Cervix ØUPD
Revision of device in
Subcutaneous Tissue and Fascia
Lower Extremity ØJWW
Trunk ØJWT
Upper Extremity ØJWV
Uterus and Cervix ØUWD
Contractility Modulation Device
Abdomen ØJH8
Chest ØJH6
Control postprocedural bleeding in
Abdominal Wall ØW3F
Ankle Region
Left ØY3L
Right ØY3K
Arm
Lower
Left ØX3F
Right ØX3D
Upper
Left ØX39
Right ØX38
Axilla
Left ØX35
Right ØX34
Back
Lower ØW3L
Upper ØW3K
Buttock
Left ØY31
Right ØY30
Cavity, Cranial ØW31
Chest Wall ØW38
Elbow Region
Left ØX3C
Right ØX3B
Extremity
Lower
Left ØY3B
Right ØY39
Upper
Left ØX37
Right ØX36
Face ØW32
Femoral Region
Left ØY38

Control postprocedural bleeding in — continued
Femoral Region — continued
Right ØY37
Foot
Left ØY3N
Right ØY3M
Gastrointestinal Tract ØW3P
Genitourinary Tract ØW3R
Hand
Left ØX3K
Right ØX3J
Head ØW30
Inguinal Region
Left ØY36
Right ØY35
Jaw
Lower ØW35
Upper ØW34
Knee Region
Left ØY3G
Right ØY3F
Leg
Lower
Left ØY3J
Right ØY3H
Upper
Left ØY3D
Right ØY3C
Mediastinum ØW3C
Neck ØW36
Oral Cavity and Throat ØW33
Pelvic Cavity ØW3J
Pericardial Cavity ØW3D
Perineum
Female ØW3N
Male ØW3M
Peritoneal Cavity ØW3G
Pleural Cavity
Left ØW3B
Right ØW39
Respiratory Tract ØW3Q
Retroperitoneum ØW3H
Shoulder Region
Left ØX33
Right ØX32
Wrist Region
Left ØX3H
Right ØX3G
Conus arteriosus *use* Ventricle, Right
Conus medullaris *use* Spinal Cord, Lumbar
Conversion
Cardiac rhythm 5A2204Z
Gastrostomy to jejunostomy feeding device *see* Insertion of device in, Jejunum ØDHA
Coracoacromial ligament
use Bursa and Ligament, Shoulder, Left
use Bursa and Ligament, Shoulder, Right
Coracobrachialis muscle
use Muscle, Upper Arm, Left
use Muscle, Upper Arm, Right
Coracoclavicular ligament
use Bursa and Ligament, Shoulder, Left
use Bursa and Ligament, Shoulder, Right
Coracohumeral ligament
use Bursa and Ligament, Shoulder, Left
use Bursa and Ligament, Shoulder, Right
Coracoid process
use Scapula, Left
use Scapula, Right
Cordotomy *see* Division, Central Nervous System ØØ8
Core needle biopsy *see* Excision with qualifier Diagnostic
Cormet Hip Resurfacing System *use* Resurfacing Device in Lower Joints
Corniculate cartilage *use* Larynx
CoRoent® XL *use* Interbody Fusion Device in Lower Joints
Coronary arteriography
see Fluoroscopy, Heart B21
see Plain Radiography, Heart B20
Corox (OTW) Bipolar Lead
use Cardiac Lead, Defibrillator in Ø2H
use Cardiac Lead, Pacemaker in Ø2H
Corpus callosum *use* Brain
Corpus cavernosum *use* Penis

Corpus spongiosum *use* Penis
Corpus striatum *use* Basal Ganglia
Corrugator supercilii muscle *use* Muscle, Facial
Cortical strip neurostimulator lead *use* Neurostimulator Lead in Central Nervous System
Costatectomy
see Excision, Upper Bones ØPB
see Resection, Upper Bones ØPT
Costectomy
see Excision, Upper Bones ØPB
see Resection, Upper Bones ØPT
Costocervical trunk
use Artery, Subclavian, Left
use Artery, Subclavian, Right
Costochondrectomy
see Excision, Upper Bones ØPB
see Resection, Upper Bones ØPT
Costoclavicular ligament
use Bursa and Ligament, Shoulder, Left
use Bursa and Ligament, Shoulder, Right
Costosternoplasty
see Repair, Upper Bones ØPQ
see Replacement, Upper Bones ØPR
see Supplement, Upper Bones ØPU
Costotomy
see Division, Upper Bones ØP8
see Drainage, Upper Bones ØP9
Costotransverse joint
use Joint, Thoracic Vertebral
use Joint, Thoracic Vertebral, 2 to 7
use Joint, Thoracic Vertebral, 8 or more
Costotransverse ligament
use Bursa and Ligament, Thorax, Left
use Bursa and Ligament, Thorax, Right
Costovertebral joint
use Joint, Thoracic Vertebral
use Joint, Thoracic Vertebral, 2 to 7
use Joint, Thoracic Vertebral, 8 or more
Costoxiphoid ligament
use Bursa and Ligament, Thorax, Left
use Bursa and Ligament, Thorax, Right
Counseling
Family, for substance abuse, Other Family Counseling HZ63ZZZ
Group
12-Step HZ43ZZZ
Behavioral HZ41ZZZ
Cognitive HZ40ZZZ
Cognitive-Behavioral HZ42ZZZ
Confrontational HZ48ZZZ
Continuing Care HZ49ZZZ
Infectious Disease
Post-Test HZ4CZZZ
Pre-Test HZ4CZZZ
Interpersonal HZ44ZZZ
Motivational Enhancement HZ47ZZZ
Psychoeducation HZ46ZZZ
Spiritual HZ4BZZZ
Vocational HZ45ZZZ
Individual
12-Step HZ33ZZZ
Behavioral HZ31ZZZ
Cognitive HZ30ZZZ
Cognitive-Behavioral HZ32ZZZ
Confrontational HZ38ZZZ
Continuing Care HZ39ZZZ
Infectious Disease
Post-Test HZ3CZZZ
Pre-Test HZ3CZZZ
Interpersonal HZ34ZZZ
Motivational Enhancement HZ37ZZZ
Psychoeducation HZ36ZZZ
Spiritual HZ3BZZZ
Vocational HZ35ZZZ
Mental Health Services
Educational GZ60ZZZ
Other Counseling GZ63ZZZ
Vocational GZ61ZZZ
Countershock, cardiac 5A2204Z
Cowper's (bulbourethral) gland *use* Urethra
CPAP (continuous positive airway pressure) *see* Assistance, Respiratory 5A09
Cranial dura mater *use* Dura Mater
Cranial epidural space *use* Epidural Space
Cranial subarachnoid space *use* Subarachnoid Space

▽ **Subterms under main terms may continue to next column or page**

Cranial subdural space *use* Subdural Space
Craniectomy
  see Excision, Head and Facial Bones ØNB
  see Resection, Head and Facial Bones ØNT
Cranioplasty
  see Repair, Head and Facial Bones ØNQ
  see Replacement, Head and Facial Bones ØNR
  see Supplement, Head and Facial Bones ØNU
Craniotomy
  see Division, Head and Facial Bones ØN8
  see Drainage, Central Nervous System ØØ9
  see Drainage, Head and Facial Bones ØN9
Creation
  Female ØW4NØ
  Male ØW4MØ
Cremaster muscle *use* Muscle, Perineum
Cribriform plate
  use Bone, Ethmoid, Left
  use Bone, Ethmoid, Right
Cricoid cartilage *use* Larynx
Cricoidectomy *see* Excision, Larynx ØCBS
Cricothyroid artery
  use Artery, Thyroid, Left
  use Artery, Thyroid, Right
Cricothyroid muscle
  use Muscle, Neck, Left
  use Muscle, Neck, Right
Crisis Intervention GZ2ZZZZ
Crural fascia
  use Subcutaneous Tissue and Fascia, Upper Leg, Left
  use Subcutaneous Tissue and Fascia, Upper Leg, Right
Crushing, nerve
  Cranial *see* Destruction, Central Nervous System ØØ5
  Peripheral *see* Destruction, Peripheral Nervous System Ø15
Cryoablation *see* Destruction
Cryotherapy *see* Destruction
Cryptorchidectomy
  see Excision, Male Reproductive System ØVB
  see Resection, Male Reproductive System ØVT
Cryptorchiectomy
  see Excision, Male Reproductive System ØVB
  see Resection, Male Reproductive System ØVT
Cryptotomy
  see Division, Gastrointestinal System ØD8
  see Drainage, Gastrointestinal System ØD9
CT scan *see* Computerized Tomography (CT Scan)
CT sialogram *see* Computerized Tomography (CT Scan), Ear, Nose, Mouth and Throat B92
Cubital lymph node
  use Lymphatic, Upper Extremity, Left
  use Lymphatic, Upper Extremity, Right
Cubital nerve *use* Nerve, Ulnar
Cuboid bone
  use Tarsal, Left
  use Tarsal, Right
Cuboideonavicular joint
  use Joint, Tarsal, Left
  use Joint, Tarsal, Right
Culdocentesis *see* Drainage, Cul-de-sac ØU9F
Culdoplasty
  see Repair, Cul-de-sac ØUQF
  see Supplement, Cul-de-sac ØUUF
Culdoscopy ØUJH8ZZ
Culdotomy *see* Drainage, Cul-de-sac ØU9F
Culmen *use* Cerebellum
Cultured epidermal cell autograft *use* Autologous Tissue Substitute
Cuneiform cartilage *use* Larynx
Cuneonavicular joint
  use Joint, Tarsal, Left
  use Joint, Tarsal, Right
Cuneonavicular ligament
  use Bursa and Ligament, Foot, Left
  use Bursa and Ligament, Foot, Right
Curettage
  see Excision
  see Extraction
Cutaneous (transverse) cervical nerve *use* Nerve, Cervical Plexus
CVP (central venous pressure) *see* Measurement, Venous 4AØ4
Cyclodiathermy *see* Destruction, Eye Ø85
Cyclophotocoagulation *see* Destruction, Eye Ø85

CYPHER® Stent *use* Intraluminal Device, Drug-eluting in Heart and Great Vessels
Cystectomy
  see Excision, Bladder ØTBB
  see Resection, Bladder ØTTB
Cystocele repair *see* Repair, Subcutaneous Tissue and Fascia, Pelvic Region ØJQC
Cystography
  see Fluoroscopy, Urinary System BT1
  see Plain Radiography, Urinary System BTØ
Cystolithotomy *see* Extirpation, Bladder ØTCB
Cystopexy
  see Repair, Bladder ØTQB
  see Reposition, Bladder ØTSB
Cystoplasty
  see Repair, Bladder ØTQB
  see Replacement, Bladder ØTRB
  see Supplement, Bladder ØTUB
Cystorrhaphy *see* Repair, Bladder ØTQB
Cystoscopy ØTJB8ZZ
Cystostomy *see* Bypass, Bladder ØT1B
Cystostomy tube *use* Drainage Device
Cystotomy *see* Drainage, Bladder ØT9B
Cystourethrography
  see Fluoroscopy, Urinary System BT1
  see Plain Radiography, Urinary System BTØ
Cystourethroplasty
  see Repair, Urinary System ØTQ
  see Replacement, Urinary System ØTR
  see Supplement, Urinary System ØTU

D

DBS lead *use* Neurostimulator Lead in Central Nervous System
DeBakey Left Ventricular Assist Device *use* Implantable Heart Assist System in Heart and Great Vessels
Debridement
  Excisional *see* Excision
  Non-excisional *see* Extraction
Decompression, Circulatory 6A15
Decortication, lung *see* Extraction, Respiratory System ØBD
Deep brain neurostimulator lead *use* Neurostimulator Lead in Central Nervous System
Deep cervical fascia *use* Subcutaneous Tissue and Fascia, Neck, Anterior
Deep cervical vein
  use Vein, Vertebral, Left
  use Vein, Vertebral, Right
Deep circumflex iliac artery
  use Artery, External Iliac, Left
  use Artery, External Iliac, Right
Deep facial vein
  use Vein, Face, Left
  use Vein, Face, Right
Deep femoral artery
  use Artery, Femoral, Left
  use Artery, Femoral, Right
Deep femoral (profunda femoris) vein
  use Vein, Femoral, Left
  use Vein, Femoral, Right
Deep Inferior Epigastric Artery Perforator Flap
  Bilateral ØHRVØ77
  Left ØHRUØ77
  Right ØHRTØ77
Deep palmar arch
  use Artery, Hand, Left
  use Artery, Hand, Right
Deep transverse perineal muscle *use* Muscle, Perineum
Deferential artery
  use Artery, Internal Iliac, Left
  use Artery, Internal Iliac, Right
Defibrillator Generator
  Abdomen ØJH8
  Chest ØJH6
Delivery
  Cesarean *see* Extraction, Products of Conception 10D0
  Forceps *see* Extraction, Products of Conception 10D0
  Manually assisted 10E0XZZ
  Products of Conception 10E0XZZ

Delivery — continued
  Vacuum assisted *see* Extraction, Products of Conception 10D0
Delta frame external fixator
  use External Fixation Device, Hybrid in ØPS
  use External Fixation Device, Hybrid in ØQH
  use External Fixation Device, Hybrid in ØQS
  use External Fixation Device, Hybrid in ØPH
Delta III Reverse shoulder prosthesis *use* Synthetic Substitute, Reverse Ball and Socket in ØRR
Deltoid fascia
  use Subcutaneous Tissue and Fascia, Upper Arm, Left
  use Subcutaneous Tissue and Fascia, Upper Arm, Right
Deltoid ligament
  use Bursa and Ligament, Ankle, Left
  use Bursa and Ligament, Ankle, Right
Deltoid muscle
  use Muscle, Shoulder, Left
  use Muscle, Shoulder, Right
Deltopectoral (infraclavicular) lymph node
  use Lymphatic, Upper Extremity, Left
  use Lymphatic, Upper Extremity, Right
Denervation
  Cranial nerve *see* Destruction, Central Nervous System ØØ5
  Peripheral nerve *see* Destruction, Peripheral Nervous System Ø15
Densitometry
  Plain Radiography
    Femur
      Left BQ04ZZ1
      Right BQ03ZZ1
    Hip
      Left BQ01ZZ1
      Right BQ00ZZ1
    Spine
      Cervical BR00ZZ1
      Lumbar BR09ZZ1
      Thoracic BR07ZZ1
      Whole BR0GZZ1
  Ultrasonography
    Elbow
      Left BP4HZZ1
      Right BP4GZZ1
    Hand
      Left BP4PZZ1
      Right BP4NZZ1
    Shoulder
      Left BP49ZZ1
      Right BP48ZZ1
    Wrist
      Left BP4MZZ1
      Right BP4LZZ1
Dentate ligament *use* Dura Mater
Denticulate ligament *use* Spinal Meninges
Depressor anguli oris muscle *use* Muscle, Facial
Depressor labii inferioris muscle *use* Muscle, Facial
Depressor septi nasi muscle *use* Muscle, Facial
Depressor supercilii muscle *use* Muscle, Facial
Dermabrasion *see* Extraction, Skin and Breast ØHD
Dermis *use* Skin
Descending genicular artery
  use Artery, Femoral, Left
  use Artery, Femoral, Right
Destruction
  Acetabulum
    Left ØQ55
    Right ØQ54
  Adenoids ØC5Q
  Ampulla of Vater ØF5C
  Anal Sphincter ØD5R
  Anterior Chamber
    Left Ø8533ZZ
    Right Ø8523ZZ
  Anus ØD5Q
  Aorta
    Abdominal Ø45Ø
    Thoracic Ø25W
  Aortic Body ØG5D
  Appendix ØD5J
  Artery
    Anterior Tibial
      Left Ø45Q
      Right Ø45P

Destruction — continued
Artery — continued
Axillary
Left 0356
Right 0355
Brachial
Left 0358
Right 0357
Celiac 0451
Colic
Left 0457
Middle 0458
Right 0456
Common Carotid
Left 035J
Right 035H
Common Iliac
Left 045D
Right 045C
External Carotid
Left 035N
Right 035M
External Iliac
Left 045J
Right 045H
Face 035R
Femoral
Left 045L
Right 045K
Foot
Left 045W
Right 045V
Gastric 0452
Hand
Left 035F
Right 035D
Hepatic 0453
Inferior Mesenteric 045B
Innominate 0352
Internal Carotid
Left 035L
Right 035K
Internal Iliac
Left 045F
Right 045E
Internal Mammary
Left 0351
Right 0350
Intracranial 035G
Lower 045Y
Peroneal
Left 045U
Right 045T
Popliteal
Left 045N
Right 045M
Posterior Tibial
Left 045S
Right 045R
Pulmonary
Left 025R
Right 025Q
Pulmonary Trunk 025P
Radial
Left 035C
Right 035B
Renal
Left 045A
Right 0459
Splenic 0454
Subclavian
Left 0354
Right 0353
Superior Mesenteric 0455
Temporal
Left 035T
Right 035S
Thyroid
Left 035V
Right 035U
Ulnar
Left 035A
Right 0359
Upper 035Y
Vertebral
Left 035Q

Destruction — continued
Artery — continued
Vertebral — continued
Right 035P
Atrium
Left 0257
Right 0256
Auditory Ossicle
Left 095A0ZZ
Right 09590ZZ
Basal Ganglia 0058
Bladder 0T5B
Bladder Neck 0T5C
Bone
Ethmoid
Left 0N5G
Right 0N5F
Frontal
Left 0N52
Right 0N51
Hyoid 0N5X
Lacrimal
Left 0N5J
Right 0N5H
Nasal 0N5B
Occipital
Left 0N58
Right 0N57
Palatine
Left 0N5L
Right 0N5K
Parietal
Left 0N54
Right 0N53
Pelvic
Left 0Q53
Right 0Q52
Sphenoid
Left 0N5D
Right 0N5C
Temporal
Left 0N56
Right 0N55
Zygomatic
Left 0N5N
Right 0N5M
Brain 0050
Breast
Bilateral 0H5V
Left 0H5U
Right 0H5T
Bronchus
Lingula 0B59
Lower Lobe
Left 0B5B
Right 0B56
Main
Left 0B57
Right 0B53
Middle Lobe, Right 0B55
Upper Lobe
Left 0B58
Right 0B54
Buccal Mucosa 0C54
Bursa and Ligament
Abdomen
Left 0M5J
Right 0M5H
Ankle
Left 0M5R
Right 0M5Q
Elbow
Left 0M54
Right 0M53
Foot
Left 0M5T
Right 0M5S
Hand
Left 0M58
Right 0M57
Head and Neck 0M50
Hip
Left 0M5M
Right 0M5L
Knee
Left 0M5P

Destruction — continued
Bursa and Ligament — continued
Knee — continued
Right 0M5N
Lower Extremity
Left 0M5W
Right 0M5V
Perineum 0M5K
Shoulder
Left 0M52
Right 0M51
Thorax
Left 0M5G
Right 0M5F
Trunk
Left 0M5D
Right 0M5C
Upper Extremity
Left 0M5B
Right 0M59
Wrist
Left 0M56
Right 0M55
Carina 0B52
Carotid Bodies, Bilateral 0G58
Carotid Body
Left 0G56
Right 0G57
Carpal
Left 0P5N
Right 0P5M
Cecum 0D5H
Cerebellum 005C
Cerebral Hemisphere 0057
Cerebral Meninges 0051
Cerebral Ventricle 0056
Cervix 0U5C
Chordae Tendineae 0259
Choroid
Left 085B
Right 085A
Cisterna Chyli 075L
Clavicle
Left 0P5B
Right 0P59
Clitoris 0U5J
Coccygeal Glomus 0G5B
Coccyx 0Q5S
Colon
Ascending 0D5K
Descending 0D5M
Sigmoid 0D5N
Transverse 0D5L
Conduction Mechanism 0258
Conjunctiva
Left 085TXZZ
Right 085SXZZ
Cord
Bilateral 0V5H
Left 0V5G
Right 0V5F
Cornea
Left 0859XZZ
Right 0858XZZ
Cul-de-sac 0U5F
Diaphragm
Left 0B5S
Right 0B5R
Disc
Cervical Vertebral 0R53
Cervicothoracic Vertebral 0R55
Lumbar Vertebral 0S52
Lumbosacral 0S54
Thoracic Vertebral 0R59
Thoracolumbar Vertebral 0R5B
Duct
Common Bile 0F59
Cystic 0F58
Hepatic
Left 0F56
Right 0F55
Lacrimal
Left 085Y
Right 085X
Pancreatic 0F5D
Accessory 0F5F

▽ **Subterms under main terms may continue to next column or page**

Destruction — continued
- Duct — continued
  - Parotid
    - Left 0C5C
    - Right 0C5B
- Duodenum 0D59
- Dura Mater 0052
- Ear
  - External
    - Left 0951
    - Right 0950
  - External Auditory Canal
    - Left 0954
    - Right 0953
  - Inner
    - Left 095E0ZZ
    - Right 095D0ZZ
  - Middle
    - Left 09560ZZ
    - Right 09550ZZ
- Endometrium 0U5B
- Epididymis
  - Bilateral 0V5L
  - Left 0V5K
  - Right 0V5J
- Epiglottis 0C5R
- Esophagogastric Junction 0D54
- Esophagus 0D55
  - Lower 0D53
  - Middle 0D52
  - Upper 0D51
- Eustachian Tube
  - Left 095G
  - Right 095F
- Eye
  - Left 0851XZZ
  - Right 0850XZZ
- Eyelid
  - Lower
    - Left 085R
    - Right 085Q
  - Upper
    - Left 085P
    - Right 085N
- Fallopian Tube
  - Left 0U56
  - Right 0U55
- Fallopian Tubes, Bilateral 0U57
- Femoral Shaft
  - Left 0Q59
  - Right 0Q58
- Femur
  - Lower
    - Left 0Q5C
    - Right 0Q5B
  - Upper
    - Left 0Q57
    - Right 0Q56
- Fibula
  - Left 0Q5K
  - Right 0Q5J
- Finger Nail 0H5QXZZ
- Gallbladder 0F54
- Gingiva
  - Lower 0C56
  - Upper 0C55
- Gland
  - Adrenal
    - Bilateral 0G54
    - Left 0G52
    - Right 0G53
  - Lacrimal
    - Left 085W
    - Right 085V
  - Minor Salivary 0C5J
  - Parotid
    - Left 0C59
    - Right 0C58
  - Pituitary 0G50
  - Sublingual
    - Left 0C5F
    - Right 0C5D
  - Submaxillary
    - Left 0C5H
    - Right 0C5G
  - Vestibular 0U5L

Destruction — continued
- Glenoid Cavity
  - Left 0P58
  - Right 0P57
- Glomus Jugulare 0G5C
- Humeral Head
  - Left 0P5D
  - Right 0P5C
- Humeral Shaft
  - Left 0P5G
  - Right 0P5F
- Hymen 0U5K
- Hypothalamus 005A
- Ileocecal Valve 0D5C
- Ileum 0D5B
- Intestine
  - Large 0D5E
    - Left 0D5G
    - Right 0D5F
  - Small 0D58
- Iris
  - Left 085D3ZZ
  - Right 085C3ZZ
- Jejunum 0D5A
- Joint
  - Acromioclavicular
    - Left 0R5H
    - Right 0R5G
  - Ankle
    - Left 0S5G
    - Right 0S5F
  - Carpal
    - Left 0R5R
    - Right 0R5Q
  - Cervical Vertebral 0R51
  - Cervicothoracic Vertebral 0R54
  - Coccygeal 0S56
  - Elbow
    - Left 0R5M
    - Right 0R5L
  - Finger Phalangeal
    - Left 0R5X
    - Right 0R5W
  - Hip
    - Left 0S5B
    - Right 0S59
  - Knee
    - Left 0S5D
    - Right 0S5C
  - Lumbar Vertebral 0S50
  - Lumbosacral 0S53
  - Metacarpocarpal
    - Left 0R5T
    - Right 0R5S
  - Metacarpophalangeal
    - Left 0R5V
    - Right 0R5U
  - Metatarsal-Phalangeal
    - Left 0S5N
    - Right 0S5M
  - Metatarsal-Tarsal
    - Left 0S5L
    - Right 0S5K
  - Occipital-cervical 0R50
  - Sacrococcygeal 0S55
  - Sacroiliac
    - Left 0S58
    - Right 0S57
  - Shoulder
    - Left 0R5K
    - Right 0R5J
  - Sternoclavicular
    - Left 0R5F
    - Right 0R5E
  - Tarsal
    - Left 0S5J
    - Right 0S5H
  - Temporomandibular
    - Left 0R5D
    - Right 0R5C
  - Thoracic Vertebral 0R56
  - Thoracolumbar Vertebral 0R5A
  - Toe Phalangeal
    - Left 0S5Q
    - Right 0S5P

Destruction — continued
- Joint — continued
  - Wrist
    - Left 0R5P
    - Right 0R5N
- Kidney
  - Left 0T51
  - Right 0T50
- Kidney Pelvis
  - Left 0T54
  - Right 0T53
- Larynx 0C5S
- Lens
  - Left 085K3ZZ
  - Right 085J3ZZ
- Lip
  - Lower 0C51
  - Upper 0C50
- Liver 0F50
  - Left Lobe 0F52
  - Right Lobe 0F51
- Lung
  - Bilateral 0B5M
  - Left 0B5L
  - Lower Lobe
    - Left 0B5J
    - Right 0B5F
  - Middle Lobe, Right 0B5D
  - Right 0B5K
  - Upper Lobe
    - Left 0B5G
    - Right 0B5C
- Lung Lingula 0B5H
- Lymphatic
  - Aortic 075D
  - Axillary
    - Left 0756
    - Right 0755
  - Head 0750
  - Inguinal
    - Left 075J
    - Right 075H
  - Internal Mammary
    - Left 0759
    - Right 0758
  - Lower Extremity
    - Left 075G
    - Right 075F
  - Mesenteric 075B
  - Neck
    - Left 0752
    - Right 0751
  - Pelvis 075C
  - Thoracic Duct 075K
  - Thorax 0757
  - Upper Extremity
    - Left 0754
    - Right 0753
- Mandible
  - Left 0N5V
  - Right 0N5T
- Maxilla
  - Left 0N5S
  - Right 0N5R
- Medulla Oblongata 005D
- Mesentery 0D5V
- Metacarpal
  - Left 0P5Q
  - Right 0P5P
- Metatarsal
  - Left 0Q5P
  - Right 0Q5N
- Muscle
  - Abdomen
    - Left 0K5L
    - Right 0K5K
  - Extraocular
    - Left 085M
    - Right 085L
  - Facial 0K51
  - Foot
    - Left 0K5W
    - Right 0K5V
  - Hand
    - Left 0K5D
    - Right 0K5C

▽ Subterms under main terms may continue to next column or page

Destruction — continued
  Tendon — continued
    Hip
      Left 0L5K
      Right 0L5J
    Knee
      Left 0L5R
      Right 0L5Q
    Lower Arm and Wrist
      Left 0L56
      Right 0L55
    Lower Leg
      Left 0L5P
      Right 0L5N
    Perineum 0L5H
    Shoulder
      Left 0L52
      Right 0L51
    Thorax
      Left 0L5D
      Right 0L5C
    Trunk
      Left 0L5B
      Right 0L59
    Upper Arm
      Left 0L54
      Right 0L53
    Upper Leg
      Left 0L5M
      Right 0L5L
  Testis
    Bilateral 0V5C
    Left 0V5B
    Right 0V59
  Thalamus 0059
  Thymus 075M
  Thyroid Gland 0G5K
    Left Lobe 0G5G
    Right Lobe 0G5H
  Tibia
    Left 0Q5H
    Right 0Q5G
  Toe Nail 0H5RXZZ
  Tongue 0C57
  Tonsils 0C5P
  Tooth
    Lower 0C5X
    Upper 0C5W
  Trachea 0B51
  Tunica Vaginalis
    Left 0V57
    Right 0V56
  Turbinate, Nasal 095L
  Tympanic Membrane
    Left 0958
    Right 0957
  Ulna
    Left 0P5L
    Right 0P5K
  Ureter
    Left 0T57
    Right 0T56
  Urethra 0T5D
  Uterine Supporting Structure 0U54
  Uterus 0U59
  Uvula 0C5N
  Vagina 0U5G
  Valve
    Aortic 025F
    Mitral 025G
    Pulmonary 025H
    Tricuspid 025J
  Vas Deferens
    Bilateral 0V5Q
    Left 0V5P
    Right 0V5N
  Vein
    Axillary
      Left 0558
      Right 0557
    Azygos 0550
    Basilic
      Left 055C
      Right 055B
    Brachial
      Left 055A

Destruction — continued
  Vein — continued
    Brachial — continued
      Right 0559
    Cephalic
      Left 055F
      Right 055D
    Colic 0657
    Common Iliac
      Left 065D
      Right 065C
    Coronary 0254
    Esophageal 0653
    External Iliac
      Left 065G
      Right 065F
    External Jugular
      Left 055Q
      Right 055P
    Face
      Left 055V
      Right 055T
    Femoral
      Left 065N
      Right 065M
    Foot
      Left 065V
      Right 065T
    Gastric 0652
    Greater Saphenous
      Left 065Q
      Right 065P
    Hand
      Left 055H
      Right 055G
    Hemiazygos 0551
    Hepatic 0654
    Hypogastric
      Left 065J
      Right 065H
    Inferior Mesenteric 0656
    Innominate
      Left 0554
      Right 0553
    Internal Jugular
      Left 055N
      Right 055M
    Intracranial 055L
    Lesser Saphenous
      Left 065S
      Right 065R
    Lower 065Y
    Portal 0658
    Pulmonary
      Left 025T
      Right 025S
    Renal
      Left 065B
      Right 0659
    Splenic 0651
    Subclavian
      Left 0556
      Right 0555
    Superior Mesenteric 0655
    Upper 055Y
    Vertebral
      Left 055S
      Right 055R
  Vena Cava
    Inferior 0650
    Superior 025V
  Ventricle
    Left 025L
    Right 025K
  Vertebra
    Cervical 0P53
    Lumbar 0Q50
    Thoracic 0P54
  Vesicle
    Bilateral 0V53
    Left 0V52
    Right 0V51
  Vitreous
    Left 08553ZZ
    Right 08543ZZ

Destruction — continued
  Vocal Cord
    Left 0C5V
    Right 0C5T
  Vulva 0U5M
Detachment
  Arm
    Lower
      Left 0X6F0Z
      Right 0X6D0Z
    Upper
      Left 0X690Z
      Right 0X680Z
  Elbow Region
    Left 0X6C0ZZ
    Right 0X6B0ZZ
  Femoral Region
    Left 0Y680ZZ
    Right 0Y670ZZ
  Finger
    Index
      Left 0X6P0Z
      Right 0X6N0Z
    Little
      Left 0X6W0Z
      Right 0X6V0Z
    Middle
      Left 0X6R0Z
      Right 0X6Q0Z
    Ring
      Left 0X6T0Z
      Right 0X6S0Z
  Foot
    Left 0Y6N0Z
    Right 0Y6M0Z
  Forequarter
    Left 0X610ZZ
    Right 0X600ZZ
  Hand
    Left 0X6K0Z
    Right 0X6J0Z
  Hindquarter
    Bilateral 0Y640ZZ
    Left 0Y630ZZ
    Right 0Y620ZZ
  Knee Region
    Left 0Y6G0ZZ
    Right 0Y6F0ZZ
  Leg
    Lower
      Left 0Y6J0Z
      Right 0Y6H0Z
    Upper
      Left 0Y6D0Z
      Right 0Y6C0Z
  Shoulder Region
    Left 0X630ZZ
    Right 0X620ZZ
  Thumb
    Left 0X6M0Z
    Right 0X6L0Z
  Toe
    1st
      Left 0Y6Q0Z
      Right 0Y6P0Z
    2nd
      Left 0Y6S0Z
      Right 0Y6R0Z
    3rd
      Left 0Y6U0Z
      Right 0Y6T0Z
    4th
      Left 0Y6W0Z
      Right 0Y6V0Z
    5th
      Left 0Y6Y0Z
      Right 0Y6X0Z
Determination, Mental status GZ14ZZZ
Detorsion
  see Release
  see Reposition
Detoxification Services, for substance abuse
  HZ2ZZZZ
Device Fitting F0DZ
Diagnostic Audiology *see* Audiology, Diagnostic
Diagnostic imaging *see* Imaging, Diagnostic

Diagnostic radiology *see* Imaging, Diagnostic
Dialysis
  Hemodialysis 5A1D00Z
  Peritoneal 3E1M39Z
Diaphragma sellae *use* Dura Mater
Diaphragmatic pacemaker generator *use* Stimulator
  Generator in Subcutaneous Tissue and Fascia
Diaphragmatic Pacemaker Lead
  Insertion of device in
    Left ØBHS
    Right ØBHR
  Removal of device from, Diaphragm ØBPT
  Revision of device in, Diaphragm ØBWT
Digital radiography, plain *see* Plain Radiography
Dilation
  Ampulla of Vater ØF7C
  Anus ØD7Q
  Aorta
    Abdominal 0470
    Thoracic 027W
  Artery
    Anterior Tibial
      Left 047Q
      Right 047P
    Axillary
      Left 0376
      Right 0375
    Brachial
      Left 0378
      Right 0377
    Celiac 0471
    Colic
      Left 0477
      Middle 0478
      Right 0476
    Common Carotid
      Left 037J
      Right 037H
    Common Iliac
      Left 047D
      Right 047C
    Coronary
      Four or More Sites 0273
      One Site 0270
      Three Sites 0272
      Two Sites 0271
    External Carotid
      Left 037N
      Right 037M
    External Iliac
      Left 047J
      Right 047H
    Face 037R
    Femoral
      Left 047L
      Right 047K
    Foot
      Left 047W
      Right 047V
    Gastric 0472
    Hand
      Left 037F
      Right 037D
    Hepatic 0473
    Inferior Mesenteric 047B
    Innominate 0372
    Internal Carotid
      Left 037L
      Right 037K
    Internal Iliac
      Left 047F
      Right 047E
    Internal Mammary
      Left 0371
      Right 0370
    Intracranial 037G
    Lower 047Y
    Peroneal
      Left 047U
      Right 047T
    Popliteal
      Left 047N
      Right 047M
    Posterior Tibial
      Left 047S
      Right 047R

Dilation — continued
  Artery — continued
    Pulmonary
      Left 027R
      Right 027Q
    Pulmonary Trunk 027P
    Radial
      Left 037C
      Right 037B
    Renal
      Left 047A
      Right 0479
    Splenic 0474
    Subclavian
      Left 0374
      Right 0373
    Superior Mesenteric 0475
    Temporal
      Left 037T
      Right 037S
    Thyroid
      Left 037V
      Right 037U
    Ulnar
      Left 037A
      Right 0379
    Upper 037Y
    Vertebral
      Left 037Q
      Right 037P
  Bladder 0T7B
  Bladder Neck 0T7C
  Bronchus
    Lingula 0B79
    Lower Lobe
      Left 0B7B
      Right 0B76
    Main
      Left 0B77
      Right 0B73
    Middle Lobe, Right 0B75
    Upper Lobe
      Left 0B78
      Right 0B74
  Carina 0B72
  Cecum 0D7H
  Cervix 0U7C
  Colon
    Ascending 0D7K
    Descending 0D7M
    Sigmoid 0D7N
    Transverse 0D7L
  Duct
    Common Bile 0F79
    Cystic 0F78
    Hepatic
      Left 0F76
      Right 0F75
    Lacrimal
      Left 087Y
      Right 087X
    Pancreatic 0F7D
      Accessory 0F7F
    Parotid
      Left 0C7C
      Right 0C7B
  Duodenum 0D79
  Esophagogastric Junction 0D74
  Esophagus 0D75
    Lower 0D73
    Middle 0D72
    Upper 0D71
  Eustachian Tube
    Left 097G
    Right 097F
  Fallopian Tube
    Left 0U76
    Right 0U75
  Fallopian Tubes, Bilateral 0U77
  Hymen 0U7K
  Ileocecal Valve 0D7C
  Ileum 0D7B
  Intestine
    Large 0D7E
      Left 0D7G
      Right 0D7F

Dilation — continued
  Intestine — continued
    Small 0D78
  Jejunum 0D7A
  Kidney Pelvis
    Left 0T74
    Right 0T73
  Larynx 0C7S
  Pharynx 0C7M
  Rectum 0D7P
  Stomach 0D76
    Pylorus 0D77
  Trachea 0B71
  Ureter
    Left 0T77
    Right 0T76
  Ureters, Bilateral 0T78
  Urethra 0T7D
  Uterus 0U79
  Vagina 0U7G
  Valve
    Aortic 027F
    Mitral 027G
    Pulmonary 027H
    Tricuspid 027J
  Vas Deferens
    Bilateral 0V7Q
    Left 0V7P
    Right 0V7N
  Vein
    Axillary
      Left 0578
      Right 0577
    Azygos 0570
    Basilic
      Left 057C
      Right 057B
    Brachial
      Left 057A
      Right 0579
    Cephalic
      Left 057F
      Right 057D
    Colic 0677
    Common Iliac
      Left 067D
      Right 067C
    Esophageal 0673
    External Iliac
      Left 067G
      Right 067F
    External Jugular
      Left 057Q
      Right 057P
    Face
      Left 057V
      Right 057T
    Femoral
      Left 067N
      Right 067M
    Foot
      Left 067V
      Right 067T
    Gastric 0672
    Greater Saphenous
      Left 067Q
      Right 067P
    Hand
      Left 057H
      Right 057G
    Hemiazygos 0571
    Hepatic 0674
    Hypogastric
      Left 067J
      Right 067H
    Inferior Mesenteric 0676
    Innominate
      Left 0574
      Right 0573
    Internal Jugular
      Left 057N
      Right 057M
    Intracranial 057L
    Lesser Saphenous
      Left 067S
      Right 067R

Dilation — continued
  Vein — continued
    Lower 067Y
    Portal 0678
    Pulmonary
      Left 027T
      Right 027S
    Renal
      Left 067B
      Right 0679
    Splenic 0671
    Subclavian
      Left 0576
      Right 0575
    Superior Mesenteric 0675
    Upper 057Y
    Vertebral
      Left 057S
      Right 057R
  Vena Cava
    Inferior 0670
    Superior 027V
  Ventricle, Right 027K
Direct Lateral Interbody Fusion (DLIF) device *use*
  Interbody Fusion Device in Lower Joints
Disarticulation *see* Detachment
Discectomy, diskectomy
  see Excision, Lower Joints 0SB
  see Excision, Upper Joints 0RB
  see Resection, Lower Joints 0ST
  see Resection, Upper Joints 0RT
Discography
  see Fluoroscopy, Axial Skeleton, Except Skull and Facial Bones BR1
  see Plain Radiography, Axial Skeleton, Except Skull and Facial Bones BR0
Distal humerus
  use Humeral Shaft, Left
  use Humeral Shaft, Right
Distal humerus, involving joint
  use Joint, Elbow, Left
  use Joint, Elbow, Right
Distal radioulnar joint
  use Joint, Wrist, Left
  use Joint, Wrist, Right
Diversion *see* Bypass
Diverticulectomy *see* Excision, Gastrointestinal System 0DB
Division
  Acetabulum
    Left 0Q85
    Right 0Q84
  Anal Sphincter 0D8R
  Basal Ganglia 0088
  Bladder Neck 0T8C
  Bone
    Ethmoid
      Left 0N8G
      Right 0N8F
    Frontal
      Left 0N82
      Right 0N81
    Hyoid 0N8X
    Lacrimal
      Left 0N8J
      Right 0N8H
    Nasal 0N8B
    Occipital
      Left 0N88
      Right 0N87
    Palatine
      Left 0N8L
      Right 0N8K
    Parietal
      Left 0N84
      Right 0N83
    Pelvic
      Left 0Q83
      Right 0Q82
    Sphenoid
      Left 0N8D
      Right 0N8C
    Temporal
      Left 0N86
      Right 0N85

Division — continued
  Bone — continued
    Zygomatic
      Left 0N8N
      Right 0N8M
  Brain 0080
  Bursa and Ligament
    Abdomen
      Left 0M8J
      Right 0M8H
    Ankle
      Left 0M8R
      Right 0M8Q
    Elbow
      Left 0M84
      Right 0M83
    Foot
      Left 0M8T
      Right 0M8S
    Hand
      Left 0M88
      Right 0M87
    Head and Neck 0M80
    Hip
      Left 0M8M
      Right 0M8L
    Knee
      Left 0M8P
      Right 0M8N
    Lower Extremity
      Left 0M8W
      Right 0M8V
    Perineum 0M8K
    Shoulder
      Left 0M82
      Right 0M81
    Thorax
      Left 0M8G
      Right 0M8F
    Trunk
      Left 0M8D
      Right 0M8C
    Upper Extremity
      Left 0M8B
      Right 0M89
    Wrist
      Left 0M86
      Right 0M85
  Carpal
    Left 0P8N
    Right 0P8M
  Cerebral Hemisphere 0087
  Chordae Tendineae 0289
  Clavicle
    Left 0P8B
    Right 0P89
  Coccyx 0Q8S
  Conduction Mechanism 0288
  Esophagogastric Junction 0D84
  Femoral Shaft
    Left 0Q89
    Right 0Q88
  Femur
    Lower
      Left 0Q8C
      Right 0Q8B
    Upper
      Left 0Q87
      Right 0Q86
  Fibula
    Left 0Q8K
    Right 0Q8J
  Gland, Pituitary 0G80
  Glenoid Cavity
    Left 0P88
    Right 0P87
  Humeral Head
    Left 0P8D
    Right 0P8C
  Humeral Shaft
    Left 0P8G
    Right 0P8F
  Hymen 0U8K
  Kidneys, Bilateral 0T82
  Mandible
    Left 0N8V

Division — continued
  Mandible — continued
    Right 0N8T
  Maxilla
    Left 0N8S
    Right 0N8R
  Metacarpal
    Left 0P8Q
    Right 0P8P
  Metatarsal
    Left 0Q8P
    Right 0Q8N
  Muscle
    Abdomen
      Left 0K8L
      Right 0K8K
    Facial 0K81
    Foot
      Left 0K8W
      Right 0K8V
    Hand
      Left 0K8D
      Right 0K8C
    Head 0K80
    Hip
      Left 0K8P
      Right 0K8N
    Lower Arm and Wrist
      Left 0K8B
      Right 0K89
    Lower Leg
      Left 0K8T
      Right 0K8S
    Neck
      Left 0K83
      Right 0K82
    Papillary 028D
    Perineum 0K8M
    Shoulder
      Left 0K86
      Right 0K85
    Thorax
      Left 0K8J
      Right 0K8H
    Tongue, Palate, Pharynx 0K84
    Trunk
      Left 0K8G
      Right 0K8F
    Upper Arm
      Left 0K88
      Right 0K87
    Upper Leg
      Left 0K8R
      Right 0K8Q
  Nerve
    Abdominal Sympathetic 018M
    Abducens 008L
    Accessory 008R
    Acoustic 008N
    Brachial Plexus 0183
    Cervical 0181
    Cervical Plexus 0180
    Facial 008M
    Femoral 018D
    Glossopharyngeal 008P
    Head and Neck Sympathetic 018K
    Hypoglossal 008S
    Lumbar 018B
    Lumbar Plexus 0189
    Lumbar Sympathetic 018N
    Lumbosacral Plexus 018A
    Median 0185
    Oculomotor 008H
    Olfactory 008F
    Optic 008G
    Peroneal 018H
    Phrenic 0182
    Pudendal 018C
    Radial 0186
    Sacral 018R
    Sacral Plexus 018Q
    Sacral Sympathetic 018P
    Sciatic 018F
    Thoracic 0188
    Thoracic Sympathetic 018L
    Tibial 018G

▼ **Subterms under main terms may continue to next column or page**

Drainage — continued
Artery — continued
Internal Carotid
Left 039L
Right 039K
Internal Iliac
Left 049F
Right 049E
Internal Mammary
Left 0391
Right 0390
Intracranial 039G
Lower 049Y
Peroneal
Left 049U
Right 049T
Popliteal
Left 049N
Right 049M
Posterior Tibial
Left 049S
Right 049R
Radial
Left 039C
Right 039B
Renal
Left 049A
Right 0499
Splenic 0494
Subclavian
Left 0394
Right 0393
Superior Mesenteric 0495
Temporal
Left 039T
Right 039S
Thyroid
Left 039V
Right 039U
Ulnar
Left 039A
Right 0399
Upper 039Y
Vertebral
Left 039Q
Right 039P
Auditory Ossicle
Left 099A
Right 0999
Axilla
Left 0X95
Right 0X94
Back
Lower 0W9L
Upper 0W9K
Basal Ganglia 0098
Bladder 0T9B
Bladder Neck 0T9C
Bone
Ethmoid
Left 0N9G
Right 0N9F
Frontal
Left 0N92
Right 0N91
Hyoid 0N9X
Lacrimal
Left 0N9J
Right 0N9H
Nasal 0N9B
Occipital
Left 0N98
Right 0N97
Palatine
Left 0N9L
Right 0N9K
Parietal
Left 0N94
Right 0N93
Pelvic
Left 0Q93
Right 0Q92
Sphenoid
Left 0N9D
Right 0N9C

Drainage — continued
Bone — continued
Temporal
Left 0N96
Right 0N95
Zygomatic
Left 0N9N
Right 0N9M
Bone Marrow 079T
Brain 0090
Breast
Bilateral 0H9V
Left 0H9U
Right 0H9T
Bronchus
Lingula 0B99
Lower Lobe
Left 0B9B
Right 0B96
Main
Left 0B97
Right 0B93
Middle Lobe, Right 0B95
Upper Lobe
Left 0B98
Right 0B94
Buccal Mucosa 0C94
Bursa and Ligament
Abdomen
Left 0M9J
Right 0M9H
Ankle
Left 0M9R
Right 0M9Q
Elbow
Left 0M94
Right 0M93
Foot
Left 0M9T
Right 0M9S
Hand
Left 0M98
Right 0M97
Head and Neck 0M90
Hip
Left 0M9M
Right 0M9L
Knee
Left 0M9P
Right 0M9N
Lower Extremity
Left 0M9W
Right 0M9V
Perineum 0M9K
Shoulder
Left 0M92
Right 0M91
Thorax
Left 0M9G
Right 0M9F
Trunk
Left 0M9D
Right 0M9C
Upper Extremity
Left 0M9B
Right 0M99
Wrist
Left 0M96
Right 0M95
Buttock
Left 0Y91
Right 0Y90
Carina 0B92
Carotid Bodies, Bilateral 0G98
Carotid Body
Left 0G96
Right 0G97
Carpal
Left 0P9N
Right 0P9M
Cavity, Cranial 0W91
Cecum 0D9H
Cerebellum 009C
Cerebral Hemisphere 0097
Cerebral Meninges 0091
Cerebral Ventricle 0096

Drainage — continued
Cervix 0U9C
Chest Wall 0W98
Choroid
Left 089B
Right 089A
Cisterna Chyli 079L
Clavicle
Left 0P9B
Right 0P99
Clitoris 0U9J
Coccygeal Glomus 0G9B
Coccyx 0Q9S
Colon
Ascending 0D9K
Descending 0D9M
Sigmoid 0D9N
Transverse 0D9L
Conjunctiva
Left 089T
Right 089S
Cord
Bilateral 0V9H
Left 0V9G
Right 0V9F
Cornea
Left 0899
Right 0898
Cul-de-sac 0U9F
Diaphragm
Left 0B9S
Right 0B9R
Disc
Cervical Vertebral 0R93
Cervicothoracic Vertebral 0R95
Lumbar Vertebral 0S92
Lumbosacral 0S94
Thoracic Vertebral 0R99
Thoracolumbar Vertebral 0R9B
Duct
Common Bile 0F99
Cystic 0F98
Hepatic
Left 0F96
Right 0F95
Lacrimal
Left 089Y
Right 089X
Pancreatic 0F9D
Accessory 0F9F
Parotid
Left 0C9C
Right 0C9B
Duodenum 0D99
Dura Mater 0092
Ear
External
Left 0991
Right 0990
External Auditory Canal
Left 0994
Right 0993
Inner
Left 099E
Right 099D
Middle
Left 0996
Right 0995
Elbow Region
Left 0X9C
Right 0X9B
Epididymis
Bilateral 0V9L
Left 0V9K
Right 0V9J
Epidural Space 0093
Epiglottis 0C9R
Esophagogastric Junction 0D94
Esophagus 0D95
Lower 0D93
Middle 0D92
Upper 0D91
Eustachian Tube
Left 099G
Right 099F

Drainage — continued
Extremity
  Lower
    Left 0Y9B
    Right 0Y99
  Upper
    Left 0X97
    Right 0X96
Eye
  Left 0891
  Right 0890
Eyelid
  Lower
    Left 089R
    Right 089Q
  Upper
    Left 089P
    Right 089N
Face 0W92
Fallopian Tube
  Left 0U96
  Right 0U95
Fallopian Tubes, Bilateral 0U97
Femoral Region
  Left 0Y98
  Right 0Y97
Femoral Shaft
  Left 0Q99
  Right 0Q98
Femur
  Lower
    Left 0Q9C
    Right 0Q9B
  Upper
    Left 0Q97
    Right 0Q96
Fibula
  Left 0Q9K
  Right 0Q9J
Finger Nail 0H9Q
Foot
  Left 0Y9N
  Right 0Y9M
Gallbladder 0F94
Gingiva
  Lower 0C96
  Upper 0C95
Gland
  Adrenal
    Bilateral 0G94
    Left 0G92
    Right 0G93
  Lacrimal
    Left 089W
    Right 089V
  Minor Salivary 0C9J
  Parotid
    Left 0C99
    Right 0C98
  Pituitary 0G90
  Sublingual
    Left 0C9F
    Right 0C9D
  Submaxillary
    Left 0C9H
    Right 0C9G
  Vestibular 0U9L
Glenoid Cavity
  Left 0P98
  Right 0P97
Glomus Jugulare 0G9C
Hand
  Left 0X9K
  Right 0X9J
Head 0W90
Humeral Head
  Left 0P9D
  Right 0P9C
Humeral Shaft
  Left 0P9G
  Right 0P9F
Hymen 0U9K
Hypothalamus 009A
Ileocecal Valve 0D9C
Ileum 0D9B

Drainage — continued
Inguinal Region
  Left 0Y96
  Right 0Y95
Intestine
  Large 0D9E
    Left 0D9G
    Right 0D9F
  Small 0D98
Iris
  Left 089D
  Right 089C
Jaw
  Lower 0W95
  Upper 0W94
Jejunum 0D9A
Joint
  Acromioclavicular
    Left 0R9H
    Right 0R9G
  Ankle
    Left 0S9G
    Right 0S9F
  Carpal
    Left 0R9R
    Right 0R9Q
  Cervical Vertebral 0R91
  Cervicothoracic Vertebral 0R94
  Coccygeal 0S96
  Elbow
    Left 0R9M
    Right 0R9L
  Finger Phalangeal
    Left 0R9X
    Right 0R9W
  Hip
    Left 0S9B
    Right 0S99
  Knee
    Left 0S9D
    Right 0S9C
  Lumbar Vertebral 0S90
  Lumbosacral 0S93
  Metacarpocarpal
    Left 0R9T
    Right 0R9S
  Metacarpophalangeal
    Left 0R9V
    Right 0R9U
  Metatarsal-Phalangeal
    Left 0S9N
    Right 0S9M
  Metatarsal-Tarsal
    Left 0S9L
    Right 0S9K
  Occipital-cervical 0R90
  Sacrococcygeal 0S95
  Sacroiliac
    Left 0S98
    Right 0S97
  Shoulder
    Left 0R9K
    Right 0R9J
  Sternoclavicular
    Left 0R9F
    Right 0R9E
  Tarsal
    Left 0S9J
    Right 0S9H
  Temporomandibular
    Left 0R9D
    Right 0R9C
  Thoracic Vertebral 0R96
  Thoracolumbar Vertebral 0R9A
  Toe Phalangeal
    Left 0S9Q
    Right 0S9P
  Wrist
    Left 0R9P
    Right 0R9N
Kidney
  Left 0T91
  Right 0T90
Kidney Pelvis
  Left 0T94
  Right 0T93

Drainage — continued
Knee Region
  Left 0Y9G
  Right 0Y9F
Larynx 0C9S
Leg
  Lower
    Left 0Y9J
    Right 0Y9H
  Upper
    Left 0Y9D
    Right 0Y9C
Lens
  Left 089K
  Right 089J
Lip
  Lower 0C91
  Upper 0C90
Liver 0F90
  Left Lobe 0F92
  Right Lobe 0F91
Lung
  Bilateral 0B9M
  Left 0B9L
  Lower Lobe
    Left 0B9J
    Right 0B9F
  Middle Lobe, Right 0B9D
  Right 0B9K
  Upper Lobe
    Left 0B9G
    Right 0B9C
Lung Lingula 0B9H
Lymphatic
  Aortic 079D
  Axillary
    Left 0796
    Right 0795
  Head 0790
  Inguinal
    Left 079J
    Right 079H
  Internal Mammary
    Left 0799
    Right 0798
  Lower Extremity
    Left 079G
    Right 079F
  Mesenteric 079B
  Neck
    Left 0792
    Right 0791
  Pelvis 079C
  Thoracic Duct 079K
  Thorax 0797
  Upper Extremity
    Left 0794
    Right 0793
Mandible
  Left 0N9V
  Right 0N9T
Maxilla
  Left 0N9S
  Right 0N9R
Mediastinum 0W9C
Medulla Oblongata 009D
Mesentery 0D9V
Metacarpal
  Left 0P9Q
  Right 0P9P
Metatarsal
  Left 0Q9P
  Right 0Q9N
Muscle
  Abdomen
    Left 0K9L
    Right 0K9K
  Extraocular
    Left 089M
    Right 089L
  Facial 0K91
  Foot
    Left 0K9W
    Right 0K9V
  Hand
    Left 0K9D

Drainage — continued
  Muscle — continued
    Hand — continued
      Right 0K9C
    Head 0K90
    Hip
      Left 0K9P
      Right 0K9N
    Lower Arm and Wrist
      Left 0K9B
      Right 0K99
    Lower Leg
      Left 0K9T
      Right 0K9S
    Neck
      Left 0K93
      Right 0K92
    Perineum 0K9M
    Shoulder
      Left 0K96
      Right 0K95
    Thorax
      Left 0K9J
      Right 0K9H
    Tongue, Palate, Pharynx 0K94
    Trunk
      Left 0K9G
      Right 0K9F
    Upper Arm
      Left 0K98
      Right 0K97
    Upper Leg
      Left 0K9R
      Right 0K9Q
  Nasopharynx 099N
  Neck 0W96
  Nerve
    Abdominal Sympathetic 019M
    Abducens 009L
    Accessory 009R
    Acoustic 009N
    Brachial Plexus 0193
    Cervical 0191
    Cervical Plexus 0190
    Facial 009M
    Femoral 019D
    Glossopharyngeal 009P
    Head and Neck Sympathetic 019K
    Hypoglossal 009S
    Lumbar 019B
    Lumbar Plexus 0199
    Lumbar Sympathetic 019N
    Lumbosacral Plexus 019A
    Median 0195
    Oculomotor 009H
    Olfactory 009F
    Optic 009G
    Peroneal 019H
    Phrenic 0192
    Pudendal 019C
    Radial 0196
    Sacral 019R
    Sacral Plexus 019Q
    Sacral Sympathetic 019P
    Sciatic 019F
    Thoracic 0198
    Thoracic Sympathetic 019L
    Tibial 019G
    Trigeminal 009K
    Trochlear 009J
    Ulnar 0194
    Vagus 009Q
  Nipple
    Left 0H9X
    Right 0H9W
  Nose 099K
  Omentum
    Greater 0D9S
    Lesser 0D9T
  Oral Cavity and Throat 0W93
  Orbit
    Left 0N9Q
    Right 0N9P
  Ovary
    Bilateral 0U92
    Left 0U91

Drainage — continued
  Ovary — continued
    Right 0U90
  Palate
    Hard 0C92
    Soft 0C93
  Pancreas 0F9G
  Para-aortic Body 0G99
  Paraganglion Extremity 0G9F
  Parathyroid Gland 0G9R
    Inferior
      Left 0G9P
      Right 0G9N
    Multiple 0G9Q
    Superior
      Left 0G9M
      Right 0G9L
  Patella
    Left 0Q9F
    Right 0Q9D
  Pelvic Cavity 0W9J
  Penis 0V9S
  Pericardial Cavity 0W9D
  Perineum
    Female 0W9N
    Male 0W9M
  Peritoneal Cavity 0W9G
  Peritoneum 0D9W
  Phalanx
    Finger
      Left 0P9V
      Right 0P9T
    Thumb
      Left 0P9S
      Right 0P9R
    Toe
      Left 0Q9R
      Right 0Q9Q
  Pharynx 0C9M
  Pineal Body 0G91
  Pleura
    Left 0B9P
    Right 0B9N
  Pleural Cavity
    Left 0W9B
    Right 0W99
  Pons 009B
  Prepuce 0V9T
  Products of Conception
    Amniotic Fluid
      Diagnostic 1090
      Therapeutic 1090
    Fetal Blood 1090
    Fetal Cerebrospinal Fluid 1090
    Fetal Fluid, Other 1090
    Fluid, Other 1090
  Prostate 0V90
  Radius
    Left 0P9J
    Right 0P9H
  Rectum 0D9P
  Retina
    Left 089F
    Right 089E
  Retinal Vessel
    Left 089H
    Right 089G
  Retroperitoneum 0W9H
  Rib
    Left 0P92
    Right 0P91
  Sacrum 0Q91
  Scapula
    Left 0P96
    Right 0P95
  Sclera
    Left 0897
    Right 0896
  Scrotum 0V95
  Septum, Nasal 099M
  Shoulder Region
    Left 0X93
    Right 0X92
  Sinus
    Accessory 099P

Drainage — continued
  Sinus — continued
    Ethmoid
      Left 099V
      Right 099U
    Frontal
      Left 099T
      Right 099S
    Mastoid
      Left 099C
      Right 099B
    Maxillary
      Left 099R
      Right 099Q
    Sphenoid
      Left 099X
      Right 099W
  Skin
    Abdomen 0H97
    Back 0H96
    Buttock 0H98
    Chest 0H95
    Ear
      Left 0H93
      Right 0H92
    Face 0H91
    Foot
      Left 0H9N
      Right 0H9M
    Genitalia 0H9A
    Hand
      Left 0H9G
      Right 0H9F
    Lower Arm
      Left 0H9E
      Right 0H9D
    Lower Leg
      Left 0H9L
      Right 0H9K
    Neck 0H94
    Perineum 0H99
    Scalp 0H90
    Upper Arm
      Left 0H9C
      Right 0H9B
    Upper Leg
      Left 0H9J
      Right 0H9H
  Skull 0N90
  Spinal Canal 009U
  Spinal Cord
    Cervical 009W
    Lumbar 009Y
    Thoracic 009X
  Spinal Meninges 009T
  Spleen 079P
  Sternum 0P90
  Stomach 0D96
    Pylorus 0D97
  Subarachnoid Space 0095
  Subcutaneous Tissue and Fascia
    Abdomen 0J98
    Back 0J97
    Buttock 0J99
    Chest 0J96
    Face 0J91
    Foot
      Left 0J9R
      Right 0J9Q
    Hand
      Left 0J9K
      Right 0J9J
    Lower Arm
      Left 0J9H
      Right 0J9G
    Lower Leg
      Left 0J9P
      Right 0J9N
    Neck
      Anterior 0J94
      Posterior 0J95
    Pelvic Region 0J9C
    Perineum 0J9B
    Scalp 0J90
    Upper Arm
      Left 0J9F

▽ **Subterms under main terms may continue to next column or page**

Duodenoenterostomy — continued
  see Drainage, Gastrointestinal System ØD9
Duodenojejunal flexure *use* Jejunum
Duodenolysis *see* Release, Duodenum ØDN9
Duodenorrhaphy *see* Repair, Duodenum ØDQ9
Duodenostomy
  see Bypass, Duodenum ØD19
  see Drainage, Duodenum ØD99
Duodenotomy *see* Drainage, Duodenum ØD99
DuraHeart Left Ventricular Assist System *use* Implantable Heart Assist System in Heart and Great Vessels
Dural venous sinus *use* Vein, Intracranial
Durata® Defibrillation Lead *use* Cardiac Lead, Defibrillator in Ø2H
Dynesys® Dynamic Stabilization System
  use Spinal Stabilization Device, Pedicle-Based in ØSH
  use Spinal Stabilization Device, Pedicle-Based in ØRH

E

E-Luminexx™ (Biliary)(Vascular) Stent *use* Intraluminal Device
Earlobe
  use Ear, External, Bilateral
  use Ear, External, Left
  use Ear, External, Right
Echocardiogram *see* Ultrasonography, Heart B24
Echography *see* Ultrasonography
ECMO *see* Performance, Circulatory 5A15
EEG (electroencephalogram) *see* Measurement, Central Nervous 4A00
EGD (esophagogastroduodenscopy) ØDJ08ZZ
Eighth cranial nerve *use* Nerve, Acoustic
Ejaculatory duct
  use Vas Deferens
  use Vas Deferens, Bilateral
  use Vas Deferens, Left
  use Vas Deferens, Right
EKG (electrocardiogram) *see* Measurement, Cardiac 4A02
Electrical bone growth stimulator (EBGS)
  use Bone Growth Stimulator in Head and Facial Bones
  use Bone Growth Stimulator in Lower Bones
  use Bone Growth Stimulator in Upper Bones
Electrical muscle stimulation (EMS) lead *use* Stimulator Lead in Muscles
Electrocautery
  Destruction *see* Destruction
  Repair *see* Repair
Electroconvulsive Therapy
  Bilateral-Multiple Seizure GZB3ZZZ
  Bilateral-Single Seizure GZB2ZZZ
  Electroconvulsive Therapy, Other GZB4ZZZ
  Unilateral-Multiple Seizure GZB1ZZZ
  Unilateral-Single Seizure GZB0ZZZ
Electroencephalogram (EEG) *see* Measurement, Central Nervous 4A00
Electromagnetic Therapy
  Central Nervous 6A22
  Urinary 6A21
Electronic muscle stimulator lead *use* Stimulator Lead in Muscles
Electrophysiologic stimulation (EPS) *see* Measurement, Cardiac 4A02
Electroshock therapy *see* Electroconvulsive Therapy
Elevation, bone fragments, skull *see* Reposition, Head and Facial Bones ØNS
Eleventh cranial nerve *use* Nerve, Accessory
Embolectomy *see* Extirpation
Embolization
  see Occlusion
  see Restriction
Embolization coil(s) *use* Intraluminal Device
EMG (electromyogram) *see* Measurement, Musculoskeletal 4A0F
Encephalon *use* Brain
Endarterectomy
  see Extirpation, Lower Arteries Ø4C
  see Extirpation, Upper Arteries Ø3C
Endeavor® (III)(IV) (Sprint) Zotarolimus-eluting Coronary Stent System *use* Intraluminal Device, Drug-eluting in Heart and Great Vessels

EndoSure® sensor *use* Monitoring Device, Pressure Sensor in Ø2H
ENDOTAK RELIANCE® (G) Defibrillation Lead *use* Cardiac Lead, Defibrillator in Ø2H
Endotracheal tube (cuffed)(double-lumen) *use* Intraluminal Device, Endotracheal Airway in Respiratory System
Endurant® Endovascular Stent Graft *use* Intraluminal Device
Enlargement
  see Dilation
  see Repair
EnRhythm *use* Pacemaker, Dual Chamber in ØJH
Enterorrhaphy *see* Repair, Gastrointestinal System ØDQ
Enterra gastric neurostimulator *use* Stimulator Generator, Multiple Array in ØJH
Enucleation
  Eyeball *see* Resection, Eye Ø8T
  Eyeball with prosthetic implant *see* Replacement, Eye Ø8R
Ependyma *use* Cerebral Ventricle
Epicel® cultured epidermal autograft *use* Autologous Tissue Substitute
Epic™ Stented Tissue Valve (aortic) *use* Zooplastic Tissue in Heart and Great Vessels
Epidermis *use* Skin
Epididymectomy
  see Excision, Male Reproductive System ØVB
  see Resection, Male Reproductive System ØVT
Epididymoplasty
  see Repair, Male Reproductive System ØVQ
  see Supplement, Male Reproductive System ØVU
Epididymorrhaphy *see* Repair, Male Reproductive System ØVQ
Epididymotomy *see* Drainage, Male Reproductive System ØV9
Epiphysiodesis
  see Fusion, Lower Joints ØSG
  see Fusion, Upper Joints ØRG
Epiploic foramen *use* Peritoneum
Epiretinal Visual Prosthesis
  use Epiretinal Visual Prosthesis in Eye
  Insertion of device in
    Left Ø8H105Z
    Right Ø8H005Z
Episiorrhaphy *see* Repair, Perineum, Female ØWQN
Episiotomy *see* Division, Perineum, Female ØW8N
Epithalamus *use* Thalamus
Epitrochlear lymph node
  use Lymphatic, Upper Extremity, Left
  use Lymphatic, Upper Extremity, Right
EPS (electrophysiologic stimulation) *see* Measurement, Cardiac 4A02
Eptifibatide, infusion *see* Introduction of Platelet Inhibitor
ERCP (endoscopic retrograde cholangiopancreatography) *see* Fluoroscopy, Hepatobiliary System and Pancreas BF1
Erector spinae muscle
  use Muscle, Trunk, Left
  use Muscle, Trunk, Right
Esophageal artery *use* Aorta, Thoracic
Esophageal obturator airway (EOA) *use* Intraluminal Device, Airway in Gastrointestinal System
Esophageal plexus *use* Nerve, Thoracic Sympathetic
Esophagectomy
  see Excision, Gastrointestinal System ØDB
  see Resection, Gastrointestinal System ØDT
Esophagocoloplasty
  see Repair, Gastrointestinal System ØDQ
  see Supplement, Gastrointestinal System ØDU
Esophagoenterostomy
  see Bypass, Gastrointestinal System ØD1
  see Drainage, Gastrointestinal System ØD9
Esophagoesophagostomy
  see Bypass, Gastrointestinal System ØD1
  see Drainage, Gastrointestinal System ØD9
Esophagogastrectomy
  see Excision, Gastrointestinal System ØDB
  see Resection, Gastrointestinal System ØDT
Esophagogastroduodenscopy (EGD) ØDJ08ZZ
Esophagogastroplasty
  see Repair, Gastrointestinal System ØDQ
  see Supplement, Gastrointestinal System ØDU

Esophagogastroscopy ØDJ68ZZ
Esophagogastrostomy
  see Bypass, Gastrointestinal System ØD1
  see Drainage, Gastrointestinal System ØD9
Esophagojejunoplasty *see* Supplement, Gastrointestinal System ØDU
Esophagojejunostomy
  see Bypass, Gastrointestinal System ØD1
  see Drainage, Gastrointestinal System ØD9
Esophagomyotomy *see* Division, Esophagogastric Junction ØD84
Esophagoplasty
  see Repair, Gastrointestinal System ØDQ
  see Replacement, Esophagus ØDR5
  see Supplement, Gastrointestinal System ØDU
Esophagoplication *see* Restriction, Gastrointestinal System ØDV
Esophagorrhaphy *see* Repair, Gastrointestinal System ØDQ
Esophagoscopy ØDJ08ZZ
Esophagotomy *see* Drainage, Gastrointestinal System ØD9
Esteem® implantable hearing system *use* Hearing Device in Ear, Nose, Sinus
ESWL (extracorporeal shock wave lithotripsy) *see* Fragmentation
Ethmoidal air cell
  use Sinus, Ethmoid, Left
  use Sinus, Ethmoid, Right
Ethmoidectomy
  see Excision, Ear, Nose, Sinus Ø9B
  see Excision, Head and Facial Bones ØNB
  see Resection, Ear, Nose, Sinus Ø9T
  see Resection, Head and Facial Bones ØNT
Ethmoidotomy *see* Drainage, Ear, Nose, Sinus Ø99
Evacuation
  Hematoma *see* Extirpation
  Other Fluid *see* Drainage
Everolimus-eluting coronary stent *use* Intraluminal Device, Drug-eluting in Heart and Great Vessels
Evisceration
  Eyeball *see* Resection, Eye Ø8T
  Eyeball with prosthetic implant *see* Replacement, Eye Ø8R
Ex-PRESS™ mini glaucoma shunt *use* Synthetic Substitute
Examination *see* Inspection
Exchange *see* Change device in
Excision
  Abdominal Wall ØWBF
  Acetabulum
    Left ØQB5
    Right ØQB4
  Adenoids ØCBQ
  Ampulla of Vater ØFBC
  Anal Sphincter ØDBR
  Ankle Region
    Left ØYBL
    Right ØYBK
  Anus ØDBQ
  Aorta
    Abdominal Ø4BØ
    Thoracic Ø2BW
  Aortic Body ØGBD
  Appendix ØDBJ
  Arm
    Lower
      Left ØXBF
      Right ØXBD
    Upper
      Left ØXB9
      Right ØXB8
  Artery
    Anterior Tibial
      Left Ø4BQ
      Right Ø4BP
    Axillary
      Left Ø3B6
      Right Ø3B5
    Brachial
      Left Ø3B8
      Right Ø3B7
    Celiac Ø4B1
    Colic
      Left Ø4B7

Excision — continued
  Artery — continued
    Colic — continued
      Middle 04B8
      Right 04B6
    Common Carotid
      Left 03BJ
      Right 03BH
    Common Iliac
      Left 04BD
      Right 04BC
    External Carotid
      Left 03BN
      Right 03BM
    External Iliac
      Left 04BJ
      Right 04BH
    Face 03BR
    Femoral
      Left 04BL
      Right 04BK
    Foot
      Left 04BW
      Right 04BV
    Gastric 04B2
    Hand
      Left 03BF
      Right 03BD
    Hepatic 04B3
    Inferior Mesenteric 04BB
    Innominate 03B2
    Internal Carotid
      Left 03BL
      Right 03BK
    Internal Iliac
      Left 04BF
      Right 04BE
    Internal Mammary
      Left 03B1
      Right 03B0
    Intracranial 03BG
    Lower 04BY
    Peroneal
      Left 04BU
      Right 04BT
    Popliteal
      Left 04BN
      Right 04BM
    Posterior Tibial
      Left 04BS
      Right 04BR
    Pulmonary
      Left 02BR
      Right 02BQ
    Pulmonary Trunk 02BP
    Radial
      Left 03BC
      Right 03BB
    Renal
      Left 04BA
      Right 04B9
    Splenic 04B4
    Subclavian
      Left 03B4
      Right 03B3
    Superior Mesenteric 04B5
    Temporal
      Left 03BT
      Right 03BS
    Thyroid
      Left 03BV
      Right 03BU
    Ulnar
      Left 03BA
      Right 03B9
    Upper 03BY
    Vertebral
      Left 03BQ
      Right 03BP
  Atrium
    Left 02B7
    Right 02B6
  Auditory Ossicle
    Left 09BA0Z
    Right 09B90Z

Excision — continued
  Axilla
    Left 0XB5
    Right 0XB4
  Back
    Lower 0WBL
    Upper 0WBK
  Basal Ganglia 00B8
  Bladder 0TBB
  Bladder Neck 0TBC
  Bone
    Ethmoid
      Left 0NBG
      Right 0NBF
    Frontal
      Left 0NB2
      Right 0NB1
    Hyoid 0NBX
    Lacrimal
      Left 0NBJ
      Right 0NBH
    Nasal 0NBB
    Occipital
      Left 0NB8
      Right 0NB7
    Palatine
      Left 0NBL
      Right 0NBK
    Parietal
      Left 0NB4
      Right 0NB3
    Pelvic
      Left 0QB3
      Right 0QB2
    Sphenoid
      Left 0NBD
      Right 0NBC
    Temporal
      Left 0NB6
      Right 0NB5
    Zygomatic
      Left 0NBN
      Right 0NBM
  Brain 00B0
  Breast
    Bilateral 0HBV
    Left 0HBU
    Right 0HBT
    Supernumerary 0HBY
  Bronchus
    Lingula 0BB9
    Lower Lobe
      Left 0BBB
      Right 0BB6
    Main
      Left 0BB7
      Right 0BB3
    Middle Lobe, Right 0BB5
    Upper Lobe
      Left 0BB8
      Right 0BB4
  Buccal Mucosa 0CB4
  Bursa and Ligament
    Abdomen
      Left 0MBJ
      Right 0MBH
    Ankle
      Left 0MBR
      Right 0MBQ
    Elbow
      Left 0MB4
      Right 0MB3
    Foot
      Left 0MBT
      Right 0MBS
    Hand
      Left 0MB8
      Right 0MB7
    Head and Neck 0MB0
    Hip
      Left 0MBM
      Right 0MBL
    Knee
      Left 0MBP
      Right 0MBN

Excision — continued
  Bursa and Ligament — continued
    Lower Extremity
      Left 0MBW
      Right 0MBV
    Perineum 0MBK
    Shoulder
      Left 0MB2
      Right 0MB1
    Thorax
      Left 0MBG
      Right 0MBF
    Trunk
      Left 0MBD
      Right 0MBC
    Upper Extremity
      Left 0MBB
      Right 0MB9
    Wrist
      Left 0MB6
      Right 0MB5
  Buttock
    Left 0YB1
    Right 0YB0
  Carina 0BB2
  Carotid Bodies, Bilateral 0GB8
  Carotid Body
    Left 0GB6
    Right 0GB7
  Carpal
    Left 0PBN
    Right 0PBM
  Cecum 0DBH
  Cerebellum 00BC
  Cerebral Hemisphere 00B7
  Cerebral Meninges 00B1
  Cerebral Ventricle 00B6
  Cervix 0UBC
  Chest Wall 0WB8
  Chordae Tendineae 02B9
  Choroid
    Left 08BB
    Right 08BA
  Cisterna Chyli 07BL
  Clavicle
    Left 0PBB
    Right 0PB9
  Clitoris 0UBJ
  Coccygeal Glomus 0GBB
  Coccyx 0QBS
  Colon
    Ascending 0DBK
    Descending 0DBM
    Sigmoid 0DBN
    Transverse 0DBL
  Conduction Mechanism 02B8
  Conjunctiva
    Left 08BTXZ
    Right 08BSXZ
  Cord
    Bilateral 0VBH
    Left 0VBG
    Right 0VBF
  Cornea
    Left 08B9XZ
    Right 08B8XZ
  Cul-de-sac 0UBF
  Diaphragm
    Left 0BBS
    Right 0BBR
  Disc
    Cervical Vertebral 0RB3
    Cervicothoracic Vertebral 0RB5
    Lumbar Vertebral 0SB2
    Lumbosacral 0SB4
    Thoracic Vertebral 0RB9
    Thoracolumbar Vertebral 0RBB
  Duct
    Common Bile 0FB9
    Cystic 0FB8
    Hepatic
      Left 0FB6
      Right 0FB5
    Lacrimal
      Left 08BY
      Right 08BX

Excision — continued
Duct — continued
Pancreatic 0FBD
Accessory 0FBF
Parotid
Left 0CBC
Right 0CBB
Duodenum 0DB9
Dura Mater 00B2
Ear
External
Left 09B1
Right 09B0
External Auditory Canal
Left 09B4
Right 09B3
Inner
Left 09BE0Z
Right 09BD0Z
Middle
Left 09B60Z
Right 09B50Z
Elbow Region
Left 0XBC
Right 0XBB
Epididymis
Bilateral 0VBL
Left 0VBK
Right 0VBJ
Epiglottis 0CBR
Esophagogastric Junction 0DB4
Esophagus 0DB5
Lower 0DB3
Middle 0DB2
Upper 0DB1
Eustachian Tube
Left 09BG
Right 09BF
Extremity
Lower
Left 0YBB
Right 0YB9
Upper
Left 0XB7
Right 0XB6
Eye
Left 08B1
Right 08B0
Eyelid
Lower
Left 08BR
Right 08BQ
Upper
Left 08BP
Right 08BN
Face 0WB2
Fallopian Tube
Left 0UB6
Right 0UB5
Fallopian Tubes, Bilateral 0UB7
Femoral Region
Left 0YB8
Right 0YB7
Femoral Shaft
Left 0QB9
Right 0QB8
Femur
Lower
Left 0QBC
Right 0QBB
Upper
Left 0QB7
Right 0QB6
Fibula
Left 0QBK
Right 0QBJ
Finger Nail 0HBQXZ
Foot
Left 0YBN
Right 0YBM
Gallbladder 0FB4
Gingiva
Lower 0CB6
Upper 0CB5

Excision — continued
Gland
Adrenal
Bilateral 0GB4
Left 0GB2
Right 0GB3
Lacrimal
Left 08BW
Right 08BV
Minor Salivary 0CBJ
Parotid
Left 0CB9
Right 0CB8
Pituitary 0GB0
Sublingual
Left 0CBF
Right 0CBD
Submaxillary
Left 0CBH
Right 0CBG
Vestibular 0UBL
Glenoid Cavity
Left 0PB8
Right 0PB7
Glomus Jugulare 0GBC
Hand
Left 0XBK
Right 0XBJ
Head 0WB0
Humeral Head
Left 0PBD
Right 0PBC
Humeral Shaft
Left 0PBG
Right 0PBF
Hymen 0UBK
Hypothalamus 00BA
Ileocecal Valve 0DBC
Ileum 0DBB
Inguinal Region
Left 0YB6
Right 0YB5
Intestine
Large 0DBE
Left 0DBG
Right 0DBF
Small 0DB8
Iris
Left 08BD3Z
Right 08BC3Z
Jaw
Lower 0WB5
Upper 0WB4
Jejunum 0DBA
Joint
Acromioclavicular
Left 0RBH
Right 0RBG
Ankle
Left 0SBG
Right 0SBF
Carpal
Left 0RBR
Right 0RBQ
Cervical Vertebral 0RB1
Cervicothoracic Vertebral 0RB4
Coccygeal 0SB6
Elbow
Left 0RBM
Right 0RBL
Finger Phalangeal
Left 0RBX
Right 0RBW
Hip
Left 0SBB
Right 0SB9
Knee
Left 0SBD
Right 0SBC
Lumbar Vertebral 0SB0
Lumbosacral 0SB3
Metacarpocarpal
Left 0RBT
Right 0RBS
Metacarpophalangeal
Left 0RBV

Excision — continued
Joint — continued
Metacarpophalangeal — continued
Right 0RBU
Metatarsal-Phalangeal
Left 0SBN
Right 0SBM
Metatarsal-Tarsal
Left 0SBL
Right 0SBK
Occipital-cervical 0RB0
Sacrococcygeal 0SB5
Sacroiliac
Left 0SB8
Right 0SB7
Shoulder
Left 0RBK
Right 0RBJ
Sternoclavicular
Left 0RBF
Right 0RBE
Tarsal
Left 0SBJ
Right 0SBH
Temporomandibular
Left 0RBD
Right 0RBC
Thoracic Vertebral 0RB6
Thoracolumbar Vertebral 0RBA
Toe Phalangeal
Left 0SBQ
Right 0SBP
Wrist
Left 0RBP
Right 0RBN
Kidney
Left 0TB1
Right 0TB0
Kidney Pelvis
Left 0TB4
Right 0TB3
Knee Region
Left 0YBG
Right 0YBF
Larynx 0CBS
Leg
Lower
Left 0YBJ
Right 0YBH
Upper
Left 0YBD
Right 0YBC
Lens
Left 08BK3Z
Right 08BJ3Z
Lip
Lower 0CB1
Upper 0CB0
Liver 0FB0
Left Lobe 0FB2
Right Lobe 0FB1
Lung
Bilateral 0BBM
Left 0BBL
Lower Lobe
Left 0BBJ
Right 0BBF
Middle Lobe, Right 0BBD
Right 0BBK
Upper Lobe
Left 0BBG
Right 0BBC
Lung Lingula 0BBH
Lymphatic
Aortic 07BD
Axillary
Left 07B6
Right 07B5
Head 07B0
Inguinal
Left 07BJ
Right 07BH
Internal Mammary
Left 07B9
Right 07B8

Excision — continued
Lymphatic — continued
Lower Extremity
Left 07BG
Right 07BF
Mesenteric 07BB
Neck
Left 07B2
Right 07B1
Pelvis 07BC
Thoracic Duct 07BK
Thorax 07B7
Upper Extremity
Left 07B4
Right 07B3
Mandible
Left 0NBV
Right 0NBT
Maxilla
Left 0NBS
Right 0NBR
Mediastinum 0WBC
Medulla Oblongata 00BD
Mesentery 0DBV
Metacarpal
Left 0PBQ
Right 0PBP
Metatarsal
Left 0QBP
Right 0QBN
Muscle
Abdomen
Left 0KBL
Right 0KBK
Extraocular
Left 08BM
Right 08BL
Facial 0KB1
Foot
Left 0KBW
Right 0KBV
Hand
Left 0KBD
Right 0KBC
Head 0KB0
Hip
Left 0KBP
Right 0KBN
Lower Arm and Wrist
Left 0KBB
Right 0KB9
Lower Leg
Left 0KBT
Right 0KBS
Neck
Left 0KB3
Right 0KB2
Papillary 02BD
Perineum 0KBM
Shoulder
Left 0KB6
Right 0KB5
Thorax
Left 0KBJ
Right 0KBH
Tongue, Palate, Pharynx 0KB4
Trunk
Left 0KBG
Right 0KBF
Upper Arm
Left 0KB8
Right 0KB7
Upper Leg
Left 0KBR
Right 0KBQ
Nasopharynx 09BN
Neck 0WB6
Nerve
Abdominal Sympathetic 01BM
Abducens 00BL
Accessory 00BR
Acoustic 00BN
Brachial Plexus 01B3
Cervical 01B1
Cervical Plexus 01B0
Facial 00BM

Excision — continued
Nerve — continued
Femoral 01BD
Glossopharyngeal 00BP
Head and Neck Sympathetic 01BK
Hypoglossal 00BS
Lumbar 01BB
Lumbar Plexus 01B9
Lumbar Sympathetic 01BN
Lumbosacral Plexus 01BA
Median 01B5
Oculomotor 00BH
Olfactory 00BF
Optic 00BG
Peroneal 01BH
Phrenic 01B2
Pudendal 01BC
Radial 01B6
Sacral 01BR
Sacral Plexus 01BQ
Sacral Sympathetic 01BP
Sciatic 01BF
Thoracic 01B8
Thoracic Sympathetic 01BL
Tibial 01BG
Trigeminal 00BK
Trochlear 00BJ
Ulnar 01B4
Vagus 00BQ
Nipple
Left 0HBX
Right 0HBW
Nose 09BK
Omentum
Greater 0DBS
Lesser 0DBT
Orbit
Left 0NBQ
Right 0NBP
Ovary
Bilateral 0UB2
Left 0UB1
Right 0UB0
Palate
Hard 0CB2
Soft 0CB3
Pancreas 0FBG
Para-aortic Body 0GB9
Paraganglion Extremity 0GBF
Parathyroid Gland 0GBR
Inferior
Left 0GBP
Right 0GBN
Multiple 0GBQ
Superior
Left 0GBM
Right 0GBL
Patella
Left 0QBF
Right 0QBD
Penis 0VBS
Pericardium 02BN
Perineum
Female 0WBN
Male 0WBM
Peritoneum 0DBW
Phalanx
Finger
Left 0PBV
Right 0PBT
Thumb
Left 0PBS
Right 0PBR
Toe
Left 0QBR
Right 0QBQ
Pharynx 0CBM
Pineal Body 0GB1
Pleura
Left 0BBP
Right 0BBN
Pons 00BB
Prepuce 0VBT
Prostate 0VB0
Radius
Left 0PBJ

Excision — continued
Radius — continued
Right 0PBH
Rectum 0DBP
Retina
Left 08BF3Z
Right 08BE3Z
Retroperitoneum 0WBH
Rib
Left 0PB2
Right 0PB1
Sacrum 0QB1
Scapula
Left 0PB6
Right 0PB5
Sclera
Left 08B7XZ
Right 08B6XZ
Scrotum 0VB5
Septum
Atrial 02B5
Nasal 09BM
Ventricular 02BM
Shoulder Region
Left 0XB3
Right 0XB2
Sinus
Accessory 09BP
Ethmoid
Left 09BV
Right 09BU
Frontal
Left 09BT
Right 09BS
Mastoid
Left 09BC
Right 09BB
Maxillary
Left 09BR
Right 09BQ
Sphenoid
Left 09BX
Right 09BW
Skin
Abdomen 0HB7XZ
Back 0HB6XZ
Buttock 0HB8XZ
Chest 0HB5XZ
Ear
Left 0HB3XZ
Right 0HB2XZ
Face 0HB1XZ
Foot
Left 0HBNXZ
Right 0HBMXZ
Genitalia 0HBAXZ
Hand
Left 0HBGXZ
Right 0HBFXZ
Lower Arm
Left 0HBEXZ
Right 0HBDXZ
Lower Leg
Left 0HBLXZ
Right 0HBKXZ
Neck 0HB4XZ
Perineum 0HB9XZ
Scalp 0HB0XZ
Upper Arm
Left 0HBCXZ
Right 0HBBXZ
Upper Leg
Left 0HBJXZ
Right 0HBHXZ
Skull 0NB0
Spinal Cord
Cervical 00BW
Lumbar 00BY
Thoracic 00BX
Spinal Meninges 00BT
Spleen 07BP
Sternum 0PB0
Stomach 0DB6
Pylorus 0DB7
Subcutaneous Tissue and Fascia
Abdomen 0JB8

Excision — continued
  Subcutaneous Tissue and Fascia — continued
    Back 0JB7
    Buttock 0JB9
    Chest 0JB6
    Face 0JB1
    Foot
      Left 0JBR
      Right 0JBQ
    Hand
      Left 0JBK
      Right 0JBJ
    Lower Arm
      Left 0JBH
      Right 0JBG
    Lower Leg
      Left 0JBP
      Right 0JBN
    Neck
      Anterior 0JB4
      Posterior 0JB5
    Pelvic Region 0JBC
    Perineum 0JBB
    Scalp 0JB0
    Upper Arm
      Left 0JBF
      Right 0JBD
    Upper Leg
      Left 0JBM
      Right 0JBL
  Tarsal
    Left 0QBM
    Right 0QBL
  Tendon
    Abdomen
      Left 0LBG
      Right 0LBF
    Ankle
      Left 0LBT
      Right 0LBS
    Foot
      Left 0LBW
      Right 0LBV
    Hand
      Left 0LB8
      Right 0LB7
    Head and Neck 0LB0
    Hip
      Left 0LBK
      Right 0LBJ
    Knee
      Left 0LBR
      Right 0LBQ
    Lower Arm and Wrist
      Left 0LB6
      Right 0LB5
    Lower Leg
      Left 0LBP
      Right 0LBN
    Perineum 0LBH
    Shoulder
      Left 0LB2
      Right 0LB1
    Thorax
      Left 0LBD
      Right 0LBC
    Trunk
      Left 0LBB
      Right 0LB9
    Upper Arm
      Left 0LB4
      Right 0LB3
    Upper Leg
      Left 0LBM
      Right 0LBL
  Testis
    Bilateral 0VBC
    Left 0VBB
    Right 0VB9
  Thalamus 00B9
  Thymus 07BM
  Thyroid Gland
    Left Lobe 0GBG
    Right Lobe 0GBH
  Tibia
    Left 0QBH

Excision — continued
  Tibia — continued
    Right 0QBG
  Toe Nail 0HBRXZ
  Tongue 0CB7
  Tonsils 0CBP
  Tooth
    Lower 0CBX
    Upper 0CBW
  Trachea 0BB1
  Tunica Vaginalis
    Left 0VB7
    Right 0VB6
  Turbinate, Nasal 09BL
  Tympanic Membrane
    Left 09B8
    Right 09B7
  Ulna
    Left 0PBL
    Right 0PBK
  Ureter
    Left 0TB7
    Right 0TB6
  Urethra 0TBD
  Uterine Supporting Structure 0UB4
  Uterus 0UB9
  Uvula 0CBN
  Vagina 0UBG
  Valve
    Aortic 02BF
    Mitral 02BG
    Pulmonary 02BH
    Tricuspid 02BJ
  Vas Deferens
    Bilateral 0VBQ
    Left 0VBP
    Right 0VBN
  Vein
    Axillary
      Left 05B8
      Right 05B7
    Azygos 05B0
    Basilic
      Left 05BC
      Right 05BB
    Brachial
      Left 05BA
      Right 05B9
    Cephalic
      Left 05BF
      Right 05BD
    Colic 06B7
    Common Iliac
      Left 06BD
      Right 06BC
    Coronary 02B4
    Esophageal 06B3
    External Iliac
      Left 06BG
      Right 06BF
    External Jugular
      Left 05BQ
      Right 05BP
    Face
      Left 05BV
      Right 05BT
    Femoral
      Left 06BN
      Right 06BM
    Foot
      Left 06BV
      Right 06BT
    Gastric 06B2
    Greater Saphenous
      Left 06BQ
      Right 06BP
    Hand
      Left 05BH
      Right 05BG
    Hemiazygos 05B1
    Hepatic 06B4
    Hypogastric
      Left 06BJ
      Right 06BH
    Inferior Mesenteric 06B6

Excision — continued
  Vein — continued
    Innominate
      Left 05B4
      Right 05B3
    Internal Jugular
      Left 05BN
      Right 05BM
    Intracranial 05BL
    Lesser Saphenous
      Left 06BS
      Right 06BR
    Lower 06BY
    Portal 06B8
    Pulmonary
      Left 02BT
      Right 02BS
    Renal
      Left 06BB
      Right 06B9
    Splenic 06B1
    Subclavian
      Left 05B6
      Right 05B5
    Superior Mesenteric 06B5
    Upper 05BY
    Vertebral
      Left 05BS
      Right 05BR
  Vena Cava
    Inferior 06B0
    Superior 02BV
  Ventricle
    Left 02BL
    Right 02BK
  Vertebra
    Cervical 0PB3
    Lumbar 0QB0
    Thoracic 0PB4
  Vesicle
    Bilateral 0VB3
    Left 0VB2
    Right 0VB1
  Vitreous
    Left 08B53Z
    Right 08B43Z
  Vocal Cord
    Left 0CBV
    Right 0CBT
  Vulva 0UBM
  Wrist Region
    Left 0XBH
    Right 0XBG
Exclusion, Left atrial appendage (LAA) *see* Occlusion, Atrium, Left 02L7
Exercise, rehabilitation *see* Motor Treatment, Rehabilitation F07
Exploration *see* Inspection
Express® Biliary SD Monorail® Premounted Stent System *use* Intraluminal Device
Express® (LD) Premounted Stent System *use* Intraluminal Device
Express® SD Renal Monorail® Premounted Stent System *use* Intraluminal Device
Extensor carpi radialis muscle
    use Muscle, Lower Arm and Wrist, Left
    use Muscle, Lower Arm and Wrist, Right
Extensor carpi ulnaris muscle
    use Muscle, Lower Arm and Wrist, Left
    use Muscle, Lower Arm and Wrist, Right
Extensor digitorum brevis muscle
    use Muscle, Foot, Left
    use Muscle, Foot, Right
Extensor digitorum longus muscle
    use Muscle, Lower Leg, Left
    use Muscle, Lower Leg, Right
Extensor hallucis brevis muscle
    use Muscle, Foot, Left
    use Muscle, Foot, Right
Extensor hallucis longus muscle
    use Muscle, Lower Leg, Left
    use Muscle, Lower Leg, Right
External anal sphincter *use* Anal Sphincter
External auditory meatus
    use Ear, External Auditory Canal, Left
    use Ear, External Auditory Canal, Right

▽ **Subterms under main terms may continue to next column or page**

External fixator
 use External Fixation Device in Head and Facial Bones
 use External Fixation Device in Lower Bones
 use External Fixation Device in Lower Joints
 use External Fixation Device in Upper Bones
 use External Fixation Device in Upper Joints
External maxillary artery *use* Artery, Face
External naris *use* Nose
External oblique aponeurosis *use* Subcutaneous Tissue and Fascia, Trunk
External oblique muscle
 use Muscle, Abdomen, Left
 use Muscle, Abdomen, Right
External popliteal nerve *use* Nerve, Peroneal
External pudendal artery
 use Artery, Femoral, Left
 use Artery, Femoral, Right
External pudendal vein
 use Vein, Greater Saphenous, Left
 use Vein, Greater Saphenous, Right
External urethral sphincter *use* Urethra
Extirpation
 Acetabulum
  Left 0QC5
  Right 0QC4
 Adenoids 0CCQ
 Ampulla of Vater 0FCC
 Anal Sphincter 0DCR
 Anterior Chamber
  Left 08C3
  Right 08C2
 Anus 0DCQ
 Aorta
  Abdominal 04C0
  Thoracic 02CW
 Aortic Body 0GCD
 Appendix 0DCJ
 Artery
  Anterior Tibial
   Left 04CQ
   Right 04CP
  Axillary
   Left 03C6
   Right 03C5
  Brachial
   Left 03C8
   Right 03C7
  Celiac 04C1
  Colic
   Left 04C7
   Middle 04C8
   Right 04C6
  Common Carotid
   Left 03CJ
   Right 03CH
  Common Iliac
   Left 04CD
   Right 04CC
  Coronary
   Four or More Sites 02C3
   One Site 02C0
   Three Sites 02C2
   Two Sites 02C1
  External Carotid
   Left 03CN
   Right 03CM
  External Iliac
   Left 04CJ
   Right 04CH
  Face 03CR
  Femoral
   Left 04CL
   Right 04CK
  Foot
   Left 04CW
   Right 04CV
  Gastric 04C2
  Hand
   Left 03CF
   Right 03CD
  Hepatic 04C3
  Inferior Mesenteric 04CB
  Innominate 03C2
  Internal Carotid
   Left 03CL
   Right 03CK

Extirpation — continued
 Artery — continued
  Internal Iliac
   Left 04CF
   Right 04CE
  Internal Mammary
   Left 03C1
   Right 03C0
  Intracranial 03CG
  Lower 04CY
  Peroneal
   Left 04CU
   Right 04CT
  Popliteal
   Left 04CN
   Right 04CM
  Posterior Tibial
   Left 04CS
   Right 04CR
  Pulmonary
   Left 02CR
   Right 02CQ
  Pulmonary Trunk 02CP
  Radial
   Left 03CC
   Right 03CB
  Renal
   Left 04CA
   Right 04C9
  Splenic 04C4
  Subclavian
   Left 03C4
   Right 03C3
  Superior Mesenteric 04C5
  Temporal
   Left 03CT
   Right 03CS
  Thyroid
   Left 03CV
   Right 03CU
  Ulnar
   Left 03CA
   Right 03C9
  Upper 03CY
  Vertebral
   Left 03CQ
   Right 03CP
 Atrium
  Left 02C7
  Right 02C6
 Auditory Ossicle
  Left 09CA0ZZ
  Right 09C90ZZ
 Basal Ganglia 00C8
 Bladder 0TCB
 Bladder Neck 0TCC
 Bone
  Ethmoid
   Left 0NCG
   Right 0NCF
  Frontal
   Left 0NC2
   Right 0NC1
  Hyoid 0NCX
  Lacrimal
   Left 0NCJ
   Right 0NCH
  Nasal 0NCB
  Occipital
   Left 0NC8
   Right 0NC7
  Palatine
   Left 0NCL
   Right 0NCK
  Parietal
   Left 0NC4
   Right 0NC3
  Pelvic
   Left 0QC3
   Right 0QC2
  Sphenoid
   Left 0NCD
   Right 0NCC
  Temporal
   Left 0NC6
   Right 0NC5

Extirpation — continued
 Bone — continued
  Zygomatic
   Left 0NCN
   Right 0NCM
 Brain 00C0
 Breast
  Bilateral 0HCV
  Left 0HCU
  Right 0HCT
 Bronchus
  Lingula 0BC9
  Lower Lobe
   Left 0BCB
   Right 0BC6
  Main
   Left 0BC7
   Right 0BC3
  Middle Lobe, Right 0BC5
  Upper Lobe
   Left 0BC8
   Right 0BC4
 Buccal Mucosa 0CC4
 Bursa and Ligament
  Abdomen
   Left 0MCJ
   Right 0MCH
  Ankle
   Left 0MCR
   Right 0MCQ
  Elbow
   Left 0MC4
   Right 0MC3
  Foot
   Left 0MCT
   Right 0MCS
  Hand
   Left 0MC8
   Right 0MC7
  Head and Neck 0MC0
  Hip
   Left 0MCM
   Right 0MCL
  Knee
   Left 0MCP
   Right 0MCN
  Lower Extremity
   Left 0MCW
   Right 0MCV
  Perineum 0MCK
  Shoulder
   Left 0MC2
   Right 0MC1
  Thorax
   Left 0MCG
   Right 0MCF
  Trunk
   Left 0MCD
   Right 0MCC
  Upper Extremity
   Left 0MCB
   Right 0MC9
  Wrist
   Left 0MC6
   Right 0MC5
 Carina 0BC2
 Carotid Bodies, Bilateral 0GC8
 Carotid Body
  Left 0GC6
  Right 0GC7
 Carpal
  Left 0PCN
  Right 0PCM
 Cavity, Cranial 0WC1
 Cecum 0DCH
 Cerebellum 00CC
 Cerebral Hemisphere 00C7
 Cerebral Meninges 00C1
 Cerebral Ventricle 00C6
 Cervix 0UCC
 Chordae Tendineae 02C9
 Choroid
  Left 08CB
  Right 08CA
 Cisterna Chyli 07CL

Extirpation — continued
- Clavicle
  - Left 0PCB
  - Right 0PC9
- Clitoris 0UCJ
- Coccygeal Glomus 0GCB
- Coccyx 0QCS
- Colon
  - Ascending 0DCK
  - Descending 0DCM
  - Sigmoid 0DCN
  - Transverse 0DCL
- Conduction Mechanism 02C8
- Conjunctiva
  - Left 08CTXZZ
  - Right 08CSXZZ
- Cord
  - Bilateral 0VCH
  - Left 0VCG
  - Right 0VCF
- Cornea
  - Left 08C9XZZ
  - Right 08C8XZZ
- Cul-de-sac 0UCF
- Diaphragm
  - Left 0BCS
  - Right 0BCR
- Disc
  - Cervical Vertebral 0RC3
  - Cervicothoracic Vertebral 0RC5
  - Lumbar Vertebral 0SC2
  - Lumbosacral 0SC4
  - Thoracic Vertebral 0RC9
  - Thoracolumbar Vertebral 0RCB
- Duct
  - Common Bile 0FC9
  - Cystic 0FC8
  - Hepatic
    - Left 0FC6
    - Right 0FC5
  - Lacrimal
    - Left 08CY
    - Right 08CX
  - Pancreatic 0FCD
    - Accessory 0FCF
  - Parotid
    - Left 0CCC
    - Right 0CCB
- Duodenum 0DC9
- Dura Mater 00C2
- Ear
  - External
    - Left 09C1
    - Right 09C0
  - External Auditory Canal
    - Left 09C4
    - Right 09C3
  - Inner
    - Left 09CE0ZZ
    - Right 09CD0ZZ
  - Middle
    - Left 09C60ZZ
    - Right 09C50ZZ
- Endometrium 0UCB
- Epididymis
  - Bilateral 0VCL
  - Left 0VCK
  - Right 0VCJ
- Epidural Space 00C3
- Epiglottis 0CCR
- Esophagogastric Junction 0DC4
- Esophagus 0DC5
  - Lower 0DC3
  - Middle 0DC2
  - Upper 0DC1
- Eustachian Tube
  - Left 09CG
  - Right 09CF
- Eye
  - Left 08C1XZZ
  - Right 08C0XZZ
- Eyelid
  - Lower
    - Left 08CR
    - Right 08CQ

Extirpation — continued
- Eyelid — continued
  - Upper
    - Left 08CP
    - Right 08CN
- Fallopian Tube
  - Left 0UC6
  - Right 0UC5
- Fallopian Tubes, Bilateral 0UC7
- Femoral Shaft
  - Left 0QC9
  - Right 0QC8
- Femur
  - Lower
    - Left 0QCC
    - Right 0QCB
  - Upper
    - Left 0QC7
    - Right 0QC6
- Fibula
  - Left 0QCK
  - Right 0QCJ
- Finger Nail 0HCQXZZ
- Gallbladder 0FC4
- Gastrointestinal Tract 0WCP
- Genitourinary Tract 0WCR
- Gingiva
  - Lower 0CC6
  - Upper 0CC5
- Gland
  - Adrenal
    - Bilateral 0GC4
    - Left 0GC2
    - Right 0GC3
  - Lacrimal
    - Left 08CW
    - Right 08CV
  - Minor Salivary 0CCJ
  - Parotid
    - Left 0CC9
    - Right 0CC8
  - Pituitary 0GC0
  - Sublingual
    - Left 0CCF
    - Right 0CCD
  - Submaxillary
    - Left 0CCH
    - Right 0CCG
  - Vestibular 0UCL
- Glenoid Cavity
  - Left 0PC8
  - Right 0PC7
- Glomus Jugulare 0GCC
- Humeral Head
  - Left 0PCD
  - Right 0PCC
- Humeral Shaft
  - Left 0PCG
  - Right 0PCF
- Hymen 0UCK
- Hypothalamus 00CA
- Ileocecal Valve 0DCC
- Ileum 0DCB
- Intestine
  - Large 0DCE
    - Left 0DCG
    - Right 0DCF
  - Small 0DC8
- Iris
  - Left 08CD
  - Right 08CC
- Jejunum 0DCA
- Joint
  - Acromioclavicular
    - Left 0RCH
    - Right 0RCG
  - Ankle
    - Left 0SCG
    - Right 0SCF
  - Carpal
    - Left 0RCR
    - Right 0RCQ
  - Cervical Vertebral 0RC1
  - Cervicothoracic Vertebral 0RC4
  - Coccygeal 0SC6

Extirpation — continued
- Joint — continued
  - Elbow
    - Left 0RCM
    - Right 0RCL
  - Finger Phalangeal
    - Left 0RCX
    - Right 0RCW
  - Hip
    - Left 0SCB
    - Right 0SC9
  - Knee
    - Left 0SCD
    - Right 0SCC
  - Lumbar Vertebral 0SC0
  - Lumbosacral 0SC3
  - Metacarpocarpal
    - Left 0RCT
    - Right 0RCS
  - Metacarpophalangeal
    - Left 0RCV
    - Right 0RCU
  - Metatarsal-Phalangeal
    - Left 0SCN
    - Right 0SCM
  - Metatarsal-Tarsal
    - Left 0SCL
    - Right 0SCK
  - Occipital-cervical 0RC0
  - Sacrococcygeal 0SC5
  - Sacroiliac
    - Left 0SC8
    - Right 0SC7
  - Shoulder
    - Left 0RCK
    - Right 0RCJ
  - Sternoclavicular
    - Left 0RCF
    - Right 0RCE
  - Tarsal
    - Left 0SCJ
    - Right 0SCH
  - Temporomandibular
    - Left 0RCD
    - Right 0RCC
  - Thoracic Vertebral 0RC6
  - Thoracolumbar Vertebral 0RCA
  - Toe Phalangeal
    - Left 0SCQ
    - Right 0SCP
  - Wrist
    - Left 0RCP
    - Right 0RCN
- Kidney
  - Left 0TC1
  - Right 0TC0
- Kidney Pelvis
  - Left 0TC4
  - Right 0TC3
- Larynx 0CCS
- Lens
  - Left 08CK
  - Right 08CJ
- Lip
  - Lower 0CC1
  - Upper 0CC0
- Liver 0FC0
  - Left Lobe 0FC2
  - Right Lobe 0FC1
- Lung
  - Bilateral 0BCM
  - Left 0BCL
  - Lower Lobe
    - Left 0BCJ
    - Right 0BCF
  - Middle Lobe, Right 0BCD
  - Right 0BCK
  - Upper Lobe
    - Left 0BCG
    - Right 0BCC
- Lung Lingula 0BCH
- Lymphatic
  - Aortic 07CD
  - Axillary
    - Left 07C6
    - Right 07C5

▽ **Subterms under main terms may continue to next column or page**

Index

Extirpation — Extirpation

Feeding Device — continued
Insertion of device in — continued
Stomach 0DH6
Removal of device from
Esophagus 0DP5
Intestinal Tract
Lower 0DPD
Upper 0DP0
Stomach 0DP6
Revision of device in
Intestinal Tract
Lower 0DWD
Upper 0DW0
Stomach 0DW6
Femoral head
use Femur, Upper, Left
use Femur, Upper, Right
Femoral lymph node
use Lymphatic, Lower Extremity, Left
use Lymphatic, Lower Extremity, Right
Femoropatellar joint
use Joint, Knee, Left
use Joint, Knee, Left, Femoral Surface
use Joint, Knee, Right
use Joint, Knee, Right, Femoral Surface
Femorotibial joint
use Joint, Knee, Left
use Joint, Knee, Left, Tibial Surface
use Joint, Knee, Right
use Joint, Knee, Right, Tibial Surface
Fibular artery
use Artery, Peroneal, Left
use Artery, Peroneal, Right
Fibularis brevis muscle
use Muscle, Lower Leg, Left
use Muscle, Lower Leg, Right
Fibularis longus muscle
use Muscle, Lower Leg, Left
use Muscle, Lower Leg, Right
Fifth cranial nerve *use* Nerve, Trigeminal
Fimbriectomy
see Excision, Female Reproductive System 0UB
see Resection, Female Reproductive System 0UT
First cranial nerve *use* Nerve, Olfactory
First intercostal nerve *use* Nerve, Brachial Plexus
Fistulization
see Bypass
see Drainage
see Repair
Fitting
Arch bars, for fracture reduction *see* Reposition, Mouth and Throat 0CS
Arch bars, for immobilization *see* Immobilization, Face 2W31
Artificial limb *see* Device Fitting, Rehabilitation F0D
Hearing aid *see* Device Fitting, Rehabilitation F0D
Ocular prosthesis F0DZ8UZ
Prosthesis, limb *see* Device Fitting, Rehabilitation F0D
Prosthesis, ocular F0DZ8UZ
Fixation, bone
External, with fracture reduction *see* Reposition
External, without fracture reduction *see* Insertion
Internal, with fracture reduction *see* Reposition
Internal, without fracture reduction *see* Insertion
FLAIR® Endovascular Stent Graft *use* Intraluminal Device
Flexible Composite Mesh *use* Synthetic Substitute
Flexor carpi radialis muscle
use Muscle, Lower Arm and Wrist, Left
use Muscle, Lower Arm and Wrist, Right
Flexor carpi ulnaris muscle
use Muscle, Lower Arm and Wrist, Left
use Muscle, Lower Arm and Wrist, Right
Flexor digitorum brevis muscle
use Muscle, Foot, Left
use Muscle, Foot, Right
Flexor digitorum longus muscle
use Muscle, Lower Leg, Left
use Muscle, Lower Leg, Right
Flexor hallucis brevis muscle
use Muscle, Foot, Left
use Muscle, Foot, Right
Flexor hallucis longus muscle
use Muscle, Lower Leg, Left

Flexor hallucis longus muscle — continued
use Muscle, Lower Leg, Right
Flexor pollicis longus muscle
use Muscle, Lower Arm and Wrist, Left
use Muscle, Lower Arm and Wrist, Right
Fluoroscopy
Abdomen and Pelvis BW11
Airway, Upper BB1DZZZ
Ankle
Left BQ1H
Right BQ1G
Aorta
Abdominal B410
Laser, Intraoperative B410
Thoracic B310
Laser, Intraoperative B310
Thoraco-Abdominal B31P
Laser, Intraoperative B31P
Aorta and Bilateral Lower Extremity Arteries B41D
Laser, Intraoperative B41D
Arm
Left BP1FZZZ
Right BP1EZZZ
Artery
Brachiocephalic-Subclavian
Laser, Intraoperative B311
Right B311
Bronchial B31L
Laser, Intraoperative B31L
Bypass Graft, Other B21F
Cervico-Cerebral Arch B31Q
Laser, Intraoperative B31Q
Common Carotid
Bilateral B315
Laser, Intraoperative B315
Left B314
Laser, Intraoperative B314
Right B313
Laser, Intraoperative B313
Coronary
Bypass Graft
Multiple B213
Laser, Intraoperative B213
Single B212
Laser, Intraoperative B212
Multiple B211
Laser, Intraoperative B211
Single B210
Laser, Intraoperative B210
External Carotid
Bilateral B31C
Laser, Intraoperative B31C
Left B31B
Laser, Intraoperative B31B
Right B319
Laser, Intraoperative B319
Hepatic B412
Laser, Intraoperative B412
Inferior Mesenteric B415
Laser, Intraoperative B415
Intercostal B31L
Laser, Intraoperative B31L
Internal Carotid
Bilateral B318
Laser, Intraoperative B318
Left B317
Laser, Intraoperative B317
Right B316
Laser, Intraoperative B316
Internal Mammary Bypass Graft
Left B218
Right B217
Intra-Abdominal
Laser, Intraoperative B41B
Other B41B
Intracranial B31R
Laser, Intraoperative B31R
Lower
Laser, Intraoperative B41J
Other B41J
Lower Extremity
Bilateral and Aorta B41D
Laser, Intraoperative B41D
Left B41G
Laser, Intraoperative B41G
Right B41F

Fluoroscopy — continued
Artery — continued
Lower Extremity — continued
Right — continued
Laser, Intraoperative B41F
Lumbar B419
Laser, Intraoperative B419
Pelvic B41C
Laser, Intraoperative B41C
Pulmonary
Left B31T
Laser, Intraoperative B31T
Right B31S
Laser, Intraoperative B31S
Renal
Bilateral B418
Laser, Intraoperative B418
Left B417
Laser, Intraoperative B417
Right B416
Laser, Intraoperative B416
Spinal B31M
Laser, Intraoperative B31M
Splenic B413
Laser, Intraoperative B413
Subclavian
Laser, Intraoperative B312
Left B312
Superior Mesenteric B414
Laser, Intraoperative B414
Upper
Laser, Intraoperative B31N
Other B31N
Upper Extremity
Bilateral B31K
Laser, Intraoperative B31K
Left B31J
Laser, Intraoperative B31J
Right B31H
Laser, Intraoperative B31H
Vertebral
Bilateral B31G
Laser, Intraoperative B31G
Left B31F
Laser, Intraoperative B31F
Right B31D
Laser, Intraoperative B31D
Bile Duct BF10
Pancreatic Duct and Gallbladder BF14
Bile Duct and Gallbladder BF13
Biliary Duct BF11
Bladder BT10
Kidney and Ureter BT14
Left BT1F
Right BT1D
Bladder and Urethra BT1B
Bowel, Small BD1
Calcaneus
Left BQ1KZZZ
Right BQ1JZZZ
Clavicle
Left BP15ZZZ
Right BP14ZZZ
Coccyx BR1F
Colon BD14
Corpora Cavernosa BV10
Dialysis Fistula B51W
Dialysis Shunt B51W
Diaphragm BB16ZZZ
Disc
Cervical BR11
Lumbar BR13
Thoracic BR12
Duodenum BD19
Elbow
Left BP1H
Right BP1G
Epiglottis B91G
Esophagus BD11
Extremity
Lower BW1C
Upper BW1J
Facet Joint
Cervical BR14
Lumbar BR16
Thoracic BR15

Fluoroscopy — continued
  Fallopian Tube
    Bilateral BU12
    Left BU11
    Right BU1Ø
  Fallopian Tube and Uterus BU18
  Femur
    Left BQ14ZZZ
    Right BQ13ZZZ
  Finger
    Left BP1SZZZ
    Right BP1RZZZ
  Foot
    Left BQ1MZZZ
    Right BQ1LZZZ
  Forearm
    Left BP1KZZZ
    Right BP1JZZZ
  Gallbladder BF12
    Bile Duct and Pancreatic Duct BF14
  Gallbladder and Bile Duct BF13
  Gastrointestinal, Upper BD1
  Hand
    Left BP1PZZZ
    Right BP1NZZZ
  Head and Neck BW19
  Heart
    Left B215
    Right B214
    Right and Left B216
  Hip
    Left BQ11
    Right BQ1Ø
  Humerus
    Left BP1BZZZ
    Right BP1AZZZ
  Ileal Diversion Loop BT1C
  Ileal Loop, Ureters and Kidney BT1G
  Intracranial Sinus B512
  Joint
    Acromioclavicular, Bilateral BP13ZZZ
    Finger
      Left BP1D
      Right BP1C
    Foot
      Left BQ1Y
      Right BQ1X
    Hand
      Left BP1D
      Right BP1C
    Lumbosacral BR1B
    Sacroiliac BR1D
    Sternoclavicular
      Bilateral BP12ZZZ
      Left BP11ZZZ
      Right BP1ØZZZ
    Temporomandibular
      Bilateral BN19
      Left BN18
      Right BN17
    Thoracolumbar BR18
    Toe
      Left BQ1Y
      Right BQ1X
  Kidney
    Bilateral BT13
    Ileal Loop and Ureter BT1G
    Left BT12
    Right BT11
    Ureter and Bladder BT14
      Left BT1F
      Right BT1D
  Knee
    Left BQ18
    Right BQ17
  Larynx B91J
  Leg
    Left BQ1FZZZ
    Right BQ1DZZZ
  Lung
    Bilateral BB14ZZZ
    Left BB13ZZZ
    Right BB12ZZZ
  Mediastinum BB1CZZZ
  Mouth BD1B
  Neck and Head BW19

Fluoroscopy — continued
  Oropharynx BD1B
  Pancreatic Duct BF1
    Gallbladder and Bile Buct BF14
  Patella
    Left BQ1WZZZ
    Right BQ1VZZZ
  Pelvis BR1C
  Pelvis and Abdomen BW11
  Pharynix B91G
  Ribs
    Left BP1YZZZ
    Right BP1XZZZ
  Sacrum BR1F
  Scapula
    Left BP17ZZZ
    Right BP16ZZZ
  Shoulder
    Left BP19
    Right BP18
  Sinus, Intracranial B512
  Spinal Cord BØ1B
  Spine
    Cervical BR1Ø
    Lumbar BR19
    Thoracic BR17
    Whole BR1G
  Sternum BR1H
  Stomach BD12
  Toe
    Left BQ1QZZZ
    Right BQ1PZZZ
  Tracheobronchial Tree
    Bilateral BB19YZZ
    Left BB18YZZ
    Right BB17YZZ
  Ureter
    Ileal Loop and Kidney BT1G
    Kidney and Bladder BT14
      Left BT1F
      Right BT1D
    Left BT17
    Right BT16
  Urethra BT15
  Urethra and Bladder BT1B
  Uterus BU16
  Uterus and Fallopian Tube BU18
  Vagina BU19
  Vasa Vasorum BV18
  Vein
    Cerebellar B511
    Cerebral B511
    Epidural B51Ø
    Jugular
      Bilateral B515
      Left B514
      Right B513
    Lower Extremity
      Bilateral B51D
      Left B51C
      Right B51B
    Other B51V
    Pelvic (Iliac)
      Left B51G
      Right B51F
    Pelvic (Iliac) Bilateral B51H
    Portal B51T
    Pulmonary
      Bilateral B51S
      Left B51R
      Right B51Q
    Renal
      Bilateral B51L
      Left B51K
      Right B51J
    Spanchnic B51T
    Subclavian
      Left B517
      Right B516
    Upper Extremity
      Bilateral B51P
      Left B51N
      Right B51M
  Vena Cava
    Inferior B519
    Superior B518

Fluoroscopy — continued
  Wrist
    Left BP1M
    Right BP1L
Flushing *see* Irrigation
Foley catheter *use* Drainage Device
Foramen magnum
  use Bone, Occipital, Left
  use Bone, Occipital, Right
Foramen of Monro (intraventricular) *use* Cerebral
  Ventricle
Foreskin *use* Prepuce
Formula™ Balloon-Expandable Renal Stent System
  use Intraluminal Device
Fossa of Rosenmuller *use* Nasopharynx
Fourth cranial nerve *use* Nerve, Trochlear
Fourth ventricle *use* Cerebral Ventricle
Fovea
  use Retina, Left
  use Retina, Right
Fragmentation
  Ampulla of Vater ØFFC
  Anus ØDFQ
  Appendix ØDFJ
  Bladder ØTFB
  Bladder Neck ØTFC
  Bronchus
    Lingula ØBF9
    Lower Lobe
      Left ØBFB
      Right ØBF6
    Main
      Left ØBF7
      Right ØBF3
    Middle Lobe, Right ØBF5
    Upper Lobe
      Left ØBF8
      Right ØBF4
  Carina ØBF2
  Cavity, Cranial ØWF1
  Cecum ØDFH
  Cerebral Ventricle ØØF6
  Colon
    Ascending ØDFK
    Descending ØDFM
    Sigmoid ØDFN
    Transverse ØDFL
  Duct
    Common Bile ØFF9
    Cystic ØFF8
    Hepatic
      Left ØFF6
      Right ØFF5
    Pancreatic ØFFD
      Accessory ØFFF
    Parotid
      Left ØCFC
      Right ØCFB
  Duodenum ØDF9
  Epidural Space ØØF3
  Esophagus ØDF5
  Fallopian Tube
    Left ØUF6
    Right ØUF5
  Fallopian Tubes, Bilateral ØUF7
  Gallbladder ØFF4
  Gastrointestinal Tract ØWFP
  Genitourinary Tract ØWFR
  Ileum ØDFB
  Intestine
    Large ØDFE
      Left ØDFG
      Right ØDFF
    Small ØDF8
  Jejunum ØDFA
  Kidney Pelvis
    Left ØTF4
    Right ØTF3
  Mediastinum ØWFC
  Oral Cavity and Throat ØWF3
  Pelvic Cavity ØWFJ
  Pericardial Cavity ØWFD
  Pericardium Ø2FN
  Peritoneal Cavity ØWFG
  Pleural Cavity
    Left ØWFB

Fragmentation — continued
  Pleural Cavity — continued
    Right ØWF9
  Rectum ØDFP
  Respiratory Tract ØWFQ
  Spinal Canal ØØFU
  Stomach ØDF6
  Subarachnoid Space ØØF5
  Subdural Space ØØF4
  Trachea ØBF1
  Ureter
    Left ØTF7
    Right ØTF6
  Urethra ØTFD
  Uterus ØUF9
  Vitreous
    Left Ø8F5
    Right Ø8F4
Freestyle (Stentless) Aortic Root Bioprosthesis *use* Zooplastic Tissue in Heart and Great Vessels
Frenectomy
  see Excision, Mouth and Throat ØCB
  see Resection, Mouth and Throat ØCT
Frenoplasty, frenuloplasty
  see Repair, Mouth and Throat ØCQ
  see Replacement, Mouth and Throat ØCR
  see Supplement, Mouth and Throat ØCU
Frenotomy
  see Drainage, Mouth and Throat ØC9
  see Release, Mouth and Throat ØCN
Frenulotomy
  see Drainage, Mouth and Throat ØC9
  see Release, Mouth and Throat ØCN
Frenulum labii inferioris *use* Lip, Lower
Frenulum labii superioris *use* Lip, Upper
Frenulum linguae *use* Tongue
Frenulumectomy
  see Excision, Mouth and Throat ØCB
  see Resection, Mouth and Throat ØCT
Frontal lobe *use* Cerebral Hemisphere
Frontal vein
  use Vein, Face, Left
  use Vein, Face, Right
Fulguration *see* Destruction
Fundoplication, gastroesophageal *see* Restriction, Esophagogastric Junction ØDV4
Fundus uteri *use* Uterus
Fusion
  Acromioclavicular
    Left ØRGH
    Right ØRGG
  Ankle
    Left ØSGG
    Right ØSGF
  Carpal
    Left ØRGR
    Right ØRGQ
  Cervical Vertebral ØRG1
    2 or more ØRG2
  Cervicothoracic Vertebral ØRG4
  Coccygeal ØSG6
  Elbow
    Left ØRGM
    Right ØRGL
  Finger Phalangeal
    Left ØRGX
    Right ØRGW
  Hip
    Left ØSGB
    Right ØSG9
  Knee
    Left ØSGD
    Right ØSGC
  Lumbar Vertebral ØSGØ
    2 or more ØSG1
  Lumbosacral ØSG3
  Metacarpocarpal
    Left ØRGT
    Right ØRGS
  Metacarpophalangeal
    Left ØRGV
    Right ØRGU
  Metatarsal-Phalangeal
    Left ØSGN
    Right ØSGM

Fusion — continued
  Metatarsal-Tarsal
    Left ØSGL
    Right ØSGK
  Occipital-cervical ØRGØ
  Sacrococcygeal ØSG5
  Sacroiliac
    Left ØSG8
    Right ØSG7
  Shoulder
    Left ØRGK
    Right ØRGJ
  Sternoclavicular
    Left ØRGF
    Right ØRGE
  Tarsal
    Left ØSGJ
    Right ØSGH
  Temporomandibular
    Left ØRGD
    Right ØRGC
  Thoracic Vertebral ØRG6
    2 to 7 ØRG7
    8 or more ØRG8
  Thoracolumbar Vertebral ØRGA
  Toe Phalangeal
    Left ØSGQ
    Right ØSGP
  Wrist
    Left ØRGP
    Right ØRGN
Fusion screw (compression)(lag)(locking)
  use Internal Fixation Device in Lower Joints
  use Internal Fixation Device in Upper Joints

G

Gait training *see* Motor Treatment, Rehabilitation FØ7
Galea aponeurotica *use* Subcutaneous Tissue and Fascia, Scalp
Ganglion impar (ganglion of Walther) *use* Nerve, Sacral Sympathetic
Ganglionectomy
  Destruction of lesion *see* Destruction
  Excision of lesion *see* Excision
Gasserian ganglion *use* Nerve, Trigeminal
Gastrectomy
  Partial *see* Excision, Stomach ØDB6
  Total *see* Resection, Stomach ØDT6
  Vertical (sleeve) *see* Excision, Stomach ØDB6
Gastric electrical stimulation (GES) lead *use* Stimulator Lead in Gastrointestinal System
Gastric lymph node *use* Lymphatic, Aortic
Gastric pacemaker lead *use* Stimulator Lead in Gastrointestinal System
Gastric plexus *use* Nerve, Abdominal Sympathetic
Gastrocnemius muscle
  use Muscle, Lower Leg, Left
  use Muscle, Lower Leg, Right
Gastrocolic ligament *use* Omentum, Greater
Gastrocolic omentum *use* Omentum, Greater
Gastrocolostomy
  see Bypass, Gastrointestinal System ØD1
  see Drainage, Gastrointestinal System ØD9
Gastroduodenal artery *use* Artery, Hepatic
Gastroduodenectomy
  see Excision, Gastrointestinal System ØDB
  see Resection, Gastrointestinal System ØDT
Gastroduodenoscopy ØDJ08ZZ
Gastroenteroplasty
  see Repair, Gastrointestinal System ØDQ
  see Supplement, Gastrointestinal System ØDU
Gastroenterostomy
  see Bypass, Gastrointestinal System ØD1
  see Drainage, Gastrointestinal System ØD9
Gastroesophageal (GE) junction *use* Esophagogastric Junction
Gastrogastrostomy
  see Bypass, Stomach ØD16
  see Drainage, Stomach ØD96
Gastrohepatic omentum *use* Omentum, Lesser
Gastrojejunostomy
  see Bypass, Stomach ØD16
  see Drainage, Stomach ØD96

Gastrolysis *see* Release, Stomach ØDN6
Gastropexy
  see Repair, Stomach ØDQ6
  see Reposition, Stomach ØDS6
Gastrophrenic ligament *use* Omentum, Greater
Gastroplasty
  see Repair, Stomach ØDQ6
  see Supplement, Stomach ØDU6
Gastroplication *see* Restriction, Stomach ØDV6
Gastropylorectomy *see* Excision, Gastrointestinal System ØDB
Gastrorrhaphy *see* Repair, Stomach ØDQ6
Gastroscopy ØDJ68ZZ
Gastrosplenic ligament *use* Omentum, Greater
Gastrostomy
  see Bypass, Stomach ØD16
  see Drainage, Stomach ØD96
Gastrotomy *see* Drainage, Stomach ØD96
Gemellus muscle
  use Muscle, Hip, Left
  use Muscle, Hip, Right
Geniculate ganglion *use* Nerve, Facial
Geniculate nucleus *use* Thalamus
Genioglossus muscle *use* Muscle, Tongue, Palate, Pharynx
Genioplasty *see* Alteration, Jaw, Lower ØWØ5
Genitofemoral nerve *use* Nerve, Lumbar Plexus
Gingivectomy *see* Excision, Mouth and Throat ØCB
Gingivoplasty
  see Repair, Mouth and Throat ØCQ
  see Replacement, Mouth and Throat ØCR
  see Supplement, Mouth and Throat ØCU
Glans penis *use* Prepuce
Glenohumeral joint
  use Joint, Shoulder, Left
  use Joint, Shoulder, Right
Glenohumeral ligament
  use Bursa and Ligament, Shoulder, Left
  use Bursa and Ligament, Shoulder, Right
Glenoid fossa (of scapula)
  use Glenoid Cavity, Left
  use Glenoid Cavity, Right
Glenoid ligament (labrum)
  use Bursa and Ligament, Shoulder, Left
  use Bursa and Ligament, Shoulder, Right
Globus pallidus *use* Basal Ganglia
Glomectomy
  see Excision, Endocrine System ØGB
  see Resection, Endocrine System ØGT
Glossectomy
  see Excision, Tongue ØCB7
  see Resection, Tongue ØCT7
Glossoepiglottic fold *use* Epiglottis
Glossopexy
  see Repair, Tongue ØCQ7
  see Reposition, Tongue ØCS7
Glossoplasty
  see Repair, Tongue ØCQ7
  see Replacement, Tongue ØCR7
  see Supplement, Tongue ØCU7
Glossorrhaphy *see* Repair, Tongue ØCQ7
Glossotomy *see* Drainage, Tongue ØC97
Glottis *use* Larynx
Gluteal Artery Perforator Flap
  Bilateral ØHRVØ79
  Left ØHRUØ79
  Right ØHRTØ79
Gluteal lymph node *use* Lymphatic, Pelvis
Gluteal vein
  use Vein, Hypogastric, Left
  use Vein, Hypogastric, Right
Gluteus maximus muscle
  use Muscle, Hip, Left
  use Muscle, Hip, Right
Gluteus medius muscle
  use Muscle, Hip, Left
  use Muscle, Hip, Right
Gluteus minimus muscle
  use Muscle, Hip, Left
  use Muscle, Hip, Right
GORE® DUALMESH® *use* Synthetic Substitute
Gracilis muscle
  use Muscle, Upper Leg, Left
  use Muscle, Upper Leg, Right

Graft
   see Replacement
   see Supplement
Great auricular nerve *use* Nerve, Cervical Plexus
Great cerebral vein *use* Vein, Intracranial
Great saphenous vein
   use Vein, Greater Saphenous, Left
   use Vein, Greater Saphenous, Right
Greater alar cartilage *use* Nose
Greater occipital nerve *use* Nerve, Cervical
Greater splanchnic nerve *use* Nerve, Thoracic Sympathetic
Greater superficial petrosal nerve *use* Nerve, Facial
Greater trochanter
   use Femur, Upper, Left
   use Femur, Upper, Right
Greater tuberosity
   use Humeral Head, Left
   use Humeral Head, Right
Greater vestibular (Bartholin's) gland *use* Gland, Vestibular
Greater wing
   use Bone, Sphenoid, Left
   use Bone, Sphenoid, Right
Guedel airway *use* Intraluminal Device, Airway in Mouth and Throat
Guidance, catheter placement
   EKG *see* Measurement, Physiological Systems 4A0
   Fluoroscopy *see* Fluoroscopy, Veins B51
   Ultrasound *use* Ultrasonography, Veins B54

H

Hallux
   use Toe, 1st, Left
   use Toe, 1st, Right
Hamate bone
   use Carpal, Left
   use Carpal, Right
Hancock Bioprosthesis (aortic) (mitral) valve *use* Zooplastic Tissue in Heart and Great Vessels
Hancock Bioprosthetic Valved Conduit *use* Zooplastic Tissue in Heart and Great Vessels
Harvesting, stem cells *see* Pheresis, Circulatory 6A55
Head of fibula
   use Fibula, Left
   use Fibula, Right
Hearing Aid Assessment F14Z
Hearing Assessment F13Z
Hearing Device
   Bone Conduction
      Left 09HE
      Right 09HD
   Insertion of device in
      Left 0NH6
      Right 0NH5
   Multiple Channel Cochlear Prosthesis
      Left 09HE
      Right 09HD
   Removal of device from, Skull 0NP0
   Revision of device in, Skull 0NW0
   Single Channel Cochlear Prosthesis
      Left 09HE
      Right 09HD
Hearing Treatment F09Z
Heart Assist System
   External
      Insertion of device in, Heart 02HA
      Removal of device from, Heart 02PA
      Revision of device in, Heart 02WA
   Implantable
      Insertion of device in, Heart 02HA
      Removal of device from, Heart 02PA
      Revision of device in, Heart 02WA
HeartMate II® Left Ventricular Assist Device (LVAD) *use* Implantable Heart Assist System in Heart and Great Vessels
HeartMate XVE® Left Ventricular Assist Device (LVAD) *use* Implantable Heart Assist System in Heart and Great Vessels
HeartMate® implantable heart assist system *see* Insertion of device in, Heart 02HA
Helix
   use Ear, External, Bilateral

Helix — continued
   use Ear, External, Left
   use Ear, External, Right
Hemicolectomy *see* Resection, Gastrointestinal System 0DT
Hemicystectomy *see* Excision, Urinary System 0TB
Hemigastrectomy *see* Excision, Gastrointestinal System 0DB
Hemiglossectomy *see* Excision, Mouth and Throat 0CB
Hemilaminectomy
   see Excision, Lower Bones 0QB
   see Excision, Upper Bones 0PB
Hemilaryngectomy *see* Excision, Larynx 0CBS
Hemimandibulectomy *see* Excision, Head and Facial Bones 0NB
Hemimaxillectomy *see* Excision, Head and Facial Bones 0NB
Hemipylorectomy *see* Excision, Gastrointestinal System 0DB
Hemispherectomy
   see Excision, Central Nervous System 00B
   see Resection, Central Nervous System 00T
Hemithyroidectomy
   see Excision, Endocrine System 0GB
   see Resection, Endocrine System 0GT
Hemodialysis 5A1D00Z
Hepatectomy
   see Excision, Hepatobiliary System and Pancreas 0FB
   see Resection, Hepatobiliary System and Pancreas 0FT
Hepatic artery proper *use* Artery, Hepatic
Hepatic flexure *use* Colon, Ascending
Hepatic lymph node *use* Lymphatic, Aortic
Hepatic plexus *use* Nerve, Abdominal Sympathetic
Hepatic portal vein *use* Vein, Portal
Hepaticoduodenostomy
   see Bypass, Hepatobiliary System and Pancreas 0F1
   see Drainage, Hepatobiliary System and Pancreas 0F9
Hepaticotomy *see* Drainage, Hepatobiliary System and Pancreas 0F9
Hepatocholedochostomy *see* Drainage, Duct, Common Bile 0F99
Hepatogastric ligament *use* Omentum, Lesser
Hepatopancreatic ampulla *use* Ampulla of Vater
Hepatopexy
   see Repair, Hepatobiliary System and Pancreas 0FQ
   see Reposition, Hepatobiliary System and Pancreas 0FS
Hepatorrhaphy *see* Repair, Hepatobiliary System and Pancreas 0FQ
Hepatotomy *see* Drainage, Hepatobiliary System and Pancreas 0F9
Herniorrhaphy
   with synthetic substitute
      see Supplement, Anatomical Regions, General 0WU
      see Supplement, Anatomical Regions, Lower Extremities 0YU
   see Repair, Anatomical Regions, General 0WQ
   see Repair, Anatomical Regions, Lower Extremities 0YQ
Hip (joint) liner *use* Liner in Lower Joints
Holter monitoring 4A12X45
Holter valve ventricular shunt *use* Synthetic Substitute
Humeroradial joint
   use Joint, Elbow, Left
   use Joint, Elbow, Right
Humeroulnar joint
   use Joint, Elbow, Left
   use Joint, Elbow, Right
Humerus, distal
   use Humeral Shaft, Left
   use Humeral Shaft, Right
Hydrocelectomy *see* Excision, Male Reproductive System 0VB
Hydrotherapy
   Assisted exercise in pool *see* Motor Treatment, Rehabilitation F07
   Whirlpool *see* Activities of Daily Living Treatment, Rehabilitation F08
Hymenectomy
   see Excision, Hymen 0UBK
   see Resection, Hymen 0UTK

Hymenoplasty
   see Repair, Hymen 0UQK
   see Supplement, Hymen 0UUK
Hymenorrhaphy *see* Repair, Hymen 0UQK
Hymenotomy
   see Division, Hymen 0U8K
   see Drainage, Hymen 0U9K
Hyoglossus muscle *use* Muscle, Tongue, Palate, Pharynx
Hyoid artery
   use Artery, Thyroid, Left
   use Artery, Thyroid, Right
Hyperalimentation *see* Introduction of substance in or on
Hyperbaric oxygenation
   Decompression sickness treatment *see* Decompression, Circulatory 6A15
   Wound treatment *see* Assistance, Circulatory 5A05
Hyperthermia
   Radiation Therapy
      Abdomen DWY38ZZ
      Adrenal Gland DGY28ZZ
      Bile Ducts DFY28ZZ
      Bladder DTY28ZZ
      Bone Marrow D7Y08ZZ
      Bone, Other DPYC8ZZ
      Brain D0Y08ZZ
      Brain Stem D0Y18ZZ
      Breast
         Left DMY08ZZ
         Right DMY18ZZ
      Bronchus DBY18ZZ
      Cervix DUY18ZZ
      Chest DWY28ZZ
      Chest Wall DBY78ZZ
      Colon DDY58ZZ
      Diaphragm DBY88ZZ
      Duodenum DDY28ZZ
      Ear D9Y08ZZ
      Esophagus DDY08ZZ
      Eye D8Y08ZZ
      Femur DPY98ZZ
      Fibula DPYB8ZZ
      Gallbladder DFY18ZZ
      Gland
         Adrenal DGY28ZZ
         Parathyroid DGY48ZZ
         Pituitary DGY08ZZ
         Thyroid DGY58ZZ
      Glands, Salivary D9Y68ZZ
      Head and Neck DWY18ZZ
      Hemibody DWY48ZZ
      Humerus DPY68ZZ
      Hypopharynx D9Y38ZZ
      Ileum DDY48ZZ
      Jejunum DDY38ZZ
      Kidney DTY08ZZ
      Larynx D9YB8ZZ
      Liver DFY08ZZ
      Lung DBY28ZZ
      Lymphatics
         Abdomen D7Y68ZZ
         Axillary D7Y48ZZ
         Inguinal D7Y88ZZ
         Neck D7Y38ZZ
         Pelvis D7Y78ZZ
         Thorax D7Y58ZZ
      Mandible DPY38ZZ
      Maxilla DPY28ZZ
      Mediastinum DBY68ZZ
      Mouth D9Y48ZZ
      Nasopharynx D9YD8ZZ
      Neck and Head DWY18ZZ
      Nerve, Peripheral D0Y78ZZ
      Nose D9Y18ZZ
      Oropharynx D9YF8ZZ
      Ovary DUY08ZZ
      Palate
         Hard D9Y88ZZ
         Soft D9Y98ZZ
      Pancreas DFY38ZZ
      Parathyroid Gland DGY48ZZ
      Pelvic Bones DPY88ZZ
      Pelvic Region DWY68ZZ
      Pineal Body DGY18ZZ
      Pituitary Gland DGY08ZZ
      Pleura DBY58ZZ

Subterms under main terms may continue to next column or page

Hyperthermia — continued
  Radiation Therapy — continued
    Prostate DVY08ZZ
    Radius DPY78ZZ
    Rectum DDY78ZZ
    Rib DPY58ZZ
    Sinuses D9Y78ZZ
    Skin
      Abdomen DHY88ZZ
      Arm DHY48ZZ
      Back DHY78ZZ
      Buttock DHY98ZZ
      Chest DHY68ZZ
      Face DHY28ZZ
      Leg DHYB8ZZ
      Neck DHY38ZZ
    Skull DPY08ZZ
    Spinal Cord D0Y68ZZ
    Spleen D7Y28ZZ
    Sternum DPY48ZZ
    Stomach DDY18ZZ
    Testis DVY18ZZ
    Thymus D7Y18ZZ
    Thyroid Gland DGY58ZZ
    Tibia DPYB8ZZ
    Tongue D9Y58ZZ
    Trachea DBY08ZZ
    Ulna DPY78ZZ
    Ureter DTY18ZZ
    Urethra DTY38ZZ
    Uterus DUY28ZZ
    Whole Body DWY58ZZ
  Whole Body 6A3Z
Hypnosis GZFZZZZ
Hypogastric artery
  use Artery, Internal Iliac, Left
  use Artery, Internal Iliac, Right
Hypopharynx *use* Pharynx
Hypophysectomy
  see Excision, Gland, Pituitary 0GB0
  see Resection, Gland, Pituitary 0GT0
Hypophysis *use* Gland, Pituitary
Hypothalamotomy *see* Destruction, Thalamus 0059
Hypothenar muscle
  use Muscle, Hand, Left
  use Muscle, Hand, Right
Hypothermia, Whole Body 6A4Z
Hysterectomy
  see Excision, Uterus 0UB9
  see Resection, Uterus 0UT9
Hysterolysis *see* Release, Uterus 0UN9
Hysteropexy
  see Repair, Uterus 0UQ9
  see Reposition, Uterus 0US9
Hysteroplasty *see* Repair, Uterus 0UQ9
Hysterorrhaphy *see* Repair, Uterus 0UQ9
Hysteroscopy 0UJD8ZZ
Hysterotomy *see* Drainage, Uterus 0U99
Hysterotrachelectomy *see* Resection, Uterus 0UT9
Hysterotracheloplasty *see* Repair, Uterus 0UQ9
Hysterotrachelorrhaphy *see* Repair, Uterus 0UQ9

I

IABP (Intra-aortic balloon pump) *see* Assistance, Cardiac 5A02
IAEMT (Intraoperative anesthetic effect monitoring and titration) *see* Monitoring, Central Nervous 4A10
Ileal artery *use* Artery, Superior Mesenteric
Ileectomy
  see Excision, Ileum 0DBB
  see Resection, Ileum 0DTB
Ileocolic artery *use* Artery, Superior Mesenteric
Ileocolic vein *use* Vein, Colic
Ileopexy
  see Repair, Ileum 0DQB
  see Reposition, Ileum 0DSB
Ileorrhaphy *see* Repair, Ileum 0DQB
Ileoscopy 0DJD8ZZ
Ileostomy
  see Bypass, Ileum 0D1B
  see Drainage, Ileum 0D9B
Ileotomy *see* Drainage, Ileum 0D9B

Ileoureterostomy *see* Bypass, Urinary System 0T1
Iliac crest
  use Bone, Pelvic, Left
  use Bone, Pelvic, Right
Iliac fascia
  use Subcutaneous Tissue and Fascia, Upper Leg, Left
  use Subcutaneous Tissue and Fascia, Upper Leg, Right
Iliac lymph node *use* Lymphatic, Pelvis
Iliacus muscle
  use Muscle, Hip, Left
  use Muscle, Hip, Right
Iliofemoral ligament
  use Bursa and Ligament, Hip, Left
  use Bursa and Ligament, Hip, Right
Iliohypogastric nerve *use* Nerve, Lumbar Plexus
Ilioinguinal nerve *use* Nerve, Lumbar Plexus
Iliolumbar artery
  use Artery, Internal Iliac, Left
  use Artery, Internal Iliac, Right
Iliolumbar ligament
  use Bursa and Ligament, Trunk, Left
  use Bursa and Ligament, Trunk, Right
Iliotibial tract (band)
  use Subcutaneous Tissue and Fascia, Upper Leg, Left
  use Subcutaneous Tissue and Fascia, Upper Leg, Right
Ilium
  use Bone, Pelvic, Left
  use Bone, Pelvic, Right
Ilizarov external fixator
  use External Fixation Device, Ring in 0PH
  use External Fixation Device, Ring in 0QS
  use External Fixation Device, Ring in 0QH
  use External Fixation Device, Ring in 0PS
Ilizarov-Vecklich device
  use External Fixation Device, Limb Lengthening in 0PH
  use External Fixation Device, Limb Lengthening in 0QH
Imaging, diagnostic
  see Computerized Tomography (CT Scan)
  see Fluoroscopy
  see Magnetic Resonance Imaging (MRI)
  see Plain Radiography
  see Ultrasonography
Immobilization
  Abdominal Wall 2W33X
  Arm
    Lower
      Left 2W3DX
      Right 2W3CX
    Upper
      Left 2W3BX
      Right 2W3AX
  Back 2W35X
  Chest Wall 2W34X
  Extremity
    Lower
      Left 2W3MX
      Right 2W3LX
    Upper
      Left 2W39X
      Right 2W38X
  Face 2W31X
  Finger
    Left 2W3KX
    Right 2W3JX
  Foot
    Left 2W3TX
    Right 2W3SX
  Hand
    Left 2W3FX
    Right 2W3EX
  Head 2W30X
  Inguinal Region
    Left 2W37X
    Right 2W36X
  Leg
    Lower
      Left 2W3RX
      Right 2W3QX
    Upper
      Left 2W3PX
      Right 2W3NX
  Neck 2W32X

Immobilization — continued
  Thumb
    Left 2W3HX
    Right 2W3GX
  Toe
    Left 2W3VX
    Right 2W3UX
Immunization *see* Introduction of Serum, Toxoid, and Vaccine
Immunotherapy *see* Introduction of Immunotherapeutic Substance
Immunotherapy, antineoplastic
  Interferon *see* Introduction of Low-dose Interleukin-2
  Interleukin-2, high-dose *see* Introduction of High-dose Interleukin-2
  Interleukin-2, low-dose *see* Introduction of Low-dose Interleukin-2
  Monoclonal antibody *see* Introduction of Monoclonal Antibody
  Proleukin, high-dose *see* Introduction of High-dose Interleukin-2
  Proleukin, low-dose *see* Introduction of Low-dose Interleukin-2
Impella® (2.5) (5.0) (LD) cardiac assist device *use* Intraluminal Device
Impeller Pump
  Continuous, Output 5A0221D
  Intermittent, Output 5A0211D
Implantable cardioverter-defibrillator (ICD) *use* Defibrillator Generator in 0JH
Implantable drug infusion pump (anti-spasmodic)(chemotherapy)(pain) *use* Infusion Device, Pump in Subcutaneous Tissue and Fascia
Implantable glucose monitoring device *use* Monitoring Device
Implantable hemodynamic monitor (IHM) *use* Monitoring Device, Hemodynamic in 0JH
Implantable hemodynamic monitoring system (IHMS) *use* Monitoring Device, Hemodynamic in 0JH
Implantable Miniature Telescope™ (IMT) *use* Synthetic Substitute, Intraocular Telescope in 08R
Implantation
  see Insertion
  see Replacement
Implanted (venous)(access) port *use* Vascular Access Device, Reservoir in Subcutaneous Tissue and Fascia
IMV (intermittent mandatory ventilation) *see* Assistance, Respiratory 5A09
In Vitro Fertilization 8E0ZXY1
Incision, abscess *see* Drainage
Incudectomy
  see Excision, Ear, Nose, Sinus 09B
  see Resection, Ear, Nose, Sinus 09T
Incudopexy
  see Repair, Ear, Nose, Sinus 09Q
  see Reposition, Ear, Nose, Sinus 09S
Incus
  use Auditory Ossicle, Left
  use Auditory Ossicle, Right
Induction of labor
  Artificial rupture of membranes *see* Drainage, Pregnancy 109
  Oxytocin *see* Introduction of Hormone
InDura, intrathecal catheter (1P) (spinal) *use* Infusion Device
Inferior cardiac nerve *use* Nerve, Thoracic Sympathetic
Inferior cerebellar vein *use* Vein, Intracranial
Inferior cerebral vein *use* Vein, Intracranial
Inferior epigastric artery
  use Artery, External Iliac, Left
  use Artery, External Iliac, Right
Inferior epigastric lymph node *use* Lymphatic, Pelvis
Inferior genicular artery
  use Artery, Popliteal, Left
  use Artery, Popliteal, Right
Inferior gluteal artery
  use Artery, Internal Iliac, Left
  use Artery, Internal Iliac, Right
Inferior gluteal nerve *use* Nerve, Sacral Plexus
Inferior hypogastric plexus *use* Nerve, Abdominal Sympathetic
Inferior labial artery *use* Artery, Face

Inferior longitudinal muscle *use* Muscle, Tongue, Palate, Pharynx
Inferior mesenteric ganglion *use* Nerve, Abdominal Sympathetic
Inferior mesenteric lymph node *use* Lymphatic, Mesenteric
Inferior mesenteric plexus *use* Nerve, Abdominal Sympathetic
Inferior oblique muscle
  use Muscle, Extraocular, Left
  use Muscle, Extraocular, Right
Inferior pancreaticoduodenal artery *use* Artery, Superior Mesenteric
Inferior phrenic artery *use* Aorta, Abdominal
Inferior rectus muscle
  use Muscle, Extraocular, Left
  use Muscle, Extraocular, Right
Inferior suprarenal artery
  use Artery, Renal, Left
  use Artery, Renal, Right
Inferior tarsal plate
  use Eyelid, Lower, Left
  use Eyelid, Lower, Right
Inferior thyroid vein
  use Vein, Innominate, Left
  use Vein, Innominate, Right
Inferior tibiofibular joint
  use Joint, Ankle, Left
  use Joint, Ankle, Right
Inferior turbinate *use* Turbinate, Nasal
Inferior ulnar collateral artery
  use Artery, Brachial, Left
  use Artery, Brachial, Right
Inferior vesical artery
  use Artery, Internal Iliac, Left
  use Artery, Internal Iliac, Right
Infraauricular lymph node *use* Lymphatic, Head
Infraclavicular (deltopectoral) lymph node
  use Lymphatic, Upper Extremity, Left
  use Lymphatic, Upper Extremity, Right
Infrahyoid muscle
  use Muscle, Neck, Left
  use Muscle, Neck, Right
Infraparotid lymph node *use* Lymphatic, Head
Infraspinatus fascia
  use Subcutaneous Tissue and Fascia, Upper Arm, Left
  use Subcutaneous Tissue and Fascia, Upper Arm, Right
Infraspinatus muscle
  use Muscle, Shoulder, Left
  use Muscle, Shoulder, Right
Infundibulopelvic ligament *use* Uterine Supporting Structure
Infusion *see* Introduction of substance in or on
Infusion Device
  Insertion of device in
    Abdomen 0JH8
    Back 0JH7
    Chest 0JH6
    Lower Arm
      Left 0JHH
      Right 0JHG
    Lower Leg
      Left 0JHP
      Right 0JHN
    Trunk 0JHT
    Upper Arm
      Left 0JHF
      Right 0JHD
    Upper Leg
      Left 0JHM
      Right 0JHL
  Removal of device from
    Lower Extremity 0JPW
    Trunk 0JPT
    Upper Extremity 0JPV
  Revision of device in
    Lower Extremity 0JWW
    Trunk 0JWT
    Upper Extremity 0JWV
Infusion, glucarpidase
  Central Vein 3E043GQ
  Peripheral Vein 3E033GQ
Inguinal canal
  use Inguinal Region, Bilateral

Inguinal canal — continued
  use Inguinal Region, Left
  use Inguinal Region, Right
Inguinal triangle
  use Inguinal Region, Bilateral
  use Inguinal Region, Left
  use Inguinal Region, Right
Injection *see* Introduction of substance in or on
Injection reservoir *use* Vascular Access Device, Reservoir in Subcutaneous Tissue and Fascia
Insemination, artificial 3E0P7LZ
Insertion
  Antimicrobial envelope *see* Introduction of Anti-infective
  Aqueous drainage shunt
    see Bypass, Eye 081
    see Drainage, Eye 089
  Products of Conception 10H0
  Spinal Stabilization Device
    see Insertion of device in, Lower Joints 0SH
    see Insertion of device in, Upper Joints 0RH
Insertion of device in
  Abdominal Wall 0WHF
  Acetabulum
    Left 0QH5
    Right 0QH4
  Anal Sphincter 0DHR
  Ankle Region
    Left 0YHL
    Right 0YHK
  Anus 0DHQ
  Aorta
    Abdominal 04H0
    Thoracic 02HW
  Arm
    Lower
      Left 0XHF
      Right 0XHD
    Upper
      Left 0XH9
      Right 0XH8
  Artery
    Anterior Tibial
      Left 04HQ
      Right 04HP
    Axillary
      Left 03H6
      Right 03H5
    Brachial
      Left 03H8
      Right 03H7
    Celiac 04H1
    Colic
      Left 04H7
      Middle 04H8
      Right 04H6
    Common Carotid
      Left 03HJ
      Right 03HH
    Common Iliac
      Left 04HD
      Right 04HC
    External Carotid
      Left 03HN
      Right 03HM
    External Iliac
      Left 04HJ
      Right 04HH
    Face 03HR
    Femoral
      Left 04HL
      Right 04HK
    Foot
      Left 04HW
      Right 04HV
    Gastric 04H2
    Hand
      Left 03HF
      Right 03HD
    Hepatic 04H3
    Inferior Mesenteric 04HB
    Innominate 03H2
    Internal Carotid
      Left 03HL
      Right 03HK

Insertion of device in — continued
  Artery — continued
    Internal Iliac
      Left 04HF
      Right 04HE
    Internal Mammary
      Left 03H1
      Right 03H0
    Intracranial 03HG
    Lower 04HY
    Peroneal
      Left 04HU
      Right 04HT
    Popliteal
      Left 04HN
      Right 04HM
    Posterior Tibial
      Left 04HS
      Right 04HR
    Pulmonary
      Left 02HR
      Right 02HQ
    Pulmonary Trunk 02HP
    Radial
      Left 03HC
      Right 03HB
    Renal
      Left 04HA
      Right 04H9
    Splenic 04H4
    Subclavian
      Left 03H4
      Right 03H3
    Superior Mesenteric 04H5
    Temporal
      Left 03HT
      Right 03HS
    Thyroid
      Left 03HV
      Right 03HU
    Ulnar
      Left 03HA
      Right 03H9
    Upper 03HY
    Vertebral
      Left 03HQ
      Right 03HP
  Atrium
    Left 02H7
    Right 02H6
  Axilla
    Left 0XH5
    Right 0XH4
  Back
    Lower 0WHL
    Upper 0WHK
  Bladder 0THB
  Bladder Neck 0THC
  Bone
    Ethmoid
      Left 0NHG
      Right 0NHF
    Facial 0NHW
    Frontal
      Left 0NH2
      Right 0NH1
    Hyoid 0NHX
    Lacrimal
      Left 0NHJ
      Right 0NHH
    Lower 0QHY
    Nasal 0NHB
    Occipital
      Left 0NH8
      Right 0NH7
    Palatine
      Left 0NHL
      Right 0NHK
    Parietal
      Left 0NH4
      Right 0NH3
    Pelvic
      Left 0QH3
      Right 0QH2
    Sphenoid
      Left 0NHD

▽ **Subterms under main terms may continue to next column or page**

Insertion of device in — continued
  Bone — continued
    Sphenoid — continued
      Right ØNHC
    Temporal
      Left ØNH6
      Right ØNH5
    Upper ØPHY
    Zygomatic
      Left ØNHN
      Right ØNHM
  Brain ØØHØ
  Breast
    Bilateral ØHHV
    Left ØHHU
    Right ØHHT
  Bronchus
    Lingula ØBH9
    Lower Lobe
      Left ØBHB
      Right ØBH6
    Main
      Left ØBH7
      Right ØBH3
    Middle Lobe, Right ØBH5
    Upper Lobe
      Left ØBH8
      Right ØBH4
  Buttock
    Left ØYH1
    Right ØYHØ
  Carpal
    Left ØPHN
    Right ØPHM
  Cavity, Cranial ØWH1
  Cerebral Ventricle ØØH6
  Cervix ØUHC
  Chest Wall ØWH8
  Cisterna Chyli Ø7HL
  Clavicle
    Left ØPHB
    Right ØPH9
  Coccyx ØQHS
  Cul-de-sac ØUHF
  Diaphragm
    Left ØBHS
    Right ØBHR
  Disc
    Cervical Vertebral ØRH3
    Cervicothoracic Vertebral ØRH5
    Lumbar Vertebral ØSH2
    Lumbosacral ØSH4
    Thoracic Vertebral ØRH9
    Thoracolumbar Vertebral ØRHB
  Duct
    Hepatobiliary ØFHB
    Pancreatic ØFHD
  Duodenum ØDH9
  Ear
    Left Ø9HE
    Right Ø9HD
  Elbow Region
    Left ØXHC
    Right ØXHB
  Epididymis and Spermatic Cord ØVHM
  Esophagus ØDH5
  Extremity
    Lower
      Left ØYHB
      Right ØYH9
    Upper
      Left ØXH7
      Right ØXH6
  Eye
    Left Ø8H1
    Right Ø8HØ
  Face ØWH2
  Fallopian Tube ØUH8
  Femoral Region
    Left ØYH8
    Right ØYH7
  Femoral Shaft
    Left ØQH9
    Right ØQH8

Insertion of device in — continued
  Femur
    Lower
      Left ØQHC
      Right ØQHB
    Upper
      Left ØQH7
      Right ØQH6
  Fibula
    Left ØQHK
    Right ØQHJ
  Foot
    Left ØYHN
    Right ØYHM
  Gallbladder ØFH4
  Gastrointestinal Tract ØWHP
  Genitourinary Tract ØWHR
  Gland, Endocrine ØGHS
  Glenoid Cavity
    Left ØPH8
    Right ØPH7
  Hand
    Left ØXHK
    Right ØXHJ
  Head ØWHØ
  Heart Ø2HA
  Humeral Head
    Left ØPHD
    Right ØPHC
  Humeral Shaft
    Left ØPHG
    Right ØPHF
  Ileum ØDHB
  Inguinal Region
    Left ØYH6
    Right ØYH5
  Intestine
    Large ØDHE
    Small ØDH8
  Jaw
    Lower ØWH5
    Upper ØWH4
  Jejunum ØDHA
  Joint
    Acromioclavicular
      Left ØRHH
      Right ØRHG
    Ankle
      Left ØSHG
      Right ØSHF
    Carpal
      Left ØRHR
      Right ØRHQ
    Cervical Vertebral ØRH1
    Cervicothoracic Vertebral ØRH4
    Coccygeal ØSH6
    Elbow
      Left ØRHM
      Right ØRHL
    Finger Phalangeal
      Left ØRHX
      Right ØRHW
    Hip
      Left ØSHB
      Right ØSH9
    Knee
      Left ØSHD
      Right ØSHC
    Lumbar Vertebral ØSHØ
    Lumbosacral ØSH3
    Metacarpocarpal
      Left ØRHT
      Right ØRHS
    Metacarpophalangeal
      Left ØRHV
      Right ØRHU
    Metatarsal-Phalangeal
      Left ØSHN
      Right ØSHM
    Metatarsal-Tarsal
      Left ØSHL
      Right ØSHK
    Occipital-cervical ØRHØ
    Sacrococcygeal ØSH5
    Sacroiliac
      Left ØSH8

Insertion of device in — continued
  Joint — continued
    Sacroiliac — continued
      Right ØSH7
    Shoulder
      Left ØRHK
      Right ØRHJ
    Sternoclavicular
      Left ØRHF
      Right ØRHE
    Tarsal
      Left ØSHJ
      Right ØSHH
    Temporomandibular
      Left ØRHD
      Right ØRHC
    Thoracic Vertebral ØRH6
    Thoracolumbar Vertebral ØRHA
    Toe Phalangeal
      Left ØSHQ
      Right ØSHP
    Wrist
      Left ØRHP
      Right ØRHN
  Kidney ØTH5
  Knee Region
    Left ØYHG
    Right ØYHF
  Leg
    Lower
      Left ØYHJ
      Right ØYHH
    Upper
      Left ØYHD
      Right ØYHC
  Liver ØFHØ
    Left Lobe ØFH2
    Right Lobe ØFH1
  Lung
    Left ØBHL
    Right ØBHK
  Lymphatic Ø7HN
    Thoracic Duct Ø7HK
  Mandible
    Left ØNHV
    Right ØNHT
  Maxilla
    Left ØNHS
    Right ØNHR
  Mediastinum ØWHC
  Metacarpal
    Left ØPHQ
    Right ØPHP
  Metatarsal
    Left ØQHP
    Right ØQHN
  Mouth and Throat ØCHY
  Muscle
    Lower ØKHY
    Upper ØKHX
  Nasopharynx Ø9HN
  Neck ØWH6
  Nerve
    Cranial ØØHE
    Peripheral Ø1HY
  Nipple
    Left ØHHX
    Right ØHHW
  Oral Cavity and Throat ØWH3
  Orbit
    Left ØNHQ
    Right ØNHP
  Ovary ØUH3
  Pancreas ØFHG
  Patella
    Left ØQHF
    Right ØQHD
  Pelvic Cavity ØWHJ
  Penis ØVHS
  Pericardial Cavity ØWHD
  Pericardium Ø2HN
  Perineum
    Female ØWHN
    Male ØWHM
  Peritoneal Cavity ØWHG

Insertion of device in — continued
  Phalanx
    Finger
      Left ØPHV
      Right ØPHT
    Thumb
      Left ØPHS
      Right ØPHR
    Toe
      Left ØQHR
      Right ØQHQ
  Pleural Cavity
    Left ØWHB
    Right ØWH9
  Prostate ØVHØ
  Prostate and Seminal Vesicles ØVH4
  Radius
    Left ØPHJ
    Right ØPHH
  Rectum ØDHP
  Respiratory Tract ØWHQ
  Retroperitoneum ØWHH
  Rib
    Left ØPH2
    Right ØPH1
  Sacrum ØQH1
  Scapula
    Left ØPH6
    Right ØPH5
  Scrotum and Tunica Vaginalis ØVH8
  Shoulder Region
    Left ØXH3
    Right ØXH2
  Skull ØNHØ
  Spinal Canal ØØHU
  Spinal Cord ØØHV
  Spleen Ø7HP
  Sternum ØPHØ
  Stomach ØDH6
  Subcutaneous Tissue and Fascia
    Abdomen ØJH8
    Back ØJH7
    Buttock ØJH9
    Chest ØJH6
    Face ØJH1
    Foot
      Left ØJHR
      Right ØJHQ
    Hand
      Left ØJHK
      Right ØJHJ
    Head and Neck ØJHS
    Lower Arm
      Left ØJHH
      Right ØJHG
    Lower Extremity ØJHW
    Lower Leg
      Left ØJHP
      Right ØJHN
    Neck
      Anterior ØJH4
      Posterior ØJH5
    Pelvic Region ØJHC
    Perineum ØJHB
    Scalp ØJHØ
    Trunk ØJHT
    Upper Arm
      Left ØJHF
      Right ØJHD
    Upper Extremity ØJHV
    Upper Leg
      Left ØJHM
      Right ØJHL
  Tarsal
    Left ØQHM
    Right ØQHL
  Testis ØVHD
  Thymus Ø7HM
  Tibia
    Left ØQHH
    Right ØQHG
  Tongue ØCH7
  Trachea ØBH1
  Tracheobronchial Tree ØBHØ
  Ulna
    Left ØPHL

Insertion of device in — continued
  Ulna — continued
    Right ØPHK
  Ureter ØTH9
  Urethra ØTHD
  Uterus ØUH9
  Uterus and Cervix ØUHD
  Vagina ØUHG
  Vagina and Cul-de-sac ØUHH
  Vas Deferens ØVHR
  Vein
    Axillary
      Left Ø5H8
      Right Ø5H7
    Azygos Ø5HØ
    Basilic
      Left Ø5HC
      Right Ø5HB
    Brachial
      Left Ø5HA
      Right Ø5H9
    Cephalic
      Left Ø5HF
      Right Ø5HD
    Colic Ø6H7
    Common Iliac
      Left Ø6HD
      Right Ø6HC
    Coronary Ø2H4
    Esophageal Ø6H3
    External Iliac
      Left Ø6HG
      Right Ø6HF
    External Jugular
      Left Ø5HQ
      Right Ø5HP
    Face
      Left Ø5HV
      Right Ø5HT
    Femoral
      Left Ø6HN
      Right Ø6HM
    Foot
      Left Ø6HV
      Right Ø6HT
    Gastric Ø6H2
    Greater Saphenous
      Left Ø6HQ
      Right Ø6HP
    Hand
      Left Ø5HH
      Right Ø5HG
    Hemiazygos Ø5H1
    Hepatic Ø6H4
    Hypogastric
      Left Ø6HJ
      Right Ø6HH
    Inferior Mesenteric Ø6H6
    Innominate
      Left Ø5H4
      Right Ø5H3
    Internal Jugular
      Left Ø5HN
      Right Ø5HM
    Intracranial Ø5HL
    Lesser Saphenous
      Left Ø6HS
      Right Ø6HR
    Lower Ø6HY
    Portal Ø6H8
    Pulmonary
      Left Ø2HT
      Right Ø2HS
    Renal
      Left Ø6HB
      Right Ø6H9
    Splenic Ø6H1
    Subclavian
      Left Ø5H6
      Right Ø5H5
    Superior Mesenteric Ø6H5
    Upper Ø5HY
    Vertebral
      Left Ø5HS
      Right Ø5HR

Insertion of device in — continued
  Vena Cava
    Inferior Ø6HØ
    Superior Ø2HV
  Ventricle
    Left Ø2HL
    Right Ø2HK
  Vertebra
    Cervical ØPH3
    Lumbar ØQHØ
    Thoracic ØPH4
  Wrist Region
    Left ØXHH
    Right ØXHG
Inspection
  Abdominal Wall ØWJF
  Ankle Region
    Left ØYJL
    Right ØYJK
  Arm
    Lower
      Left ØXJF
      Right ØXJD
    Upper
      Left ØXJ9
      Right ØXJ8
  Artery
    Lower Ø4JY
    Upper Ø3JY
  Axilla
    Left ØXJ5
    Right ØXJ4
  Back
    Lower ØWJL
    Upper ØWJK
  Bladder ØTJB
  Bone
    Facial ØNJW
    Lower ØQJY
    Nasal ØNJB
    Upper ØPJY
  Bone Marrow Ø7JT
  Brain ØØJØ
  Breast
    Left ØHJU
    Right ØHJT
  Bursa and Ligament
    Lower ØMJY
    Upper ØMJX
  Buttock
    Left ØYJ1
    Right ØYJØ
  Cavity, Cranial ØWJ1
  Chest Wall ØWJ8
  Cisterna Chyli Ø7JL
  Diaphragm ØBJT
  Disc
    Cervical Vertebral ØRJ3
    Cervicothoracic Vertebral ØRJ5
    Lumbar Vertebral ØSJ2
    Lumbosacral ØSJ4
    Thoracic Vertebral ØRJ9
    Thoracolumbar Vertebral ØRJB
  Duct
    Hepatobiliary ØFJB
    Pancreatic ØFJD
  Ear
    Inner
      Left Ø9JE
      Right Ø9JD
    Left Ø9JJ
    Right Ø9JH
  Elbow Region
    Left ØXJC
    Right ØXJB
  Epididymis and Spermatic Cord ØVJM
  Extremity
    Lower
      Left ØYJB
      Right ØYJ9
    Upper
      Left ØXJ7
      Right ØXJ6
  Eye
    Left Ø8J1XZZ
    Right Ø8JØXZZ

▼ **Subterms under main terms may continue to next column or page**

Inspection — continued
  Face ØWJ2
  Fallopian Tube ØUJ8
  Femoral Region
    Bilateral ØYJE
    Left ØYJ8
    Right ØYJ7
  Finger Nail ØHJQXZZ
  Foot
    Left ØYJN
    Right ØYJM
  Gallbladder ØFJ4
  Gastrointestinal Tract ØWJP
  Genitourinary Tract ØWJR
  Gland
    Adrenal ØGJ5
    Endocrine ØGJS
    Pituitary ØGJØ
    Salivary ØCJA
  Great Vessel Ø2JY
  Hand
    Left ØXJK
    Right ØXJJ
  Head ØWJØ
  Heart Ø2JA
  Inguinal Region
    Bilateral ØYJA
    Left ØYJ6
    Right ØYJ5
  Intestinal Tract
    Lower ØDJD
    Upper ØDJØ
  Jaw
    Lower ØWJ5
    Upper ØWJ4
  Joint
    Acromioclavicular
      Left ØRJH
      Right ØRJG
    Ankle
      Left ØSJG
      Right ØSJF
    Carpal
      Left ØRJR
      Right ØRJQ
    Cervical Vertebral ØRJ1
    Cervicothoracic Vertebral ØRJ4
    Coccygeal ØSJ6
    Elbow
      Left ØRJM
      Right ØRJL
    Finger Phalangeal
      Left ØRJX
      Right ØRJW
    Hip
      Left ØSJB
      Right ØSJ9
    Knee
      Left ØSJD
      Right ØSJC
    Lumbar Vertebral ØSJØ
    Lumbosacral ØSJ3
    Metacarpocarpal
      Left ØRJT
      Right ØRJS
    Metacarpophalangeal
      Left ØRJV
      Right ØRJU
    Metatarsal-Phalangeal
      Left ØSJN
      Right ØSJM
    Metatarsal-Tarsal
      Left ØSJL
      Right ØSJK
    Occipital-cervical ØRJØ
    Sacrococcygeal ØSJ5
    Sacroiliac
      Left ØSJ8
      Right ØSJ7
    Shoulder
      Left ØRJK
      Right ØRJJ
    Sternoclavicular
      Left ØRJF
      Right ØRJE

Inspection — continued
  Joint — continued
    Tarsal
      Left ØSJJ
      Right ØSJH
    Temporomandibular
      Left ØRJD
      Right ØRJC
    Thoracic Vertebral ØRJ6
    Thoracolumbar Vertebral ØRJA
    Toe Phalangeal
      Left ØSJQ
      Right ØSJP
    Wrist
      Left ØRJP
      Right ØRJN
  Kidney ØTJ5
  Knee Region
    Left ØYJG
    Right ØYJF
  Larynx ØCJS
  Leg
    Lower
      Left ØYJJ
      Right ØYJH
    Upper
      Left ØYJD
      Right ØYJC
  Lens
    Left Ø8JKXZZ
    Right Ø8JJXZZ
  Liver ØFJØ
  Lung
    Left ØBJL
    Right ØBJK
  Lymphatic Ø7JN
    Thoracic Duct Ø7JK
  Mediastinum ØWJC
  Mesentery ØDJV
  Mouth and Throat ØCJY
  Muscle
    Extraocular
      Left Ø8JM
      Right Ø8JL
    Lower ØKJY
    Upper ØKJX
  Neck ØWJ6
  Nerve
    Cranial ØØJE
    Peripheral Ø1JY
  Nose Ø9JK
  Omentum ØDJU
  Oral Cavity and Throat ØWJ3
  Ovary ØUJ3
  Pancreas ØFJG
  Parathyroid Gland ØGJR
  Pelvic Cavity ØWJJ
  Penis ØVJS
  Pericardial Cavity ØWJD
  Perineum
    Female ØWJN
    Male ØWJM
  Peritoneal Cavity ØWJG
  Peritoneum ØDJW
  Pineal Body ØGJ1
  Pleura ØBJQ
  Pleural Cavity
    Left ØWJB
    Right ØWJ9
  Products of Conception 1ØJØ
    Ectopic 1ØJ2
    Retained 1ØJ1
  Prostate and Seminal Vesicles ØVJ4
  Respiratory Tract ØWJQ
  Retroperitoneum ØWJH
  Scrotum and Tunica Vaginalis ØVJ8
  Shoulder Region
    Left ØXJ3
    Right ØXJ2
  Sinus Ø9JY
  Skin ØHJPXZZ
  Skull ØNJØ
  Spinal Canal ØØJU
  Spinal Cord ØØJV
  Spleen Ø7JP
  Stomach ØDJ6

Inspection — continued
  Subcutaneous Tissue and Fascia
    Head and Neck ØJJS
    Lower Extremity ØJJW
    Trunk ØJJT
    Upper Extremity ØJJV
  Tendon
    Lower ØLJY
    Upper ØLJX
  Testis ØVJD
  Thymus Ø7JM
  Thyroid Gland ØGJK
  Toe Nail ØHJRXZZ
  Trachea ØBJ1
  Tracheobronchial Tree ØBJØ
  Tympanic Membrane
    Left Ø9J8
    Right Ø9J7
  Ureter ØTJ9
  Urethra ØTJD
  Uterus and Cervix ØUJD
  Vagina and Cul-de-sac ØUJH
  Vas Deferens ØVJR
  Vein
    Lower Ø6JY
    Upper Ø5JY
  Vulva ØUJM
  Wrist Region
    Left ØXJH
    Right ØXJG
Instillation see Introduction of substance in or on
Insufflation see Introduction of substance in or on
Interatrial septum use Septum, Atrial
Interbody fusion (spine) cage
  use Interbody Fusion Device in Lower Joints
  use Interbody Fusion Device in Upper Joints
Intercarpal joint
  use Joint, Carpal, Left
  use Joint, Carpal, Right
Intercarpal ligament
  use Bursa and Ligament, Hand, Left
  use Bursa and Ligament, Hand, Right
Interclavicular ligament
  use Bursa and Ligament, Shoulder, Left
  use Bursa and Ligament, Shoulder, Right
Intercostal lymph node use Lymphatic, Thorax
Intercostal muscle
  use Muscle, Thorax, Left
  use Muscle, Thorax, Right
Intercostal nerve use Nerve, Thoracic
Intercostobrachial nerve use Nerve, Thoracic
Intercuneiform joint
  use Joint, Tarsal, Left
  use Joint, Tarsal, Right
Intercuneiform ligament
  use Bursa and Ligament, Foot, Left
  use Bursa and Ligament, Foot, Right
Intermediate cuneiform bone
  use Tarsal, Left
  use Tarsal, Right
Intermittent mandatory ventilation see Assistance,
  Respiratory 5AØ9
Intermittent Negative Airway Pressure
  24-96 Consecutive Hours, Ventilation 5AØ945B
  Greater than 96 Consecutive Hours, Ventilation
    5AØ955B
  Less than 24 Consecutive Hours, Ventilation 5AØ935B
Intermittent Positive Airway Pressure
  24-96 Consecutive Hours, Ventilation 5AØ9458
  Greater than 96 Consecutive Hours, Ventilation
    5AØ9558
  Less than 24 Consecutive Hours, Ventilation 5AØ9358
Intermittent positive pressure breathing see Assis-
  tance, Respiratory 5AØ9
Internal anal sphincter use Anal Sphincter
Internal carotid plexus use Nerve, Head and Neck
  Sympathetic
Internal (basal) cerebral vein use Vein, Intracranial
Internal iliac vein
  use Vein, Hypogastric, Left
  use Vein, Hypogastric, Right
Internal maxillary artery
  use Artery, External Carotid, Left
  use Artery, External Carotid, Right
Internal naris use Nose

Internal oblique muscle
use Muscle, Abdomen, Left
use Muscle, Abdomen, Right
Internal pudendal artery
use Artery, Internal Iliac, Left
use Artery, Internal Iliac, Right
Internal pudendal vein
use Vein, Hypogastric, Left
use Vein, Hypogastric, Right
Internal thoracic artery
use Artery, Internal Mammary, Left
use Artery, Internal Mammary, Right
use Artery, Subclavian, Left
use Artery, Subclavian, Right
Internal urethral sphincter use Urethra
Interphalangeal (IP) joint
use Joint, Finger Phalangeal, Left
use Joint, Finger Phalangeal, Right
use Joint, Toe Phalangeal, Left
use Joint, Toe Phalangeal, Right
Interphalangeal ligament
use Bursa and Ligament, Foot, Left
use Bursa and Ligament, Foot, Right
use Bursa and Ligament, Hand, Left
use Bursa and Ligament, Hand, Right
Interrogation, cardiac rhythm related device
With cardiac function testing see Measurement, Cardiac 4A02
Interrogation only see Measurement, Cardiac 4B02
Interruption see Occlusion
Interspinalis muscle
use Muscle, Trunk, Left
use Muscle, Trunk, Right
Interspinous ligament
use Bursa and Ligament, Trunk, Left
use Bursa and Ligament, Trunk, Right
Interspinous process spinal stabilization device
use Spinal Stabilization Device, Interspinous Process in ØRH
use Spinal Stabilization Device, Interspinous Process in ØSH
InterStim® Therapy lead use Neurostimulator Lead in Peripheral Nervous System
InterStim® Therapy neurostimulator use Stimulator Generator, Single Array in ØJH
Intertransversarius muscle
use Muscle, Trunk, Left
use Muscle, Trunk, Right
Intertransverse ligament
use Bursa and Ligament, Trunk, Left
use Bursa and Ligament, Trunk, Right
Interventricular foramen (Monro) use Cerebral Ventricle
Interventricular septum use Septum, Ventricular
Intestinal lymphatic trunk use Cisterna Chyli
Intraluminal Device
Airway
Esophagus ØDH5
Mouth and Throat ØCHY
Nasopharynx Ø9HN
Bioactive
Occlusion
Common Carotid
Left Ø3LJ
Right Ø3LH
External Carotid
Left Ø3LN
Right Ø3LM
Internal Carotid
Left Ø3LL
Right Ø3LK
Intracranial Ø3LG
Vertebral
Left Ø3LQ
Right Ø3LP
Restriction
Common Carotid
Left Ø3VJ
Right Ø3VH
External Carotid
Left Ø3VN
Right Ø3VM
Internal Carotid
Left Ø3VL
Right Ø3VK

Intraluminal Device — continued
Bioactive — continued
Restriction — continued
Intracranial Ø3VG
Vertebral
Left Ø3VQ
Right Ø3VP
Endobronchial Valve
Lingula ØBH9
Lower Lobe
Left ØBHB
Right ØBH6
Main
Left ØBH7
Right ØBH3
Middle Lobe, Right ØBH5
Upper Lobe
Left ØBH8
Right ØBH4
Endotracheal Airway
Change device in, Trachea ØB21XEZ
Insertion of device in, Trachea ØBH1
Pessary
Change device in, Vagina and Cul-de-sac ØU2HXGZ
Insertion of device in
Cul-de-sac ØUHF
Vagina ØUHG
Intramedullary (IM) rod (nail)
use Internal Fixation Device, Intramedullary in Lower Bones
use Internal Fixation Device, Intramedullary in Upper Bones
Intramedullary skeletal kinetic distractor (ISKD)
use Internal Fixation Device, Intramedullary in Lower Bones
use Internal Fixation Device, Intramedullary in Upper Bones
Intraocular Telescope
Left Ø8RK3ØZ
Right Ø8RJ3ØZ
Intraoperative Radiation Therapy (IORT)
Anus DDY8CZZ
Bile Ducts DFY2CZZ
Bladder DTY2CZZ
Cervix DUY1CZZ
Colon DDY5CZZ
Duodenum DDY2CZZ
Gallbladder DFY1CZZ
Ileum DDY4CZZ
Jejunum DDY3CZZ
Kidney DTYØCZZ
Larynx D9YBCZZ
Liver DFYØCZZ
Mouth D9Y4CZZ
Nasopharynx D9YDCZZ
Ovary DUYØCZZ
Pancreas DFY3CZZ
Pharynx D9YCCZZ
Prostate DVYØCZZ
Rectum DDY7CZZ
Stomach DDY1CZZ
Ureter DTY1CZZ
Urethra DTY3CZZ
Uterus DUY2CZZ
Intrauterine Device (IUD) use Contraceptive Device in Female Reproductive System
Introduction of substance in or on
Artery
Central 3E06
Analgesics 3E06
Anesthetic, Intracirculatory 3E06
Anti-infective 3E06
Anti-inflammatory 3E06
Antiarrhythmic 3E06
Antineoplastic 3E06
Destructive Agent 3E06
Diagnostic Substance, Other 3E06
Electrolytic Substance 3E06
Hormone 3E06
Hypnotics 3E06
Immunotherapeutic 3E06
Nutritional Substance 3E06
Platelet Inhibitor 3E06
Radioactive Substance 3E06
Sedatives 3E06

Introduction of substance in or on — continued
Artery — continued
Central — continued
Serum 3E06
Thrombolytic 3E06
Toxoid 3E06
Vaccine 3E06
Vasopressor 3E06
Water Balance Substance 3E06
Coronary 3E07
Diagnostic Substance, Other 3E07
Platelet Inhibitor 3E07
Thrombolytic 3E07
Peripheral 3E05
Analgesics 3E05
Anesthetic, Intracirculatory 3E05
Anti-infective 3E05
Anti-inflammatory 3E05
Antiarrhythmic 3E05
Antineoplastic 3E05
Destructive Agent 3E05
Diagnostic Substance, Other 3E05
Electrolytic Substance 3E05
Hormone 3E05
Hypnotics 3E05
Immunotherapeutic 3E05
Nutritional Substance 3E05
Platelet Inhibitor 3E05
Radioactive Substance 3E05
Sedatives 3E05
Serum 3E05
Thrombolytic 3E05
Toxoid 3E05
Vaccine 3E05
Vasopressor 3E05
Water Balance Substance 3E05
Biliary Tract 3EØJ
Analgesics 3EØJ
Anesthetic, Local 3EØJ
Anti-infective 3EØJ
Anti-inflammatory 3EØJ
Antineoplastic 3EØJ
Destructive Agent 3EØJ
Diagnostic Substance, Other 3EØJ
Electrolytic Substance 3EØJ
Gas 3EØJ
Hypnotics 3EØJ
Islet Cells, Pancreatic 3EØJ
Nutritional Substance 3EØJ
Radioactive Substance 3EØJ
Sedatives 3EØJ
Water Balance Substance 3EØJ
Bone 3EØV
Analgesics 3EØV3NZ
Anesthetic, Local 3EØV3BZ
Anti-infective 3EØV32
Anti-inflammatory 3EØV33Z
Antineoplastic 3EØV3Ø
Destructive Agent 3EØV3TZ
Diagnostic Substance, Other 3EØV3KZ
Electrolytic Substance 3EØV37Z
Hypnotics 3EØV3NZ
Nutritional Substance 3EØV36Z
Radioactive Substance 3EØV3HZ
Sedatives 3EØV3NZ
Water Balance Substance 3EØV37Z
Bone Marrow 3EØA3GC
Antineoplastic 3EØA3Ø
Brain 3EØQ3GC
Analgesics 3EØQ3NZ
Anesthetic, Local 3EØQ3BZ
Anti-infective 3EØQ32
Anti-inflammatory 3EØQ33Z
Antineoplastic 3EØQ
Destructive Agent 3EØQ3TZ
Diagnostic Substance, Other 3EØQ3KZ
Electrolytic Substance 3EØQ37Z
Gas 3EØQ
Hypnotics 3EØQ3NZ
Nutritional Substance 3EØQ36Z
Radioactive Substance 3EØQ3HZ
Sedatives 3EØQ3NZ
Stem Cells
Embryonic 3EØQ
Somatic 3EØQ
Water Balance Substance 3EØQ37Z

Introduction of substance in or on — continued
Cranial Cavity 3E0Q3GC
  Analgesics 3E0Q3NZ
  Anesthetic, Local 3E0Q3BZ
  Anti-infective 3E0Q32
  Anti-inflammatory 3E0Q33Z
  Antineoplastic 3E0Q
  Destructive Agent 3E0Q3TZ
  Diagnostic Substance, Other 3E0Q3KZ
  Electrolytic Substance 3E0Q37Z
  Gas 3E0Q
  Hypnotics 3E0Q3NZ
  Nutritional Substance 3E0Q36Z
  Radioactive Substance 3E0Q3HZ
  Sedatives 3E0Q3NZ
  Stem Cells
    Embryonic 3E0Q
    Somatic 3E0Q
  Water Balance Substance 3E0Q37Z
Ear 3E0B
  Analgesics 3E0B
  Anesthetic, Local 3E0B
  Anti-infective 3E0B
  Anti-inflammatory 3E0B
  Antineoplastic 3E0B
  Destructive Agent 3E0B
  Diagnostic Substance, Other 3E0B
  Hypnotics 3E0B
  Radioactive Substance 3E0B
  Sedatives 3E0B
Epidural Space 3E0S3GC
  Analgesics 3E0S3NZ
  Anesthetic
    Local 3E0S3BZ
    Regional 3E0S3CZ
  Anti-infective 3E0S32
  Anti-inflammatory 3E0S33Z
  Antineoplastic 3E0S30
  Destructive Agent 3E0S3TZ
  Diagnostic Substance, Other 3E0S3KZ
  Electrolytic Substance 3E0S37Z
  Gas 3E0S
  Hypnotics 3E0S3NZ
  Nutritional Substance 3E0S36Z
  Radioactive Substance 3E0S3HZ
  Sedatives 3E0S3NZ
  Water Balance Substance 3E0S37Z
Eye 3E0C
  Analgesics 3E0C
  Anesthetic, Local 3E0C
  Anti-infective 3E0C
  Anti-inflammatory 3E0C
  Antineoplastic 3E0C
  Destructive Agent 3E0C
  Diagnostic Substance, Other 3E0C
  Gas 3E0C
  Hypnotics 3E0C
  Pigment 3E0C
  Radioactive Substance 3E0C
  Sedatives 3E0C
Gastrointestinal Tract
  Lower 3E0H
    Analgesics 3E0H
    Anesthetic, Local 3E0H
    Anti-infective 3E0H
    Anti-inflammatory 3E0H
    Antineoplastic 3E0H
    Destructive Agent 3E0H
    Diagnostic Substance, Other 3E0H
    Electrolytic Substance 3E0H
    Gas 3E0H
    Hypnotics 3E0H
    Nutritional Substance 3E0H
    Radioactive Substance 3E0H
    Sedatives 3E0H
    Water Balance Substance 3E0H
  Upper 3E0G
    Analgesics 3E0G
    Anesthetic, Local 3E0G
    Anti-infective 3E0G
    Anti-inflammatory 3E0G
    Antineoplastic 3E0G
    Destructive Agent 3E0G
    Diagnostic Substance, Other 3E0G
    Electrolytic Substance 3E0G
    Gas 3E0G

Introduction of substance in or on — continued
Gastrointestinal Tract — continued
  Upper — continued
    Hypnotics 3E0G
    Nutritional Substance 3E0G
    Radioactive Substance 3E0G
    Sedatives 3E0G
    Water Balance Substance 3E0G
Genitourinary Tract 3E0K
  Analgesics 3E0K
  Anesthetic, Local 3E0K
  Anti-infective 3E0K
  Anti-inflammatory 3E0K
  Antineoplastic 3E0K
  Destructive Agent 3E0K
  Diagnostic Substance, Other 3E0K
  Electrolytic Substance 3E0K
  Gas 3E0K
  Hypnotics 3E0K
  Nutritional Substance 3E0K
  Radioactive Substance 3E0K
  Sedatives 3E0K
  Water Balance Substance 3E0K
Heart 3E08
  Diagnostic Substance, Other 3E08
  Platelet Inhibitor 3E08
  Thrombolytic 3E08
Joint 3E0U
  Analgesics 3E0U3NZ
  Anesthetic, Local 3E0U3BZ
  Anti-infective 3E0U
  Anti-inflammatory 3E0U33Z
  Antineoplastic 3E0U30
  Destructive Agent 3E0U3TZ
  Diagnostic Substance, Other 3E0U3KZ
  Electrolytic Substance 3E0U37Z
  Gas 3E0U3SF
  Hypnotics 3E0U3NZ
  Nutritional Substance 3E0U36Z
  Radioactive Substance 3E0U3HZ
  Sedatives 3E0U3NZ
  Water Balance Substance 3E0U37Z
Lymphatic 3E0W3GC
  Analgesics 3E0W3NZ
  Anesthetic, Local 3E0W3BZ
  Anti-infective 3E0W32
  Anti-inflammatory 3E0W33Z
  Antineoplastic 3E0W30
  Destructive Agent 3E0W3TZ
  Diagnostic Substance, Other 3E0W3KZ
  Electrolytic Substance 3E0W37Z
  Hypnotics 3E0W3NZ
  Nutritional Substance 3E0W36Z
  Radioactive Substance 3E0W3HZ
  Sedatives 3E0W3NZ
  Water Balance Substance 3E0W37Z
Mouth 3E0D
  Analgesics 3E0D
  Anesthetic, Local 3E0D
  Anti-infective 3E0D
  Anti-inflammatory 3E0D
  Antiarrhythmic 3E0D
  Antineoplastic 3E0D
  Destructive Agent 3E0D
  Diagnostic Substance, Other 3E0D
  Electrolytic Substance 3E0D
  Hypnotics 3E0D
  Nutritional Substance 3E0D
  Radioactive Substance 3E0D
  Sedatives 3E0D
  Serum 3E0D
  Toxoid 3E0D
  Vaccine 3E0D
  Water Balance Substance 3E0D
Mucous Membrane 3E00XGC
  Analgesics 3E00XNZ
  Anesthetic, Local 3E00XBZ
  Anti-infective 3E00X2
  Anti-inflammatory 3E00X3Z
  Antineoplastic 3E00X0
  Destructive Agent 3E00XTZ
  Diagnostic Substance, Other 3E00XKZ
  Hypnotics 3E00XNZ
  Pigment 3E00XMZ
  Sedatives 3E00XNZ
  Serum 3E00X4Z

Introduction of substance in or on — continued
Mucous Membrane — continued
  Toxoid 3E00X4Z
  Vaccine 3E00X4Z
Muscle 3E023GC
  Analgesics 3E023NZ
  Anesthetic, Local 3E023BZ
  Anti-infective 3E0232
  Anti-inflammatory 3E0233Z
  Antineoplastic 3E0230
  Destructive Agent 3E023TZ
  Diagnostic Substance, Other 3E023KZ
  Electrolytic Substance 3E0237Z
  Hypnotics 3E023NZ
  Nutritional Substance 3E0236Z
  Radioactive Substance 3E023HZ
  Sedatives 3E023NZ
  Serum 3E0234Z
  Toxoid 3E0234Z
  Vaccine 3E0234Z
  Water Balance Substance 3E0237Z
Nerve
  Cranial 3E0X3GC
    Anesthetic
      Local 3E0X3BZ
      Regional 3E0X3CZ
    Anti-inflammatory 3E0X33Z
    Destructive Agent 3E0X3TZ
  Peripheral 3E0T3GC
    Anesthetic
      Local 3E0T3BZ
      Regional 3E0T3CZ
    Anti-inflammatory 3E0T33Z
    Destructive Agent 3E0T3TZ
  Plexus 3E0T3GC
    Anesthetic
      Local 3E0T3BZ
      Regional 3E0T3CZ
    Anti-inflammatory 3E0T33Z
    Destructive Agent 3E0T3TZ
Nose 3E09
  Analgesics 3E09
  Anesthetic, Local 3E09
  Anti-infective 3E09
  Anti-inflammatory 3E09
  Antineoplastic 3E09
  Destructive Agent 3E09
  Diagnostic Substance, Other 3E09
  Hypnotics 3E09
  Radioactive Substance 3E09
  Sedatives 3E09
  Serum 3E09
  Toxoid 3E09
  Vaccine 3E09
Pancreatic Tract 3E0J
  Analgesics 3E0J
  Anesthetic, Local 3E0J
  Anti-infective 3E0J
  Anti-inflammatory 3E0J
  Antineoplastic 3E0J
  Destructive Agent 3E0J
  Diagnostic Substance, Other 3E0J
  Electrolytic Substance 3E0J
  Gas 3E0J
  Hypnotics 3E0J
  Islet Cells, Pancreatic 3E0J
  Nutritional Substance 3E0J
  Radioactive Substance 3E0J
  Sedatives 3E0J
  Water Balance Substance 3E0J
Pericardial Cavity 3E0Y3GC
  Analgesics 3E0Y3NZ
  Anesthetic, Local 3E0Y3BZ
  Anti-infective 3E0Y32
  Anti-inflammatory 3E0Y33Z
  Antineoplastic 3E0Y
  Destructive Agent 3E0Y3TZ
  Diagnostic Substance, Other 3E0Y3KZ
  Electrolytic Substance 3E0Y37Z
  Gas 3E0Y
  Hypnotics 3E0Y3NZ
  Nutritional Substance 3E0Y36Z
  Radioactive Substance 3E0Y3HZ
  Sedatives 3E0Y3NZ
  Water Balance Substance 3E0Y37Z
Peritoneal Cavity 3E0M3GC

Introduction of substance in or on — continued
  Peritoneal Cavity — continued
    Adhesion Barrier 3E0M05Z
    Analgesics 3E0M3NZ
    Anesthetic, Local 3E0M3BZ
    Anti-infective 3E0M32
    Anti-inflammatory 3E0M33Z
    Antineoplastic 3E0M
    Destructive Agent 3E0M3TZ
    Diagnostic Substance, Other 3E0M3KZ
    Electrolytic Substance 3E0M37Z
    Gas 3E0M
    Hypnotics 3E0M3NZ
    Nutritional Substance 3E0M36Z
    Radioactive Substance 3E0M3HZ
    Sedatives 3E0M3NZ
    Water Balance Substance 3E0M37Z
  Pharynx 3E0D
    Analgesics 3E0D
    Anesthetic, Local 3E0D
    Anti-infective 3E0D
    Anti-inflammatory 3E0D
    Antiarrhythmic 3E0D
    Antineoplastic 3E0D
    Destructive Agent 3E0D
    Diagnostic Substance, Other 3E0D
    Electrolytic Substance 3E0D
    Hypnotics 3E0D
    Nutritional Substance 3E0D
    Radioactive Substance 3E0D
    Sedatives 3E0D
    Serum 3E0D
    Toxoid 3E0D
    Vaccine 3E0D
    Water Balance Substance 3E0D
  Pleural Cavity 3E0L3GC
    Adhesion Barrier 3E0L05Z
    Analgesics 3E0L3NZ
    Anesthetic, Local 3E0L3BZ
    Anti-infective 3E0L32
    Anti-inflammatory 3E0L33Z
    Antineoplastic 3E0L
    Destructive Agent 3E0L3TZ
    Diagnostic Substance, Other 3E0L3KZ
    Electrolytic Substance 3E0L37Z
    Gas 3E0L
    Hypnotics 3E0L3NZ
    Nutritional Substance 3E0L36Z
    Radioactive Substance 3E0L3HZ
    Sedatives 3E0L3NZ
    Water Balance Substance 3E0L37Z
  Products of Conception 3E0E
    Analgesics 3E0E
    Anesthetic, Local 3E0E
    Anti-infective 3E0E
    Anti-inflammatory 3E0E
    Antineoplastic 3E0E
    Destructive Agent 3E0E
    Diagnostic Substance, Other 3E0E
    Electrolytic Substance 3E0E
    Gas 3E0E
    Hypnotics 3E0E
    Nutritional Substance 3E0E
    Radioactive Substance 3E0E
    Sedatives 3E0E
    Water Balance Substance 3E0E
  Reproductive
    Female 3E0P
      Adhesion Barrier 3E0P05Z
      Analgesics 3E0P
      Anesthetic, Local 3E0P
      Anti-infective 3E0P
      Anti-inflammatory 3E0P
      Antineoplastic 3E0P
      Destructive Agent 3E0P
      Diagnostic Substance, Other 3E0P
      Electrolytic Substance 3E0P
      Gas 3E0P
      Hypnotics 3E0P
      Nutritional Substance 3E0P
      Ovum, Fertilized 3E0P
      Radioactive Substance 3E0P
      Sedatives 3E0P
      Sperm 3E0P
      Water Balance Substance 3E0P
    Male 3E0N

Introduction of substance in or on — continued
  Reproductive — continued
    Male — continued
      Analgesics 3E0N
      Anesthetic, Local 3E0N
      Anti-infective 3E0N
      Anti-inflammatory 3E0N
      Antineoplastic 3E0N
      Destructive Agent 3E0N
      Diagnostic Substance, Other 3E0N
      Electrolytic Substance 3E0N
      Gas 3E0N
      Hypnotics 3E0N
      Nutritional Substance 3E0N
      Radioactive Substance 3E0N
      Sedatives 3E0N
      Water Balance Substance 3E0N
  Respiratory Tract 3E0F
    Analgesics 3E0F
    Anesthetic
      Inhalation 3E0F
      Local 3E0F
    Anti-infective 3E0F
    Anti-inflammatory 3E0F
    Antineoplastic 3E0F
    Destructive Agent 3E0F
    Diagnostic Substance, Other 3E0F
    Electrolytic Substance 3E0F
    Gas 3E0F
    Hypnotics 3E0F
    Nutritional Substance 3E0F
    Radioactive Substance 3E0F
    Sedatives 3E0F
    Water Balance Substance 3E0F
  Skin 3E00XGC
    Analgesics 3E00XNZ
    Anesthetic, Local 3E00XBZ
    Anti-infective 3E00X2
    Anti-inflammatory 3E00X3Z
    Antineoplastic 3E00X0
    Destructive Agent 3E00XTZ
    Diagnostic Substance, Other 3E00XKZ
    Hypnotics 3E00XNZ
    Pigment 3E00XMZ
    Sedatives 3E00XNZ
    Serum 3E00X4Z
    Toxoid 3E00X4Z
    Vaccine 3E00X4Z
  Spinal Canal 3E0R3GC
    Analgesics 3E0R3NZ
    Anesthetic
      Local 3E0R3BZ
      Regional 3E0R3CZ
    Anti-infective 3E0R32
    Anti-inflammatory 3E0R33Z
    Antineoplastic 3E0R30
    Destructive Agent 3E0R3TZ
    Diagnostic Substance, Other 3E0R3KZ
    Electrolytic Substance 3E0R37Z
    Gas 3E0R
    Hypnotics 3E0R3NZ
    Nutritional Substance 3E0R36Z
    Radioactive Substance 3E0R3HZ
    Sedatives 3E0R3NZ
    Stem Cells
      Embryonic 3E0R
      Somatic 3E0R
    Water Balance Substance 3E0R37Z
  Subcutaneous Tissue 3E013GC
    Analgesics 3E013NZ
    Anesthetic, Local 3E013BZ
    Anti-infective 3E01
    Anti-inflammatory 3E0133Z
    Antineoplastic 3E0130
    Destructive Agent 3E013TZ
    Diagnostic Substance, Other 3E013KZ
    Electrolytic Substance 3E0137Z
    Hormone 3E013V
    Hypnotics 3E013NZ
    Nutritional Substance 3E0136Z
    Radioactive Substance 3E013HZ
    Sedatives 3E013NZ
    Serum 3E0134Z
    Toxoid 3E0134Z
    Vaccine 3E0134Z
    Water Balance Substance 3E0137Z

Introduction of substance in or on — continued
  Vein
    Central 3E04
      Analgesics 3E04
      Anesthetic, Intracirculatory 3E04
      Anti-infective 3E04
      Anti-inflammatory 3E04
      Antiarrhythmic 3E04
      Antineoplastic 3E04
      Destructive Agent 3E04
      Diagnostic Substance, Other 3E04
      Electrolytic Substance 3E04
      Hormone 3E04
      Hypnotics 3E04
      Immunotherapeutic 3E04
      Nutritional Substance 3E04
      Platelet Inhibitor 3E04
      Radioactive Substance 3E04
      Sedatives 3E04
      Serum 3E04
      Thrombolytic 3E04
      Toxoid 3E04
      Vaccine 3E04
      Vasopressor 3E04
      Water Balance Substance 3E04
    Peripheral 3E03
      Analgesics 3E03
      Anesthetic, Intracirculatory 3E03
      Anti-infective 3E03
      Anti-inflammatory 3E03
      Antiarrhythmic 3E03
      Antineoplastic 3E03
      Destructive Agent 3E03
      Diagnostic Substance, Other 3E03
      Electrolytic Substance 3E03
      Hormone 3E03
      Hypnotics 3E03
      Immunotherapeutic 3E03
      Islet Cells, Pancreatic 3E03
      Nutritional Substance 3E03
      Platelet Inhibitor 3E03
      Radioactive Substance 3E03
      Sedatives 3E03
      Serum 3E03
      Thrombolytic 3E03
      Toxoid 3E03
      Vaccine 3E03
      Vasopressor 3E03
      Water Balance Substance 3E03
Intubation
  Airway
    see Insertion of device in, Esophagus 0DH5
    see Insertion of device in, Mouth and Throat 0CHY
    see Insertion of device in, Trachea 0BH1
  Drainage device *see* Drainage
  Feeding Device *see* Insertion of device in, Gastrointestinal System 0DH
IPPB (intermittent positive pressure breathing) *see* Assistance, Respiratory 5A09
Iridectomy
  see Excision, Eye 08B
  see Resection, Eye 08T
Iridoplasty
  see Repair, Eye 08Q
  see Replacement, Eye 08R
  see Supplement, Eye 08U
Iridotomy *see* Drainage, Eye 089
Irrigation
  Biliary Tract, Irrigating Substance 3E1J
  Brain, Irrigating Substance 3E1Q38Z
  Cranial Cavity, Irrigating Substance 3E1Q38Z
  Ear, Irrigating Substance 3E1B
  Epidural Space, Irrigating Substance 3E1S38Z
  Eye, Irrigating Substance 3E1C
  Gastrointestinal Tract
    Lower, Irrigating Substance 3E1H
    Upper, Irrigating Substance 3E1G
  Genitourinary Tract, Irrigating Substance 3E1K
  Irrigating Substance 3C1ZX8Z
  Joint, Irrigating Substance 3E1U38Z
  Mucous Membrane, Irrigating Substance 3E10
  Nose, Irrigating Substance 3E19
  Pancreatic Tract, Irrigating Substance 3E1J
  Pericardial Cavity, Irrigating Substance 3E1Y38Z
  Peritoneal Cavity
    Dialysate 3E1M39Z

Irrigation — continued
  Peritoneal Cavity — continued
    Irrigating Substance 3E1M38Z
  Pleural Cavity, Irrigating Substance 3E1L38Z
  Reproductive
    Female, Irrigating Substance 3E1P
    Male, Irrigating Substance 3E1N
  Respiratory Tract, Irrigating Substance 3E1F
  Skin, Irrigating Substance 3E10
  Spinal Canal, Irrigating Substance 3E1R38Z
Ischiatic nerve use Nerve, Sciatic
Ischiocavernosus muscle use Muscle, Perineum
Ischiofemoral ligament
  use Bursa and Ligament, Hip, Left
  use Bursa and Ligament, Hip, Right
Ischium
  use Bone, Pelvic, Left
  use Bone, Pelvic, Right
Isolation 8E0ZXY6
Isotope Administration, Whole Body DWY5G
Itrel(3)(4)neurostimulator use Stimulator Generator, Single Array 0JH

J

Jejunal artery use Artery, Superior Mesenteric
Jejunectomy
  see Excision, Jejunum 0DBA
  see Resection, Jejunum 0DTA
Jejunocolostomy
  see Bypass, Gastrointestinal System 0D1
  see Drainage, Gastrointestinal System 0D9
Jejunopexy
  see Repair, Jejunum 0DQA
  see Reposition, Jejunum 0DSA
Jejunostomy
  see Bypass, Jejunum 0D1A
  see Drainage, Jejunum 0D9A
Jejunotomy see Drainage, Jejunum 0D9A
Joint fixation plate
  use Internal Fixation Device in Lower Joints
  use Internal Fixation Device in Upper Joints
Joint liner (insert) use Liner in Lower Joints
Joint spacer (antibiotic)
  use Spacer in Lower Joints
  use Spacer in Upper Joints
Jugular body use Glomus Jugulare
Jugular lymph node
  use Lymphatic, Neck, Left
  use Lymphatic, Neck, Right

K

Kappa use Pacemaker, Dual Chamber in 0JH
Keratectomy, kerectomy
  see Excision, Eye 08B
  see Resection, Eye 08T
Keratocentesis see Drainage, Eye 089
Keratoplasty
  see Repair, Eye 08Q
  see Replacement, Eye 08R
  see Supplement, Eye 08U
Keratotomy
  see Drainage, Eye 089
  see Repair, Eye 08Q
Kinetra® multiple-channel neurostimulator use Stimulator Generator, Multiple Array in 0JH
Kirschner wire (K-wire)
  use Internal Fixation Device in Head and Facial Bones
  use Internal Fixation Device in Lower Bones
  use Internal Fixation Device in Lower Joints
  use Internal Fixation Device in Upper Bones
  use Internal Fixation Device in Upper Joints
Knee (implant) insert use Liner in Lower Joints
KUB x-ray see Plain Radiography, Kidney, Ureter and Bladder BT04
Kuntscher nail
  use Internal Fixation Device, Intramedullary in Lower Bones
  use Internal Fixation Device, Intramedullary in Upper Bones

L

Labia majora use Vulva
Labia minora use Vulva
Labial gland
  use Lip, Lower
  use Lip, Upper
Labiectomy
  see Excision, Female Reproductive System 0UB
  see Resection, Female Reproductive System 0UT
Lacrimal canaliculus
  use Duct, Lacrimal, Left
  use Duct, Lacrimal, Right
Lacrimal punctum
  use Duct, Lacrimal, Left
  use Duct, Lacrimal, Right
Lacrimal sac
  use Duct, Lacrimal, Left
  use Duct, Lacrimal, Right
Laminectomy
  see Excision, Lower Bones 0QB
  see Excision, Upper Bones 0PB
Laminotomy
  see Drainage, Lower Joints 0S9
  see Drainage, Upper Joints 0R9
  see Release, Central Nervous System 00N
  see Release, Lower Joints 0SN
  see Release, Peripheral Nervous System 01N
  see Release, Upper Joints 0RN
LAP-BAND® Adjustable Gastric Banding System use Extraluminal Device
Laparoscopy see Inspection
Laparotomy
  Drainage see Drainage, Peritoneal Cavity 0W9G
  Exploratory see Inspection, Peritoneal Cavity 0WJG
Laryngectomy
  see Excision, Larynx 0CBS
  see Resection, Larynx 0CTS
Laryngocentesis see Drainage, Larynx 0C9S
Laryngogram see Fluoroscopy, Larynx B91J
Laryngopexy see Repair, Larynx 0CQS
Laryngopharynx use Pharynx
Laryngoplasty
  see Repair, Larynx 0CQS
  see Replacement, Larynx 0CRS
  see Supplement, Larynx 0CUS
Laryngorrhaphy see Repair, Larynx 0CQS
Laryngoscopy 0CJS8ZZ
Laryngotomy see Drainage, Larynx 0C9S
Laser Interstitial Thermal Therapy
  Adrenal Gland DGY2KZZ
  Anus DDY8KZZ
  Bile Ducts DFY2KZZ
  Brain D0Y0KZZ
  Brain Stem D0Y1KZZ
  Breast
    Left DMY0KZZ
    Right DMY1KZZ
  Bronchus DBY1KZZ
  Chest Wall DBY7KZZ
  Colon DDY5KZZ
  Diaphragm DBY8KZZ
  Duodenum DDY2KZZ
  Esophagus DDY0KZZ
  Gallbladder DFY1KZZ
  Gland
    Adrenal DGY2KZZ
    Parathyroid DGY4KZZ
    Pituitary DGY0KZZ
    Thyroid DGY5KZZ
  Ileum DDY4KZZ
  Jejunum DDY3KZZ
  Liver DFY0KZZ
  Lung DBY2KZZ
  Mediastinum DBY6KZZ
  Nerve, Peripheral D0Y7KZZ
  Pancreas DFY3KZZ
  Parathyroid Gland DGY4KZZ
  Pineal Body DGY1KZZ
  Pituitary Gland DGY0KZZ
  Pleura DBY5KZZ
  Prostate DVY0KZZ
  Rectum DDY7KZZ
  Spinal Cord D0Y6KZZ

Laser Interstitial Thermal Therapy — continued
  Stomach DDY1KZZ
  Thyroid Gland DGY5KZZ
  Trachea DBY0KZZ
Lateral canthus
  use Eyelid, Upper, Left
  use Eyelid, Upper, Right
Lateral collateral ligament (LCL)
  use Bursa and Ligament, Knee, Left
  use Bursa and Ligament, Knee, Right
Lateral condyle of femur
  use Femur, Lower, Left
  use Femur, Lower, Right
Lateral condyle of tibia
  use Tibia, Left
  use Tibia, Right
Lateral cuneiform bone
  use Tarsal, Left
  use Tarsal, Right
Lateral epicondyle of femur
  use Femur, Lower, Left
  use Femur, Lower, Right
Lateral epicondyle of humerus
  use Humeral Shaft, Left
  use Humeral Shaft, Right
Lateral femoral cutaneous nerve use Nerve, Lumbar Plexus
Lateral (brachial) lymph node
  use Lymphatic, Axillary, Left
  use Lymphatic, Axillary, Right
Lateral malleolus
  use Fibula, Left
  use Fibula, Right
Lateral meniscus
  use Joint, Knee, Left
  use Joint, Knee, Right
Lateral nasal cartilage use Nose
Lateral plantar artery
  use Artery, Foot, Left
  use Artery, Foot, Right
Lateral plantar nerve use Nerve, Tibial
Lateral rectus muscle
  use Muscle, Extraocular, Left
  use Muscle, Extraocular, Right
Lateral sacral artery
  use Artery, Internal Iliac, Left
  use Artery, Internal Iliac, Right
Lateral sacral vein
  use Vein, Hypogastric, Left
  use Vein, Hypogastric, Right
Lateral sural cutaneous nerve use Nerve, Peroneal
Lateral tarsal artery
  use Artery, Foot, Left
  use Artery, Foot, Right
Lateral temporomandibular ligament use Bursa and Ligament, Head and Neck
Lateral thoracic artery
  use Artery, Axillary, Left
  use Artery, Axillary, Right
Latissimus dorsi muscle
  use Muscle, Trunk, Left
  use Muscle, Trunk, Right
Latissimus Dorsi Myocutaneous Flap
  Bilateral 0HRV075
  Left 0HRU075
  Right 0HRT075
Lavage
  see Irrigation
  Bronchial alveolar, diagnostic see Drainage, Respiratory System 0B9
Least splanchnic nerve use Nerve, Thoracic Sympathetic
Left ascending lumbar vein use Vein, Hemiazygos
Left atrioventricular valve use Valve, Mitral
Left auricular appendix use Atrium, Left
Left colic vein use Vein, Colic
Left coronary sulcus use Heart, Left
Left gastric artery use Artery, Gastric
Left gastroepiploic artery use Artery, Splenic
Left gastroepiploic vein use Vein, Splenic
Left inferior phrenic vein use Vein, Renal, Left
Left inferior pulmonary vein use Vein, Pulmonary, Left
Left jugular trunk use Lymphatic, Thoracic Duct

Left lateral ventricle *use* Cerebral Ventricle
Left ovarian vein *use* Vein, Renal, Left
Left second lumbar vein *use* Vein, Renal, Left
Left subclavian trunk *use* Lymphatic, Thoracic Duct
Left subcostal vein *use* Vein, Hemiazygos
Left superior pulmonary vein *use* Vein, Pulmonary, Left
Left suprarenal vein *use* Vein, Renal, Left
Left testicular vein *use* Vein, Renal, Left
Lengthening
    Bone, with device *see* Insertion of Limb Lengthening Device
    Muscle, by incision *see* Division, Muscles ØK8
    Tendon, by incision *see* Division, Tendons ØL8
Leptomeninges
    use Cerebral Meninges
    use Spinal Meninges
Lesser alar cartilage *use* Nose
Lesser occipital nerve *use* Nerve, Cervical Plexus
Lesser splanchnic nerve *use* Nerve, Thoracic Sympathetic
Lesser trochanter
    use Femur, Upper, Left
    use Femur, Upper, Right
Lesser tuberosity
    use Humeral Head, Left
    use Humeral Head, Right
Lesser wing
    use Bone, Sphenoid, Left
    use Bone, Sphenoid, Right
Leukopheresis, therapeutic *see* Pheresis, Circulatory 6A55
Levator anguli oris muscle *use* Muscle, Facial
Levator ani muscle
    use Muscle, Trunk, Left
    use Muscle, Trunk, Right
Levator labii superioris alaeque nasi muscle *use* Muscle, Facial
Levator labii superioris muscle *use* Muscle, Facial
Levator palpebrae superioris muscle
    use Eyelid, Upper, Left
    use Eyelid, Upper, Right
Levator scapulae muscle
    use Muscle, Neck, Left
    use Muscle, Neck, Right
Levator veli palatini muscle *use* Muscle, Tongue, Palate, Pharynx
Levatores costarum muscle
    use Muscle, Thorax, Left
    use Muscle, Thorax, Right
LifeStent® (Flexstar)(XL) Vascular Stent System *use* Intraluminal Device
Ligament of head of fibula
    use Bursa and Ligament, Knee, Left
    use Bursa and Ligament, Knee, Right
Ligament of the lateral malleolus
    use Bursa and Ligament, Ankle, Left
    use Bursa and Ligament, Ankle, Right
Ligamentum flavum
    use Bursa and Ligament, Trunk, Left
    use Bursa and Ligament, Trunk, Right
Ligation *see* Occlusion
Ligation, hemorrhoid *see* Occlusion, Lower Veins, Hemorrhoidal Plexus
Light Therapy GZJZZZZ
Liner
    Removal of device from
        Hip
            Left ØSPBØ9Z
            Right ØSP9Ø9Z
        Knee
            Left ØSPDØ9Z
            Right ØSPCØ9Z
    Revision of device in
        Hip
            Left ØSWBØ9Z
            Right ØSW9Ø9Z
        Knee
            Left ØSWDØ9Z
            Right ØSWCØ9Z
    Supplement
        Hip
            Left ØSUBØ9Z
                Acetabular Surface ØSUEØ9Z
                Femoral Surface ØSUSØ9Z

Liner — continued
    Supplement — continued
        Hip — continued
            Right ØSU9Ø9Z
                Acetabular Surface ØSUAØ9Z
                Femoral Surface ØSURØ9Z
        Knee
            Left ØSUDØ9
                Femoral Surface ØSUUØ9Z
                Tibial Surface ØSUWØ9Z
            Right ØSUCØ9
                Femoral Surface ØSUTØ9Z
                Tibial Surface ØSUVØ9Z
Lingual artery
    use Artery, External Carotid, Left
    use Artery, External Carotid, Right
Lingual tonsil *use* Tongue
Lingulectomy, lung
    see Excision, Lung Lingula ØBBH
    see Resection, Lung Lingula ØBTH
Lithotripsy
    With removal of fragments *see* Extirpation
    see Fragmentation
LIVIAN™ CRT-D *use* Cardiac Resynchronization Defibrillator Pulse Generator in ØJH
Lobectomy
    see Excision, Central Nervous System ØØB
    see Excision, Endocrine System ØGB
    see Excision, Hepatobiliary System and Pancreas ØFB
    see Excision, Respiratory System ØBB
    see Resection, Endocrine System ØGT
    see Resection, Hepatobiliary System and Pancreas ØFT
    see Resection, Respiratory System ØBT
Lobotomy *see* Division, Brain ØØ8Ø
Localization
    see Imaging
    see Map
Locus ceruleus *use* Pons
Long thoracic nerve *use* Nerve, Brachial Plexus
Loop ileostomy *see* Bypass, Ileum ØD1B
Loop recorder, implantable *use* Monitoring Device
Lower GI series *see* Fluoroscopy, Colon BD14
Lumbar artery *use* Aorta, Abdominal
Lumbar facet joint
    use Joint, Lumbar Vertebral
    use Joint, Lumbar Vertebral, 2 or more
Lumbar ganglion *use* Nerve, Lumbar Sympathetic
Lumbar lymph node *use* Lymphatic, Aortic
Lumbar lymphatic trunk *use* Cisterna Chyli
Lumbar splanchnic nerve *use* Nerve, Lumbar Sympathetic
Lumbosacral facet joint *use* Joint, Lumbosacral
Lumbosacral trunk *use* Nerve, Lumbar
Lumpectomy *see* Excision
Lunate bone
    use Carpal, Left
    use Carpal, Right
Lunotriquetral ligament
    use Bursa and Ligament, Hand, Left
    use Bursa and Ligament, Hand, Right
Lymphadenectomy
    see Excision, Lymphatic and Hemic Systems Ø7B
    see Resection, Lymphatic and Hemic Systems Ø7T
Lymphadenotomy *see* Drainage, Lymphatic and Hemic Systems Ø79
Lymphangiectomy
    see Excision, Lymphatic and Hemic Systems Ø7B
    see Resection, Lymphatic and Hemic Systems Ø7T
Lymphangiogram *see* Plain Radiography, Lymphatic System B7Ø
Lymphangioplasty
    see Repair, Lymphatic and Hemic Systems Ø7Q
    see Supplement, Lymphatic and Hemic Systems Ø7U
Lymphangiorrhaphy *see* Repair, Lymphatic and Hemic Systems Ø7Q
Lymphangiotomy *see* Drainage, Lymphatic and Hemic Systems Ø79
Lysis *see* Release

M

Macula
    use Retina, Left

Macula — continued
    use Retina, Right
Magnet extraction, ocular foreign body *see* Extirpation, Eye Ø8C
Magnetic Resonance Imaging (MRI)
    Abdomen BW3Ø
    Ankle
        Left BQ3H
        Right BQ3G
    Aorta
        Abdominal B43Ø
        Thoracic B33Ø
    Arm
        Left BP3F
        Right BP3E
    Artery
        Celiac B431
        Cervico-Cerebral Arch B33Q
        Common Carotid, Bilateral B335
        Coronary
            Bypass Graft, Multiple B233
                Multiple B231
        Internal Carotid, Bilateral B338
        Intracranial B33R
        Lower Extremity
            Bilateral B43H
            Left B43G
            Right B43F
        Pelvic B43C
        Renal, Bilateral B438
        Spinal B33M
        Superior Mesenteric B434
        Upper Extremity
            Bilateral B33K
            Left B33J
            Right B33H
        Vertebral, Bilateral B33G
    Bladder BT3Ø
    Brachial Plexus BW3P
    Brain BØ3Ø
    Breast
        Bilateral BH32
        Left BH31
        Right BH3Ø
    Calcaneus
        Left BQ3K
        Right BQ3J
    Chest BW33Y
    Coccyx BR3F
    Connective Tissue
        Lower Extremity BL31
        Upper Extremity BL3Ø
    Corpora Cavernosa BV3Ø
    Disc
        Cervical BR31
        Lumbar BR33
        Thoracic BR32
    Ear B93Ø
    Elbow
        Left BP3H
        Right BP3G
    Eye
        Bilateral B837
        Left B836
        Right B835
    Femur
        Left BQ34
        Right BQ33
    Fetal Abdomen BY33
    Fetal Extremity BY35
    Fetal Head BY3Ø
    Fetal Heart BY31
    Fetal Spine BY34
    Fetal Thorax BY32
    Fetus, Whole BY36
    Foot
        Left BQ3M
        Right BQ3L
    Forearm
        Left BP3K
        Right BP3J
    Gland
        Adrenal, Bilateral BG32
        Parathyroid BG33
        Parotid, Bilateral B936
        Salivary, Bilateral B93D

Magnetic Resonance Imaging (MRI) — continued
Gland — continued
  Submandibular, Bilateral B939
  Thyroid BG34
Head BW38
Heart, Right and Left B236
Hip
  Left BQ31
  Right BQ30
Intracranial Sinus B532
Joint
  Finger
    Left BP3D
    Right BP3C
  Hand
    Left BP3D
    Right BP3C
  Temporomandibular, Bilateral BN39
Kidney
  Bilateral BT33
  Left BT32
  Right BT31
  Transplant BT39
Knee
  Left BQ38
  Right BQ37
Larynx B93J
Leg
  Left BQ3F
  Right BQ3D
Liver BF35
Liver and Spleen BF36
Lung Apices BB3G
Nasopharynx B93F
Neck BW3F
Nerve
  Acoustic B03C
  Brachial Plexus BW3P
Oropharynx B93F
Ovary
  Bilateral BU35
  Left BU34
  Right BU33
Ovary and Uterus BU3C
Pancreas BF37
Patella
  Left BQ3W
  Right BQ3V
Pelvic Region BW3G
Pelvis BR3C
Pituitary Gland B039
Plexus, Brachial BW3P
Prostate BV33
Retroperitoneum BW3H
Sacrum BR3F
Scrotum BV34
Sella Turcica B039
Shoulder
  Left BP39
  Right BP38
Sinus
  Intracranial B532
  Paranasal B932
Spinal Cord B03B
Spine
  Cervical BR30
  Lumbar BR39
  Thoracic BR37
Spleen and Liver BF36
Subcutaneous Tissue
  Abdomen BH3H
  Extremity
    Lower BH3J
    Upper BH3F
  Head BH3D
  Neck BH3D
  Pelvis BH3H
  Thorax BH3G
Tendon
  Lower Extremity BL33
  Upper Extremity BL32
Testicle
  Bilateral BV37
  Left BV36
  Right BV35

Magnetic Resonance Imaging (MRI) — continued
Toe
  Left BQ3Q
  Right BQ3P
Uterus BU36
  Pregnant BU3B
Uterus and Ovary BU3C
Vagina BU39
Vein
  Cerebellar B531
  Cerebral B531
  Jugular, Bilateral B535
  Lower Extremity
    Bilateral B53D
    Left B53C
    Right B53B
  Other B53V
  Pelvic (Iliac) Bilateral B53H
  Portal B53T
  Pulmonary, Bilateral B53S
  Renal, Bilateral B53L
  Spanchnic B53T
  Upper Extremity
    Bilateral B53P
    Left B53N
    Right B53M
Vena Cava
  Inferior B539
  Superior B538
Wrist
  Left BP3M
  Right BP3L
Malleotomy see Drainage, Ear, Nose, Sinus 099
Malleus
  use Auditory Ossicle, Left
  use Auditory Ossicle, Right
Mammaplasty, mammoplasty
  see Alteration, Skin and Breast 0H0
  see Repair, Skin and Breast 0HQ
  see Replacement, Skin and Breast 0HR
  see Supplement, Skin and Breast 0HU
Mammary duct
  use Breast, Bilateral
  use Breast, Left
  use Breast, Right
Mammary gland
  use Breast, Bilateral
  use Breast, Left
  use Breast, Right
Mammectomy
  see Excision, Skin and Breast 0HB
  see Resection, Skin and Breast 0HT
Mammillary body use Hypothalamus
Mammography see Plain Radiography, Skin, Subcutaneous Tissue and Breast BH0
Mammotomy see Drainage, Skin and Breast 0H9
Mandibular nerve use Nerve, Trigeminal
Mandibular notch
  use Mandible, Left
  use Mandible, Right
Mandibulectomy
  see Excision, Head and Facial Bones 0NB
  see Resection, Head and Facial Bones 0NT
Manipulation
  Adhesions see Release
  Chiropractic see Chiropractic Manipulation
Manubrium use Sternum
Map
  Basal Ganglia 00K8
  Brain 00K0
  Cerebellum 00KC
  Cerebral Hemisphere 00K7
  Conduction Mechanism 02K8
  Hypothalamus 00KA
  Medulla Oblongata 00KD
  Pons 00KB
  Thalamus 00K9
Mapping
  Doppler ultrasound see Ultrasonography
  Electrocardiogram only see Measurement, Cardiac 4A02
Mark IV Breathing Pacemaker System use Stimulator Generator in Subcutaneous Tissue and Fascia
Marsupialization
  see Drainage

Marsupialization — continued
  see Excision
Massage, cardiac
  External 5A12012
  Open 02QA0ZZ
Masseter muscle use Muscle, Head
Masseteric fascia use Subcutaneous Tissue and Fascia, Face
Mastectomy
  see Excision, Skin and Breast 0HB
  see Resection, Skin and Breast 0HT
Mastoid air cells
  use Sinus, Mastoid, Left
  use Sinus, Mastoid, Right
Mastoid (postauricular) lymph node
  use Lymphatic, Neck, Left
  use Lymphatic, Neck, Right
Mastoid process
  use Bone, Temporal, Left
  use Bone, Temporal, Right
Mastoidectomy
  see Excision, Ear, Nose, Sinus 09B
  see Resection, Ear, Nose, Sinus 09T
Mastoidotomy see Drainage, Ear, Nose, Sinus 099
Mastopexy
  see Repair, Skin and Breast 0HQ
  see Reposition, Skin and Breast 0HS
Mastorrhaphy see Repair, Skin and Breast 0HQ
Mastotomy see Drainage, Skin and Breast 0H9
Maxillary artery
  use Artery, External Carotid, Left
  use Artery, External Carotid, Right
Maxillary nerve use Nerve, Trigeminal
Maximo II DR (VR) use Defibrillator Generator in 0JH
Maximo II DR CRT-D use Cardiac Resynchronization Defibrillator Pulse Generator in 0JH
Measurement
Arterial
  Flow
    Coronary 4A03
    Peripheral 4A03
    Pulmonary 4A03
  Pressure
    Coronary 4A03
    Peripheral 4A03
    Pulmonary 4A03
    Thoracic, Other 4A03
  Pulse
    Coronary 4A03
    Peripheral 4A03
    Pulmonary 4A03
  Saturation, Peripheral 4A03
  Sound, Peripheral 4A03
Biliary
  Flow 4A0C
  Pressure 4A0C
Cardiac
  Action Currents 4A02
  Defibrillator 4B02XTZ
  Electrical Activity 4A02
    Guidance 4A02X4A
    No Qualifier 4A02X4Z
  Output 4A02
  Pacemaker 4B02XSZ
  Rate 4A02
  Rhythm 4A02
  Sampling and Pressure
    Bilateral 4A02
    Left Heart 4A02
    Right Heart 4A02
  Sound 4A02
  Total Activity, Stress 4A02XM4
Central Nervous
  Conductivity 4A00
  Electrical Activity 4A00
  Pressure 4A000BZ
    Intracranial 4A00
  Saturation, Intracranial 4A00
  Stimulator 4B00XVZ
  Temperature, Intracranial 4A00
Circulatory, Volume 4A05XLZ
Gastrointestinal
  Motility 4A0B
  Pressure 4A0B
  Secretion 4A0B

Monitoring — continued
  Products of Conception — continued
    Nervous — continued
      Pressure 4A1J
    Respiratory
      Capacity 4A19
      Flow 4A19
      Rate 4A19
      Resistance 4A19
      Volume 4A19
    Sleep 4A1ZXQZ
    Temperature 4A1Z
    Urinary
      Contractility 4A1D73Z
      Flow 4A1D75Z
      Pressure 4A1D7BZ
      Resistance 4A1D7DZ
      Volume 4A1D7LZ
    Venous
      Flow
        Central 4A14
        Peripheral 4A14
        Portal 4A14
        Pulmonary 4A14
      Pressure
        Central 4A14
        Peripheral 4A14
        Portal 4A14
        Pulmonary 4A14
      Pulse
        Central 4A14
        Peripheral 4A14
        Portal 4A14
        Pulmonary 4A14
      Saturation
        Central 4A14
        Portal 4A14
        Pulmonary 4A14
Monitoring Device
  Abdomen ØJH8
  Chest ØJH6
Motor Function Assessment F01
Motor Treatment F07
MR Angiography
  see Magnetic Resonance Imaging (MRI), Heart B23
  see Magnetic Resonance Imaging (MRI), Lower Arteries B43
  see Magnetic Resonance Imaging (MRI), Upper Arteries B33
Multiple sleep latency test 4A0ZXQZ
Musculocutaneous nerve *use* Nerve, Brachial Plexus
Musculopexy
  see Repair, Muscles ØKQ
  see Reposition, Muscles ØKS
Musculophrenic artery
  use Artery, Internal Mammary, Left
  use Artery, Internal Mammary, Right
Musculoplasty
  see Repair, Muscles ØKQ
  see Supplement, Muscles ØKU
Musculorrhaphy *see* Repair, Muscles ØKQ
Musculospiral nerve *use* Nerve, Radial
Myectomy
  see Excision, Muscles ØKB
  see Resection, Muscles ØKT
Myelencephalon *use* Medulla Oblongata
Myelogram
  CT *see* Computerized Tomography (CT Scan), Central Nervous System B02
  MRI *see* Magnetic Resonance Imaging (MRI), Central Nervous System B03
Myenteric (Auerbach's) plexus *use* Nerve, Abdominal Sympathetic
Myomectomy *see* Excision, Female Reproductive System ØUB
Myometrium *use* Uterus
Myopexy
  see Repair, Muscles ØKQ
  see Reposition, Muscles ØKS
Myoplasty
  see Repair, Muscles ØKQ
  see Supplement, Muscles ØKU
Myorrhaphy *see* Repair, Muscles ØKQ
Myoscopy *see* Inspection, Muscles ØKJ

Myotomy
  see Division, Muscles ØK8
  see Drainage, Muscles ØK9
Myringectomy
  see Excision, Ear, Nose, Sinus Ø9B
  see Resection, Ear, Nose, Sinus Ø9T
Myringoplasty
  see Repair, Ear, Nose, Sinus Ø9Q
  see Replacement, Ear, Nose, Sinus Ø9R
  see Supplement, Ear, Nose, Sinus Ø9U
Myringostomy *see* Drainage, Ear, Nose, Sinus Ø99
Myringotomy *see* Drainage, Ear, Nose, Sinus Ø99

N

Nail bed
  use Finger Nail
  use Toe Nail
Nail plate
  use Finger Nail
  use Toe Nail
Narcosynthesis GZGZZZZ
Nasal cavity *use* Nose
Nasal concha *use* Turbinate, Nasal
Nasalis muscle *use* Muscle, Facial
Nasolacrimal duct
  use Duct, Lacrimal, Left
  use Duct, Lacrimal, Right
Nasopharyngeal airway (NPA) *use* Intraluminal Device, Airway in Ear, Nose, Sinus
Navicular bone
  use Tarsal, Left
  use Tarsal, Right
Near Infrared Spectroscopy, Circulatory System 8E023DZ
Neck of femur
  use Femur, Upper, Left
  use Femur, Upper, Right
Neck of humerus (anatomical)(surgical)
  use Humeral Head, Left
  use Humeral Head, Right
Nephrectomy
  see Excision, Urinary System ØTB
  see Resection, Urinary System ØTT
Nephrolithotomy *see* Extirpation, Urinary System ØTC
Nephrolysis *see* Release, Urinary System ØTN
Nephropexy
  see Repair, Urinary System ØTQ
  see Reposition, Urinary System ØTS
Nephroplasty
  see Repair, Urinary System ØTQ
  see Supplement, Urinary System ØTU
Nephropyeloureterostomy
  see Bypass, Urinary System ØT1
  see Drainage, Urinary System ØT9
Nephrorrhaphy *see* Repair, Urinary System ØTQ
Nephroscopy, transurethral ØTJ58ZZ
Nephrostomy
  see Bypass, Urinary System ØT1
  see Drainage, Urinary System ØT9
Nephrotomography
  see Fluoroscopy, Urinary System BT1
  see Plain Radiography, Urinary System BT0
Nephrotomy
  see Division, Urinary System ØT8
  see Drainage, Urinary System ØT9
Nerve conduction study
  see Measurement, Central Nervous 4A00
  see Measurement, Peripheral Nervous 4A01
Nerve Function Assessment F01
Nerve to the stapedius *use* Nerve, Facial
Neurectomy
  see Excision, Central Nervous System 00B
  see Excision, Peripheral Nervous System 01B
Neurexeresis
  see Extraction, Central Nervous System 00D
  see Extraction, Peripheral Nervous System 01D
Neurohypophysis *use* Gland, Pituitary
Neurolysis
  see Release, Central Nervous System 00N
  see Release, Peripheral Nervous System 01N
Neuromuscular electrical stimulation (NEMS) lead
  use Stimulator Lead in Muscles

Neurophysiologic monitoring *see* Monitoring, Central Nervous 4A10
Neuroplasty
  see Repair, Central Nervous System 00Q
  see Repair, Peripheral Nervous System 01Q
  see Supplement, Central Nervous System 00U
  see Supplement, Peripheral Nervous System 01U
Neurorrhaphy
  see Repair, Central Nervous System 00Q
  see Repair, Peripheral Nervous System 01Q
Neurostimulator Generator
  Insertion of device in, Skull 0NH00NZ
  Removal of device from, Skull 0NP00NZ
  Revision of device in, Skull 0NW00NZ
Neurostimulator generator, multiple channel *use* Stimulator Generator, Multiple Array in 0JH
Neurostimulator generator, multiple channel rechargeable *use* Stimulator Generator, Multiple Array Rechargeable in 0JH
Neurostimulator generator, single channel *use* Stimulator Generator, Single Array in 0JH
Neurostimulator generator, single channel rechargeable *use* Stimulator Generator, Single Array Rechargeable in 0JH
Neurostimulator Lead
  Insertion of device in
    Brain 00H0
    Cerebral Ventricle 00H6
    Nerve
      Cranial 00HE
      Peripheral 01HY
    Spinal Canal 00HU
    Spinal Cord 00HV
  Removal of device from
    Brain 00P0
    Cerebral Ventricle 00P6
    Nerve
      Cranial 00PE
      Peripheral 01PY
    Spinal Canal 00PU
    Spinal Cord 00PV
  Revision of device in
    Brain 00W0
    Cerebral Ventricle 00W6
    Nerve
      Cranial 00WE
      Peripheral 01WY
    Spinal Canal 00WU
    Spinal Cord 00WV
Neurotomy
  see Division, Central Nervous System 008
  see Division, Peripheral Nervous System 018
Neurotripsy
  see Destruction, Central Nervous System 005
  see Destruction, Peripheral Nervous System 015
Neutralization plate
  use Internal Fixation Device in Head and Facial Bones
  use Internal Fixation Device in Lower Bones
  use Internal Fixation Device in Upper Bones
Ninth cranial nerve *use* Nerve, Glossopharyngeal
Nitinol framed polymer mesh *use* Synthetic Substitute
Non-tunneled central venous catheter *use* Infusion Device
Nonimaging Nuclear Medicine Assay
  Bladder, Kidneys and Ureters CT63
  Blood C763
  Kidneys, Ureters and Bladder CT63
  Lymphatics and Hematologic System C76YYZZ
  Ureters, Kidneys and Bladder CT63
  Urinary System CT6YYZZ
Nonimaging Nuclear Medicine Probe CP5YYZZ
  Abdomen CW50
  Abdomen and Chest CW54
  Abdomen and Pelvis CW51
  Brain C050
  Central Nervous System C05YYZZ
  Chest CW53
  Chest and Abdomen CW54
  Chest and Neck CW56
  Extremity
    Lower CP5
    Upper CP5
  Head and Neck CW5B
  Heart C25YYZZ
    Right and Left C256

Nonimaging Nuclear Medicine Probe —
continued
Lymphatics
Head C75J
Head and Neck C755
Lower Extremity C75P
Neck C75K
Pelvic C75D
Trunk C75M
Upper Chest C75L
Upper Extremity C75N
Lymphatics and Hematologic System C75YYZZ
Neck and Chest CW56
Neck and Head CW5B
Pelvic Region CW5J
Pelvis and Abdomen CW51
Spine CP55ZZZ
Nonimaging Nuclear Medicine Uptake
Endocrine System CG4YYZZ
Gland, Thyroid CG42
Nostril *use* Nose
Novacor Left Ventricular Assist Device *use* Implantable Heart Assist System in Heart and Great Vessels
Novation® Ceramic AHS® (Articulation Hip System) *use* Synthetic Substitute, Ceramic in ØSR
Nuclear medicine
see Nonimaging Nuclear Medicine Assay
see Nonimaging Nuclear Medicine Probe
see Nonimaging Nuclear Medicine Uptake
see Planar Nuclear Medicine Imaging
see Positron Emission Tomographic (PET) Imaging
see Systemic Nuclear Medicine Therapy
see Tomographic (Tomo) Nuclear Medicine Imaging
Nuclear scintigraphy *see* Nuclear Medicine
Nutrition, concentrated substances
Enteral infusion 3E0G36Z
Parenteral (peripheral) infusion *see* Introduction of Nutritional Substance

O

Obliteration *see* Destruction
Obturator artery
use Artery, Internal Iliac, Left
use Artery, Internal Iliac, Right
Obturator lymph node *use* Lymphatic, Pelvis
Obturator muscle
use Muscle, Hip, Left
use Muscle, Hip, Right
Obturator nerve *use* Nerve, Lumbar Plexus
Obturator vein
use Vein, Hypogastric, Left
use Vein, Hypogastric, Right
Obtuse margin *use* Heart, Left
Occipital artery
use Artery, External Carotid, Left
use Artery, External Carotid, Right
Occipital lobe *use* Cerebral Hemisphere
Occipital lymph node
use Lymphatic, Neck, Left
use Lymphatic, Neck, Right
Occipitofrontalis muscle *use* Muscle, Facial
Occlusion
Ampulla of Vater ØFLC
Anus ØDLQ
Aorta, Abdominal 04L0
Artery
Anterior Tibial
Left 04LQ
Right 04LP
Axillary
Left 03L6
Right 03L5
Brachial
Left 03L8
Right 03L7
Celiac 04L1
Colic
Left 04L7
Middle 04L8
Right 04L6
Common Carotid
Left 03LJ

Occlusion — continued
Artery — continued
Common Carotid — continued
Right 03LH
Common Iliac
Left 04LD
Right 04LC
External Carotid
Left 03LN
Right 03LM
External Iliac
Left 04LJ
Right 04LH
Face 03LR
Femoral
Left 04LL
Right 04LK
Foot
Left 04LW
Right 04LV
Gastric 04L2
Hand
Left 03LF
Right 03LD
Hepatic 04L3
Inferior Mesenteric 04LB
Innominate 03L2
Internal Carotid
Left 03LL
Right 03LK
Internal Iliac
Left, Uterine Artery, Left 04LF
Right, Uterine Artery, Right 04LE
Internal Mammary
Left 03L1
Right 03L0
Intracranial 03LG
Lower 04LY
Peroneal
Left 04LU
Right 04LT
Popliteal
Left 04LN
Right 04LM
Posterior Tibial
Left 04LS
Right 04LR
Pulmonary, Left 02LR
Radial
Left 03LC
Right 03LB
Renal
Left 04LA
Right 04L9
Splenic 04L4
Subclavian
Left 03L4
Right 03L3
Superior Mesenteric 04L5
Temporal
Left 03LT
Right 03LS
Thyroid
Left 03LV
Right 03LU
Ulnar
Left 03LA
Right 03L9
Upper 03LY
Vertebral
Left 03LQ
Right 03LP
Atrium, Left 02L7
Bladder ØTLB
Bladder Neck ØTLC
Bronchus
Lingula ØBL9
Lower Lobe
Left ØBLB
Right ØBL6
Main
Left ØBL7
Right ØBL3
Middle Lobe, Right ØBL5
Upper Lobe
Left ØBL8

Occlusion — continued
Bronchus — continued
Upper Lobe — continued
Right ØBL4
Carina ØBL2
Cecum ØDLH
Cisterna Chyli 07LL
Colon
Ascending ØDLK
Descending ØDLM
Sigmoid ØDLN
Transverse ØDLL
Cord
Bilateral ØVLH
Left ØVLG
Right ØVLF
Cul-de-sac ØULF
Duct
Common Bile ØFL9
Cystic ØFL8
Hepatic
Left ØFL6
Right ØFL5
Lacrimal
Left 08LY
Right 08LX
Pancreatic ØFLD
Accessory ØFLF
Parotid
Left ØCLC
Right ØCLB
Duodenum ØDL9
Esophagogastric Junction ØDL4
Esophagus ØDL5
Lower ØDL3
Middle ØDL2
Upper ØDL1
Fallopian Tube
Left ØUL6
Right ØUL5
Fallopian Tubes, Bilateral ØUL7
Ileocecal Valve ØDLC
Ileum ØDLB
Intestine
Large ØDLE
Left ØDLG
Right ØDLF
Small ØDL8
Jejunum ØDLA
Kidney Pelvis
Left ØTL4
Right ØTL3
Left atrial appendage (LAA) *see* Occlusion, Atrium, Left 02L7
Lymphatic
Aortic 07LD
Axillary
Left 07L6
Right 07L5
Head 07L0
Inguinal
Left 07LJ
Right 07LH
Internal Mammary
Left 07L9
Right 07L8
Lower Extremity
Left 07LG
Right 07LF
Mesenteric 07LB
Neck
Left 07L2
Right 07L1
Pelvis 07LC
Thoracic Duct 07LK
Thorax 07L7
Upper Extremity
Left 07L4
Right 07L3
Rectum ØDLP
Stomach ØDL6
Pylorus ØDL7
Trachea ØBL1
Ureter
Left ØTL7
Right ØTL6

Occlusion — continued
 Urethra ØTLD
 Vagina ØULG
 Vas Deferens
  Bilateral ØVLQ
  Left ØVLP
  Right ØVLN
 Vein
  Axillary
   Left Ø5L8
   Right Ø5L7
  Azygos Ø5LØ
  Basilic
   Left Ø5LC
   Right Ø5LB
  Brachial
   Left Ø5LA
   Right Ø5L9
  Cephalic
   Left Ø5LF
   Right Ø5LD
  Colic Ø6L7
  Common Iliac
   Left Ø6LD
   Right Ø6LC
  Esophageal Ø6L3
  External Iliac
   Left Ø6LG
   Right Ø6LF
  External Jugular
   Left Ø5LQ
   Right Ø5LP
  Face
   Left Ø5LV
   Right Ø5LT
  Femoral
   Left Ø6LN
   Right Ø6LM
  Foot
   Left Ø6LV
   Right Ø6LT
  Gastric Ø6L2
  Greater Saphenous
   Left Ø6LQ
   Right Ø6LP
  Hand
   Left Ø5LH
   Right Ø5LG
  Hemiazygos Ø5L1
  Hepatic Ø6L4
  Hypogastric
   Left Ø6LJ
   Right Ø6LH
  Inferior Mesenteric Ø6L6
  Innominate
   Left Ø5L4
   Right Ø5L3
  Internal Jugular
   Left Ø5LN
   Right Ø5LM
  Intracranial Ø5LL
  Lesser Saphenous
   Left Ø6LS
   Right Ø6LR
  Lower Ø6LY
  Portal Ø6L8
  Pulmonary
   Left Ø2LT
   Right Ø2LS
  Renal
   Left Ø6LB
   Right Ø6L9
  Splenic Ø6L1
  Subclavian
   Left Ø5L6
   Right Ø5L5
  Superior Mesenteric Ø6L5
  Upper Ø5LY
  Vertebral
   Left Ø5LS
   Right Ø5LR
 Vena Cava
  Inferior Ø6LØ
  Superior Ø2LV
Occupational therapy see Activities of Daily Living
 Treatment, Rehabilitation FØ8

Odentectomy
 see Excision, Mouth and Throat ØCB
 see Resection, Mouth and Throat ØCT
Olecranon bursa
 use Bursa and Ligament, Elbow, Left
 use Bursa and Ligament, Elbow, Right
Olecranon process
 use Ulna, Left
 use Ulna, Right
Olfactory bulb use Nerve, Olfactory
Omentectomy, omentumectomy
 see Excision, Gastrointestinal System ØDB
 see Resection, Gastrointestinal System ØDT
Omentofixation see Repair, Gastrointestinal System
 ØDQ
Omentoplasty
 see Repair, Gastrointestinal System ØDQ
 see Replacement, Gastrointestinal System ØDR
 see Supplement, Gastrointestinal System ØDU
Omentorrhaphy see Repair, Gastrointestinal System
 ØDQ
Omentotomy see Drainage, Gastrointestinal System
 ØD9
Onychectomy
 see Excision, Skin and Breast ØHB
 see Resection, Skin and Breast ØHT
Onychoplasty
 see Repair, Skin and Breast ØHQ
 see Replacement, Skin and Breast ØHR
Onychotomy see Drainage, Skin and Breast ØH9
Oophorectomy
 see Excision, Female Reproductive System ØUB
 see Resection, Female Reproductive System ØUT
Oophoropexy
 see Repair, Female Reproductive System ØUQ
 see Reposition, Female Reproductive System ØUS
Oophoroplasty
 see Repair, Female Reproductive System ØUQ
 see Supplement, Female Reproductive System ØUU
Oophororrhaphy see Repair, Female Reproductive
 System ØUQ
Oophorostomy see Drainage, Female Reproductive
 System ØU9
Oophorotomy
 see Division, Female Reproductive System ØU8
 see Drainage, Female Reproductive System ØU9
Oophorrhaphy see Repair, Female Reproductive System
 ØUQ
Ophthalmic artery
 use Artery, Internal Carotid, Left
 use Artery, Internal Carotid, Right
Ophthalmic nerve use Nerve, Trigeminal
Ophthalmic vein use Vein, Intracranial
Opponensplasty
 Tendon replacement see Replacement, Tendons ØLR
 Tendon transfer see Transfer, Tendons ØLX
Optic chiasma use Nerve, Optic
Optic disc
 use Retina, Left
 use Retina, Right
Optic foramen
 use Bone, Sphenoid, Left
 use Bone, Sphenoid, Right
Optical coherence tomography, intravascular see
 Computerized Tomography (CT Scan)
Optimizer™ III implantable pulse generator use
 Contractility Modulation Device in ØJH
Orbicularis oculi muscle
 use Eyelid, Upper, Left
 use Eyelid, Upper, Right
Orbicularis oris muscle use Muscle, Facial
Orbital fascia use Subcutaneous Tissue and Fascia, Face
Orbital portion of ethmoid bone
 use Orbit, Left
 use Orbit, Right
Orbital portion of frontal bone
 use Orbit, Left
 use Orbit, Right
Orbital portion of lacrimal bone
 use Orbit, Left
 use Orbit, Right
Orbital portion of maxilla
 use Orbit, Left
 use Orbit, Right

Orbital portion of palatine bone
 use Orbit, Left
 use Orbit, Right
Orbital portion of sphenoid bone
 use Orbit, Left
 use Orbit, Right
Orbital portion of zygomatic bone
 use Orbit, Left
 use Orbit, Right
Orchectomy, orchidectomy, orchiectomy
 see Excision, Male Reproductive System ØVB
 see Resection, Male Reproductive System ØVT
Orchidoplasty, orchioplasty
 see Repair, Male Reproductive System ØVQ
 see Replacement, Male Reproductive System ØVR
 see Supplement, Male Reproductive System ØVU
Orchidorrhaphy, orchiorrhaphy see Repair, Male Reproductive System ØVQ
Orchidotomy, orchiotomy, orchotomy see Drainage,
 Male Reproductive System ØV9
Orchiopexy
 see Repair, Male Reproductive System ØVQ
 see Reposition, Male Reproductive System ØVS
Oropharyngeal airway (OPA) use Intraluminal Device,
 Airway in Mouth and Throat
Oropharynx use Pharynx
Ossicular chain
 use Auditory Ossicle, Left
 use Auditory Ossicle, Right
Ossiculectomy
 see Excision, Ear, Nose, Sinus Ø9B
 see Resection, Ear, Nose, Sinus Ø9T
Ossiculotomy see Drainage, Ear, Nose, Sinus Ø99
Ostectomy
 see Excision, Head and Facial Bones ØNB
 see Excision, Lower Bones ØQB
 see Excision, Upper Bones ØPB
 see Resection, Head and Facial Bones ØNT
 see Resection, Lower Bones ØQT
 see Resection, Upper Bones ØPT
Osteoclasis
 see Division, Head and Facial Bones ØN8
 see Division, Lower Bones ØQ8
 see Division, Upper Bones ØP8
Osteolysis
 see Release, Head and Facial Bones ØNN
 see Release, Lower Bones ØQN
 see Release, Upper Bones ØPN
Osteopathic Treatment
 Abdomen 7WØ9X
 Cervical 7WØ1X
 Extremity
  Lower 7WØ6X
  Upper 7WØ7X
 Head 7WØØX
 Lumbar 7WØ3X
 Pelvis 7WØ5X
 Rib Cage 7WØ8X
 Sacrum 7WØ4X
 Thoracic 7WØ2X
Osteopexy
 see Repair, Head and Facial Bones ØNQ
 see Repair, Lower Bones ØQQ
 see Repair, Upper Bones ØPQ
 see Reposition, Head and Facial Bones ØNS
 see Reposition, Lower Bones ØQS
 see Reposition, Upper Bones ØPS
Osteoplasty
 see Repair, Head and Facial Bones ØNQ
 see Repair, Lower Bones ØQQ
 see Repair, Upper Bones ØPQ
 see Replacement, Head and Facial Bones ØNR
 see Replacement, Lower Bones ØQR
 see Replacement, Upper Bones ØPR
 see Supplement, Head and Facial Bones ØNU
 see Supplement, Lower Bones ØQU
 see Supplement, Upper Bones ØPU
Osteorrhaphy
 see Repair, Head and Facial Bones ØNQ
 see Repair, Lower Bones ØQQ
 see Repair, Upper Bones ØPQ
Osteotomy, ostotomy
 see Division, Head and Facial Bones ØN8
 see Division, Lower Bones ØQ8

Osteotomy, ostotomy — continued
  see Division, Upper Bones ØP8
  see Drainage, Head and Facial Bones ØN9
  see Drainage, Lower Bones ØQ9
  see Drainage, Upper Bones ØP9
Otic ganglion *use* Nerve, Head and Neck Sympathetic
Otoplasty
  see Repair, Ear, Nose, Sinus Ø9Q
  see Replacement, Ear, Nose, Sinus Ø9R
  see Supplement, Ear, Nose, Sinus Ø9U
Otoscopy *see* Inspection, Ear, Nose, Sinus Ø9J
Oval window
  use Ear, Middle, Left
  use Ear, Middle, Right
Ovarian artery *use* Aorta, Abdominal
Ovarian ligament *use* Uterine Supporting Structure
Ovariectomy
  see Excision, Female Reproductive System ØUB
  see Resection, Female Reproductive System ØUT
Ovariocentesis *see* Drainage, Female Reproductive
  System ØU9
Ovariopexy
  see Repair, Female Reproductive System ØUQ
  see Reposition, Female Reproductive System ØUS
Ovariotomy
  see Division, Female Reproductive System ØU8
  see Drainage, Female Reproductive System ØU9
Ovatio™ CRT-D *use* Cardiac Resynchronization Defibril-
  lator Pulse Generator in ØJH
Oversewing
  Gastrointestinal ulcer *see* Repair, Gastrointestinal
    System ØDQ
  Pleural bleb *see* Repair, Respiratory System ØBQ
Oviduct
  use Fallopian Tube, Left
  use Fallopian Tube, Right
Oxidized zirconium ceramic hip bearing surface
  use Synthetic Substitute, Ceramic on Polyethylene
    in ØSR
Oximetry, Fetal pulse 1ØH073Z
Oxygenation
  Extracorporeal membrane (ECMO) *see* Assistance,
    Circulatory 5AØ5
  Hyperbaric *see* Assistance, Circulatory 5AØ5
  Supersaturated *see* Assistance, Circulatory 5AØ5

P

Pacemaker
  Dual Chamber
    Abdomen ØJH8
    Chest ØJH6
  Single Chamber
    Abdomen ØJH8
    Chest ØJH6
  Single Chamber Rate Responsive
    Abdomen ØJH8
    Chest ØJH6
Packing
  Abdominal Wall 2W43X5Z
  Anorectal 2Y43X5Z
  Arm
    Lower
      Left 2W4DX5Z
      Right 2W4CX5Z
    Upper
      Left 2W4BX5Z
      Right 2W4AX5Z
  Back 2W45X5Z
  Chest Wall 2W44X5Z
  Ear 2Y42X5Z
  Extremity
    Lower
      Left 2W4MX5Z
      Right 2W4LX5Z
    Upper
      Left 2W49X5Z
      Right 2W48X5Z
  Face 2W41X5Z
  Finger
    Left 2W4KX5Z
    Right 2W4JX5Z
  Foot
    Left 2W4TX5Z

Packing — continued
  Foot — continued
    Right 2W4SX5Z
  Genital Tract, Female 2Y44X5Z
  Hand
    Left 2W4FX5Z
    Right 2W4EX5Z
  Head 2W40X5Z
  Inguinal Region
    Left 2W47X5Z
    Right 2W46X5Z
  Leg
    Lower
      Left 2W4RX5Z
      Right 2W4QX5Z
    Upper
      Left 2W4PX5Z
      Right 2W4NX5Z
  Mouth and Pharynx 2Y40X5Z
  Nasal 2Y41X5Z
  Neck 2W42X5Z
  Thumb
    Left 2W4HX5Z
    Right 2W4GX5Z
  Toe
    Left 2W4VX5Z
    Right 2W4UX5Z
  Urethra 2Y45X5Z
Paclitaxel-eluting coronary stent *use* Intraluminal
  Device, Drug-eluting in Heart and Great Vessels
Paclitaxel-eluting peripheral stent
  use Intraluminal Device, Drug-eluting in Lower Arter-
    ies
  use Intraluminal Device, Drug-eluting in Upper Arter-
    ies
Palatine gland *use* Buccal Mucosa
Palatine tonsil *use* Tonsils
Palatine uvula *use* Uvula
Palatoglossal muscle *use* Muscle, Tongue, Palate,
  Pharynx
Palatopharyngeal muscle *use* Muscle, Tongue, Palate,
  Pharynx
Palatoplasty
  see Repair, Mouth and Throat ØCQ
  see Replacement, Mouth and Throat ØCR
  see Supplement, Mouth and Throat ØCU
Palatorrhaphy *see* Repair, Mouth and Throat ØCQ
Palmar cutaneous nerve
  use Nerve, Median
  use Nerve, Radial
Palmar (volar) digital vein
  use Vein, Hand, Left
  use Vein, Hand, Right
Palmar fascia (aponeurosis)
  use Subcutaneous Tissue and Fascia, Hand, Left
  use Subcutaneous Tissue and Fascia, Hand, Right
Palmar interosseous muscle
  use Muscle, Hand, Left
  use Muscle, Hand, Right
Palmar (volar) metacarpal vein
  use Vein, Hand, Left
  use Vein, Hand, Right
Palmar ulnocarpal ligament
  use Bursa and Ligament, Wrist, Left
  use Bursa and Ligament, Wrist, Right
Palmaris longus muscle
  use Muscle, Lower Arm and Wrist, Left
  use Muscle, Lower Arm and Wrist, Right
Pancreatectomy
  see Excision, Pancreas ØFBG
  see Resection, Pancreas ØFTG
Pancreatic artery *use* Artery, Splenic
Pancreatic plexus *use* Nerve, Abdominal Sympathetic
Pancreatic vein *use* Vein, Splenic
Pancreaticoduodenostomy *see* Bypass, Hepatobiliary
  System and Pancreas ØF1
Pancreaticosplenic lymph node *use* Lymphatic, Aortic
Pancreatogram, endoscopic retrograde *see* Fluo-
  roscopy, Pancreatic Duct BF18
Pancreatolithotomy *see* Extirpation, Pancreas ØFCG
Pancreatotomy
  see Division, Pancreas ØF8G
  see Drainage, Pancreas ØF9G
Panniculectomy
  see Excision, Abdominal Wall ØWBF

Panniculectomy — continued
  see Excision, Skin, Abdomen ØHB7
Paraaortic lymph node *use* Lymphatic, Aortic
Paracentesis
  Eye *see* Drainage, Eye Ø89
  Peritoneal Cavity *see* Drainage, Peritoneal Cavity
    ØW9G
  Tympanum *see* Drainage, Ear, Nose, Sinus Ø99
Pararectal lymph node *use* Lymphatic, Mesenteric
Parasternal lymph node *use* Lymphatic, Thorax
Parathyroidectomy
  see Excision, Endocrine System ØGB
  see Resection, Endocrine System ØGT
Paratracheal lymph node *use* Lymphatic, Thorax
Paraurethral (Skene's) gland *use* Gland, Vestibular
Parenteral nutrition, total *see* Introduction of Nutri-
  tional Substance
Parietal lobe *use* Cerebral Hemisphere
Parotid lymph node *use* Lymphatic, Head
Parotid plexus *use* Nerve, Facial
Parotidectomy
  see Excision, Mouth and Throat ØCB
  see Resection, Mouth and Throat ØCT
Pars flaccida
  use Tympanic Membrane, Left
  use Tympanic Membrane, Right
Partial joint replacement
  Hip *see* Replacement, Lower Joints ØSR
  Knee *see* Replacement, Lower Joints ØSR
  Shoulder *see* Replacement, Upper Joints ØRR
Partially absorbable mesh *use* Synthetic Substitute
Patch, blood, spinal 3EØS3GC
Patellapexy
  see Repair, Lower Bones ØQQ
  see Reposition, Lower Bones ØQS
Patellaplasty
  see Repair, Lower Bones ØQQ
  see Replacement, Lower Bones ØQR
  see Supplement, Lower Bones ØQU
Patellar ligament
  use Bursa and Ligament, Knee, Left
  use Bursa and Ligament, Knee, Right
Patellar tendon
  use Tendon, Knee, Left
  use Tendon, Knee, Right
Patellectomy
  see Excision, Lower Bones ØQB
  see Resection, Lower Bones ØQT
Patellofemoral joint
  use Joint, Knee, Left
  use Joint, Knee, Left, Femoral Surface
  use Joint, Knee, Right
  use Joint, Knee, Right, Femoral Surface
Pectineus muscle
  use Muscle, Upper Leg, Left
  use Muscle, Upper Leg, Right
Pectoral fascia *use* Subcutaneous Tissue and Fascia,
  Chest
Pectoral (anterior) lymph node
  use Lymphatic, Axillary, Left
  use Lymphatic, Axillary, Right
Pectoralis major muscle
  use Muscle, Thorax, Left
  use Muscle, Thorax, Right
Pectoralis minor muscle
  use Muscle, Thorax, Left
  use Muscle, Thorax, Right
Pedicle-based dynamic stabilization device
  use Spinal Stabilization Device, Pedicle-Based in ØRH
  use Spinal Stabilization Device, Pedicle-Based in ØSH
PEEP (positive end expiratory pressure) *see* Assistance, Respiratory 5AØ9
PEG (percutaneous endoscopic gastrostomy)
  ØDH64UZ
PEJ (percutaneous endoscopic jejunostomy)
  ØDHA4UZ
Pelvic splanchnic nerve
  use Nerve, Abdominal Sympathetic
  use Nerve, Sacral Sympathetic
Penectomy
  see Excision, Male Reproductive System ØVB
  see Resection, Male Reproductive System ØVT
Penile urethra *use* Urethra

Percutaneous endoscopic gastrojejunostomy (PEG/J) tube *use* Feeding Device in Gastrointestinal System
Percutaneous endoscopic gastrostomy (PEG) tube *use* Feeding Device in Gastrointestinal System
Percutaneous nephrostomy catheter *use* Drainage Device
Percutaneous transluminal coronary angioplasty (PTCA) *see* Dilation, Heart and Great Vessels 027
Performance
  Biliary
    Multiple, Filtration 5A1C60Z
    Single, Filtration 5A1C00Z
  Cardiac
    Continuous
        Output 5A1221Z
        Pacing 5A1223Z
      Intermittent, Pacing 5A1213Z
      Single, Output, Manual 5A12012
  Circulatory, Continuous, Oxygenation, Membrane 5A15223
  Respiratory
    24-96 Consecutive Hours, Ventilation 5A1945Z
    Greater than 96 Consecutive Hours, Ventilation 5A1955Z
    Less than 24 Consecutive Hours, Ventilation 5A1935Z
    Single, Ventilation, Nonmechanical 5A19054
  Urinary
    Multiple, Filtration 5A1D60Z
    Single, Filtration 5A1D00Z
Perfusion *see* Introduction of substance in or on
Pericardiectomy
  see Excision, Pericardium 02BN
  see Resection, Pericardium 02TN
Pericardiocentesis *see* Drainage, Pericardial Cavity 0W9D
Pericardiolysis *see* Release, Pericardium 02NN
Pericardiophrenic artery
  use Artery, Internal Mammary, Left
  use Artery, Internal Mammary, Right
Pericardioplasty
  see Repair, Pericardium 02QN
  see Replacement, Pericardium 02RN
  see Supplement, Pericardium 02UN
Pericardiorrhaphy *see* Repair, Pericardium 02QN
Pericardiostomy *see* Drainage, Pericardial Cavity 0W9D
Pericardiotomy *see* Drainage, Pericardial Cavity 0W9D
Perimetrium *use* Uterus
Peripheral parenteral nutrition *see* Introduction of Nutritional Substance
Peripherally inserted central catheter (PICC) *use* Infusion Device
Peritoneal dialysis 3E1M39Z
Peritoneocentesis
  see Drainage, Peritoneal Cavity 0W9G
  see Drainage, Peritoneum 0D9W
Peritoneoplasty
  see Repair, Peritoneum 0DQW
  see Replacement, Peritoneum 0DRW
  see Supplement, Peritoneum 0DUW
Peritoneoscopy 0DJW4ZZ
Peritoneotomy *see* Drainage, Peritoneum 0D9W
Peritoneumectomy *see* Excision, Peritoneum 0DBW
Peroneus brevis muscle
  use Muscle, Lower Leg, Left
  use Muscle, Lower Leg, Right
Peroneus longus muscle
  use Muscle, Lower Leg, Left
  use Muscle, Lower Leg, Right
Pessary ring *use* Intraluminal Device, Pessary in Female Reproductive System
PET scan *see* Positron Emission Tomographic (PET) Imaging
Petrous part of temoporal bone
  use Bone, Temporal, Left
  use Bone, Temporal, Right
Phacoemulsification, lens
  With IOL implant *see* Replacement, Eye 08R
  Without IOL implant *see* Extraction, Eye 08D
Phalangectomy
  see Excision, Lower Bones 0QB
  see Excision, Upper Bones 0PB
  see Resection, Lower Bones 0QT
  see Resection, Upper Bones 0PT

Phallectomy
  see Excision, Penis 0VBS
  see Resection, Penis 0VTS
Phalloplasty
  see Repair, Penis 0VQS
  see Supplement, Penis 0VUS
Phallotomy *see* Drainage, Penis 0V9S
Pharmacotherapy
  Antabuse HZ93ZZZ
  Bupropion HZ97ZZZ
  Clonidine HZ96ZZZ
  Levo-alpha-acetyl-methadol (LAAM) HZ92ZZZ
  Methadone Maintenance HZ91ZZZ
  Naloxone HZ95ZZZ
  Naltrexone HZ94ZZZ
  Nicotine Replacement HZ90ZZZ
  Psychiatric Medication HZ98ZZZ
  Replacement Medication, Other HZ99ZZZ
Pharyngeal constrictor muscle *use* Muscle, Tongue, Palate, Pharynx
Pharyngeal plexus *use* Nerve, Vagus
Pharyngeal recess *use* Nasopharynx
Pharyngeal tonsil *use* Adenoids
Pharyngogram *see* Fluoroscopy, Pharynix B91G
Pharyngoplasty
  see Repair, Mouth and Throat 0CQ
  see Replacement, Mouth and Throat 0CR
  see Supplement, Mouth and Throat 0CU
Pharyngorrhaphy *see* Repair, Mouth and Throat 0CQ
Pharyngotomy *see* Drainage, Mouth and Throat 0C9
Pharyngotympanic tube
  use Eustachian Tube, Left
  use Eustachian Tube, Right
Pheresis
  Erythrocytes 6A55
  Leukocytes 6A55
  Plasma 6A55
  Platelets 6A55
  Stem Cells
    Cord Blood 6A55
    Hematopoietic 6A55
Phlebectomy
  see Excision, Lower Veins 06B
  see Excision, Upper Veins 05B
  see Extraction, Lower Veins 06D
  see Extraction, Upper Veins 05D
Phlebography
  see Plain Radiography, Veins B50
  Impedance 4A04X51
Phleborrhaphy
  see Repair, Lower Veins 06Q
  see Repair, Upper Veins 05Q
Phlebotomy
  see Drainage, Lower Veins 069
  see Drainage, Upper Veins 059
Photocoagulation
  for Destruction *see* Destruction
  for Repair *see* Repair
Photopheresis, therapeutic *see* Phototherapy, Circulatory 6A65
Phototherapy
  Circulatory 6A65
  Skin 6A60
Phrenectomy, phrenoneurectomy *see* Excision, Nerve, Phrenic 01B2
Phrenemphraxis *see* Destruction, Nerve, Phrenic 0152
Phrenic nerve stimulator generator *use* Stimulator Generator in Subcutaneous Tissue and Fascia
Phrenic nerve stimulator lead *use* Diaphragmatic Pacemaker Lead in Respiratory System
Phreniclasis *see* Destruction, Nerve, Phrenic 0152
Phrenicoexeresis *see* Extraction, Nerve, Phrenic 01D2
Phrenicotomy *see* Division, Nerve, Phrenic 0182
Phrenicotripsy *see* Destruction, Nerve, Phrenic 0152
Phrenoplasty
  see Repair, Respiratory System 0BQ
  see Supplement, Respiratory System 0BU
Phrenotomy *see* Drainage, Respiratory System 0B9
Physiatry *see* Motor Treatment, Rehabilitation F07
Physical medicine *see* Motor Treatment, Rehabilitation F07
Physical therapy *see* Motor Treatment, Rehabilitation F07
PHYSIOMESH™ Flexible Composite Mesh *use* Synthetic Substitute

Pia mater
  use Cerebral Meninges
  use Spinal Meninges
Pinealectomy
  see Excision, Pineal Body 0GB1
  see Resection, Pineal Body 0GT1
Pinealoscopy 0GJ14ZZ
Pinealotomy *see* Drainage, Pineal Body 0G91
Pinna
  use Ear, External, Bilateral
  use Ear, External, Left
  use Ear, External, Right
Pipeline™ Embolization device (PED) *use* Intraluminal Device
Piriform recess (sinus) *use* Pharynx
Piriformis muscle
  use Muscle, Hip, Left
  use Muscle, Hip, Right
Pisiform bone
  use Carpal, Left
  use Carpal, Right
Pisohamate ligament
  use Bursa and Ligament, Hand, Left
  use Bursa and Ligament, Hand, Right
Pisometacarpal ligament
  use Bursa and Ligament, Hand, Left
  use Bursa and Ligament, Hand, Right
Pituitectomy
  see Excision, Gland, Pituitary 0GB0
  see Resection, Gland, Pituitary 0GT0
Plain film radiology *see* Plain Radiography
Plain Radiography
  Abdomen BW00ZZZ
  Abdomen and Pelvis BW01ZZZ
  Abdominal Lymphatic
    Bilateral B701
    Unilateral B700
  Airway, Upper BB0DZZZ
  Ankle
    Left BQ0H
    Right BQ0G
  Aorta
    Abdominal B400
    Thoracic B300
    Thoraco-Abdominal B30P
  Aorta and Bilateral Lower Extremity Arteries B40D
  Arch
    Bilateral BN0DZZZ
    Left BN0CZZZ
    Right BN0BZZZ
  Arm
    Left BP0FZZZ
    Right BP0EZZZ
  Artery
    Brachiocephalic-Subclavian, Right B301
    Bronchial B30L
    Bypass Graft, Other B20F
    Cervico-Cerebral Arch B30Q
    Common Carotid
      Bilateral B305
      Left B304
      Right B303
    Coronary
      Bypass Graft
        Multiple B203
        Single B202
      Multiple B201
      Single B200
    External Carotid
      Bilateral B30C
      Left B30B
      Right B309
    Hepatic B402
    Inferior Mesenteric B405
    Intercostal B30L
    Internal Carotid
      Bilateral B308
      Left B307
      Right B306
    Internal Mammary Bypass Graft
      Left B208
      Right B207
    Intra-Abdominal, Other B40B
    Intracranial B30R
    Lower Extremity
      Bilateral and Aorta B40D

Plain Radiography — continued
Vein — continued
  Jugular — continued
    Right B503
  Lower Extremity
    Bilateral B50D
    Left B50C
    Right B50B
  Other B50V
  Pelvic (Iliac)
    Left B50G
    Right B50F
  Pelvic (Iliac) Bilateral B50H
  Portal B50T
  Pulmonary
    Bilateral B50S
    Left B50R
    Right B50Q
  Renal
    Bilateral B50L
    Left B50K
    Right B50J
  Spanchnic B50T
  Subclavian
    Left B507
    Right B506
  Upper Extremity
    Bilateral B50P
    Left B50N
    Right B50M
Vena Cava
  Inferior B509
  Superior B508
Whole Body BW0KZZZ
  Infant BW0MZZZ
Whole Skeleton BW0LZZZ
Wrist
  Left BP0M
  Right BP0L

Planar Nuclear Medicine Imaging CP1
Abdomen CW10
Abdomen and Chest CW14
Abdomen and Pelvis CW11
Anatomical Regions, Multiple CW1YYZZ
Bladder and Ureters CT1H
Bladder, Kidneys and Ureters CT13
Blood C713
Bone Marrow C710
Brain C010
Breast CH1YYZZ
  Bilateral CH12
  Left CH11
  Right CH10
Bronchi and Lungs CB12
Central Nervous System C01YYZZ
Cerebrospinal Fluid C015
Chest CW13
Chest and Abdomen CW14
Chest and Neck CW16
Digestive System CD1YYZZ
Ducts, Lacrimal, Bilateral C819
Ear, Nose, Mouth and Throat C91YYZZ
Endocrine System CG1YYZZ
Extremity
  Lower CW1D
    Bilateral CP1F
    Left CP1D
    Right CP1C
  Upper CW1M
    Bilateral CP1B
    Left CP19
    Right CP18
Eye C81YYZZ
Gallbladder CF14
Gastrointestinal Tract CD17
  Upper CD15
Gland
  Adrenal, Bilateral CG14
  Parathyroid CG11
  Thyroid CG12
Glands, Salivary, Bilateral C91B
Head and Neck CW1B
Heart C21YYZZ
  Right and Left C216
Hepatobiliary System, All CF1C
Hepatobiliary System and Pancreas CF1YYZZ

Planar Nuclear Medicine Imaging — continued
Kidneys, Ureters and Bladder CT13
Liver CF15
Liver and Spleen CF16
Lungs and Bronchi CB12
Lymphatics
  Head C71J
  Head and Neck C715
  Lower Extremity C71P
  Neck C71K
  Pelvic C71D
  Trunk C71M
  Upper Chest C71L
  Upper Extremity C71N
Lymphatics and Hematologic System C71YYZZ
Musculoskeletal System, All CP1Z
Myocardium C21G
Neck and Chest CW16
Neck and Head CW1B
Pancreas and Hepatobiliary System CF1YYZZ
Pelvic Region CW1J
Pelvis CP16
Pelvis and Abdomen CW11
Pelvis and Spine CP17
Reproductive System, Male CV1YYZZ
Respiratory System CB1YYZZ
Skin CH1YYZZ
Skull CP11
Spine CP15
Spine and Pelvis CP17
Spleen C712
Spleen and Liver CF16
Subcutaneous Tissue CH1YYZZ
Testicles, Bilateral CV19
Thorax CP14
Ureters and Bladder CT1H
Ureters, Kidneys and Bladder CT13
Urinary System CT1YYZZ
Veins C51YYZZ
  Central C51R
  Lower Extremity
    Bilateral C51D
    Left C51C
    Right C51B
  Upper Extremity
    Bilateral C51Q
    Left C51P
    Right C51N
Whole Body CW1N

Plantar digital vein
  use Vein, Foot, Left
  use Vein, Foot, Right
Plantar fascia (aponeurosis)
  use Subcutaneous Tissue and Fascia, Foot, Left
  use Subcutaneous Tissue and Fascia, Foot, Right
Plantar metatarsal vein
  use Vein, Foot, Left
  use Vein, Foot, Right
Plantar venous arch
  use Vein, Foot, Left
  use Vein, Foot, Right
Plaque Radiation
Abdomen DWY3FZZ
Adrenal Gland DGY2FZZ
Anus DDY8FZZ
Bile Ducts DFY2FZZ
Bladder DTY2FZZ
Bone Marrow D7Y0FZZ
Bone, Other DPYCFZZ
Brain D0Y0FZZ
Brain Stem D0Y1FZZ
Breast
  Left DMY0FZZ
  Right DMY1FZZ
Bronchus DBY1FZZ
Cervix DUY1FZZ
Chest DWY2FZZ
Chest Wall DBY7FZZ
Colon DDY5FZZ
Diaphragm DBY8FZZ
Duodenum DDY2FZZ
Ear D9Y0FZZ
Esophagus DDY0FZZ
Eye D8Y0FZZ
Femur DPY9FZZ
Fibula DPYBFZZ

Plaque Radiation — continued
Gallbladder DFY1FZZ
Gland
  Adrenal DGY2FZZ
  Parathyroid DGY4FZZ
  Pituitary DGY0FZZ
  Thyroid DGY5FZZ
Glands, Salivary D9Y6FZZ
Head and Neck DWY1FZZ
Hemibody DWY4FZZ
Humerus DPY6FZZ
Ileum DDY4FZZ
Jejunum DDY3FZZ
Kidney DTY0FZZ
Larynx D9YBFZZ
Liver DFY0FZZ
Lung DBY2FZZ
Lymphatics
  Abdomen D7Y6FZZ
  Axillary D7Y4FZZ
  Inguinal D7Y8FZZ
  Neck D7Y3FZZ
  Pelvis D7Y7FZZ
  Thorax D7Y5FZZ
Mandible DPY3FZZ
Maxilla DPY2FZZ
Mediastinum DBY6FZZ
Mouth D9Y4FZZ
Nasopharynx D9YDFZZ
Neck and Head DWY1FZZ
Nerve, Peripheral D0Y7FZZ
Nose D9Y1FZZ
Ovary DUY0FZZ
Palate
  Hard D9Y8FZZ
  Soft D9Y9FZZ
Pancreas DFY3FZZ
Parathyroid Gland DGY4FZZ
Pelvic Bones DPY8FZZ
Pelvic Region DWY6FZZ
Pharynx D9YCFZZ
Pineal Body DGY1FZZ
Pituitary Gland DGY0FZZ
Pleura DBY5FZZ
Prostate DVY0FZZ
Radius DPY7FZZ
Rectum DDY7FZZ
Rib DPY5FZZ
Sinuses D9Y7FZZ
Skin
  Abdomen DHY8FZZ
  Arm DHY4FZZ
  Back DHY7FZZ
  Buttock DHY9FZZ
  Chest DHY6FZZ
  Face DHY2FZZ
  Foot DHYCFZZ
  Hand DHY5FZZ
  Leg DHYBFZZ
  Neck DHY3FZZ
Skull DPY0FZZ
Spinal Cord D0Y6FZZ
Spleen D7Y2FZZ
Sternum DPY4FZZ
Stomach DDY1FZZ
Testis DVY1FZZ
Thymus D7Y1FZZ
Thyroid Gland DGY5FZZ
Tibia DPYBFZZ
Tongue D9Y5FZZ
Trachea DBY0FZZ
Ulna DPY7FZZ
Ureter DTY1FZZ
Urethra DTY3FZZ
Uterus DUY2FZZ
Whole Body DWY5FZZ
Plasmapheresis, therapeutic 6A550Z3
Plateletpheresis, therapeutic 6A550Z2
Platysma muscle
  use Muscle, Neck, Left
  use Muscle, Neck, Right
Pleurectomy
  see Excision, Respiratory System 0BB
  see Resection, Respiratory System 0BT
Pleurocentesis *see* Drainage, Anatomical Regions, General 0W9

▽ **Subterms under main terms may continue to next column or page**

Pterygopalatine (sphenopalatine) ganglion *use* Nerve, Head and Neck Sympathetic

Pubic ligament
use Bursa and Ligament, Trunk, Left
use Bursa and Ligament, Trunk, Right

Pubis
use Bone, Pelvic, Left
use Bone, Pelvic, Right

Pubofemoral ligament
use Bursa and Ligament, Hip, Left
use Bursa and Ligament, Hip, Right

Pudendal nerve *use* Nerve, Sacral Plexus

Pull-through, rectal *see* Resection, Rectum ØDTP

Pulmoaortic canal *use* Artery, Pulmonary, Left

Pulmonary annulus *use* Valve, Pulmonary

Pulmonary artery wedge monitoring *see* Monitoring, Arterial 4A13

Pulmonary plexus
use Nerve, Thoracic Sympathetic
use Nerve, Vagus

Pulmonic valve *use* Valve, Pulmonary

Pulpectomy *see* Excision, Mouth and Throat ØCB

Pulverization *see* Fragmentation

Pulvinar *use* Thalamus

Pump reservoir *use* Infusion Device, Pump in Subcutaneous Tissue and Fascia

Punch biopsy *see* Excision with qualifier Diagnostic

Puncture *see* Drainage

Puncture, lumbar *see* Drainage, Spinal Canal ØØ9U

Pyelography
see Fluoroscopy, Urinary System BT1
see Plain Radiography, Urinary System BTØ

Pyeloileostomy, urinary diversion *see* Bypass, Urinary System ØT1

Pyeloplasty
see Repair, Urinary System ØTQ
see Replacement, Urinary System ØTR
see Supplement, Urinary System ØTU

Pyelorrhaphy *see* Repair, Urinary System ØTQ

Pyeloscopy ØTJ58ZZ

Pyelostomy
see Bypass, Urinary System ØT1
see Drainage, Urinary System ØT9

Pyelotomy *see* Drainage, Urinary System ØT9

Pylorectomy
see Excision, Stomach, Pylorus ØDB7
see Resection, Stomach, Pylorus ØDT7

Pyloric antrum *use* Stomach, Pylorus

Pyloric canal *use* Stomach, Pylorus

Pyloric sphincter *use* Stomach, Pylorus

Pylorodiosis *see* Dilation, Stomach, Pylorus ØD77

Pylorogastrectomy
see Excision, Gastrointestinal System ØDB
see Resection, Gastrointestinal System ØDT

Pyloroplasty
see Repair, Stomach, Pylorus ØDQ7
see Supplement, Stomach, Pylorus ØDU7

Pyloroscopy ØDJ68ZZ

Pylorotomy *see* Drainage, Stomach, Pylorus ØD97

Pyramidalis muscle
use Muscle, Abdomen, Left
use Muscle, Abdomen, Right

Q

Quadrangular cartilage *use* Septum, Nasal

Quadrant resection of breast *see* Excision, Skin and Breast ØHB

Quadrate lobe *use* Liver

Quadratus femoris muscle
use Muscle, Hip, Left
use Muscle, Hip, Right

Quadratus lumborum muscle
use Muscle, Trunk, Left
use Muscle, Trunk, Right

Quadratus plantae muscle
use Muscle, Foot, Left
use Muscle, Foot, Right

Quadriceps (femoris)
use Muscle, Upper Leg, Left
use Muscle, Upper Leg, Right

Quarantine 8EØZXY6

R

Radial collateral carpal ligament
use Bursa and Ligament, Wrist, Left
use Bursa and Ligament, Wrist, Right

Radial collateral ligament
use Bursa and Ligament, Elbow, Left
use Bursa and Ligament, Elbow, Right

Radial notch
use Ulna, Left
use Ulna, Right

Radial recurrent artery
use Artery, Radial, Left
use Artery, Radial, Right

Radial vein
use Vein, Brachial, Left
use Vein, Brachial, Right

Radialis indicis
use Artery, Hand, Left
use Artery, Hand, Right

Radiation Therapy
see Beam Radiation
see Brachytherapy

Radiation treatment *see* Radiation Therapy

Radiocarpal joint
use Joint, Wrist, Left
use Joint, Wrist, Right

Radiocarpal ligament
use Bursa and Ligament, Wrist, Left
use Bursa and Ligament, Wrist, Right

Radiography *see* Plain Radiography

Radiology, analog *see* Plain Radiography

Radiology, diagnostic *see* Imaging, Diagnostic

Radioulnar ligament
use Bursa and Ligament, Wrist, Left
use Bursa and Ligament, Wrist, Right

Range of motion testing *see* Motor Function Assessment, Rehabilitation FØ1

REALIZE® Adjustable Gastric Band *use* Extraluminal Device

Reattachment
Abdominal Wall ØWMFØZZ
Ampulla of Vater ØFMC
Ankle Region
  Left ØYMLØZZ
  Right ØYMKØZZ
Arm
  Lower
    Left ØXMFØZZ
    Right ØXMDØZZ
  Upper
    Left ØXM9ØZZ
    Right ØXM8ØZZ
Axilla
  Left ØXM5ØZZ
  Right ØXM4ØZZ
Back
  Lower ØWMLØZZ
  Upper ØWMKØZZ
Bladder ØTMB
Bladder Neck ØTMC
Breast
  Bilateral ØHMVXZZ
  Left ØHMUXZZ
  Right ØHMTXZZ
Bronchus
  Lingula ØBM9ØZZ
  Lower Lobe
    Left ØBMBØZZ
    Right ØBM6ØZZ
  Main
    Left ØBM7ØZZ
    Right ØBM3ØZZ
  Middle Lobe, Right ØBM5ØZZ
  Upper Lobe
    Left ØBM8ØZZ
    Right ØBM4ØZZ
Bursa and Ligament
  Abdomen
    Left ØMMJ
    Right ØMMH
  Ankle
    Left ØMMR
    Right ØMMQ

Reattachment — continued
Bursa and Ligament — continued
  Elbow
    Left ØMM4
    Right ØMM3
  Foot
    Left ØMMT
    Right ØMMS
  Hand
    Left ØMM8
    Right ØMM7
  Head and Neck ØMMØ
  Hip
    Left ØMMM
    Right ØMML
  Knee
    Left ØMMP
    Right ØMMN
  Lower Extremity
    Left ØMMW
    Right ØMMV
  Perineum ØMMK
  Shoulder
    Left ØMM2
    Right ØMM1
  Thorax
    Left ØMMG
    Right ØMMF
  Trunk
    Left ØMMD
    Right ØMMC
  Upper Extremity
    Left ØMMB
    Right ØMM9
  Wrist
    Left ØMM6
    Right ØMM5
Buttock
  Left ØYM1ØZZ
  Right ØYMØZZ
Carina ØBM2ØZZ
Cecum ØDMH
Cervix ØUMC
Chest Wall ØWM8ØZZ
Clitoris ØUMJXZZ
Colon
  Ascending ØDMK
  Descending ØDMM
  Sigmoid ØDMN
  Transverse ØDML
Cord
  Bilateral ØVMH
  Left ØVMG
  Right ØVMF
Cul-de-sac ØUMF
Diaphragm
  Left ØBMSØZZ
  Right ØBMRØZZ
Duct
  Common Bile ØFM9
  Cystic ØFM8
  Hepatic
    Left ØFM6
    Right ØFM5
  Pancreatic ØFMD
    Accessory ØFMF
Duodenum ØDM9
Ear
  Left Ø9M1XZZ
  Right Ø9MØXZZ
Elbow Region
  Left ØXMCØZZ
  Right ØXMBØZZ
Esophagus ØDM5
Extremity
  Lower
    Left ØYMBØZZ
    Right ØYM9ØZZ
  Upper
    Left ØXM7ØZZ
    Right ØXM6ØZZ
Eyelid
  Lower
    Left Ø8MRXZZ
    Right Ø8MQXZZ

Reattachment — continued
Eyelid — continued
  Upper
    Left 08MPXZZ
    Right 08MNXZZ
Face 0WM20ZZ
Fallopian Tube
  Left 0UM6
  Right 0UM5
Fallopian Tubes, Bilateral 0UM7
Femoral Region
  Left 0YM80ZZ
  Right 0YM70ZZ
Finger
  Index
    Left 0XMP0ZZ
    Right 0XMN0ZZ
  Little
    Left 0XMW0ZZ
    Right 0XMV0ZZ
  Middle
    Left 0XMR0ZZ
    Right 0XMQ0ZZ
  Ring
    Left 0XMT0ZZ
    Right 0XMS0ZZ
Foot
  Left 0YMN0ZZ
  Right 0YMM0ZZ
Forequarter
  Left 0XM10ZZ
  Right 0XM00ZZ
Gallbladder 0FM4
Gland
  Left 0GM2
  Right 0GM3
Hand
  Left 0XMK0ZZ
  Right 0XMJ0ZZ
Hindquarter
  Bilateral 0YM40ZZ
  Left 0YM30ZZ
  Right 0YM20ZZ
Hymen 0UMK
Ileum 0DMB
Inguinal Region
  Left 0YM60ZZ
  Right 0YM50ZZ
Intestine
  Large 0DME
    Left 0DMG
    Right 0DMF
  Small 0DM8
Jaw
  Lower 0WM50ZZ
  Upper 0WM40ZZ
Jejunum 0DMA
Kidney
  Left 0TM1
  Right 0TM0
Kidney Pelvis
  Left 0TM4
  Right 0TM3
Kidneys, Bilateral 0TM2
Knee Region
  Left 0YMG0ZZ
  Right 0YMF0ZZ
Leg
  Lower
    Left 0YMJ0ZZ
    Right 0YMH0ZZ
  Upper
    Left 0YMD0ZZ
    Right 0YMC0ZZ
Lip
  Lower 0CM10ZZ
  Upper 0CM00ZZ
Liver 0FM0
  Left Lobe 0FM2
  Right Lobe 0FM1
Lung
  Left 0BML0ZZ
  Lower Lobe
    Left 0BMJ0ZZ
    Right 0BMF0ZZ
  Middle Lobe, Right 0BMD0ZZ

Reattachment — continued
Lung — continued
  Right 0BMK0ZZ
  Upper Lobe
    Left 0BMG0ZZ
    Right 0BMC0ZZ
Lung Lingula 0BMH0ZZ
Muscle
  Abdomen
    Left 0KML
    Right 0KMK
  Facial 0KM1
  Foot
    Left 0KMW
    Right 0KMV
  Hand
    Left 0KMD
    Right 0KMC
  Head 0KM0
  Hip
    Left 0KMP
    Right 0KMN
  Lower Arm and Wrist
    Left 0KMB
    Right 0KM9
  Lower Leg
    Left 0KMT
    Right 0KMS
  Neck
    Left 0KM3
    Right 0KM2
  Perineum 0KMM
  Shoulder
    Left 0KM6
    Right 0KM5
  Thorax
    Left 0KMJ
    Right 0KMH
  Tongue, Palate, Pharynx 0KM4
  Trunk
    Left 0KMG
    Right 0KMF
  Upper Arm
    Left 0KM8
    Right 0KM7
  Upper Leg
    Left 0KMR
    Right 0KMQ
Neck 0WM60ZZ
Nipple
  Left 0HMXXZZ
  Right 0HMWXZZ
Nose 09MKXZZ
Ovary
  Bilateral 0UM2
  Left 0UM1
  Right 0UM0
Palate, Soft 0CM30ZZ
Pancreas 0FMG
Parathyroid Gland 0GMR
  Inferior
    Left 0GMP
    Right 0GMN
  Multiple 0GMQ
  Superior
    Left 0GMM
    Right 0GML
Penis 0VMSXZZ
Perineum
  Female 0WMN0ZZ
  Male 0WMM0ZZ
Rectum 0DMP
Scrotum 0VM5XZZ
Shoulder Region
  Left 0XM30ZZ
  Right 0XM20ZZ
Skin
  Abdomen 0HM7XZZ
  Back 0HM6XZZ
  Buttock 0HM8XZZ
  Chest 0HM5XZZ
  Ear
    Left 0HM3XZZ
    Right 0HM2XZZ
  Face 0HM1XZZ

Reattachment — continued
Skin — continued
  Foot
    Left 0HMNXZZ
    Right 0HMMXZZ
  Genitalia 0HMAXZZ
  Hand
    Left 0HMGXZZ
    Right 0HMFXZZ
  Lower Arm
    Left 0HMEXZZ
    Right 0HMDXZZ
  Lower Leg
    Left 0HMLXZZ
    Right 0HMKXZZ
  Neck 0HM4XZZ
  Perineum 0HM9XZZ
  Scalp 0HM0XZZ
  Upper Arm
    Left 0HMCXZZ
    Right 0HMBXZZ
  Upper Leg
    Left 0HMJXZZ
    Right 0HMHXZZ
Stomach 0DM6
Tendon
  Abdomen
    Left 0LMG
    Right 0LMF
  Ankle
    Left 0LMT
    Right 0LMS
  Foot
    Left 0LMW
    Right 0LMV
  Hand
    Left 0LM8
    Right 0LM7
  Head and Neck 0LM0
  Hip
    Left 0LMK
    Right 0LMJ
  Knee
    Left 0LMR
    Right 0LMQ
  Lower Arm and Wrist
    Left 0LM6
    Right 0LM5
  Lower Leg
    Left 0LMP
    Right 0LMN
  Perineum 0LMH
  Shoulder
    Left 0LM2
    Right 0LM1
  Thorax
    Left 0LMD
    Right 0LMC
  Trunk
    Left 0LMB
    Right 0LM9
  Upper Arm
    Left 0LM4
    Right 0LM3
  Upper Leg
    Left 0LMM
    Right 0LML
Testis
  Bilateral 0VMC
  Left 0VMB
  Right 0VM9
Thumb
  Left 0XMM0ZZ
  Right 0XML0ZZ
Thyroid Gland
  Left Lobe 0GMG
  Right Lobe 0GMH
Toe
  1st
    Left 0YMQ0ZZ
    Right 0YMP0ZZ
  2nd
    Left 0YMS0ZZ
    Right 0YMR0ZZ
  3rd
    Left 0YMU0ZZ

Subterms under main terms may continue to next column or page

Reattachment — continued
  Toe — continued
    3rd — continued
      Right ØYMTØZZ
    4th
      Left ØYMWØZZ
      Right ØYMVØZZ
    5th
      Left ØYMYØZZ
      Right ØYMXØZZ
  Tongue ØCM7ØZZ
  Tooth
    Lower ØCMX
    Upper ØCMW
  Trachea ØBM1ØZZ
  Tunica Vaginalis
    Left ØVM7
    Right ØVM6
  Ureter
    Left ØTM7
    Right ØTM6
  Ureters, Bilateral ØTM8
  Urethra ØTMD
  Uterine Supporting Structure ØUM4
  Uterus ØUM9
  Uvula ØCMNØZZ
  Vagina ØUMG
  Vulva ØUMMXZZ
  Wrist Region
    Left ØXMHØZZ
    Right ØXMGØZZ
Rebound HRD® (Hernia Repair Device) use Synthetic
  Substitute
Recession
  see Repair
  see Reposition
Reclosure, disrupted abdominal wall ØWQFXZZ
Reconstruction
  see Repair
  see Replacement
  see Supplement
Rectectomy
  see Excision, Rectum ØDBP
  see Resection, Rectum ØDTP
Rectocele repair see Repair, Subcutaneous Tissue and
  Fascia, Pelvic Region ØJQC
Rectopexy
  see Repair, Gastrointestinal System ØDQ
  see Reposition, Gastrointestinal System ØDS
Rectoplasty
  see Repair, Gastrointestinal System ØDQ
  see Supplement, Gastrointestinal System ØDU
Rectorrhaphy see Repair, Gastrointestinal System ØDQ
Rectoscopy ØDJD8ZZ
Rectosigmoid junction use Colon, Sigmoid
Rectosigmoidectomy
  see Excision, Gastrointestinal System ØDB
  see Resection, Gastrointestinal System ØDT
Rectostomy see Drainage, Rectum ØD9P
Rectotomy see Drainage, Rectum ØD9P
Rectus abdominis muscle
  use Muscle, Abdomen, Left
  use Muscle, Abdomen, Right
Rectus femoris muscle
  use Muscle, Upper Leg, Left
  use Muscle, Upper Leg, Right
Recurrent laryngeal nerve use Nerve, Vagus
Reduction
  Dislocation see Reposition
  Fracture see Reposition
  Intussusception, intestinal see Reposition, Gastroin-
    testinal System ØDS
  Mammoplasty see Excision, Skin and Breast ØHB
  Prolapse see Reposition
  Torsion see Reposition
  Volvulus, gastrointestinal see Reposition, Gastroin-
    testinal System ØDS
Refusion see Fusion
Reimplantation
  see Reattachment
  see Reposition
  see Transfer
Reinforcement
  see Repair
  see Supplement

Relaxation, scar tissue see Release
Release
  Acetabulum
    Left ØQN5
    Right ØQN4
  Adenoids ØCNQ
  Ampulla of Vater ØFNC
  Anal Sphincter ØDNR
  Anterior Chamber
    Left Ø8N33ZZ
    Right Ø8N23ZZ
  Anus ØDNQ
  Aorta
    Abdominal Ø4NØ
    Thoracic Ø2NW
  Aortic Body ØGND
  Appendix ØDNJ
  Artery
    Anterior Tibial
      Left Ø4NQ
      Right Ø4NP
    Axillary
      Left Ø3N6
      Right Ø3N5
    Brachial
      Left Ø3N8
      Right Ø3N7
    Celiac Ø4N1
    Colic
      Left Ø4N7
      Middle Ø4N8
      Right Ø4N9
    Common Carotid
      Left Ø3NJ
      Right Ø3NH
    Common Iliac
      Left Ø4ND
      Right Ø4NC
    External Carotid
      Left Ø3NN
      Right Ø3NM
    External Iliac
      Left Ø4NJ
      Right Ø4NH
    Face Ø3NR
    Femoral
      Left Ø4NL
      Right Ø4NK
    Foot
      Left Ø4NW
      Right Ø4NV
    Gastric Ø4N2
    Hand
      Left Ø3NF
      Right Ø3ND
    Hepatic Ø4N3
    Inferior Mesenteric Ø4NB
    Innominate Ø3N2
    Internal Carotid
      Left Ø3NL
      Right Ø3NK
    Internal Iliac
      Left Ø4NF
      Right Ø4NE
    Internal Mammary
      Left Ø3N1
      Right Ø3NØ
    Intracranial Ø3NG
    Lower Ø4NY
    Peroneal
      Left Ø4NU
      Right Ø4NT
    Popliteal
      Left Ø4NN
      Right Ø4NM
    Posterior Tibial
      Left Ø4NS
      Right Ø4NR
    Pulmonary
      Left Ø2NR
      Right Ø2NQ
    Pulmonary Trunk Ø2NP
    Radial
      Left Ø3NC
      Right Ø3NB

Release — continued
  Artery — continued
    Renal
      Left Ø4NA
      Right Ø4N9
    Splenic Ø4N4
    Subclavian
      Left Ø3N4
      Right Ø3N3
    Superior Mesenteric Ø4N5
    Temporal
      Left Ø3NT
      Right Ø3NS
    Thyroid
      Left Ø3NV
      Right Ø3NU
    Ulnar
      Left Ø3NA
      Right Ø3N9
    Upper Ø3NY
    Vertebral
      Left Ø3NQ
      Right Ø3NP
  Atrium
    Left Ø2N7
    Right Ø2N6
  Auditory Ossicle
    Left Ø9NAØZZ
    Right Ø9N9ØZZ
  Basal Ganglia ØØN8
  Bladder ØTNB
  Bladder Neck ØTNC
  Bone
    Ethmoid
      Left ØNNG
      Right ØNNF
    Frontal
      Left ØNN2
      Right ØNN1
    Hyoid ØNNX
    Lacrimal
      Left ØNNJ
      Right ØNNH
    Nasal ØNNB
    Occipital
      Left ØNN8
      Right ØNN7
    Palatine
      Left ØNNL
      Right ØNNK
    Parietal
      Left ØNN4
      Right ØNN3
    Pelvic
      Left ØQN3
      Right ØQN2
    Sphenoid
      Left ØNND
      Right ØNNC
    Temporal
      Left ØNN6
      Right ØNN5
    Zygomatic
      Left ØNNN
      Right ØNNM
  Brain ØØNØ
  Breast
    Bilateral ØHNV
    Left ØHNU
    Right ØHNT
  Bronchus
    Lingula ØBN9
    Lower Lobe
      Left ØBNB
      Right ØBN6
    Main
      Left ØBN7
      Right ØBN3
    Middle Lobe, Right ØBN5
    Upper Lobe
      Left ØBN8
      Right ØBN4
  Buccal Mucosa ØCN4
  Bursa and Ligament
    Abdomen
      Left ØMNJ

Release — continued
  Bursa and Ligament — continued
    Abdomen — continued
      Right ØMNH
    Ankle
      Left ØMNR
      Right ØMNQ
    Elbow
      Left ØMN4
      Right ØMN3
    Foot
      Left ØMNT
      Right ØMNS
    Hand
      Left ØMN8
      Right ØMN7
    Head and Neck ØMNØ
    Hip
      Left ØMNM
      Right ØMNL
    Knee
      Left ØMNP
      Right ØMNN
    Lower Extremity
      Left ØMNW
      Right ØMNV
    Perineum ØMNK
    Shoulder
      Left ØMN2
      Right ØMN1
    Thorax
      Left ØMNG
      Right ØMNF
    Trunk
      Left ØMND
      Right ØMNC
    Upper Extremity
      Left ØMNB
      Right ØMN9
    Wrist
      Left ØMN6
      Right ØMN5
  Carina ØBN2
  Carotid Bodies, Bilateral ØGN8
  Carotid Body
    Left ØGN6
    Right ØGN7
  Carpal
    Left ØPNN
    Right ØPNM
  Cecum ØDNH
  Cerebellum ØØNC
  Cerebral Hemisphere ØØN7
  Cerebral Meninges ØØN1
  Cerebral Ventricle ØØN6
  Cervix ØUNC
  Chordae Tendineae Ø2N9
  Choroid
    Left Ø8NB
    Right Ø8NA
  Cisterna Chyli Ø7NL
  Clavicle
    Left ØPNB
    Right ØPN9
  Clitoris ØUNJ
  Coccygeal Glomus ØGNB
  Coccyx ØQNS
  Colon
    Ascending ØDNK
    Descending ØDNM
    Sigmoid ØDNN
    Transverse ØDNL
  Conduction Mechanism Ø2N8
  Conjunctiva
    Left Ø8NTXZZ
    Right Ø8NSXZZ
  Cord
    Bilateral ØVNH
    Left ØVNG
    Right ØVNF
  Cornea
    Left Ø8N9XZZ
    Right Ø8N8XZZ
  Cul-de-sac ØUNF
  Diaphragm
    Left ØBNS

Release — continued
  Diaphragm — continued
    Right ØBNR
  Disc
    Cervical Vertebral ØRN3
    Cervicothoracic Vertebral ØRN5
    Lumbar Vertebral ØSN2
    Lumbosacral ØSN4
    Thoracic Vertebral ØRN9
    Thoracolumbar Vertebral ØRNB
  Duct
    Common Bile ØFN9
    Cystic ØFN8
    Hepatic
      Left ØFN6
      Right ØFN5
    Lacrimal
      Left Ø8NY
      Right Ø8NX
    Pancreatic ØFND
      Accessory ØFNF
    Parotid
      Left ØCNC
      Right ØCNB
  Duodenum ØDN9
  Dura Mater ØØN2
  Ear
    External
      Left Ø9N1
      Right Ø9NØ
    External Auditory Canal
      Left Ø9N4
      Right Ø9N3
    Inner
      Left Ø9NEØZZ
      Right Ø9NDØZZ
    Middle
      Left Ø9N6ØZZ
      Right Ø9N5ØZZ
  Epididymis
    Bilateral ØVNL
    Left ØVNK
    Right ØVNJ
  Epiglottis ØCNR
  Esophagogastric Junction ØDN4
  Esophagus ØDN5
    Lower ØDN3
    Middle ØDN2
    Upper ØDN1
  Eustachian Tube
    Left Ø9NG
    Right Ø9NF
  Eye
    Left Ø8N1XZZ
    Right Ø8NØXZZ
  Eyelid
    Lower
      Left Ø8NR
      Right Ø8NQ
    Upper
      Left Ø8NP
      Right Ø8NN
  Fallopian Tube
    Left ØUN6
    Right ØUN5
  Fallopian Tubes, Bilateral ØUN7
  Femoral Shaft
    Left ØQN9
    Right ØQN8
  Femur
    Lower
      Left ØQNC
      Right ØQNB
    Upper
      Left ØQN7
      Right ØQN6
  Fibula
    Left ØQNK
    Right ØQNJ
  Finger Nail ØHNQXZZ
  Gallbladder ØFN4
  Gingiva
    Lower ØCN6
    Upper ØCN5

Release — continued
  Gland
    Adrenal
      Bilateral ØGN4
      Left ØGN2
      Right ØGN3
    Lacrimal
      Left Ø8NW
      Right Ø8NV
    Minor Salivary ØCNJ
    Parotid
      Left ØCN9
      Right ØCN8
    Pituitary ØGNØ
    Sublingual
      Left ØCNF
      Right ØCND
    Submaxillary
      Left ØCNH
      Right ØCNG
    Vestibular ØUNL
  Glenoid Cavity
    Left ØPN8
    Right ØPN7
  Glomus Jugulare ØGNC
  Humeral Head
    Left ØPND
    Right ØPNC
  Humeral Shaft
    Left ØPNG
    Right ØPNF
  Hymen ØUNK
  Hypothalamus ØØNA
  Ileocecal Valve ØDNC
  Ileum ØDNB
  Intestine
    Large ØDNE
      Left ØDNG
      Right ØDNF
    Small ØDN8
  Iris
    Left Ø8ND3ZZ
    Right Ø8NC3ZZ
  Jejunum ØDNA
  Joint
    Acromioclavicular
      Left ØRNH
      Right ØRNG
    Ankle
      Left ØSNG
      Right ØSNF
    Carpal
      Left ØRNR
      Right ØRNQ
    Cervical Vertebral ØRN1
    Cervicothoracic Vertebral ØRN4
    Coccygeal ØSN6
    Elbow
      Left ØRNM
      Right ØRNL
    Finger Phalangeal
      Left ØRNX
      Right ØRNW
    Hip
      Left ØSNB
      Right ØSN9
    Knee
      Left ØSND
      Right ØSNC
    Lumbar Vertebral ØSNØ
    Lumbosacral ØSN3
    Metacarpocarpal
      Left ØRNT
      Right ØRNS
    Metacarpophalangeal
      Left ØRNV
      Right ØRNU
    Metatarsal-Phalangeal
      Left ØSNN
      Right ØSNM
    Metatarsal-Tarsal
      Left ØSNL
      Right ØSNK
    Occipital-cervical ØRNØ
    Sacrococcygeal ØSN5

Release — continued
  Joint — continued
    Sacroiliac
      Left 0SN8
      Right 0SN7
    Shoulder
      Left 0RNK
      Right 0RNJ
    Sternoclavicular
      Left 0RNF
      Right 0RNE
    Tarsal
      Left 0SNJ
      Right 0SNH
    Temporomandibular
      Left 0RND
      Right 0RNC
    Thoracic Vertebral 0RN6
    Thoracolumbar Vertebral 0RNA
    Toe Phalangeal
      Left 0SNQ
      Right 0SNP
    Wrist
      Left 0RNP
      Right 0RNN
  Kidney
    Left 0TN1
    Right 0TN0
  Kidney Pelvis
    Left 0TN4
    Right 0TN3
  Larynx 0CNS
  Lens
    Left 08NK3ZZ
    Right 08NJ3ZZ
  Lip
    Lower 0CN1
    Upper 0CN0
  Liver 0FN0
    Left Lobe 0FN2
    Right Lobe 0FN1
  Lung
    Bilateral 0BNM
    Left 0BNL
    Lower Lobe
      Left 0BNJ
      Right 0BNF
    Middle Lobe, Right 0BND
    Right 0BNK
    Upper Lobe
      Left 0BNG
      Right 0BNC
  Lung Lingula 0BNH
  Lymphatic
    Aortic 07ND
    Axillary
      Left 07N6
      Right 07N5
    Head 07N0
    Inguinal
      Left 07NJ
      Right 07NH
    Internal Mammary
      Left 07N9
      Right 07N8
    Lower Extremity
      Left 07NG
      Right 07NF
    Mesenteric 07NB
    Neck
      Left 07N2
      Right 07N1
    Pelvis 07NC
    Thoracic Duct 07NK
    Thorax 07N7
    Upper Extremity
      Left 07N4
      Right 07N3
  Mandible
    Left 0NNV
    Right 0NNT
  Maxilla
    Left 0NNS
    Right 0NNR
  Medulla Oblongata 00ND
  Mesentery 0DNV

Release — continued
  Metacarpal
    Left 0PNQ
    Right 0PNP
  Metatarsal
    Left 0QNP
    Right 0QNN
  Muscle
    Abdomen
      Left 0KNL
      Right 0KNK
    Extraocular
      Left 08NM
      Right 08NL
    Facial 0KN1
    Foot
      Left 0KNW
      Right 0KNV
    Hand
      Left 0KND
      Right 0KNC
    Head 0KN0
    Hip
      Left 0KNP
      Right 0KNN
    Lower Arm and Wrist
      Left 0KNB
      Right 0KN9
    Lower Leg
      Left 0KNT
      Right 0KNS
    Neck
      Left 0KN3
      Right 0KN2
    Papillary 02ND
    Perineum 0KNM
    Shoulder
      Left 0KN6
      Right 0KN5
    Thorax
      Left 0KNJ
      Right 0KNH
    Tongue, Palate, Pharynx 0KN4
    Trunk
      Left 0KNG
      Right 0KNF
    Upper Arm
      Left 0KN8
      Right 0KN7
    Upper Leg
      Left 0KNR
      Right 0KNQ
  Nasopharynx 09NN
  Nerve
    Abdominal Sympathetic 01NM
    Abducens 00NL
    Accessory 00NR
    Acoustic 00NN
    Brachial Plexus 01N3
    Cervical 01N1
    Cervical Plexus 01N0
    Facial 00NM
    Femoral 01ND
    Glossopharyngeal 00NP
    Head and Neck Sympathetic 01NK
    Hypoglossal 00NS
    Lumbar 01NB
    Lumbar Plexus 01N9
    Lumbar Sympathetic 01NN
    Lumbosacral Plexus 01NA
    Median 01N5
    Oculomotor 00NH
    Olfactory 00NF
    Optic 00NG
    Peroneal 01NH
    Phrenic 01N2
    Pudendal 01NC
    Radial 01N6
    Sacral 01NR
    Sacral Plexus 01NQ
    Sacral Sympathetic 01NP
    Sciatic 01NF
    Thoracic 01N8
    Thoracic Sympathetic 01NL
    Tibial 01NG
    Trigeminal 00NK

Release — continued
  Nerve — continued
    Trochlear 00NJ
    Ulnar 01N4
    Vagus 00NQ
  Nipple
    Left 0HNX
    Right 0HNW
  Nose 09NK
  Omentum
    Greater 0DNS
    Lesser 0DNT
  Orbit
    Left 0NNQ
    Right 0NNP
  Ovary
    Bilateral 0UN2
    Left 0UN1
    Right 0UN0
  Palate
    Hard 0CN2
    Soft 0CN3
  Pancreas 0FNG
  Para-aortic Body 0GN9
  Paraganglion Extremity 0GNF
  Parathyroid Gland 0GNR
    Inferior
      Left 0GNP
      Right 0GNN
    Multiple 0GNQ
    Superior
      Left 0GNM
      Right 0GNL
  Patella
    Left 0QNF
    Right 0QND
  Penis 0VNS
  Pericardium 02NN
  Peritoneum 0DNW
  Phalanx
    Finger
      Left 0PNV
      Right 0PNT
    Thumb
      Left 0PNS
      Right 0PNR
    Toe
      Left 0QNR
      Right 0QNQ
  Pharynx 0CNM
  Pineal Body 0GN1
  Pleura
    Left 0BNP
    Right 0BNN
  Pons 00NB
  Prepuce 0VNT
  Prostate 0VN0
  Radius
    Left 0PNJ
    Right 0PNH
  Rectum 0DNP
  Retina
    Left 08NF3ZZ
    Right 08NE3ZZ
  Retinal Vessel
    Left 08NH3ZZ
    Right 08NG3ZZ
  Rib
    Left 0PN2
    Right 0PN1
  Sacrum 0QN1
  Scapula
    Left 0PN6
    Right 0PN5
  Sclera
    Left 08N7XZZ
    Right 08N6XZZ
  Scrotum 0VN5
  Septum
    Atrial 02N5
    Nasal 09NM
    Ventricular 02NM
  Sinus
    Accessory 09NP
    Ethmoid
      Left 09NV

⬮ **Subterms under main terms may continue to next column or page**

Release — continued
  Sinus — continued
    Ethmoid — continued
      Right Ø9NU
    Frontal
      Left Ø9NT
      Right Ø9NS
    Mastoid
      Left Ø9NC
      Right Ø9NB
    Maxillary
      Left Ø9NR
      Right Ø9NQ
    Sphenoid
      Left Ø9NX
      Right Ø9NW
  Skin
    Abdomen ØHN7XZZ
    Back ØHN6XZZ
    Buttock ØHN8XZZ
    Chest ØHN5XZZ
    Ear
      Left ØHN3XZZ
      Right ØHN2XZZ
    Face ØHN1XZZ
    Foot
      Left ØHNNXZZ
      Right ØHNMXZZ
    Genitalia ØHNAXZZ
    Hand
      Left ØHNGXZZ
      Right ØHNFXZZ
    Lower Arm
      Left ØHNEXZZ
      Right ØHNDXZZ
    Lower Leg
      Left ØHNLXZZ
      Right ØHNKXZZ
    Neck ØHN4XZZ
    Perineum ØHN9XZZ
    Scalp ØHNØXZZ
    Upper Arm
      Left ØHNCXZZ
      Right ØHNBXZZ
    Upper Leg
      Left ØHNJXZZ
      Right ØHNHXZZ
  Spinal Cord
    Cervical ØØNW
    Lumbar ØØNY
    Thoracic ØØNX
  Spinal Meninges ØØNT
  Spleen Ø7NP
  Sternum ØPNØ
  Stomach ØDN6
    Pylorus ØDN7
  Subcutaneous Tissue and Fascia
    Abdomen ØJN8
    Back ØJN7
    Buttock ØJN9
    Chest ØJN6
    Face ØJN1
    Foot
      Left ØJNR
      Right ØJNQ
    Hand
      Left ØJNK
      Right ØJNJ
    Lower Arm
      Left ØJNH
      Right ØJNG
    Lower Leg
      Left ØJNP
      Right ØJNN
    Neck
      Anterior ØJN4
      Posterior ØJN5
    Pelvic Region ØJNC
    Perineum ØJNB
    Scalp ØJNØ
    Upper Arm
      Left ØJNF
      Right ØJND
    Upper Leg
      Left ØJNM
      Right ØJNL

Release — continued
  Tarsal
    Left ØQNM
    Right ØQNL
  Tendon
    Abdomen
      Left ØLNG
      Right ØLNF
    Ankle
      Left ØLNT
      Right ØLNS
    Foot
      Left ØLNW
      Right ØLNV
    Hand
      Left ØLN8
      Right ØLN7
    Head and Neck ØLNØ
    Hip
      Left ØLNK
      Right ØLNJ
    Knee
      Left ØLNR
      Right ØLNQ
    Lower Arm and Wrist
      Left ØLN6
      Right ØLN5
    Lower Leg
      Left ØLNP
      Right ØLNN
    Perineum ØLNH
    Shoulder
      Left ØLN2
      Right ØLN1
    Thorax
      Left ØLND
      Right ØLNC
    Trunk
      Left ØLNB
      Right ØLN9
    Upper Arm
      Left ØLN4
      Right ØLN3
    Upper Leg
      Left ØLNM
      Right ØLNL
  Testis
    Bilateral ØVNC
    Left ØVNB
    Right ØVN9
  Thalamus ØØN9
  Thymus Ø7NM
  Thyroid Gland ØGNK
    Left Lobe ØGNG
    Right Lobe ØGNH
  Tibia
    Left ØQNH
    Right ØQNG
  Toe Nail ØHNRXZZ
  Tongue ØCN7
  Tonsils ØCNP
  Tooth
    Lower ØCNX
    Upper ØCNW
  Trachea ØBN1
  Tunica Vaginalis
    Left ØVN7
    Right ØVN6
  Turbinate, Nasal Ø9NL
  Tympanic Membrane
    Left Ø9N8
    Right Ø9N7
  Ulna
    Left ØPNL
    Right ØPNK
  Ureter
    Left ØTN7
    Right ØTN6
  Urethra ØTND
  Uterine Supporting Structure ØUN4
  Uterus ØUN9
  Uvula ØCNN
  Vagina ØUNG
  Valve
    Aortic Ø2NF
    Mitral Ø2NG

Release — continued
  Valve — continued
    Pulmonary Ø2NH
    Tricuspid Ø2NJ
  Vas Deferens
    Bilateral ØVNQ
    Left ØVNP
    Right ØVNN
  Vein
    Axillary
      Left Ø5N8
      Right Ø5N7
    Azygos Ø5NØ
    Basilic
      Left Ø5NC
      Right Ø5NB
    Brachial
      Left Ø5NA
      Right Ø5N9
    Cephalic
      Left Ø5NF
      Right Ø5ND
    Colic Ø6N7
    Common Iliac
      Left Ø6ND
      Right Ø6NC
    Coronary Ø2N4
    Esophageal Ø6N3
    External Iliac
      Left Ø6NG
      Right Ø6NF
    External Jugular
      Left Ø5NQ
      Right Ø5NP
    Face
      Left Ø5NV
      Right Ø5NT
    Femoral
      Left Ø6NN
      Right Ø6NM
    Foot
      Left Ø6NV
      Right Ø6NT
    Gastric Ø6N2
    Greater Saphenous
      Left Ø6NQ
      Right Ø6NP
    Hand
      Left Ø5NH
      Right Ø5NG
    Hemiazygos Ø5N1
    Hepatic Ø6N4
    Hypogastric
      Left Ø6NJ
      Right Ø6NH
    Inferior Mesenteric Ø6N6
    Innominate
      Left Ø5N4
      Right Ø5N3
    Internal Jugular
      Left Ø5NN
      Right Ø5NM
    Intracranial Ø5NL
    Lesser Saphenous
      Left Ø6NS
      Right Ø6NR
    Lower Ø6NY
    Portal Ø6N8
    Pulmonary
      Left Ø2NT
      Right Ø2NS
    Renal
      Left Ø6NB
      Right Ø6N9
    Splenic Ø6N1
    Subclavian
      Left Ø5N6
      Right Ø5N5
    Superior Mesenteric Ø6N5
    Upper Ø5NY
    Vertebral
      Left Ø5NS
      Right Ø5NR
  Vena Cava
    Inferior Ø6NØ
    Superior Ø2NV

Removal of device from — continued
Lung
  Left ØBPL
  Right ØBPK
Lymphatic Ø7PN
  Thoracic Duct Ø7PK
Mediastinum ØWPC
Mesentery ØDPV
Metacarpal
  Left ØPPQ
  Right ØPPP
Metatarsal
  Left ØQPP
  Right ØQPN
Mouth and Throat ØCPY
Muscle
  Extraocular
    Left Ø8PM
    Right Ø8PL
  Lower ØKPY
  Upper ØKPX
Neck ØWP6
Nerve
  Cranial ØØPE
  Peripheral Ø1PY
Nose Ø9PK
Omentum ØDPU
Ovary ØUP3
Pancreas ØFPG
Parathyroid Gland ØGPR
Patella
  Left ØQPF
  Right ØQPD
Pelvic Cavity ØWPJ
Penis ØVPS
Pericardial Cavity ØWPD
Perineum
  Female ØWPN
  Male ØWPM
Peritoneal Cavity ØWPG
Peritoneum ØDPW
Phalanx
  Finger
    Left ØPPV
    Right ØPPT
  Thumb
    Left ØPPS
    Right ØPPR
  Toe
    Left ØQPR
    Right ØQPQ
Pineal Body ØGP1
Pleura ØBPQ
Pleural Cavity
  Left ØWPB
  Right ØWP9
Products of Conception 1ØPØ
Prostate and Seminal Vesicles ØVP4
Radius
  Left ØPPJ
  Right ØPPH
Rectum ØDPP
Respiratory Tract ØWPQ
Retroperitoneum ØWPH
Rib
  Left ØPP2
  Right ØPP1
Sacrum ØQP1
Scapula
  Left ØPP6
  Right ØPP5
Scrotum and Tunica Vaginalis ØVP8
Sinus Ø9PY
Skin ØHPPX
Skull ØNPØ
Spinal Canal ØØPU
Spinal Cord ØØPV
Spleen Ø7PP
Sternum ØPPØ
Stomach ØDP6
Subcutaneous Tissue and Fascia
  Head and Neck ØJPS
  Lower Extremity ØJPW
  Trunk ØJPT
  Upper Extremity ØJPV

Removal of device from — continued
Tarsal
  Left ØQPM
  Right ØQPL
Tendon
  Lower ØLPY
  Upper ØLPX
Testis ØVPD
Thymus Ø7PM
Thyroid Gland ØGPK
Tibia
  Left ØQPH
  Right ØQPG
Toe Nail ØHPRX
Trachea ØBP1
Tracheobronchial Tree ØBPØ
Tympanic Membrane
  Left Ø9P8
  Right Ø9P7
Ulna
  Left ØPPL
  Right ØPPK
Ureter ØTP9
Urethra ØTPD
Uterus and Cervix ØUPD
Vagina and Cul-de-sac ØUPH
Vas Deferens ØVPR
Vein
  Lower Ø6PY
  Upper Ø5PY
Vertebra
  Cervical ØPP3
  Lumbar ØQPØ
  Thoracic ØPP4
Vulva ØUPM
Renal calyx
  use Kidney
  use Kidney, Left
  use Kidney, Right
  use Kidneys, Bilateral
Renal capsule
  use Kidney
  use Kidney, Left
  use Kidney, Right
  use Kidneys, Bilateral
Renal cortex
  use Kidney
  use Kidney, Left
  use Kidney, Right
  use Kidneys, Bilateral
Renal dialysis *see* Performance, Urinary 5A1D
Renal plexus *use* Nerve, Abdominal Sympathetic
Renal segment
  use Kidney
  use Kidney, Left
  use Kidney, Right
  use Kidneys, Bilateral
Renal segmental artery
  use Artery, Renal, Left
  use Artery, Renal, Right
Reopening, operative site
  Control of bleeding *see* Control postprocedural
    bleeding in
  Inspection only *see* Inspection
Repair
Abdominal Wall ØWQF
Acetabulum
  Left ØQQ5
  Right ØQQ4
Adenoids ØCQQ
Ampulla of Vater ØFQC
Anal Sphincter ØDQR
Ankle Region
  Left ØYQL
  Right ØYQK
Anterior Chamber
  Left Ø8Q33ZZ
  Right Ø8Q23ZZ
Anus ØDQQ
Aorta
  Abdominal Ø4QØ
  Thoracic Ø2QW
Aortic Body ØGQD
Appendix ØDQJ

Repair — continued
Arm
  Lower
    Left ØXQF
    Right ØXQD
  Upper
    Left ØXQ9
    Right ØXQ8
Artery
  Anterior Tibial
    Left Ø4QQ
    Right Ø4QP
  Axillary
    Left Ø3Q6
    Right Ø3Q5
  Brachial
    Left Ø3Q8
    Right Ø3Q7
  Celiac Ø4Q1
  Colic
    Left Ø4Q7
    Middle Ø4Q8
    Right Ø4Q6
  Common Carotid
    Left Ø3QJ
    Right Ø3QH
  Common Iliac
    Left Ø4QD
    Right Ø4QC
  Coronary
    Four or More Sites Ø2Q3
    One Site Ø2QØ
    Three Sites Ø2Q2
    Two Sites Ø2Q1
  External Carotid
    Left Ø3QN
    Right Ø3QM
  External Iliac
    Left Ø4QJ
    Right Ø4QH
  Face Ø3QR
  Femoral
    Left Ø4QL
    Right Ø4QK
  Foot
    Left Ø4QW
    Right Ø4QV
  Gastric Ø4Q2
  Hand
    Left Ø3QF
    Right Ø3QD
  Hepatic Ø4Q3
  Inferior Mesenteric Ø4QB
  Innominate Ø3Q2
  Internal Carotid
    Left Ø3QL
    Right Ø3QK
  Internal Iliac
    Left Ø4QF
    Right Ø4QE
  Internal Mammary
    Left Ø3Q1
    Right Ø3QØ
  Intracranial Ø3QG
  Lower Ø4QY
  Peroneal
    Left Ø4QU
    Right Ø4QT
  Popliteal
    Left Ø4QN
    Right Ø4QM
  Posterior Tibial
    Left Ø4QS
    Right Ø4QR
  Pulmonary
    Left Ø2QR
    Right Ø2QQ
  Pulmonary Trunk Ø2QP
  Radial
    Left Ø3QC
    Right Ø3QB
  Renal
    Left Ø4QA
    Right Ø4Q9
  Splenic Ø4Q4

Repair — continued
  Femoral Region — continued
    Right 0YQ7
  Femoral Shaft
    Left 0QQ9
    Right 0QQ8
  Femur
    Lower
      Left 0QQC
      Right 0QQB
    Upper
      Left 0QQ7
      Right 0QQ6
  Fibula
    Left 0QQK
    Right 0QQJ
  Finger
    Index
      Left 0XQP
      Right 0XQN
    Little
      Left 0XQW
      Right 0XQV
    Middle
      Left 0XQR
      Right 0XQQ
    Ring
      Left 0XQT
      Right 0XQS
  Finger Nail 0HQQXZZ
  Foot
    Left 0YQN
    Right 0YQM
  Gallbladder 0FQ4
  Gingiva
    Lower 0CQ6
    Upper 0CQ5
  Gland
    Adrenal
      Bilateral 0GQ4
      Left 0GQ2
      Right 0GQ3
    Lacrimal
      Left 08QW
      Right 08QV
    Minor Salivary 0CQJ
    Parotid
      Left 0CQ9
      Right 0CQ8
    Pituitary 0GQ0
    Sublingual
      Left 0CQF
      Right 0CQD
    Submaxillary
      Left 0CQH
      Right 0CQG
    Vestibular 0UQL
  Glenoid Cavity
    Left 0PQ8
    Right 0PQ7
  Glomus Jugulare 0GQC
  Hand
    Left 0XQK
    Right 0XQJ
  Head 0WQ0
  Heart 02QA
    Left 02QC
    Right 02QB
  Humeral Head
    Left 0PQD
    Right 0PQC
  Humeral Shaft
    Left 0PQG
    Right 0PQF
  Hymen 0UQK
  Hypothalamus 00QA
  Ileocecal Valve 0DQC
  Ileum 0DQB
  Inguinal Region
    Bilateral 0YQA
    Left 0YQ6
    Right 0YQ5
  Intestine
    Large 0DQE
      Left 0DQG
      Right 0DQF

Repair — continued
  Intestine — continued
    Small 0DQ8
  Iris
    Left 08QD3ZZ
    Right 08QC3ZZ
  Jaw
    Lower 0WQ5
    Upper 0WQ4
  Jejunum 0DQA
  Joint
    Acromioclavicular
      Left 0RQH
      Right 0RQG
    Ankle
      Left 0SQG
      Right 0SQF
    Carpal
      Left 0RQR
      Right 0RQQ
    Cervical Vertebral 0RQ1
    Cervicothoracic Vertebral 0RQ4
    Coccygeal 0SQ6
    Elbow
      Left 0RQM
      Right 0RQL
    Finger Phalangeal
      Left 0RQX
      Right 0RQW
    Hip
      Left 0SQB
      Right 0SQ9
    Knee
      Left 0SQD
      Right 0SQC
    Lumbar Vertebral 0SQ0
    Lumbosacral 0SQ3
    Metacarpocarpal
      Left 0RQT
      Right 0RQS
    Metacarpophalangeal
      Left 0RQV
      Right 0RQU
    Metatarsal-Phalangeal
      Left 0SQN
      Right 0SQM
    Metatarsal-Tarsal
      Left 0SQL
      Right 0SQK
    Occipital-cervical 0RQ0
    Sacrococcygeal 0SQ5
    Sacroiliac
      Left 0SQ8
      Right 0SQ7
    Shoulder
      Left 0RQK
      Right 0RQJ
    Sternoclavicular
      Left 0RQF
      Right 0RQE
    Tarsal
      Left 0SQJ
      Right 0SQH
    Temporomandibular
      Left 0RQD
      Right 0RQC
    Thoracic Vertebral 0RQ6
    Thoracolumbar Vertebral 0RQA
    Toe Phalangeal
      Left 0SQQ
      Right 0SQP
    Wrist
      Left 0RQP
      Right 0RQN
  Kidney
    Left 0TQ1
    Right 0TQ0
  Kidney Pelvis
    Left 0TQ4
    Right 0TQ3
  Knee Region
    Left 0YQG
    Right 0YQF
  Larynx 0CQS

Repair — continued
  Leg
    Lower
      Left 0YQJ
      Right 0YQH
    Upper
      Left 0YQD
      Right 0YQC
  Lens
    Left 08QK3ZZ
    Right 08QJ3ZZ
  Lip
    Lower 0CQ1
    Upper 0CQ0
  Liver 0FQ0
    Left Lobe 0FQ2
    Right Lobe 0FQ1
  Lung
    Bilateral 0BQM
    Left 0BQL
    Lower Lobe
      Left 0BQJ
      Right 0BQF
    Middle Lobe, Right 0BQD
    Right 0BQK
    Upper Lobe
      Left 0BQG
      Right 0BQC
  Lung Lingula 0BQH
  Lymphatic
    Aortic 07QD
    Axillary
      Left 07Q6
      Right 07Q5
    Head 07Q0
    Inguinal
      Left 07QJ
      Right 07QH
    Internal Mammary
      Left 07Q9
      Right 07Q8
    Lower Extremity
      Left 07QG
      Right 07QF
    Mesenteric 07QB
    Neck
      Left 07Q2
      Right 07Q1
    Pelvis 07QC
    Thoracic Duct 07QK
    Thorax 07Q7
    Upper Extremity
      Left 07Q4
      Right 07Q3
  Mandible
    Left 0NQV
    Right 0NQT
  Maxilla
    Left 0NQS
    Right 0NQR
  Mediastinum 0WQC
  Medulla Oblongata 00QD
  Mesentery 0DQV
  Metacarpal
    Left 0PQQ
    Right 0PQP
  Metatarsal
    Left 0QQP
    Right 0QQN
  Muscle
    Abdomen
      Left 0KQL
      Right 0KQK
    Extraocular
      Left 08QM
      Right 08QL
    Facial 0KQ1
    Foot
      Left 0KQW
      Right 0KQV
    Hand
      Left 0KQD
      Right 0KQC
    Head 0KQ0
    Hip
      Left 0KQP

Repair — continued
Muscle — continued
Hip — continued
Right 0KQN
Lower Arm and Wrist
Left 0KQB
Right 0KQ9
Lower Leg
Left 0KQT
Right 0KQS
Neck
Left 0KQ3
Right 0KQ2
Papillary 02QD
Perineum 0KQM
Shoulder
Left 0KQ6
Right 0KQ5
Thorax
Left 0KQJ
Right 0KQH
Tongue, Palate, Pharynx 0KQ4
Trunk
Left 0KQG
Right 0KQF
Upper Arm
Left 0KQ8
Right 0KQ7
Upper Leg
Left 0KQR
Right 0KQQ
Nasopharynx 09QN
Neck 0WQ6
Nerve
Abdominal Sympathetic 01QM
Abducens 00QL
Accessory 00QR
Acoustic 00QN
Brachial Plexus 01Q3
Cervical 01Q1
Cervical Plexus 01Q0
Facial 00QM
Femoral 01QD
Glossopharyngeal 00QP
Head and Neck Sympathetic 01QK
Hypoglossal 00QS
Lumbar 01QB
Lumbar Plexus 01Q9
Lumbar Sympathetic 01QN
Lumbosacral Plexus 01QA
Median 01Q5
Oculomotor 00QH
Olfactory 00QF
Optic 00QG
Peroneal 01QH
Phrenic 01Q2
Pudendal 01QC
Radial 01Q6
Sacral 01QR
Sacral Plexus 01QQ
Sacral Sympathetic 01QP
Sciatic 01QF
Thoracic 01Q8
Thoracic Sympathetic 01QL
Tibial 01QG
Trigeminal 00QK
Trochlear 00QJ
Ulnar 01Q4
Vagus 00QQ
Nipple
Left 0HQX
Right 0HQW
Nose 09QK
Omentum
Greater 0DQS
Lesser 0DQT
Orbit
Left 0NQQ
Right 0NQP
Ovary
Bilateral 0UQ2
Left 0UQ1
Right 0UQ0
Palate
Hard 0CQ2
Soft 0CQ3

Repair — continued
Pancreas 0FQG
Para-aortic Body 0GQ9
Paraganglion Extremity 0GQF
Parathyroid Gland 0GQR
Inferior
Left 0GQP
Right 0GQN
Multiple 0GQQ
Superior
Left 0GQM
Right 0GQL
Patella
Left 0QQF
Right 0QQD
Penis 0VQS
Pericardium 02QN
Perineum
Female 0WQN
Male 0WQM
Peritoneum 0DQW
Phalanx
Finger
Left 0PQV
Right 0PQT
Thumb
Left 0PQS
Right 0PQR
Toe
Left 0QQR
Right 0QQQ
Pharynx 0CQM
Pineal Body 0GQ1
Pleura
Left 0BQP
Right 0BQN
Pons 00QB
Prepuce 0VQT
Products of Conception 10Q0
Prostate 0VQ0
Radius
Left 0PQJ
Right 0PQH
Rectum 0DQP
Retina
Left 08QF3ZZ
Right 08QE3ZZ
Retinal Vessel
Left 08QH3ZZ
Right 08QG3ZZ
Rib
Left 0PQ2
Right 0PQ1
Sacrum 0QQ1
Scapula
Left 0PQ6
Right 0PQ5
Sclera
Left 08Q7XZZ
Right 08Q6XZZ
Scrotum 0VQ5
Septum
Atrial 02Q5
Nasal 09QM
Ventricular 02QM
Shoulder Region
Left 0XQ3
Right 0XQ2
Sinus
Accessory 09QP
Ethmoid
Left 09QV
Right 09QU
Frontal
Left 09QT
Right 09QS
Mastoid
Left 09QC
Right 09QB
Maxillary
Left 09QR
Right 09QQ
Sphenoid
Left 09QX
Right 09QW

Repair — continued
Skin
Abdomen 0HQ7XZZ
Back 0HQ6XZZ
Buttock 0HQ8XZZ
Chest 0HQ5XZZ
Ear
Left 0HQ3XZZ
Right 0HQ2XZZ
Face 0HQ1XZZ
Foot
Left 0HQNXZZ
Right 0HQMXZZ
Genitalia 0HQAXZZ
Hand
Left 0HQGXZZ
Right 0HQFXZZ
Lower Arm
Left 0HQEXZZ
Right 0HQDXZZ
Lower Leg
Left 0HQLXZZ
Right 0HQKXZZ
Neck 0HQ4XZZ
Perineum 0HQ9XZZ
Scalp 0HQ0XZZ
Upper Arm
Left 0HQCXZZ
Right 0HQBXZZ
Upper Leg
Left 0HQJXZZ
Right 0HQHXZZ
Skull 0NQ0
Spinal Cord
Cervical 00QW
Lumbar 00QY
Thoracic 00QX
Spinal Meninges 00QT
Spleen 07QP
Sternum 0PQ0
Stomach 0DQ6
Pylorus 0DQ7
Subcutaneous Tissue and Fascia
Abdomen 0JQ8
Back 0JQ7
Buttock 0JQ9
Chest 0JQ6
Face 0JQ1
Foot
Left 0JQR
Right 0JQQ
Hand
Left 0JQK
Right 0JQJ
Lower Arm
Left 0JQH
Right 0JQG
Lower Leg
Left 0JQP
Right 0JQN
Neck
Anterior 0JQ4
Posterior 0JQ5
Pelvic Region 0JQC
Perineum 0JQB
Scalp 0JQ0
Upper Arm
Left 0JQF
Right 0JQD
Upper Leg
Left 0JQM
Right 0JQL
Tarsal
Left 0QQM
Right 0QQL
Tendon
Abdomen
Left 0LQG
Right 0LQF
Ankle
Left 0LQT
Right 0LQS
Foot
Left 0LQW
Right 0LQV

▼ **Subterms under main terms may continue to next column or page**

Replacement — continued
- Artery — continued
  - Internal Mammary
    - Left Ø3R1
    - Right Ø3RØ
  - Intracranial Ø3RG
  - Lower Ø4RY
  - Peroneal
    - Left Ø4RU
    - Right Ø4RT
  - Popliteal
    - Left Ø4RN
    - Right Ø4RM
  - Posterior Tibial
    - Left Ø4RS
    - Right Ø4RR
  - Pulmonary
    - Left Ø2RR
    - Right Ø2RQ
  - Pulmonary Trunk Ø2RP
  - Radial
    - Left Ø3RC
    - Right Ø3RB
  - Renal
    - Left Ø4RA
    - Right Ø4R9
  - Splenic Ø4R4
  - Subclavian
    - Left Ø3R4
    - Right Ø3R3
  - Superior Mesenteric Ø4R5
  - Temporal
    - Left Ø3RT
    - Right Ø3RS
  - Thyroid
    - Left Ø3RV
    - Right Ø3RU
  - Ulnar
    - Left Ø3RA
    - Right Ø3R9
  - Upper Ø3RY
  - Vertebral
    - Left Ø3RQ
    - Right Ø3RP
- Atrium
  - Left Ø2R7
  - Right Ø2R6
- Auditory Ossicle
  - Left Ø9RAØ
  - Right Ø9R9Ø
- Bladder ØTRB
- Bladder Neck ØTRC
- Bone
  - Ethmoid
    - Left ØNRG
    - Right ØNRF
  - Frontal
    - Left ØNR2
    - Right ØNR1
  - Hyoid ØNRX
  - Lacrimal
    - Left ØNRJ
    - Right ØNRH
  - Nasal ØNRB
  - Occipital
    - Left ØNR8
    - Right ØNR7
  - Palatine
    - Left ØNRL
    - Right ØNRK
  - Parietal
    - Left ØNR4
    - Right ØNR3
  - Pelvic
    - Left ØQR3
    - Right ØQR2
  - Sphenoid
    - Left ØNRD
    - Right ØNRC
  - Temporal
    - Left ØNR6
    - Right ØNR5
  - Zygomatic
    - Left ØNRN
    - Right ØNRM

Replacement — continued
- Breast
  - Bilateral ØHRV
  - Left ØHRU
  - Right ØHRT
- Buccal Mucosa ØCR4
- Carpal
  - Left ØPRN
  - Right ØPRM
- Chordae Tendineae Ø2R9
- Choroid
  - Left Ø8RB
  - Right Ø8RA
- Clavicle
  - Left ØPRB
  - Right ØPR9
- Coccyx ØQRS
- Conjunctiva
  - Left Ø8RTX
  - Right Ø8RSX
- Cornea
  - Left Ø8R9
  - Right Ø8R8
- Disc
  - Cervical Vertebral ØRR3Ø
  - Cervicothoracic Vertebral ØRR5Ø
  - Lumbar Vertebral ØSR2Ø
  - Lumbosacral ØSR4Ø
  - Thoracic Vertebral ØRR9Ø
  - Thoracolumbar Vertebral ØRRBØ
- Duct
  - Common Bile ØFR9
  - Cystic ØFR8
  - Hepatic
    - Left ØFR6
    - Right ØFR5
  - Lacrimal
    - Left Ø8RY
    - Right Ø8RX
  - Pancreatic ØFRD
    - Accessory ØFRF
  - Parotid
    - Left ØCRC
    - Right ØCRB
- Ear
  - External
    - Bilateral Ø9R2
    - Left Ø9R1
    - Right Ø9RØ
  - Inner
    - Left Ø9REØ
    - Right Ø9RDØ
  - Middle
    - Left Ø9R6Ø
    - Right Ø9R5Ø
- Epiglottis ØCRR
- Esophagus ØDR5
- Eye
  - Left Ø8R1
  - Right Ø8RØ
- Eyelid
  - Lower
    - Left Ø8RR
    - Right Ø8RQ
  - Upper
    - Left Ø8RP
    - Right Ø8RN
- Femoral Shaft
  - Left ØQR9
  - Right ØQR8
- Femur
  - Lower
    - Left ØQRC
    - Right ØQRB
  - Upper
    - Left ØQR7
    - Right ØQR6
- Fibula
  - Left ØQRK
  - Right ØQRJ
- Finger Nail ØHRQX
- Gingiva
  - Lower ØCR6
  - Upper ØCR5
- Glenoid Cavity
  - Left ØPR8

Replacement — continued
- Glenoid Cavity — continued
  - Right ØPR7
- Hair ØHRSX
- Humeral Head
  - Left ØPRD
  - Right ØPRC
- Humeral Shaft
  - Left ØPRG
  - Right ØPRF
- Iris
  - Left Ø8RD3
  - Right Ø8RC3
- Joint
  - Acromioclavicular
    - Left ØRRHØ
    - Right ØRRGØ
  - Ankle
    - Left ØSRG
    - Right ØSRF
  - Carpal
    - Left ØRRRØ
    - Right ØRRQØ
  - Cervical Vertebral ØRR1Ø
  - Cervicothoracic Vertebral ØRR4Ø
  - Coccygeal ØSR6Ø
  - Elbow
    - Left ØRRMØ
    - Right ØRRLØ
  - Finger Phalangeal
    - Left ØRRXØ
    - Right ØRRWØ
  - Hip
    - Left ØSRB
      - Acetabular Surface ØSRE
      - Femoral Surface ØSRS
    - Right ØSR9
      - Acetabular Surface ØSRA
      - Femoral Surface ØSRR
  - Knee
    - Left ØSRD
      - Femoral Surface ØSRU
      - Tibial Surface ØSRW
    - Right ØSRC
      - Femoral Surface ØSRT
      - Tibial Surface ØSRV
  - Lumbar Vertebral ØSRØØ
  - Lumbosacral ØSR3Ø
  - Metacarpocarpal
    - Left ØRRTØ
    - Right ØRRSØ
  - Metacarpophalangeal
    - Left ØRRVØ
    - Right ØRRUØ
  - Metatarsal-Phalangeal
    - Left ØSRNØ
    - Right ØSRMØ
  - Metatarsal-Tarsal
    - Left ØSRLØ
    - Right ØSRKØ
  - Occipital-cervical ØRRØØ
  - Sacrococcygeal ØSR5Ø
  - Sacroiliac
    - Left ØSR8Ø
    - Right ØSR7Ø
  - Shoulder
    - Left ØRRK
    - Right ØRRJ
  - Sternoclavicular
    - Left ØRRFØ
    - Right ØRREØ
  - Tarsal
    - Left ØSRJØ
    - Right ØSRHØ
  - Temporomandibular
    - Left ØRRDØ
    - Right ØRRCØ
  - Thoracic Vertebral ØRR6Ø
  - Thoracolumbar Vertebral ØRRAØ
  - Toe Phalangeal
    - Left ØSRQØ
    - Right ØSRPØ
  - Wrist
    - Left ØRRPØ
    - Right ØRRNØ

Replacement — continued
Kidney Pelvis
   Left 0TR4
   Right 0TR3
Larynx 0CRS
Lens
   Left 08RK30Z
   Right 08RJ30Z
Lip
   Lower 0CR1
   Upper 0CR0
Mandible
   Left 0NRV
   Right 0NRT
Maxilla
   Left 0NRS
   Right 0NRR
Mesentery 0DRV
Metacarpal
   Left 0PRQ
   Right 0PRP
Metatarsal
   Left 0QRP
   Right 0QRN
Muscle, Papillary 02RD
Nasopharynx 09RN
Nipple
   Left 0HRX
   Right 0HRW
Nose 09RK
Omentum
   Greater 0DRS
   Lesser 0DRT
Orbit
   Left 0NRQ
   Right 0NRP
Palate
   Hard 0CR2
   Soft 0CR3
Patella
   Left 0QRF
   Right 0QRD
Pericardium 02RN
Peritoneum 0DRW
Phalanx
   Finger
      Left 0PRV
      Right 0PRT
   Thumb
      Left 0PRS
      Right 0PRR
   Toe
      Left 0QRR
      Right 0QRQ
Pharynx 0CRM
Radius
   Left 0PRJ
   Right 0PRH
Retinal Vessel
   Left 08RH3
   Right 08RG3
Rib
   Left 0PR2
   Right 0PR1
Sacrum 0QR1
Scapula
   Left 0PR6
   Right 0PR5
Sclera
   Left 08R7X
   Right 08R6X
Septum
   Atrial 02R5
   Nasal 09RM
   Ventricular 02RM
Skin
   Abdomen 0HR7
   Back 0HR6
   Buttock 0HR8
   Chest 0HR5
   Ear
      Left 0HR3
      Right 0HR2
   Face 0HR1
   Foot
      Left 0HRN

Replacement — continued
Skin — continued
   Foot — continued
      Right 0HRM
   Genitalia 0HRA
   Hand
      Left 0HRG
      Right 0HRF
   Lower Arm
      Left 0HRE
      Right 0HRD
   Lower Leg
      Left 0HRL
      Right 0HRK
   Neck 0HR4
   Perineum 0HR9
   Scalp 0HR0
   Upper Arm
      Left 0HRC
      Right 0HRB
   Upper Leg
      Left 0HRJ
      Right 0HRH
Skull 0NR0
Sternum 0PR0
Subcutaneous Tissue and Fascia
   Abdomen 0JR8
   Back 0JR7
   Buttock 0JR9
   Chest 0JR6
   Face 0JR1
   Foot
      Left 0JRR
      Right 0JRQ
   Hand
      Left 0JRK
      Right 0JRJ
   Lower Arm
      Left 0JRH
      Right 0JRG
   Lower Leg
      Left 0JRP
      Right 0JRN
   Neck
      Anterior 0JR4
      Posterior 0JR5
   Pelvic Region 0JRC
   Perineum 0JRB
   Scalp 0JR0
   Upper Arm
      Left 0JRF
      Right 0JRD
   Upper Leg
      Left 0JRM
      Right 0JRL
Tarsal
   Left 0QRM
   Right 0QRL
Tendon
   Abdomen
      Left 0LRG
      Right 0LRF
   Ankle
      Left 0LRT
      Right 0LRS
   Foot
      Left 0LRW
      Right 0LRV
   Hand
      Left 0LR8
      Right 0LR7
   Head and Neck 0LR0
   Hip
      Left 0LRK
      Right 0LRJ
   Knee
      Left 0LRR
      Right 0LRQ
   Lower Arm and Wrist
      Left 0LR6
      Right 0LR5
   Lower Leg
      Left 0LRP
      Right 0LRN
   Perineum 0LRH

Replacement — continued
Tendon — continued
   Shoulder
      Left 0LR2
      Right 0LR1
   Thorax
      Left 0LRD
      Right 0LRC
   Trunk
      Left 0LRB
      Right 0LR9
   Upper Arm
      Left 0LR4
      Right 0LR3
   Upper Leg
      Left 0LRM
      Right 0LRL
Testis
   Bilateral 0VRC0JZ
   Left 0VRB0JZ
   Right 0VR90JZ
Thumb
   Left 0XRM
   Right 0XRL
Tibia
   Left 0QRH
   Right 0QRG
Toe Nail 0HRRX
Tongue 0CR7
Tooth
   Lower 0CRX
   Upper 0CRW
Turbinate, Nasal 09RL
Tympanic Membrane
   Left 09R8
   Right 09R7
Ulna
   Left 0PRL
   Right 0PRK
Ureter
   Left 0TR7
   Right 0TR6
Urethra 0TRD
Uvula 0CRN
Valve
   Aortic 02RF
   Mitral 02RG
   Pulmonary 02RH
   Tricuspid 02RJ
Vein
   Axillary
      Left 05R8
      Right 05R7
   Azygos 05R0
   Basilic
      Left 05RC
      Right 05RB
   Brachial
      Left 05RA
      Right 05R9
   Cephalic
      Left 05RF
      Right 05RD
   Colic 06R7
   Common Iliac
      Left 06RD
      Right 06RC
   Esophageal 06R3
   External Iliac
      Left 06RG
      Right 06RF
   External Jugular
      Left 05RQ
      Right 05RP
   Face
      Left 05RV
      Right 05RT
   Femoral
      Left 06RN
      Right 06RM
   Foot
      Left 06RV
      Right 06RT
   Gastric 06R2
   Greater Saphenous
      Left 06RQ

Replacement — continued
 Vein — continued
  Greater Saphenous — continued
   Right 06RP
  Hand
   Left 05RH
   Right 05RG
  Hemiazygos 05R1
  Hepatic 06R4
  Hypogastric
   Left 06RJ
   Right 06RH
  Inferior Mesenteric 06R6
  Innominate
   Left 05R4
   Right 05R3
  Internal Jugular
   Left 05RN
   Right 05RM
  Intracranial 05RL
  Lesser Saphenous
   Left 06RS
   Right 06RR
  Lower 06RY
  Portal 06R8
  Pulmonary
   Left 02RT
   Right 02RS
  Renal
   Left 06RB
   Right 06R9
  Splenic 06R1
  Subclavian
   Left 05R6
   Right 05R5
  Superior Mesenteric 06R5
  Upper 05RY
  Vertebral
   Left 05RS
   Right 05RR
 Vena Cava
  Inferior 06R0
  Superior 02RV
 Ventricle
  Left 02RL
  Right 02RK
 Vertebra
  Cervical 0PR3
  Lumbar 0QR0
  Thoracic 0PR4
 Vitreous
  Left 08R53
  Right 08R43
 Vocal Cord
  Left 0CRV
  Right 0CRT
Replantation *see* Reposition
Replantation, scalp *see* Reattachment, Skin, Scalp
 0HM0
Reposition
 Acetabulum
  Left 0QS5
  Right 0QS4
 Ampulla of Vater 0FSC
 Anus 0DSQ
 Aorta
  Abdominal 04S0
  Thoracic 02SW0ZZ
 Artery
  Anterior Tibial
   Left 04SQ
   Right 04SP
  Axillary
   Left 03S6
   Right 03S5
  Brachial
   Left 03S8
   Right 03S7
  Celiac 04S1
  Colic
   Left 04S7
   Middle 04S8
   Right 04S6
  Common Carotid
   Left 03SJ
   Right 03SH

Reposition — continued
 Artery — continued
  Common Iliac
   Left 04SD
   Right 04SC
  External Carotid
   Left 03SN
   Right 03SM
  External Iliac
   Left 04SJ
   Right 04SH
  Face 03SR
  Femoral
   Left 04SL
   Right 04SK
  Foot
   Left 04SW
   Right 04SV
  Gastric 04S2
  Hand
   Left 03SF
   Right 03SD
  Hepatic 04S3
  Inferior Mesenteric 04SB
  Innominate 03S2
  Internal Carotid
   Left 03SL
   Right 03SK
  Internal Iliac
   Left 04SF
   Right 04SE
  Internal Mammary
   Left 03S1
   Right 03S0
  Intracranial 03SG
  Lower 04SY
  Peroneal
   Left 04SU
   Right 04ST
  Popliteal
   Left 04SN
   Right 04SM
  Posterior Tibial
   Left 04SS
   Right 04SR
  Pulmonary
   Left 02SR0ZZ
   Right 02SQ0ZZ
  Pulmonary Trunk 02SP0ZZ
  Radial
   Left 03SC
   Right 03SB
  Renal
   Left 04SA
   Right 04S9
  Splenic 04S4
  Subclavian
   Left 03S4
   Right 03S3
  Superior Mesenteric 04S5
  Temporal
   Left 03ST
   Right 03SS
  Thyroid
   Left 03SV
   Right 03SU
  Ulnar
   Left 03SA
   Right 03S9
  Upper 03SY
  Vertebral
   Left 03SQ
   Right 03SP
 Auditory Ossicle
  Left 09SA
  Right 09S9
 Bladder 0TSB
 Bladder Neck 0TSC
 Bone
  Ethmoid
   Left 0NSG
   Right 0NSF
  Frontal
   Left 0NS2
   Right 0NS1
  Hyoid 0NSX

Reposition — continued
 Bone — continued
  Lacrimal
   Left 0NSJ
   Right 0NSH
  Nasal 0NSB
  Occipital
   Left 0NS8
   Right 0NS7
  Palatine
   Left 0NSL
   Right 0NSK
  Parietal
   Left 0NS4
   Right 0NS3
  Pelvic
   Left 0QS3
   Right 0QS2
  Sphenoid
   Left 0NSD
   Right 0NSC
  Temporal
   Left 0NS6
   Right 0NS5
  Zygomatic
   Left 0NSN
   Right 0NSM
 Breast
  Bilateral 0HSV0ZZ
  Left 0HSU0ZZ
  Right 0HST0ZZ
 Bronchus
  Lingula 0BS90ZZ
  Lower Lobe
   Left 0BSB0ZZ
   Right 0BS60ZZ
  Main
   Left 0BS70ZZ
   Right 0BS30ZZ
  Middle Lobe, Right 0BS50ZZ
  Upper Lobe
   Left 0BS80ZZ
   Right 0BS40ZZ
 Bursa and Ligament
  Abdomen
   Left 0MSJ
   Right 0MSH
  Ankle
   Left 0MSR
   Right 0MSQ
  Elbow
   Left 0MS4
   Right 0MS3
  Foot
   Left 0MST
   Right 0MSS
  Hand
   Left 0MS8
   Right 0MS7
  Head and Neck 0MS0
  Hip
   Left 0MSM
   Right 0MSL
  Knee
   Left 0MSP
   Right 0MSN
  Lower Extremity
   Left 0MSW
   Right 0MSV
  Perineum 0MSK
  Shoulder
   Left 0MS2
   Right 0MS1
  Thorax
   Left 0MSG
   Right 0MSF
  Trunk
   Left 0MSD
   Right 0MSC
  Upper Extremity
   Left 0MSB
   Right 0MS9
  Wrist
   Left 0MS6
   Right 0MS5
 Carina 0BS20ZZ

Reposition — continued
- Carpal
  - Left 0PSN
  - Right 0PSM
- Cecum 0DSH
- Cervix 0USC
- Clavicle
  - Left 0PSB
  - Right 0PS9
- Coccyx 0QSS
- Colon
  - Ascending 0DSK
  - Descending 0DSM
  - Sigmoid 0DSN
  - Transverse 0DSL
- Cord
  - Bilateral 0VSH
  - Left 0VSG
  - Right 0VSF
- Cul-de-sac 0USF
- Diaphragm
  - Left 0BSS0ZZ
  - Right 0BSR0ZZ
- Duct
  - Common Bile 0FS9
  - Cystic 0FS8
  - Hepatic
    - Left 0FS6
    - Right 0FS5
  - Lacrimal
    - Left 08SY
    - Right 08SX
  - Pancreatic 0FSD
    - Accessory 0FSF
  - Parotid
    - Left 0CSC
    - Right 0CSB
- Duodenum 0DS9
- Ear
  - Bilateral 09S2
  - Left 09S1
  - Right 09S0
- Epiglottis 0CSR
- Esophagus 0DS5
- Eustachian Tube
  - Left 09SG
  - Right 09SF
- Eyelid
  - Lower
    - Left 08SR
    - Right 08SQ
  - Upper
    - Left 08SP
    - Right 08SN
- Fallopian Tube
  - Left 0US6
  - Right 0US5
- Fallopian Tubes, Bilateral 0US7
- Femoral Shaft
  - Left 0QS9
  - Right 0QS8
- Femur
  - Lower
    - Left 0QSC
    - Right 0QSB
  - Upper
    - Left 0QS7
    - Right 0QS6
- Fibula
  - Left 0QSK
  - Right 0QSJ
- Gallbladder 0FS4
- Gland
  - Adrenal
    - Left 0GS2
    - Right 0GS3
  - Lacrimal
    - Left 08SW
    - Right 08SV
- Glenoid Cavity
  - Left 0PS8
  - Right 0PS7
- Hair 0HSSXZZ
- Humeral Head
  - Left 0PSD
  - Right 0PSC

Reposition — continued
- Humeral Shaft
  - Left 0PSG
  - Right 0PSF
- Ileum 0DSB
- Iris
  - Left 08SD3ZZ
  - Right 08SC3ZZ
- Jejunum 0DSA
- Joint
  - Acromioclavicular
    - Left 0RSH
    - Right 0RSG
  - Ankle
    - Left 0SSG
    - Right 0SSF
  - Carpal
    - Left 0RSR
    - Right 0RSQ
  - Cervical Vertebral 0RS1
  - Cervicothoracic Vertebral 0RS4
  - Coccygeal 0SS6
  - Elbow
    - Left 0RSM
    - Right 0RSL
  - Finger Phalangeal
    - Left 0RSX
    - Right 0RSW
  - Hip
    - Left 0SSB
    - Right 0SS9
  - Knee
    - Left 0SSD
    - Right 0SSC
  - Lumbar Vertebral 0SS0
  - Lumbosacral 0SS3
  - Metacarpocarpal
    - Left 0RST
    - Right 0RSS
  - Metacarpophalangeal
    - Left 0RSV
    - Right 0RSU
  - Metatarsal-Phalangeal
    - Left 0SSN
    - Right 0SSM
  - Metatarsal-Tarsal
    - Left 0SSL
    - Right 0SSK
  - Occipital-cervical 0RS0
  - Sacrococcygeal 0SS5
  - Sacroiliac
    - Left 0SS8
    - Right 0SS7
  - Shoulder
    - Left 0RSK
    - Right 0RSJ
  - Sternoclavicular
    - Left 0RSF
    - Right 0RSE
  - Tarsal
    - Left 0SSJ
    - Right 0SSH
  - Temporomandibular
    - Left 0RSD
    - Right 0RSC
  - Thoracic Vertebral 0RS6
  - Thoracolumbar Vertebral 0RSA
  - Toe Phalangeal
    - Left 0SSQ
    - Right 0SSP
  - Wrist
    - Left 0RSP
    - Right 0RSN
- Kidney
  - Left 0TS1
  - Right 0TS0
- Kidney Pelvis
  - Left 0TS4
  - Right 0TS3
- Kidneys, Bilateral 0TS2
- Lens
  - Left 08SK3ZZ
  - Right 08SJ3ZZ
- Lip
  - Lower 0CS1
  - Upper 0CS0

Reposition — continued
- Liver 0FS0
- Lung
  - Left 0BSL0ZZ
  - Lower Lobe
    - Left 0BSJ0ZZ
    - Right 0BSF0ZZ
  - Middle Lobe, Right 0BSD0ZZ
  - Right 0BSK0ZZ
  - Upper Lobe
    - Left 0BSG0ZZ
    - Right 0BSC0ZZ
- Lung Lingula 0BSH0ZZ
- Mandible
  - Left 0NSV
  - Right 0NST
- Maxilla
  - Left 0NSS
  - Right 0NSR
- Metacarpal
  - Left 0PSQ
  - Right 0PSP
- Metatarsal
  - Left 0QSP
  - Right 0QSN
- Muscle
  - Abdomen
    - Left 0KSL
    - Right 0KSK
  - Extraocular
    - Left 08SM
    - Right 08SL
  - Facial 0KS1
  - Foot
    - Left 0KSW
    - Right 0KSV
  - Hand
    - Left 0KSD
    - Right 0KSC
  - Head 0KS0
  - Hip
    - Left 0KSP
    - Right 0KSN
  - Lower Arm and Wrist
    - Left 0KSB
    - Right 0KS9
  - Lower Leg
    - Left 0KST
    - Right 0KSS
  - Neck
    - Left 0KS3
    - Right 0KS2
  - Perineum 0KSM
  - Shoulder
    - Left 0KS6
    - Right 0KS5
  - Thorax
    - Left 0KSJ
    - Right 0KSH
  - Tongue, Palate, Pharynx 0KS4
  - Trunk
    - Left 0KSG
    - Right 0KSF
  - Upper Arm
    - Left 0KS8
    - Right 0KS7
  - Upper Leg
    - Left 0KSR
    - Right 0KSQ
- Nerve
  - Abducens 00SL
  - Accessory 00SR
  - Acoustic 00SN
  - Brachial Plexus 01S3
  - Cervical 01S1
  - Cervical Plexus 01S0
  - Facial 00SM
  - Femoral 01SD
  - Glossopharyngeal 00SP
  - Hypoglossal 00SS
  - Lumbar 01SB
  - Lumbar Plexus 01S9
  - Lumbosacral Plexus 01SA
  - Median 01S5
  - Oculomotor 00SH
  - Olfactory 00SF

Subterms under main terms may continue to next column or page

Reposition — continued
  Nerve — continued
    Optic 00SG
    Peroneal 01SH
    Phrenic 01S2
    Pudendal 01SC
    Radial 01S6
    Sacral 01SR
    Sacral Plexus 01SQ
    Sciatic 01SF
    Thoracic 01S8
    Tibial 01SG
    Trigeminal 00SK
    Trochlear 00SJ
    Ulnar 01S4
    Vagus 00SQ
  Nipple
    Left 0HSXXZZ
    Right 0HSWXZZ
  Nose 09SK
  Orbit
    Left 0NSQ
    Right 0NSP
  Ovary
    Bilateral 0US2
    Left 0US1
    Right 0US0
  Palate
    Hard 0CS2
    Soft 0CS3
  Pancreas 0FSG
  Parathyroid Gland 0GSR
    Inferior
      Left 0GSP
      Right 0GSN
    Multiple 0GSQ
    Superior
      Left 0GSM
      Right 0GSL
  Patella
    Left 0QSF
    Right 0QSD
  Phalanx
    Finger
      Left 0PSV
      Right 0PST
    Thumb
      Left 0PSS
      Right 0PSR
    Toe
      Left 0QSR
      Right 0QSQ
  Products of Conception 10S0
    Ectopic 10S2
  Radius
    Left 0PSJ
    Right 0PSH
  Rectum 0DSP
  Retinal Vessel
    Left 08SH3ZZ
    Right 08SG3ZZ
  Rib
    Left 0PS2
    Right 0PS1
  Sacrum 0QS1
  Scapula
    Left 0PS6
    Right 0PS5
  Septum, Nasal 09SM
  Skull 0NS0
  Spinal Cord
    Cervical 00SW
    Lumbar 00SY
    Thoracic 00SX
  Spleen 07SP0ZZ
  Sternum 0PS0
  Stomach 0DS6
  Tarsal
    Left 0QSM
    Right 0QSL
  Tendon
    Abdomen
      Left 0LSG
      Right 0LSF
    Ankle
      Left 0LST

Reposition — continued
  Tendon — continued
    Ankle — continued
      Right 0LSS
    Foot
      Left 0LSW
      Right 0LSV
    Hand
      Left 0LS8
      Right 0LS7
    Head and Neck 0LS0
    Hip
      Left 0LSK
      Right 0LSJ
    Knee
      Left 0LSR
      Right 0LSQ
    Lower Arm and Wrist
      Left 0LS6
      Right 0LS5
    Lower Leg
      Left 0LSP
      Right 0LSN
    Perineum 0LSH
    Shoulder
      Left 0LS2
      Right 0LS1
    Thorax
      Left 0LSD
      Right 0LSC
    Trunk
      Left 0LSB
      Right 0LS9
    Upper Arm
      Left 0LS4
      Right 0LS3
    Upper Leg
      Left 0LSM
      Right 0LSL
  Testis
    Bilateral 0VSC
    Left 0VSB
    Right 0VS9
  Thymus 07SM0ZZ
  Thyroid Gland
    Left Lobe 0GSG
    Right Lobe 0GSH
  Tibia
    Left 0QSH
    Right 0QSG
  Tongue 0CS7
  Tooth
    Lower 0CSX
    Upper 0CSW
  Trachea 0BS10ZZ
  Turbinate, Nasal 09SL
  Tympanic Membrane
    Left 09S8
    Right 09S7
  Ulna
    Left 0PSL
    Right 0PSK
  Ureter
    Left 0TS7
    Right 0TS6
  Ureters, Bilateral 0TS8
  Urethra 0TSD
  Uterine Supporting Structure 0US4
  Uterus 0US9
  Uvula 0CSN
  Vagina 0USG
  Vein
    Axillary
      Left 05S8
      Right 05S7
    Azygos 05S0
    Basilic
      Left 05SC
      Right 05SB
    Brachial
      Left 05SA
      Right 05S9
    Cephalic
      Left 05SF
      Right 05SD
    Colic 06S7

Reposition — continued
  Vein — continued
    Common Iliac
      Left 06SD
      Right 06SC
    Esophageal 06S3
    External Iliac
      Left 06SG
      Right 06SF
    External Jugular
      Left 05SQ
      Right 05SP
    Face
      Left 05SV
      Right 05ST
    Femoral
      Left 06SN
      Right 06SM
    Foot
      Left 06SV
      Right 06ST
    Gastric 06S2
    Greater Saphenous
      Left 06SQ
      Right 06SP
    Hand
      Left 05SH
      Right 05SG
    Hemiazygos 05S1
    Hepatic 06S4
    Hypogastric
      Left 06SJ
      Right 06SH
    Inferior Mesenteric 06S6
    Innominate
      Left 05S4
      Right 05S3
    Internal Jugular
      Left 05SN
      Right 05SM
    Intracranial 05SL
    Lesser Saphenous
      Left 06SS
      Right 06SR
    Lower 06SY
    Portal 06S8
    Pulmonary
      Left 02ST0ZZ
      Right 02SS0ZZ
    Renal
      Left 06SB
      Right 06S9
    Splenic 06S1
    Subclavian
      Left 05S6
      Right 05S5
    Superior Mesenteric 06S5
    Upper 05SY
    Vertebral
      Left 05SS
      Right 05SR
  Vena Cava
    Inferior 06S0
    Superior 02SV0ZZ
  Vertebra
    Cervical 0PS3
    Lumbar 0QS0
    Thoracic 0PS4
  Vocal Cord
    Left 0CSV
    Right 0CST

Resection
  Acetabulum
    Left 0QT50ZZ
    Right 0QT40ZZ
  Adenoids 0CTQ
  Ampulla of Vater 0FTC
  Anal Sphincter 0DTR
  Anus 0DTQ
  Aortic Body 0GTD
  Appendix 0DTJ
  Auditory Ossicle
    Left 09TA0ZZ
    Right 09T90ZZ
  Bladder 0TTB
  Bladder Neck 0TTC

▽ **Subterms under main terms may continue to next column or page**

Resection — continued
  Joint — continued
    Carpal
      Left ØRTRØZZ
      Right ØRTQØZZ
    Cervicothoracic Vertebral ØRT4ØZZ
    Coccygeal ØST6ØZZ
    Elbow
      Left ØRTMØZZ
      Right ØRTLØZZ
    Finger Phalangeal
      Left ØRTXØZZ
      Right ØRTWØZZ
    Hip
      Left ØSTBØZZ
      Right ØST9ØZZ
    Knee
      Left ØSTDØZZ
      Right ØSTCØZZ
    Metacarpocarpal
      Left ØRTTØZZ
      Right ØRTSØZZ
    Metacarpophalangeal
      Left ØRTVØZZ
      Right ØRTUØZZ
    Metatarsal-Phalangeal
      Left ØSTNØZZ
      Right ØSTMØZZ
    Metatarsal-Tarsal
      Left ØSTLØZZ
      Right ØSTKØZZ
    Sacrococcygeal ØST5ØZZ
    Sacroiliac
      Left ØST8ØZZ
      Right ØST7ØZZ
    Shoulder
      Left ØRTKØZZ
      Right ØRTJØZZ
    Sternoclavicular
      Left ØRTFØZZ
      Right ØRTEØZZ
    Tarsal
      Left ØSTJØZZ
      Right ØSTHØZZ
    Temporomandibular
      Left ØRTDØZZ
      Right ØRTCØZZ
    Toe Phalangeal
      Left ØSTQØZZ
      Right ØSTPØZZ
    Wrist
      Left ØRTPØZZ
      Right ØRTNØZZ
  Kidney
    Left ØTT1
    Right ØTTØ
  Kidney Pelvis
    Left ØTT4
    Right ØTT3
  Kidneys, Bilateral ØTT2
  Larynx ØCTS
  Lens
    Left Ø8TK3ZZ
    Right Ø8TJ3ZZ
  Lip
    Lower ØCT1
    Upper ØCTØ
  Liver ØFTØ
    Left Lobe ØFT2
    Right Lobe ØFT1
  Lung
    Bilateral ØBTM
    Left ØBTL
    Lower Lobe
      Left ØBTJ
      Right ØBTF
    Middle Lobe, Right ØBTD
    Right ØBTK
    Upper Lobe
      Left ØBTG
      Right ØBTC
  Lung Lingula ØBTH
  Lymphatic
    Aortic Ø7TD
    Axillary
      Left Ø7T6

Resection — continued
  Lymphatic — continued
    Axillary — continued
      Right Ø7T5
    Head Ø7TØ
    Inguinal
      Left Ø7TJ
      Right Ø7TH
    Internal Mammary
      Left Ø7T9
      Right Ø7T8
    Lower Extremity
      Left Ø7TG
      Right Ø7TF
    Mesenteric Ø7TB
    Neck
      Left Ø7T2
      Right Ø7T1
    Pelvis Ø7TC
    Thoracic Duct Ø7TK
    Thorax Ø7T7
    Upper Extremity
      Left Ø7T4
      Right Ø7T3
  Mandible
    Left ØNTVØZZ
    Right ØNTTØZZ
  Maxilla
    Left ØNTSØZZ
    Right ØNTRØZZ
  Metacarpal
    Left ØPTQØZZ
    Right ØPTPØZZ
  Metatarsal
    Left ØQTPØZZ
    Right ØQTNØZZ
  Muscle
    Abdomen
      Left ØKTL
      Right ØKTK
    Extraocular
      Left Ø8TM
      Right Ø8TL
    Facial ØKT1
    Foot
      Left ØKTW
      Right ØKTV
    Hand
      Left ØKTD
      Right ØKTC
    Head ØKTØ
    Hip
      Left ØKTP
      Right ØKTN
    Lower Arm and Wrist
      Left ØKTB
      Right ØKT9
    Lower Leg
      Left ØKTT
      Right ØKTS
    Neck
      Left ØKT3
      Right ØKT2
    Papillary Ø2TD
    Perineum ØKTM
    Shoulder
      Left ØKT6
      Right ØKT5
    Thorax
      Left ØKTJ
      Right ØKTH
    Tongue, Palate, Pharynx ØKT4
    Trunk
      Left ØKTG
      Right ØKTF
    Upper Arm
      Left ØKT8
      Right ØKT7
    Upper Leg
      Left ØKTR
      Right ØKTQ
  Nasopharynx Ø9TN
  Nipple
    Left ØHTXXZZ
    Right ØHTWXZZ
  Nose Ø9TK

Resection — continued
  Omentum
    Greater ØDTS
    Lesser ØDTT
  Orbit
    Left ØNTQØZZ
    Right ØNTPØZZ
  Ovary
    Bilateral ØUT2
    Left ØUT1
    Right ØUTØ
  Palate
    Hard ØCT2
    Soft ØCT3
  Pancreas ØFTG
  Para-aortic Body ØGT9
  Paraganglion Extremity ØGTF
  Parathyroid Gland ØGTR
    Inferior
      Left ØGTP
      Right ØGTN
    Multiple ØGTQ
    Superior
      Left ØGTM
      Right ØGTL
  Patella
    Left ØQTFØZZ
    Right ØQTDØZZ
  Penis ØVTS
  Pericardium Ø2TN
  Phalanx
    Finger
      Left ØPTVØZZ
      Right ØPTTØZZ
    Thumb
      Left ØPTSØZZ
      Right ØPTRØZZ
    Toe
      Left ØQTRØZZ
      Right ØQTQØZZ
  Pharynx ØCTM
  Pineal Body ØGT1
  Prepuce ØVTT
  Products of Conception, Ectopic 1ØT2
  Prostate ØVTØ
  Radius
    Left ØPTJØZZ
    Right ØPTHØZZ
  Rectum ØDTP
  Rib
    Left ØPT2ØZZ
    Right ØPT1ØZZ
  Scapula
    Left ØPT6ØZZ
    Right ØPT5ØZZ
  Scrotum ØVT5
  Septum
    Atrial Ø2T5
    Nasal Ø9TM
    Ventricular Ø2TM
  Sinus
    Accessory Ø9TP
    Ethmoid
      Left Ø9TV
      Right Ø9TU
    Frontal
      Left Ø9TT
      Right Ø9TS
    Mastoid
      Left Ø9TC
      Right Ø9TB
    Maxillary
      Left Ø9TR
      Right Ø9TQ
    Sphenoid
      Left Ø9TX
      Right Ø9TW
  Spleen Ø7TP
  Sternum ØPTØØZZ
  Stomach ØDT6
    Pylorus ØDT7
  Tarsal
    Left ØQTMØZZ
    Right ØQTLØZZ

Resection — continued
  Tendon
    Abdomen
      Left 0LTG
      Right 0LTF
    Ankle
      Left 0LTT
      Right 0LTS
    Foot
      Left 0LTW
      Right 0LTV
    Hand
      Left 0LT8
      Right 0LT7
    Head and Neck 0LT0
    Hip
      Left 0LTK
      Right 0LTJ
    Knee
      Left 0LTR
      Right 0LTQ
    Lower Arm and Wrist
      Left 0LT6
      Right 0LT5
    Lower Leg
      Left 0LTP
      Right 0LTN
    Perineum 0LTH
    Shoulder
      Left 0LT2
      Right 0LT1
    Thorax
      Left 0LTD
      Right 0LTC
    Trunk
      Left 0LTB
      Right 0LT9
    Upper Arm
      Left 0LT4
      Right 0LT3
    Upper Leg
      Left 0LTM
      Right 0LTL
  Testis
    Bilateral 0VTC
    Left 0VTB
    Right 0VT9
  Thymus 07TM
  Thyroid Gland 0GTK
    Left Lobe 0GTG
    Right Lobe 0GTH
  Tibia
    Left 0QTH0ZZ
    Right 0QTG0ZZ
  Toe Nail 0HTRXZZ
  Tongue 0CT7
  Tonsils 0CTP
  Tooth
    Lower 0CTX0Z
    Upper 0CTW0Z
  Trachea 0BT1
  Tunica Vaginalis
    Left 0VT7
    Right 0VT6
  Turbinate, Nasal 09TL
  Tympanic Membrane
    Left 09T8
    Right 09T7
  Ulna
    Left 0PTL0ZZ
    Right 0PTK0ZZ
  Ureter
    Left 0TT7
    Right 0TT6
  Urethra 0TTD
  Uterine Supporting Structure 0UT4
  Uterus 0UT9
  Uvula 0CTN
  Vagina 0UTG
  Valve, Pulmonary 02TH
  Vas Deferens
    Bilateral 0VTQ
    Left 0VTP
    Right 0VTN
  Vesicle
    Bilateral 0VT3

Resection — continued
  Vesicle — continued
    Left 0VT2
    Right 0VT1
  Vitreous
    Left 08T53ZZ
    Right 08T43ZZ
  Vocal Cord
    Left 0CTV
    Right 0CTT
  Vulva 0UTM
Restoration, Cardiac, Single, Rhythm 5A2204Z
RestoreAdvanced neurostimulator use Stimulator
  Generator, Multiple Array Rechargeable in 0JH
RestoreSensor neurostimulator use Stimulator Gen-
  erator, Multiple Array Rechargeable in 0JH
RestoreUltra neurostimulator use Simulator Genera-
  tor, Multiple Array Rechargeable in 0JH
Restriction
  Ampulla of Vater 0FVC
  Anus 0DVQ
  Aorta
    Abdominal 04V0
    Thoracic 02VW
  Artery
    Anterior Tibial
      Left 04VQ
      Right 04VP
    Axillary
      Left 03V6
      Right 03V5
    Brachial
      Left 03V8
      Right 03V7
    Celiac 04V1
    Colic
      Left 04V7
      Middle 04V8
      Right 04V6
    Common Carotid
      Left 03VJ
      Right 03VH
    Common Iliac
      Left 04VD
      Right 04VC
    External Carotid
      Left 03VN
      Right 03VM
    External Iliac
      Left 04VJ
      Right 04VH
    Face 03VR
    Femoral
      Left 04VL
      Right 04VK
    Foot
      Left 04VW
      Right 04VV
    Gastric 04V2
    Hand
      Left 03VF
      Right 03VD
    Hepatic 04V3
    Inferior Mesenteric 04VB
    Innominate 03V2
    Internal Carotid
      Left 03VL
      Right 03VK
    Internal Iliac
      Left 04VF
      Right 04VE
    Internal Mammary
      Left 03V1
      Right 03V0
    Intracranial 03VG
    Lower 04VY
    Peroneal
      Left 04VU
      Right 04VT
    Popliteal
      Left 04VN
      Right 04VM
    Posterior Tibial
      Left 04VS
      Right 04VR

Restriction — continued
  Artery — continued
    Pulmonary
      Left 02VR
      Right 02VQ
    Pulmonary Trunk 02VP
    Radial
      Left 03VC
      Right 03VB
    Renal
      Left 04VA
      Right 04V9
    Splenic 04V4
    Subclavian
      Left 03V4
      Right 03V3
    Superior Mesenteric 04V5
    Temporal
      Left 03VT
      Right 03VS
    Thyroid
      Left 03VV
      Right 03VU
    Ulnar
      Left 03VA
      Right 03V9
    Upper 03VY
    Vertebral
      Left 03VQ
      Right 03VP
  Bladder 0TVB
  Bladder Neck 0TVC
  Bronchus
    Lingula 0BV9
    Lower Lobe
      Left 0BVB
      Right 0BV6
    Main
      Left 0BV7
      Right 0BV3
    Middle Lobe, Right 0BV5
    Upper Lobe
      Left 0BV8
      Right 0BV4
  Carina 0BV2
  Cecum 0DVH
  Cervix 0UVC
  Cisterna Chyli 07VL
  Colon
    Ascending 0DVK
    Descending 0DVM
    Sigmoid 0DVN
    Transverse 0DVL
  Duct
    Common Bile 0FV9
    Cystic 0FV8
    Hepatic
      Left 0FV6
      Right 0FV5
    Lacrimal
      Left 08VY
      Right 08VX
    Pancreatic 0FVD
      Accessory 0FVF
    Parotid
      Left 0CVC
      Right 0CVB
  Duodenum 0DV9
  Esophagogastric Junction 0DV4
  Esophagus 0DV5
    Lower 0DV3
    Middle 0DV2
    Upper 0DV1
  Heart 02VA
  Ileocecal Valve 0DVC
  Ileum 0DVB
  Intestine
    Large 0DVE
      Left 0DVG
      Right 0DVF
    Small 0DV8
  Jejunum 0DVA
  Kidney Pelvis
    Left 0TV4
    Right 0TV3

⚐ **Subterms under main terms may continue to next column or page**

Revision of device in — continued
Head ØWWØ
Heart Ø2WA
Humeral Head
  Left ØPWD
  Right ØPWC
Humeral Shaft
  Left ØPWG
  Right ØPWF
Intestinal Tract
  Lower ØDWD
  Upper ØDWØ
Intestine
  Large ØDWE
  Small ØDW8
Jaw
  Lower ØWW5
  Upper ØWW4
Joint
  Acromioclavicular
    Left ØRWH
    Right ØRWG
  Ankle
    Left ØSWG
    Right ØSWF
  Carpal
    Left ØRWR
    Right ØRWQ
  Cervical Vertebral ØRW1
  Cervicothoracic Vertebral ØRW4
  Coccygeal ØSW6
  Elbow
    Left ØRWM
    Right ØRWL
  Finger Phalangeal
    Left ØRWX
    Right ØRWW
  Hip
    Left ØSWB
    Right ØSW9
  Knee
    Left ØSWD
    Right ØSWC
  Lumbar Vertebral ØSWØ
  Lumbosacral ØSW3
  Metacarpocarpal
    Left ØRWT
    Right ØRWS
  Metacarpophalangeal
    Left ØRWV
    Right ØRWU
  Metatarsal-Phalangeal
    Left ØSWN
    Right ØSWM
  Metatarsal-Tarsal
    Left ØSWL
    Right ØSWK
  Occipital-cervical ØRWØ
  Sacrococcygeal ØSW5
  Sacroiliac
    Left ØSW8
    Right ØSW7
  Shoulder
    Left ØRWK
    Right ØRWJ
  Sternoclavicular
    Left ØRWF
    Right ØRWE
  Tarsal
    Left ØSWJ
    Right ØSWH
  Temporomandibular
    Left ØRWD
    Right ØRWC
  Thoracic Vertebral ØRW6
  Thoracolumbar Vertebral ØRWA
  Toe Phalangeal
    Left ØSWQ
    Right ØSWP
  Wrist
    Left ØRWP
    Right ØRWN
Kidney ØTW5
Larynx ØCWS
Lens
  Left Ø8WK

Revision of device in — continued
Lens — continued
  Right Ø8WJ
Liver ØFWØ
Lung
  Left ØBWL
  Right ØBWK
Lymphatic Ø7WN
  Thoracic Duct Ø7WK
Mediastinum ØWWC
Mesentery ØDWV
Metacarpal
  Left ØPWQ
  Right ØPWP
Metatarsal
  Left ØQWP
  Right ØQWN
Mouth and Throat ØCWY
Muscle
  Extraocular
    Left Ø8WM
    Right Ø8WL
  Lower ØKWY
  Upper ØKWX
Neck ØWW6
Nerve
  Cranial ØØWE
  Peripheral Ø1WY
Nose Ø9WK
Omentum ØDWU
Ovary ØUW3
Pancreas ØFWG
Parathyroid Gland ØGWR
Patella
  Left ØQWF
  Right ØQWD
Pelvic Cavity ØWWJ
Penis ØVWS
Pericardial Cavity ØWWD
Perineum
  Female ØWWN
  Male ØWWM
Peritoneal Cavity ØWWG
Peritoneum ØDWW
Phalanx
  Finger
    Left ØPWV
    Right ØPWT
  Thumb
    Left ØPWS
    Right ØPWR
  Toe
    Left ØQWR
    Right ØQWQ
Pineal Body ØGW1
Pleura ØBWQ
Pleural Cavity
  Left ØWWB
  Right ØWW9
Prostate and Seminal Vesicles ØVW4
Radius
  Left ØPWJ
  Right ØPWH
Respiratory Tract ØWWQ
Retroperitoneum ØWWH
Rib
  Left ØPW2
  Right ØPW1
Sacrum ØQW1
Scapula
  Left ØPW6
  Right ØPW5
Scrotum and Tunica Vaginalis ØVW8
Septum
  Atrial Ø2W5
  Ventricular Ø2WM
Sinus Ø9WY
Skin ØHWPX
Skull ØNWØ
Spinal Canal ØØWU
Spinal Cord ØØWV
Spleen Ø7WP
Sternum ØPWØ
Stomach ØDW6
Subcutaneous Tissue and Fascia
  Head and Neck ØJWS

Revision of device in — continued
Subcutaneous Tissue and Fascia — continued
  Lower Extremity ØJWW
  Trunk ØJWT
  Upper Extremity ØJWV
Tarsal
  Left ØQWM
  Right ØQWL
Tendon
  Lower ØLWY
  Upper ØLWX
Testis ØVWD
Thymus Ø7WM
Thyroid Gland ØGWK
Tibia
  Left ØQWH
  Right ØQWG
Toe Nail ØHWRX
Trachea ØBW1
Tracheobronchial Tree ØBWØ
Tympanic Membrane
  Left Ø9W8
  Right Ø9W7
Ulna
  Left ØPWL
  Right ØPWK
Ureter ØTW9
Urethra ØTWD
Uterus and Cervix ØUWD
Vagina and Cul-de-sac ØUWH
Valve
  Aortic Ø2WF
  Mitral Ø2WG
  Pulmonary Ø2WH
  Tricuspid Ø2WJ
Vas Deferens ØVWR
Vein
  Lower Ø6WY
  Upper Ø5WY
Vertebra
  Cervical ØPW3
  Lumbar ØQWØ
  Thoracic ØPW4
Vulva ØUWM
Revo MRI™ SureScan® pacemaker *use* Pacemaker, Dual Chamber in ØJH
Rheos® System device *use* Cardiac Rhythm Related Device in Subcutaneous Tissue and Fascia
Rheos® System lead *use* Stimulator Lead in Upper Arteries
Rhinopharynx *use* Nasopharynx
Rhinoplasty
  see Alteration, Nose Ø9ØK
  see Repair, Nose Ø9QK
  see Replacement, Nose Ø9RK
  see Supplement, Nose Ø9UK
Rhinorrhaphy *see* Repair, Nose Ø9QK
Rhinoscopy Ø9JKXZZ
Rhizotomy
  see Division, Central Nervous System ØØ8
  see Division, Peripheral Nervous System Ø18
Rhomboid major muscle
  use Muscle, Trunk, Left
  use Muscle, Trunk, Right
Rhomboid minor muscle
  use Muscle, Trunk, Left
  use Muscle, Trunk, Right
Rhythm electrocardiogram *see* Measurement, Cardiac 4AØ2
Rhytidectomy *see* Face lift
Right ascending lumbar vein *use* Vein, Azygos
Right atrioventricular valve *use* Valve, Tricuspid
Right auricular appendix *use* Atrium, Right
Right colic vein *use* Vein, Colic
Right coronary sulcus *use* Heart, Right
Right gastric artery *use* Artery, Gastric
Right gastroepiploic vein *use* Vein, Superior Mesenteric
Right inferior phrenic vein *use* Vena Cava, Inferior
Right inferior pulmonary vein *use* Vein, Pulmonary, Right
Right jugular trunk *use* Lymphatic, Neck, Right
Right lateral ventricle *use* Cerebral Ventricle
Right lymphatic duct *use* Lymphatic, Neck, Right
Right ovarian vein *use* Vena Cava, Inferior

Right second lumbar vein *use* Vena Cava, Inferior
Right subclavian trunk *use* Lymphatic, Neck, Right
Right subcostal vein *use* Vein, Azygos
Right superior pulmonary vein *use* Vein, Pulmonary, Right
Right suprarenal vein *use* Vena Cava, Inferior
Right testicular vein *use* Vena Cava, Inferior
Rima glottidis *use* Larynx
Risorius muscle *use* Muscle, Facial
RNS System lead *use* Neurostimulator Lead in Central Nervous System
RNS system neurostimulator generator *use* Neurostimulator Generator in Head and Facial Bones
Robotic Assisted Procedure
    Extremity
        Lower 8E0Y
        Upper 8E0X
    Head and Neck Region 8E09
    Trunk Region 8E0W
Rotation of fetal head
    Forceps 10S07ZZ
    Manual 10S0XZZ
Round ligament of uterus *use* Uterine Supporting Structure
Round window
    use Ear, Inner, Left
    use Ear, Inner, Right
Roux-en-Y operation
    see Bypass, Gastrointestinal System 0D1
    see Bypass, Hepatobiliary System and Pancreas 0F1
Rupture
    Adhesions *see* Release
    Fluid collection *see* Drainage

S

Sacral ganglion *use* Nerve, Sacral Sympathetic
Sacral lymph node *use* Lymphatic, Pelvis
Sacral nerve modulation (SNM) lead *use* Stimulator Lead in Urinary System
Sacral neuromodulation lead *use* Stimulator Lead in Urinary System
Sacral splanchnic nerve *use* Nerve, Sacral Sympathetic
Sacrectomy *see* Excision, Lower Bones 0QB
Sacrococcygeal ligament
    use Bursa and Ligament, Trunk, Left
    use Bursa and Ligament, Trunk, Right
Sacrococcygeal symphysis *use* Joint, Sacrococcygeal
Sacroiliac ligament
    use Bursa and Ligament, Trunk, Left
    use Bursa and Ligament, Trunk, Right
Sacrospinous ligament
    use Bursa and Ligament, Trunk, Left
    use Bursa and Ligament, Trunk, Right
Sacrotuberous ligament
    use Bursa and Ligament, Trunk, Left
    use Bursa and Ligament, Trunk, Right
Salpingectomy
    see Excision, Female Reproductive System 0UB
    see Resection, Female Reproductive System 0UT
Salpingolysis *see* Release, Female Reproductive System 0UN
Salpingopexy
    see Repair, Female Reproductive System 0UQ
    see Reposition, Female Reproductive System 0US
Salpingopharyngeus muscle *use* Muscle, Tongue, Palate, Pharynx
Salpingoplasty
    see Repair, Female Reproductive System 0UQ
    see Supplement, Female Reproductive System 0UU
Salpingorrhaphy *see* Repair, Female Reproductive System 0UQ
Salpingoscopy 0UJ88ZZ
Salpingostomy *see* Drainage, Female Reproductive System 0U9
Salpingotomy *see* Drainage, Female Reproductive System 0U9
Salpinx
    use Fallopian Tube, Left
    use Fallopian Tube, Right
Saphenous nerve *use* Nerve, Femoral
SAPIEN transcatheter aortic valve *use* Zooplastic Tissue in Heart and Great Vessels

Sartorius muscle
    use Muscle, Upper Leg, Left
    use Muscle, Upper Leg, Right
Scalene muscle
    use Muscle, Neck, Left
    use Muscle, Neck, Right
Scan
    Computerized Tomography (CT) *see* Computerized Tomography (CT Scan)
    Radioisotope *see* Planar Nuclear Medicine Imaging
Scaphoid bone
    use Carpal, Left
    use Carpal, Right
Scapholunate ligament
    use Bursa and Ligament, Hand, Left
    use Bursa and Ligament, Hand, Right
Scaphotrapezium ligament
    use Bursa and Ligament, Hand, Left
    use Bursa and Ligament, Hand, Right
Scapulectomy
    see Excision, Upper Bones 0PB
    see Resection, Upper Bones 0PT
Scapulopexy
    see Repair, Upper Bones 0PQ
    see Reposition, Upper Bones 0PS
Scarpa's (vestibular) ganglion *use* Nerve, Acoustic
Sclerectomy *see* Excision, Eye 08B
Sclerotherapy, mechanical *see* Destruction
Sclerotomy *see* Drainage, Eye 089
Scrotectomy
    see Excision, Male Reproductive System 0VB
    see Resection, Male Reproductive System 0VT
Scrotoplasty
    see Repair, Male Reproductive System 0VQ
    see Supplement, Male Reproductive System 0VU
Scrotorrhaphy *see* Repair, Male Reproductive System 0VQ
Scrototomy *see* Drainage, Male Reproductive System 0V9
Sebaceous gland *use* Skin
Second cranial nerve *use* Nerve, Optic
Section, cesarean *see* Extraction, Pregnancy 10D
Secura (DR) (VR) *use* Defibrillator Generator in 0JH
Sella Turcica
    use Bone, Sphenoid, Left
    use Bone, Sphenoid, Right
Semicircular canal
    use Ear, Inner, Left
    use Ear, Inner, Right
Semimembranosus muscle
    use Muscle, Upper Leg, Left
    use Muscle, Upper Leg, Right
Semitendinosus muscle
    use Muscle, Upper Leg, Left
    use Muscle, Upper Leg, Right
Septal cartilage *use* Septum, Nasal
Septectomy
    see Excision, Ear, Nose, Sinus 09B
    see Excision, Heart and Great Vessels 02B
    see Resection, Ear, Nose, Sinus 09T
    see Resection, Heart and Great Vessels 02T
Septoplasty
    see Repair, Ear, Nose, Sinus 09Q
    see Repair, Heart and Great Vessels 02Q
    see Replacement, Ear, Nose, Sinus 09R
    see Replacement, Heart and Great Vessels 02R
    see Reposition, Ear, Nose, Sinus 09S
    see Supplement, Ear, Nose, Sinus 09U
    see Supplement, Heart and Great Vessels 02U
Septotomy *see* Drainage, Ear, Nose, Sinus 099
Sequestrectomy, bone *see* Extirpation
Serratus anterior muscle
    use Muscle, Thorax, Left
    use Muscle, Thorax, Right
Serratus posterior muscle
    use Muscle, Trunk, Left
    use Muscle, Trunk, Right
Seventh cranial nerve *use* Nerve, Facial
Sheffield hybrid external fixator
    use External Fixation Device, Hybrid in 0QH
    use External Fixation Device, Hybrid in 0QS
    use External Fixation Device, Hybrid in 0PS
    use External Fixation Device, Hybrid in 0PH

Sheffield ring external fixator
    use External Fixation Device, Ring in 0PS
    use External Fixation Device, Ring in 0QS
    use External Fixation Device, Ring in 0QH
    use External Fixation Device, Ring in 0PH
Shirodkar cervical cerclage 0UVC7ZZ
Shock Wave Therapy, Musculoskeletal 6A93
Short gastric artery *use* Artery, Splenic
Shortening
    see Excision
    see Repair
    see Reposition
Shunt creation *see* Bypass
Sialoadenectomy
    Complete *see* Resection, Mouth and Throat 0CT
    Partial *see* Excision, Mouth and Throat 0CB
Sialodochoplasty
    see Repair, Mouth and Throat 0CQ
    see Replacement, Mouth and Throat 0CR
    see Supplement, Mouth and Throat 0CU
Sialoectomy
    see Excision, Mouth and Throat 0CB
    see Resection, Mouth and Throat 0CT
Sialography *see* Plain Radiography, Ear, Nose, Mouth and Throat B90
Sialolithotomy *see* Extirpation, Mouth and Throat 0CC
Sigmoid artery *use* Artery, Inferior Mesenteric
Sigmoid flexure *use* Colon, Sigmoid
Sigmoid vein *use* Vein, Inferior Mesenteric
Sigmoidectomy
    see Excision, Gastrointestinal System 0DB
    see Resection, Gastrointestinal System 0DT
Sigmoidorrhaphy *see* Repair, Gastrointestinal System 0DQ
Sigmoidoscopy 0DJD8ZZ
Sigmoidotomy *see* Drainage, Gastrointestinal System 0D9
Single lead pacemaker (atrium)(ventricle) *use* Pacemaker, Single Chamber in 0JH
Single lead rate responsive pacemaker (atrium)(ventricle) *use* Pacemaker, Single Chamber Rate Responsive in 0JH
Sinoatrial node *use* Conduction Mechanism
Sinogram
    Abdominal Wall *see* Fluoroscopy, Abdomen and Pelvis BW11
    Chest Wall *see* Plain Radiography, Chest BW03
    Retroperitoneum *see* Fluoroscopy, Abdomen and Pelvis BW11
Sinus venosus *use* Atrium, Right
Sinusectomy
    see Excision, Ear, Nose, Sinus 09B
    see Resection, Ear, Nose, Sinus 09T
Sinusoscopy 09JY4ZZ
Sinusotomy *see* Drainage, Ear, Nose, Sinus 099
Sirolimus-eluting coronary stent *use* Intraluminal Device, Drug-eluting in Heart and Great Vessels
Sixth cranial nerve *use* Nerve, Abducens
Size reduction, breast *see* Excision, Skin and Breast 0HB
SJM Biocor® Stented Valve System *use* Zooplastic Tissue in Heart and Great Vessels
Skene's (paraurethral) gland *use* Gland, Vestibular
Sling
    Fascial, orbicularis muscle (mouth) *see* Supplement, Muscle, Facial 0KU1
    Levator muscle, for urethral suspension *see* Reposition, Bladder Neck 0TSC
    Pubococcygeal, for urethral suspension *see* Reposition, Bladder Neck 0TSC
    Rectum *see* Reposition, Rectum 0DSP
Small bowel series *see* Fluoroscopy, Bowel, Small BD13
Small saphenous vein
    use Vein, Lesser Saphenous, Left
    use Vein, Lesser Saphenous, Right
Snaring, polyp, colon *see* Excision, Gastrointestinal System 0DB
Solar (celiac) plexus *use* Nerve, Abdominal Sympathetic
Soletra® single-channel neurostimulator *use* Stimulator Generator, Single Array in 0JH
Soleus muscle
    use Muscle, Lower Leg, Left
    use Muscle, Lower Leg, Right

Spacer
  Insertion of device in
    Disc
      Lumbar Vertebral ØSH2
      Lumbosacral ØSH4
    Joint
      Acromioclavicular
        Left ØRHH
        Right ØRHG
      Ankle
        Left ØSHG
        Right ØSHF
      Carpal
        Left ØRHR
        Right ØRHQ
      Cervical Vertebral ØRH1
      Cervicothoracic Vertebral ØRH4
      Coccygeal ØSH6
      Elbow
        Left ØRHM
        Right ØRHL
      Finger Phalangeal
        Left ØRHX
        Right ØRHW
      Hip
        Left ØSHB
        Right ØSH9
      Knee
        Left ØSHD
        Right ØSHC
      Lumbar Vertebral ØSH0
      Lumbosacral ØSH3
      Metacarpocarpal
        Left ØRHT
        Right ØRHS
      Metacarpophalangeal
        Left ØRHV
        Right ØRHU
      Metatarsal-Phalangeal
        Left ØSHN
        Right ØSHM
      Metatarsal-Tarsal
        Left ØSHL
        Right ØSHK
      Occipital-cervical ØRH0
      Sacrococcygeal ØSH5
      Sacroiliac
        Left ØSH8
        Right ØSH7
      Shoulder
        Left ØRHK
        Right ØRHJ
      Sternoclavicular
        Left ØRHF
        Right ØRHE
      Tarsal
        Left ØSHJ
        Right ØSHH
      Temporomandibular
        Left ØRHD
        Right ØRHC
      Thoracic Vertebral ØRH6
      Thoracolumbar Vertebral ØRHA
      Toe Phalangeal
        Left ØSHQ
        Right ØSHP
      Wrist
        Left ØRHP
        Right ØRHN
  Removal of device from
    Acromioclavicular
      Left ØRPH
      Right ØRPG
    Ankle
      Left ØSPG
      Right ØSPF
    Carpal
      Left ØRPR
      Right ØRPQ
    Cervical Vertebral ØRP1
    Cervicothoracic Vertebral ØRP4
    Coccygeal ØSP6
    Elbow
      Left ØRPM
      Right ØRPL

Spacer — continued
  Removal of device from — continued
    Finger Phalangeal
      Left ØRPX
      Right ØRPW
    Hip
      Left ØSPB
      Right ØSP9
    Knee
      Left ØSPD
      Right ØSPC
    Lumbar Vertebral ØSP0
    Lumbosacral ØSP3
    Metacarpocarpal
      Left ØRPT
      Right ØRPS
    Metacarpophalangeal
      Left ØRPV
      Right ØRPU
    Metatarsal-Phalangeal
      Left ØSPN
      Right ØSPM
    Metatarsal-Tarsal
      Left ØSPL
      Right ØSPK
    Occipital-cervical ØRP0
    Sacrococcygeal ØSP5
    Sacroiliac
      Left ØSP8
      Right ØSP7
    Shoulder
      Left ØRPK
      Right ØRPJ
    Sternoclavicular
      Left ØRPF
      Right ØRPE
    Tarsal
      Left ØSPJ
      Right ØSPH
    Temporomandibular
      Left ØRPD
      Right ØRPC
    Thoracic Vertebral ØRP6
    Thoracolumbar Vertebral ØRPA
    Toe Phalangeal
      Left ØSPQ
      Right ØSPP
    Wrist
      Left ØRPP
      Right ØRPN
  Revision of device in
    Acromioclavicular
      Left ØRWH
      Right ØRWG
    Ankle
      Left ØSWG
      Right ØSWF
    Carpal
      Left ØRWR
      Right ØRWQ
    Cervical Vertebral ØRW1
    Cervicothoracic Vertebral ØRW4
    Coccygeal ØSW6
    Elbow
      Left ØRWM
      Right ØRWL
    Finger Phalangeal
      Left ØRWX
      Right ØRWW
    Hip
      Left ØSWB
      Right ØSW9
    Knee
      Left ØSWD
      Right ØSWC
    Lumbar Vertebral ØSW0
    Lumbosacral ØSW3
    Metacarpocarpal
      Left ØRWT
      Right ØRWS
    Metacarpophalangeal
      Left ØRWV
      Right ØRWU
    Metatarsal-Phalangeal
      Left ØSWN
      Right ØSWM

Spacer — continued
  Revision of device in — continued
    Metatarsal-Tarsal
      Left ØSWL
      Right ØSWK
    Occipital-cervical ØRW0
    Sacrococcygeal ØSW5
    Sacroiliac
      Left ØSW8
      Right ØSW7
    Shoulder
      Left ØRWK
      Right ØRWJ
    Sternoclavicular
      Left ØRWF
      Right ØRWE
    Tarsal
      Left ØSWJ
      Right ØSWH
    Temporomandibular
      Left ØRWD
      Right ØRWC
    Thoracic Vertebral ØRW6
    Thoracolumbar Vertebral ØRWA
    Toe Phalangeal
      Left ØSWQ
      Right ØSWP
    Wrist
      Left ØRWP
      Right ØRWN
Spectroscopy
  Intravascular 8E023DZ
  Near infrared 8E023DZ
Speech Assessment F00
Speech therapy *see* Speech Treatment, Rehabilitation
  F06
Speech Treatment F06
Sphenoidectomy
  see Excision, Ear, Nose, Sinus 09B
  see Excision, Head and Facial Bones ØNB
  see Resection, Ear, Nose, Sinus 09T
  see Resection, Head and Facial Bones ØNT
Sphenoidotomy *see* Drainage, Ear, Nose, Sinus 099
Sphenomandibular ligament *use* Bursa and Ligament,
  Head and Neck
Sphenopalatine (pterygopalatine) ganglion *use*
  Nerve, Head and Neck Sympathetic
Sphincterorrhaphy, anal *see* Repair, Anal Sphincter
  ØDQR
Sphincterotomy, anal
  see Division, Anal Sphincter ØD8R
  see Drainage, Anal Sphincter ØD9R
Spinal cord neurostimulator lead *use* Neurostimulator
  Lead in Central Nervous System
Spinal dura mater *use* Dura Mater
Spinal epidural space *use* Epidural Space
Spinal nerve, cervical *use* Nerve, Cervical
Spinal nerve, lumbar *use* Nerve, Lumbar
Spinal nerve, sacral *use* Nerve, Sacral
Spinal nerve, thoracic *use* Nerve, Thoracic
Spinal Stabilization Device
  Facet Replacement
    Cervical Vertebral ØRH1
    Cervicothoracic Vertebral ØRH4
    Lumbar Vertebral ØSH0
    Lumbosacral ØSH3
    Occipital-cervical ØRH0
    Thoracic Vertebral ØRH6
    Thoracolumbar Vertebral ØRHA
  Interspinous Process
    Cervical Vertebral ØRH1
    Cervicothoracic Vertebral ØRH4
    Lumbar Vertebral ØSH0
    Lumbosacral ØSH3
    Occipital-cervical ØRH0
    Thoracic Vertebral ØRH6
    Thoracolumbar Vertebral ØRHA
  Pedicle-Based
    Cervical Vertebral ØRH1
    Cervicothoracic Vertebral ØRH4
    Lumbar Vertebral ØSH0
    Lumbosacral ØSH3
    Occipital-cervical ØRH0
    Thoracic Vertebral ØRH6
    Thoracolumbar Vertebral ØRHA
Spinal subarachnoid space *use* Subarachnoid Space

Spinal subdural space *use* Subdural Space
Spinous process
  use Vertebra, Cervical
  use Vertebra, Lumbar
  use Vertebra, Thoracic
Spiral ganglion *use* Nerve, Acoustic
Spiration IBV™ Valve System *use* Intraluminal Device, Endobronchial Valve in Respiratory System
Splenectomy
  see Excision, Lymphatic and Hemic Systems 07B
  see Resection, Lymphatic and Hemic Systems 07T
Splenic flexure *use* Colon, Transverse
Splenic plexus *use* Nerve, Abdominal Sympathetic
Splenius capitis muscle *use* Muscle, Head
Splenius cervicis muscle
  use Muscle, Neck, Left
  use Muscle, Neck, Right
Splenolysis *see* Release, Lymphatic and Hemic Systems 07N
Splenopexy
  see Repair, Lymphatic and Hemic Systems 07Q
  see Reposition, Lymphatic and Hemic Systems 07S
Splenoplasty *see* Repair, Lymphatic and Hemic Systems 07Q
Splenorrhaphy *see* Repair, Lymphatic and Hemic Systems 07Q
Splenotomy *see* Drainage, Lymphatic and Hemic Systems 079
Splinting, musculoskeletal *see* Immobilization, Anatomical Regions 2W3
Stapedectomy
  see Excision, Ear, Nose, Sinus 09B
  see Resection, Ear, Nose, Sinus 09T
Stapediolysis *see* Release, Ear, Nose, Sinus 09N
Stapedioplasty
  see Repair, Ear, Nose, Sinus 09Q
  see Replacement, Ear, Nose, Sinus 09R
  see Supplement, Ear, Nose, Sinus 09U
Stapedotomy *see* Drainage, Ear, Nose, Sinus 099
Stapes
  use Auditory Ossicle, Left
  use Auditory Ossicle, Right
Stellate ganglion *use* Nerve, Head and Neck Sympathetic
Stensen's duct
  use Duct, Parotid, Left
  use Duct, Parotid, Right
Stent (angioplasty)(embolization) *use* Intraluminal Device
Stented tissue valve *use* Zooplastic Tissue in Heart and Great Vessels
Stereotactic Radiosurgery
  Gamma Beam
    Abdomen DW23JZZ
    Adrenal Gland DG22JZZ
    Bile Ducts DF22JZZ
    Bladder DT22JZZ
    Bone Marrow D720JZZ
    Brain D020JZZ
    Brain Stem D021JZZ
    Breast
      Left DM20JZZ
      Right DM21JZZ
    Bronchus DB21JZZ
    Cervix DU21JZZ
    Chest DW22JZZ
    Chest Wall DB27JZZ
    Colon DD25JZZ
    Diaphragm DB28JZZ
    Duodenum DD22JZZ
    Ear D920JZZ
    Esophagus DD20JZZ
    Eye D820JZZ
    Gallbladder DF21JZZ
    Gland
      Adrenal DG22JZZ
      Parathyroid DG24JZZ
      Pituitary DG20JZZ
      Thyroid DG25JZZ
    Glands, Salivary D926JZZ
    Head and Neck DW21JZZ
    Ileum DD24JZZ
    Jejunum DD23JZZ
    Kidney DT20JZZ
    Larynx D92BJZZ

Stereotactic Radiosurgery — continued
  Gamma Beam — continued
    Liver DF20JZZ
    Lung DB22JZZ
    Lymphatics
      Abdomen D726JZZ
      Axillary D724JZZ
      Inguinal D728JZZ
      Neck D723JZZ
      Pelvis D727JZZ
      Thorax D725JZZ
    Mediastinum DB26JZZ
    Mouth D924JZZ
    Nasopharynx D92DJZZ
    Neck and Head DW21JZZ
    Nerve, Peripheral D027JZZ
    Nose D921JZZ
    Ovary DU20JZZ
    Palate
      Hard D928JZZ
      Soft D929JZZ
    Pancreas DF23JZZ
    Parathyroid Gland DG24JZZ
    Pelvic Region DW26JZZ
    Pharynx D92CJZZ
    Pineal Body DG21JZZ
    Pituitary Gland DG20JZZ
    Pleura DB25JZZ
    Prostate DV20JZZ
    Rectum DD27JZZ
    Sinuses D927JZZ
    Spinal Cord D026JZZ
    Spleen D722JZZ
    Stomach DD21JZZ
    Testis DV21JZZ
    Thymus D721JZZ
    Thyroid Gland DG25JZZ
    Tongue D925JZZ
    Trachea DB20JZZ
    Ureter DT21JZZ
    Urethra DT23JZZ
    Uterus DU22JZZ
  Other Photon
    Abdomen DW23DZZ
    Adrenal Gland DG22DZZ
    Bile Ducts DF22DZZ
    Bladder DT22DZZ
    Bone Marrow D720DZZ
    Brain D020DZZ
    Brain Stem D021DZZ
    Breast
      Left DM20DZZ
      Right DM21DZZ
    Bronchus DB21DZZ
    Cervix DU21DZZ
    Chest DW22DZZ
    Chest Wall DB27DZZ
    Colon DD25DZZ
    Diaphragm DB28DZZ
    Duodenum DD22DZZ
    Ear D920DZZ
    Esophagus DD20DZZ
    Eye D820DZZ
    Gallbladder DF21DZZ
    Gland
      Adrenal DG22DZZ
      Parathyroid DG24DZZ
      Pituitary DG20DZZ
      Thyroid DG25DZZ
    Glands, Salivary D926DZZ
    Head and Neck DW21DZZ
    Ileum DD24DZZ
    Jejunum DD23DZZ
    Kidney DT20DZZ
    Larynx D92BDZZ
    Liver DF20DZZ
    Lung DB22DZZ
    Lymphatics
      Abdomen D726DZZ
      Axillary D724DZZ
      Inguinal D728DZZ
      Neck D723DZZ
      Pelvis D727DZZ
      Thorax D725DZZ
    Mediastinum DB26DZZ
    Mouth D924DZZ

Stereotactic Radiosurgery — continued
  Other Photon — continued
    Nasopharynx D92DDZZ
    Neck and Head DW21DZZ
    Nerve, Peripheral D027DZZ
    Nose D921DZZ
    Ovary DU20DZZ
    Palate
      Hard D928DZZ
      Soft D929DZZ
    Pancreas DF23DZZ
    Parathyroid Gland DG24DZZ
    Pelvic Region DW26DZZ
    Pharynx D92CDZZ
    Pineal Body DG21DZZ
    Pituitary Gland DG20DZZ
    Pleura DB25DZZ
    Prostate DV20DZZ
    Rectum DD27DZZ
    Sinuses D927DZZ
    Spinal Cord D026DZZ
    Spleen D722DZZ
    Stomach DD21DZZ
    Testis DV21DZZ
    Thymus D721DZZ
    Thyroid Gland DG25DZZ
    Tongue D925DZZ
    Trachea DB20DZZ
    Ureter DT21DZZ
    Urethra DT23DZZ
    Uterus DU22DZZ
  Particulate
    Abdomen DW23HZZ
    Adrenal Gland DG22HZZ
    Bile Ducts DF22HZZ
    Bladder DT22HZZ
    Bone Marrow D720HZZ
    Brain D020HZZ
    Brain Stem D021HZZ
    Breast
      Left DM20HZZ
      Right DM21HZZ
    Bronchus DB21HZZ
    Cervix DU21HZZ
    Chest DW22HZZ
    Chest Wall DB27HZZ
    Colon DD25HZZ
    Diaphragm DB28HZZ
    Duodenum DD22HZZ
    Ear D920HZZ
    Esophagus DD20HZZ
    Eye D820HZZ
    Gallbladder DF21HZZ
    Gland
      Adrenal DG22HZZ
      Parathyroid DG24HZZ
      Pituitary DG20HZZ
      Thyroid DG25HZZ
    Glands, Salivary D926HZZ
    Head and Neck DW21HZZ
    Ileum DD24HZZ
    Jejunum DD23HZZ
    Kidney DT20HZZ
    Larynx D92BHZZ
    Liver DF20HZZ
    Lung DB22HZZ
    Lymphatics
      Abdomen D726HZZ
      Axillary D724HZZ
      Inguinal D728HZZ
      Neck D723HZZ
      Pelvis D727HZZ
      Thorax D725HZZ
    Mediastinum DB26HZZ
    Mouth D924HZZ
    Nasopharynx D92DHZZ
    Neck and Head DW21HZZ
    Nerve, Peripheral D027HZZ
    Nose D921HZZ
    Ovary DU20HZZ
    Palate
      Hard D928HZZ
      Soft D929HZZ
    Pancreas DF23HZZ
    Parathyroid Gland DG24HZZ
    Pelvic Region DW26HZZ

Stereotactic Radiosurgery — continued
   Particulate — continued
      Pharynx D92CHZZ
      Pineal Body DG20HZZ
      Pituitary Gland DG20HZZ
      Pleura DB25HZZ
      Prostate DV20HZZ
      Rectum DD27HZZ
      Sinuses D927HZZ
      Spinal Cord D026HZZ
      Spleen D722HZZ
      Stomach DD21HZZ
      Testis DV21HZZ
      Thymus D721HZZ
      Thyroid Gland DG25HZZ
      Tongue D925HZZ
      Trachea DB20HZZ
      Ureter DT21HZZ
      Urethra DT23HZZ
      Uterus DU22HZZ
Sternoclavicular ligament
   use Bursa and Ligament, Shoulder, Left
   use Bursa and Ligament, Shoulder, Right
Sternocleidomastoid artery
   use Artery, Thyroid, Left
   use Artery, Thyroid, Right
Sternocleidomastoid muscle
   use Muscle, Neck, Left
   use Muscle, Neck, Right
Sternocostal ligament
   use Bursa and Ligament, Thorax, Left
   use Bursa and Ligament, Thorax, Right
Sternotomy
   see Division, Sternum 0P80
   see Drainage, Sternum 0P90
Stimulation, cardiac
   Cardioversion 5A2204Z
   Electrophysiologic testing *see* Measurement, Cardiac 4A02
Stimulator Generator
   Insertion of device in
      Abdomen 0JH8
      Back 0JH7
      Chest 0JH6
      Multiple Array
         Abdomen 0JH8
         Back 0JH7
         Chest 0JH6
      Multiple Array Rechargeable
         Abdomen 0JH8
         Back 0JH7
         Chest 0JH6
      Removal of device from, Subcutaneous Tissue and Fascia, Trunk 0JPT
      Revision of device in, Subcutaneous Tissue and Fascia, Trunk 0JWT
      Single Array
         Abdomen 0JH8
         Back 0JH7
         Chest 0JH6
      Single Array Rechargeable
         Abdomen 0JH8
         Back 0JH7
         Chest 0JH6
Stimulator Lead
   Insertion of device in
      Anal Sphincter 0DHR
      Artery
         Left 03HL
         Right 03HK
      Bladder 0THB
      Muscle
         Lower 0KHY
         Upper 0KHX
      Stomach 0DH6
      Ureter 0TH9
   Removal of device from
      Anal Sphincter 0DPR
      Artery, Upper 03PY
      Bladder 0TPB
      Muscle
         Lower 0KPY
         Upper 0KPX
      Stomach 0DP6
      Ureter 0TP9

Stimulator Lead — continued
   Revision of device in
      Anal Sphincter 0DWR
      Artery, Upper 03WY
      Bladder 0TWB
      Muscle
         Lower 0KWY
         Upper 0KWX
      Stomach 0DW6
      Ureter 0TW9
Stoma
   Excision
      Abdominal Wall 0WBFXZ2
      Neck 0WB6XZ2
   Repair
      Abdominal Wall 0WQFXZ2
      Neck 0WQ6XZ2
Stomatoplasty
   see Repair, Mouth and Throat 0CQ
   see Replacement, Mouth and Throat 0CR
   see Supplement, Mouth and Throat 0CU
Stomatorrhaphy *see* Repair, Mouth and Throat 0CQ
Stratos LV *use* Cardiac Resynchronization Pacemaker Pulse Generator in 0JH
Stress test 4A12XM4
Stripping *see* Extraction
Study
   Electrophysiologic stimulation, cardiac *see* Measurement, Cardiac 4A02
   Ocular motility 4A07X7Z
   Pulmonary airway flow measurement *see* Measurement, Respiratory 4A09
   Visual acuity 4A07X0Z
Styloglossus muscle *use* Muscle, Tongue, Palate, Pharynx
Stylomandibular ligament *use* Bursa and Ligament, Head and Neck
Stylopharyngeus muscle *use* Muscle, Tongue, Palate, Pharynx
Subacromial bursa
   use Bursa and Ligament, Shoulder, Left
   use Bursa and Ligament, Shoulder, Right
Subaortic (common iliac) lymph node *use* Lymphatic, Pelvis
Subclavicular (apical) lymph node
   use Lymphatic, Axillary, Left
   use Lymphatic, Axillary, Right
Subclavius muscle
   use Muscle, Thorax, Left
   use Muscle, Thorax, Right
Subclavius nerve *use* Nerve, Brachial Plexus
Subcostal artery *use* Aorta, Thoracic
Subcostal muscle
   use Muscle, Thorax, Left
   use Muscle, Thorax, Right
Subcostal nerve *use* Nerve, Thoracic
Subcutaneous injection reservoir, port *use* Vascular Access Device, Reservoir in Subcutaneous Tissue and Fascia
Subcutaneous injection reservoir, pump *use* Infusion Device, Pump in Subcutaneous Tissue and Fascia
Subdermal progesterone implant *use* Contraceptive Device in Subcutaneous Tissue and Fascia
Submandibular ganglion
   use Nerve, Facial
   use Nerve, Head and Neck Sympathetic
Submandibular gland
   use Gland, Submaxillary, Left
   use Gland, Submaxillary, Right
Submandibular lymph node *use* Lymphatic, Head
Submaxillary ganglion *use* Nerve, Head and Neck Sympathetic
Submaxillary lymph node *use* Lymphatic, Head
Submental artery *use* Artery, Face
Submental lymph node *use* Lymphatic, Head
Submucous (Meissner's) plexus *use* Nerve, Abdominal Sympathetic
Suboccipital nerve *use* Nerve, Cervical
Suboccipital venous plexus
   use Vein, Vertebral, Left
   use Vein, Vertebral, Right
Subparotid lymph node *use* Lymphatic, Head
Subscapular aponeurosis
   use Subcutaneous Tissue and Fascia, Upper Arm, Left

Subscapular aponeurosis — continued
   use Subcutaneous Tissue and Fascia, Upper Arm, Right
Subscapular artery
   use Artery, Axillary, Left
   use Artery, Axillary, Right
Subscapular (posterior) lymph node
   use Lymphatic, Axillary, Left
   use Lymphatic, Axillary, Right
Subscapularis muscle
   use Muscle, Shoulder, Left
   use Muscle, Shoulder, Right
Substance Abuse Treatment
   Counseling
      Family, for substance abuse, Other Family Counseling HZ63ZZZ
      Group
         12-Step HZ43ZZZ
         Behavioral HZ41ZZZ
         Cognitive HZ40ZZZ
         Cognitive-Behavioral HZ42ZZZ
         Confrontational HZ48ZZZ
         Continuing Care HZ49ZZZ
         Infectious Disease
            Post-Test HZ4CZZZ
            Pre-Test HZ4CZZZ
         Interpersonal HZ44ZZZ
         Motivational Enhancement HZ47ZZZ
         Psychoeducation HZ46ZZZ
         Spiritual HZ4BZZZ
         Vocational HZ45ZZZ
      Individual
         12-Step HZ33ZZZ
         Behavioral HZ31ZZZ
         Cognitive HZ30ZZZ
         Cognitive-Behavioral HZ32ZZZ
         Confrontational HZ38ZZZ
         Continuing Care HZ39ZZZ
         Infectious Disease
            Post-Test HZ3CZZZ
            Pre-Test HZ3CZZZ
         Interpersonal HZ34ZZZ
         Motivational Enhancement HZ37ZZZ
         Psychoeducation HZ36ZZZ
         Spiritual HZ3BZZZ
         Vocational HZ35ZZZ
   Detoxification Services, for substance abuse HZ2ZZZZ
   Medication Management
      Antabuse HZ83ZZZ
      Bupropion HZ87ZZZ
      Clonidine HZ86ZZZ
      Levo-alpha-acetyl-methadol (LAAM) HZ82ZZZ
      Methadone Maintenance HZ81ZZZ
      Naloxone HZ85ZZZ
      Naltrexone HZ84ZZZ
      Nicotine Replacement HZ80ZZZ
      Other Replacement Medication HZ89ZZZ
      Psychiatric Medication HZ88ZZZ
   Pharmacotherapy
      Antabuse HZ93ZZZ
      Bupropion HZ97ZZZ
      Clonidine HZ96ZZZ
      Levo-alpha-acetyl-methadol (LAAM) HZ92ZZZ
      Methadone Maintenance HZ91ZZZ
      Naloxone HZ95ZZZ
      Naltrexone HZ94ZZZ
      Nicotine Replacement HZ90ZZZ
      Psychiatric Medication HZ98ZZZ
      Replacement Medication, Other HZ99ZZZ
   Psychotherapy
      12-Step HZ53ZZZ
      Behavioral HZ51ZZZ
      Cognitive HZ50ZZZ
      Cognitive-Behavioral HZ52ZZZ
      Confrontational HZ58ZZZ
      Interactive HZ55ZZZ
      Interpersonal HZ54ZZZ
      Motivational Enhancement HZ57ZZZ
      Psychoanalysis HZ5BZZZ
      Psychodynamic HZ5CZZZ
      Psychoeducation HZ56ZZZ
      Psychophysiological HZ5DZZZ
      Supportive HZ59ZZZ
Substantia nigra *use* Basal Ganglia
Subtalar (talocalcaneal) joint
   use Joint, Tarsal, Left

Subtalar (talocalcaneal) joint — continued
  use Joint, Tarsal, Right
Subtalar ligament
  use Bursa and Ligament, Foot, Left
  use Bursa and Ligament, Foot, Right
Subthalamic nucleus *use* Basal Ganglia
Suction *see* Drainage
Suction curettage (D&C), nonobstetric *see* Extraction, Endometrium ØUDB
Suction curettage, obstetric post-delivery *see* Extraction, Products of Conception, Retained 1ØD1
Superficial circumflex iliac vein
  use Vein, Greater Saphenous, Left
  use Vein, Greater Saphenous, Right
Superficial epigastric artery
  use Artery, Femoral, Left
  use Artery, Femoral, Right
Superficial epigastric vein
  use Vein, Greater Saphenous, Left
  use Vein, Greater Saphenous, Right
Superficial Inferior Epigastric Artery Flap
  Bilateral ØHRVØ78
  Left ØHRUØ78
  Right ØHRTØ78
Superficial palmar arch
  use Artery, Hand, Left
  use Artery, Hand, Right
Superficial palmar venous arch
  use Vein, Hand, Left
  use Vein, Hand, Right
Superficial temporal artery
  use Artery, Temporal, Left
  use Artery, Temporal, Right
Superficial transverse perineal muscle *use* Muscle, Perineum
Superior cardiac nerve *use* Nerve, Thoracic Sympathetic
Superior cerebellar vein *use* Vein, Intracranial
Superior cerebral vein *use* Vein, Intracranial
Superior clunic (cluneal) nerve *use* Nerve, Lumbar
Superior epigastric artery
  use Artery, Internal Mammary, Left
  use Artery, Internal Mammary, Right
Superior genicular artery
  use Artery, Popliteal, Left
  use Artery, Popliteal, Right
Superior gluteal artery
  use Artery, Internal Iliac, Left
  use Artery, Internal Iliac, Right
Superior gluteal nerve *use* Nerve, Lumbar Plexus
Superior hypogastric plexus *use* Nerve, Abdominal Sympathetic
Superior labial artery *use* Artery, Face
Superior laryngeal artery
  use Artery, Thyroid, Left
  use Artery, Thyroid, Right
Superior laryngeal nerve *use* Nerve, Vagus
Superior longitudinal muscle *use* Muscle, Tongue, Palate, Pharynx
Superior mesenteric ganglion *use* Nerve, Abdominal Sympathetic
Superior mesenteric lymph node *use* Lymphatic, Mesenteric
Superior mesenteric plexus *use* Nerve, Abdominal Sympathetic
Superior oblique muscle
  use Muscle, Extraocular, Left
  use Muscle, Extraocular, Right
Superior olivary nucleus *use* Pons
Superior rectal artery *use* Artery, Inferior Mesenteric
Superior rectal vein *use* Vein, Inferior Mesenteric
Superior rectus muscle
  use Muscle, Extraocular, Left
  use Muscle, Extraocular, Right
Superior tarsal plate
  use Eyelid, Upper, Left
  use Eyelid, Upper, Right
Superior thoracic artery
  use Artery, Axillary, Left
  use Artery, Axillary, Right
Superior thyroid artery
  use Artery, External Carotid, Left
  use Artery, External Carotid, Right
  use Artery, Thyroid, Left

Superior thyroid artery — continued
  use Artery, Thyroid, Right
Superior turbinate *use* Turbinate, Nasal
Superior ulnar collateral artery
  use Artery, Brachial, Left
  use Artery, Brachial, Right
Supplement
  Abdominal Wall ØWUF
  Acetabulum
    Left ØQU5
    Right ØQU4
  Ampulla of Vater ØFUC
  Anal Sphincter ØDUR
  Ankle Region
    Left ØYUL
    Right ØYUK
  Anus ØDUQ
  Aorta
    Abdominal Ø4UØ
    Thoracic Ø2UW
  Arm
    Lower
      Left ØXUF
      Right ØXUD
    Upper
      Left ØXU9
      Right ØXU8
  Artery
    Anterior Tibial
      Left Ø4UQ
      Right Ø4UP
    Axillary
      Left Ø3U6
      Right Ø3U5
    Brachial
      Left Ø3U8
      Right Ø3U7
    Celiac Ø4U1
    Colic
      Left Ø4U7
      Middle Ø4U8
      Right Ø4U6
    Common Carotid
      Left Ø3UJ
      Right Ø3UH
    Common Iliac
      Left Ø4UD
      Right Ø4UC
    External Carotid
      Left Ø3UN
      Right Ø3UM
    External Iliac
      Left Ø4UJ
      Right Ø4UH
    Face Ø3UR
    Femoral
      Left Ø4UL
      Right Ø4UK
    Foot
      Left Ø4UW
      Right Ø4UV
    Gastric Ø4U2
    Hand
      Left Ø3UF
      Right Ø3UD
    Hepatic Ø4U3
    Inferior Mesenteric Ø4UB
    Innominate Ø3U2
    Internal Carotid
      Left Ø3UL
      Right Ø3UK
    Internal Iliac
      Left Ø4UF
      Right Ø4UE
    Internal Mammary
      Left Ø3U1
      Right Ø3UØ
    Intracranial Ø3UG
    Lower Ø4UY
    Peroneal
      Left Ø4UU
      Right Ø4UT
    Popliteal
      Left Ø4UN
      Right Ø4UM

Supplement — continued
  Artery — continued
    Posterior Tibial
      Left Ø4US
      Right Ø4UR
    Pulmonary
      Left Ø2UR
      Right Ø2UQ
    Pulmonary Trunk Ø2UP
    Radial
      Left Ø3UC
      Right Ø3UB
    Renal
      Left Ø4UA
      Right Ø4U9
    Splenic Ø4U4
    Subclavian
      Left Ø3U4
      Right Ø3U3
    Superior Mesenteric Ø4U5
    Temporal
      Left Ø3UT
      Right Ø3US
    Thyroid
      Left Ø3UV
      Right Ø3UU
    Ulnar
      Left Ø3UA
      Right Ø3U9
    Upper Ø3UY
    Vertebral
      Left Ø3UQ
      Right Ø3UP
  Atrium
    Left Ø2U7
    Right Ø2U6
  Auditory Ossicle
    Left Ø9UAØ
    Right Ø9U9Ø
  Axilla
    Left ØXU5
    Right ØXU4
  Back
    Lower ØWUL
    Upper ØWUK
  Bladder ØTUB
  Bladder Neck ØTUC
  Bone
    Ethmoid
      Left ØNUG
      Right ØNUF
    Frontal
      Left ØNU2
      Right ØNU1
    Hyoid ØNUX
    Lacrimal
      Left ØNUJ
      Right ØNUH
    Nasal ØNUB
    Occipital
      Left ØNU8
      Right ØNU7
    Palatine
      Left ØNUL
      Right ØNUK
    Parietal
      Left ØNU4
      Right ØNU3
    Pelvic
      Left ØQU3
      Right ØQU2
    Sphenoid
      Left ØNUD
      Right ØNUC
    Temporal
      Left ØNU6
      Right ØNU5
    Zygomatic
      Left ØNUN
      Right ØNUM
  Breast
    Bilateral ØHUV
    Left ØHUU
    Right ØHUT
  Bronchus
    Lingula ØBU9

⌂ **Subterms under main terms may continue to next column or page**

Supplement — continued
  Subcutaneous Tissue and Fascia — continued
    Lower Leg
      Left ØJUP
      Right ØJUN
    Neck
      Anterior ØJU4
      Posterior ØJU5
    Pelvic Region ØJUC
    Perineum ØJUB
    Scalp ØJUØ
    Upper Arm
      Left ØJUF
      Right ØJUD
    Upper Leg
      Left ØJUM
      Right ØJUL
  Tarsal
    Left ØQUM
    Right ØQUL
  Tendon
    Abdomen
      Left ØLUG
      Right ØLUF
    Ankle
      Left ØLUT
      Right ØLUS
    Foot
      Left ØLUW
      Right ØLUV
    Hand
      Left ØLU8
      Right ØLU7
    Head and Neck ØLUØ
    Hip
      Left ØLUK
      Right ØLUJ
    Knee
      Left ØLUR
      Right ØLUQ
    Lower Arm and Wrist
      Left ØLU6
      Right ØLU5
    Lower Leg
      Left ØLUP
      Right ØLUN
    Perineum ØLUH
    Shoulder
      Left ØLU2
      Right ØLU1
    Thorax
      Left ØLUD
      Right ØLUC
    Trunk
      Left ØLUB
      Right ØLU9
    Upper Arm
      Left ØLU4
      Right ØLU3
    Upper Leg
      Left ØLUM
      Right ØLUL
  Testis
    Bilateral ØVUCØ
    Left ØVUBØ
    Right ØVU9Ø
  Thumb
    Left ØXUM
    Right ØXUL
  Tibia
    Left ØQUH
    Right ØQUG
  Toe
    1st
      Left ØYUQ
      Right ØYUP
    2nd
      Left ØYUS
      Right ØYUR
    3rd
      Left ØYUU
      Right ØYUT
    4th
      Left ØYUW
      Right ØYUV

Supplement — continued
  Toe — continued
    5th
      Left ØYUY
      Right ØYUX
  Tongue ØCU7
  Trachea ØBU1
  Tunica Vaginalis
    Left ØVU7
    Right ØVU6
  Turbinate, Nasal Ø9UL
  Tympanic Membrane
    Left Ø9U8
    Right Ø9U7
  Ulna
    Left ØPUL
    Right ØPUK
  Ureter
    Left ØTU7
    Right ØTU6
  Urethra ØTUD
  Uterine Supporting Structure ØUU4
  Uvula ØCUN
  Vagina ØUUG
  Valve
    Aortic Ø2UF
    Mitral Ø2UG
    Pulmonary Ø2UH
    Tricuspid Ø2UJ
  Vas Deferens
    Bilateral ØVUQ
    Left ØVUP
    Right ØVUN
  Vein
    Axillary
      Left Ø5U8
      Right Ø5U7
    Azygos Ø5UØ
    Basilic
      Left Ø5UC
      Right Ø5UB
    Brachial
      Left Ø5UA
      Right Ø5U9
    Cephalic
      Left Ø5UF
      Right Ø5UD
    Colic Ø6U7
    Common Iliac
      Left Ø6UD
      Right Ø6UC
    Esophageal Ø6U3
    External Iliac
      Left Ø6UG
      Right Ø6UF
    External Jugular
      Left Ø5UQ
      Right Ø5UP
    Face
      Left Ø5UV
      Right Ø5UT
    Femoral
      Left Ø6UN
      Right Ø6UM
    Foot
      Left Ø6UV
      Right Ø6UT
    Gastric Ø6U2
    Greater Saphenous
      Left Ø6UQ
      Right Ø6UP
    Hand
      Left Ø5UH
      Right Ø5UG
    Hemiazygos Ø5U1
    Hepatic Ø6U4
    Hypogastric
      Left Ø6UJ
      Right Ø6UH
    Inferior Mesenteric Ø6U6
    Innominate
      Left Ø5U4
      Right Ø5U3
    Internal Jugular
      Left Ø5UN
      Right Ø5UM

Supplement — continued
  Vein — continued
    Intracranial Ø5UL
    Lesser Saphenous
      Left Ø6US
      Right Ø6UR
    Lower Ø6UY
    Portal Ø6U8
    Pulmonary
      Left Ø2UT
      Right Ø2US
    Renal
      Left Ø6UB
      Right Ø6U9
    Splenic Ø6U1
    Subclavian
      Left Ø5U6
      Right Ø5U5
    Superior Mesenteric Ø6U5
    Upper Ø5UY
    Vertebral
      Left Ø5US
      Right Ø5UR
  Vena Cava
    Inferior Ø6UØ
    Superior Ø2UV
  Ventricle
    Left Ø2UL
    Right Ø2UK
  Vertebra
    Cervical ØPU3
    Lumbar ØQUØ
    Thoracic ØPU4
  Vesicle
    Bilateral ØVU3
    Left ØVU2
    Right ØVU1
  Vocal Cord
    Left ØCUV
    Right ØCUT
  Vulva ØUUM
  Wrist Region
    Left ØXUH
    Right ØXUG
Supraclavicular (Virchow's) lymph node
  use Lymphatic, Neck, Left
  use Lymphatic, Neck, Right
Supraclavicular nerve *use* Nerve, Cervical Plexus
Suprahyoid lymph node *use* Lymphatic, Head
Suprahyoid muscle
  use Muscle, Neck, Left
  use Muscle, Neck, Right
Suprainguinal lymph node *use* Lymphatic, Pelvis
Supraorbital vein
  use Vein, Face, Left
  use Vein, Face, Right
Suprarenal gland
  use Gland, Adrenal
  use Gland, Adrenal, Bilateral
  use Gland, Adrenal, Left
  use Gland, Adrenal, Right
Suprarenal plexus *use* Nerve, Abdominal Sympathetic
Suprascapular nerve *use* Nerve, Brachial Plexus
Supraspinatus fascia
  use Subcutaneous Tissue and Fascia, Upper Arm, Left
  use Subcutaneous Tissue and Fascia, Upper Arm, Right
Supraspinatus muscle
  use Muscle, Shoulder, Left
  use Muscle, Shoulder, Right
Supraspinous ligament
  use Bursa and Ligament, Trunk, Left
  use Bursa and Ligament, Trunk, Right
Suprasternal notch *use* Sternum
Supratrochlear lymph node
  use Lymphatic, Upper Extremity, Left
  use Lymphatic, Upper Extremity, Right
Sural artery
  use Artery, Popliteal, Left
  use Artery, Popliteal, Right
Suspension
  Bladder Neck *see* Reposition, Bladder Neck ØTSC
  Kidney *see* Reposition, Urinary System ØTS
  Urethra *see* Reposition, Urinary System ØTS
  Urethrovesical *see* Reposition, Bladder Neck ØTSC

Suspension — continued
  Uterus *see* Reposition, Uterus ØUS9
  Vagina *see* Reposition, Vagina ØUSG
Suture
  Laceration repair *see* Repair
  Ligation *see* Occlusion
Suture Removal
  Extremity
    Lower 8EØYXY8
    Upper 8EØXXY8
  Head and Neck Region 8EØ9XY8
  Trunk Region 8EØWXY8
Sweat gland *use* Skin
Sympathectomy *see* Excision, Peripheral Nervous System Ø1B
SynCardia Total Artificial Heart *use* Synthetic Substitute
Synchra CRT-P *use* Cardiac Resynchronization Pacemaker Pulse Generator in ØJH
Synechiotomy, iris *see* Release, Eye Ø8N
Synovectomy
  Lower joint *see* Excision, Lower Joints ØSB
  Upper joint *see* Excision, Upper Joints ØRB
Systemic Nuclear Medicine Therapy
  Abdomen CW7Ø
  Anatomical Regions, Multiple CW7YYZZ
  Chest CW73
  Thyroid CW7G
  Whole Body CW7N

T

Takedown
  Arteriovenous shunt *see* Removal of device from, Upper Arteries Ø3P
  Arteriovenous shunt, with creation of new shunt *see* Bypass, Upper Arteries Ø31
  Stoma *see* Repair
Talent® Converter *use* Intraluminal Device
Talent® Occluder *use* Intraluminal Device
Talent® Stent Graft (abdominal)(thoracic) *use* Intraluminal Device
Talocalcaneal (subtalar) joint
  use Joint, Tarsal, Left
  use Joint, Tarsal, Right
Talocalcaneal ligament
  use Bursa and Ligament, Foot, Left
  use Bursa and Ligament, Foot, Right
Talocalcaneonavicular joint
  use Joint, Tarsal, Left
  use Joint, Tarsal, Right
Talocalcaneonavicular ligament
  use Bursa and Ligament, Foot, Left
  use Bursa and Ligament, Foot, Right
Talocrural joint
  use Joint, Ankle, Left
  use Joint, Ankle, Right
Talofibular ligament
  use Bursa and Ligament, Ankle, Left
  use Bursa and Ligament, Ankle, Right
Talus bone
  use Tarsal, Left
  use Tarsal, Right
TandemHeart® System *use* External Heart Assist System in Heart and Great Vessels
Tarsectomy
  see Excision, Lower Bones ØQB
  see Resection, Lower Bones ØQT
Tarsometatarsal joint
  use Joint, Metatarsal-Tarsal, Left
  use Joint, Metatarsal-Tarsal, Right
Tarsometatarsal ligament
  use Bursa and Ligament, Foot, Left
  use Bursa and Ligament, Foot, Right
Tarsorrhaphy *see* Repair, Eye Ø8Q
Tattooing
  Cornea 3EØCXMZ
  Skin *see* Introduction of substance in or on, Skin 3EØØ
TAXUS® Liberté® Paclitaxel-eluting Coronary Stent System *use* Intraluminal Device, Drug-eluting in Heart and Great Vessels
TBNA (transbronchial needle aspiration) *see* Drainage, Respiratory System ØB9
Telemetry 4A12X4Z

Telemetry — continued
  Ambulatory 4A12X45
Temperature gradient study 4AØZXKZ
Temporal lobe *use* Cerebral Hemisphere
Temporalis muscle *use* Muscle, Head
Temporoparietalis muscle *use* Muscle, Head
Tendolysis *see* Release, Tendons ØLN
Tendonectomy
  see Excision, Tendons ØLB
  see Resection, Tendons ØLT
Tendonoplasty, tenoplasty
  see Repair, Tendons ØLQ
  see Replacement, Tendons ØLR
  see Supplement, Tendons ØLU
Tendorrhaphy *see* Repair, Tendons ØLQ
Tendototomy
  see Division, Tendons ØL8
  see Drainage, Tendons ØL9
Tenectomy, tenonectomy
  see Excision, Tendons ØLB
  see Resection, Tendons ØLT
Tenolysis *see* Release, Tendons ØLN
Tenontorrhaphy *see* Repair, Tendons ØLQ
Tenontotomy
  see Division, Tendons ØL8
  see Drainage, Tendons ØL9
Tenorrhaphy *see* Repair, Tendons ØLQ
Tenosynovectomy
  see Excision, Tendons ØLB
  see Resection, Tendons ØLT
Tenotomy
  see Division, Tendons ØL8
  see Drainage, Tendons ØL9
Tensor fasciae latae muscle
  use Muscle, Hip, Left
  use Muscle, Hip, Right
Tensor veli palatini muscle *use* Muscle, Tongue, Palate, Pharynx
Tenth cranial nerve *use* Nerve, Vagus
Tentorium cerebelli *use* Dura Mater
Teres major muscle
  use Muscle, Shoulder, Left
  use Muscle, Shoulder, Right
Teres minor muscle
  use Muscle, Shoulder, Left
  use Muscle, Shoulder, Right
Termination of pregnancy
  Aspiration curettage 10A07ZZ
  Dilation and curettage 10A07ZZ
  Hysterotomy 10A00ZZ
  Intra-amniotic injection 10A03ZZ
  Laminaria 10A07ZW
  Vacuum 10A07Z6
Testectomy
  see Excision, Male Reproductive System ØVB
  see Resection, Male Reproductive System ØVT
Testicular artery *use* Aorta, Abdominal
Testing
  Glaucoma 4A07XBZ
  Hearing *see* Hearing Assessment, Diagnostic Audiology F13
  Mental health *see* Psychological Tests
  Muscle function, electromyography (EMG) *see* Measurement, Musculoskeletal 4AØF
  Muscle function, manual *see* Motor Function Assessment, Rehabilitation FØ1
  Neurophysiologic monitoring, intra-operative *see* Monitoring, Physiological Systems 4A1
  Range of motion *see* Motor Function Assessment, Rehabilitation FØ1
  Vestibular function *see* Vestibular Assessment, Diagnostic Audiology F15
Thalamectomy *see* Excision, Thalamus 00B9
Thalamotomy *see* Drainage, Thalamus 0099
Thenar muscle
  use Muscle, Hand, Left
  use Muscle, Hand, Right
Therapeutic Massage
  Musculoskeletal System 8EØKX1Z
  Reproductive System
    Prostate 8EØVX1C
    Rectum 8EØVX1D
Therapeutic occlusion coil(s) *use* Intraluminal Device
Thermography 4AØZXKZ

Thermotherapy, prostate *see* Destruction, Prostate ØV5Ø
Third cranial nerve *use* Nerve, Oculomotor
Third occipital nerve *use* Nerve, Cervical
Third ventricle *use* Cerebral Ventricle
Thoracectomy *see* Excision, Anatomical Regions, General ØWB
Thoracentesis *see* Drainage, Anatomical Regions, General ØW9
Thoracic aortic plexus *use* Nerve, Thoracic Sympathetic
Thoracic esophagus *use* Esophagus, Middle
Thoracic facet joint
  use Joint, Thoracic Vertebral
  use Joint, Thoracic Vertebral, 2 to 7
  use Joint, Thoracic Vertebral, 8 or more
Thoracic ganglion *use* Nerve, Thoracic Sympathetic
Thoracoacromial artery
  use Artery, Axillary, Left
  use Artery, Axillary, Right
Thoracocentesis *see* Drainage, Anatomical Regions, General ØW9
Thoracolumbar facet joint *use* Joint, Thoracolumbar Vertebral
Thoracoplasty
  see Repair, Anatomical Regions, General ØWQ
  see Supplement, Anatomical Regions, General ØWU
Thoracostomy, for lung collapse *see* Drainage, Respiratory System ØB9
Thoracostomy tube *use* Drainage Device
Thoracotomy *see* Drainage, Anatomical Regions, General ØW9
Thoratec IVAD (Implantable Ventricular Assist Device) *use* Implantable Heart Assist System in Heart and Great Vessels
Thoratec Paracorporeal Ventricular Assist Device *use* External Heart Assist System in Heart and Great Vessels
Thrombectomy *see* Extirpation
Thymectomy
  see Excision, Lymphatic and Hemic Systems Ø7B
  see Resection, Lymphatic and Hemic Systems Ø7T
Thymopexy
  see Repair, Lymphatic and Hemic Systems Ø7Q
  see Reposition, Lymphatic and Hemic Systems Ø7S
Thymus gland *use* Thymus
Thyroarytenoid muscle
  use Muscle, Neck, Left
  use Muscle, Neck, Right
Thyrocervical trunk
  use Artery, Thyroid, Left
  use Artery, Thyroid, Right
Thyroid cartilage *use* Larynx
Thyroidectomy
  see Excision, Endocrine System ØGB
  see Resection, Endocrine System ØGT
Thyroidorrhaphy *see* Repair, Endocrine System ØGQ
Thyroidoscopy ØGJK4ZZ
Thyroidotomy *see* Drainage, Endocrine System ØG9
Tibialis anterior muscle
  use Muscle, Lower Leg, Left
  use Muscle, Lower Leg, Right
Tibialis posterior muscle
  use Muscle, Lower Leg, Left
  use Muscle, Lower Leg, Right
Tibiofemoral joint
  use Joint, Knee, Left
  use Joint, Knee, Left, Tibial Surface
  use Joint, Knee, Right
  use Joint, Knee, Right, Tibial Surface
TigerPaw® system for closure of left atrial appendage *use* Extraluminal Device
Tissue bank graft *use* Nonautologous Tissue Substitute
Tissue Expander
  Insertion of device in
    Breast
      Bilateral ØHHV
      Left ØHHU
      Right ØHHT
    Nipple
      Left ØHHX
      Right ØHHW
    Subcutaneous Tissue and Fascia
      Abdomen ØJH8
      Back ØJH7

Tissue Expander — continued
  Insertion of device in — continued
    Subcutaneous Tissue and Fascia — continued
      Buttock ØJH9
      Chest ØJH6
      Face ØJH1
      Foot
        Left ØJHR
        Right ØJHQ
      Hand
        Left ØJHK
        Right ØJHJ
      Lower Arm
        Left ØJHH
        Right ØJHG
      Lower Leg
        Left ØJHP
        Right ØJHN
      Neck
        Anterior ØJH4
        Posterior ØJH5
      Pelvic Region ØJHC
      Perineum ØJHB
      Scalp ØJHØ
      Upper Arm
        Left ØJHF
        Right ØJHD
      Upper Leg
        Left ØJHM
        Right ØJHL
  Removal of device from
    Breast
      Left ØHPU
      Right ØHPT
    Subcutaneous Tissue and Fascia
      Head and Neck ØJPS
      Lower Extremity ØJPW
      Trunk ØJPT
      Upper Extremity ØJPV
  Revision of device in
    Breast
      Left ØHWU
      Right ØHWT
    Subcutaneous Tissue and Fascia
      Head and Neck ØJWS
      Lower Extremity ØJWW
      Trunk ØJWT
      Upper Extremity ØJWV
Tissue expander (inflatable)(injectable)
  use Tissue Expander in Skin and Breast
  use Tissue Expander in Subcutaneous Tissue and
    Fascia
Titanium Sternal Fixation System (TSFS)
  use Internal Fixation Device, Rigid Plate in ØPS
  use Internal Fixation Device, Rigid Plate in ØPH
Tomographic (Tomo) Nuclear Medicine Imaging
  CP2YYZZ
  Abdomen CW2Ø
  Abdomen and Chest CW24
  Abdomen and Pelvis CW21
  Anatomical Regions, Multiple CW2YYZZ
  Bladder, Kidneys and Ureters CT23
  Brain CØ2Ø
  Breast CH2YYZZ
    Bilateral CH22
    Left CH21
    Right CH2Ø
  Bronchi and Lungs CB22
  Central Nervous System CØ2YYZZ
  Cerebrospinal Fluid CØ25
  Chest CW23
  Chest and Abdomen CW24
  Chest and Neck CW26
  Digestive System CD2YYZZ
  Endocrine System CG2YYZZ
  Extremity
    Lower CW2D
      Bilateral CP2F
      Left CP2D
      Right CP2C
    Upper CW2M
      Bilateral CP2B
      Left CP29
      Right CP28
  Gallbladder CF24
  Gastrointestinal Tract CD27

Tomographic (Tomo) Nuclear Medicine Imaging —
  continued
  Gland, Parathyroid CG21
  Head and Neck CW2B
  Heart C22YYZZ
    Right and Left C226
  Hepatobiliary System and Pancreas CF2YYZZ
  Kidneys, Ureters and Bladder CT23
  Liver CF25
  Liver and Spleen CF26
  Lungs and Bronchi CB22
  Lymphatics and Hematologic System C72YYZZ
  Myocardium C22G
  Neck and Chest CW26
  Neck and Head CW2B
  Pancreas and Hepatobiliary System CF2YYZZ
  Pelvic Region CW2J
  Pelvis CP26
  Pelvis and Abdomen CW21
  Pelvis and Spine CP27
  Respiratory System CB2YYZZ
  Skin CH2YYZZ
  Skull CP21
  Skull and Cervical Spine CP23
  Spine
    Cervical CP22
    Cervical and Skull CP23
    Lumbar CP2H
    Thoracic CP2G
    Thoracolumbar CP2J
  Spine and Pelvis CP27
  Spleen C722
  Spleen and Liver CF26
  Subcutaneous Tissue CH2YYZZ
  Thorax CP24
  Ureters, Kidneys and Bladder CT23
  Urinary System CT2YYZZ
Tomography, computerized *see* Computerized Tomog-
  raphy (CT Scan)
Tonometry 4AØ7XBZ
Tonsillectomy
  see Excision, Mouth and Throat ØCB
  see Resection, Mouth and Throat ØCT
Tonsillotomy *see* Drainage, Mouth and Throat ØC9
Total artificial (replacement) heart *use* Synthetic
  Substitute
Total parenteral nutrition (TPN) *see* Introduction of
  Nutritional Substance
Trachectomy
  see Excision, Trachea ØBB1
  see Resection, Trachea ØBT1
Trachelectomy
  see Excision, Cervix ØUBC
  see Resection, Cervix ØUTC
Trachelopexy
  see Repair, Cervix ØUQC
  see Reposition, Cervix ØUSC
Tracheloplasty *see* Repair, Cervix ØUQC
Trachelorrhaphy *see* Repair, Cervix ØUQC
Trachelotomy *see* Drainage, Cervix ØU9C
Tracheobronchial lymph node *use* Lymphatic, Thorax
Tracheoesophageal fistulization ØB11ØD6
Tracheolysis *see* Release, Respiratory System ØBN
Tracheoplasty
  see Repair, Respiratory System ØBQ
  see Supplement, Respiratory System ØBU
Tracheorrhaphy *see* Repair, Respiratory System ØBQ
Tracheoscopy ØBJ18ZZ
Tracheostomy *see* Bypass, Respiratory System ØB1
Tracheostomy Device
  Bypass, Trachea ØB11
  Change device in, Trachea ØB21XFZ
  Removal of device from, Trachea ØBP1
  Revision of device in, Trachea ØBW1
Tracheostomy tube *use* Tracheostomy Device in Respi-
  ratory System
Tracheotomy *see* Drainage, Respiratory System ØB9
Traction
  Abdominal Wall 2W63X
  Arm
    Lower
      Left 2W6DX
      Right 2W6CX
    Upper
      Left 2W6BX

Traction — continued
  Arm — continued
    Upper — continued
      Right 2W6AX
  Back 2W65X
  Chest Wall 2W64X
  Extremity
    Lower
      Left 2W6MX
      Right 2W6LX
    Upper
      Left 2W69X
      Right 2W68X
  Face 2W61X
  Finger
    Left 2W6KX
    Right 2W6JX
  Foot
    Left 2W6TX
    Right 2W6SX
  Hand
    Left 2W6FX
    Right 2W6EX
  Head 2W6ØX
  Inguinal Region
    Left 2W67X
    Right 2W66X
  Leg
    Lower
      Left 2W6RX
      Right 2W6QX
    Upper
      Left 2W6PX
      Right 2W6NX
  Neck 2W62X
  Thumb
    Left 2W6HX
    Right 2W6GX
  Toe
    Left 2W6VX
    Right 2W6UX
Tractotomy *see* Division, Central Nervous System ØØ8
Tragus
  use Ear, External, Bilateral
  use Ear, External, Left
  use Ear, External, Right
Training, caregiver *see* Caregiver Training
TRAM (transverse rectus abdominis myocutaneous)
  flap reconstruction
  Free *see* Replacement, Skin and Breast ØHR
  Pedicled *see* Transfer, Muscles ØKX
Transection *see* Division
Transfer
  Buccal Mucosa ØCX4
  Bursa and Ligament
    Abdomen
      Left ØMXJ
      Right ØMXH
    Ankle
      Left ØMXR
      Right ØMXQ
    Elbow
      Left ØMX4
      Right ØMX3
    Foot
      Left ØMXT
      Right ØMXS
    Hand
      Left ØMX8
      Right ØMX7
    Head and Neck ØMXØ
    Hip
      Left ØMXM
      Right ØMXL
    Knee
      Left ØMXP
      Right ØMXN
    Lower Extremity
      Left ØMXW
      Right ØMXV
    Perineum ØMXK
    Shoulder
      Left ØMX2
      Right ØMX1
    Thorax
      Left ØMXG

Transfer — continued
- Bursa and Ligament — continued
  - Thorax — continued
    - Right 0MXF
  - Trunk
    - Left 0MXD
    - Right 0MXC
  - Upper Extremity
    - Left 0MXB
    - Right 0MX9
  - Wrist
    - Left 0MX6
    - Right 0MX5
- Finger
  - Left 0XXP0ZM
  - Right 0XXN0ZL
- Gingiva
  - Lower 0CX6
  - Upper 0CX5
- Intestine
  - Large 0DXE
  - Small 0DX8
- Lip
  - Lower 0CX1
  - Upper 0CX0
- Muscle
  - Abdomen
    - Left 0KXL
    - Right 0KXK
  - Extraocular
    - Left 08XM
    - Right 08XL
  - Facial 0KX1
  - Foot
    - Left 0KXW
    - Right 0KXV
  - Hand
    - Left 0KXD
    - Right 0KXC
  - Head 0KX0
  - Hip
    - Left 0KXP
    - Right 0KXN
  - Lower Arm and Wrist
    - Left 0KXB
    - Right 0KX9
  - Lower Leg
    - Left 0KXT
    - Right 0KXS
  - Neck
    - Left 0KX3
    - Right 0KX2
  - Perineum 0KXM
  - Shoulder
    - Left 0KX6
    - Right 0KX5
  - Thorax
    - Left 0KXJ
    - Right 0KXH
  - Tongue, Palate, Pharynx 0KX4
  - Trunk
    - Left 0KXG
    - Right 0KXF
  - Upper Arm
    - Left 0KX8
    - Right 0KX7
  - Upper Leg
    - Left 0KXR
    - Right 0KXQ
- Nerve
  - Abducens 00XL
  - Accessory 00XR
  - Acoustic 00XN
  - Cervical 01X1
  - Facial 00XM
  - Femoral 01XD
  - Glossopharyngeal 00XP
  - Hypoglossal 00XS
  - Lumbar 01XB
  - Median 01X5
  - Oculomotor 00XH
  - Olfactory 00XF
  - Optic 00XG
  - Peroneal 01XH
  - Phrenic 01X2
  - Pudendal 01XC

Transfer — continued
- Nerve — continued
  - Radial 01X6
  - Sciatic 01XF
  - Thoracic 01X8
  - Tibial 01XG
  - Trigeminal 00XK
  - Trochlear 00XJ
  - Ulnar 01X4
  - Vagus 00XQ
- Palate, Soft 0CX3
- Skin
  - Abdomen 0HX7XZZ
  - Back 0HX6XZZ
  - Buttock 0HX8XZZ
  - Chest 0HX5XZZ
  - Ear
    - Left 0HX3XZZ
    - Right 0HX2XZZ
  - Face 0HX1XZZ
  - Foot
    - Left 0HXNXZZ
    - Right 0HXMXZZ
  - Genitalia 0HXAXZZ
  - Hand
    - Left 0HXGXZZ
    - Right 0HXFXZZ
  - Lower Arm
    - Left 0HXEXZZ
    - Right 0HXDXZZ
  - Lower Leg
    - Left 0HXLXZZ
    - Right 0HXKXZZ
  - Neck 0HX4XZZ
  - Perineum 0HX9XZZ
  - Scalp 0HX0XZZ
  - Upper Arm
    - Left 0HXCXZZ
    - Right 0HXBXZZ
  - Upper Leg
    - Left 0HXJXZZ
    - Right 0HXHXZZ
- Stomach 0DX6
- Subcutaneous Tissue and Fascia
  - Abdomen 0JX8
  - Back 0JX7
  - Buttock 0JX9
  - Chest 0JX6
  - Face 0JX1
  - Foot
    - Left 0JXR
    - Right 0JXQ
  - Hand
    - Left 0JXK
    - Right 0JXJ
  - Lower Arm
    - Left 0JXH
    - Right 0JXG
  - Lower Leg
    - Left 0JXP
    - Right 0JXN
  - Neck
    - Anterior 0JX4
    - Posterior 0JX5
  - Pelvic Region 0JXC
  - Perineum 0JXB
  - Scalp 0JX0
  - Upper Arm
    - Left 0JXF
    - Right 0JXD
  - Upper Leg
    - Left 0JXM
    - Right 0JXL
- Tendon
  - Abdomen
    - Left 0LXG
    - Right 0LXF
  - Ankle
    - Left 0LXT
    - Right 0LXS
  - Foot
    - Left 0LXW
    - Right 0LXV
  - Hand
    - Left 0LX8
    - Right 0LX7

Transfer — continued
- Tendon — continued
  - Head and Neck 0LX0
  - Hip
    - Left 0LXK
    - Right 0LXJ
  - Knee
    - Left 0LXR
    - Right 0LXQ
  - Lower Arm and Wrist
    - Left 0LX6
    - Right 0LX5
  - Lower Leg
    - Left 0LXP
    - Right 0LXN
  - Perineum 0LXH
  - Shoulder
    - Left 0LX2
    - Right 0LX1
  - Thorax
    - Left 0LXD
    - Right 0LXC
  - Trunk
    - Left 0LXB
    - Right 0LX9
  - Upper Arm
    - Left 0LX4
    - Right 0LX3
  - Upper Leg
    - Left 0LXM
    - Right 0LXL
- Tongue 0CX7

Transfusion
- Artery
  - Central
    - Antihemophilic Factors 3026
    - Blood
      - Platelets 3026
      - Red Cells 3026
        - Frozen 3026
      - White Cells 3026
      - Whole 3026
    - Bone Marrow 3026
    - Factor IX 3026
    - Fibrinogen 3026
    - Globulin 3026
    - Plasma
      - Fresh 3026
      - Frozen 3026
    - Plasma Cryoprecipitate 3026
    - Serum Albumin 3026
    - Stem Cells
      - Cord Blood 3026
      - Hematopoietic 3026
  - Peripheral
    - Antihemophilic Factors 3025
    - Blood
      - Platelets 3025
      - Red Cells 3025
        - Frozen 3025
      - White Cells 3025
      - Whole 3025
    - Bone Marrow 3025
    - Factor IX 3025
    - Fibrinogen 3025
    - Globulin 3025
    - Plasma
      - Fresh 3025
      - Frozen 3025
    - Plasma Cryoprecipitate 3025
    - Serum Albumin 3025
    - Stem Cells
      - Cord Blood 3025
      - Hematopoietic 3025
- Products of Conception
  - Antihemophilic Factors 3027
  - Blood
    - Platelets 3027
    - Red Cells 3027
      - Frozen 3027
    - White Cells 3027
    - Whole 3027
  - Factor IX 3027
  - Fibrinogen 3027
  - Globulin 3027

▼ Subterms under main terms may continue to next column or page

Index

Ultrasonography — Uterine Artery

Ultrasonography — continued
- Artery — continued
  - Renal
    - Bilateral, Intravascular B448ZZ3
    - Left, Intravascular B447ZZ3
    - Right, Intravascular B446ZZ3
  - Subclavian, Left, Intravascular B342ZZ3
  - Superior Mesenteric, Intravascular B444ZZ3
  - Upper Extremity
    - Bilateral, Intravascular B34KZZ3
    - Left, Intravascular B34JZZ3
    - Right, Intravascular B34HZZ3
- Bile Duct BF40ZZZ
- Bile Duct and Gallbladder BF43ZZZ
- Bladder BT40ZZZ
  - and Kidney BT4JZZZ
- Brain B040ZZZ
- Breast
  - Bilateral BH42ZZZ
  - Left BH41ZZZ
  - Right BH40ZZZ
- Chest Wall BH4BZZZ
- Coccyx BR4FZZZ
- Connective Tissue
  - Lower Extremity BL41ZZZ
  - Upper Extremity BL40ZZZ
- Duodenum BD49ZZZ
- Elbow
  - Left, Densitometry BP4HZZ1
  - Right, Densitometry BP4GZZ1
- Esophagus BD41ZZZ
- Extremity
  - Lower BH48ZZZ
  - Upper BH47ZZZ
- Eye
  - Bilateral B847ZZZ
  - Left B846ZZZ
  - Right B845ZZZ
- Fallopian Tube
  - Bilateral BU42
  - Left BU41
  - Right BU40
- Fetal Umbilical Cord BY47ZZZ
- Fetus
  - First Trimester, Multiple Gestation BY4BZZZ
  - Second Trimester, Multiple Gestation BY4DZZZ
  - Single
    - First Trimester BY49ZZZ
    - Second Trimester BY4CZZZ
    - Third Trimester BY4FZZZ
  - Third Trimester, Multiple Gestation BY4GZZZ
- Gallbladder BF42ZZZ
- Gallbladder and Bile Duct BF43ZZZ
- Gastrointestinal Tract BD47ZZZ
- Gland
  - Adrenal
    - Bilateral BG42ZZZ
    - Left BG41ZZZ
    - Right BG40ZZZ
  - Parathyroid BG43ZZZ
  - Thyroid BG44ZZZ
- Hand
  - Left, Densitometry BP4PZZ1
  - Right, Densitometry BP4NZZ1
- Head and Neck BH4CZZZ
- Heart
  - Left B245YZZ
    - Intravascular B245ZZ3
    - Transesophageal B245ZZ4
  - Pediatric B24DYZZ
    - Intravascular B24DZZ3
    - Transesophageal B24DZZ4
  - Right B244YZZ
    - Intravascular B244ZZ3
    - Transesophageal B244ZZ4
  - Right and Left B246YZZ
    - Intravascular B246ZZ3
    - Transesophageal B246ZZ4
  - Heart with Aorta B24BYZZ
    - Intravascular B24BZZ3
    - Transesophageal B24BZZ4
- Hepatobiliary System, All BF4CZZZ
- Hip
  - Bilateral BQ42ZZZ
  - Left BQ41ZZZ
  - Right BQ40ZZZ

Ultrasonography — continued
- Kidney
  - and Bladder BT4JZZZ
  - Bilateral BT43ZZZ
  - Left BT42ZZZ
  - Right BT41ZZZ
  - Transplant BT49ZZZ
- Knee
  - Bilateral BQ49ZZZ
  - Left BQ48ZZZ
  - Right BQ47ZZZ
- Liver BF45ZZZ
- Liver and Spleen BF46ZZZ
- Mediastinum BB4CZZZ
- Neck BW4FZZZ
- Ovary
  - Bilateral BU45
  - Left BU44
  - Right BU43
- Ovary and Uterus BU4C
- Pancreas BF47ZZZ
- Pelvic Region BW4GZZZ
- Pelvis and Abdomen BW41ZZZ
- Penis BV4BZZZ
- Pericardium B24CYZZ
  - Intravascular B24CZZ3
  - Transesophageal B24CZZ4
- Placenta BY48ZZZ
- Pleura BB4BZZZ
- Prostate and Seminal Vesicle BV49ZZZ
- Rectum BD4CZZZ
- Sacrum BR4FZZZ
- Scrotum BV44ZZZ
- Seminal Vesicle and Prostate BV49ZZZ
- Shoulder
  - Left, Densitometry BP49ZZ1
  - Right, Densitometry BP48ZZ1
- Spinal Cord B04BZZZ
- Spine
  - Cervical BR40ZZZ
  - Lumbar BR49ZZZ
  - Thoracic BR47ZZZ
- Spleen and Liver BF46ZZZ
- Stomach BD42ZZZ
- Tendon
  - Lower Extremity BL43ZZZ
  - Upper Extremity BL42ZZZ
- Ureter
  - Bilateral BT48ZZZ
  - Left BT47ZZZ
  - Right BT46ZZZ
- Urethra BT45ZZZ
- Uterus BU46
- Uterus and Ovary BU4C
- Vein
  - Jugular
    - Left, Intravascular B544ZZ3
    - Right, Intravascular B543ZZ3
  - Lower Extremity
    - Bilateral, Intravascular B54DZZ3
    - Left, Intravascular B54CZZ3
    - Right, Intravascular B54BZZ3
  - Portal, Intravascular B54TZZ3
  - Renal
    - Bilateral, Intravascular B54LZZ3
    - Left, Intravascular B54KZZ3
    - Right, Intravascular B54JZZ3
  - Spanchnic, Intravascular B54TZZ3
  - Subclavian
    - Left, Intravascular B547ZZ3
    - Right, Intravascular B546ZZ3
  - Upper Extremity
    - Bilateral, Intravascular B54PZZ3
    - Left, Intravascular B54NZZ3
    - Right, Intravascular B54MZZ3
  - Vena Cava
    - Inferior, Intravascular B549ZZ3
    - Superior, Intravascular B548ZZ3
- Wrist
  - Left, Densitometry BP4MZZ1
  - Right, Densitometry BP4LZZ1

Ultrasound bone healing system
- *use* Bone Growth Stimulator in Head and Facial Bones
- *use* Bone Growth Stimulator in Lower Bones
- *use* Bone Growth Stimulator in Upper Bones

Ultrasound Therapy
- Heart 6A75
- No Qualifier 6A75
- Vessels
  - Head and Neck 6A75
  - Other 6A75
  - Peripheral 6A75

Ultraviolet Light Therapy, Skin 6A80

Umbilical artery
- *use* Artery, Internal Iliac, Left
- *use* Artery, Internal Iliac, Right

Uniplanar external fixator
- *use* External Fixation Device, Monoplanar in 0QS
- *use* External Fixation Device, Monoplanar in 0QH
- *use* External Fixation Device, Monoplanar in 0PH
- *use* External Fixation Device, Monoplanar in 0PS

Upper GI series *see* Fluoroscopy, Gastrointestinal, Upper BD15

Ureteral orifice
- *use* Ureter
- *use* Ureter, Left
- *use* Ureter, Right
- *use* Ureters, Bilateral

Ureterectomy
- *see* Excision, Urinary System 0TB
- *see* Resection, Urinary System 0TT

Ureterocolostomy *see* Bypass, Urinary System 0T1
Ureterocystostomy *see* Bypass, Urinary System 0T1
Ureteroenterostomy *see* Bypass, Urinary System 0T1
Ureteroileostomy *see* Bypass, Urinary System 0T1
Ureterolithotomy *see* Extirpation, Urinary System 0TC
Ureterolysis *see* Release, Urinary System 0TN
Ureteroneocystostomy
- *see* Bypass, Urinary System 0T1
- *see* Reposition, Urinary System 0TS

Ureteropelvic junction (UPJ)
- *use* Kidney Pelvis, Left
- *use* Kidney Pelvis, Right

Ureteropexy
- *see* Repair, Urinary System 0TQ
- *see* Reposition, Urinary System 0TS

Ureteroplasty
- *see* Repair, Urinary System 0TQ
- *see* Replacement, Urinary System 0TR
- *see* Supplement, Urinary System 0TU

Ureteroplication *see* Restriction, Urinary System 0TV
Ureteropyelography *see* Fluoroscopy, Urinary System BT1
Ureterorrhaphy *see* Repair, Urinary System 0TQ
Ureteroscopy 0TJ98ZZ
Ureterostomy
- *see* Bypass, Urinary System 0T1
- *see* Drainage, Urinary System 0T9

Ureterotomy *see* Drainage, Urinary System 0T9
Ureteroureterostomy *see* Bypass, Urinary System 0T1
Ureterovesical orifice
- *use* Ureter
- *use* Ureter, Left
- *use* Ureter, Right
- *use* Ureters, Bilateral

Urethral catheterization, indwelling 0T9B70Z
Urethrectomy
- *see* Excision, Urethra 0TBD
- *see* Resection, Urethra 0TTD

Urethrolithotomy *see* Extirpation, Urethra 0TCD
Urethrolysis *see* Release, Urethra 0TND
Urethropexy
- *see* Repair, Urethra 0TQD
- *see* Reposition, Urethra 0TSD

Urethroplasty
- *see* Repair, Urethra 0TQD
- *see* Replacement, Urethra 0TRD
- *see* Supplement, Urethra 0TUD

Urethrorrhaphy *see* Repair, Urethra 0TQD
Urethroscopy 0TJD8ZZ
Urethrotomy *see* Drainage, Urethra 0T9D
Urinary incontinence stimulator lead *use* Stimulator Lead in Urinary System
Urography *see* Fluoroscopy, Urinary System BT1
Uterine Artery
- *use* Artery, Internal Iliac, Left
- *use* Artery, Internal Iliac, Right
- Left, Occlusion, Artery, Internal Iliac, Left 04LF
- Right, Occlusion, Artery, Internal Iliac, Right 04LE

Uterine artery embolization (UAE) *see* Occlusion, Lower Arteries Ø4L
Uterine cornu *use* Uterus
Uterine tube
　use Fallopian Tube, Left
　use Fallopian Tube, Right
Uterine vein
　use Vein, Hypogastric, Left
　use Vein, Hypogastric, Right
Uvulectomy
　see Excision, Uvula ØCBN
　see Resection, Uvula ØCTN
Uvulorrhaphy *see* Repair, Uvula ØCQN
Uvulotomy *see* Drainage, Uvula ØC9N

V

Vaccination *see* Introduction of Serum, Toxoid, and Vaccine
Vacuum extraction, obstetric 1ØDØ7Z6
Vaginal artery
　use Artery, Internal Iliac, Left
　use Artery, Internal Iliac, Right
Vaginal pessary *use* Intraluminal Device, Pessary in Female Reproductive System
Vaginal vein
　use Vein, Hypogastric, Left
　use Vein, Hypogastric, Right
Vaginectomy
　see Excision, Vagina ØUBG
　see Resection, Vagina ØUTG
Vaginofixation
　see Repair, Vagina ØUQG
　see Reposition, Vagina ØUSG
Vaginoplasty
　see Repair, Vagina ØUQG
　see Supplement, Vagina ØUUG
Vaginorrhaphy *see* Repair, Vagina ØUQG
Vaginoscopy ØUJH8ZZ
Vaginotomy *see* Drainage, Female Reproductive System ØU9
Vagotomy *see* Division, Nerve, Vagus ØØ8Q
Valiant Thoracic Stent Graft *use* Synthetic Substitute
Valvotomy, valvulotomy
　see Division, Heart and Great Vessels Ø28
　see Release, Heart and Great Vessels Ø2N
Valvuloplasty
　see Repair, Heart and Great Vessels Ø2Q
　see Replacement, Heart and Great Vessels Ø2R
　see Supplement, Heart and Great Vessels Ø2U
Vascular Access Device
　Insertion of device in
　　Abdomen ØJH8
　　Chest ØJH6
　　Lower Arm
　　　Left ØJHH
　　　Right ØJHG
　　Lower Leg
　　　Left ØJHP
　　　Right ØJHN
　　Upper Arm
　　　Left ØJHF
　　　Right ØJHD
　　Upper Leg
　　　Left ØJHM
　　　Right ØJHL
　Removal of device from
　　Lower Extremity ØJPW
　　Trunk ØJPT
　　Upper Extremity ØJPV
　Reservoir
　　Insertion of device in
　　　Abdomen ØJH8
　　　Chest ØJH6
　　　Lower Arm
　　　　Left ØJHH
　　　　Right ØJHG
　　　Lower Leg
　　　　Left ØJHP
　　　　Right ØJHN
　　　Upper Arm
　　　　Left ØJHF
　　　　Right ØJHD

Vascular Access Device — continued
　Reservoir — continued
　　Insertion of device in — continued
　　　Upper Leg
　　　　Left ØJHM
　　　　Right ØJHL
　　Removal of device from
　　　Lower Extremity ØJPW
　　　Trunk ØJPT
　　　Upper Extremity ØJPV
　　Revision of device in
　　　Lower Extremity ØJWW
　　　Trunk ØJWT
　　　Upper Extremity ØJWV
　Revision of device in
　　Lower Extremity ØJWW
　　Trunk ØJWT
　　Upper Extremity ØJWV
Vasectomy *see* Excision, Male Reproductive System ØVB
Vasography
　see Fluoroscopy, Male Reproductive System BV1
　see Plain Radiography, Male Reproductive System BVØ
Vasoligation *see* Occlusion, Male Reproductive System ØVL
Vasorrhaphy *see* Repair, Male Reproductive System ØVQ
Vasostomy *see* Bypass, Male Reproductive System ØV1
Vasotomy
　With ligation *see* Occlusion, Male Reproductive System ØVL
　Drainage *see* Drainage, Male Reproductive System ØV9
Vasovasostomy *see* Repair, Male Reproductive System ØVQ
Vastus intermedius muscle
　use Muscle, Upper Leg, Left
　use Muscle, Upper Leg, Right
Vastus lateralis muscle
　use Muscle, Upper Leg, Left
　use Muscle, Upper Leg, Right
Vastus medialis muscle
　use Muscle, Upper Leg, Left
　use Muscle, Upper Leg, Right
VCG (vectorcardiogram) *see* Measurement, Cardiac 4AØ2
Vectra® Vascular Access Graft *use* Vascular Access Device in Subcutaneous Tissue and Fascia
Venectomy
　see Excision, Lower Veins Ø6B
　see Excision, Upper Veins Ø5B
Venography
　see Fluoroscopy, Veins B51
　see Plain Radiography, Veins B5Ø
Venorrhaphy
　see Repair, Lower Veins Ø6Q
　see Repair, Upper Veins Ø5Q
Venotripsy
　see Occlusion, Lower Veins Ø6L
　see Occlusion, Upper Veins Ø5L
Ventricular fold *use* Larynx
Ventriculoatriostomy *see* Bypass, Central Nervous System ØØ1
Ventriculocisternostomy *see* Bypass, Central Nervous System ØØ1
Ventriculogram, cardiac
　Combined left and right heart *see* Fluoroscopy, Heart, Right and Left B216
　Left ventricle *see* Fluoroscopy, Heart, Left B215
　Right ventricle *see* Fluoroscopy, Heart, Right B214
Ventriculopuncture, through previously implanted catheter 8CØ1X6J
Ventriculoscopy ØØJØ4ZZ
Ventriculostomy
　External drainage *see* Drainage, Cerebral Ventricle ØØ96
　Internal shunt *see* Bypass, Cerebral Ventricle ØØ16
Ventriculovenostomy *see* Bypass, Cerebral Ventricle ØØ16
Ventrio™ Hernia Patch *use* Synthetic Substitute
VEP (visual evoked potential) 4AØ7XØZ
Vermiform appendix *use* Appendix
Vermilion border
　use Lip, Lower
　use Lip, Upper
Versa *use* Pacemaker, Dual Chamber in ØJH

Version, obstetric
　External 1ØSØXZZ
　Internal 1ØSØ7ZZ
Vertebral arch
　use Vertebra, Cervical
　use Vertebra, Lumbar
　use Vertebra, Thoracic
Vertebral canal *use* Spinal Canal
Vertebral foramen
　use Vertebra, Cervical
　use Vertebra, Lumbar
　use Vertebra, Thoracic
Vertebral lamina
　use Vertebra, Cervical
　use Vertebra, Lumbar
　use Vertebra, Thoracic
Vertebral pedicle
　use Vertebra, Cervical
　use Vertebra, Lumbar
　use Vertebra, Thoracic
Vesical vein
　use Vein, Hypogastric, Left
　use Vein, Hypogastric, Right
Vesicotomy *see* Drainage, Urinary System ØT9
Vesiculectomy
　see Excision, Male Reproductive System ØVB
　see Resection, Male Reproductive System ØVT
Vesiculogram, seminal *see* Plain Radiography, Male Reproductive System BVØ
Vesiculotomy *see* Drainage, Male Reproductive System ØV9
Vestibular Assessment F15Z
Vestibular (Scarpa's) ganglion *use* Nerve, Acoustic
Vestibular nerve *use* Nerve, Acoustic
Vestibular Treatment FØC
Vestibulocochlear nerve *use* Nerve, Acoustic
Virchow's (supraclavicular) lymph node
　use Lymphatic, Neck, Left
　use Lymphatic, Neck, Right
Virtuoso (II) (DR) (VR) *use* Defibrillator Generator in ØJH
Vitrectomy
　see Excision, Eye Ø8B
　see Resection, Eye Ø8T
Vitreous body
　use Vitreous, Left
　use Vitreous, Right
Vocal fold
　use Vocal Cord, Left
　use Vocal Cord, Right
Vocational
　Assessment *see* Activities of Daily Living Assessment, Rehabilitation FØ2
　Retraining *see* Activities of Daily Living Treatment, Rehabilitation FØ8
Volar (palmar) digital vein
　use Vein, Hand, Left
　use Vein, Hand, Right
Volar (palmar) metacarpal vein
　use Vein, Hand, Left
　use Vein, Hand, Right
Vomer bone *use* Septum, Nasal
Vomer of nasal septum *use* Bone, Nasal
Vulvectomy
　see Excision, Female Reproductive System ØUB
　see Resection, Female Reproductive System ØUT

W

WALLSTENT® Endoprosthesis *use* Intraluminal Device
Washing *see* Irrigation
Wedge resection, pulmonary *see* Excision, Respiratory System ØBB
Window *see* Drainage
Wiring, dental 2W31X9Z

X

X-ray *see* Plain Radiography
X-STOP® Spacer
　use Spinal Stabilization Device, Interspinous Process in ØRH

 Subterms under main terms may continue to next column or page

X-STOP® Spacer — continued
use Spinal Stabilization Device, Interspinous Process in ØSH
Xenograft *use* Zooplastic Tissue in Heart and Great Vessels
XIENCE V Everolimus Eluting Coronary Stent System *use* Intraluminal Device, Drug-eluting in Heart and Great Vessels
Xiphoid process *use* Sternum
XLIF® System *use* Interbody Fusion Device in Lower Joints

Y

Yoga Therapy 8E0ZXY4

Z

Z-plasty, skin for scar contracture *see* Release, Skin and Breast ØHN
Zenith Flex® AAA Endovascular Graft *use* Intraluminal Device
Zenith TX2® TAA Endovascular Graft *use* Intraluminal Device
Zenith® Renu™ AAA Ancillary Graft *use* Intraluminal Device
Zilver® PTX® (paclitaxel) Drug-Eluting Peripheral Stent
use Intraluminal Device, Drug-eluting in Lower Arteries
use Intraluminal Device, Drug-eluting in Upper Arteries

Zimmer® NexGen® LPS Mobile Bearing Knee *use* Synthetic Substitute
Zimmer® NexGen® LPS-Flex Mobile Knee *use* Synthetic Substitute
Zonule of Zinn
use Lens, Left
use Lens, Right
Zotarolimus-eluting coronary stent *use* Intraluminal Device, Drug-eluting in Heart and Great Vessels
Zygomatic process of frontal bone
use Bone, Frontal, Left
use Bone, Frontal, Right
Zygomatic process of temporal bone
use Bone, Temporal, Left
use Bone, Temporal, Right
Zygomaticus muscle *use* Muscle, Facial

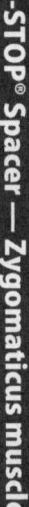

X-STOP® Spacer — Zygomaticus muscle

ICD-10-PCS Tables

Central Nervous System 001–00X

0   Medical and Surgical
0   Central Nervous System
1   Bypass   Altering the route of passage of the contents of a tubular body part

Body Part Character 4	Approach Character 5	Device Character 6	Qualifier Character 7
6 Cerebral Ventricle	0 Open 3 Percutaneous	7 Autologous Tissue Substitute J Synthetic Substitute K Nonautologous Tissue Substitute	0 Nasopharynx 1 Mastoid Sinus 2 Atrium 3 Blood Vessel 4 Pleural Cavity 5 Intestine 6 Peritoneal Cavity 7 Urinary Tract 8 Bone Marrow B Cerebral Cisterns
U Spinal Canal	0 Open 3 Percutaneous	7 Autologous Tissue Substitute J Synthetic Substitute K Nonautologous Tissue Substitute	4 Pleural Cavity 6 Peritoneal Cavity 7 Urinary Tract 9 Fallopian Tube

0   Medical and Surgical
0   Central Nervous System
2   Change   Taking out or off a device from a body part and putting back an identical or similar device in or on the same body part without cutting or puncturing the skin or a mucous membrane

Body Part Character 4	Approach Character 5	Device Character 6	Qualifier Character 7
0 Brain E Cranial Nerve U Spinal Canal	X External	0 Drainage Device Y Other Device	Z No Qualifier

Non-OR   For all body part, approach, device, and qualifier values

0   Medical and Surgical
0   Central Nervous System
5   Destruction   Physical eradication of all or a portion of a body part by the direct use of energy, force, or a destructive agent

Body Part Character 4	Approach Character 5	Device Character 6	Qualifier Character 7
0 Brain 1 Cerebral Meninges 2 Dura Mater 6 Cerebral Ventricle 7 Cerebral Hemisphere 8 Basal Ganglia 9 Thalamus A Hypothalamus B Pons C Cerebellum D Medulla Oblongata F Olfactory Nerve G Optic Nerve H Oculomotor Nerve J Trochlear Nerve K Trigeminal Nerve L Abducens Nerve M Facial Nerve N Acoustic Nerve P Glossopharyngeal Nerve Q Vagus Nerve R Accessory Nerve S Hypoglossal Nerve T Spinal Meninges W Cervical Spinal Cord X Thoracic Spinal Cord Y Lumbar Spinal Cord	0 Open 3 Percutaneous 4 Percutaneous Endoscopic	Z No Device	Z No Qualifier

Non-OR   005[F,G,H,J,K,L,M,N,P,Q,R,S][0,3,4]ZZ

[LC] Limited Coverage   [NC] Noncovered   HAC associated procedure   Combination Only   DRG Non-OR   Non-OR   Revised Text in **GREEN**

ICD-10-PCS 2014 (Draft)   131

Ø   Medical and Surgical
Ø   Central Nervous System
8   Division   Cutting into a body part without draining fluids and/or gases from the body part in order to separate or transect a body part

Body Part Character 4	Approach Character 5	Device Character 6	Qualifier Character 7
Ø Brain	Ø Open	Z No Device	Z No Qualifier
7 Cerebral Hemisphere	3 Percutaneous		
8 Basal Ganglia	4 Percutaneous Endoscopic		
F Olfactory Nerve			
G Optic Nerve			
H Oculomotor Nerve			
J Trochlear Nerve			
K Trigeminal Nerve			
L Abducens Nerve			
M Facial Nerve			
N Acoustic Nerve			
P Glossopharyngeal Nerve			
Q Vagus Nerve			
R Accessory Nerve			
S Hypoglossal Nerve			
W Cervical Spinal Cord			
X Thoracic Spinal Cord			
Y Lumbar Spinal Cord			

Ø   Medical and Surgical
Ø   Central Nervous System
9   Drainage   Taking or letting out fluids and/or gases from a body part

Body Part Character 4	Approach Character 5	Device Character 6	Qualifier Character 7
Ø Brain	Ø Open	Ø Drainage Device	Z No Qualifier
1 Cerebral Meninges	3 Percutaneous		
2 Dura Mater	4 Percutaneous Endoscopic		
3 Epidural Space			
4 Subdural Space			
5 Subarachnoid Space			
6 Cerebral Ventricle			
7 Cerebral Hemisphere			
8 Basal Ganglia			
9 Thalamus			
A Hypothalamus			
B Pons			
C Cerebellum			
D Medulla Oblongata			
F Olfactory Nerve			
G Optic Nerve			
H Oculomotor Nerve			
J Trochlear Nerve			
K Trigeminal Nerve			
L Abducens Nerve			
M Facial Nerve			
N Acoustic Nerve			
P Glossopharyngeal Nerve			
Q Vagus Nerve			
R Accessory Nerve			
S Hypoglossal Nerve			
T Spinal Meninges			
U Spinal Canal			
W Cervical Spinal Cord			
X Thoracic Spinal Cord			
Y Lumbar Spinal Cord			

009 Continued on next page

Non-OR   009[1,2,4,5,U][3,4]ØZ

Ø   **Medical and Surgical**   *009 Continued*
Ø   **Central Nervous System**
9   **Drainage**   Taking or letting out fluids and/or gases from a body part

Body Part Character 4	Approach Character 5	Device Character 6	Qualifier Character 7
Ø Brain	Ø Open	Z No Device	X Diagnostic
1 Cerebral Meninges	3 Percutaneous		Z No Qualifier
2 Dura Mater	4 Percutaneous Endoscopic		
3 Epidural Space			
4 Subdural Space			
5 Subarachnoid Space			
6 Cerebral Ventricle			
7 Cerebral Hemisphere			
8 Basal Ganglia			
9 Thalamus			
A Hypothalamus			
B Pons			
C Cerebellum			
D Medulla Oblongata			
F Olfactory Nerve			
G Optic Nerve			
H Oculomotor Nerve			
J Trochlear Nerve			
K Trigeminal Nerve			
L Abducens Nerve			
M Facial Nerve			
N Acoustic Nerve			
P Glossopharyngeal Nerve			
Q Vagus Nerve			
R Accessory Nerve			
S Hypoglossal Nerve			
T Spinal Meninges			
U Spinal Canal			
W Cervical Spinal Cord			
X Thoracic Spinal Cord			
Y Lumbar Spinal Cord			

Non-OR   009[Ø,1,2,3,4,5,6,7,8,9,A,B,C,D,F,G,H,J,K,L,M,N,P,Q,R,S,U][3,4]Z[X,Z]

Ø   **Medical and Surgical**
Ø   **Central Nervous System**
B   **Excision**   Cutting out or off, without replacement, a portion of a body part

Body Part Character 4	Approach Character 5	Device Character 6	Qualifier Character 7
Ø Brain	Ø Open	Z No Device	X Diagnostic
1 Cerebral Meninges	3 Percutaneous		Z No Qualifier
2 Dura Mater	4 Percutaneous Endoscopic		
6 Cerebral Ventricle			
7 Cerebral Hemisphere			
8 Basal Ganglia			
9 Thalamus			
A Hypothalamus			
B Pons			
C Cerebellum			
D Medulla Oblongata			
F Olfactory Nerve			
G Optic Nerve			
H Oculomotor Nerve			
J Trochlear Nerve			
K Trigeminal Nerve			
L Abducens Nerve			
M Facial Nerve			
N Acoustic Nerve			
P Glossopharyngeal Nerve			
Q Vagus Nerve			
R Accessory Nerve			
S Hypoglossal Nerve			
T Spinal Meninges			
W Cervical Spinal Cord			
X Thoracic Spinal Cord			
Y Lumbar Spinal Cord			

Non-OR   00B[Ø,1,2,6,7,8,9,A,B,C,D,F,G,H,J,K,L,M,N,P,Q,R,S][3,4]ZX

LC Limited Coverage   **NC** Noncovered   HAC associated procedure   Combination Only   DRG Non-OR   Non-OR   Revised Text in **GREEN**

Central Nervous System

Ø   **Medical and Surgical**
Ø   **Central Nervous System**
C   **Extirpation**   Taking or cutting out solid matter from a body part

Body Part Character 4	Approach Character 5	Device Character 6	Qualifier Character 7
Ø Brain	**Ø** Open	**Z** No Device	**Z** No Qualifier
1 Cerebral Meninges	**3** Percutaneous		
2 Dura Mater	**4** Percutaneous Endoscopic		
3 Epidural Space			
4 Subdural Space			
5 Subarachnoid Space			
6 Cerebral Ventricle			
7 Cerebral Hemisphere			
8 Basal Ganglia			
9 Thalamus			
A Hypothalamus			
B Pons			
C Cerebellum			
D Medulla Oblongata			
F Olfactory Nerve			
G Optic Nerve			
H Oculomotor Nerve			
J Trochlear Nerve			
K Trigeminal Nerve			
L Abducens Nerve			
M Facial Nerve			
N Acoustic Nerve			
P Glossopharyngeal Nerve			
Q Vagus Nerve			
R Accessory Nerve			
S Hypoglossal Nerve			
T Spinal Meninges			
W Cervical Spinal Cord			
X Thoracic Spinal Cord			
Y Lumbar Spinal Cord			

Ø   **Medical and Surgical**
Ø   **Central Nervous System**
D   **Extraction**   Pulling or stripping out or off all or a portion of a body part by the use of force

Body Part Character 4	Approach Character 5	Device Character 6	Qualifier Character 7
1 Cerebral Meninges	**Ø** Open	**Z** No Device	**Z** No Qualifier
2 Dura Mater	**3** Percutaneous		
F Olfactory Nerve	**4** Percutaneous Endoscopic		
G Optic Nerve			
H Oculomotor Nerve			
J Trochlear Nerve			
K Trigeminal Nerve			
L Abducens Nerve			
M Facial Nerve			
N Acoustic Nerve			
P Glossopharyngeal Nerve			
Q Vagus Nerve			
R Accessory Nerve			
S Hypoglossal Nerve			
T Spinal Meninges			

Ø   **Medical and Surgical**
Ø   **Central Nervous System**
F   **Fragmentation**   Breaking solid matter in a body part into pieces

Body Part Character 4	Approach Character 5	Device Character 6	Qualifier Character 7
3 Epidural Space NC	**Ø** Open	**Z** No Device	**Z** No Qualifier
4 Subdural Space NC	**3** Percutaneous		
5 Subarachnoid Space NC	**4** Percutaneous Endoscopic		
6 Cerebral Ventricle NC	**X** External		
U Spinal Canal			

    NC   ØØF[3,4,5,6]XZZ
    Non-OR   ØØF[3,4,5,6]XZZ

LC Limited Coverage   **NC** Noncovered   HAC associated procedure   Combination Only   DRG Non-OR   Non-OR   Revised Text in **GREEN**

134   ICD-10-PCS 2014 (Draft)

0   **Medical and Surgical**
0   **Central Nervous System**
H   **Insertion**   Putting in a nonbiological appliance that monitors, assists, performs, or prevents a physiological function but does not physically take the place of a body part

Body Part Character 4	Approach Character 5	Device Character 6	Qualifier Character 7
0 Brain **6** Cerebral Ventricle **E** Cranial Nerve **U** Spinal Canal **V** Spinal Cord	**0** Open **3** Percutaneous **4** Percutaneous Endoscopic	**2** Monitoring Device **3** Infusion Device **M** Neurostimulator Lead	**Z** No Qualifier

Non-OR   00H[U,V][0,3,4]3Z
Combination Only
   Major Brain Implant
     One of 00H[0,6][0,3,4]MZ with one of 0JH[6,7,8][0,3][D,E]Z or 0NH00NZ

Neurotransmitter/Neurostimulator
One of 00HE[0,3,4]MZ with one of 0JH[6,7,8][0,3][B,C,D,E] Z
Or
One of 00H[U,V][0,3,4]MZ with one of 0JH[6,7,8][0,3][B,C,D,E]Z

0   **Medical and Surgical**
0   **Central Nervous System**
J   **Inspection**   Visually and/or manually exploring a body part

Body Part Character 4	Approach Character 5	Device Character 6	Qualifier Character 7
0 Brain **E** Cranial Nerve **U** Spinal Canal **V** Spinal Cord	**0** Open **3** Percutaneous **4** Percutaneous Endoscopic	**Z** No Device	**Z** No Qualifier

0   **Medical and Surgical**
0   **Central Nervous System**
K   **Map**   Locating the route of passage of electrical impulses and/or locating functional areas in a body part

Body Part Character 4	Approach Character 5	Device Character 6	Qualifier Character 7
0 Brain **7** Cerebral Hemisphere **8** Basal Ganglia **9** Thalamus **A** Hypothalamus **B** Pons **C** Cerebellum **D** Medulla Oblongata	**0** Open **3** Percutaneous **4** Percutaneous Endoscopic	**Z** No Device	**Z** No Qualifier

0   **Medical and Surgical**
0   **Central Nervous System**
N   **Release**   Freeing a body part from an abnormal physical constraint

Body Part Character 4	Approach Character 5	Device Character 6	Qualifier Character 7
0 Brain **1** Cerebral Meninges **2** Dura Mater **6** Cerebral Ventricle **7** Cerebral Hemisphere **8** Basal Ganglia **9** Thalamus **A** Hypothalamus **B** Pons **C** Cerebellum **D** Medulla Oblongata **F** Olfactory Nerve **G** Optic Nerve **H** Oculomotor Nerve **J** Trochlear Nerve **K** Trigeminal Nerve **L** Abducens Nerve **M** Facial Nerve **N** Acoustic Nerve **P** Glossopharyngeal Nerve **Q** Vagus Nerve **R** Accessory Nerve **S** Hypoglossal Nerve **T** Spinal Meninges **W** Cervical Spinal Cord **X** Thoracic Spinal Cord **Y** Lumbar Spinal Cord	**0** Open **3** Percutaneous **4** Percutaneous Endoscopic	**Z** No Device	**Z** No Qualifier

Central Nervous System

0   **Medical and Surgical**
0   **Central Nervous System**
P   **Removal**   Taking out or off a device from a body part

Body Part Character 4	Approach Character 5	Device Character 6	Qualifier Character 7
0 Brain **6** Cerebral Ventricle **E** Cranial Nerve **U** Spinal Canal **V** Spinal Cord	**X** External	**0** Drainage Device **2** Monitoring Device **3** Infusion Device **M** Neurostimulator Lead	**Z** No Qualifier
0 Brain **V** Spinal Cord	**0** Open **3** Percutaneous **4** Percutaneous Endoscopic	**0** Drainage Device **2** Monitoring Device **3** Infusion Device **7** Autologous Tissue Substitute **J** Synthetic Substitute **K** Nonautologous Tissue Substitute **M** Neurostimulator Lead	**Z** No Qualifier
6 Cerebral Ventricle **U** Spinal Canal	**0** Open **3** Percutaneous **4** Percutaneous Endoscopic	**0** Drainage Device **2** Monitoring Device **3** Infusion Device **J** Synthetic Substitute **M** Neurostimulator Lead	**Z** No Qualifier
E Cranial Nerve	**0** Open **3** Percutaneous **4** Percutaneous Endoscopic	**0** Drainage Device **2** Monitoring Device **3** Infusion Device **7** Autologous Tissue Substitute **M** Neurostimulator Lead	**Z** No Qualifier

Non-OR   00P[0,U,V]X[0,2,3,M]Z
Non-OR   00P6X[0,3]Z
Non-OR   00PEX[0,2,3]Z

0   **Medical and Surgical**
0   **Central Nervous System**
Q   **Repair**   Restoring, to the extent possible, a body part to its normal anatomic structure and function

Body Part Character 4	Approach Character 5	Device Character 6	Qualifier Character 7
0 Brain **1** Cerebral Meninges **2** Dura Mater **6** Cerebral Ventricle **7** Cerebral Hemisphere **8** Basal Ganglia **9** Thalamus **A** Hypothalamus **B** Pons **C** Cerebellum **D** Medulla Oblongata **F** Olfactory Nerve **G** Optic Nerve **H** Oculomotor Nerve **J** Trochlear Nerve **K** Trigeminal Nerve **L** Abducens Nerve **M** Facial Nerve **N** Acoustic Nerve **P** Glossopharyngeal Nerve **Q** Vagus Nerve **R** Accessory Nerve **S** Hypoglossal Nerve **T** Spinal Meninges **W** Cervical Spinal Cord **X** Thoracic Spinal Cord **Y** Lumbar Spinal Cord	**0** Open **3** Percutaneous **4** Percutaneous Endoscopic	**Z** No Device	**Z** No Qualifier

LC Limited Coverage   **NC** Noncovered   HAC associated procedure   Combination Only   DRG Non-OR   Non-OR   Revised Text in **GREEN**

136   ICD-10-PCS 2014 (Draft)

0　**Medical and Surgical**
0　**Central Nervous System**
S　**Reposition**　　Moving to its normal location or other suitable location all or a portion of a body part

Body Part Character 4	Approach Character 5	Device Character 6	Qualifier Character 7
F Olfactory Nerve **G** Optic Nerve **H** Oculomotor Nerve **J** Trochlear Nerve **K** Trigeminal Nerve **L** Abducens Nerve **M** Facial Nerve **N** Acoustic Nerve **P** Glossopharyngeal Nerve **Q** Vagus Nerve **R** Accessory Nerve **S** Hypoglossal Nerve **W** Cervical Spinal Cord **X** Thoracic Spinal Cord **Y** Lumbar Spinal Cord	**0** Open **3** Percutaneous **4** Percutaneous Endoscopic	**Z** No Device	**Z** No Qualifier

0　**Medical and Surgical**
0　**Central Nervous System**
T　**Resection**　　Cutting out or off, without replacement, all of a body part

Body Part Character 4	Approach Character 5	Device Character 6	Qualifier Character 7
7 Cerebral Hemisphere	**0** Open **3** Percutaneous **4** Percutaneous Endoscopic	**Z** No Device	**Z** No Qualifier

0　**Medical and Surgical**
0　**Central Nervous System**
U　**Supplement**　　Putting in or on biological or synthetic material that physically reinforces and/or augments the function of a portion of a body part

Body Part Character 4	Approach Character 5	Device Character 6	Qualifier Character 7
1 Cerebral Meninges **2** Dura Mater **T** Spinal Meninges	**0** Open **3** Percutaneous **4** Percutaneous Endoscopic	**7** Autologous Tissue Substitute **J** Synthetic Substitute **K** Nonautologous Tissue Substitute	**Z** No Qualifier
F Olfactory Nerve **G** Optic Nerve **H** Oculomotor Nerve **J** Trochlear Nerve **K** Trigeminal Nerve **L** Abducens Nerve **M** Facial Nerve **N** Acoustic Nerve **P** Glossopharyngeal Nerve **Q** Vagus Nerve **R** Accessory Nerve **S** Hypoglossal Nerve	**0** Open **3** Percutaneous **4** Percutaneous Endoscopic	**7** Autologous Tissue Substitute	**Z** No Qualifier

Central Nervous System

0   **Medical and Surgical**
0   **Central Nervous System**
W   **Revision**   Correcting, to the extent possible, a portion of a malfunctioning device or the position of a displaced device

Body Part Character 4	Approach Character 5	Device Character 6	Qualifier Character 7
0 Brain **V** Spinal Cord	**0** Open **3** Percutaneous **4** Percutaneous Endoscopic **X** External	**0** Drainage Device **2** Monitoring Device **3** Infusion Device **7** Autologous Tissue Substitute **J** Synthetic Substitute **K** Nonautologous Tissue Substitute **M** Neurostimulator Lead	**Z** No Qualifier
6 Cerebral Ventricle **U** Spinal Canal	**0** Open **3** Percutaneous **4** Percutaneous Endoscopic **X** External	**0** Drainage Device **2** Monitoring Device **3** Infusion Device **J** Synthetic Substitute **M** Neurostimulator Lead	**Z** No Qualifier
E Cranial Nerve	**0** Open **3** Percutaneous **4** Percutaneous Endoscopic **X** External	**0** Drainage Device **2** Monitoring Device **3** Infusion Device **7** Autologous Tissue Substitute **M** Neurostimulator Lead	**Z** No Qualifier

Non-OR	00WEX[0,2,3,7,M]Z
Non-OR	00W[6,U]X[0,2,3,J,M]Z
Non-OR	00W[0,V]X[0,2,3,7,J,K,M]Z

0   **Medical and Surgical**
0   **Central Nervous System**
X   **Transfer**   Moving, without taking out, all or a portion of a body part to another location to take over the function of all or a portion of a body part

Body Part Character 4	Approach Character 5	Device Character 6	Qualifier Character 7
F Olfactory Nerve **G** Optic Nerve **H** Oculomotor Nerve **J** Trochlear Nerve **K** Trigeminal Nerve **L** Abducens Nerve **M** Facial Nerve **N** Acoustic Nerve **P** Glossopharyngeal Nerve **Q** Vagus Nerve **R** Accessory Nerve **S** Hypoglossal Nerve	**0** Open **4** Percutaneous Endoscopic	**Z** No Device	**F** Olfactory Nerve **G** Optic Nerve **H** Oculomotor Nerve **J** Trochlear Nerve **K** Trigeminal Nerve **L** Abducens Nerve **M** Facial Nerve **N** Acoustic Nerve **P** Glossopharyngeal Nerve **Q** Vagus Nerve **R** Accessory Nerve **S** Hypoglossal Nerve

Peripheral Nervous System 012-01X

0 **Medical and Surgical**
1 **Peripheral Nervous System**
2 **Change** Taking out or off a device from a body part and putting back an identical or similar device in or on the same body part without cutting or puncturing the skin or a mucous membrane

Body Part Character 4	Approach Character 5	Device Character 6	Qualifier Character 7
Y Peripheral Nerve	**X** External	**0** Drainage Device **Y** Other Device	**Z** No Qualifier

Non-OR For all body part, approach, device, and qualifier values

0 **Medical and Surgical**
1 **Peripheral Nervous System**
5 **Destruction** Physical eradication of all or a portion of a body part by the direct use of energy, force, or a destructive agent

Body Part Character 4	Approach Character 5	Device Character 6	Qualifier Character 7
0 Cervical Plexus **1** Cervical Nerve **2** Phrenic Nerve **3** Brachial Plexus **4** Ulnar Nerve **5** Median Nerve **6** Radial Nerve **8** Thoracic Nerve **9** Lumbar Plexus **A** Lumbosacral Plexus **B** Lumbar Nerve **C** Pudendal Nerve **D** Femoral Nerve **F** Sciatic Nerve **G** Tibial Nerve **H** Peroneal Nerve **K** Head and Neck Sympathetic Nerve **L** Thoracic Sympathetic Nerve **M** Abdominal Sympathetic Nerve **N** Lumbar Sympathetic Nerve **P** Sacral Sympathetic Nerve **Q** Sacral Plexus **R** Sacral Nerve	**0** Open **3** Percutaneous **4** Percutaneous Endoscopic	**Z** No Device	**Z** No Qualifier

Non-OR 015[0,2,3,4,5,6,9,A,C,D,F,G,H,Q][0,3,4]ZZ
Non-OR 015[1,8,B,R]3ZZ

0 **Medical and Surgical**
1 **Peripheral Nervous System**
8 **Division** Cutting into a body part without draining fluids and/or gases from the body part in order to separate or transect a body part

Body Part Character 4	Approach Character 5	Device Character 6	Qualifier Character 7
0 Cervical Plexus **1** Cervical Nerve **2** Phrenic Nerve **3** Brachial Plexus **4** Ulnar Nerve **5** Median Nerve **6** Radial Nerve **8** Thoracic Nerve **9** Lumbar Plexus **A** Lumbosacral Plexus **B** Lumbar Nerve **C** Pudendal Nerve **D** Femoral Nerve **F** Sciatic Nerve **G** Tibial Nerve **H** Peroneal Nerve **K** Head and Neck Sympathetic Nerve **L** Thoracic Sympathetic Nerve **M** Abdominal Sympathetic Nerve **N** Lumbar Sympathetic Nerve **P** Sacral Sympathetic Nerve **Q** Sacral Plexus **R** Sacral Nerve	**0** Open **3** Percutaneous **4** Percutaneous Endoscopic	**Z** No Device	**Z** No Qualifier

Peripheral Nervous System

019–019

0   Medical and Surgical
1   Peripheral Nervous System
9   Drainage   Taking or letting out fluids and/or gases from a body part

Body Part Character 4	Approach Character 5	Device Character 6	Qualifier Character 7
0 Cervical Plexus **1** Cervical Nerve **2** Phrenic Nerve **3** Brachial Plexus **4** Ulnar Nerve **5** Median Nerve **6** Radial Nerve **8** Thoracic Nerve **9** Lumbar Plexus **A** Lumbosacral Plexus **B** Lumbar Nerve **C** Pudendal Nerve **D** Femoral Nerve **F** Sciatic Nerve **G** Tibial Nerve **H** Peroneal Nerve **K** Head and Neck Sympathetic Nerve **L** Thoracic Sympathetic Nerve **M** Abdominal Sympathetic Nerve **N** Lumbar Sympathetic Nerve **P** Sacral Sympathetic Nerve **Q** Sacral Plexus **R** Sacral Nerve	**0** Open **3** Percutaneous **4** Percutaneous Endoscopic	**0** Drainage Device	**Z** No Qualifier
0 Cervical Plexus **1** Cervical Nerve **2** Phrenic Nerve **3** Brachial Plexus **4** Ulnar Nerve **5** Median Nerve **6** Radial Nerve **8** Thoracic Nerve **9** Lumbar Plexus **A** Lumbosacral Plexus **B** Lumbar Nerve **C** Pudendal Nerve **D** Femoral Nerve **F** Sciatic Nerve **G** Tibial Nerve **H** Peroneal Nerve **K** Head and Neck Sympathetic Nerve **L** Thoracic Sympathetic Nerve **M** Abdominal Sympathetic Nerve **N** Lumbar Sympathetic Nerve **P** Sacral Sympathetic Nerve **Q** Sacral Plexus **R** Sacral Nerve	**0** Open **3** Percutaneous **4** Percutaneous Endoscopic	**Z** No Device	**X** Diagnostic **Z** No Qualifier

Non-OR   019[0,1,2,3,4,5,6,8,9,A,B,C,D,F,G,H,Q,R][3,4]ZX

LC Limited Coverage   **NC** Noncovered   HAC associated procedure   Combination Only   DRG Non-OR   Non-OR   Revised Text in **GREEN**

140   ICD-10-PCS 2014 (Draft)

0   **Medical and Surgical**
1   **Peripheral Nervous System**
B   **Excision**   Cutting out or off, without replacement, a portion of a body part

Body Part Character 4	Approach Character 5	Device Character 6	Qualifier Character 7
0 Cervical Plexus **1** Cervical Nerve **2** Phrenic Nerve **3** Brachial Plexus **4** Ulnar Nerve **5** Median Nerve **6** Radial Nerve **8** Thoracic Nerve **9** Lumbar Plexus **A** Lumbosacral Plexus **B** Lumbar Nerve **C** Pudendal Nerve **D** Femoral Nerve **F** Sciatic Nerve **G** Tibial Nerve **H** Peroneal Nerve **K** Head and Neck Sympathetic Nerve **L** Thoracic Sympathetic Nerve **M** Abdominal Sympathetic Nerve **N** Lumbar Sympathetic Nerve **P** Sacral Sympathetic Nerve **Q** Sacral Plexus **R** Sacral Nerve	**0** Open **3** Percutaneous **4** Percutaneous Endoscopic	**Z** No Device	**X** Diagnostic **Z** No Qualifier

Non-OR   01B[0,1,2,3,4,5,6,8,9,A,B,C,D,F,G,H,Q,R][3,4]ZX

0   **Medical and Surgical**
1   **Peripheral Nervous System**
C   **Extirpation**   Taking or cutting out solid matter from a body part

Body Part Character 4	Approach Character 5	Device Character 6	Qualifier Character 7
0 Cervical Plexus **1** Cervical Nerve **2** Phrenic Nerve **3** Brachial Plexus **4** Ulnar Nerve **5** Median Nerve **6** Radial Nerve **8** Thoracic Nerve **9** Lumbar Plexus **A** Lumbosacral Plexus **B** Lumbar Nerve **C** Pudendal Nerve **D** Femoral Nerve **F** Sciatic Nerve **G** Tibial Nerve **H** Peroneal Nerve **K** Head and Neck Sympathetic Nerve **L** Thoracic Sympathetic Nerve **M** Abdominal Sympathetic Nerve **N** Lumbar Sympathetic Nerve **P** Sacral Sympathetic Nerve **Q** Sacral Plexus **R** Sacral Nerve	**0** Open **3** Percutaneous **4** Percutaneous Endoscopic	**Z** No Device	**Z** No Qualifier

LC Limited Coverage   **NC** Noncovered   HAC associated procedure   Combination Only   DRG Non-OR   Non-OR   Revised Text in **GREEN**

ICD-10-PCS 2014 (Draft)   **141**

0   Medical and Surgical
1   Peripheral Nervous System
D   Extraction   Pulling or stripping out or off all or a portion of a body part by the use of force

Body Part Character 4	Approach Character 5	Device Character 6	Qualifier Character 7
0 Cervical Plexus	0 Open	Z No Device	Z No Qualifier
1 Cervical Nerve	3 Percutaneous		
2 Phrenic Nerve	4 Percutaneous Endoscopic		
3 Brachial Plexus			
4 Ulnar Nerve			
5 Median Nerve			
6 Radial Nerve			
8 Thoracic Nerve			
9 Lumbar Plexus			
A Lumbosacral Plexus			
B Lumbar Nerve			
C Pudendal Nerve			
D Femoral Nerve			
F Sciatic Nerve			
G Tibial Nerve			
H Peroneal Nerve			
K Head and Neck Sympathetic Nerve			
L Thoracic Sympathetic Nerve			
M Abdominal Sympathetic Nerve			
N Lumbar Sympathetic Nerve			
P Sacral Sympathetic Nerve			
Q Sacral Plexus			
R Sacral Nerve			

0   Medical and Surgical
1   Peripheral Nervous System
H   Insertion   Putting in a nonbiological appliance that monitors, assists, performs, or prevents a physiological function but does not physically take the place of a body part

Body Part Character 4	Approach Character 5	Device Character 6	Qualifier Character 7
Y Peripheral Nerve	0 Open	2 Monitoring Device	Z No Qualifier
	3 Percutaneous	M Neurostimulator Lead	
	4 Percutaneous Endoscopic		

Combination Only
  Neurotransmitter/Neurostimulator
  One of 01HY[0,3,4]MZ with one of 0JH[6,7,8][0,3][B,C,D,E] Z

0   Medical and Surgical
1   Peripheral Nervous System
J   Inspection   Visually and/or manually exploring a body part

Body Part Character 4	Approach Character 5	Device Character 6	Qualifier Character 7
Y Peripheral Nerve	0 Open	Z No Device	Z No Qualifier
	3 Percutaneous		
	4 Percutaneous Endoscopic		

Ø **Medical and Surgical**
1 **Peripheral Nervous System**
N **Release**　　　　Freeing a body part from an abnormal physical constraint

Body Part Character 4	Approach Character 5	Device Character 6	Qualifier Character 7
Ø Cervical Plexus	Ø Open	Z No Device	Z No Qualifier
1 Cervical Nerve	3 Percutaneous		
2 Phrenic Nerve	4 Percutaneous Endoscopic		
3 Brachial Plexus			
4 Ulnar Nerve			
5 Median Nerve			
6 Radial Nerve			
8 Thoracic Nerve			
9 Lumbar Plexus			
A Lumbosacral Plexus			
B Lumbar Nerve			
C Pudendal Nerve			
D Femoral Nerve			
F Sciatic Nerve			
G Tibial Nerve			
H Peroneal Nerve			
K Head and Neck Sympathetic Nerve			
L Thoracic Sympathetic Nerve			
M Abdominal Sympathetic Nerve			
N Lumbar Sympathetic Nerve			
P Sacral Sympathetic Nerve			
Q Sacral Plexus			
R Sacral Nerve			

Ø **Medical and Surgical**
1 **Peripheral Nervous System**
P **Removal**　　　　Taking out or off a device from a body part

Body Part Character 4	Approach Character 5	Device Character 6	Qualifier Character 7
Y Peripheral Nerve	Ø Open	Ø Drainage Device	Z No Qualifier
	3 Percutaneous	2 Monitoring Device	
	4 Percutaneous Endoscopic	7 Autologous Tissue Substitute	
		M Neurostimulator Lead	
Y Peripheral Nerve	X External	Ø Drainage Device	Z No Qualifier
		2 Monitoring Device	
		M Neurostimulator Lead	

Non-OR Ø1PYX[Ø,2]Z

Ø **Medical and Surgical**
1 **Peripheral Nervous System**
Q **Repair**　　　　Restoring, to the extent possible, a body part to its normal anatomic structure and function

Body Part Character 4	Approach Character 5	Device Character 6	Qualifier Character 7
Ø Cervical Plexus	Ø Open	Z No Device	Z No Qualifier
1 Cervical Nerve	3 Percutaneous		
2 Phrenic Nerve	4 Percutaneous Endoscopic		
3 Brachial Plexus			
4 Ulnar Nerve			
5 Median Nerve			
6 Radial Nerve			
8 Thoracic Nerve			
9 Lumbar Plexus			
A Lumbosacral Plexus			
B Lumbar Nerve			
C Pudendal Nerve			
D Femoral Nerve			
F Sciatic Nerve			
G Tibial Nerve			
H Peroneal Nerve			
K Head and Neck Sympathetic Nerve			
L Thoracic Sympathetic Nerve			
M Abdominal Sympathetic Nerve			
N Lumbar Sympathetic Nerve			
P Sacral Sympathetic Nerve			
Q Sacral Plexus			
R Sacral Nerve			

LC Limited Coverage　**NC** Noncovered　HAC associated procedure　Combination Only　DRG Non-OR　Non-OR　Revised Text in **GREEN**

ICD-10-PCS 2014 (Draft)　　　　　　143

Peripheral Nervous System

0 **Medical and Surgical**
1 **Peripheral Nervous System**
S **Reposition** Moving to its normal location or other suitable location all or a portion of a body part

Body Part Character 4	Approach Character 5	Device Character 6	Qualifier Character 7
0 Cervical Plexus	**0** Open	**Z** No Device	**Z** No Qualifier
1 Cervical Nerve	**3** Percutaneous		
2 Phrenic Nerve	**4** Percutaneous Endoscopic		
3 Brachial Plexus			
4 Ulnar Nerve			
5 Median Nerve			
6 Radial Nerve			
8 Thoracic Nerve			
9 Lumbar Plexus			
A Lumbosacral Plexus			
B Lumbar Nerve			
C Pudendal Nerve			
D Femoral Nerve			
F Sciatic Nerve			
G Tibial Nerve			
H Peroneal Nerve			
Q Sacral Plexus			
R Sacral Nerve			

0 **Medical and Surgical**
1 **Peripheral Nervous System**
U **Supplement** Putting in or on biological or synthetic material that physically reinforces and/or augments the function of a portion of a body part

Body Part Character 4	Approach Character 5	Device Character 6	Qualifier Character 7
1 Cervical Nerve	**0** Open	**7** Autologous Tissue Substitute	**Z** No Qualifier
2 Phrenic Nerve	**3** Percutaneous		
4 Ulnar Nerve	**4** Percutaneous Endoscopic		
5 Median Nerve			
6 Radial Nerve			
8 Thoracic Nerve			
B Lumbar Nerve			
C Pudendal Nerve			
D Femoral Nerve			
F Sciatic Nerve			
G Tibial Nerve			
H Peroneal Nerve			
R Sacral Nerve			

0 **Medical and Surgical**
1 **Peripheral Nervous System**
W **Revision** Correcting, to the extent possible, a portion of a malfunctioning device or the position of a displaced device

Body Part Character 4	Approach Character 5	Device Character 6	Qualifier Character 7
Y Peripheral Nerve	**0** Open	**0** Drainage Device	**Z** No Qualifier
	3 Percutaneous	**2** Monitoring Device	
	4 Percutaneous Endoscopic	**7** Autologous Tissue Substitute	
	X External	**M** Neurostimulator Lead	

Non-OR 01WYX[0,2,7,M]Z

0 **Medical and Surgical**
1 **Peripheral Nervous System**
X **Transfer** Moving, without taking out, all or a portion of a body part to another location to take over the function of all or a portion of a body part

Body Part Character 4	Approach Character 5	Device Character 6	Qualifier Character 7
1 Cervical Nerve	**0** Open	**Z** No Device	**1** Cervical Nerve
2 Phrenic Nerve	**4** Percutaneous Endoscopic		**2** Phrenic Nerve
4 Ulnar Nerve	**0** Open	**Z** No Device	**4** Ulnar Nerve
5 Median Nerve	**4** Percutaneous Endoscopic		**5** Median Nerve
6 Radial Nerve			**6** Radial Nerve
8 Thoracic Nerve	**0** Open	**Z** No Device	**8** Thoracic Nerve
	4 Percutaneous Endoscopic		
B Lumbar Nerve	**0** Open	**Z** No Device	**B** Lumbar Nerve
C Pudendal Nerve	**4** Percutaneous Endoscopic		**C** Perineal Nerve
D Femoral Nerve	**0** Open	**Z** No Device	**D** Femoral Nerve
F Sciatic Nerve	**4** Percutaneous Endoscopic		**F** Sciatic Nerve
G Tibial Nerve			**G** Tibial Nerve
H Peroneal Nerve			**H** Peroneal Nerve

Heart and Great Vessels Ø21–Ø2Y

Ø   **Medical and Surgical**
2   **Heart and Great Vessels**
1   **Bypass**   Altering the route of passage of the contents of a tubular body part

Body Part Character 4	Approach Character 5	Device Character 6	Qualifier Character 7
Ø Coronary Artery, One Site 1 Coronary Artery, Two Sites 2 Coronary Artery, Three Sites 3 Coronary Artery, Four or More Sites	Ø Open 4 Percutaneous Endoscopic	9 Autologous Venous Tissue A Autologous Arterial Tissue J Synthetic Substitute K Nonautologous Tissue Substitute	3 Coronary Artery 8 Internal Mammary, Right 9 Internal Mammary, Left C Thoracic Artery F Abdominal Artery W Aorta
Ø Coronary Artery, One Site 1 Coronary Artery, Two Sites 2 Coronary Artery, Three Sites 3 Coronary Artery, Four or More Sites	Ø Open 4 Percutaneous Endoscopic	Z No Device	3 Coronary Artery 8 Internal Mammary, Right 9 Internal Mammary, Left C Thoracic Artery F Abdominal Artery
Ø Coronary Artery, One Site 1 Coronary Artery, Two Sites 2 Coronary Artery, Three Sites 3 Coronary Artery, Four or More Sites	3 Percutaneous 4 Percutaneous Endoscopic	4 Drug-eluting Intraluminal Device D Intraluminal Device	4 Coronary Vein
6 Atrium, Right	Ø Open 4 Percutaneous Endoscopic	Z No Device	7 Atrium, Left P Pulmonary Trunk Q Pulmonary Artery, Right R Pulmonary Artery, Left
6 Atrium, Right K Ventricle, Right L Ventricle, Left	Ø Open 4 Percutaneous Endoscopic	9 Autologous Venous Tissue A Autologous Arterial Tissue J Synthetic Substitute K Nonautologous Tissue Substitute	P Pulmonary Trunk Q Pulmonary Artery, Right R Pulmonary Artery, Left
7 Atrium, Left V Superior Vena Cava	Ø Open 4 Percutaneous Endoscopic	9 Autologous Venous Tissue A Autologous Arterial Tissue J Synthetic Substitute K Nonautologous Tissue Substitute Z No Device	P Pulmonary Trunk Q Pulmonary Artery, Right R Pulmonary Artery, Left
K Ventricle, Right L Ventricle, Left	Ø Open 4 Percutaneous Endoscopic	Z No Device	5 Coronary Circulation 8 Internal Mammary, Right 9 Internal Mammary, Left C Thoracic Artery F Abdominal Artery P Pulmonary Trunk Q Pulmonary Artery, Right R Pulmonary Artery, Left W Aorta
W Thoracic Aorta	Ø Open 4 Percutaneous Endoscopic	9 Autologous Venous Tissue A Autologous Arterial Tissue J Synthetic Substitute K Nonautologous Tissue Substitute Z No Device	B Subclavian D Carotid P Pulmonary Trunk Q Pulmonary Artery, Right R Pulmonary Artery, Left

Non-OR   Ø21[Ø,1,2,3][3,4][4,D]4
HAC   Ø21[Ø,1,2,3][Ø,4][9,A,J,K][3,8,9,C,F,W] when reported with SDx J98.5
HAC   Ø21[Ø,1,2,3][Ø,4]Z[3,8,9,C,F] when reported with SDx J98.5

Heart and Great Vessels

Ø   **Medical and Surgical**
2   **Heart and Great Vessels**
5   **Destruction**   Physical eradication of all or a portion of a body part by the direct use of energy, force, or a destructive agent

Body Part Character 4	Approach Character 5	Device Character 6	Qualifier Character 7
4 Coronary Vein **5** Atrial Septum **6** Atrium, Right **8** Conduction Mechanism **9** Chordae Tendineae **D** Papillary Muscle **F** Aortic Valve **G** Mitral Valve **H** Pulmonary Valve **J** Tricuspid Valve **K** Ventricle, Right **L** Ventricle, Left **M** Ventricular Septum **N** Pericardium **P** Pulmonary Trunk **Q** Pulmonary Artery, Right **R** Pulmonary Artery, Left **S** Pulmonary Vein, Right **T** Pulmonary Vein, Left **V** Superior Vena Cava **W** Thoracic Aorta	**Ø** Open **3** Percutaneous **4** Percutaneous Endoscopic	**Z** No Device	**Z** No Qualifier
7 Atrium, Left	**Ø** Open **3** Percutaneous **4** Percutaneous Endoscopic	**Z** No Device	**K** Left Atrial Appendage **Z** No Qualifier

DRG Non-OR   Ø257[Ø,3,4]ZK

Ø   **Medical and Surgical**
2   **Heart and Great Vessels**
7   **Dilation**   Expanding an orifice or the lumen of a tubular body part

Body Part Character 4	Approach Character 5	Device Character 6	Qualifier Character 7
Ø Coronary Artery, One Site **1** Coronary Artery, Two Sites **2** Coronary Artery, Three Sites **3** Coronary Artery, Four or More Sites	**Ø** Open **3** Percutaneous **4** Percutaneous Endoscopic	**4** Intraluminal Device, Drug-eluting **D** Intraluminal Device **T** Radioactive Intraluminal Device **Z** No Device	**6** Bifurcation **Z** No Qualifier
F Aortic Valve **G** Mitral Valve **H** Pulmonary Valve **J** Tricuspid Valve **K** Ventricle, Right **P** Pulmonary Trunk **Q** Pulmonary Artery, Right **S** Pulmonary Vein, Right **T** Pulmonary Vein, Left **V** Superior Vena Cava **W** Thoracic Aorta	**Ø** Open **3** Percutaneous **4** Percutaneous Endoscopic	**4** Intraluminal Device, Drug-eluting **D** Intraluminal Device **Z** No Device	**Z** No Qualifier
R Pulmonary Artery, Left	**Ø** Open **3** Percutaneous **4** Percutaneous Endoscopic	**4** Intraluminal Device, Drug-eluting **D** Intraluminal Device **Z** No Device	**T** Ductus Arteriosus **Z** No Qualifier

Ø   **Medical and Surgical**
2   **Heart and Great Vessels**
8   **Division**   Cutting into a body part without draining fluids and/or gases from the body part in order to separate or transect a body part

Body Part Character 4	Approach Character 5	Device Character 6	Qualifier Character 7
8 Conduction Mechanism **9** Chordae Tendineae **D** Papillary Muscle	**Ø** Open **3** Percutaneous **4** Percutaneous Endoscopic	**Z** No Device	**Z** No Qualifier

LC Limited Coverage   **NC** Noncovered   HAC associated procedure   Combination Only   DRG Non-OR   Non-OR   Revised Text in **GREEN**

146   ICD-10-PCS 2014 (Draft)

0 **Medical and Surgical**
2 **Heart and Great Vessels**
B **Excision**   Cutting out or off, without replacement, a portion of a body part

Body Part Character 4	Approach Character 5	Device Character 6	Qualifier Character 7
4 Coronary Vein 5 Atrial Septum 6 Atrium, Right 7 Atrium, Left 8 Conduction Mechanism 9 Chordae Tendineae D Papillary Muscle F Aortic Valve G Mitral Valve H Pulmonary Valve J Tricuspid Valve K Ventricle, Right ᴺᶜ L Ventricle, Left ᴺᶜ M Ventricular Septum N Pericardium P Pulmonary Trunk Q Pulmonary Artery, Right R Pulmonary Artery, Left S Pulmonary Vein, Right T Pulmonary Vein, Left V Superior Vena Cava W Thoracic Aorta	0 Open 3 Percutaneous 4 Percutaneous Endoscopic	Z No Device	X Diagnostic Z No Qualifier
7 Atrium, Left	0 Open 3 Percutaneous 4 Percutaneous Endoscopic	Z No Device	K Left Atrial Appendage

ᴺᶜ	02BK[0,3,4]ZZ
ᴺᶜ	02BL[0,3,4]ZZ
DRG Non-OR	02B7[0,3,4]ZK
Non-OR	02B[4,5,6,7,8,9,D,F,G,H,J,K,L,M][0,3,4]ZX

0 **Medical and Surgical**
2 **Heart and Great Vessels**
C **Extirpation**   Taking or cutting out solid matter from a body part

Body Part Character 4	Approach Character 5	Device Character 6	Qualifier Character 7
0 Coronary Artery, One Site 1 Coronary Artery, Two Sites 2 Coronary Artery, Three Sites 3 Coronary Artery, Four or More Sites 4 Coronary Vein 5 Atrial Septum 6 Atrium, Right 7 Atrium, Left 8 Conduction Mechanism 9 Chordae Tendineae D Papillary Muscle F Aortic Valve G Mitral Valve H Pulmonary Valve J Tricuspid Valve K Ventricle, Right L Ventricle, Left M Ventricular Septum N Pericardium P Pulmonary Trunk Q Pulmonary Artery, Right R Pulmonary Artery, Left S Pulmonary Vein, Right T Pulmonary Vein, Left V Superior Vena Cava W Thoracic Aorta	0 Open 3 Percutaneous 4 Percutaneous Endoscopic	Z No Device	Z No Qualifier

ᴸᶜ Limited Coverage	ᴺᶜ Noncovered	HAC associated procedure	Combination Only	DRG Non-OR	Non-OR	Revised Text in **GREEN**

Heart and Great Vessels

02F–02H

Ø Medical and Surgical
2 Heart and Great Vessels
F Fragmentation   Breaking solid matter in a body part into pieces

Body Part Character 4	Approach Character 5	Device Character 6	Qualifier Character 7
N Pericardium **NC**	Ø Open 3 Percutaneous 4 Percutaneous Endoscopic X External	Z No Device	Z No Qualifier

NC	Ø2FNXZZ
Non-OR	Ø2FNXZZ

Ø Medical and Surgical
2 Heart and Great Vessels
H Insertion   Putting in a nonbiological appliance that monitors, assists, performs, or prevents a physiological function but does not physically take the place of a body part

Body Part Character 4	Approach Character 5	Device Character 6	Qualifier Character 7
4 Coronary Vein 6 Atrium, Right 7 Atrium, Left K Ventricle, Right L Ventricle, Left	Ø Open 3 Percutaneous 4 Percutaneous Endoscopic	Ø Monitoring Device, Pressure Sensor 2 Monitoring Device 3 Infusion Device D Intraluminal Device J Cardiac Lead, Pacemaker K Cardiac Lead, Defibrillator M Cardiac Lead	Z No Qualifier
A Heart **LC**	Ø Open 3 Percutaneous 4 Percutaneous Endoscopic	Q Implantable Heart Assist System	Z No Qualifier
A Heart	Ø Open 3 Percutaneous 4 Percutaneous Endoscopic	R External Heart Assist System	S Biventricular Z No Qualifier
N Pericardium	Ø Open 3 Percutaneous 4 Percutaneous Endoscopic	Ø Monitoring Device, Pressure Sensor 2 Monitoring Device J Cardiac Lead, Pacemaker K Cardiac Lead, Defibrillator M Cardiac Lead	Z No Qualifier
P Pulmonary Trunk Q Pulmonary Artery, Right R Pulmonary Artery, Left S Pulmonary Vein, Right T Pulmonary Vein, Left V Superior Vena Cava W Thoracic Aorta	Ø Open 3 Percutaneous 4 Percutaneous Endoscopic	Ø Monitoring Device, Pressure Sensor 2 Monitoring Device 3 Infusion Device D Intraluminal Device	Z No Qualifier

Combinations Only

Pacemaker Lead/Device
One of Ø2H[4,6,7][Ø,4][J,M]Z with one of ØJH[6,8][Ø,3][4,5,6]Z with one of ØJPT[Ø,3]PZ
Or
One of Ø2H[6,7]3JZ with one of ØJH[6,8][Ø,3][4,5,6]Z with one of ØJPT[Ø,3]PZ
Or
One of Ø2H[K,L][Ø,3,4][J,M]Z with one of ØJH[6,8][Ø,3][4,5,6]Z with one of ØJPT[Ø,3]PZ
Or
One of Ø2H[4,6,7][Ø,4][J,M]Z with one of ØJH[6,8][Ø,3][4,5,P]Z
Or
One of Ø2H[6,7]3JZ with one of ØJH[6,8][Ø,3][4,5,P]Z
Or
One of Ø2H[K,L][Ø,3,4][J,M]Z with one of ØJH[6,8][Ø,3][4,5,P]Z
Or
Ø2H[6,7]3JZ with one of ØJH[6,8][Ø,3][4,5,6]Z with one of ØJPT[Ø,3]PZ
Or
One of Ø2H64[J,M]Z with one of ØJH[6,8][Ø,3][4,5,6]Z with one of ØJPT[Ø,3]PZ
Or
One of Ø2H7[Ø,4][J,M]Z with one of ØJH[6,8][Ø,3][4,5,6]Z with one of ØJPT[Ø,3]PZ
Or
One of Ø2H[K,L][Ø,3,4][J,M]Z with one of ØJH[6,8][Ø,3][4,5,6]Z with one of ØJPT[Ø,3]PZ
Or
One of Ø2H[6,7,K,L]3JZ with one of Ø2PA[Ø,3,4,X]MZ with one of ØJH[6,8][Ø,3][4,5,6]Z with one of ØJPT[Ø,3]PZ
Or
One of Ø2H[6,7,K,L]3JZ with one of Ø2PA[Ø,3,4,X]MZ with one of ØJH[6,8][Ø,3]PZ

Or
One of Ø2H[6,7]3MZ with one of ØJH[6,8][Ø,3][4,5,6]Z and one of ØJPT[Ø,3]PZ
Or
One of Ø2H[6,7]3MZ with one of ØJH[6,8][Ø,3]PZ
Or
One of Ø2HK[3,4][J,M]Z with one of ØJH[6,8][Ø,3][4,5,6]Z with one of ØJPT[Ø,3]PZ
Or
One of Ø2HL[Ø,3,4][J,M]Z with one of ØJH[6,8][Ø,3][4,5,6]Z with one of ØJPT[Ø,3]PZ
Or
One of Ø2H[K,L]3JZ with one of ØJH[6,8][Ø,3][6,P]Z
Or
One of Ø2HN[Ø,3,4][J,M]Z with one of ØJH[6,8][Ø,3][4,5,6,P]Z
Or
One of Ø2HN[Ø,3,4][J,M]Z with one of ØJH[6,8][Ø,3][4,5,6]Z with one of ØJPT[Ø,2]PZ

Heart Assist System
One of Ø2HA[Ø,3,4]R[S,Z] with one of Ø2PA[Ø,3,4]RZ

Intracardiac Lead/Device
One of Ø2HK[Ø,3,4][Ø,2]Z with one of ØJH[6,8][Ø,3]ØZ

LC	Ø2HA[Ø,3,4]QZ
Non-OR	Ø2H[4,6,7,K,L][Ø,4][J,M]Z
Non-OR	Ø2H[K,L]3MZ
Non-OR	Ø2H[P,Q,R][Ø,3,4][Ø,2,3]Z
Non-OR	Ø2H[S,T,V,W][Ø,3,4]3Z
Non-OR	Ø2HW[Ø,3,4][Ø,3]Z
DRG Non-OR	Ø2H[6,7,K,L]3JZ

LC Limited Coverage   **NC** Noncovered   HAC associated procedure   Combination Only   DRG Non-OR   Non-OR   Revised Text in **GREEN**

148   ICD-10-PCS 2014 (Draft)

0   **Medical and Surgical**
2   **Heart and Great Vessels**
J   **Inspection**   Visually and/or manually exploring a body part

Body Part Character 4	Approach Character 5	Device Character 6	Qualifier Character 7
A Heart Y Great Vessel	0 Open 3 Percutaneous 4 Percutaneous Endoscopic	Z No Device	Z No Qualifier

Non-OR   02J[A,Y]3ZZ

0   **Medical and Surgical**
2   **Heart and Great Vessels**
K   **Map**   Locating the route of passage of electrical impulses and/or locating functional areas in a body part

Body Part Character 4	Approach Character 5	Device Character 6	Qualifier Character 7
8 Conduction Mechanism	0 Open 3 Percutaneous 4 Percutaneous Endoscopic	Z No Device	Z No Qualifier

DRG Non-OR   02K8[0,3,4]ZZ

0   **Medical and Surgical**
2   **Heart and Great Vessels**
L   **Occlusion**   Completely closing an orifice or the lumen of a tubular body part

Body Part Character 4	Approach Character 5	Device Character 6	Qualifier Character 7
7 Atrium, Left	0 Open 3 Percutaneous 4 Percutaneous Endoscopic	C Extraluminal Device D Intraluminal Device Z No Device	K Left Atrial Appendage
R Pulmonary Artery, Left	0 Open 3 Percutaneous 4 Percutaneous Endoscopic	C Extraluminal Device D Intraluminal Device Z No Device	T Ductus Arteriosus
S Pulmonary Vein, Right T Pulmonary Vein, Left V Superior Vena Cava	0 Open 3 Percutaneous 4 Percutaneous Endoscopic	C Extraluminal Device D Intraluminal Device Z No Device	Z No Qualifier

DRG Non-OR   02L7[0,3,4][C,D,Z]K

0   **Medical and Surgical**
2   **Heart and Great Vessels**
N   **Release**   Freeing a body part from an abnormal physical constraint

Body Part Character 4	Approach Character 5	Device Character 6	Qualifier Character 7
4 Coronary Vein 5 Atrial Septum 6 Atrium, Right 7 Atrium, Left 8 Conduction Mechanism 9 Chordae Tendineae D Papillary Muscle F Aortic Valve G Mitral Valve H Pulmonary Valve J Tricuspid Valve K Ventricle, Right L Ventricle, Left M Ventricular Septum N Pericardium P Pulmonary Trunk Q Pulmonary Artery, Right R Pulmonary Artery, Left S Pulmonary Vein, Right T Pulmonary Vein, Left V Superior Vena Cava W Thoracic Aorta	0 Open 3 Percutaneous 4 Percutaneous Endoscopic	Z No Device	Z No Qualifier

LC Limited Coverage   **NC** Noncovered   HAC associated procedure   Combination Only   DRG Non-OR   Non-OR   Revised Text in **GREEN**

ICD-10-PCS 2014 (Draft)   149

Heart and Great Vessels

0	Medical and Surgical
2	Heart and Great Vessels
P	Removal Taking out or off a device from a body part

Body Part Character 4	Approach Character 5	Device Character 6	Qualifier Character 7
A Heart	0 Open 3 Percutaneous 4 Percutaneous Endoscopic	2 Monitoring Device 3 Infusion Device 7 Autologous Tissue Substitute 8 Zooplastic Tissue C Extraluminal Device D Intraluminal Device J Synthetic Substitute K Nonautologous Tissue Substitute M Cardiac Lead Q Implantable Heart Assist System R External Heart Assist System	Z No Qualifier
A Heart	X External	2 Monitoring Device 3 Infusion Device D Intraluminal Device M Cardiac Lead	Z No Qualifier
Y Great Vessel	0 Open 3 Percutaneous 4 Percutaneous Endoscopic	2 Monitoring Device 3 Infusion Device 7 Autologous Tissue Substitute 8 Zooplastic Tissue C Extraluminal Device D Intraluminal Device J Synthetic Substitute K Nonautologous Tissue Substitute	Z No Qualifier
Y Great Vessel	X External	2 Monitoring Device 3 Infusion Device D Intraluminal Device	Z No Qualifier

Non-OR   02PAX[2,3,D]Z
Non-OR   02PYX[2,3,D]Z

0	Medical and Surgical
2	Heart and Great Vessels
Q	Repair Restoring, to the extent possible, a body part to its normal anatomic structure and function

Body Part Character 4	Approach Character 5	Device Character 6	Qualifier Character 7
0 Coronary Artery, One Site 1 Coronary Artery, Two Sites 2 Coronary Artery, Three Sites 3 Coronary Artery, Four or More Sites 4 Coronary Vein 5 Atrial Septum 6 Atrium, Right 7 Atrium, Left 8 Conduction Mechanism 9 Chordae Tendineae A Heart B Heart, Right C Heart, Left D Papillary Muscle F Aortic Valve G Mitral Valve H Pulmonary Valve J Tricuspid Valve K Ventricle, Right L Ventricle, Left M Ventricular Septum N Pericardium P Pulmonary Trunk Q Pulmonary Artery, Right R Pulmonary Artery, Left S Pulmonary Vein, Right T Pulmonary Vein, Left V Superior Vena Cava W Thoracic Aorta	0 Open 3 Percutaneous 4 Percutaneous Endoscopic	Z No Device	Z No Qualifier

Ø Medical and Surgical
2 Heart and Great Vessels
R Replacement　　Putting in or on biological or synthetic material that physically takes the place and/or function of all or a portion of a body part

Body Part Character 4	Approach Character 5	Device Character 6	Qualifier Character 7
5　Atrial Septum 6　Atrium, Right 7　Atrium, Left 9　Chordae Tendineae D　Papillary Muscle J　Tricuspid Valve K　Ventricle, Right　NC LC L　Ventricle, Left　NC LC M　Ventricular Septum N　Pericardium P　Pulmonary Trunk Q　Pulmonary Artery, Right R　Pulmonary Artery, Left S　Pulmonary Vein, Right T　Pulmonary Vein, Left V　Superior Vena Cava W　Thoracic Aorta	Ø　Open 4　Percutaneous Endoscopic	7　Autologous Tissue Substitute 8　Zooplastic Tissue J　Synthetic Substitute K　Nonautologous Tissue Substitute	Z　No Qualifier
F　Aortic Valve G　Mitral Valve H　Pulmonary Valve	Ø　Open 4　Percutaneous Endoscopic	7　Autologous Tissue Substitute 8　Zooplastic Tissue J　Synthetic Substitute K　Nonautologous Tissue Substitute	Z　No Qualifier
F　Aortic Valve G　Mitral Valve H　Pulmonary Valve	3　Percutaneous	7　Autologous Tissue Substitute 8　Zooplastic Tissue J　Synthetic Substitute K　Nonautologous Tissue Substitute	H　Transapical Z　No Qualifier

LC	Ø2RKØJZ with Ø2RLØJZ when reported with diagnosis code ZØØ.6
NC	Ø2RKØJZ except when reported with Ø2RLØJZ and diagnosis code ZØØ.6
NC	Ø2RLØJZ except when reported with Ø2RRØJZ and diagnosis code ZØØ.6

Ø Medical and Surgical
2 Heart and Great Vessels
S Reposition　　Moving to its normal location or other suitable location all or a portion of a body part

Body Part Character 4	Approach Character 5	Device Character 6	Qualifier Character 7
P　Pulmonary Trunk Q　Pulmonary Artery, Right R　Pulmonary Artery, Left S　Pulmonary Vein, Right T　Pulmonary Vein, Left V　Superior Vena Cava W　Thoracic Aorta	Ø　Open	Z　No Device	Z　No Qualifier

Ø Medical and Surgical
2 Heart and Great Vessels
T Resection　　Cutting out or off, without replacement, all of a body part

Body Part Character 4	Approach Character 5	Device Character 6	Qualifier Character 7
5　Atrial Septum 8　Conduction Mechanism 9　Chordae Tendineae D　Papillary Muscle H　Pulmonary Valve M　Ventricular Septum N　Pericardium	Ø　Open 3　Percutaneous 4　Percutaneous Endoscopic	Z　No Device	Z　No Qualifier

---

LC Limited Coverage　　　NC Noncovered　　　HAC associated procedure　　　Combination Only　　　DRG Non-OR　　　Non-OR　　　Revised Text in **GREEN**

0 Medical and Surgical
2 Heart and Great Vessels
U Supplement   Putting in or on biological or synthetic material that physically reinforces and/or augments the function of a portion of a body part

Body Part Character 4	Approach Character 5	Device Character 6	Qualifier Character 7
5 Atrial Septum **6** Atrium, Right **7** Atrium, Left **9** Chordae Tendineae **A** Heart **D** Papillary Muscle **F** Aortic Valve **G** Mitral Valve **H** Pulmonary Valve **J** Tricuspid Valve **K** Ventricle, Right **L** Ventricle, Left **M** Ventricular Septum **N** Pericardium **P** Pulmonary Trunk **Q** Pulmonary Artery, Right **R** Pulmonary Artery, Left **S** Pulmonary Vein, Right **T** Pulmonary Vein, Left **V** Superior Vena Cava **W** Thoracic Aorta	**0** Open **3** Percutaneous **4** Percutaneous Endoscopic	**7** Autologous Tissue Substitute **8** Zooplastic Tissue **J** Synthetic Substitute **K** Nonautologous Tissue Substitute	**Z** No Qualifier

DRG Non-OR 02U7[3,4]JZ

0 Medical and Surgical
2 Heart and Great Vessels
V Restriction   Partially closing an orifice or the lumen of a tubular body part

Body Part Character 4	Approach Character 5	Device Character 6	Qualifier Character 7
A Heart	**0** Open **3** Percutaneous **4** Percutaneous Endoscopic	**C** Extraluminal Device **Z** No Device	**Z** No Qualifier
P Pulmonary Trunk **Q** Pulmonary Artery, Right **S** Pulmonary Vein, Right **T** Pulmonary Vein, Left **V** Superior Vena Cava **W** Thoracic Aorta	**0** Open **3** Percutaneous **4** Percutaneous Endoscopic	**C** Extraluminal Device **D** Intraluminal Device **Z** No Device	**Z** No Qualifier
R Pulmonary Artery, Left	**0** Open **3** Percutaneous **4** Percutaneous Endoscopic	**C** Extraluminal Device **D** Intraluminal Device **Z** No Device	**T** Ductus Arteriosus **Z** No Qualifier

0   **Medical and Surgical**
2   **Heart and Great Vessels**
W   **Revision**   Correcting, to the extent possible, a portion of a malfunctioning device or the position of a displaced device

Body Part Character 4	Approach Character 5	Device Character 6	Qualifier Character 7
5 Atrial Septum **M** Ventricular Septum	**0** Open **4** Percutaneous Endoscopic	**J** Synthetic Substitute	**Z** No Qualifier
A Heart **NC**	**0** Open **3** Percutaneous **4** Percutaneous Endoscopic **X** External	**2** Monitoring Device **3** Infusion Device **7** Autologous Tissue Substitute **8** Zooplastic Tissue **C** Extraluminal Device **D** Intraluminal Device **J** Synthetic Substitute **K** Nonautologous Tissue Substitute **M** Cardiac Lead **Q** Implantable Heart Assist System **R** External Heart Assist System	**Z** No Qualifier
F Aortic Valve **G** Mitral Valve **H** Pulmonary Valve **J** Tricuspid Valve	**0** Open **4** Percutaneous Endoscopic	**7** Autologous Tissue Substitute **8** Zooplastic Tissue **J** Synthetic Substitute **K** Nonautologous Tissue Substitute	**Z** No Qualifier
Y Great Vessel	**0** Open **3** Percutaneous **4** Percutaneous Endoscopic **X** External	**2** Monitoring Device **3** Infusion Device **7** Autologous Tissue Substitute **8** Zooplastic Tissue **C** Extraluminal Device **D** Intraluminal Device **J** Synthetic Substitute **K** Nonautologous Tissue Substitute	**Z** No Qualifier

Combinations Only
    Heart Assist System
        02WA[0,3,4][R,Q]Z and 02PA[0,3,4]RZ

    NC   02WA0[J,Q]Z
    NC   02WA[3,4]QZ
    Non-OR 02WAX[2,3,7,8,C,D,J,K,M,Q,R]Z
    Non-OR 02WYX[2,3,7,8,C,D,J,K]Z

0   **Medical and Surgical**
2   **Heart and Great Vessels**
Y   **Transplantation**   Putting in or on all or a portion of a living body part taken from another individual or animal to physically take the place and/or function of all or a portion of a similar body part

Body Part Character 4	Approach Character 5	Device Character 6	Qualifier Character 7
A Heart **LC**	**0** Open	**Z** No Device	**0** Allogeneic **1** Syngeneic **2** Zooplastic

    LC   02YA0Z[0,1,2]

Upper Arteries Ø31–Ø3W

Ø	**Medical and Surgical**
3	**Upper Arteries**
1	**Bypass**	Altering the route of passage of the contents of a tubular body part

Body Part Character 4	Approach Character 5	Device Character 6	Qualifier Character 7
2 Innominate Artery 5 Axillary Artery, Right 6 Axillary Artery, Left	Ø Open	9 Autologous Venous Tissue A Autologous Arterial Tissue J Synthetic Substitute K Nonautologous Tissue Substitute Z No Device	Ø Upper Arm Artery, Right 1 Upper Arm Artery, Left 2 Upper Arm Artery, Bilateral 3 Lower Arm Artery, Right 4 Lower Arm Artery, Left 5 Lower Arm Artery, Bilateral 6 Upper Leg Artery, Right 7 Upper Leg Artery, Left 8 Upper Leg Artery, Bilateral 9 Lower Leg Artery, Right B Lower Leg Artery, Left C Lower Leg Artery, Bilateral D Upper Arm Vein F Lower Arm Vein J Extracranial Artery, Right K Extracranial Artery, Left
3 Subclavian Artery, Right 4 Subclavian Artery, Left	Ø Open	9 Autologous Venous Tissue A Autologous Arterial Tissue J Synthetic Substitute K Nonautologous Tissue Substitute Z No Device	Ø Upper Arm Artery, Right 1 Upper Arm Artery, Left 2 Upper Arm Artery, Bilateral 3 Lower Arm Artery, Right 4 Lower Arm Artery, Left 5 Lower Arm Artery, Bilateral 6 Upper Leg Artery, Right 7 Upper Leg Artery, Left 8 Upper Leg Artery, Bilateral 9 Lower Leg Artery, Right B Lower Leg Artery, Left C Lower Leg Artery, Bilateral D Upper Arm Vein F Lower Arm Vein J Extracranial Artery, Right K Extracranial Artery, Left M Pulmonary Artery, Right N Pulmonary Artery, Left
7 Brachial Artery, Right	Ø Open	9 Autologous Venous Tissue A Autologous Arterial Tissue J Synthetic Substitute K Nonautologous Tissue Substitute Z No Device	Ø Upper Arm Artery, Right 3 Lower Arm Artery, Right D Upper Arm Vein F Lower Arm Vein
8 Brachial Artery, Left	Ø Open	9 Autologous Venous Tissue A Autologous Arterial Tissue J Synthetic Substitute K Nonautologous Tissue Substitute Z No Device	1 Upper Arm Artery, Left 4 Lower Arm Artery, Left D Upper Arm Vein F Lower Arm Vein
9 Ulnar Artery, Right B Radial Artery, Right	Ø Open	9 Autologous Venous Tissue A Autologous Arterial Tissue J Synthetic Substitute K Nonautologous Tissue Substitute Z No Device	3 Lower Arm Artery, Right F Lower Arm Vein
A Ulnar Artery, Left C Radial Artery, Left	Ø Open	9 Autologous Venous Tissue A Autologous Arterial Tissue J Synthetic Substitute K Nonautologous Tissue Substitute Z No Device	4 Lower Arm Artery, Left F Lower Arm Vein
G Intracranial Artery S Temporal Artery, Right `NC` T Temporal Artery, Left `NC`	Ø Open	9 Autologous Venous Tissue A Autologous Arterial Tissue J Synthetic Substitute K Nonautologous Tissue Substitute Z No Device	G Intracranial Artery

Ø31 Continued on next page

`NC`	Ø31SØ[9,A,J,K,Z]G
`NC`	Ø31TØ[9,A,J,K,Z]G

`LC` Limited Coverage　　`NC` Noncovered　　HAC associated procedure　　Combination Only　　DRG Non-OR　　Non-OR　　Revised Text in **GREEN**

154　　　　　　　　　　　　　　　　　　　　　　　　　　　　　　ICD-10-PCS 2014 (Draft)

Ø Medical and Surgical
3 Upper Arteries
1 Bypass   Altering the route of passage of the contents of a tubular body part

Ø31 Continued

Body Part Character 4	Approach Character 5	Device Character 6	Qualifier Character 7
H Common Carotid Artery, Right NC	**Ø** Open	**9** Autologous Venous Tissue **A** Autologous Arterial Tissue **J** Synthetic Substitute **K** Nonautologous Tissue Substitute **Z** No Device	**G** Intracranial Artery **J** Extracranial Artery, Right
J Common Carotid Artery, Left NC	**Ø** Open	**9** Autologous Venous Tissue **A** Autologous Arterial Tissue **J** Synthetic Substitute **K** Nonautologous Tissue Substitute **Z** No Device	**G** Intracranial Artery **J** Extracranial Artery, Left
K Internal Carotid Artery, Right NC **M** External Carotid Artery, Right NC	**Ø** Open	**9** Autologous Venous Tissue **A** Autologous Arterial Tissue **J** Synthetic Substitute **K** Nonautologous Tissue Substitute **Z** No Device	**J** Extracranial Artery, Right
L Internal Carotid Artery, Left NC **N** External Carotid Artery, Left NC	**Ø** Open	**9** Autologous Venous Tissue **A** Autologous Arterial Tissue **J** Synthetic Substitute **K** Nonautologous Tissue Substitute **Z** No Device	**K** Extracranial Artery, Left

NC   Ø31HØ[9,A,J,K,Z]J   NC   Ø31LØ[9,A,J,K,Z]K
NC   Ø31JØ[9,A,J,K,Z]K   NC   Ø31MØ[9,A,J,K,Z]J
NC   Ø31KØ[9,A,J,K,Z]J   NC   Ø31NØ[9,A,J,K,Z]K

Ø Medical and Surgical
3 Upper Arteries
5 Destruction   Physical eradication of all or a portion of a body part by the direct use of energy, force, or a destructive agent

Body Part Character 4	Approach Character 5	Device Character 6	Qualifier Character 7
Ø Internal Mammary Artery, Right **1** Internal Mammary Artery, Left **2** Innominate Artery **3** Subclavian Artery, Right **4** Subclavian Artery, Left **5** Axillary Artery, Right **6** Axillary Artery, Left **7** Brachial Artery, Right **8** Brachial Artery, Left **9** Ulnar Artery, Right **A** Ulnar Artery, Left **B** Radial Artery, Right **C** Radial Artery, Left **D** Hand Artery, Right **F** Hand Artery, Left **G** Intracranial Artery **H** Common Carotid Artery, Right **J** Common Carotid Artery, Left **K** Internal Carotid Artery, Right **L** Internal Carotid Artery, Left **M** External Carotid Artery, Right **N** External Carotid Artery, Left **P** Vertebral Artery, Right **Q** Vertebral Artery, Left **R** Face Artery **S** Temporal Artery, Right **T** Temporal Artery, Left **U** Thyroid Artery, Right **V** Thyroid Artery, Left **Y** Upper Artery	**Ø** Open **3** Percutaneous **4** Percutaneous Endoscopic	**Z** No Device	**Z** No Qualifier

0 Medical and Surgical
3 Upper Arteries
7 Dilation   Expanding an orifice or the lumen of a tubular body part

Body Part Character 4	Approach Character 5	Device Character 6	Qualifier Character 7
0 Internal Mammary Artery, Right	0 Open	4 Drug-eluting Intraluminal Device	Z No Qualifier
1 Internal Mammary Artery, Left	3 Percutaneous	D Intraluminal Device	
2 Innominate Artery	4 Percutaneous Endoscopic	Z No Device	
3 Subclavian Artery, Right			
4 Subclavian Artery, Left			
5 Axillary Artery, Right			
6 Axillary Artery, Left			
7 Brachial Artery, Right			
8 Brachial Artery, Left			
9 Ulnar Artery, Right			
A Ulnar Artery, Left			
B Radial Artery, Right			
C Radial Artery, Left			
D Hand Artery, Right			
F Hand Artery, Left			
G Intracranial Artery NC			
H Common Carotid Artery, Right			
J Common Carotid Artery, Left			
K Internal Carotid Artery, Right			
L Internal Carotid Artery, Left			
M External Carotid Artery, Right			
N External Carotid Artery, Left			
P Vertebral Artery, Right			
Q Vertebral Artery, Left			
R Face Artery			
S Temporal Artery, Right			
T Temporal Artery, Left			
U Thyroid Artery, Right			
V Thyroid Artery, Left			
Y Upper Artery			

NC   037G[3,4]ZZ Noncovered without stent placement

0 Medical and Surgical
3 Upper Arteries
9 Drainage   Taking or letting out fluids and/or gases from a body part

Body Part Character 4	Approach Character 5	Device Character 6	Qualifier Character 7
0 Internal Mammary Artery, Right	0 Open	0 Drainage Device	Z No Qualifier
1 Internal Mammary Artery, Left	3 Percutaneous		
2 Innominate Artery	4 Percutaneous Endoscopic		
3 Subclavian Artery, Right			
4 Subclavian Artery, Left			
5 Axillary Artery, Right			
6 Axillary Artery, Left			
7 Brachial Artery, Right			
8 Brachial Artery, Left			
9 Ulnar Artery, Right			
A Ulnar Artery, Left			
B Radial Artery, Right			
C Radial Artery, Left			
D Hand Artery, Right			
F Hand Artery, Left			
G Intracranial Artery			
H Common Carotid Artery, Right			
J Common Carotid Artery, Left			
K Internal Carotid Artery, Right			
L Internal Carotid Artery, Left			
M External Carotid Artery, Right			
N External Carotid Artery, Left			
P Vertebral Artery, Right			
Q Vertebral Artery, Left			
R Face Artery			
S Temporal Artery, Right			
T Temporal Artery, Left			
U Thyroid Artery, Right			
V Thyroid Artery, Left			
Y Upper Artery			

039 Continued on next page

Non-OR   039[0,1,2,3,4,5,6,7,8,9,A,B,C,D,F,G,H,J,K,L,M,N,P,Q,R,S,T,U,V,Y][0,3,4]0Z

0 Medical and Surgical   *039 Continued*
3 Upper Arteries
9 Drainage   Taking or letting out fluids and/or gases from a body part

Body Part Character 4	Approach Character 5	Device Character 6	Qualifier Character 7
0 Internal Mammary Artery, Right **1** Internal Mammary Artery, Left **2** Innominate Artery **3** Subclavian Artery, Right **4** Subclavian Artery, Left **5** Axillary Artery, Right **6** Axillary Artery, Left **7** Brachial Artery, Right **8** Brachial Artery, Left **9** Ulnar Artery, Right **A** Ulnar Artery, Left **B** Radial Artery, Right **C** Radial Artery, Left **D** Hand Artery, Right **F** Hand Artery, Left **G** Intracranial Artery **H** Common Carotid Artery, Right **J** Common Carotid Artery, Left **K** Internal Carotid Artery, Right **L** Internal Carotid Artery, Left **M** External Carotid Artery, Right **N** External Carotid Artery, Left **P** Vertebral Artery, Right **Q** Vertebral Artery, Left **R** Face Artery **S** Temporal Artery, Right **T** Temporal Artery, Left **U** Thyroid Artery, Right **V** Thyroid Artery, Left **Y** Upper Artery	**0** Open **3** Percutaneous **4** Percutaneous Endoscopic	**Z** No Device	**X** Diagnostic **Z** No Qualifier

Non-OR 039[0,1,2,3,4,5,6,7,8,9,A,B,C,D,F,G,H,J,K,L,M,N,P,Q,R,S,T,U,V,Y][0,3,4]ZZ

0 Medical and Surgical
3 Upper Arteries
B Excision   Cutting out or off, without replacement, a portion of a body part

Body Part Character 4	Approach Character 5	Device Character 6	Qualifier Character 7
0 Internal Mammary Artery, Right **1** Internal Mammary Artery, Left **2** Innominate Artery **3** Subclavian Artery, Right **4** Subclavian Artery, Left **5** Axillary Artery, Right **6** Axillary Artery, Left **7** Brachial Artery, Right **8** Brachial Artery, Left **9** Ulnar Artery, Right **A** Ulnar Artery, Left **B** Radial Artery, Right **C** Radial Artery, Left **D** Hand Artery, Right **F** Hand Artery, Left **G** Intracranial Artery **H** Common Carotid Artery, Right **J** Common Carotid Artery, Left **K** Internal Carotid Artery, Right **L** Internal Carotid Artery, Left **M** External Carotid Artery, Right **N** External Carotid Artery, Left **P** Vertebral Artery, Right **Q** Vertebral Artery, Left **R** Face Artery **S** Temporal Artery, Right **T** Temporal Artery, Left **U** Thyroid Artery, Right **V** Thyroid Artery, Left **Y** Upper Artery	**0** Open **3** Percutaneous **4** Percutaneous Endoscopic	**Z** No Device	**X** Diagnostic **Z** No Qualifier

---

LC Limited Coverage   **NC** Noncovered   HAC associated procedure   Combination Only   DRG Non-OR   Non-OR   Revised Text in **GREEN**

Upper Arteries

0   **Medical and Surgical**
3   **Upper Arteries**
C   **Extirpation**   Taking or cutting out solid matter from a body part

Body Part Character 4	Approach Character 5	Device Character 6	Qualifier Character 7
0 Internal Mammary Artery, Right	**0** Open	**Z** No Device	**Z** No Qualifier
1 Internal Mammary Artery, Left	**3** Percutaneous		
2 Innominate Artery	**4** Percutaneous Endoscopic		
3 Subclavian Artery, Right			
4 Subclavian Artery, Left			
5 Axillary Artery, Right			
6 Axillary Artery, Left			
7 Brachial Artery, Right			
8 Brachial Artery, Left			
9 Ulnar Artery, Right			
A Ulnar Artery, Left			
B Radial Artery, Right			
C Radial Artery, Left			
D Hand Artery, Right			
F Hand Artery, Left			
G Intracranial Artery `NC`			
H Common Carotid Artery, Right			
J Common Carotid Artery, Left			
K Internal Carotid Artery, Right			
L Internal Carotid Artery, Left			
M External Carotid Artery, Right			
N External Carotid Artery, Left			
P Vertebral Artery, Right			
Q Vertebral Artery, Left			
R Face Artery			
S Temporal Artery, Right			
T Temporal Artery, Left			
U Thyroid Artery, Right			
V Thyroid Artery, Left			
Y Upper Artery			

`NC`   03CG[3,4]ZZ Noncovered without stent placement

0   **Medical and Surgical**
3   **Upper Arteries**
H   **Insertion**   Putting in a nonbiological appliance that monitors, assists, performs, or prevents a physiological function but does not physically take the place of a body part

Body Part Character 4	Approach Character 5	Device Character 6	Qualifier Character 7
0 Internal Mammary Artery, Right	**0** Open	**3** Infusion Device	**Z** No Qualifier
1 Internal Mammary Artery, Left	**3** Percutaneous	**D** Intraluminal Device	
2 Innominate Artery	**4** Percutaneous Endoscopic		
3 Subclavian Artery, Right			
4 Subclavian Artery, Left			
5 Axillary Artery, Right			
6 Axillary Artery, Left			
7 Brachial Artery, Right			
8 Brachial Artery, Left			
9 Ulnar Artery, Right			
A Ulnar Artery, Left			
B Radial Artery, Right			
C Radial Artery, Left			
D Hand Artery, Right			
F Hand Artery, Left			
G Intracranial Artery			
H Common Carotid Artery, Right			
J Common Carotid Artery, Left			
M External Carotid Artery, Right			
N External Carotid Artery, Left			
P Vertebral Artery, Right			
Q Vertebral Artery, Left			
R Face Artery			
S Temporal Artery, Right			
T Temporal Artery, Left			
U Thyroid Artery, Right			
V Thyroid Artery, Left			

03H Continued on next page

Non-OR   03H[0,1,2,3,4,5,6,7,8,9,A,B,C,D,F,G,H,J,M,N,P,Q,R,S,T,U,V][0,3,4]3Z

`LC` Limited Coverage   `NC` Noncovered   HAC associated procedure   Combination Only   DRG Non-OR   Non-OR   Revised Text in **GREEN**

03H Continued

0　**Medical and Surgical**
3　**Upper Arteries**
H　**Insertion**　　Putting in a nonbiological appliance that monitors, assists, performs, or prevents a physiological function but does not physically take the place of a body part

Body Part Character 4	Approach Character 5	Device Character 6	Qualifier Character 7
K　Internal Carotid Artery, Right L　Internal Carotid Artery, Left	0　Open 3　Percutaneous 4　Percutaneous Endoscope	3　Infusion Device D　Intraluminal Device M　Stimulator Lead	Z　No Qualifier
Y　Upper Artery	0　Open 3　Percutaneous 4　Percutaneous Endoscopic	2　Monitoring Device 3　Infusion Device D　Intraluminal Device	Z　No Qualifier

Non-OR　03H[K,L][0,3,4]3Z
Non-OR　03HY[0,3,4]3Z

0　**Medical and Surgical**
3　**Upper Arteries**
J　**Inspection**　　Visually and/or manually exploring a body part

Body Part Character 4	Approach Character 5	Device Character 6	Qualifier Character 7
Y　Upper Artery	0　Open 3　Percutaneous 4　Percutaneous Endoscopic X　External	Z　No Device	Z　No Qualifier

Non-OR　03JY[4,X]ZZ

0　**Medical and Surgical**
3　**Upper Arteries**
L　**Occlusion**　　Completely closing an orifice or the lumen of a tubular body part

Body Part Character 4	Approach Character 5	Device Character 6	Qualifier Character 7
0　Internal Mammary Artery, Right 1　Internal Mammary Artery, Left 2　Innominate Artery 3　Subclavian Artery, Right 4　Subclavian Artery, Left 5　Axillary Artery, Right 6　Axillary Artery, Left 7　Brachial Artery, Right 8　Brachial Artery, Left 9　Ulnar Artery, Right A　Ulnar Artery, Left B　Radial Artery, Right C　Radial Artery, Left D　Hand Artery, Right F　Hand Artery, Left R　Face Artery S　Temporal Artery, Right T　Temporal Artery, Left U　Thyroid Artery, Right V　Thyroid Artery, Left Y　Upper Artery	0　Open 3　Percutaneous 4　Percutaneous Endoscopic	C　Extraluminal Device D　Intraluminal Device Z　No Device	Z　No Qualifier
G　Intracranial Artery H　Common Carotid Artery, Right J　Common Carotid Artery, Left K　Internal Carotid Artery, Right L　Internal Carotid Artery, Left M　External Carotid Artery, Right N　External Carotid Artery, Left P　Vertebral Artery, Right Q　Vertebral Artery, Left	0　Open 3　Percutaneous 4　Percutaneous Endoscopic	B　Bioactive Intraluminal Device C　Extraluminal Device D　Intraluminal Device Z　No Device	Z　No Qualifier

Upper Arteries *(side tab)*

Ø Medical and Surgical
3 Upper Arteries
N Release   Freeing a body part from an abnormal physical constraint

Body Part Character 4	Approach Character 5	Device Character 6	Qualifier Character 7
Ø Internal Mammary Artery, Right 1 Internal Mammary Artery, Left 2 Innominate Artery 3 Subclavian Artery, Right 4 Subclavian Artery, Left 5 Axillary Artery, Right 6 Axillary Artery, Left 7 Brachial Artery, Right 8 Brachial Artery, Left 9 Ulnar Artery, Right A Ulnar Artery, Left B Radial Artery, Right C Radial Artery, Left D Hand Artery, Right F Hand Artery, Left G Intracranial Artery H Common Carotid Artery, Right J Common Carotid Artery, Left K Internal Carotid Artery, Right L Internal Carotid Artery, Left M External Carotid Artery, Right N External Carotid Artery, Left P Vertebral Artery, Right Q Vertebral Artery, Left R Face Artery S Temporal Artery, Right T Temporal Artery, Left U Thyroid Artery, Right V Thyroid Artery, Left Y Upper Artery	Ø Open 3 Percutaneous 4 Percutaneous Endoscopic	Z No Device	Z No Qualifier

Ø Medical and Surgical
3 Upper Arteries
P Removal   Taking out or off a device from a body part

Body Part Character 4	Approach Character 5	Device Character 6	Qualifier Character 7
Y Upper Artery	Ø Open 3 Percutaneous 4 Percutaneous Endoscopic	Ø Drainage Device 2 Monitoring Device 3 Infusion Device 7 Autologous Tissue Substitute C Extraluminal Device D Intraluminal Device J Synthetic Substitute K Nonautologous Tissue Substitute M Stimulator Lead	Z No Qualifier
Y Upper Artery	X External	Ø Drainage Device 2 Monitoring Device 3 Infusion Device D Intraluminal Device M Stimulator Lead	Z No Qualifier

Non-OR   Ø3PYX[Ø,2,3,D,M]Z

0 Medical and Surgical
3 Upper Arteries
Q Repair Restoring, to the extent possible, a body part to its normal anatomic structure and function

Body Part Character 4	Approach Character 5	Device Character 6	Qualifier Character 7
0 Internal Mammary Artery, Right	0 Open	Z No Device	Z No Qualifier
1 Internal Mammary Artery, Left	3 Percutaneous		
2 Innominate Artery	4 Percutaneous Endoscopic		
3 Subclavian Artery, Right			
4 Subclavian Artery, Left			
5 Axillary Artery, Right			
6 Axillary Artery, Left			
7 Brachial Artery, Right			
8 Brachial Artery, Left			
9 Ulnar Artery, Right			
A Ulnar Artery, Left			
B Radial Artery, Right			
C Radial Artery, Left			
D Hand Artery, Right			
F Hand Artery, Left			
G Intracranial Artery			
H Common Carotid Artery, Right			
J Common Carotid Artery, Left			
K Internal Carotid Artery, Right			
L Internal Carotid Artery, Left			
M External Carotid Artery, Right			
N External Carotid Artery, Left			
P Vertebral Artery, Right			
Q Vertebral Artery, Left			
R Face Artery			
S Temporal Artery, Right			
T Temporal Artery, Left			
U Thyroid Artery, Right			
V Thyroid Artery, Left			
Y Upper Artery			

0 Medical and Surgical
3 Upper Arteries
R Replacement Putting in or on biological or synthetic material that physically takes the place and/or function of all or a portion of a body part

Body Part Character 4	Approach Character 5	Device Character 6	Qualifier Character 7
0 Internal Mammary Artery, Right	0 Open	7 Autologous Tissue Substitute	Z No Qualifier
1 Internal Mammary Artery, Left	4 Percutaneous Endoscopic	J Synthetic Substitute	
2 Innominate Artery		K Nonautologous Tissue Substitute	
3 Subclavian Artery, Right			
4 Subclavian Artery, Left			
5 Axillary Artery, Right			
6 Axillary Artery, Left			
7 Brachial Artery, Right			
8 Brachial Artery, Left			
9 Ulnar Artery, Right			
A Ulnar Artery, Left			
B Radial Artery, Right			
C Radial Artery, Left			
D Hand Artery, Right			
F Hand Artery, Left			
G Intracranial Artery			
H Common Carotid Artery, Right			
J Common Carotid Artery, Left			
K Internal Carotid Artery, Right			
L Internal Carotid Artery, Left			
M External Carotid Artery, Right			
N External Carotid Artery, Left			
P Vertebral Artery, Right			
Q Vertebral Artery, Left			
R Face Artery			
S Temporal Artery, Right			
T Temporal Artery, Left			
U Thyroid Artery, Right			
V Thyroid Artery, Left			
Y Upper Artery			

Upper Arteries

03S–03U

0   **Medical and Surgical**
3   **Upper Arteries**
S   **Reposition**   Moving to its normal location or other suitable location all or a portion of a body part

Body Part Character 4	Approach Character 5	Device Character 6	Qualifier Character 7
0 Internal Mammary Artery, Right **1** Internal Mammary Artery, Left **2** Innominate Artery **3** Subclavian Artery, Right **4** Subclavian Artery, Left **5** Axillary Artery, Right **6** Axillary Artery, Left **7** Brachial Artery, Right **8** Brachial Artery, Left **9** Ulnar Artery, Right **A** Ulnar Artery, Left **B** Radial Artery, Right **C** Radial Artery, Left **D** Hand Artery, Right **F** Hand Artery, Left **G** Intracranial Artery **H** Common Carotid Artery, Right **J** Common Carotid Artery, Left **K** Internal Carotid Artery, Right **L** Internal Carotid Artery, Left **M** External Carotid Artery, Right **N** External Carotid Artery, Left **P** Vertebral Artery, Right **Q** Vertebral Artery, Left **R** Face Artery **S** Temporal Artery, Right **T** Temporal Artery, Left **U** Thyroid Artery, Right **V** Thyroid Artery, Left **Y** Upper Artery	**0** Open **3** Percutaneous **4** Percutaneous Endoscopic	**Z** No Device	**Z** No Qualifier

0   **Medical and Surgical**
3   **Upper Arteries**
U   **Supplement**   Putting in or on biological or synthetic material that physically reinforces and/or augments the function of a portion of a body part

Body Part Character 4	Approach Character 5	Device Character 6	Qualifier Character 7
0 Internal Mammary Artery, Right **1** Internal Mammary Artery, Left **2** Innominate Artery **3** Subclavian Artery, Right **4** Subclavian Artery, Left **5** Axillary Artery, Right **6** Axillary Artery, Left **7** Brachial Artery, Right **8** Brachial Artery, Left **9** Ulnar Artery, Right **A** Ulnar Artery, Left **B** Radial Artery, Right **C** Radial Artery, Left **D** Hand Artery, Right **F** Hand Artery, Left **G** Intracranial Artery **H** Common Carotid Artery, Right **J** Common Carotid Artery, Left **K** Internal Carotid Artery, Right **L** Internal Carotid Artery, Left **M** External Carotid Artery, Right **N** External Carotid Artery, Left **P** Vertebral Artery, Right **Q** Vertebral Artery, Left **R** Face Artery **S** Temporal Artery, Right **T** Temporal Artery, Left **U** Thyroid Artery, Right **V** Thyroid Artery, Left **Y** Upper Artery	**0** Open **3** Percutaneous **4** Percutaneous Endoscopic	**7** Autologous Tissue Substitute **J** Synthetic Substitute **K** Nonautologous Tissue Substitute	**Z** No Qualifier

LC Limited Coverage   **NC** Noncovered   HAC associated procedure   Combination Only   DRG Non-OR   Non-OR   Revised Text in **GREEN**

162   ICD-10-PCS 2014 (Draft)

Ø   Medical and Surgical
3   Upper Arteries
V   Restriction   Partially closing an orifice or the lumen of a tubular body part

Body Part Character 4	Approach Character 5	Device Character 6	Qualifier Character 7
Ø Internal Mammary Artery, Right **1** Internal Mammary Artery, Left **2** Innominate Artery **3** Subclavian Artery, Right **4** Subclavian Artery, Left **5** Axillary Artery, Right **6** Axillary Artery, Left **7** Brachial Artery, Right **8** Brachial Artery, Left **9** Ulnar Artery, Right **A** Ulnar Artery, Left **B** Radial Artery, Right **C** Radial Artery, Left **D** Hand Artery, Right **F** Hand Artery, Left **R** Face Artery **S** Temporal Artery, Right **T** Temporal Artery, Left **U** Thyroid Artery, Right **V** Thyroid Artery, Left **Y** Upper Artery	**Ø** Open **3** Percutaneous **4** Percutaneous Endoscopic	**C** Extraluminal Device **D** Intraluminal Device **Z** No Device	**Z** No Qualifier
G Intracranial Artery **H** Common Carotid Artery, Right **J** Common Carotid Artery, Left **K** Internal Carotid Artery, Right **L** Internal Carotid Artery, Left **M** External Carotid Artery, Right **N** External Carotid Artery, Left **P** Vertebral Artery, Right **Q** Vertebral Artery, Left	**Ø** Open **3** Percutaneous **4** Percutaneous Endoscopic	**B** Bioactive Intraluminal Device **C** Extraluminal Device **D** Intraluminal Device **Z** No Device	**Z** No Qualifier

Ø   Medical and Surgical
3   Upper Arteries
W   Revision   Correcting, to the extent possible, a portion of a malfunctioning device or the position of a displaced device

Body Part Character 4	Approach Character 5	Device Character 6	Qualifier Character 7
Y Upper Artery	**Ø** Open **3** Percutaneous **4** Percutaneous Endoscopic **X** External	**Ø** Drainage Device **2** Monitoring Device **3** Infusion Device **7** Autologous Tissue Substitute **C** Extraluminal Device **D** Intraluminal Device **J** Synthetic Substitute **K** Nonautologous Tissue Substitute **M** Stimulator Lead	**Z** No Qualifier

Non-OR   Ø3WYX[Ø,2,3,7,C,D,J,K,M]Z

Lower Arteries

041–041

Lower Arteries 041–04W

0   **Medical and Surgical**
4   **Lower Arteries**
1   **Bypass**   Altering the route of passage of the contents of a tubular body part

Body Part Character 4	Approach Character 5	Device Character 6	Qualifier Character 7
0 Abdominal Aorta **C** Common Iliac Artery, Right **D** Common Iliac Artery, Left	**0** Open **4** Percutaneous Endoscopic	**9** Autologous Venous Tissue **A** Autologous Arterial Tissue **J** Synthetic Substitute **K** Nonautologous Tissue Substitute **Z** No Device	**0** Abdominal Aorta **1** Celiac Artery **2** Mesenteric Artery **3** Renal Artery, Right **4** Renal Artery, Left **5** Renal Artery, Bilateral **6** Common Iliac Artery, Right **7** Common Iliac Artery, Left **8** Common Iliac Arteries, Bilateral **9** Internal Iliac Artery, Right **B** Internal Iliac Artery, Left **C** Internal Iliac Arteries, Bilateral **D** External Iliac Artery, Right **F** External Iliac Artery, Left **G** External Iliac Arteries, Bilateral **H** Femoral Artery, Right **J** Femoral Artery, Left **K** Femoral Arteries, Bilateral **Q** Lower Extremity Artery **R** Lower Artery
4 Splenic Artery	**0** Open **4** Percutaneous Endoscopic	**9** Autologous Venous Tissue **A** Autologous Arterial Tissue **J** Synthetic Substitute **K** Nonautologous Tissue Substitute **Z** No Device	**3** Renal Artery, Right **4** Renal Artery, Left **5** Renal Artery, Bilateral
E Internal Iliac Artery, Right **F** Internal Iliac Artery, Left **H** External Iliac Artery, Right **J** External Iliac Artery, Left	**0** Open **4** Percutaneous Endoscopic	**9** Autologous Venous Tissue **A** Autologous Arterial Tissue **J** Synthetic Substitute **K** Nonautologous Tissue Substitute **Z** No Device	**9** Internal Iliac Artery, Right **B** Internal Iliac Artery, Left **C** Internal Iliac Arteries, Bilateral **D** External Iliac Artery, Right **F** External Iliac Artery, Left **G** External Iliac Arteries, Bilateral **H** Femoral Artery, Right **J** Femoral Artery, Left **K** Femoral Arteries, Bilateral **P** Foot Artery **Q** Lower Extremity Artery
K Femoral Artery, Right **L** Femoral Artery, Left	**0** Open **4** Percutaneous Endoscopic	**9** Autologous Venous Tissue **A** Autologous Arterial Tissue **J** Synthetic Substitute **K** Nonautologous Tissue Substitute **Z** No Device	**H** Femoral Artery, Right **J** Femoral Artery, Left **K** Femoral Arteries, Bilateral **L** Popliteal Artery **M** Peroneal Artery **N** Posterior Tibial Artery **P** Foot Artery **Q** Lower Extremity Artery **S** Lower Extremity Vein
M Popliteal Artery, Right **N** Popliteal Artery, Left	**0** Open **4** Percutaneous Endoscopic	**9** Autologous Venous Tissue **A** Autologous Arterial Tissue **J** Synthetic Substitute **K** Nonautologous Tissue Substitute **Z** No Device	**L** Popliteal Artery **M** Peroneal Artery **P** Foot Artery **Q** Lower Extremity Artery **S** Lower Extremity Vein

LC Limited Coverage   **NC** Noncovered   HAC associated procedure   Combination Only   DRG Non-OR   Non-OR   Revised Text in **GREEN**

164   ICD-10-PCS 2014 (Draft)

Lower Arteries

0 Medical and Surgical
4 Lower Arteries
5 Destruction   Physical eradication of all or a portion of a body part by the direct use of energy, force, or a destructive agent

Body Part Character 4	Approach Character 5	Device Character 6	Qualifier Character 7
0 Abdominal Aorta	0 Open	Z No Device	Z No Qualifier
1 Celiac Artery	3 Percutaneous		
2 Gastric Artery	4 Percutaneous Endoscopic		
3 Hepatic Artery			
4 Splenic Artery			
5 Superior Mesenteric Artery			
6 Colic Artery, Right			
7 Colic Artery, Left			
8 Colic Artery, Middle			
9 Renal Artery, Right			
A Renal Artery, Left			
B Inferior Mesenteric Artery			
C Common Iliac Artery, Right			
D Common Iliac Artery, Left			
E Internal Iliac Artery, Right			
F Internal Iliac Artery, Left			
H External Iliac Artery, Right			
J External Iliac Artery, Left			
K Femoral Artery, Right			
L Femoral Artery, Left			
M Popliteal Artery, Right			
N Popliteal Artery, Left			
P Anterior Tibial Artery, Right			
Q Anterior Tibial Artery, Left			
R Posterior Tibial Artery, Right			
S Posterior Tibial Artery, Left			
T Peroneal Artery, Right			
U Peroneal Artery, Left			
V Foot Artery, Right			
W Foot Artery, Left			
Y Lower Artery			

0 Medical and Surgical
4 Lower Arteries
7 Dilation   Expanding an orifice or the lumen of a tubular body part

Body Part Character 4	Approach Character 5	Device Character 6	Qualifier Character 7
0 Abdominal Aorta	0 Open	4 Drug-eluting Intraluminal Device	Z No Qualifier
1 Celiac Artery	3 Percutaneous	D Intraluminal Device	
2 Gastric Artery	4 Percutaneous Endoscopic	Z No Device	
3 Hepatic Artery			
4 Splenic Artery			
5 Superior Mesenteric Artery			
6 Colic Artery, Right			
7 Colic Artery, Left			
8 Colic Artery, Middle			
9 Renal Artery, Right			
A Renal Artery, Left			
B Inferior Mesenteric Artery			
C Common Iliac Artery, Right			
D Common Iliac Artery, Left			
E Internal Iliac Artery, Right			
F Internal Iliac Artery, Left			
H External Iliac Artery, Right			
J External Iliac Artery, Left			
K Femoral Artery, Right			
L Femoral Artery, Left			
M Popliteal Artery, Right			
N Popliteal Artery, Left			
P Anterior Tibial Artery, Right			
Q Anterior Tibial Artery, Left			
R Posterior Tibial Artery, Right			
S Posterior Tibial Artery, Left			
T Peroneal Artery, Right			
U Peroneal Artery, Left			
V Foot Artery, Right			
W Foot Artery, Left			
Y Lower Artery			

LC Limited Coverage   NC Noncovered   HAC associated procedure   Combination Only   DRG Non-OR   Non-OR   Revised Text in **GREEN**

Lower Arteries

049–049

Ø　Medical and Surgical
4　Lower Arteries
9　Drainage　　　Taking or letting out fluids and/or gases from a body part

Body Part Character 4	Approach Character 5	Device Character 6	Qualifier Character 7
Ø　Abdominal Aorta 1　Celiac Artery 2　Gastric Artery 3　Hepatic Artery 4　Splenic Artery 5　Superior Mesenteric Artery 6　Colic Artery, Right 7　Colic Artery, Left 8　Colic Artery, Middle 9　Renal Artery, Right A　Renal Artery, Left B　Inferior Mesenteric Artery C　Common Iliac Artery, Right D　Common Iliac Artery, Left E　Internal Iliac Artery, Right F　Internal Iliac Artery, Left H　External Iliac Artery, Right J　External Iliac Artery, Left K　Femoral Artery, Right L　Femoral Artery, Left M　Popliteal Artery, Right N　Popliteal Artery, Left P　Anterior Tibial Artery, Right Q　Anterior Tibial Artery, Left R　Posterior Tibial Artery, Right S　Posterior Tibial Artery, Left T　Peroneal Artery, Right U　Peroneal Artery, Left V　Foot Artery, Right W　Foot Artery, Left Y　Lower Artery	Ø　Open 3　Percutaneous 4　Percutaneous Endoscopic	Ø　Drainage Device	Z　No Qualifier
Ø　Abdominal Aorta 1　Celiac Artery 2　Gastric Artery 3　Hepatic Artery 4　Splenic Artery 5　Superior Mesenteric Artery 6　Colic Artery, Right 7　Colic Artery, Left 8　Colic Artery, Middle 9　Renal Artery, Right A　Renal Artery, Left B　Inferior Mesenteric Artery C　Common Iliac Artery, Right D　Common Iliac Artery, Left E　Internal Iliac Artery, Right F　Internal Iliac Artery, Left H　External Iliac Artery, Right J　External Iliac Artery, Left K　Femoral Artery, Right L　Femoral Artery, Left M　Popliteal Artery, Right N　Popliteal Artery, Left P　Anterior Tibial Artery, Right Q　Anterior Tibial Artery, Left R　Posterior Tibial Artery, Right S　Posterior Tibial Artery, Left T　Peroneal Artery, Right U　Peroneal Artery, Left V　Foot Artery, Right W　Foot Artery, Left Y　Lower Artery	Ø　Open 3　Percutaneous 4　Percutaneous Endoscopic	Z　No Device	X　Diagnostic Z　No Qualifier

Non-OR　049[Ø,1,2,3,4,5,6,7,8,9,A,B,C,D,E,F,H,J,K,L,M,N,P,Q,R,S,T,U,V,W,Y][Ø,3,4]ØZ
Non-OR　049[Ø,1,2,3,4,5,6,7,8,9,A,B,C,D,E,F,H,J,K,L,M,N,P,Q,R,S,T,U,V,W,Y][Ø,3,4]ZZ

0 Medical and Surgical
4 Lower Arteries
B Excision   Cutting out or off, without replacement, a portion of a body part

Body Part Character 4	Approach Character 5	Device Character 6	Qualifier Character 7
0 Abdominal Aorta	0 Open	Z No Device	X Diagnostic
1 Celiac Artery	3 Percutaneous		Z No Qualifier
2 Gastric Artery	4 Percutaneous Endoscopic		
3 Hepatic Artery			
4 Splenic Artery			
5 Superior Mesenteric Artery			
6 Colic Artery, Right			
7 Colic Artery, Left			
8 Colic Artery, Middle			
9 Renal Artery, Right			
A Renal Artery, Left			
B Inferior Mesenteric Artery			
C Common Iliac Artery, Right			
D Common Iliac Artery, Left			
E Internal Iliac Artery, Right			
F Internal Iliac Artery, Left			
H External Iliac Artery, Right			
J External Iliac Artery, Left			
K Femoral Artery, Right			
L Femoral Artery, Left			
M Popliteal Artery, Right			
N Popliteal Artery, Left			
P Anterior Tibial Artery, Right			
Q Anterior Tibial Artery, Left			
R Posterior Tibial Artery, Right			
S Posterior Tibial Artery, Left			
T Peroneal Artery, Right			
U Peroneal Artery, Left			
V Foot Artery, Right			
W Foot Artery, Left			
Y Lower Artery			

0 Medical and Surgical
4 Lower Arteries
C Extirpation   Taking or cutting out solid matter from a body part

Body Part Character 4	Approach Character 5	Device Character 6	Qualifier Character 7
0 Abdominal Aorta	0 Open	Z No Device	Z No Qualifier
1 Celiac Artery	3 Percutaneous		
2 Gastric Artery	4 Percutaneous Endoscopic		
3 Hepatic Artery			
4 Splenic Artery			
5 Superior Mesenteric Artery			
6 Colic Artery, Right			
7 Colic Artery, Left			
8 Colic Artery, Middle			
9 Renal Artery, Right			
A Renal Artery, Left			
B Inferior Mesenteric Artery			
C Common Iliac Artery, Right			
D Common Iliac Artery, Left			
E Internal Iliac Artery, Right			
F Internal Iliac Artery, Left			
H External Iliac Artery, Right			
J External Iliac Artery, Left			
K Femoral Artery, Right			
L Femoral Artery, Left			
M Popliteal Artery, Right			
N Popliteal Artery, Left			
P Anterior Tibial Artery, Right			
Q Anterior Tibial Artery, Left			
R Posterior Tibial Artery, Right			
S Posterior Tibial Artery, Left			
T Peroneal Artery, Right			
U Peroneal Artery, Left			
V Foot Artery, Right			
W Foot Artery, Left			
Y Lower Artery			

0   Medical and Surgical
4   Lower Arteries
H   Insertion   Putting in a nonbiological appliance that monitors, assists, performs, or prevents a physiological function but does not physically take the place of a body part

Body Part Character 4	Approach Character 5	Device Character 6	Qualifier Character 7
0 Abdominal Aorta **Y** Lower Artery	**0** Open **3** Percutaneous **4** Percutaneous Endoscopic	**2** Monitoring Device **3** Infusion Device **D** Intraluminal Device	**Z** No Qualifier
1 Celiac Artery **2** Gastric Artery **3** Hepatic Artery **4** Splenic Artery **5** Superior Mesenteric Artery **6** Colic Artery, Right **7** Colic Artery, Left **8** Colic Artery, Middle **9** Renal Artery, Right **A** Renal Artery, Left **B** Inferior Mesenteric Artery **C** Common Iliac Artery, Right **D** Common Iliac Artery, Left **E** Internal Iliac Artery, Right **F** Internal Iliac Artery, Left **H** External Iliac Artery, Right **J** External Iliac Artery, Left **K** Femoral Artery, Right **L** Femoral Artery, Left **M** Popliteal Artery, Right **N** Popliteal Artery, Left **P** Anterior Tibial Artery, Right **Q** Anterior Tibial Artery, Left **R** Posterior Tibial Artery, Right **S** Posterior Tibial Artery, Left **T** Peroneal Artery, Right **U** Peroneal Artery, Left **V** Foot Artery, Right **W** Foot Artery, Left	**0** Open **3** Percutaneous **4** Percutaneous Endoscopic	**3** Infusion Device **D** Intraluminal Device	**Z** No Qualifier

Non-OR   04H0[0,3,4][2,3]Z
Non-OR   04HY[0,3,4]3Z
Non-OR   04H[1,2,3,4,5,6,7,8,9,A,B,C,D,E,F,H,J,K,L,M,N,P,Q,R,S,T,U,V,W][0,3,4]3Z

0   Medical and Surgical
4   Lower Arteries
J   Inspection   Visually and/or manually exploring a body part

Body Part Character 4	Approach Character 5	Device Character 6	Qualifier Character 7
Y Lower Artery	**0** Open **3** Percutaneous **4** Percutaneous Endoscopic **X** External	**Z** No Device	**Z** No Qualifier

Non-OR   04JY[4,X]ZZ

0　Medical and Surgical
4　Lower Arteries
L　Occlusion　　　　　Completely closing an orifice or the lumen of a tubular body part

Body Part Character 4	Approach Character 5	Device Character 6	Qualifier Character 7
0 Abdominal Aorta	**0** Open	**C** Extraluminal Device	**Z** No Qualifier
1 Celiac Artery	**3** Percutaneous	**D** Intraluminal Device	
2 Gastric Artery	**4** Percutaneous Endoscopic	**Z** No Device	
3 Hepatic Artery			
4 Splenic Artery			
5 Superior Mesenteric Artery			
6 Colic Artery, Right			
7 Colic Artery, Left			
8 Colic Artery, Middle			
9 Renal Artery, Right			
A Renal Artery, Left			
B Inferior Mesenteric Artery			
C Common Iliac Artery, Right			
D Common Iliac Artery, Left			
H External Iliac Artery, Right			
J External Iliac Artery, Left			
K Femoral Artery, Right			
L Femoral Artery, Left			
M Popliteal Artery, Right			
N Popliteal Artery, Left			
P Anterior Tibial Artery, Right			
Q Anterior Tibial Artery, Left			
R Posterior Tibial Artery, Right			
S Posterior Tibial Artery, Left			
T Peroneal Artery, Right			
U Peroneal Artery, Left			
V Foot Artery, Right			
W Foot Artery, Left			
Y Lower Artery			
E Internal Iliac Artery, Right	**0** Open	**C** Extraluminal Device	**T** Uterine Artery, Right ♀
	3 Percutaneous	**D** Intraluminal Device	**Z** No Qualifier
	4 Percutaneous Endoscopic	**Z** No Device	
F Internal Iliac Artery, Left	**0** Open	**C** Extraluminal Device	**U** Uterine Artery, Left ♀
	3 Percutaneous	**D** Intraluminal Device	**Z** No Qualifier
	4 Percutaneous Endoscopic	**Z** No Device	

Non-OR　04L23DZ

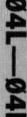

LC Limited Coverage　　**NC** Noncovered　　　HAC associated procedure　　　Combination Only　　　DRG Non-OR　　　Non-OR　　　Revised Text in **GREEN**

Ø   **Medical and Surgical**
4   **Lower Arteries**
N   **Release**   Freeing a body part from an abnormal physical constraint

Body Part Character 4	Approach Character 5	Device Character 6	Qualifier Character 7
Ø Abdominal Aorta **1** Celiac Artery **2** Gastric Artery **3** Hepatic Artery **4** Splenic Artery **5** Superior Mesenteric Artery **6** Colic Artery, Right **7** Colic Artery, Left **8** Colic Artery, Middle **9** Renal Artery, Right **A** Renal Artery, Left **B** Inferior Mesenteric Artery **C** Common Iliac Artery, Right **D** Common Iliac Artery, Left **E** Internal Iliac Artery, Right **F** Internal Iliac Artery, Left **H** External Iliac Artery, Right **J** External Iliac Artery, Left **K** Femoral Artery, Right **L** Femoral Artery, Left **M** Popliteal Artery, Right **N** Popliteal Artery, Left **P** Anterior Tibial Artery, Right **Q** Anterior Tibial Artery, Left **R** Posterior Tibial Artery, Right **S** Posterior Tibial Artery, Left **T** Peroneal Artery, Right **U** Peroneal Artery, Left **V** Foot Artery, Right **W** Foot Artery, Left **Y** Lower Artery	**Ø** Open **3** Percutaneous **4** Percutaneous Endoscopic	**Z** No Device	**Z** No Qualifier

Ø   **Medical and Surgical**
4   **Lower Arteries**
P   **Removal**   Taking out or off a device from a body part

Body Part Character 4	Approach Character 5	Device Character 6	Qualifier Character 7
Y Lower Artery	**Ø** Open **3** Percutaneous **4** Percutaneous Endoscopic	**Ø** Drainage Device **2** Monitoring Device **3** Infusion Device **7** Autologous Tissue Substitute **C** Extraluminal Device **D** Intraluminal Device **J** Synthetic Substitute **K** Nonautologous Tissue Substitute	**Z** No Qualifier
Y Lower Artery	**X** External	**Ø** Drainage Device **1** Radioactive Element **2** Monitoring Device **3** Infusion Device **D** Intraluminal Device	**Z** No Qualifier

Non-OR   Ø4PYX[Ø,1,2,3,D]Z

Ø   Medical and Surgical
4   Lower Arteries
Q   Repair   Restoring, to the extent possible, a body part to its normal anatomic structure and function

Body Part Character 4	Approach Character 5	Device Character 6	Qualifier Character 7
Ø Abdominal Aorta	Ø Open	Z No Device	Z No Qualifier
1 Celiac Artery	3 Percutaneous		
2 Gastric Artery	4 Percutaneous Endoscopic		
3 Hepatic Artery			
4 Splenic Artery			
5 Superior Mesenteric Artery			
6 Colic Artery, Right			
7 Colic Artery, Left			
8 Colic Artery, Middle			
9 Renal Artery, Right			
A Renal Artery, Left			
B Inferior Mesenteric Artery			
C Common Iliac Artery, Right			
D Common Iliac Artery, Left			
E Internal Iliac Artery, Right			
F Internal Iliac Artery, Left			
H External Iliac Artery, Right			
J External Iliac Artery, Left			
K Femoral Artery, Right			
L Femoral Artery, Left			
M Popliteal Artery, Right			
N Popliteal Artery, Left			
P Anterior Tibial Artery, Right			
Q Anterior Tibial Artery, Left			
R Posterior Tibial Artery, Right			
S Posterior Tibial Artery, Left			
T Peroneal Artery, Right			
U Peroneal Artery, Left			
V Foot Artery, Right			
W Foot Artery, Left			
Y Lower Artery			

Ø   Medical and Surgical
4   Lower Arteries
R   Replacement   Putting in or on biological or synthetic material that physically takes the place and/or function of all or a portion of a body part

Body Part Character 4	Approach Character 5	Device Character 6	Qualifier Character 7
Ø Abdominal Aorta	Ø Open	7 Autologous Tissue Substitute	Z No Qualifier
1 Celiac Artery	4 Percutaneous Endoscopic	J Synthetic Substitute	
2 Gastric Artery		K Nonautologous Tissue Substitute	
3 Hepatic Artery			
4 Splenic Artery			
5 Superior Mesenteric Artery			
6 Colic Artery, Right			
7 Colic Artery, Left			
8 Colic Artery, Middle			
9 Renal Artery, Right			
A Renal Artery, Left			
B Inferior Mesenteric Artery			
C Common Iliac Artery, Right			
D Common Iliac Artery, Left			
E Internal Iliac Artery, Right			
F Internal Iliac Artery, Left			
H External Iliac Artery, Right			
J External Iliac Artery, Left			
K Femoral Artery, Right			
L Femoral Artery, Left			
M Popliteal Artery, Right			
N Popliteal Artery, Left			
P Anterior Tibial Artery, Right			
Q Anterior Tibial Artery, Left			
R Posterior Tibial Artery, Right			
S Posterior Tibial Artery, Left			
T Peroneal Artery, Right			
U Peroneal Artery, Left			
V Foot Artery, Right			
W Foot Artery, Left			
Y Lower Artery			

Lower Arteries

04S–04U

Ø Medical and Surgical
4 Lower Arteries
S Reposition Moving to its normal location or other suitable location all or a portion of a body part

Body Part Character 4	Approach Character 5	Device Character 6	Qualifier Character 7
Ø Abdominal Aorta	**Ø** Open	**Z** No Device	**Z** No Qualifier
1 Celiac Artery	**3** Percutaneous		
2 Gastric Artery	**4** Percutaneous Endoscopic		
3 Hepatic Artery			
4 Splenic Artery			
5 Superior Mesenteric Artery			
6 Colic Artery, Right			
7 Colic Artery, Left			
8 Colic Artery, Middle			
9 Renal Artery, Right			
A Renal Artery, Left			
B Inferior Mesenteric Artery			
C Common Iliac Artery, Right			
D Common Iliac Artery, Left			
E Internal Iliac Artery, Right			
F Internal Iliac Artery, Left			
H External Iliac Artery, Right			
J External Iliac Artery, Left			
K Femoral Artery, Right			
L Femoral Artery, Left			
M Popliteal Artery, Right			
N Popliteal Artery, Left			
P Anterior Tibial Artery, Right			
Q Anterior Tibial Artery, Left			
R Posterior Tibial Artery, Right			
S Posterior Tibial Artery, Left			
T Peroneal Artery, Right			
U Peroneal Artery, Left			
V Foot Artery, Right			
W Foot Artery, Left			
Y Lower Artery			

Ø Medical and Surgical
4 Lower Arteries
U Supplement Putting in or on biological or synthetic material that physically reinforces and/or augments the function of a portion of a body part

Body Part Character 4	Approach Character 5	Device Character 6	Qualifier Character 7
Ø Abdominal Aorta	**Ø** Open	**7** Autologous Tissue Substitute	**Z** No Qualifier
1 Celiac Artery	**3** Percutaneous	**J** Synthetic Substitute	
2 Gastric Artery	**4** Percutaneous Endoscopic	**K** Nonautologous Tissue Substitute	
3 Hepatic Artery			
4 Splenic Artery			
5 Superior Mesenteric Artery			
6 Colic Artery, Right			
7 Colic Artery, Left			
8 Colic Artery, Middle			
9 Renal Artery, Right			
A Renal Artery, Left			
B Inferior Mesenteric Artery			
C Common Iliac Artery, Right			
D Common Iliac Artery, Left			
E Internal Iliac Artery, Right			
F Internal Iliac Artery, Left			
H External Iliac Artery, Right			
J External Iliac Artery, Left			
K Femoral Artery, Right			
L Femoral Artery, Left			
M Popliteal Artery, Right			
N Popliteal Artery, Left			
P Anterior Tibial Artery, Right			
Q Anterior Tibial Artery, Left			
R Posterior Tibial Artery, Right			
S Posterior Tibial Artery, Left			
T Peroneal Artery, Right			
U Peroneal Artery, Left			
V Foot Artery, Right			
W Foot Artery, Left			
Y Lower Artery			

LC Limited Coverage **NC** Noncovered HAC associated procedure Combination Only DRG Non-OR Non-OR Revised Text in **GREEN**

172   ICD-10-PCS 2014 (Draft)

0　Medical and Surgical
4　Lower Arteries
V　Restriction　　Partially closing an orifice or the lumen of a tubular body part

Body Part Character 4	Approach Character 5	Device Character 6	Qualifier Character 7
0 Abdominal Aorta	0 Open 3 Percutaneous 4 Percutaneous Endoscopic	C Extraluminal Device Z No Device	Z No Qualifier
0 Abdominal Aorta	0 Open 3 Percutaneous 4 Percutaneous Endoscopic	D Intraluminal Device	J Temporary Z No Qualifier
1 Celiac Artery 2 Gastric Artery 3 Hepatic Artery 4 Splenic Artery 5 Superior Mesenteric Artery 6 Colic Artery, Right 7 Colic Artery, Left 8 Colic Artery, Middle 9 Renal Artery, Right A Renal Artery, Left B Inferior Mesenteric Artery C Common Iliac Artery, Right D Common Iliac Artery, Left E Internal Iliac Artery, Right F Internal Iliac Artery, Left H External Iliac Artery, Right J External Iliac Artery, Left K Femoral Artery, Right L Femoral Artery, Left M Popliteal Artery, Right N Popliteal Artery, Left P Anterior Tibial Artery, Right Q Anterior Tibial Artery, Left R Posterior Tibial Artery, Right S Posterior Tibial Artery, Left T Peroneal Artery, Right U Peroneal Artery, Left V Foot Artery, Right W Foot Artery, Left Y Lower Artery	0 Open 3 Percutaneous 4 Percutaneous Endoscopic	C Extraluminal Device D Intraluminal Device Z No Device	Z No Qualifier

0　Medical and Surgical
4　Lower Arteries
W　Revision　　Correcting, to the extent possible, a portion of a malfunctioning device or the position of a displaced device

Body Part Character 4	Approach Character 5	Device Character 6	Qualifier Character 7
Y Lower Artery	0 Open 3 Percutaneous 4 Percutaneous Endoscopic X External	0 Drainage Device 2 Monitoring Device 3 Infusion Device 7 Autologous Tissue Substitute C Extraluminal Device D Intraluminal Device J Synthetic Substitute K Nonautologous Tissue Substitute	Z No Qualifier

Non-OR　04WYX[0,2,3,7,C,D,J,K]Z

Upper Veins Ø51–Ø5W

Ø   **Medical and Surgical**
5   **Upper Veins**
1   **Bypass**   Altering the route of passage of the contents of a tubular body part

Body Part Character 4	Approach Character 5	Device Character 6	Qualifier Character 7
Ø Azygos Vein 1 Hemiazygos Vein 3 Innominate Vein, Right 4 Innominate Vein, Left 5 Subclavian Vein, Right 6 Subclavian Vein, Left 7 Axillary Vein, Right 8 Axillary Vein, Left 9 Brachial Vein, Right A Brachial Vein, Left B Basilic Vein, Right C Basilic Vein, Left D Cephalic Vein, Right F Cephalic Vein, Left G Hand Vein, Right H Hand Vein, Left L Intracranial Vein M Internal Jugular Vein, Right N Internal Jugular Vein, Left P External Jugular Vein, Right Q External Jugular Vein, Left R Vertebral Vein, Right S Vertebral Vein, Left T Face Vein, Right V Face Vein, Left	Ø Open 4 Percutaneous Endoscopic	7 Autologous Tissue Substitute 9 Autologous Venous Tissue A Autologous Arterial Tissue J Synthetic Substitute K Nonautologous Tissue Substitute Z No Device	Y Upper Vein

Ø   **Medical and Surgical**
5   **Upper Veins**
5   **Destruction**   Physical eradication of all or a portion of a body part by the direct use of energy, force, or a destructive agent

Body Part Character 4	Approach Character 5	Device Character 6	Qualifier Character 7
Ø Azygos Vein 1 Hemiazygos Vein 3 Innominate Vein, Right 4 Innominate Vein, Left 5 Subclavian Vein, Right 6 Subclavian Vein, Left 7 Axillary Vein, Right 8 Axillary Vein, Left 9 Brachial Vein, Right A Brachial Vein, Left B Basilic Vein, Right C Basilic Vein, Left D Cephalic Vein, Right F Cephalic Vein, Left G Hand Vein, Right H Hand Vein, Left L Intracranial Vein M Internal Jugular Vein, Right N Internal Jugular Vein, Left P External Jugular Vein, Right Q External Jugular Vein, Left R Vertebral Vein, Right S Vertebral Vein, Left T Face Vein, Right V Face Vein, Left Y Upper Vein	Ø Open 3 Percutaneous 4 Percutaneous Endoscopic	Z No Device	Z No Qualifier

Upper Veins

Ø51–Ø55

Ø   **Medical and Surgical**
5   **Upper Veins**
7   **Dilation**   Expanding an orifice or the lumen of a tubular body part

Body Part Character 4	Approach Character 5	Device Character 6	Qualifier Character 7
Ø Azygos Vein	**Ø** Open	**D** Intraluminal Device	**Z** No Qualifier
1 Hemiazygos Vein	**3** Percutaneous	**Z** No Device	
3 Innominate Vein, Right	**4** Percutaneous Endoscopic		
4 Innominate Vein, Left			
5 Subclavian Vein, Right			
6 Subclavian Vein, Left			
7 Axillary Vein, Right			
8 Axillary Vein, Left			
9 Brachial Vein, Right			
A Brachial Vein, Left			
B Basilic Vein, Right			
C Basilic Vein, Left			
D Cephalic Vein, Right			
F Cephalic Vein, Left			
G Hand Vein, Right			
H Hand Vein, Left			
L Intracranial Vein NC			
M Internal Jugular Vein, Right			
N Internal Jugular Vein, Left			
P External Jugular Vein, Right			
Q External Jugular Vein, Left			
R Vertebral Vein, Right			
S Vertebral Vein, Left			
T Face Vein, Right			
V Face Vein, Left			
Y Upper Vein			

NC   057L[3,4]ZZ

Ø   **Medical and Surgical**
5   **Upper Veins**
9   **Drainage**   Taking or letting out fluids and/or gases from a body part

Body Part Character 4	Approach Character 5	Device Character 6	Qualifier Character 7
Ø Azygos Vein	**Ø** Open	**Ø** Drainage Device	**Z** No Qualifier
1 Hemiazygos Vein	**3** Percutaneous		
3 Innominate Vein, Right	**4** Percutaneous Endoscopic		
4 Innominate Vein, Left			
5 Subclavian Vein, Right			
6 Subclavian Vein, Left			
7 Axillary Vein, Right			
8 Axillary Vein, Left			
9 Brachial Vein, Right			
A Brachial Vein, Left			
B Basilic Vein, Right			
C Basilic Vein, Left			
D Cephalic Vein, Right			
F Cephalic Vein, Left			
G Hand Vein, Right			
H Hand Vein, Left			
L Intracranial Vein			
M Internal Jugular Vein, Right			
N Internal Jugular Vein, Left			
P External Jugular Vein, Right			
Q External Jugular Vein, Left			
R Vertebral Vein, Right			
S Vertebral Vein, Left			
T Face Vein, Right			
V Face Vein, Left			
Y Upper Vein			

Ø59 Continued on next page

Non-OR   Ø59[Ø,1,3,4,5,6,7,8,9,A,B,C,D,F,G,H,L,M,N,P,Q,R,S,T,V,Y][Ø,3,4]ØZ

LC Limited Coverage   NC Noncovered   HAC associated procedure   Combination Only   DRG Non-OR   Non-OR   Revised Text in **GREEN**

Ø Medical and Surgical
5 Upper Veins
9 Drainage   Taking or letting out fluids and/or gases from a body part

Ø59 Continued

Body Part Character 4	Approach Character 5	Device Character 6	Qualifier Character 7
Ø Azygos Vein **1** Hemiazygos Vein **3** Innominate Vein, Right **4** Innominate Vein, Left **5** Subclavian Vein, Right **6** Subclavian Vein, Left **7** Axillary Vein, Right **8** Axillary Vein, Left **9** Brachial Vein, Right **A** Brachial Vein, Left **B** Basilic Vein, Right **C** Basilic Vein, Left **D** Cephalic Vein, Right **F** Cephalic Vein, Left **G** Hand Vein, Right **H** Hand Vein, Left **L** Intracranial Vein **M** Internal Jugular Vein, Right **N** Internal Jugular Vein, Left **P** External Jugular Vein, Right **Q** External Jugular Vein, Left **R** Vertebral Vein, Right **S** Vertebral Vein, Left **T** Face Vein, Right **V** Face Vein, Left **Y** Upper Vein	**Ø** Open **3** Percutaneous **4** Percutaneous Endoscopic	**Z** No Device	**X** Diagnostic **Z** No Qualifier

Non-OR Ø59[Ø,1,3,4,5,6,7,8,9,A,B,C,D,F,G,H,L,M,N,P,Q,R,S,T,V,Y][Ø,3,4]ZZ

Ø Medical and Surgical
5 Upper Veins
B Excision   Cutting out or off, without replacement, a portion of a body part

Body Part Character 4	Approach Character 5	Device Character 6	Qualifier Character 7
Ø Azygos Vein **1** Hemiazygos Vein **3** Innominate Vein, Right **4** Innominate Vein, Left **5** Subclavian Vein, Right **6** Subclavian Vein, Left **7** Axillary Vein, Right **8** Axillary Vein, Left **9** Brachial Vein, Right **A** Brachial Vein, Left **B** Basilic Vein, Right **C** Basilic Vein, Left **D** Cephalic Vein, Right **F** Cephalic Vein, Left **G** Hand Vein, Right **H** Hand Vein, Left **L** Intracranial Vein **M** Internal Jugular Vein, Right **N** Internal Jugular Vein, Left **P** External Jugular Vein, Right **Q** External Jugular Vein, Left **R** Vertebral Vein, Right **S** Vertebral Vein, Left **T** Face Vein, Right **V** Face Vein, Left **Y** Upper Vein	**Ø** Open **3** Percutaneous **4** Percutaneous Endoscopic	**Z** No Device	**X** Diagnostic **Z** No Qualifier

LC Limited Coverage   **NC** Noncovered   HAC associated procedure   Combination Only   DRG Non-OR   Non-OR   Revised Text in **GREEN**

176   ICD-1Ø-PCS 2Ø14 (Draft)

0　Medical and Surgical
5　Upper Veins
C　Extirpation　　Taking or cutting out solid matter from a body part

Body Part Character 4	Approach Character 5	Device Character 6	Qualifier Character 7
0 Azygos Vein	**0** Open	**Z** No Device	**Z** No Qualifier
1 Hemiazygos Vein	**3** Percutaneous		
3 Innominate Vein, Right	**4** Percutaneous Endoscopic		
4 Innominate Vein, Left			
5 Subclavian Vein, Right			
6 Subclavian Vein, Left			
7 Axillary Vein, Right			
8 Axillary Vein, Left			
9 Brachial Vein, Right			
A Brachial Vein, Left			
B Basilic Vein, Right			
C Basilic Vein, Left			
D Cephalic Vein, Right			
F Cephalic Vein, Left			
G Hand Vein, Right			
H Hand Vein, Left			
L Intracranial Vein NC			
M Internal Jugular Vein, Right			
N Internal Jugular Vein, Left			
P External Jugular Vein, Right			
Q External Jugular Vein, Left			
R Vertebral Vein, Right			
S Vertebral Vein, Left			
T Face Vein, Right			
V Face Vein, Left			
Y Upper Vein			

NC　05CL[3,4]ZZ

0　Medical and Surgical
5　Upper Veins
D　Extraction　　Pulling or stripping out or off all or a portion of a body part by the use of force

Body Part Character 4	Approach Character 5	Device Character 6	Qualifier Character 7
9 Brachial Vein, Right	**0** Open	**Z** No Device	**Z** No Qualifier
A Brachial Vein, Left	**3** Percutaneous		
B Basilic Vein, Right			
C Basilic Vein, Left			
D Cephalic Vein, Right			
F Cephalic Vein, Left			
G Hand Vein, Right			
H Hand Vein, Left			
Y Upper Vein			

Upper Veins (side tab)

0 Medical and Surgical
5 Upper Veins
H Insertion Putting in a nonbiological appliance that monitors, assists, performs, or prevents a physiological function but does not physically take the place of a body part

Body Part Character 4	Approach Character 5	Device Character 6	Qualifier Character 7
0 Azygos Vein 1 Hemiazygos Vein 3 Innominate Vein, Right 4 Innominate Vein, Left 5 Subclavian Vein, Right 6 Subclavian Vein, Left 7 Axillary Vein, Right 8 Axillary Vein, Left 9 Brachial Vein, Right A Brachial Vein, Left B Basilic Vein, Right C Basilic Vein, Left D Cephalic Vein, Right F Cephalic Vein, Left G Hand Vein, Right H Hand Vein, Left L Intracranial Vein M Internal Jugular Vein, Right N Internal Jugular Vein, Left P External Jugular Vein, Right Q External Jugular Vein, Left R Vertebral Vein, Right S Vertebral Vein, Left T Face Vein, Right V Face Vein, Left	0 Open 3 Percutaneous 4 Percutaneous Endoscopic	3 Infusion Device D Intraluminal Device	Z No Qualifier
Y Upper Vein	0 Open 3 Percutaneous 4 Percutaneous Endoscopic	2 Monitoring Device 3 Infusion Device D Intraluminal Device	Z No Qualifier

Non-OR 05H[0,1,3,4,5,6,7,8,9,A,B,C,D,F,G,H,L,M,N,P,Q,R,S,T,V][0,3,4]3Z
Non-OR 05HY[0,3,4]3Z

0 Medical and Surgical
5 Upper Veins
J Inspection Visually and/or manually exploring a body part

Body Part Character 4	Approach Character 5	Device Character 6	Qualifier Character 7
Y Upper Vein	0 Open 3 Percutaneous 4 Percutaneous Endoscopic X External	Z No Device	Z No Qualifier

Non-OR 05JYXZZ

Ø　Medical and Surgical
5　Upper Veins
L　Occlusion　　Completely closing an orifice or the lumen of a tubular body part

Body Part Character 4	Approach Character 5	Device Character 6	Qualifier Character 7
Ø Azygos Vein	**Ø** Open	**C** Extraluminal Device	**Z** No Qualifier
1 Hemiazygos Vein	**3** Percutaneous	**D** Intraluminal Device	
3 Innominate Vein, Right	**4** Percutaneous Endoscopic	**Z** No Device	
4 Innominate Vein, Left			
5 Subclavian Vein, Right			
6 Subclavian Vein, Left			
7 Axillary Vein, Right			
8 Axillary Vein, Left			
9 Brachial Vein, Right			
A Brachial Vein, Left			
B Basilic Vein, Right			
C Basilic Vein, Left			
D Cephalic Vein, Right			
F Cephalic Vein, Left			
G Hand Vein, Right			
H Hand Vein, Left			
L Intracranial Vein			
M Internal Jugular Vein, Right			
N Internal Jugular Vein, Left			
P External Jugular Vein, Right			
Q External Jugular Vein, Left			
R Vertebral Vein, Right			
S Vertebral Vein, Left			
T Face Vein, Right			
V Face Vein, Left			
Y Upper Vein			

Ø　Medical and Surgical
5　Upper Veins
N　Release　　Freeing a body part from an abnormal physical constraint

Body Part Character 4	Approach Character 5	Device Character 6	Qualifier Character 7
Ø Azygos Vein	**Ø** Open	**Z** No Device	**Z** No Qualifier
1 Hemiazygos Vein	**3** Percutaneous		
3 Innominate Vein, Right	**4** Percutaneous Endoscopic		
4 Innominate Vein, Left			
5 Subclavian Vein, Right			
6 Subclavian Vein, Left			
7 Axillary Vein, Right			
8 Axillary Vein, Left			
9 Brachial Vein, Right			
A Brachial Vein, Left			
B Basilic Vein, Right			
C Basilic Vein, Left			
D Cephalic Vein, Right			
F Cephalic Vein, Left			
G Hand Vein, Right			
H Hand Vein, Left			
L Intracranial Vein			
M Internal Jugular Vein, Right			
N Internal Jugular Vein, Left			
P External Jugular Vein, Right			
Q External Jugular Vein, Left			
R Vertebral Vein, Right			
S Vertebral Vein, Left			
T Face Vein, Right			
V Face Vein, Left			
Y Upper Vein			

Ø   **Medical and Surgical**
5   **Upper Veins**
P   **Removal**   Taking out or off a device from a body part

Body Part Character 4	Approach Character 5	Device Character 6	Qualifier Character 7
Y Upper Vein	**Ø** Open **3** Percutaneous **4** Percutaneous Endoscopic	**Ø** Drainage Device **2** Monitoring Device **3** Infusion Device **7** Autologous Tissue Substitute **C** Extraluminal Device **D** Intraluminal Device **J** Synthetic Substitute **K** Nonautologous Tissue Substitute	**Z** No Qualifier
Y Upper Vein	**X** External	**Ø** Drainage Device **2** Monitoring Device **3** Infusion Device **D** Intraluminal Device	**Z** No Qualifier

Non-OR   Ø5PYX[Ø,2,3,D]Z

Ø   **Medical and Surgical**
5   **Upper Veins**
Q   **Repair**   Restoring, to the extent possible, a body part to its normal anatomic structure and function

Body Part Character 4	Approach Character 5	Device Character 6	Qualifier Character 7
Ø Azygos Vein **1** Hemiazygos Vein **3** Innominate Vein, Right **4** Innominate Vein, Left **5** Subclavian Vein, Right **6** Subclavian Vein, Left **7** Axillary Vein, Right **8** Axillary Vein, Left **9** Brachial Vein, Right **A** Brachial Vein, Left **B** Basilic Vein, Right **C** Basilic Vein, Left **D** Cephalic Vein, Right **F** Cephalic Vein, Left **G** Hand Vein, Right **H** Hand Vein, Left **L** Intracranial Vein **M** Internal Jugular Vein, Right **N** Internal Jugular Vein, Left **P** External Jugular Vein, Right **Q** External Jugular Vein, Left **R** Vertebral Vein, Right **S** Vertebral Vein, Left **T** Face Vein, Right **V** Face Vein, Left **Y** Upper Vein	**Ø** Open **3** Percutaneous **4** Percutaneous Endoscopic	**Z** No Device	**Z** No Qualifier

LC Limited Coverage   **NC** Noncovered   HAC associated procedure   Combination Only   DRG Non-OR   Non-OR   Revised Text in **GREEN**

180   ICD-1Ø-PCS 2Ø14 (Draft)

0   **Medical and Surgical**
5   **Upper Veins**
R   **Replacement**   Putting in or on biological or synthetic material that physically takes the place and/or function of all or a portion of a body part

Body Part Character 4	Approach Character 5	Device Character 6	Qualifier Character 7
0 Azygos Vein **1** Hemiazygos Vein **3** Innominate Vein, Right **4** Innominate Vein, Left **5** Subclavian Vein, Right **6** Subclavian Vein, Left **7** Axillary Vein, Right **8** Axillary Vein, Left **9** Brachial Vein, Right **A** Brachial Vein, Left **B** Basilic Vein, Right **C** Basilic Vein, Left **D** Cephalic Vein, Right **F** Cephalic Vein, Left **G** Hand Vein, Right **H** Hand Vein, Left **L** Intracranial Vein **M** Internal Jugular Vein, Right **N** Internal Jugular Vein, Left **P** External Jugular Vein, Right **Q** External Jugular Vein, Left **R** Vertebral Vein, Right **S** Vertebral Vein, Left **T** Face Vein, Right **V** Face Vein, Left **Y** Upper Vein	**0** Open **4** Percutaneous Endoscopic	**7** Autologous Tissue Substitute **J** Synthetic Substitute **K** Nonautologous Tissue Substitute	**Z** No Qualifier

0   **Medical and Surgical**
5   **Upper Veins**
S   **Reposition**   Moving to its normal location or other suitable location all or a portion of a body part

Body Part Character 4	Approach Character 5	Device Character 6	Qualifier Character 7
0 Azygos Vein **1** Hemiazygos Vein **3** Innominate Vein, Right **4** Innominate Vein, Left **5** Subclavian Vein, Right **6** Subclavian Vein, Left **7** Axillary Vein, Right **8** Axillary Vein, Left **9** Brachial Vein, Right **A** Brachial Vein, Left **B** Basilic Vein, Right **C** Basilic Vein, Left **D** Cephalic Vein, Right **F** Cephalic Vein, Left **G** Hand Vein, Right **H** Hand Vein, Left **L** Intracranial Vein **M** Internal Jugular Vein, Right **N** Internal Jugular Vein, Left **P** External Jugular Vein, Right **Q** External Jugular Vein, Left **R** Vertebral Vein, Right **S** Vertebral Vein, Left **T** Face Vein, Right **V** Face Vein, Left **Y** Upper Vein	**0** Open **3** Percutaneous **4** Percutaneous Endoscopic	**Z** No Device	**Z** No Qualifier

05R—05S

0   Medical and Surgical
5   Upper Veins
U   Supplement   Putting in or on biological or synthetic material that physically reinforces and/or augments the function of a portion of a body part

Body Part Character 4	Approach Character 5	Device Character 6	Qualifier Character 7
0 Azygos Vein	0 Open	7 Autologous Tissue Substitute	Z No Qualifier
1 Hemiazygos Vein	3 Percutaneous	J Synthetic Substitute	
3 Innominate Vein, Right	4 Percutaneous Endoscopic	K Nonautologous Tissue Substitute	
4 Innominate Vein, Left			
5 Subclavian Vein, Right			
6 Subclavian Vein, Left			
7 Axillary Vein, Right			
8 Axillary Vein, Left			
9 Brachial Vein, Right			
A Brachial Vein, Left			
B Basilic Vein, Right			
C Basilic Vein, Left			
D Cephalic Vein, Right			
F Cephalic Vein, Left			
G Hand Vein, Right			
H Hand Vein, Left			
L Intracranial Vein			
M Internal Jugular Vein, Right			
N Internal Jugular Vein, Left			
P External Jugular Vein, Right			
Q External Jugular Vein, Left			
R Vertebral Vein, Right			
S Vertebral Vein, Left			
T Face Vein, Right			
V Face Vein, Left			
Y Upper Vein			

0   Medical and Surgical
5   Upper Veins
V   Restriction   Partially closing an orifice or the lumen of a tubular body part

Body Part Character 4	Approach Character 5	Device Character 6	Qualifier Character 7
0 Azygos Vein	0 Open	C Extraluminal Device	Z No Qualifier
1 Hemiazygos Vein	3 Percutaneous	D Intraluminal Device	
3 Innominate Vein, Right	4 Percutaneous Endoscopic	Z No Device	
4 Innominate Vein, Left			
5 Subclavian Vein, Right			
6 Subclavian Vein, Left			
7 Axillary Vein, Right			
8 Axillary Vein, Left			
9 Brachial Vein, Right			
A Brachial Vein, Left			
B Basilic Vein, Right			
C Basilic Vein, Left			
D Cephalic Vein, Right			
F Cephalic Vein, Left			
G Hand Vein, Right			
H Hand Vein, Left			
L Intracranial Vein			
M Internal Jugular Vein, Right			
N Internal Jugular Vein, Left			
P External Jugular Vein, Right			
Q External Jugular Vein, Left			
R Vertebral Vein, Right			
S Vertebral Vein, Left			
T Face Vein, Right			
V Face Vein, Left			
Y Upper Vein			

0 **Medical and Surgical**
5 **Upper Veins**
W **Revision**　　Correcting, to the extent possible, a portion of a malfunctioning device or the position of a displaced device

Body Part Character 4	Approach Character 5	Device Character 6	Qualifier Character 7
Y Upper Vein	**0** Open **3** Percutaneous **4** Percutaneous Endoscopic **X** External	**0** Drainage Device **2** Monitoring Device **3** Infusion Device **7** Autologous Tissue Substitute **C** Extraluminal Device **D** Intraluminal Device **J** Synthetic Substitute **K** Nonautologous Tissue Substitute	**Z** No Qualifier

Non-OR　　05WYX[0,2,3,7,C,D,J,K]Z

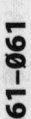

Lower Veins Lower Veins 061–061

Lower Veins 061–06W

0	**Medical and Surgical**
6	**Lower Veins**
1	**Bypass** Altering the route of passage of the contents of a tubular body part

Body Part Character 4	Approach Character 5	Device Character 6	Qualifier Character 7
0 Inferior Vena Cava	**0** Open **4** Percutaneous Endoscopic	**7** Autologous Tissue Substitute **9** Autologous Venous Tissue **A** Autologous Arterial Tissue **J** Synthetic Substitute **K** Nonautologous Tissue Substitute **Z** No Device	**5** Superior Mesenteric Vein **6** Inferior Mesenteric Vein **Y** Lower Vein
1 Splenic Vein **8** Portal Vein	**0** Open **4** Percutaneous Endoscopic	**7** Autologous Tissue Substitute **9** Autologous Venous Tissue **A** Autologous Arterial Tissue **J** Synthetic Substitute **K** Nonautologous Tissue Substitute **Z** No Device	**9** Renal Vein, Right **B** Renal Vein, Left **Y** Lower Vein
2 Gastric Vein **3** Esophageal Vein **4** Hepatic Vein **5** Superior Mesenteric Vein **6** Inferior Mesenteric Vein **7** Colic Vein **9** Renal Vein, Right **B** Renal Vein, Left **C** Common Iliac Vein, Right **D** Common Iliac Vein, Left **F** External Iliac Vein, Right **G** External Iliac Vein, Left **H** Hypogastric Vein, Right **J** Hypogastric Vein, Left **M** Femoral Vein, Right **N** Femoral Vein, Left **P** Greater Saphenous Vein, Right **Q** Greater Saphenous Vein, Left **R** Lesser Saphenous Vein, Right **S** Lesser Saphenous Vein, Left **T** Foot Vein, Right **V** Foot Vein, Left	**0** Open **4** Percutaneous Endoscopic	**7** Autologous Tissue Substitute **9** Autologous Venous Tissue **A** Autologous Arterial Tissue **J** Synthetic Substitute **K** Nonautologous Tissue Substitute **Z** No Device	**Y** Lower Vein
8 Portal Vein	**3** Percutaneous **4** Percutaneous Endoscopic	**D** Intraluminal Device	**Y** Lower Vein

Ø   **Medical and Surgical**
6   **Lower Veins**
5   **Destruction**   Physical eradication of all or a portion of a body part by the direct use of energy, force, or a destructive agent

Body Part Character 4	Approach Character 5	Device Character 6	Qualifier Character 7
Ø Inferior Vena Cava **1** Splenic Vein **2** Gastric Vein **3** Esophageal Vein **4** Hepatic Vein **5** Superior Mesenteric Vein **6** Inferior Mesenteric Vein **7** Colic Vein **8** Portal Vein **9** Renal Vein, Right **B** Renal Vein, Left **C** Common Iliac Vein, Right **D** Common Iliac Vein, Left **F** External Iliac Vein, Right **G** External Iliac Vein, Left **H** Hypogastric Vein, Right **J** Hypogastric Vein, Left **M** Femoral Vein, Right **N** Femoral Vein, Left **P** Greater Saphenous Vein, Right **Q** Greater Saphenous Vein, Left **R** Lesser Saphenous Vein, Right **S** Lesser Saphenous Vein, Left **T** Foot Vein, Right **V** Foot Vein, Left	**Ø** Open **3** Percutaneous **4** Percutaneous Endoscopic	**Z** No Device	**Z** No Qualifier
Y Lower Vein	**Ø** Open **3** Percutaneous **4** Percutaneous Endoscopic	**Z** No Device	**C** Hemorrhoidal Plexus **Z** No Qualifier

Ø   **Medical and Surgical**
6   **Lower Veins**
7   **Dilation**   Expanding an orifice or the lumen of a tubular body part

Body Part Character 4	Approach Character 5	Device Character 6	Qualifier Character 7
Ø Inferior Vena Cava **1** Splenic Vein **2** Gastric Vein **3** Esophageal Vein **4** Hepatic Vein **5** Superior Mesenteric Vein **6** Inferior Mesenteric Vein **7** Colic Vein **8** Portal Vein **9** Renal Vein, Right **B** Renal Vein, Left **C** Common Iliac Vein, Right **D** Common Iliac Vein, Left **F** External Iliac Vein, Right **G** External Iliac Vein, Left **H** Hypogastric Vein, Right **J** Hypogastric Vein, Left **M** Femoral Vein, Right **N** Femoral Vein, Left **P** Greater Saphenous Vein, Right **Q** Greater Saphenous Vein, Left **R** Lesser Saphenous Vein, Right **S** Lesser Saphenous Vein, Left **T** Foot Vein, Right **V** Foot Vein, Left **Y** Lower Vein	**Ø** Open **3** Percutaneous **4** Percutaneous Endoscopic	**D** Intraluminal Device **Z** No Device	**Z** No Qualifier

LC Limited Coverage   **NC** Noncovered   HAC associated procedure   Combination Only   DRG Non-OR   Non-OR   Revised Text in **GREEN**

ICD-10-PCS 2014 (Draft)   185

0   Medical and Surgical
6   Lower Veins
9   Drainage   Taking or letting out fluids and/or gases from a body part

Body Part Character 4	Approach Character 5	Device Character 6	Qualifier Character 7
0 Inferior Vena Cava 1 Splenic Vein 2 Gastric Vein 3 Esophageal Vein 4 Hepatic Vein 5 Superior Mesenteric Vein 6 Inferior Mesenteric Vein 7 Colic Vein 8 Portal Vein 9 Renal Vein, Right B Renal Vein, Left C Common Iliac Vein, Right D Common Iliac Vein, Left F External Iliac Vein, Right G External Iliac Vein, Left H Hypogastric Vein, Right J Hypogastric Vein, Left M Femoral Vein, Right N Femoral Vein, Left P Greater Saphenous Vein, Right Q Greater Saphenous Vein, Left R Lesser Saphenous Vein, Right S Lesser Saphenous Vein, Left T Foot Vein, Right V Foot Vein, Left Y Lower Vein	0 Open 3 Percutaneous 4 Percutaneous Endoscopic	0 Drainage Device	Z No Qualifier
0 Inferior Vena Cava 1 Splenic Vein 2 Gastric Vein 3 Esophageal Vein 4 Hepatic Vein 5 Superior Mesenteric Vein 6 Inferior Mesenteric Vein 7 Colic Vein 8 Portal Vein 9 Renal Vein, Right B Renal Vein, Left C Common Iliac Vein, Right D Common Iliac Vein, Left F External Iliac Vein, Right G External Iliac Vein, Left H Hypogastric Vein, Right J Hypogastric Vein, Left M Femoral Vein, Right N Femoral Vein, Left P Greater Saphenous Vein, Right Q Greater Saphenous Vein, Left R Lesser Saphenous Vein, Right S Lesser Saphenous Vein, Left T Foot Vein, Right V Foot Vein, Left Y Lower Vein	0 Open 3 Percutaneous 4 Percutaneous Endoscopic	Z No Device	X Diagnostic Z No Qualifier

Non-OR   069[0,1,2,4,5,6,7,8,9,B,C,D,F,G,H,J,M,N,P,Q,R,S,T,V,Y][0,3,4]0Z
Non-OR   069[0,1,2,4,5,6,7,8,9,B,C,D,F,G,H,J,M,N,P,Q,R,S,T,V,Y][0,3,4]ZZ

Ø　Medical and Surgical
6　Lower Veins
B　Excision　　　Cutting out or off, without replacement, a portion of a body part

Body Part Character 4	Approach Character 5	Device Character 6	Qualifier Character 7
Ø Inferior Vena Cava 1 Splenic Vein 2 Gastric Vein 3 Esophageal Vein 4 Hepatic Vein 5 Superior Mesenteric Vein 6 Inferior Mesenteric Vein 7 Colic Vein 8 Portal Vein 9 Renal Vein, Right B Renal Vein, Left C Common Iliac Vein, Right D Common Iliac Vein, Left F External Iliac Vein, Right G External Iliac Vein, Left H Hypogastric Vein, Right J Hypogastric Vein, Left M Femoral Vein, Right N Femoral Vein, Left P Greater Saphenous Vein, Right Q Greater Saphenous Vein, Left R Lesser Saphenous Vein, Right S Lesser Saphenous Vein, Left T Foot Vein, Right V Foot Vein, Left	Ø Open 3 Percutaneous 4 Percutaneous Endoscopic	Z No Device	X Diagnostic Z No Qualifier
Y Lower Vein	Ø Open 3 Percutaneous 4 Percutaneous Endoscopic	Z No Device	C Hemorrhoidal Plexus X Diagnostic Z No Qualifier

Ø　Medical and Surgical
6　Lower Veins
C　Extirpation　　　Taking or cutting out solid matter from a body part

Body Part Character 4	Approach Character 5	Device Character 6	Qualifier Character 7
Ø Inferior Vena Cava 1 Splenic Vein 2 Gastric Vein 3 Esophageal Vein 4 Hepatic Vein 5 Superior Mesenteric Vein 6 Inferior Mesenteric Vein 7 Colic Vein 8 Portal Vein 9 Renal Vein, Right B Renal Vein, Left C Common Iliac Vein, Right D Common Iliac Vein, Left F External Iliac Vein, Right G External Iliac Vein, Left H Hypogastric Vein, Right J Hypogastric Vein, Left M Femoral Vein, Right N Femoral Vein, Left P Greater Saphenous Vein, Right Q Greater Saphenous Vein, Left R Lesser Saphenous Vein, Right S Lesser Saphenous Vein, Left T Foot Vein, Right V Foot Vein, Left Y Lower Vein	Ø Open 3 Percutaneous 4 Percutaneous Endoscopic	Z No Device	Z No Qualifier

Lower Veins

06D–06J   Lower Veins   ICD-10-PCS (2014 Draft)

Ø   Medical and Surgical
6   Lower Veins
D   Extraction Pulling or stripping out or off all or a portion of a body part by the use of force

Body Part Character 4	Approach Character 5	Device Character 6	Qualifier Character 7
M Femoral Vein, Right **N** Femoral Vein, Left **P** Greater Saphenous Vein, Right **Q** Greater Saphenous Vein, Left **R** Lesser Saphenous Vein, Right **S** Lesser Saphenous Vein, Left **T** Foot Vein, Right **V** Foot Vein, Left **Y** Lower Vein	**Ø** Open **3** Percutaneous **4** Percutaneous Endoscopic	**Z** No Device	**Z** No Qualifier

Ø   Medical and Surgical
6   Lower Veins
H   Insertion Putting in a nonbiological appliance that monitors, assists, performs, or prevents a physiological function but does not physically take the place of a body part

Body Part Character 4	Approach Character 5	Device Character 6	Qualifier Character 7
Ø Inferior Vena Cava	**Ø** Open **3** Percutaneous	**3** Infusion Device	**T** Via Umbilical Vein **Z** No Qualifier
Ø Inferior Vena Cava	**Ø** Open **3** Percutaneous	**D** Intraluminal Device	**Z** No Qualifier
Ø Inferior Vena Cava	**4** Percutaneous Endoscopic	**3** Infusion Device **D** Intraluminal Device	**Z** No Qualifier
1 Splenic Vein **2** Gastric Vein **3** Esophageal Vein **4** Hepatic Vein **5** Superior Mesenteric Vein **6** Inferior Mesenteric Vein **7** Colic Vein **8** Portal Vein **9** Renal Vein, Right **B** Renal Vein, Left **C** Common Iliac Vein, Right **D** Common Iliac Vein, Left **F** External Iliac Vein, Right **G** External Iliac Vein, Left **H** Hypogastric Vein, Right **J** Hypogastric Vein, Left **M** Femoral Vein, Right **N** Femoral Vein, Left **P** Greater Saphenous Vein, Right **Q** Greater Saphenous Vein, Left **R** Lesser Saphenous Vein, Right **S** Lesser Saphenous Vein, Left **T** Foot Vein, Right **V** Foot Vein, Left	**Ø** Open **3** Percutaneous **4** Percutaneous Endoscopic	**3** Infusion Device **D** Intraluminal Device	**Z** No Qualifier
Y Lower Vein	**Ø** Open **3** Percutaneous **4** Percutaneous Endoscopic	**2** Monitoring Device **3** Infusion Device **D** Intraluminal Device	**Z** No Qualifier

Non-OR 06HØ[Ø,3]3[T,Z]
Non-OR 06HØ43Z
Non-OR 06H[1,2,3,4,5,6,7,8,9,B,C,D,F,G,H,J,M,N,P,Q,R,S,T,V][Ø,3,4]3Z
Non-OR 06HY[Ø,3,4]3Z

Ø   Medical and Surgical
6   Lower Veins
J   Inspection Visually and/or manually exploring a body part

Body Part Character 4	Approach Character 5	Device Character 6	Qualifier Character 7
Y Lower Vein	**Ø** Open **3** Percutaneous **4** Percutaneous Endoscopic **X** External	**Z** No Device	**Z** No Qualifier

Non-OR 06JYXZZ

LC Limited Coverage **NC** Noncovered HAC associated procedure Combination Only DRG Non-OR Non-OR Revised Text in **GREEN**

188   ICD-10-PCS 2014 (Draft)

Ø   **Medical and Surgical**
6   **Lower Veins**
L   **Occlusion**   Completely closing an orifice or the lumen of a tubular body part

Body Part Character 4	Approach Character 5	Device Character 6	Qualifier Character 7
Ø Inferior Vena Cava 1 Splenic Vein 2 Gastric Vein 3 Esophageal Vein 4 Hepatic Vein 5 Superior Mesenteric Vein 6 Inferior Mesenteric Vein 7 Colic Vein 8 Portal Vein 9 Renal Vein, Right B Renal Vein, Left C Common Iliac Vein, Right D Common Iliac Vein, Left F External Iliac Vein, Right G External Iliac Vein, Left H Hypogastric Vein, Right J Hypogastric Vein, Left M Femoral Vein, Right N Femoral Vein, Left P Greater Saphenous Vein, Right Q Greater Saphenous Vein, Left R Lesser Saphenous Vein, Right S Lesser Saphenous Vein, Left T Foot Vein, Right V Foot Vein, Left	Ø Open 3 Percutaneous 4 Percutaneous Endoscopic	C Extraluminal Device D Intraluminal Device Z No Device	Z No Qualifier
Y Lower Vein	Ø Open 3 Percutaneous 4 Percutaneous Endoscopic	C Extraluminal Device D Intraluminal Device Z No Device	C Hemorrhoidal Plexus Z No Qualifier

Ø   **Medical and Surgical**
6   **Lower Veins**
N   **Release**   Freeing a body part from an abnormal physical constraint

Body Part Character 4	Approach Character 5	Device Character 6	Qualifier Character 7
Ø Inferior Vena Cava 1 Splenic Vein 2 Gastric Vein 3 Esophageal Vein 4 Hepatic Vein 5 Superior Mesenteric Vein 6 Inferior Mesenteric Vein 7 Colic Vein 8 Portal Vein 9 Renal Vein, Right B Renal Vein, Left C Common Iliac Vein, Right D Common Iliac Vein, Left F External Iliac Vein, Right G External Iliac Vein, Left H Hypogastric Vein, Right J Hypogastric Vein, Left M Femoral Vein, Right N Femoral Vein, Left P Greater Saphenous Vein, Right Q Greater Saphenous Vein, Left R Lesser Saphenous Vein, Right S Lesser Saphenous Vein, Left T Foot Vein, Right V Foot Vein, Left Y Lower Vein	Ø Open 3 Percutaneous 4 Percutaneous Endoscopic	Z No Device	Z No Qualifier

LC Limited Coverage   **NC** Noncovered   HAC associated procedure   **Combination Only**   DRG Non-OR   Non-OR   Revised Text in **GREEN**

ICD-10-PCS 2014 (Draft)   **189**

06L—06N

0   **Medical and Surgical**
6   **Lower Veins**
P   **Removal**   Taking out or off a device from a body part

Body Part Character 4	Approach Character 5	Device Character 6	Qualifier Character 7
Y Lower Vein	0 Open 3 Percutaneous 4 Percutaneous Endoscopic	0 Drainage Device 2 Monitoring Device 3 Infusion Device 7 Autologous Tissue Substitute C Extraluminal Device D Intraluminal Device J Synthetic Substitute K Nonautologous Tissue Substitute	Z No Qualifier
Y Lower Vein	X External	0 Drainage Device 2 Monitoring Device 3 Infusion Device D Intraluminal Device	Z No Qualifier

Non-OR   06PYX[0,2,3,D]Z

0   **Medical and Surgical**
6   **Lower Veins**
Q   **Repair**   Restoring, to the extent possible, a body part to its normal anatomic structure and function

Body Part Character 4	Approach Character 5	Device Character 6	Qualifier Character 7
0 Inferior Vena Cava 1 Splenic Vein 2 Gastric Vein 3 Esophageal Vein 4 Hepatic Vein 5 Superior Mesenteric Vein 6 Inferior Mesenteric Vein 7 Colic Vein 8 Portal Vein 9 Renal Vein, Right B Renal Vein, Left C Common Iliac Vein, Right D Common Iliac Vein, Left F External Iliac Vein, Right G External Iliac Vein, Left H Hypogastric Vein, Right J Hypogastric Vein, Left M Femoral Vein, Right N Femoral Vein, Left P Greater Saphenous Vein, Right Q Greater Saphenous Vein, Left R Lesser Saphenous Vein, Right S Lesser Saphenous Vein, Left T Foot Vein, Right V Foot Vein, Left Y Lower Vein	0 Open 3 Percutaneous 4 Percutaneous Endoscopic	Z No Device	Z No Qualifier

Ø   **Medical and Surgical**
6   **Lower Veins**
R   **Replacement**   Putting in or on biological or synthetic material that physically takes the place and/or function of all or a portion of a body part

Body Part Character 4	Approach Character 5	Device Character 6	Qualifier Character 7
Ø Inferior Vena Cava 1 Splenic Vein 2 Gastric Vein 3 Esophageal Vein 4 Hepatic Vein 5 Superior Mesenteric Vein 6 Inferior Mesenteric Vein 7 Colic Vein 8 Portal Vein 9 Renal Vein, Right B Renal Vein, Left C Common Iliac Vein, Right D Common Iliac Vein, Left F External Iliac Vein, Right G External Iliac Vein, Left H Hypogastric Vein, Right J Hypogastric Vein, Left M Femoral Vein, Right N Femoral Vein, Left P Greater Saphenous Vein, Right Q Greater Saphenous Vein, Left R Lesser Saphenous Vein, Right S Lesser Saphenous Vein, Left T Foot Vein, Right V Foot Vein, Left Y Lower Vein	Ø Open 4 Percutaneous Endoscopic	7 Autologous Tissue Substitute J Synthetic Substitute K Nonautologous Tissue Substitute	Z No Qualifier

Ø   **Medical and Surgical**
6   **Lower Veins**
S   **Reposition**   Moving to its normal location or other suitable location all or a portion of a body part

Body Part Character 4	Approach Character 5	Device Character 6	Qualifier Character 7
Ø Inferior Vena Cava 1 Splenic Vein 2 Gastric Vein 3 Esophageal Vein 4 Hepatic Vein 5 Superior Mesenteric Vein 6 Inferior Mesenteric Vein 7 Colic Vein 8 Portal Vein 9 Renal Vein, Right B Renal Vein, Left C Common Iliac Vein, Right D Common Iliac Vein, Left F External Iliac Vein, Right G External Iliac Vein, Left H Hypogastric Vein, Right J Hypogastric Vein, Left M Femoral Vein, Right N Femoral Vein, Left P Greater Saphenous Vein, Right Q Greater Saphenous Vein, Left R Lesser Saphenous Vein, Right S Lesser Saphenous Vein, Left T Foot Vein, Right V Foot Vein, Left Y Lower Vein	Ø Open 3 Percutaneous 4 Percutaneous Endoscopic	Z No Device	Z No Qualifier

Ø   **Medical and Surgical**
6   **Lower Veins**
U   **Supplement**   Putting in or on biological or synthetic material that physically reinforces and/or augments the function of a portion of a body part

Body Part Character 4	Approach Character 5	Device Character 6	Qualifier Character 7
Ø Inferior Vena Cava **1** Splenic Vein **2** Gastric Vein **3** Esophageal Vein **4** Hepatic Vein **5** Superior Mesenteric Vein **6** Inferior Mesenteric Vein **7** Colic Vein **8** Portal Vein **9** Renal Vein, Right **B** Renal Vein, Left **C** Common Iliac Vein, Right **D** Common Iliac Vein, Left **F** External Iliac Vein, Right **G** External Iliac Vein, Left **H** Hypogastric Vein, Right **J** Hypogastric Vein, Left **M** Femoral Vein, Right **N** Femoral Vein, Left **P** Greater Saphenous Vein, Right **Q** Greater Saphenous Vein, Left **R** Lesser Saphenous Vein, Right **S** Lesser Saphenous Vein, Left **T** Foot Vein, Right **V** Foot Vein, Left **Y** Lower Vein	**Ø** Open **3** Percutaneous **4** Percutaneous Endoscopic	**7** Autologous Tissue Substitute **J** Synthetic Substitute **K** Nonautologous Tissue Substitute	**Z** No Qualifier

Ø   **Medical and Surgical**
6   **Lower Veins**
V   **Restriction**   Partially closing an orifice or the lumen of a tubular body part

Body Part Character 4	Approach Character 5	Device Character 6	Qualifier Character 7
Ø Inferior Vena Cava **1** Splenic Vein **2** Gastric Vein **3** Esophageal Vein **4** Hepatic Vein **5** Superior Mesenteric Vein **6** Inferior Mesenteric Vein **7** Colic Vein **8** Portal Vein **9** Renal Vein, Right **B** Renal Vein, Left **C** Common Iliac Vein, Right **D** Common Iliac Vein, Left **F** External Iliac Vein, Right **G** External Iliac Vein, Left **H** Hypogastric Vein, Right **J** Hypogastric Vein, Left **M** Femoral Vein, Right **N** Femoral Vein, Left **P** Greater Saphenous Vein, Right **Q** Greater Saphenous Vein, Left **R** Lesser Saphenous Vein, Right **S** Lesser Saphenous Vein, Left **T** Foot Vein, Right **V** Foot Vein, Left **Y** Lower Vein	**Ø** Open **3** Percutaneous **4** Percutaneous Endoscopic	**C** Extraluminal Device **D** Intraluminal Device **Z** No Device	**Z** No Qualifier

LC Limited Coverage   **NC** Noncovered   HAC associated procedure   Combination Only   DRG Non-OR   Non-OR   Revised Text in **GREEN**

192   ICD-10-PCS 2014 (Draft)

0　Medical and Surgical
6　Lower Veins
W　Revision　　Correcting, to the extent possible, a portion of a malfunctioning device or the position of a displaced device

Body Part Character 4	Approach Character 5	Device Character 6	Qualifier Character 7
Y　Lower Vein	**0**　Open **3**　Percutaneous **4**　Percutaneous Endoscopic **X**　External	**0**　Drainage Device **2**　Monitoring Device **3**　Infusion Device **7**　Autologous Tissue Substitute **C**　Extraluminal Device **D**　Intraluminal Device **J**　Synthetic Substitute **K**　Nonautologous Tissue Substitute	**Z**　No Qualifier

Non-OR　　06WYX[0,2,3,7,C,D,J,K]Z

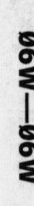

Lymphatic and Hemic Systems 072–07Y

0   **Medical and Surgical**
7   **Lymphatic and Hemic Systems**
2   **Change**   Taking out or off a device from a body part and putting back an identical or similar device in or on the same body part without cutting or puncturing the skin or a mucous membrane

Body Part Character 4	Approach Character 5	Device Character 6	Qualifier Character 7
K Thoracic Duct **L** Cisterna Chyli **M** Thymus **N** Lymphatic **P** Spleen **T** Bone Marrow	**X** External	**0** Drainage Device **Y** Other Device	**Z** No Qualifier

Non-OR   For all body part, approach, device, and qualifier values

0   **Medical and Surgical**
7   **Lymphatic and Hemic Systems**
5   **Destruction**   Physical eradication of all or a portion of a body part by the direct use of energy, force, or a destructive agent

Body Part Character 4	Approach Character 5	Device Character 6	Qualifier Character 7
0 Lymphatic, Head **1** Lymphatic, Right Neck **2** Lymphatic, Left Neck **3** Lymphatic, Right Upper Extremity **4** Lymphatic, Left Upper Extremity **5** Lymphatic, Right Axillary **6** Lymphatic, Left Axillary **7** Lymphatic, Thorax **8** Lymphatic, Internal Mammary, Right **9** Lymphatic, Internal Mammary, Left **B** Lymphatic, Mesenteric **C** Lymphatic, Pelvis **D** Lymphatic, Aortic **F** Lymphatic, Right Lower Extremity **G** Lymphatic, Left Lower Extremity **H** Lymphatic, Right Inguinal **J** Lymphatic, Left Inguinal **K** Thoracic Duct **L** Cisterna Chyli **M** Thymus **P** Spleen	**0** Open **3** Percutaneous **4** Percutaneous Endoscopic	**Z** No Device	**Z** No Qualifier

0   **Medical and Surgical**
7   **Lymphatic and Hemic Systems**
9   **Drainage**   Taking or letting out fluids and/or gases from a body part

Body Part Character 4	Approach Character 5	Device Character 6	Qualifier Character 7
0 Lymphatic, Head **1** Lymphatic, Right Neck **2** Lymphatic, Left Neck **3** Lymphatic, Right Upper Extremity **4** Lymphatic, Left Upper Extremity **5** Lymphatic, Right Axillary **6** Lymphatic, Left Axillary **7** Lymphatic, Thorax **8** Lymphatic, Internal Mammary, Right **9** Lymphatic, Internal Mammary, Left **B** Lymphatic, Mesenteric **C** Lymphatic, Pelvis **D** Lymphatic, Aortic **F** Lymphatic, Right Lower Extremity **G** Lymphatic, Left Lower Extremity **H** Lymphatic, Right Inguinal **J** Lymphatic, Left Inguinal **K** Thoracic Duct **L** Cisterna Chyli	**0** Open **3** Percutaneous **4** Percutaneous Endoscopic	**0** Drainage Device	**Z** No Qualifier

079 Continued on next page

LC Limited Coverage   **NC** Noncovered   HAC associated procedure   Combination Only   DRG Non-OR   Non-OR   Revised Text in **GREEN**

194   ICD-10-PCS 2014 (Draft)

Ø Medical and Surgical
7 Lymphatic and Hemic Systems
9 Drainage Taking or letting out fluids and/or gases from a body part

Body Part Character 4	Approach Character 5	Device Character 6	Qualifier Character 7
M Thymus P Spleen T Bone Marrow	Ø Open 3 Percutaneous 4 Percutaneous Endoscopic	Ø Drainage Device	Z No Qualifier
Ø Lymphatic, Head 1 Lymphatic, Right Neck 2 Lymphatic, Left Neck 3 Lymphatic, Right Upper Extremity 4 Lymphatic, Left Upper Extremity 5 Lymphatic, Right Axillary 6 Lymphatic, Left Axillary 7 Lymphatic, Thorax 8 Lymphatic, Internal Mammary, Right 9 Lymphatic, Internal Mammary, Left B Lymphatic, Mesenteric C Lymphatic, Pelvis D Lymphatic, Aortic F Lymphatic, Right Lower Extremity G Lymphatic, Left Lower Extremity H Lymphatic, Right Inguinal J Lymphatic, Left Inguinal K Thoracic Duct L Cisterna Chyli M Thymus P Spleen T Bone Marrow	Ø Open 3 Percutaneous 4 Percutaneous Endoscopic	Z No Device	X Diagnostic Z No Qualifier

Non-OR	079P[3,4]0Z
Non-OR	079T[0,3,4]0Z
Non-OR	079P[3,4]Z[X,Z]
Non-OR	079T[0,3,4]Z[X,Z]

Ø Medical and Surgical
7 Lymphatic and Hemic Systems
B Excision Cutting out or off, without replacement, a portion of a body part

Body Part Character 4	Approach Character 5	Device Character 6	Qualifier Character 7
Ø Lymphatic, Head 1 Lymphatic, Right Neck 2 Lymphatic, Left Neck 3 Lymphatic, Right Upper Extremity 4 Lymphatic, Left Upper Extremity 5 Lymphatic, Right Axillary 6 Lymphatic, Left Axillary 7 Lymphatic, Thorax 8 Lymphatic, Internal Mammary, Right 9 Lymphatic, Internal Mammary, Left B Lymphatic, Mesenteric C Lymphatic, Pelvis D Lymphatic, Aortic F Lymphatic, Right Lower Extremity G Lymphatic, Left Lower Extremity H Lymphatic, Right Inguinal J Lymphatic, Left Inguinal K Thoracic Duct L Cisterna Chyli M Thymus P Spleen	Ø Open 3 Percutaneous 4 Percutaneous Endoscopic	Z No Device	X Diagnostic Z No Qualifier

Non-OR	07BP[3,4]ZX

LC Limited Coverage   NC Noncovered   HAC associated procedure   Combination Only   DRG Non-OR   Non-OR   Revised Text in GREEN

Lymphatic and Hemic Systems

0   Medical and Surgical
7   Lymphatic and Hemic Systems
C   Extirpation   Taking or cutting out solid matter from a body part

Body Part Character 4	Approach Character 5	Device Character 6	Qualifier Character 7
0 Lymphatic, Head **1** Lymphatic, Right Neck **2** Lymphatic, Left Neck **3** Lymphatic, Right Upper Extremity **4** Lymphatic, Left Upper Extremity **5** Lymphatic, Right Axillary **6** Lymphatic, Left Axillary **7** Lymphatic, Thorax **8** Lymphatic, Internal Mammary, Right **9** Lymphatic, Internal Mammary, Left **B** Lymphatic, Mesenteric **C** Lymphatic, Pelvis **D** Lymphatic, Aortic **F** Lymphatic, Right Lower Extremity **G** Lymphatic, Left Lower Extremity **H** Lymphatic, Right Inguinal **J** Lymphatic, Left Inguinal **K** Thoracic Duct **L** Cisterna Chyli **M** Thymus **P** Spleen	**0** Open **3** Percutaneous **4** Percutaneous Endoscopic	**Z** No Device	**Z** No Qualifier

Non-OR   07CP[3,4]ZZ

0   Medical and Surgical
7   Lymphatic and Hemic Systems
D   Extraction   Pulling or stripping out or off all or a portion of a body part by the use of force

Body Part Character 4	Approach Character 5	Device Character 6	Qualifier Character 7
Q Bone Marrow, Sternum **R** Bone Marrow, Iliac **S** Bone Marrow, Vertebral	**0** Open **3** Percutaneous	**Z** No Device	**X** Diagnostic **Z** No Qualifier

Non-OR   For all body part, approach, device, and qualifier values

0   Medical and Surgical
7   Lymphatic and Hemic Systems
H   Insertion   Putting in a nonbiological appliance that monitors, assists, performs, or prevents a physiological function but does not physically take the place of a body part

Body Part Character 4	Approach Character 5	Device Character 6	Qualifier Character 7
K Thoracic Duct **L** Cisterna Chyli **M** Thymus **N** Lymphatic **P** Spleen	**0** Open **3** Percutaneous **4** Percutaneous Endoscopic	**3** Infusion Device	**Z** No Qualifier

Non-OR   For all body part, approach, device, and qualifier values

0   Medical and Surgical
7   Lymphatic and Hemic Systems
J   Inspection   Visually and/or manually exploring a body part

Body Part Character 4	Approach Character 5	Device Character 6	Qualifier Character 7
K Thoracic Duct **L** Cisterna Chyli **M** Thymus **T** Bone Marrow	**0** Open **3** Percutaneous **4** Percutaneous Endoscopic	**Z** No Device	**Z** No Qualifier
N Lymphatic **P** Spleen	**0** Open **3** Percutaneous **4** Percutaneous Endoscopic **X** External	**Z** No Device	**Z** No Qualifier

Non-OR   07JT[0,3,4]ZZ
Non-OR   07JNXZZ
Non-OR   07JP[3,4,X]ZZ

0 **Medical and Surgical**
7 **Lymphatic and Hemic Systems**
L **Occlusion** Completely closing an orifice or the lumen of a tubular body part

Body Part Character 4	Approach Character 5	Device Character 6	Qualifier Character 7
0 Lymphatic, Head **1** Lymphatic, Right Neck **2** Lymphatic, Left Neck **3** Lymphatic, Right Upper Extremity **4** Lymphatic, Left Upper Extremity **5** Lymphatic, Right Axillary **6** Lymphatic, Left Axillary **7** Lymphatic, Thorax **8** Lymphatic, Internal Mammary, Right **9** Lymphatic, Internal Mammary, Left **B** Lymphatic, Mesenteric **C** Lymphatic, Pelvis **D** Lymphatic, Aortic **F** Lymphatic, Right Lower Extremity **G** Lymphatic, Left Lower Extremity **H** Lymphatic, Right Inguinal **J** Lymphatic, Left Inguinal **K** Thoracic Duct **L** Cisterna Chyli	**0** Open **3** Percutaneous **4** Percutaneous Endoscopic	**C** Extraluminal Device **D** Intraluminal Device **Z** No Device	**Z** No Qualifier

0 **Medical and Surgical**
7 **Lymphatic and Hemic Systems**
N **Release** Freeing a body part from an abnormal physical constraint

Body Part Character 4	Approach Character 5	Device Character 6	Qualifier Character 7
0 Lymphatic, Head **1** Lymphatic, Right Neck **2** Lymphatic, Left Neck **3** Lymphatic, Right Upper Extremity **4** Lymphatic, Left Upper Extremity **5** Lymphatic, Right Axillary **6** Lymphatic, Left Axillary **7** Lymphatic, Thorax **8** Lymphatic, Internal Mammary, Right **9** Lymphatic, Internal Mammary, Left **B** Lymphatic, Mesenteric **C** Lymphatic, Pelvis **D** Lymphatic, Aortic **F** Lymphatic, Right Lower Extremity **G** Lymphatic, Left Lower Extremity **H** Lymphatic, Right Inguinal **J** Lymphatic, Left Inguinal **K** Thoracic Duct **L** Cisterna Chyli **M** Thymus **P** Spleen	**0** Open **3** Percutaneous **4** Percutaneous Endoscopic	**Z** No Device	**Z** No Qualifier

0 **Medical and Surgical**
7 **Lymphatic and Hemic Systems**
P **Removal** Taking out or off a device from a body part

Body Part Character 4	Approach Character 5	Device Character 6	Qualifier Character 7
K Thoracic Duct **L** Cisterna Chyli **N** Lymphatic	**0** Open **3** Percutaneous **4** Percutaneous Endoscopic	**0** Drainage Device **3** Infusion Device **7** Autologous Tissue Substitute **C** Extraluminal Device **D** Intraluminal Device **J** Synthetic Substitute **K** Nonautologous Tissue Substitute	**Z** No Qualifier
K Thoracic Duct **L** Cisterna Chyli **N** Lymphatic	**X** External	**0** Drainage Device **3** Infusion Device **D** Intraluminal Device	**Z** No Qualifier

07P Continued on next page

Non-OR 07P[K,L,N]X[0,3,D]Z

Lymphatic and Hemic Systems

07P–07S

0 Medical and Surgicall
7 Lymphatic and Hemic Systems
P Removal   Taking out or off a device from a body part

Body Part Character 4	Approach Character 5	Device Character 6	Qualifier Character 7
M Thymus **P** Spleen	**0** Open **3** Percutaneous **4** Percutaneous Endoscopic **X** External	**0** Drainage Device **3** Infusion Device	**Z** No Qualifier
T Bone Marrow	**0** Open **3** Percutaneous **4** Percutaneous Endoscopic **X** External	**0** Drainage Device	**Z** No Qualifier

Non-OR   07P[M,P]X[0,3]Z
Non-OR   07PT[0,3,4,X]0Z

0 Medical and Surgical
7 Lymphatic and Hemic Systems
Q Repair   Restoring, to the extent possible, a body part to its normal anatomic structure and function

Body Part Character 4	Approach Character 5	Device Character 6	Qualifier Character 7
0 Lymphatic, Head **1** Lymphatic, Right Neck **2** Lymphatic, Left Neck **3** Lymphatic, Right Upper Extremity **4** Lymphatic, Left Upper Extremity **5** Lymphatic, Right Axillary **6** Lymphatic, Left Axillary **7** Lymphatic, Thorax **8** Lymphatic, Internal Mammary, Right **9** Lymphatic, Internal Mammary, Left **B** Lymphatic, Mesenteric **C** Lymphatic, Pelvis **D** Lymphatic, Aortic **F** Lymphatic, Right Lower Extremity **G** Lymphatic, Left Lower Extremity **H** Lymphatic, Right Inguinal **J** Lymphatic, Left Inguinal **K** Thoracic Duct **L** Cisterna Chyli **M** Thymus **P** Spleen	**0** Open **3** Percutaneous **4** Percutaneous Endoscopic	**Z** No Device	**Z** No Qualifier

0 Medical and Surgical
7 Lymphatic and Hemic Systems
S Reposition   Moving to its normal location or other suitable location all or a portion of a body part

Body Part Character 4	Approach Character 5	Device Character 6	Qualifier Character 7
M Thymus **P** Spleen	**0** Open	**Z** No Device	**Z** No Qualifier

0   **Medical and Surgical**
7   **Lymphatic and Hemic Systems**
T   **Resection**   Cutting out or off, without replacement, all of a body part

Body Part Character 4	Approach Character 5	Device Character 6	Qualifier Character 7
0 Lymphatic, Head	**0** Open	**Z** No Device	**Z** No Qualifier
1 Lymphatic, Right Neck	**4** Percutaneous Endoscopic		
2 Lymphatic, Left Neck			
3 Lymphatic, Right Upper Extremity			
4 Lymphatic, Left Upper Extremity			
5 Lymphatic, Right Axillary			
6 Lymphatic, Left Axillary			
7 Lymphatic, Thorax			
8 Lymphatic, Internal Mammary, Right			
9 Lymphatic, Internal Mammary, Left			
B Lymphatic, Mesenteric			
C Lymphatic, Pelvis			
D Lymphatic, Aortic			
F Lymphatic, Right Lower Extremity			
G Lymphatic, Left Lower Extremity			
H Lymphatic, Right Inguinal			
J Lymphatic, Left Inguinal			
K Thoracic Duct			
L Cisterna Chyli			
M Thymus			
P Spleen			

0   **Medical and Surgical**
7   **Lymphatic and Hemic Systems**
U   **Supplement**   Putting in or on biological or synthetic material that physically reinforces and/or augments the function of a portion of a body part

Body Part Character 4	Approach Character 5	Device Character 6	Qualifier Character 7
0 Lymphatic, Head	**0** Open	**7** Autologous Tissue Substitute	**Z** No Qualifier
1 Lymphatic, Right Neck	**4** Percutaneous Endoscopic	**J** Synthetic Substitute	
2 Lymphatic, Left Neck		**K** Nonautologous Tissue Substitute	
3 Lymphatic, Right Upper Extremity			
4 Lymphatic, Left Upper Extremity			
5 Lymphatic, Right Axillary			
6 Lymphatic, Left Axillary			
7 Lymphatic, Thorax			
8 Lymphatic, Internal Mammary, Right			
9 Lymphatic, Internal Mammary, Left			
B Lymphatic, Mesenteric			
C Lymphatic, Pelvis			
D Lymphatic, Aortic			
F Lymphatic, Right Lower Extremity			
G Lymphatic, Left Lower Extremity			
H Lymphatic, Right Inguinal			
J Lymphatic, Left Inguinal			
K Thoracic Duct			
L Cisterna Chyli			

Ø **Medical and Surgical**
7 **Lymphatic and Hemic Systems**
V **Restriction**   Partially closing an orifice or the lumen of a tubular body part

Body Part Character 4	Approach Character 5	Device Character 6	Qualifier Character 7
Ø Lymphatic, Head	Ø Open	C Extraluminal Device	Z No Qualifier
1 Lymphatic, Right Neck	3 Percutaneous	D Intraluminal Device	
2 Lymphatic, Left Neck	4 Percutaneous Endoscopic	Z No Device	
3 Lymphatic, Right Upper Extremity			
4 Lymphatic, Left Upper Extremity			
5 Lymphatic, Right Axillary			
6 Lymphatic, Left Axillary			
7 Lymphatic, Thorax			
8 Lymphatic, Internal Mammary, Right			
9 Lymphatic, Internal Mammary, Left			
B Lymphatic, Mesenteric			
C Lymphatic, Pelvis			
D Lymphatic, Aortic			
F Lymphatic, Right Lower Extremity			
G Lymphatic, Left Lower Extremity			
H Lymphatic, Right Inguinal			
J Lymphatic, Left Inguinal			
K Thoracic Duct			
L Cisterna Chyli			

Ø **Medical and Surgical**
7 **Lymphatic and Hemic Systems**
W **Revision**   Correcting, to the extent possible, a portion of a malfunctioning device or the position of a displaced device

Body Part Character 4	Approach Character 5	Device Character 6	Qualifier Character 7
K Thoracic Duct	Ø Open	Ø Drainage Device	Z No Qualifier
L Cisterna Chyli	3 Percutaneous	3 Infusion Device	
N Lymphatic	4 Percutaneous Endoscopic	7 Autologous Tissue Substitute	
	X External	C Extraluminal Device	
		D Intraluminal Device	
		J Synthetic Substitute	
		K Nonautologous Tissue Substitute	
M Thymus	Ø Open	Ø Drainage Device	Z No Qualifier
P Spleen	3 Percutaneous	3 Infusion Device	
	4 Percutaneous Endoscopic		
	X External		
T Bone Marrow	Ø Open	Ø Drainage Device	Z No Qualifier
	3 Percutaneous		
	4 Percutaneous Endoscopic		
	X External		

Non-OR   Ø7W[K,L,N]X[Ø,3,7,C,D,J,K]Z
Non-OR   Ø7W[M,P]X[Ø,3]Z
Non-OR   Ø7WT[Ø,3,4,X]ØZ

Ø **Medical and Surgical**
7 **Lymphatic and Hemic Systems**
Y **Transplantation** Putting in or on all or a portion of a living body part taken from another individual or animal to physically take the place and/or function of
all or a portion of a similar body part

Body Part Character 4	Approach Character 5	Device Character 6	Qualifier Character 7
M Thymus	Ø Open	Z No Device	Ø Allogeneic
P Spleen			1 Syngeneic
			2 Zooplastic

Eye 080–08X

0　Medical and Surgical
8　Eye
0　Alteration　　Modifying the anatomic structure of a body part without affecting the function of the body part

Body Part Character 4	Approach Character 5	Device Character 6	Qualifier Character 7
N Upper Eyelid, Right P Upper Eyelid, Left Q Lower Eyelid, Right R Lower Eyelid, Left	0 Open 3 Percutaneous X External	7 Autologous Tissue Substitute J Synthetic Substitute K Nonautologous Tissue Substitute Z No Device	Z No Qualifier

Non-OR　For all body part, approach, device, and qualifier values

0　Medical and Surgical
8　Eye
1　Bypass　　Altering the route of passage of the contents of a tubular body part

Body Part Character 4	Approach Character 5	Device Character 6	Qualifier Character 7
2 Anterior Chamber, Right 3 Anterior Chamber, Left	3 Percutaneous	J Synthetic Substitute K Nonautologous Tissue Substitute Z No Device	4 Sclera
X Lacrimal Duct, Right Y Lacrimal Duct, Left	0 Open 3 Percutaneous	J Synthetic Substitute K Nonautologous Tissue Substitute Z No Device	3 Nasal Cavity

0　Medical and Surgical
8　Eye
2　Change　　Taking out or off a device from a body part and putting back an identical or similar device in or on the same body part without cutting or puncturing the skin or a mucous membrane

Body Part Character 4	Approach Character 5	Device Character 6	Qualifier Character 7
0 Eye, Right 1 Eye, Left	X External	0 Drainage Device Y Other Device	Z No Qualifier

Non-OR　For all body part, approach, device, and qualifier values

0　Medical and Surgical
8　Eye
5　Destruction　　Physical eradication of all or a portion of a body part by the direct use of energy, force, or a destructive agent

Body Part Character 4	Approach Character 5	Device Character 6	Qualifier Character 7
0 Eye, Right 1 Eye, Left 6 Sclera, Right 7 Sclera, Left 8 Cornea, Right 9 Cornea, Left S Conjunctiva, Right T Conjunctiva, Left	X External	Z No Device	Z No Qualifier
2 Anterior Chamber, Right 3 Anterior Chamber, Left 4 Vitreous, Right 5 Vitreous, Left C Iris, Right D Iris, Left E Retina, Right F Retina, Left G Retinal Vessel, Right H Retinal Vessel, Left J Lens, Right K Lens, Left	3 Percutaneous	Z No Device	Z No Qualifier
A Choroid, Right B Choroid, Left L Extraocular Muscle, Right M Extraocular Muscle, Left V Lacrimal Gland, Right W Lacrimal Gland, Left	0 Open 3 Percutaneous	Z No Device	Z No Qualifier
N Upper Eyelid, Right P Upper Eyelid, Left Q Lower Eyelid, Right R Lower Eyelid, Left	0 Open 3 Percutaneous X External	Z No Device	Z No Qualifier

085 Continued on next page

LC Limited Coverage　　NC Noncovered　　HAC associated procedure　　Combination Only　　DRG Non-OR　　Non-OR　　Revised Text in GREEN

Ø   Medical and Surgical
8   Eye   *Ø85 Continued*
5   Destruction   Physical eradication of all or a portion of a body part by the direct use of energy, force, or a destructive agent

Body Part Character 4	Approach Character 5	Device Character 6	Qualifier Character 7
X Lacrimal Duct, Right Y Lacrimal Duct, Left	Ø Open 3 Percutaneous 7 Via Natural or Artificial Opening 8 Via Natural or Artificial Opening Endoscopic	Z No Device	Z No Qualifier

Ø   Medical and Surgical
8   Eye
7   Dilation   Expanding an orifice or the lumen of a tubular body part

Body Part Character 4	Approach Character 5	Device Character 6	Qualifier Character 7
X Lacrimal Duct, Right Y Lacrimal Duct, Left	Ø Open 3 Percutaneous 7 Via Natural or Artificial Opening 8 Via Natural or Artificial Opening Endoscopic	D Intraluminal Device Z No Device	Z No Qualifier

Ø   Medical and Surgical
8   Eye
9   Drainage   Taking or letting out fluids and/or gases from a body part

Body Part Character 4	Approach Character 5	Device Character 6	Qualifier Character 7
Ø Eye, Right 1 Eye, Left 6 Sclera, Right 7 Sclera, Left 8 Cornea, Right 9 Cornea, Left S Conjunctiva, Right T Conjunctiva, Left	X External	Ø Drainage Device	Z No Qualifier
Ø Eye, Right 1 Eye, Left 6 Sclera, Right 7 Sclera, Left 8 Cornea, Right 9 Cornea, Left S Conjunctiva, Right T Conjunctiva, Left	X External	Z No Device	X Diagnostic Z No Qualifier
2 Anterior Chamber, Right 3 Anterior Chamber, Left 4 Vitreous, Right 5 Vitreous, Left C Iris, Right D Iris, Left E Retina, Right F Retina, Left G Retinal Vessel, Right H Retinal Vessel, Left J Lens, Right K Lens, Left	3 Percutaneous	Ø Drainage Device	Z No Qualifier
2 Anterior Chamber, Right 3 Anterior Chamber, Left 4 Vitreous, Right 5 Vitreous, Left C Iris, Right D Iris, Left E Retina, Right F Retina, Left G Retinal Vessel, Right H Retinal Vessel, Left J Lens, Right K Lens, Left	3 Percutaneous	Z No Device	X Diagnostic Z No Qualifier

Ø89 Continued on next page

0 Medical and Surgical
8 Eye
9 Drainage   Taking or letting out fluids and/or gases from a body part

089 Continued

Body Part Character 4	Approach Character 5	Device Character 6	Qualifier Character 7
A Choroid, Right B Choroid, Left L Extraocular Muscle, Right M Extraocular Muscle, Left V Lacrimal Gland, Right W Lacrimal Gland, Left	0 Open 3 Percutaneous	0 Drainage Device	Z No Qualifier
A Choroid, Right B Choroid, Left L Extraocular Muscle, Right M Extraocular Muscle, Left V Lacrimal Gland, Right W Lacrimal Gland, Left	0 Open 3 Percutaneous	Z No Device	X Diagnostic Z No Qualifier
N Upper Eyelid, Right P Upper Eyelid, Left Q Lower Eyelid, Right R Lower Eyelid, Left	0 Open 3 Percutaneous X External	0 Drainage Device	Z No Qualifier
N Upper Eyelid, Right P Upper Eyelid, Left Q Lower Eyelid, Right R Lower Eyelid, Left	0 Open 3 Percutaneous X External	Z No Device	X Diagnostic Z No Qualifier
X Lacrimal Duct, Right Y Lacrimal Duct, Left	0 Open 3 Percutaneous 7 Via Natural or Artificial Opening 8 Via Natural or Artificial Opening Endoscopic	0 Drainage Device	Z No Qualifier
X Lacrimal Duct, Right Y Lacrimal Duct, Left	0 Open 3 Percutaneous 7 Via Natural or Artificial Opening 8 Via Natural or Artificial Opening Endoscopic	Z No Device	X Diagnostic Z No Qualifier

Non-OR   089[N,P,Q,R][0,3,X]0Z
Non-OR   089[N,P,Q,R][0,3,X]ZZ

0 Medical and Surgical
8 Eye
B Excision   Cutting out or off, without replacement, a portion of a body part

Body Part Character 4	Approach Character 5	Device Character 6	Qualifier Character 7
0 Eye, Right 1 Eye, Left N Upper Eyelid, Right P Upper Eyelid, Left Q Lower Eyelid, Right R Lower Eyelid, Left	0 Open 3 Percutaneous X External	Z No Device	X Diagnostic Z No Qualifier
4 Vitreous, Right 5 Vitreous, Left C Iris, Right D Iris, Left E Retina, Right F Retina, Left J Lens, Right K Lens, Left	3 Percutaneous	Z No Device	X Diagnostic Z No Qualifier
6 Sclera, Right 7 Sclera, Left 8 Cornea, Right 9 Cornea, Left S Conjunctiva, Right T Conjunctiva, Left	X External	Z No Device	X Diagnostic Z No Qualifier
A Choroid, Right B Choroid, Left L Extraocular Muscle, Right M Extraocular Muscle, Left V Lacrimal Gland, Right W Lacrimal Gland, Left	0 Open 3 Percutaneous	Z No Device	X Diagnostic Z No Qualifier
X Lacrimal Duct, Right Y Lacrimal Duct, Left	0 Open 3 Percutaneous 7 Via Natural or Artificial Opening 8 Via Natural or Artificial Opening Endoscopic	Z No Device	X Diagnostic Z No Qualifier

LC Limited Coverage   NC Noncovered   HAC associated procedure   Combination Only   DRG Non-OR   Non-OR   Revised Text in GREEN

Eye

08C–08F

0   **Medical and Surgical**
8   **Eye**
C   **Extirpation**   Taking or cutting out solid matter from a body part

Body Part Character 4	Approach Character 5	Device Character 6	Qualifier Character 7
0 Eye, Right **1** Eye, Left **6** Sclera, Right **7** Sclera, Left **8** Cornea, Right **9** Cornea, Left **S** Conjunctiva, Right **T** Conjunctiva, Left	**X** External	**Z** No Device	**Z** No Qualifier
2 Anterior Chamber, Right **3** Anterior Chamber, Left **4** Vitreous, Right **5** Vitreous, Left **C** Iris, Right **D** Iris, Left **E** Retina, Right **F** Retina, Left **G** Retinal Vessel, Right **H** Retinal Vessel, Left **J** Lens, Right **K** Lens, Left	**3** Percutaneous **X** External	**Z** No Device	**Z** No Qualifier
A Choroid, Right **B** Choroid, Left **L** Extraocular Muscle, Right **M** Extraocular Muscle, Left **N** Upper Eyelid, Right **P** Upper Eyelid, Left **Q** Lower Eyelid, Right **R** Lower Eyelid, Left **V** Lacrimal Gland, Right **W** Lacrimal Gland, Left	**0** Open **3** Percutaneous **X** External	**Z** No Device	**Z** No Qualifier
X Lacrimal Duct, Right **Y** Lacrimal Duct, Left	**0** Open **3** Percutaneous **7** Via Natural or Artificial Opening **8** Via Natural or Artificial Opening Endoscopic	**Z** No Device	**Z** No Qualifier

Non-OR   08C[6,7]XZZ
Non-OR   08C[2,3]XZZ
Non-OR   08C[N,P,Q,R][0,3,X]ZZ

0   **Medical and Surgical**
8   **Eye**
D   **Extraction**   Pulling or stripping out or off all or a portion of a body part by the use of force

Body Part Character 4	Approach Character 5	Device Character 6	Qualifier Character 7
8 Cornea, Right **9** Cornea, Left	**X** External	**Z** No Device	**X** Diagnostic **Z** No Qualifier
J Lens, Right **K** Lens, Left	**3** Percutaneous	**Z** No Device	**Z** No Qualifier

0   **Medical and Surgical**
8   **Eye**
F   **Fragmentation**   Breaking solid matter in a body part into pieces

Body Part Character 4	Approach Character 5	Device Character 6	Qualifier Character 7
4 Vitreous, Right NC **5** Vitreous, Left NC	**3** Percutaneous **X** External	**Z** No Device	**Z** No Qualifier

NC   08F[4,5]XZZ
Non-OR   08F[4,5]XZZ

LC Limited Coverage   **NC** Noncovered   HAC associated procedure   Combination Only   DRG Non-OR   Non-OR   Revised Text in **GREEN**

204   ICD-10-PCS 2014 (Draft)

0 Medical and Surgical
8 Eye
H Insertion Putting in a nonbiological appliance that monitors, assists, performs, or prevents a physiological function but does not physically take the place of a body part

Body Part Character 4	Approach Character 5	Device Character 6	Qualifier Character 7
0 Eye, Right 1 Eye, Left	0 Open	5 Epiretinal Visual Prosthesis	Z No Qualifier
0 Eye, Right 1 Eye, Left	3 Percutaneous X External	1 Radioactive Element 3 Infusion Device	Z No Qualifier

0 Medical and Surgical
8 Eye
J Inspection Visually and/or manually exploring a body part

Body Part Character 4	Approach Character 5	Device Character 6	Qualifier Character 7
0 Eye, Right 1 Eye, Left J Lens, Right K Lens, Left	X External	Z No Device	Z No Qualifier
L Extraocular Muscle, Right M Extraocular Muscle, Left	0 Open X External	Z No Device	Z No Qualifier

0 Medical and Surgical
8 Eye
L Occlusion Completely closing an orifice or the lumen of a tubular body part

Body Part Character 4	Approach Character 5	Device Character 6	Qualifier Character 7
X Lacrimal Duct, Right Y Lacrimal Duct, Left	0 Open 3 Percutaneous	C Extraluminal Device D Intraluminal Device Z No Device	Z No Qualifier
X Lacrimal Duct, Right Y Lacrimal Duct, Left	7 Via Natural or Artificial Opening 8 Via Natural or Artificial Opening Endoscopic	D Intraluminal Device Z No Device	Z No Qualifier

0 Medical and Surgical
8 Eye
M Reattachment Putting back in or on all or a portion of a separated body part to its normal location or other suitable location

Body Part Character 4	Approach Character 5	Device Character 6	Qualifier Character 7
N Upper Eyelid, Right P Upper Eyelid, Left Q Lower Eyelid, Right R Lower Eyelid, Left	X External	Z No Device	Z No Qualifier

0 Medical and Surgical
8 Eye
N Release Freeing a body part from an abnormal physical constraint

Body Part Character 4	Approach Character 5	Device Character 6	Qualifier Character 7
0 Eye, Right 1 Eye, Left 6 Sclera, Right 7 Sclera, Left 8 Cornea, Right 9 Cornea, Left S Conjunctiva, Right T Conjunctiva, Left	X External	Z No Device	Z No Qualifier
2 Anterior Chamber, Right 3 Anterior Chamber, Left 4 Vitreous, Right 5 Vitreous, Left C Iris, Right D Iris, Left E Retina, Right F Retina, Left G Retinal Vessel, Right H Retinal Vessel, Left J Lens, Right K Lens, Left	3 Percutaneous	Z No Device	Z No Qualifier

08N Continued on next page

Ø **Medical and Surgical**

Ø8N Continued

8 **Eye**

N **Release** Freeing a body part from an abnormal physical constraint

Body Part Character 4	Approach Character 5	Device Character 6	Qualifier Character 7
A Choroid, Right **B** Choroid, Left **L** Extraocular Muscle, Right **M** Extraocular Muscle, Left **V** Lacrimal Gland, Right **W** Lacrimal Gland, Left	**Ø** Open **3** Percutaneous	**Z** No Device	**Z** No Qualifier
N Upper Eyelid, Right **P** Upper Eyelid, Left **Q** Lower Eyelid, Right **R** Lower Eyelid, Left	**Ø** Open **3** Percutaneous **X** External	**Z** No Device	**Z** No Qualifier
X Lacrimal Duct, Right **Y** Lacrimal Duct, Left	**Ø** Open **3** Percutaneous **7** Via Natural or Artificial Opening **8** Via Natural or Artificial Opening Endoscopic	**Z** No Device	**Z** No Qualifier

Ø **Medical and Surgical**

8 **Eye**

P **Removal** Taking out or off a device from a body part

Body Part Character 4	Approach Character 5	Device Character 6	Qualifier Character 7
Ø Eye, Right **1** Eye, Left	**Ø** Open **3** Percutaneous **7** Via Natural or Artificial Opening **8** Via Natural or Artificial Opening Endoscopic **X** External	**Ø** Drainage Device **1** Radioactive Element **3** Infusion Device **7** Autologous Tissue Substitute **C** Extraluminal Device **D** Intraluminal Device **J** Synthetic Substitute **K** Nonautologous Tissue Substitute	**Z** No Qualifier
J Lens, Right **K** Lens, Left	**3** Percutaneous	**J** Synthetic Substitute	**Z** No Qualifier
L Extraocular Muscle, Right **M** Extraocular Muscle, Left	**Ø** Open **3** Percutaneous	**Ø** Drainage Device **7** Autologous Tissue Substitute **J** Synthetic Substitute **K** Nonautologous Tissue Substitute	**Z** No Qualifier

Non-OR Ø8P[Ø,1]X[Ø,1,3,C,D]Z

Ø **Medical and Surgical**

8 **Eye**

Q **Repair** Restoring, to the extent possible, a body part to its normal anatomic structure and function

Body Part Character 4	Approach Character 5	Device Character 6	Qualifier Character 7
Ø Eye, Right **1** Eye, Left **6** Sclera, Right **7** Sclera, Left **8** Cornea, Right NC **9** Cornea, Left NC **S** Conjunctiva, Right **T** Conjunctiva, Left	**X** External	**Z** No Device	**Z** No Qualifier
2 Anterior Chamber, Right **3** Anterior Chamber, Left **4** Vitreous, Right **5** Vitreous, Left **C** Iris, Right **D** Iris, Left **E** Retina, Right **F** Retina, Left **G** Retinal Vessel, Right **H** Retinal Vessel, Left **J** Lens, Right **K** Lens, Left	**3** Percutaneous	**Z** No Device	**Z** No Qualifier

Ø8Q Continued on next page

NC	Ø8Q[8,9]XZZ
Non-OR	Ø8Q[N,P,Q,R][Ø,3,X]ZZ

LC Limited Coverage   **NC** Noncovered   HAC associated procedure   Combination Only   DRG Non-OR   Non-OR   Revised Text in **GREEN**

206   ICD-1Ø-PCS 2014 (Draft)

Ø Medical and Surgical
8 Eye
Q Repair   Restoring, to the extent possible, a body part to its normal anatomic structure and function

Ø8Q Continued

Body Part Character 4	Approach Character 5	Device Character 6	Qualifier Character 7
A Choroid, Right B Choroid, Left L Extraocular Muscle, Right M Extraocular Muscle, Left V Lacrimal Gland, Right W Lacrimal Gland, Left	Ø Open 3 Percutaneous	Z No Device	Z No Qualifier
N Upper Eyelid, Right P Upper Eyelid, Left Q Lower Eyelid, Right R Lower Eyelid, Left	Ø Open 3 Percutaneous X External	Z No Device	Z No Qualifier
X Lacrimal Duct, Right Y Lacrimal Duct, Left	Ø Open 3 Percutaneous 7 Via Natural or Artificial Opening 8 Via Natural or Artificial Opening Endoscopic	Z No Device	Z No Qualifier

Ø Medical and Surgical
8 Eye
R Replacement   Putting in or on biological or synthetic material that physically takes the place and/or function of all or a portion of a body part

Body Part Character 4	Approach Character 5	Device Character 6	Qualifier Character 7
Ø Eye, Right 1 Eye, Left A Choroid, Right B Choroid, Left	Ø Open 3 Percutaneous	7 Autologous Tissue Substitute J Synthetic Substitute K Nonautologous Tissue Substitute	Z No Qualifier
4 Vitreous, Right 5 Vitreous, Left C Iris, Right D Iris, Left G Retinal Vessel, Right H Retinal Vessel, Left	3 Percutaneous	7 Autologous Tissue Substitute J Synthetic Substitute K Nonautologous Tissue Substitute	Z No Qualifier
6 Sclera, Right 7 Sclera, Left S Conjunctiva, Right T Conjunctiva, Left	X External	7 Autologous Tissue Substitute J Synthetic Substitute K Nonautologous Tissue Substitute	Z No Qualifier
8 Cornea, Right 9 Cornea, Left	3 Percutaneous X External	7 Autologous Tissue Substitute J Synthetic Substitute K Nonautologous Tissue Substitute	Z No Qualifier
J Lens, Right K Lens, Left	3 Percutaneous	Ø Synthetic Substitute, Intraocular Telescope 7 Autologous Tissue Substitute J Synthetic Substitute K Nonautologous Tissue Substitute	Z No Qualifier
N Upper Eyelid, Right P Upper Eyelid, Left Q Lower Eyelid, Right R Lower Eyelid, Left	Ø Open 3 Percutaneous X External	7 Autologous Tissue Substitute J Synthetic Substitute K Nonautologous Tissue Substitute	Z No Qualifier
X Lacrimal Duct, Right Y Lacrimal Duct, Left	Ø Open 3 Percutaneous 7 Via Natural or Artificial Opening 8 Via Natural or Artificial Opening Endoscopic	7 Autologous Tissue Substitute J Synthetic Substitute K Nonautologous Tissue Substitute	Z No Qualifier

Ø Medical and Surgical
8 Eye
S Reposition   Moving to its normal location or other suitable location all or a portion of a body part

Body Part Character 4	Approach Character 5	Device Character 6	Qualifier Character 7
C Iris, Right D Iris, Left G Retinal Vessel, Right H Retinal Vessel, Left J Lens, Right K Lens, Left	3 Percutaneous	Z No Device	Z No Qualifier

Ø8S Continued on next page

Ø   **Medical and Surgical**   *Ø8S Continued*
8   **Eye**
S   **Reposition**   Moving to its normal location or other suitable location all or a portion of a body part

Body Part Character 4	Approach Character 5	Device Character 6	Qualifier Character 7
L Extraocular Muscle, Right **M** Extraocular Muscle, Left **V** Lacrimal Gland, Right **W** Lacrimal Gland, Left	**Ø** Open **3** Percutaneous	**Z** No Device	**Z** No Qualifier
N Upper Eyelid, Right **P** Upper Eyelid, Left **Q** Lower Eyelid, Right **R** Lower Eyelid, Left	**Ø** Open **3** Percutaneous **X** External	**Z** No Device	**Z** No Qualifier
X Lacrimal Duct, Right **Y** Lacrimal Duct, Left	**Ø** Open **3** Percutaneous **7** Via Natural or Artificial Opening **8** Via Natural or Artificial Opening Endoscopic	**Z** No Device	**Z** No Qualifier

Ø   **Medical and Surgical**
8   **Eye**
T   **Resection**   Cutting out or off, without replacement, all of a body part

Body Part Character 4	Approach Character 5	Device Character 6	Qualifier Character 7
Ø Eye, Right **1** Eye, Left **8** Cornea, Right **9** Cornea, Left	**X** External	**Z** No Device	**Z** No Qualifier
4 Vitreous, Right **5** Vitreous, Left **C** Iris, Right **D** Iris, Left **J** Lens, Right **K** Lens, Left	**3** Percutaneous	**Z** No Device	**Z** No Qualifier
L Extraocular Muscle, Right **M** Extraocular Muscle, Left **V** Lacrimal Gland, Right **W** Lacrimal Gland, Left	**Ø** Open **3** Percutaneous	**Z** No Device	**Z** No Qualifier
N Upper Eyelid, Right **P** Upper Eyelid, Left **Q** Lower Eyelid, Right **R** Lower Eyelid, Left	**Ø** Open **X** External	**Z** No Device	**Z** No Qualifier
X Lacrimal Duct, Right **Y** Lacrimal Duct, Left	**Ø** Open **3** Percutaneous **7** Via Natural or Artificial Opening **8** Via Natural or Artificial Opening Endoscopic	**Z** No Device	**Z** No Qualifier

LC Limited Coverage   **NC** Noncovered   HAC associated procedure   Combination Only   DRG Non-OR   Non-OR   Revised Text in **GREEN**

208   ICD-10-PCS 2014 (Draft)

0　Medical and Surgical
8　Eye
U　Supplement　　　Putting in or on biological or synthetic material that physically reinforces and/or augments the function of a portion of a body part

Body Part Character 4	Approach Character 5	Device Character 6	Qualifier Character 7
0 Eye, Right 1 Eye, Left C Iris, Right D Iris, Left E Retina, Right F Retina, Left G Retinal Vessel, Right H Retinal Vessel, Left L Extraocular Muscle, Right M Extraocular Muscle, Left	0 Open 3 Percutaneous	7 Autologous Tissue Substitute J Synthetic Substitute K Nonautologous Tissue Substitute	Z No Qualifier
8 Cornea, Right　NC 9 Cornea, Left　NC N Upper Eyelid, Right P Upper Eyelid, Left Q Lower Eyelid, Right R Lower Eyelid, Left	0 Open 3 Percutaneous X External	7 Autologous Tissue Substitute J Synthetic Substitute K Nonautologous Tissue Substitute	Z No Qualifier
X Lacrimal Duct, Right Y Lacrimal Duct, Left	0 Open 3 Percutaneous 7 Via Natural or Artificial Opening 8 Via Natural or Artificial Opening 　 Endoscopic	7 Autologous Tissue Substitute J Synthetic Substitute K Nonautologous Tissue Substitute	Z No Qualifier

NC　08U8[0,3,X]KZ
NC　08U9[0,3,X]KZ

0　Medical and Surgical
8　Eye
V　Restriction　　　Partially closing an orifice or the lumen of a tubular body part

Body Part Character 4	Approach Character 5	Device Character 6	Qualifier Character 7
X Lacrimal Duct, Right Y Lacrimal Duct, Left	0 Open 3 Percutaneous	C Extraluminal Device D Intraluminal Device Z No Device	Z No Qualifier
X Lacrimal Duct, Right Y Lacrimal Duct, Left	7 Via Natural or Artificial Opening 8 Via Natural or Artificial Opening 　 Endoscopic	D Intraluminal Device Z No Device	Z No Qualifier

0　Medical and Surgical
8　Eye
W　Revision　　　Correcting, to the extent possible, a portion of a malfunctioning device or the position of a displaced device

Body Part Character 4	Approach Character 5	Device Character 6	Qualifier Character 7
0 Eye, Right 1 Eye, Left	0 Open 3 Percutaneous 7 Via Natural or Artificial Opening 8 Via Natural or Artificial Opening 　 Endoscopic X External	0 Drainage Device 3 Infusion Device 7 Autologous Tissue Substitute C Extraluminal Device D Intraluminal Device J Synthetic Substitute K Nonautologous Tissue Substitute	Z No Qualifier
J Lens, Right K Lens, Left	3 Percutaneous X External	J Synthetic Substitute	Z No Qualifier
L Extraocular Muscle, Right M Extraocular Muscle, Left	0 Open 3 Percutaneous	0 Drainage Device 7 Autologous Tissue Substitute J Synthetic Substitute K Nonautologous Tissue Substitute	Z No Qualifier

Non-OR　08W[0,1]X[0,3,7,C,D,J,K]Z
Non-OR　08W[J,K]XJZ

0　Medical and Surgical
8　Eye
X　Transfer　　　Moving, without taking out, all or a portion of a body part to another location to take over the function of all or a portion of a body part

Body Part Character 4	Approach Character 5	Device Character 6	Qualifier Character 7
L Extraocular Muscle, Right M Extraocular Muscle, Left	0 Open 3 Percutaneous	Z No Device	Z No Qualifier

Ear, Nose, Sinus 090–09W

0   **Medical and Surgical**
9   **Ear, Nose, Sinus**
0   **Alteration**   Modifying the anatomic structure of a body part without affecting the function of the body part

Body Part Character 4	Approach Character 5	Device Character 6	Qualifier Character 7
0 External Ear, Right **1** External Ear, Left **2** External Ear, Bilateral **K** Nose	**0** Open **3** Percutaneous **4** Percutaneous Endoscopic **X** External	**7** Autologous Tissue Substitute **J** Synthetic Substitute **K** Nonautologous Tissue Substitute **Z** No Device	**Z** No Qualifier

0   **Medical and Surgical**
9   **Ear, Nose, Sinus**
1   **Bypass**   Altering the route of passage of the contents of a tubular body part

Body Part Character 4	Approach Character 5	Device Character 6	Qualifier Character 7
D Inner Ear, Right **E** Inner Ear, Left	**0** Open	**7** Autologous Tissue Substitute **J** Synthetic Substitute **K** Nonautologous Tissue Substitute **Z** No Device	**0** Endolymphatic

0   **Medical and Surgical**
9   **Ear, Nose, Sinus**
2   **Change**   Taking out or off a device from a body part and putting back an identical or similar device in or on the same body part without cutting or puncturing the skin or a mucous membrane

Body Part Character 4	Approach Character 5	Device Character 6	Qualifier Character 7
H Ear, Right **J** Ear, Left **K** Nose **Y** Sinus	**X** External	**0** Drainage Device **Y** Other Device	**Z** No Qualifier

Non-OR   For all body part, approach, device, and qualifier values

0   **Medical and Surgical**
9   **Ear, Nose, Sinus**
5   **Destruction**   Physical eradication of all or a portion of a body part by the direct use of energy, force, or a destructive agent

Body Part Character 4	Approach Character 5	Device Character 6	Qualifier Character 7
0 External Ear, Right **1** External Ear, Left **K** Nose	**0** Open **3** Percutaneous **4** Percutaneous Endoscopic **X** External	**Z** No Device	**Z** No Qualifier
3 External Auditory Canal, Right **4** External Auditory Canal, Left	**0** Open **3** Percutaneous **4** Percutaneous Endoscopic **7** Via Natural or Artificial Opening **8** Via Natural or Artificial Opening Endoscopic **X** External	**Z** No Device	**Z** No Qualifier
5 Middle Ear, Right **6** Middle Ear, Left **9** Auditory Ossicle, Right **A** Auditory Ossicle, Left **D** Inner Ear, Right **E** Inner Ear, Left	**0** Open	**Z** No Device	**Z** No Qualifier
7 Tympanic Membrane, Right **8** Tympanic Membrane, Left **F** Eustachian Tube, Right **G** Eustachian Tube, Left **L** Nasal Turbinate **N** Nasopharynx	**0** Open **3** Percutaneous **4** Percutaneous Endoscopic **7** Via Natural or Artificial Opening **8** Via Natural or Artificial Opening Endoscopic	**Z** No Device	**Z** No Qualifier

095 Continued on next page

Non-OR   095[0,1,K][0,3,4,X]ZZ
Non-OR   095[3,4][0,3,4,7,8,X]ZZ
Non-OR   095[F,G][0,3,4,7,8]ZZ

Ø95 Continued

Ø   **Medical and Surgical**
9   **Ear, Nose, Sinus**
5   **Destruction**   Physical eradication of all or a portion of a body part by the direct use of energy, force, or a destructive agent

Body Part Character 4	Approach Character 5	Device Character 6	Qualifier Character 7
B Mastoid Sinus, Right **C** Mastoid Sinus, Left **M** Nasal Septum **P** Accessory Sinus **Q** Maxillary Sinus, Right **R** Maxillary Sinus, Left **S** Frontal Sinus, Right **T** Frontal Sinus, Left **U** Ethmoid Sinus, Right **V** Ethmoid Sinus, Left **W** Sphenoid Sinus, Right **X** Sphenoid Sinus, Left	**Ø** Open **3** Percutaneous **4** Percutaneous Endoscopic	**Z** No Device	**Z** No Qualifier

Non-OR   Ø95M[Ø,3,4]ZZ

Ø   **Medical and Surgical**
9   **Ear, Nose, Sinus**
7   **Dilation**   Expanding an orifice or the lumen of a tubular body part

Body Part Character 4	Approach Character 5	Device Character 6	Qualifier Character 7
F Eustachian Tube, Right **G** Eustachian Tube, Left	**Ø** Open **7** Via Natural or Artificial Opening **8** Via Natural or Artificial Opening Endoscopic	**D** Intraluminal Device **Z** No Device	**Z** No Qualifier
F Eustachian Tube, Right **G** Eustachian Tube, Left	**3** Percutaneous **4** Percutaneous Endoscopic	**Z** No Device	**Z** No Qualifier

Non-OR   For all body part, approach, device, and qualifier values

Ø   **Medical and Surgical**
9   **Ear, Nose, Sinus**
8   **Division**   Cutting into a body part without draining fluids and/or gases from the body part in order to separate or transect a body part

Body Part Character 4	Approach Character 5	Device Character 6	Qualifier Character 7
L Nasal Turbinate	**Ø** Open **3** Percutaneous **4** Percutaneous Endoscopic **7** Via Natural or Artificial Opening **8** Via Natural or Artificial Opening Endoscopic	**Z** No Device	**Z** No Qualifier

Ø   **Medical and Surgical**
9   **Ear, Nose, Sinus**
9   **Drainage**   Taking or letting out fluids and/or gases from a body part

Body Part Character 4	Approach Character 5	Device Character 6	Qualifier Character 7
Ø External Ear, Right **1** External Ear, Left **K** Nose	**Ø** Open **3** Percutaneous **4** Percutaneous Endoscopic **X** External	**Ø** Drainage Device	**Z** No Qualifier
Ø External Ear, Right **1** External Ear, Left **K** Nose	**Ø** Open **3** Percutaneous **4** Percutaneous Endoscopic **X** External	**Z** No Device	**X** Diagnostic **Z** No Qualifier
3 External Auditory Canal, Right **4** External Auditory Canal, Left	**Ø** Open **3** Percutaneous **4** Percutaneous Endoscopic **7** Via Natural or Artificial Opening **8** Via Natural or Artificial Opening Endoscopic **X** External	**Ø** Drainage Device	**Z** No Qualifier

Ø99 Continued on next page

Non-OR   Ø99[Ø,1,K][Ø,3,4,X]ØZ
Non-OR   Ø99[Ø,1,K][Ø,3,4,X]Z[X,Z]
Non-OR   Ø99[3,4][Ø,3,4,7,8,X]ØZ

LC Limited Coverage   **NC** Noncovered   HAC associated procedure   Combination Only   DRG Non-OR   Non-OR   Revised Text in **GREEN**

ICD-10-PCS 2014 (Draft)

211

Ear, Nose, Sinus

099–099

0   **Medical and Surgical**   *099 Continued*
9   **Ear, Nose, Sinus**
9   **Drainage**   Taking or letting out fluids and/or gases from a body part

Body Part Character 4	Approach Character 5	Device Character 6	Qualifier Character 7
3 External Auditory Canal, Right 4 External Auditory Canal, Left	0 Open 3 Percutaneous 4 Percutaneous Endoscopic 7 Via Natural or Artificial Opening 8 Via Natural or Artificial Opening Endoscopic X External	Z No Device	X Diagnostic Z No Qualifier
5 Middle Ear, Right 6 Middle Ear, Left 9 Auditory Ossicle, Right A Auditory Ossicle, Left D Inner Ear, Right E Inner Ear, Left	0 Open	0 Drainage Device	Z No Qualifier
5 Middle Ear, Right 6 Middle Ear, Left 9 Auditory Ossicle, Right A Auditory Ossicle, Left D Inner Ear, Right E Inner Ear, Left	0 Open	Z No Device	X Diagnostic Z No Qualifier
7 Tympanic Membrane, Right 8 Tympanic Membrane, Left F Eustachian Tube, Right G Eustachian Tube, Left L Nasal Turbinate N Nasopharynx	0 Open 3 Percutaneous 4 Percutaneous Endoscopic 7 Via Natural or Artificial Opening 8 Via Natural or Artificial Opening Endoscopic	0 Drainage Device	Z No Qualifier
7 Tympanic Membrane, Right 8 Tympanic Membrane, Left F Eustachian Tube, Right G Eustachian Tube, Left L Nasal Turbinate N Nasopharynx	0 Open 3 Percutaneous 4 Percutaneous Endoscopic 7 Via Natural or Artificial Opening 8 Via Natural or Artificial Opening Endoscopic	Z No Device	X Diagnostic Z No Qualifier
B Mastoid Sinus, Right C Mastoid Sinus, Left M Nasal Septum P Accessory Sinus Q Maxillary Sinus, Right R Maxillary Sinus, Left S Frontal Sinus, Right T Frontal Sinus, Left U Ethmoid Sinus, Right V Ethmoid Sinus, Left W Sphenoid Sinus, Right X Sphenoid Sinus, Left	0 Open 3 Percutaneous 4 Percutaneous Endoscopic	0 Drainage Device	Z No Qualifier
B Mastoid Sinus, Right C Mastoid Sinus, Left M Nasal Septum P Accessory Sinus Q Maxillary Sinus, Right R Maxillary Sinus, Left S Frontal Sinus, Right T Frontal Sinus, Left U Ethmoid Sinus, Right V Ethmoid Sinus, Left W Sphenoid Sinus, Right X Sphenoid Sinus, Left	0 Open 3 Percutaneous 4 Percutaneous Endoscopic	Z No Device	X Diagnostic Z No Qualifier

Non-OR   099[3,4][0,3,4,7,8,X]Z[X,Z]
Non-OR   099[5,6]0ZZ
Non-OR   099[F,G,L][0,3,4,7,8]0Z
Non-OR   099[7,8,F,G,L,N][0,3,4,7,8]Z[X,Z]
Non-OR   099[M,P,Q,R,S,T,U,V,W,X][0,3,4]0Z
Non-OR   099[M,P,Q,R,S,T,U,V,W,X][0,3,4]Z[X,Z]

Ø **Medical and Surgical**
9 **Ear, Nose, Sinus**
B **Excision**　　　Cutting out or off, without replacement, a portion of a body part

Body Part Character 4		Approach Character 5		Device Character 6		Qualifier Character 7	
Ø	External Ear, Right	**Ø**	Open	**Z**	No Device	**X**	Diagnostic
1	External Ear, Left	**3**	Percutaneous			**Z**	No Qualifier
K	Nose	**4**	Percutaneous Endoscopic				
		X	External				
3	External Auditory Canal, Right	**Ø**	Open	**Z**	No Device	**X**	Diagnostic
4	External Auditory Canal, Left	**3**	Percutaneous			**Z**	No Qualifier
		4	Percutaneous Endoscopic				
		7	Via Natural or Artificial Opening				
		8	Via Natural or Artificial Opening Endoscopic				
		X	External				
5	Middle Ear, Right	**Ø**	Open	**Z**	No Device	**X**	Diagnostic
6	Middle Ear, Left					**Z**	No Qualifier
9	Auditory Ossicle, Right						
A	Auditory Ossicle, Left						
D	Inner Ear, Right						
E	Inner Ear, Left						
7	Tympanic Membrane, Right	**Ø**	Open	**Z**	No Device	**X**	Diagnostic
8	Tympanic Membrane, Left	**3**	Percutaneous			**Z**	No Qualifier
F	Eustachian Tube, Right	**4**	Percutaneous Endoscopic				
G	Eustachian Tube, Left	**7**	Via Natural or Artificial Opening				
L	Nasal Turbinate	**8**	Via Natural or Artificial Opening Endoscopic				
N	Nasopharynx						
B	Mastoid Sinus, Right	**Ø**	Open	**Z**	No Device	**X**	Diagnostic
C	Mastoid Sinus, Left	**3**	Percutaneous			**Z**	No Qualifier
M	Nasal Septum	**4**	Percutaneous Endoscopic				
P	Accessory Sinus						
Q	Maxillary Sinus, Right						
R	Maxillary Sinus, Left						
S	Frontal Sinus, Right						
T	Frontal Sinus, Left						
U	Ethmoid Sinus, Right						
V	Ethmoid Sinus, Left						
W	Sphenoid Sinus, Right						
X	Sphenoid Sinus, Left						

Non-OR　09B[Ø,1,K][Ø,3,4,X]Z[X,Z]
Non-OR　09B[3,4][Ø,3,4,7,8,X]Z[X,Z]
Non-OR　09B[F,G,L,N][Ø,3,4,7,8]ZX
Non-OR　09B[F,G][Ø,3,4,7,8]ZZ
Non-OR　09BM[Ø,3,4]ZX
Non-OR　09B[P,Q,R,S,T,U,V,W,X][3,4]ZX

Ø **Medical and Surgical**
9 **Ear, Nose, Sinus**
C **Extirpation**　　　Taking or cutting out solid matter from a body part

Body Part Character 4		Approach Character 5		Device Character 6		Qualifier Character 7	
Ø	External Ear, Right	**Ø**	Open	**Z**	No Device	**Z**	No Qualifier
1	External Ear, Left	**3**	Percutaneous				
K	Nose	**4**	Percutaneous Endoscopic				
		X	External				
3	External Auditory Canal, Right	**Ø**	Open	**Z**	No Device	**Z**	No Qualifier
4	External Auditory Canal, Left	**3**	Percutaneous				
		4	Percutaneous Endoscopic				
		7	Via Natural or Artificial Opening				
		8	Via Natural or Artificial Opening Endoscopic				
		X	External				
5	Middle Ear, Right	**Ø**	Open	**Z**	No Device	**Z**	No Qualifier
6	Middle Ear, Left						
9	Auditory Ossicle, Right						
A	Auditory Ossicle, Left						
D	Inner Ear, Right						
E	Inner Ear, Left						

09C Continued on next page

Non-OR　09C[Ø,1,3,K][Ø,3,4,X]ZZ
Non-OR　09C[3,4][Ø,3,4,7,8,X]ZZ

Ear, Nose, Sinus

09C Continued

0   Medical and Surgical
9   Ear, Nose, Sinus
C   Extirpation   Taking or cutting out solid matter from a body part

Body Part Character 4	Approach Character 5	Device Character 6	Qualifier Character 7
7 Tympanic Membrane, Right 8 Tympanic Membrane, Left F Eustachian Tube, Right G Eustachian Tube, Left L Nasal Turbinate N Nasopharynx	0 Open 3 Percutaneous 4 Percutaneous Endoscopic 7 Via Natural or Artificial Opening 8 Via Natural or Artificial Opening Endoscopic	Z No Device	Z No Qualifier
B Mastoid Sinus, Right C Mastoid Sinus, Left M Nasal Septum P Accessory Sinus Q Maxillary Sinus, Right R Maxillary Sinus, Left S Frontal Sinus, Right T Frontal Sinus, Left U Ethmoid Sinus, Right V Ethmoid Sinus, Left W Sphenoid Sinus, Right X Sphenoid Sinus, Left	0 Open 3 Percutaneous 4 Percutaneous Endoscopic	Z No Device	Z No Qualifier

Non-OR   09C[7,8,F,G,L][0,3,4,7,8]ZZ
Non-OR   09CM[0,3,4]ZZ

0   Medical and Surgical
9   Ear, Nose, Sinus
D   Extraction   Pulling or stripping out or off all or a portion of a body part by the use of force

Body Part Character 4	Approach Character 5	Device Character 6	Qualifier Character 7
7 Tympanic Membrane, Right 8 Tympanic Membrane, Left L Nasal Turbinate	0 Open 3 Percutaneous 4 Percutaneous Endoscopic 7 Via Natural or Artificial Opening 8 Via Natural or Artificial Opening Endoscopic	Z No Device	Z No Qualifier
9 Auditory Ossicle, Right A Auditory Ossicle, Left	0 Open	Z No Device	Z No Qualifier
B Mastoid Sinus, Right C Mastoid Sinus, Left M Nasal Septum P Accessory Sinus Q Maxillary Sinus, Right R Maxillary Sinus, Left S Frontal Sinus, Right T Frontal Sinus, Left U Ethmoid Sinus, Right V Ethmoid Sinus, Left W Sphenoid Sinus, Right X Sphenoid Sinus, Left	0 Open 3 Percutaneous 4 Percutaneous Endoscopic	Z No Device	Z No Qualifier

0   Medical and Surgical
9   Ear, Nose, Sinus
H   Insertion   Putting in a nonbiological appliance that monitors, assists, performs, or prevents a physiological function but does not physically take the place of a body part

Body Part Character 4	Approach Character 5	Device Character 6	Qualifier Character 7
D Inner Ear, Right E Inner Ear, Left	0 Open 3 Percutaneous 4 Percutaneous Endoscopic	4 Hearing Device, Bone Conduction 5 Hearing Device, Single Channel Cochlear Prosthesis 6 Hearing Device, Multiple Channel Cochlear Prosthesis S Hearing Device	Z No Qualifier
N Nasopharynx	7 Via Natural or Artificial Opening 8 Via Natural or Artificial Opening Endoscopic	B Intraluminal Device, Airway	Z No Qualifier

Non-OR   09HN[7,8]BZ

LC Limited Coverage   **NC** Noncovered   HAC associated procedure   Combination Only   DRG Non-OR   Non-OR   Revised Text in **GREEN**

214   ICD-10-PCS 2014 (Draft)

0　Medical and Surgical
9　Ear, Nose, Sinus
J　Inspection　　Visually and/or manually exploring a body part

Body Part Character 4	Approach Character 5	Device Character 6	Qualifier Character 7
7　Tympanic Membrane, Right 8　Tympanic Membrane, Left H　Ear, Right J　Ear, Left	0　Open 3　Percutaneous 4　Percutaneous Endoscopic 7　Via Natural or Artificial Opening 8　Via Natural or Artificial Opening 　　Endoscopic X　External	Z　No Device	Z　No Qualifier
D　Inner Ear, Right E　Inner Ear, Left K　Nose Y　Sinus	0　Open 3　Percutaneous 4　Percutaneous Endoscopic X　External	Z　No Device	Z　No Qualifier

Non-OR　09J[7,8]8ZZ
Non-OR　09J[H,J][0,3,4,7,8,X]ZZ
Non-OR　09J[K,Y][0,3,4,X]ZZ

0　Medical and Surgical
9　Ear, Nose, Sinus
M　Reattachment　　Putting back in or on all or a portion of a separated body part to its normal location or other suitable location

Body Part Character 4	Approach Character 5	Device Character 6	Qualifier Character 7
0　External Ear, Right 1　External Ear, Left K　Nose	X　External	Z　No Device	Z　No Qualifier

0　Medical and Surgical
9　Ear, Nose, Sinus
N　Release　　Freeing a body part from an abnormal physical constraint

Body Part Character 4	Approach Character 5	Device Character 6	Qualifier Character 7
0　External Ear, Right 1　External Ear, Left K　Nose	0　Open 3　Percutaneous 4　Percutaneous Endoscopic X　External	Z　No Device	Z　No Qualifier
3　External Auditory Canal, Right 4　External Auditory Canal, Left	0　Open 3　Percutaneous 4　Percutaneous Endoscopic 7　Via Natural or Artificial Opening 8　Via Natural or Artificial Opening 　　Endoscopic X　External	Z　No Device	Z　No Qualifier
5　Middle Ear, Right 6　Middle Ear, Left 9　Auditory Ossicle, Right A　Auditory Ossicle, Left D　Inner Ear, Right E　Inner Ear, Left	0　Open	Z　No Device	Z　No Qualifier
7　Tympanic Membrane, Right 8　Tympanic Membrane, Left F　Eustachian Tube, Right G　Eustachian Tube, Left L　Nasal Turbinate N　Nasopharynx	0　Open 3　Percutaneous 4　Percutaneous Endoscopic 7　Via Natural or Artificial Opening 8　Via Natural or Artificial Opening 　　Endoscopic	Z　No Device	Z　No Qualifier
B　Mastoid Sinus, Right C　Mastoid Sinus, Left M　Nasal Septum P　Accessory Sinus Q　Maxillary Sinus, Right R　Maxillary Sinus, Left S　Frontal Sinus, Right T　Frontal Sinus, Left U　Ethmoid Sinus, Right V　Ethmoid Sinus, Left W　Sphenoid Sinus, Right X　Sphenoid Sinus, Left	0　Open 3　Percutaneous 4　Percutaneous Endoscopic	Z　No Device	Z　No Qualifier

Non-OR　09NK[0,3,4,X]ZZ
Non-OR　09N[F,G,L][0,3,4,7,8]ZZ
Non-OR　09NM[0,3,4]ZZ

LC Limited Coverage　　　**NC** Noncovered　　　HAC associated procedure　　　Combination Only　　　DRG Non-OR　　　Non-OR　　　Revised Text in **GREEN**

Ear, Nose, Sinus

09P–09Q

Ø Medical and Surgical
9 Ear, Nose, Sinus
P Removal   Taking out or off a device from a body part

Body Part Character 4	Approach Character 5	Device Character 6	Qualifier Character 7
7 Tympanic Membrane, Right 8 Tympanic Membrane, Left	Ø Open 7 Via Natural or Artificial Opening 8 Via Natural or Artificial Opening Endoscopic X External	Ø Drainage Device	Z No Qualifier
D Inner Ear, Right E Inner Ear, Left	Ø Open 7 Via Natural or Artificial Opening 8 Via Natural or Artificial Opening Endoscopic	S Hearing Device	Z No Qualifier
H Ear, Right J Ear, Left K Nose	Ø Open 3 Percutaneous 4 Percutaneous Endoscopic 7 Via Natural or Artificial Opening 8 Via Natural or Artificial Opening Endoscopic X External	Ø Drainage Device 7 Autologous Tissue Substitute D Intraluminal Device J Synthetic Substitute K Nonautologous Tissue Substitute	Z No Qualifier
Y Sinus	Ø Open 3 Percutaneous 4 Percutaneous Endoscopic X External	Ø Drainage Device	Z No Qualifier

Non-OR   09P[7,8][0,7,8,X]0Z
Non-OR   09P[H,J][3,4][0,J,K]Z
Non-OR   09P[H,J]X[0,7,D,J,K]Z

Non-OR   09P[H,J][7,8][0,D]Z
Non-OR   09PK[0,3,4,7,8,X][0,7,D,J,K]Z
Non-OR   09PYX0Z

Ø Medical and Surgical
9 Ear, Nose, Sinus
Q Repair   Restoring, to the extent possible, a body part to its normal anatomic structure and function

Body Part Character 4	Approach Character 5	Device Character 6	Qualifier Character 7
Ø External Ear, Right 1 External Ear, Left 2 External Ear, Bilateral K Nose	Ø Open 3 Percutaneous 4 Percutaneous Endoscopic X External	Z No Device	Z No Qualifier
3 External Auditory Canal, Right 4 External Auditory Canal, Left F Eustachian Tube, Right G Eustachian Tube, Left	Ø Open 3 Percutaneous 4 Percutaneous Endoscopic 7 Via Natural or Artificial Opening 8 Via Natural or Artificial Opening Endoscopic X External	Z No Device	Z No Qualifier
5 Middle Ear, Right 6 Middle Ear, Left 9 Auditory Ossicle, Right A Auditory Ossicle, Left D Inner Ear, Right E Inner Ear, Left	Ø Open	Z No Device	Z No Qualifier
7 Tympanic Membrane, Right 8 Tympanic Membrane, Left L Nasal Turbinate N Nasopharynx	Ø Open 3 Percutaneous 4 Percutaneous Endoscopic 7 Via Natural or Artificial Opening 8 Via Natural or Artificial Opening Endoscopic	Z No Device	Z No Qualifier
B Mastoid Sinus, Right C Mastoid Sinus, Left M Nasal Septum P Accessory Sinus Q Maxillary Sinus, Right R Maxillary Sinus, Left S Frontal Sinus, Right T Frontal Sinus, Left U Ethmoid Sinus, Right V Ethmoid Sinus, Left W Sphenoid Sinus, Right X Sphenoid Sinus, Left	Ø Open 3 Percutaneous 4 Percutaneous Endoscopic	Z No Device	Z No Qualifier

Non-OR   09Q[0,1,2]XZZ
Non-OR   09Q[3,4,F,G][0,3,4,7,8,X]ZZ

0 Medical and Surgical
9 Ear, Nose, Sinus
R Replacement Putting in or on biological or synthetic material that physically takes the place and/or function of all or a portion of a body part

Body Part Character 4	Approach Character 5	Device Character 6	Qualifier Character 7
0 External Ear, Right 1 External Ear, Left 2 External Ear, Bilateral K Nose	0 Open X External	7 Autologous Tissue Substitute J Synthetic Substitute K Nonautologous Tissue Substitute	Z No Qualifier
5 Middle Ear, Right 6 Middle Ear, Left 9 Auditory Ossicle, Right A Auditory Ossicle, Left D Inner Ear, Right E Inner Ear, Left	0 Open	7 Autologous Tissue Substitute J Synthetic Substitute K Nonautologous Tissue Substitute	Z No Qualifier
7 Tympanic Membrane, Right 8 Tympanic Membrane, Left N Nasopharynx	0 Open 7 Via Natural or Artificial Opening 8 Via Natural or Artificial Opening Endoscopic	7 Autologous Tissue Substitute J Synthetic Substitute K Nonautologous Tissue Substitute	Z No Qualifier
L Nasal Turbinate	0 Open 3 Percutaneous 4 Percutaneous Endoscopic 7 Via Natural or Artificial Opening 8 Via Natural or Artificial Opening Endoscopic	7 Autologous Tissue Substitute J Synthetic Substitute K Nonautologous Tissue Substitute	Z No Qualifier
M Nasal Septum	0 Open 3 Percutaneous 4 Percutaneous Endoscopic	7 Autologous Tissue Substitute J Synthetic Substitute K Nonautologous Tissue Substitute	Z No Qualifier

0 Medical and Surgical
9 Ear, Nose, Sinus
S Reposition Moving to its normal location or other suitable location all or a portion of a body part

Body Part Character 4	Approach Character 5	Device Character 6	Qualifier Character 7
0 External Ear, Right 1 External Ear, Left 2 External Ear, Bilateral K Nose	0 Open 4 Percutaneous Endoscopic X External	Z No Device	Z No Qualifier
7 Tympanic Membrane, Right 8 Tympanic Membrane, Left F Eustachian Tube, Right G Eustachian Tube, Left L Nasal Turbinate	0 Open 4 Percutaneous Endoscopic 7 Via Natural or Artificial Opening 8 Via Natural or Artificial Opening Endoscopic	Z No Device	Z No Qualifier
9 Auditory Ossicle, Right A Auditory Ossicle, Left M Nasal Septum	0 Open 4 Percutaneous Endoscopic	Z No Device	Z No Qualifier

Non-OR 09S[F,G][0,4,7,8]ZZ

0 Medical and Surgical
9 Ear, Nose, Sinus
T Resection Cutting out or off, without replacement, all of a body part

Body Part Character 4	Approach Character 5	Device Character 6	Qualifier Character 7
0 External Ear, Right 1 External Ear, Left K Nose	0 Open 4 Percutaneous Endoscopic X External	Z No Device	Z No Qualifier
5 Middle Ear, Right 6 Middle Ear, Left 9 Auditory Ossicle, Right A Auditory Ossicle, Left D Inner Ear, Right E Inner Ear, Left	0 Open	Z No Device	Z No Qualifier
7 Tympanic Membrane, Right 8 Tympanic Membrane, Left F Eustachian Tube, Right G Eustachian Tube, Left L Nasal Turbinate N Nasopharynx	0 Open 4 Percutaneous Endoscopic 7 Via Natural or Artificial Opening 8 Via Natural or Artificial Opening Endoscopic	Z No Device	Z No Qualifier

09T Continued on next page

Non-OR 09T[F,G][0,4,7,8]ZZ

Ear, Nose, Sinus

09T–09U

09T Continued

Ø   **Medical and Surgical**
9   **Ear, Nose, Sinus**
T   **Resection**   Cutting out or off, without replacement, all of a body part

Body Part Character 4	Approach Character 5	Device Character 6	Qualifier Character 7
B Mastoid Sinus, Right **C** Mastoid Sinus, Left **M** Nasal Septum **P** Accessory Sinus **Q** Maxillary Sinus, Right **R** Maxillary Sinus, Left **S** Frontal Sinus, Right **T** Frontal Sinus, Left **U** Ethmoid Sinus, Right **V** Ethmoid Sinus, Left **W** Sphenoid Sinus, Right **X** Sphenoid Sinus, Left	**Ø** Open **4** Percutaneous Endoscopic	**Z** No Device	**Z** No Qualifier

Ø   **Medical and Surgical**
9   **Ear, Nose, Sinus**
U   **Supplement**   Putting in or on biological or synthetic material that physically reinforces and/or augments the function of a portion of a body part

Body Part Character 4	Approach Character 5	Device Character 6	Qualifier Character 7
Ø External Ear, Right **1** External Ear, Left **2** External Ear, Bilateral **K** Nose	**Ø** Open **X** External	**7** Autologous Tissue Substitute **J** Synthetic Substitute **K** Nonautologous Tissue Substitute	**Z** No Qualifier
5 Middle Ear, Right **6** Middle Ear, Left **9** Auditory Ossicle, Right **A** Auditory Ossicle, Left **D** Inner Ear, Right **E** Inner Ear, Left	**Ø** Open	**7** Autologous Tissue Substitute **J** Synthetic Substitute **K** Nonautologous Tissue Substitute	**Z** No Qualifier
7 Tympanic Membrane, Right **8** Tympanic Membrane, Left **N** Nasopharynx	**Ø** Open **7** Via Natural or Artificial Opening **8** Via Natural or Artificial Opening Endoscopic	**7** Autologous Tissue Substitute **J** Synthetic Substitute **K** Nonautologous Tissue Substitute	**Z** No Qualifier
L Nasal Turbinate	**Ø** Open **3** Percutaneous **4** Percutaneous Endoscopic **7** Via Natural or Artificial Opening **8** Via Natural or Artificial Opening Endoscopic	**7** Autologous Tissue Substitute **J** Synthetic Substitute **K** Nonautologous Tissue Substitute	**Z** No Qualifier
M Nasal Septum	**Ø** Open **3** Percutaneous **4** Percutaneous Endoscopic	**7** Autologous Tissue Substitute **J** Synthetic Substitute **K** Nonautologous Tissue Substitute	**Z** No Qualifier

LC Limited Coverage   **NC** Noncovered   HAC associated procedure   Combination Only   DRG Non-OR   Non-OR   Revised Text in **GREEN**

218   ICD-10-PCS 2014 (Draft)

0　Medical and Surgical
9　Ear, Nose, Sinus
W　Revision　　Correcting, to the extent possible, a portion of a malfunctioning device or the position of a displaced device

Body Part Character 4	Approach Character 5	Device Character 6	Qualifier Character 7
7 Tympanic Membrane, Right **8** Tympanic Membrane, Left **9** Auditory Ossicle, Right **A** Auditory Ossicle, Left	**0** Open **7** Via Natural or Artificial Opening **8** Via Natural or Artificial Opening Endoscopic	**7** Autologous Tissue Substitute **J** Synthetic Substitute **K** Nonautologous Tissue Substitute	**Z** No Qualifier
D Inner Ear, Right **E** Inner Ear, Left	**0** Open **7** Via Natural or Artificial Opening **8** Via Natural or Artificial Opening Endoscopic	**S** Hearing Device	**Z** No Qualifier
H Ear, Right **J** Ear, Left **K** Nose	**0** Open **3** Percutaneous **4** Percutaneous Endoscopic **7** Via Natural or Artificial Opening **8** Via Natural or Artificial Opening Endoscopic **X** External	**0** Drainage Device **7** Autologous Tissue Substitute **D** Intraluminal Device **J** Synthetic Substitute **K** Nonautologous Tissue Substitute	**Z** No Qualifier
Y Sinus	**0** Open **3** Percutaneous **4** Percutaneous Endoscopic **X** External	**0** Drainage Device	**Z** No Qualifier

Non-OR　09W[H,J][3,4][J,K]Z
Non-OR　09WK[0,3,4,7,8,X][0,7,D,J,K]Z
Non-OR　09W[H,J,K][7,8]DZ
Non-OR　09W[H,J]X[0,7,D,J,K]Z
Non-OR　09WYX0Z

LC Limited Coverage　　　**NC** Noncovered　　　HAC associated procedure　　　Combination Only　　　DRG Non-OR　　　Non-OR　　　Revised Text in **GREEN**

ICD-10-PCS 2014 (Draft)　　219

Ear, Nose, Sinus

09W—09W

Respiratory System ØB1–ØBY

Ø   **Medical and Surgical**
B   **Respiratory System**
1   **Bypass**   Altering the route of passage of the contents of a tubular body part

Body Part Character 4	Approach Character 5	Device Character 6	Qualifier Character 7
1 Trachea	Ø Open	D Intraluminal Device	6 Esophagus
1 Trachea	Ø Open 3 Percutaneous 4 Percutaneous Endoscopic	F Tracheostomy Device Z No Device	4 Cutaneous

DRG Non-OR ØB113[F,Z]4
Non-OR   ØB110D6

Ø   **Medical and Surgical**
B   **Respiratory System**
2   **Change**   Taking out or off a device from a body part and putting back an identical or similar device in or on the same body part without cutting or puncturing the skin or a mucous membrane

Body Part Character 4	Approach Character 5	Device Character 6	Qualifier Character 7
Ø Tracheobronchial Tree K Lung, Right L Lung, Left Q Pleura T Diaphragm	X External	Ø Drainage Device Y Other Device	Z No Qualifier
1 Trachea	X External	Ø Drainage Device E Intraluminal Device, Endotracheal Airway F Tracheostomy Device Y Other Device	Z No Qualifier

Non-OR   For all body part, approach, device, and qualifier values

Ø   **Medical and Surgical**
B   **Respiratory System**
5   **Destruction**   Physical eradication of all or a portion of a body part by the direct use of energy, force, or a destructive agent

Body Part Character 4	Approach Character 5	Device Character 6	Qualifier Character 7
1 Trachea 2 Carina 3 Main Bronchus, Right 4 Upper Lobe Bronchus, Right 5 Middle Lobe Bronchus, Right 6 Lower Lobe Bronchus, Right 7 Main Bronchus, Left 8 Upper Lobe Bronchus, Left 9 Lingula Bronchus B Lower Lobe Bronchus, Left C Upper Lung Lobe, Right D Middle Lung Lobe, Right F Lower Lung Lobe, Right G Upper Lung Lobe, Left H Lung Lingula J Lower Lung Lobe, Left K Lung, Right L Lung, Left M Lungs, Bilateral	Ø Open 3 Percutaneous 4 Percutaneous Endoscopic 7 Via Natural or Artificial Opening 8 Via Natural or Artificial Opening Endoscopic	Z No Device	Z No Qualifier
N Pleura, Right P Pleura, Left R Diaphragm, Right S Diaphragm, Left	Ø Open 3 Percutaneous 4 Percutaneous Endoscopic	Z No Device	Z No Qualifier

Non-OR   ØB5[3,4,5,6,7,8,9,B]4ZZ
Non-OR   ØB5[C,D,F,G,H,J,K,L,M]8ZZ

220   ICD-10-PCS 2014 (Draft)

0　Medical and Surgical
B　Respiratory System
7　Dilation　　　Expanding an orifice or the lumen of a tubular body part

Body Part Character 4	Approach Character 5	Device Character 6	Qualifier Character 7
1　Trachea 2　Carina 3　Main Bronchus, Right 4　Upper Lobe Bronchus, Right 5　Middle Lobe Bronchus, Right 6　Lower Lobe Bronchus, Right 7　Main Bronchus, Left 8　Upper Lobe Bronchus, Left 9　Lingula Bronchus B　Lower Lobe Bronchus, Left	0　Open 3　Percutaneous 4　Percutaneous Endoscopic 7　Via Natural or Artificial Opening 8　Via Natural or Artificial Opening Endoscopic	D　Intraluminal Device Z　No Device	Z　No Qualifier

Non-OR　0B7[3,4,5,6,7,8,9,B][0,3,4,7,8][D,Z]Z

0　Medical and Surgical
B　Respiratory System
9　Drainage　　　Taking or letting out fluids and/or gases from a body part

Body Part Character 4	Approach Character 5	Device Character 6	Qualifier Character 7
1　Trachea 2　Carina 3　Main Bronchus, Right 4　Upper Lobe Bronchus, Right 5　Middle Lobe Bronchus, Right 6　Lower Lobe Bronchus, Right 7　Main Bronchus, Left 8　Upper Lobe Bronchus, Left 9　Lingula Bronchus B　Lower Lobe Bronchus, Left C　Upper Lung Lobe, Right D　Middle Lung Lobe, Right F　Lower Lung Lobe, Right G　Upper Lung Lobe, Left H　Lung Lingula J　Lower Lung Lobe, Left K　Lung, Right L　Lung, Left M　Lungs, Bilateral	0　Open 3　Percutaneous 4　Percutaneous Endoscopic 7　Via Natural or Artificial Opening 8　Via Natural or Artificial Opening Endoscopic	0　Drainage Device	Z　No Qualifier
1　Trachea 2　Carina 3　Main Bronchus, Right 4　Upper Lobe Bronchus, Right 5　Middle Lobe Bronchus, Right 6　Lower Lobe Bronchus, Right 7　Main Bronchus, Left 8　Upper Lobe Bronchus, Left 9　Lingula Bronchus B　Lower Lobe Bronchus, Left C　Upper Lung Lobe, Right D　Middle Lung Lobe, Right F　Lower Lung Lobe, Right G　Upper Lung Lobe, Left H　Lung Lingula J　Lower Lung Lobe, Left K　Lung, Right L　Lung, Left M　Lungs, Bilateral	0　Open 3　Percutaneous 4　Percutaneous Endoscopic 7　Via Natural or Artificial Opening 8　Via Natural or Artificial Opening Endoscopic	Z　No Device	X　Diagnostic Z　No Qualifier
N　Pleura, Right P　Pleura, Left R　Diaphragm, Right S　Diaphragm, Left	0　Open 3　Percutaneous 4　Percutaneous Endoscopic	0　Drainage Device	Z　No Qualifier
N　Pleura, Right P　Pleura, Left R　Diaphragm, Right S　Diaphragm, Left	0　Open 3　Percutaneous 4　Percutaneous Endoscopic	Z　No Device	X　Diagnostic Z　No Qualifier

Non-OR　0B9[1,2,3,4,5,6,7,8,9,B][3,4,7,8]ZX
Non-OR　0B9[C,D,F,G,H,J,K,L,M][3,4,7]ZX
Non-OR　0B9[N,P][0,3]0Z
Non-OR　0B9[N,P][0,3,4]ZX

[LC] Limited Coverage　　[NC] Noncovered　　HAC associated procedure　　Combination Only　　DRG Non-OR　　Non-OR　　Revised Text in **GREEN**

ICD-10-PCS 2014 (Draft)　　　　　　　　　　　　　　　　　　　　　　　　　　　　221

Respiratory System

Ø **Medical and Surgical**
B **Respiratory System**
B **Excision**   Cutting out or off, without replacement, a portion of a body part

Body Part Character 4	Approach Character 5	Device Character 6	Qualifier Character 7
1 Trachea **2** Carina **3** Main Bronchus, Right **4** Upper Lobe Bronchus, Right **5** Middle Lobe Bronchus, Right **6** Lower Lobe Bronchus, Right **7** Main Bronchus, Left **8** Upper Lobe Bronchus, Left **9** Lingula Bronchus **B** Lower Lobe Bronchus, Left **C** Upper Lung Lobe, Right **D** Middle Lung Lobe, Right **F** Lower Lung Lobe, Right **G** Upper Lung Lobe, Left **H** Lung Lingula **J** Lower Lung Lobe, Left **K** Lung, Right **L** Lung, Left **M** Lungs, Bilateral	**Ø** Open **3** Percutaneous **4** Percutaneous Endoscopic **7** Via Natural or Artificial Opening **8** Via Natural or Artificial Opening Endoscopic	**Z** No Device	**X** Diagnostic **Z** No Qualifier
N Pleura, Right **P** Pleura, Left **R** Diaphragm, Right **S** Diaphragm, Left	**Ø** Open **3** Percutaneous **4** Percutaneous Endoscopic	**Z** No Device	**X** Diagnostic **Z** No Qualifier

Non-OR ØBB[1,2,3,4,5,6,7,8,9,B][3,4,7,8]ZX
Non-OR ØBB[3,4,5,6,7,8,9,B][4,8]ZZ
Non-OR ØBB[C,D,F,G,H,J,K,L,M]3ZX

Non-OR ØBB[C,D,F,G,H,J,K,L,M]8ZZ
Non-OR ØBBM4ZZ
Non-OR ØBB[N,P][Ø,3]ZX

Ø **Medical and Surgical**
B **Respiratory System**
C **Extirpation**   Taking or cutting out solid matter from a body part

Body Part Character 4	Approach Character 5	Device Character 6	Qualifier Character 7
1 Trachea **2** Carina **3** Main Bronchus, Right **4** Upper Lobe Bronchus, Right **5** Middle Lobe Bronchus, Right **6** Lower Lobe Bronchus, Right **7** Main Bronchus, Left **8** Upper Lobe Bronchus, Left **9** Lingula Bronchus **B** Lower Lobe Bronchus, Left **C** Upper Lung Lobe, Right **D** Middle Lung Lobe, Right **F** Lower Lung Lobe, Right **G** Upper Lung Lobe, Left **H** Lung Lingula **J** Lower Lung Lobe, Left **K** Lung, Right **L** Lung, Left **M** Lungs, Bilateral	**Ø** Open **3** Percutaneous **4** Percutaneous Endoscopic **7** Via Natural or Artificial Opening **8** Via Natural or Artificial Opening Endoscopic	**Z** No Device	**Z** No Qualifier
N Pleura, Right **P** Pleura, Left **R** Diaphragm, Right **S** Diaphragm, Left	**Ø** Open **3** Percutaneous **4** Percutaneous Endoscopic	**Z** No Device	**Z** No Qualifier

Non-OR ØBC[1,2,3,4,5,6,7,8,9,B][7,8]ZZ
Non-OR ØBC[N,P][Ø,3,4]ZZ

Ø **Medical and Surgical**
B **Respiratory System**
D **Extraction**   Pulling or stripping out or off all or a portion of a body part by the use of force

Body Part Character 4	Approach Character 5	Device Character 6	Qualifier Character 7
N Pleura, Right **P** Pleura, Left	**Ø** Open **3** Percutaneous **4** Percutaneous Endoscopic	**Z** No Device	**X** Diagnostic **Z** No Qualifier

0   **Medical and Surgical**
B   **Respiratory System**
F   **Fragmentation**   Breaking solid matter in a body part into pieces

Body Part Character 4	Approach Character 5	Device Character 6	Qualifier Character 7
1 Trachea **NC** **2** Carina **NC** **3** Main Bronchus, Right **NC** **4** Upper Lobe Bronchus, Right **NC** **5** Middle Lobe Bronchus, Right **NC** **6** Lower Lobe Bronchus, Right **NC** **7** Main Bronchus, Left **NC** **8** Upper Lobe Bronchus, Left **NC** **9** Lingula Bronchus **NC** **B** Lower Lobe Bronchus, Left **NC**	**0** Open **3** Percutaneous **4** Percutaneous Endoscopic **7** Via Natural or Artificial Opening **8** Via Natural or Artificial Opening Endoscopic **X** External	**Z** No Device	**Z** No Qualifier

    NC   0BF[1,2,3,4,5,6,7,8,9,B]XZZ
    Non-OR   0BF[1,2,3,4,5,6,7,8,9,B]XZZ

0   **Medical and Surgical**
B   **Respiratory System**
H   **Insertion**   Putting in a nonbiological appliance that monitors, assists, performs, or prevents a physiological function but does not physically take the place of a body part

Body Part Character 4	Approach Character 5	Device Character 6	Qualifier Character 7
0 Tracheobronchial Tree	**0** Open **3** Percutaneous **4** Percutaneous Endoscopic **7** Via Natural or Artificial Opening **8** Via Natural or Artificial Opening Endoscopic	**1** Radioactive Element **2** Monitoring Device **3** Infusion Device **D** Intraluminal Device	**Z** No Qualifier
1 Trachea	**0** Open	**2** Monitoring Device **D** Intraluminal Device	**Z** No Qualifier
1 Trachea	**3** Percutaneous	**D** Intraluminal Device **E** Intraluminal Device, Endotracheal Airway	**Z** No Qualifier
1 Trachea	**4** Percutaneous Endoscopic	**D** Intraluminal Device	**Z** No Qualifier

1 Trachea	**7** Via Natural or Artificial Opening
	8 Via Natural or Artificial Opening
	   Endoscopic
		2 Monitoring Device
		D Intraluminal Device
		E Intraluminal Device, Endotracheal
		   Airway
			Z No Qualifier

3 Main Bronchus, Right **4** Upper Lobe Bronchus, Right **5** Middle Lobe Bronchus, Right **6** Lower Lobe Bronchus, Right **7** Main Bronchus, Left **8** Upper Lobe Bronchus, Left **9** Lingula Bronchus **B** Lower Lobe Bronchus, Left	**0** Open **3** Percutaneous **4** Percutaneous Endoscopic **7** Via Natural or Artificial Opening **8** Via Natural or Artificial Opening Endoscopic	**G** Endobronchial Valve	**Z** No Qualifier
K Lung, Right **L** Lung, Left	**0** Open **3** Percutaneous **4** Percutaneous Endoscopic **7** Via Natural or Artificial Opening **8** Via Natural or Artificial Opening Endoscopic	**1** Radioactive Element **2** Monitoring Device **3** Infusion Device	**Z** No Qualifier
R Diaphragm, Right **S** Diaphragm, Left	**0** Open **3** Percutaneous **4** Percutaneous Endoscopic	**2** Monitoring Device **M** Diaphragmatic Pacemaker Lead	**Z** No Qualifier

    Non-OR   0BH0[7,8][2,3,D]Z
    Non-OR   0BH13EZ
    Non-OR   0BH1[7,8]EZ
    Non-OR   0BH[3,4,5,6,7,8,9,B]8GZ

LC Limited Coverage   **NC** Noncovered   HAC associated procedure   Combination Only   DRG Non-OR   Non-OR   Revised Text in **GREEN**

ICD-10-PCS 2014 (Draft)   223

Ø   Medical and Surgical
B   Respiratory System
J   Inspection   Visually and/or manually exploring a body part

Body Part Character 4	Approach Character 5	Device Character 6	Qualifier Character 7
Ø Tracheobronchial Tree	Ø Open	Z No Device	Z No Qualifier
1 Trachea	3 Percutaneous		
K Lung, Right	4 Percutaneous Endoscopic		
L Lung, Left	7 Via Natural or Artificial Opening		
Q Pleura	8 Via Natural or Artificial Opening Endoscopic		
T Diaphragm	X External		

Non-OR	ØBJ[Ø,K,L]8ZZ
Non-OR	ØBJ1[3,4,7,8,X]ZZ

Ø   Medical and Surgical
B   Respiratory System
L   Occlusion   Completely closing an orifice or the lumen of a tubular body part

Body Part Character 4	Approach Character 5	Device Character 6	Qualifier Character 7
1 Trachea	Ø Open	C Extraluminal Device	Z No Qualifier
2 Carina	3 Percutaneous	D Intraluminal Device	
3 Main Bronchus, Right	4 Percutaneous Endoscopic	Z No Device	
4 Upper Lobe Bronchus, Right			
5 Middle Lobe Bronchus, Right			
6 Lower Lobe Bronchus, Right			
7 Main Bronchus, Left			
8 Upper Lobe Bronchus, Left			
9 Lingula Bronchus			
B Lower Lobe Bronchus, Left			
1 Trachea	7 Via Natural or Artificial Opening	D Intraluminal Device	Z No Qualifier
2 Carina	8 Via Natural or Artificial Opening Endoscopic	Z No Device	
3 Main Bronchus, Right			
4 Upper Lobe Bronchus, Right			
5 Middle Lobe Bronchus, Right			
6 Lower Lobe Bronchus, Right			
7 Main Bronchus, Left			
8 Upper Lobe Bronchus, Left			
9 Lingula Bronchus			
B Lower Lobe Bronchus, Left			

Ø   Medical and Surgical
B   Respiratory System
M   Reattachment   Putting back in or on all or a portion of a separated body part to its normal location or other suitable location

Body Part Character 4	Approach Character 5	Device Character 6	Qualifier Character 7
1 Trachea	Ø Open	Z No Device	Z No Qualifier
2 Carina			
3 Main Bronchus, Right			
4 Upper Lobe Bronchus, Right			
5 Middle Lobe Bronchus, Right			
6 Lower Lobe Bronchus, Right			
7 Main Bronchus, Left			
8 Upper Lobe Bronchus, Left			
9 Lingula Bronchus			
B Lower Lobe Bronchus, Left			
C Upper Lung Lobe, Right			
D Middle Lung Lobe, Right			
F Lower Lung Lobe, Right			
G Upper Lung Lobe, Left			
H Lung Lingula			
J Lower Lung Lobe, Left			
K Lung, Right			
L Lung, Left			
R Diaphragm, Right			
S Diaphragm, Left			

Ø Medical and Surgical
B Respiratory System
N Release   Freeing a body part from an abnormal physical constraint

Body Part Character 4	Approach Character 5	Device Character 6	Qualifier Character 7
1 Trachea 2 Carina 3 Main Bronchus, Right 4 Upper Lobe Bronchus, Right 5 Middle Lobe Bronchus, Right 6 Lower Lobe Bronchus, Right 7 Main Bronchus, Left 8 Upper Lobe Bronchus, Left 9 Lingula Bronchus B Lower Lobe Bronchus, Left C Upper Lung Lobe, Right D Middle Lung Lobe, Right F Lower Lung Lobe, Right G Upper Lung Lobe, Left H Lung Lingula J Lower Lung Lobe, Left K Lung, Right L Lung, Left M Lungs, Bilateral	Ø Open 3 Percutaneous 4 Percutaneous Endoscopic 7 Via Natural or Artificial Opening 8 Via Natural or Artificial Opening Endoscopic	Z No Device	Z No Qualifier
N Pleura, Right P Pleura, Left R Diaphragm, Right S Diaphragm, Left	Ø Open 3 Percutaneous 4 Percutaneous Endoscopic	Z No Device	Z No Qualifier

Ø Medical and Surgical
B Respiratory System
P Removal   Taking out or off a device from a body part

Body Part Character 4	Approach Character 5	Device Character 6	Qualifier Character 7
Ø Tracheobronchial Tree	Ø Open 3 Percutaneous 4 Percutaneous Endoscopic 7 Via Natural or Artificial Opening 8 Via Natural or Artificial Opening Endoscopic	Ø Drainage Device 1 Radioactive Element 2 Monitoring Device 3 Infusion Device 7 Autologous Tissue Substitute C Extraluminal Device D Intraluminal Device J Synthetic Substitute K Nonautologous Tissue Substitute	Z No Qualifier
Ø Tracheobronchial Tree	X External	Ø Drainage Device 1 Radioactive Element 2 Monitoring Device 3 Infusion Device D Intraluminal Device	Z No Qualifier
1 Trachea	Ø Open 3 Percutaneous 4 Percutaneous Endoscopic 7 Via Natural or Artificial Opening 8 Via Natural or Artificial Opening Endoscopic	Ø Drainage Device 2 Monitoring Device 7 Autologous Tissue Substitute C Extraluminal Device D Intraluminal Device F Tracheostomy Device J Synthetic Substitute K Nonautologous Tissue Substitute	Z No Qualifier
1 Trachea	X External	Ø Drainage Device 2 Monitoring Device D Intraluminal Device F Tracheostomy Device	Z No Qualifier
K Lung, Right L Lung, Left	Ø Open 3 Percutaneous 4 Percutaneous Endoscopic 7 Via Natural or Artificial Opening 8 Via Natural or Artificial Opening Endoscopic X External	Ø Drainage Device 1 Radioactive Element 2 Monitoring Device 3 Infusion Device	Z No Qualifier

ØBP Continued on next page

Non-OR   ØBPØX[Ø,1,2,3,D]Z
Non-OR   ØBP1X[Ø,2,D,F]Z
Non-OR   ØBP[K,L]X[Ø,1,2,3]Z

LC Limited Coverage   NC Noncovered   HAC associated procedure   Combination Only   DRG Non-OR   Non-OR   Revised Text in GREEN

Respiratory System

Ø Medical and Surgical
B Respiratory System
P Removal   Taking out or off a device from a body part

ØBP Continued

Body Part Character 4	Approach Character 5	Device Character 6	Qualifier Character 7
Q Pleura	**Ø** Open **3** Percutaneous **4** Percutaneous Endoscopic **7** Via Natural or Artificial Opening **8** Via Natural or Artificial Opening Endoscopic **X** External	**Ø** Drainage Device **1** Radioactive Element **2** Monitoring Device	**Z** No Qualifier
T Diaphragm	**Ø** Open **3** Percutaneous **4** Percutaneous Endoscopic **7** Via Natural or Artificial Opening **8** Via Natural or Artificial Opening Endoscopic	**Ø** Drainage Device **2** Monitoring Device **7** Autologous Tissue Substitute **J** Synthetic Substitute **K** Nonautologous Tissue Substitute **M** Diaphragmatic Pacemaker Lead	**Z** No Qualifier
T Diaphragm	**X** External	**Ø** Drainage Device **2** Monitoring Device **M** Diaphragmatic Pacemaker Lead	**Z** No Qualifier

Non-OR   ØBPQ[Ø,3,4,7,8,X][Ø,1,2]Z
Non-OR   ØBPTX[Ø,2,M]Z

Ø Medical and Surgical
B Respiratory System
Q Repair   Restoring, to the extent possible, a body part to its normal anatomic structure and function

Body Part Character 4	Approach Character 5	Device Character 6	Qualifier Character 7
1 Trachea **2** Carina **3** Main Bronchus, Right **4** Upper Lobe Bronchus, Right **5** Middle Lobe Bronchus, Right **6** Lower Lobe Bronchus, Right **7** Main Bronchus, Left **8** Upper Lobe Bronchus, Left **9** Lingula Bronchus **B** Lower Lobe Bronchus, Left **C** Upper Lung Lobe, Right **D** Middle Lung Lobe, Right **F** Lower Lung Lobe, Right **G** Upper Lung Lobe, Left **H** Lung Lingula **J** Lower Lung Lobe, Left **K** Lung, Right **L** Lung, Left **M** Lungs, Bilateral	**Ø** Open **3** Percutaneous **4** Percutaneous Endoscopic **7** Via Natural or Artificial Opening **8** Via Natural or Artificial Opening Endoscopic	**Z** No Device	**Z** No Qualifier
N Pleura, Right **P** Pleura, Left **R** Diaphragm, Right **S** Diaphragm, Left	**Ø** Open **3** Percutaneous **4** Percutaneous Endoscopic	**Z** No Device	**Z** No Qualifier

LC Limited Coverage   **NC** Noncovered   HAC associated procedure   Combination Only   DRG Non-OR   Non-OR   Revised Text in **GREEN**

226   ICD-10-PCS 2014 (Draft)

Ø **Medical and Surgical**
B **Respiratory System**
S **Reposition**　　　Moving to its normal location or other suitable location all or a portion of a body part

Body Part Character 4	Approach Character 5	Device Character 6	Qualifier Character 7
1 Trachea	**Ø** Open	**Z** No Device	**Z** No Qualifier
2 Carina			
3 Main Bronchus, Right			
4 Upper Lobe Bronchus, Right			
5 Middle Lobe Bronchus, Right			
6 Lower Lobe Bronchus, Right			
7 Main Bronchus, Left			
8 Upper Lobe Bronchus, Left			
9 Lingula Bronchus			
B Lower Lobe Bronchus, Left			
C Upper Lung Lobe, Right			
D Middle Lung Lobe, Right			
F Lower Lung Lobe, Right			
G Upper Lung Lobe, Left			
H Lung Lingula			
J Lower Lung Lobe, Left			
K Lung, Right			
L Lung, Left			
R Diaphragm, Right			
S Diaphragm, Left			

Ø **Medical and Surgical**
B **Respiratory System**
T **Resection**　　　Cutting out or off, without replacement, all of a body part

Body Part Character 4	Approach Character 5	Device Character 6	Qualifier Character 7
1 Trachea	**Ø** Open	**Z** No Device	**Z** No Qualifier
2 Carina	**4** Percutaneous Endoscopic		
3 Main Bronchus, Right			
4 Upper Lobe Bronchus, Right			
5 Middle Lobe Bronchus, Right			
6 Lower Lobe Bronchus, Right			
7 Main Bronchus, Left			
8 Upper Lobe Bronchus, Left			
9 Lingula Bronchus			
B Lower Lobe Bronchus, Left			
C Upper Lung Lobe, Right			
D Middle Lung Lobe, Right			
F Lower Lung Lobe, Right			
G Upper Lung Lobe, Left			
H Lung Lingula			
J Lower Lung Lobe, Left			
K Lung, Right			
L Lung, Left			
M Lungs, Bilateral			
R Diaphragm, Right			
S Diaphragm, Left			

Ø **Medical and Surgical**
B **Respiratory System**
U **Supplement**　　　Putting in or on biological or synthetic material that physically reinforces and/or augments the function of a portion of a body part

Body Part Character 4	Approach Character 5	Device Character 6	Qualifier Character 7
1 Trachea	**Ø** Open	**7** Autologous Tissue Substitute	**Z** No Qualifier
2 Carina	**4** Percutaneous Endoscopic	**J** Synthetic Substitute	
3 Main Bronchus, Right		**K** Nonautologous Tissue Substitute	
4 Upper Lobe Bronchus, Right			
5 Middle Lobe Bronchus, Right			
6 Lower Lobe Bronchus, Right			
7 Main Bronchus, Left			
8 Upper Lobe Bronchus, Left			
9 Lingula Bronchus			
B Lower Lobe Bronchus, Left			
R Diaphragm, Right			
S Diaphragm, Left			

LC Limited Coverage　　　**NC** Noncovered　　　HAC associated procedure　　　Combination Only　　　DRG Non-OR　　　Non-OR　　　Revised Text in **GREEN**

ICD-10-PCS 2014 (Draft)　　　　　　　　　　　　　　　　　　　　　　　　　　　　　　　　227

Respiratory System

Ø BV–ØBW

Ø   **Medical and Surgical**
B   **Respiratory System**
V   **Restriction**   Partially closing an orifice or the lumen of a tubular body part

Body Part Character 4	Approach Character 5	Device Character 6	Qualifier Character 7
1 Trachea 2 Carina 3 Main Bronchus, Right 4 Upper Lobe Bronchus, Right 5 Middle Lobe Bronchus, Right 6 Lower Lobe Bronchus, Right 7 Main Bronchus, Left 8 Upper Lobe Bronchus, Left 9 Lingula Bronchus B Lower Lobe Bronchus, Left	Ø Open 3 Percutaneous 4 Percutaneous Endoscopic	C Extraluminal Device D Intraluminal Device Z No Device	Z No Qualifier
1 Trachea 2 Carina 3 Main Bronchus, Right 4 Upper Lobe Bronchus, Right 5 Middle Lobe Bronchus, Right 6 Lower Lobe Bronchus, Right 7 Main Bronchus, Left 8 Upper Lobe Bronchus, Left 9 Lingula Bronchus B Lower Lobe Bronchus, Left	7 Via Natural or Artificial Opening 8 Via Natural or Artificial Opening Endoscopic	D Intraluminal Device Z No Device	Z No Qualifier

Ø   **Medical and Surgical**
B   **Respiratory System**
W   **Revision**   Correcting, to the extent possible, a portion of a malfunctioning device or the position of a displaced device

Body Part Character 4	Approach Character 5	Device Character 6	Qualifier Character 7
Ø Tracheobronchial Tree	Ø Open 3 Percutaneous 4 Percutaneous Endoscopic 7 Via Natural or Artificial Opening 8 Via Natural or Artificial Opening Endoscopic X External	Ø Drainage Device 2 Monitoring Device 3 Infusion Device 7 Autologous Tissue Substitute C Extraluminal Device D Intraluminal Device J Synthetic Substitute K Nonautologous Tissue Substitute	Z No Qualifier
1 Trachea	Ø Open 3 Percutaneous 4 Percutaneous Endoscopic 7 Via Natural or Artificial Opening 8 Via Natural or Artificial Opening Endoscopic X External	Ø Drainage Device 2 Monitoring Device 7 Autologous Tissue Substitute C Extraluminal Device D Intraluminal Device F Tracheostomy Device J Synthetic Substitute K Nonautologous Tissue Substitute	Z No Qualifier
K Lung, Right L Lung, Left	Ø Open 3 Percutaneous 4 Percutaneous Endoscopic 7 Via Natural or Artificial Opening 8 Via Natural or Artificial Opening Endoscopic X External	Ø Drainage Device 2 Monitoring Device 3 Infusion Device	Z No Qualifier
Q Pleura	Ø Open 3 Percutaneous 4 Percutaneous Endoscopic 7 Via Natural or Artificial Opening 8 Via Natural or Artificial Opening Endoscopic X External	Ø Drainage Device 2 Monitoring Device	Z No Qualifier
T Diaphragm	Ø Open 3 Percutaneous 4 Percutaneous Endoscopic 7 Via Natural or Artificial Opening 8 Via Natural or Artificial Opening Endoscopic X External	Ø Drainage Device 2 Monitoring Device 7 Autologous Tissue Substitute J Synthetic Substitute K Nonautologous Tissue Substitute M Diaphragmatic Pacemaker Lead	Z No Qualifier

Non-OR   ØBWØX[Ø,2,3,7,C,D,J,K]Z
Non-OR   ØBW1X[Ø,2,7,C,D,F,J,K]Z
Non-OR   ØBW[K,L]X[Ø,2,3]Z
Non-OR   ØBWQ[Ø,3,4,7,8,X][Ø,2]Z
Non-OR   ØBWTX[Ø,2,7,J,K,M]Z

LC Limited Coverage   NC Noncovered   HAC associated procedure   Combination Only   DRG Non-OR   Non-OR   Revised Text in **GREEN**

0 **Medical and Surgical**
B **Respiratory System**
Y **Transplantation** Putting in or on all or a portion of a living body part taken from another individual or animal to physically take the place and/or function of all or a portion of a similar body part

Body Part Character 4	Approach Character 5	Device Character 6	Qualifier Character 7
C Upper Lung Lobe, Right **LC** **D** Middle Lung Lobe, Right **LC** **F** Lower Lung Lobe, Right **LC** **G** Upper Lung Lobe, Left **LC** **H** Lung Lingula **LC** **J** Lower Lung Lobe, Left **LC** **K** Lung, Right **LC** **L** Lung, Left **LC** **M** Lungs, Bilateral **LC**	**0** Open	**Z** No Device	**0** Allogeneic **1** Syngeneic **2** Zooplastic

LC 0BY[C,D,F,G,H,J,K,L,M]0Z[0,1,2]

Mouth and Throat ØCØ–ØCX

Ø	Medical and Surgical
C	Mouth and Throat
Ø	Alteration	Modifying the anatomic structure of a body part without affecting the function of the body part

Body Part Character 4	Approach Character 5	Device Character 6	Qualifier Character 7
Ø Upper Lip 1 Lower Lip	X External	7 Autologous Tissue Substitute J Synthetic Substitute K Nonautologous Tissue Substitute Z No Device	Z No Qualifier

Ø	Medical and Surgical
C	Mouth and Throat
2	Change	Taking out or off a device from a body part and putting back an identical or similar device in or on the same body part without cutting or puncturing the skin or a mucous membrane

Body Part Character 4	Approach Character 5	Device Character 6	Qualifier Character 7
A Salivary Gland S Larynx Y Mouth and Throat	X External	Ø Drainage Device Y Other Device	Z No Qualifier

Non-OR For all body part, approach, device, and qualifier values

Ø	Medical and Surgical
C	Mouth and Throat
5	Destruction	Physical eradication of all or a portion of a body part by the direct use of energy, force, or a destructive agent

Body Part Character 4	Approach Character 5	Device Character 6	Qualifier Character 7
Ø Upper Lip 1 Lower Lip 2 Hard Palate 3 Soft Palate 4 Buccal Mucosa 5 Upper Gingiva 6 Lower Gingiva 7 Tongue N Uvula P Tonsils Q Adenoids	Ø Open 3 Percutaneous X External	Z No Device	Z No Qualifier
8 Parotid Gland, Right 9 Parotid Gland, Left B Parotid Duct, Right C Parotid Duct, Left D Sublingual Gland, Right F Sublingual Gland, Left G Submaxillary Gland, Right H Submaxillary Gland, Left J Minor Salivary Gland	Ø Open 3 Percutaneous	Z No Device	Z No Qualifier
M Pharynx R Epiglottis S Larynx T Vocal Cord, Right V Vocal Cord, Left	Ø Open 3 Percutaneous 4 Percutaneous Endoscopic 7 Via Natural or Artificial Opening 8 Via Natural or Artificial Opening Endoscopic	Z No Device	Z No Qualifier
W Upper Tooth X Lower Tooth	Ø Open X External	Z No Device	Ø Single 1 Multiple 2 All

Non-OR ØC5[5,6][Ø,3,X]ZZ
Non-OR ØC5[W,X][Ø,X]Z[Ø,1,2]

0   **Medical and Surgical**
C   **Mouth and Throat**
7   **Dilation**   Expanding an orifice or the lumen of a tubular body part

Body Part Character 4	Approach Character 5	Device Character 6	Qualifier Character 7
B Parotid Duct, Right **C** Parotid Duct, Left	**0** Open **3** Percutaneous **7** Via Natural or Artificial Opening	**D** Intraluminal Device **Z** No Device	**Z** No Qualifier
M Pharynx	**7** Via Natural or Artificial Opening **8** Via Natural or Artificial Opening Endoscopic	**D** Intraluminal Device **Z** No Device	**Z** No Qualifier
S Larynx	**0** Open **3** Percutaneous **4** Percutaneous Endoscopic **7** Via Natural or Artificial Opening **8** Via Natural or Artificial Opening Endoscopic	**D** Intraluminal Device **Z** No Device	**Z** No Qualifier

Non-OR   0C7[B,C][0,3,7][D,Z]Z
Non-OR   0C7M[7,8][D,Z]Z

0   **Medical and Surgical**
C   **Mouth and Throat**
9   **Drainage**   Taking or letting out fluids and/or gases from a body part

Body Part Character 4	Approach Character 5	Device Character 6	Qualifier Character 7
0 Upper Lip **1** Lower Lip **2** Hard Palate **3** Soft Palate **4** Buccal Mucosa **5** Upper Gingiva **6** Lower Gingiva **7** Tongue **N** Uvula **P** Tonsils **Q** Adenoids	**0** Open **3** Percutaneous **X** External	**0** Drainage Device	**Z** No Qualifier
0 Upper Lip **1** Lower Lip **2** Hard Palate **3** Soft Palate **4** Buccal Mucosa **5** Upper Gingiva **6** Lower Gingiva **7** Tongue **N** Uvula **P** Tonsils **Q** Adenoids	**0** Open **3** Percutaneous **X** External	**Z** No Device	**X** Diagnostic **Z** No Qualifier
8 Parotid Gland, Right **9** Parotid Gland, Left **B** Parotid Duct, Right **C** Parotid Duct, Left **D** Sublingual Gland, Right **F** Sublingual Gland, Left **G** Submaxillary Gland, Right **H** Submaxillary Gland, Left **J** Minor Salivary Gland	**0** Open **3** Percutaneous	**0** Drainage Device	**Z** No Qualifier
8 Parotid Gland, Right **9** Parotid Gland, Left **B** Parotid Duct, Right **C** Parotid Duct, Left **D** Sublingual Gland, Right **F** Sublingual Gland, Left **G** Submaxillary Gland, Right **H** Submaxillary Gland, Left **J** Minor Salivary Gland	**0** Open **3** Percutaneous	**Z** No Device	**X** Diagnostic **Z** No Qualifier

0C9 Continued on next page

Non-OR   0C9[5,6][0,3,X]0Z
Non-OR   0C9[0,1,4,5,6][0,3,X]ZX
Non-OR   0C9[5,6][0,3,X]ZZ
Non-OR   0C9[8,9,B,C,D,F,G,H,J]3ZX
Non-OR   0C9[8,9,B,C,D,F,G,H,J][0,3]0Z
Non-OR   0C9[8,9,B,C,D,F,G,H,J][0,3]ZZ

LC Limited Coverage   **NC** Noncovered   HAC associated procedure   Combination Only   DRG Non-OR   Non-OR   Revised Text in **GREEN**

ICD-10-PCS 2014 (Draft)   231

0C9 Continued

0	**Medical and Surgical**
C	**Mouth and Throat**
9	**Drainage** Taking or letting out fluids and/or gases from a body part

Body Part Character 4	Approach Character 5	Device Character 6	Qualifier Character 7
M Pharynx R Epiglottis S Larynx T Vocal Cord, Right V Vocal Cord, Left	0 Open 3 Percutaneous 4 Percutaneous Endoscopic 7 Via Natural or Artificial Opening 8 Via Natural or Artificial Opening Endoscopic	0 Drainage Device	Z No Qualifier
M Pharynx R Epiglottis S Larynx T Vocal Cord, Right V Vocal Cord, Left	0 Open 3 Percutaneous 4 Percutaneous Endoscopic 7 Via Natural or Artificial Opening 8 Via Natural or Artificial Opening Endoscopic	Z No Device	X Diagnostic Z No Qualifier
W Upper Tooth X Lower Tooth	0 Open X External	0 Drainage Device Z No Device	0 Single 1 Multiple 2 All

Non-OR   0C9[R,S,T,V][3,4,7,8]ZX
Non-OR   0C9[W,X][0,X][0,Z][0,1,2]

0	**Medical and Surgical**
C	**Mouth and Throat**
B	**Excision** Cutting out or off, without replacement, a portion of a body part

Body Part Character 4	Approach Character 5	Device Character 6	Qualifier Character 7
0 Upper Lip 1 Lower Lip 2 Hard Palate 3 Soft Palate 4 Buccal Mucosa 5 Upper Gingiva 6 Lower Gingiva 7 Tongue N Uvula P Tonsils Q Adenoids	0 Open 3 Percutaneous X External	Z No Device	X Diagnostic Z No Qualifier
8 Parotid Gland, Right 9 Parotid Gland, Left B Parotid Duct, Right C Parotid Duct, Left D Sublingual Gland, Right F Sublingual Gland, Left G Submaxillary Gland, Right H Submaxillary Gland, Left J Minor Salivary Gland	0 Open 3 Percutaneous	Z No Device	X Diagnostic Z No Qualifier
M Pharynx R Epiglottis S Larynx T Vocal Cord, Right V Vocal Cord, Left	0 Open 3 Percutaneous 4 Percutaneous Endoscopic 7 Via Natural or Artificial Opening 8 Via Natural or Artificial Opening Endoscopic	Z No Device	X Diagnostic Z No Qualifier
W Upper Tooth X Lower Tooth	0 Open X External	Z No Device	0 Single 1 Multiple 2 All

Non-OR   0CB[0,1,4,5,6][0,3,X]ZX
Non-OR   0CB[5,6][0,3,X]ZZ
Non-OR   0CB7[3,X]ZX
Non-OR   0CB[8,9,B,C,D,F,G,H,J]3ZX
Non-OR   0CBM[0,3,4,7,8]ZX
Non-OR   0CB[R,S,T,V][3,4,7,8]ZX
Non-OR   0CB[W,X][0,X]Z[0,1,2]

0 **Medical and Surgical**
C **Mouth and Throat**
C **Extirpation**   Taking or cutting out solid matter from a body part

Body Part Character 4	Approach Character 5	Device Character 6	Qualifier Character 7
0 Upper Lip **1** Lower Lip **2** Hard Palate **3** Soft Palate **4** Buccal Mucosa **5** Upper Gingiva **6** Lower Gingiva **7** Tongue **N** Uvula **P** Tonsils **Q** Adenoids	**0** Open **3** Percutaneous **X** External	**Z** No Device	**Z** No Qualifier
8 Parotid Gland, Right **9** Parotid Gland, Left **B** Parotid Duct, Right **C** Parotid Duct, Left **D** Sublingual Gland, Right **F** Sublingual Gland, Left **G** Submaxillary Gland, Right **H** Submaxillary Gland, Left **J** Minor Salivary Gland	**0** Open **3** Percutaneous	**Z** No Device	**Z** No Qualifier
M Pharynx **R** Epiglottis **S** Larynx **T** Vocal Cord, Right **V** Vocal Cord, Left	**0** Open **3** Percutaneous **4** Percutaneous Endoscopic **7** Via Natural or Artificial Opening **8** Via Natural or Artificial Opening Endoscopic	**Z** No Device	**Z** No Qualifier
W Upper Tooth **X** Lower Tooth	**0** Open **X** External	**Z** No Device	**0** Single **1** Multiple **2** All

Non-OR   0CC[0,1,2,3,4,7,N,P,Q]XZZ
Non-OR   0CC[5,6][0,3,X]ZZ
Non-OR   0CC[8,9,B,C,D,F,G,H,J][0,3]ZZ
Non-OR   0CC[M,S][7,8]ZZ
Non-OR   0CC[W,X][0,X]Z[0,1,2]

0 **Medical and Surgical**
C **Mouth and Throat**
D **Extraction**   Pulling or stripping out or off all or a portion of a body part by the use of force

Body Part Character 4	Approach Character 5	Device Character 6	Qualifier Character 7
T Vocal Cord, Right **V** Vocal Cord, Left	**0** Open **3** Percutaneous **4** Percutaneous Endoscopic **7** Via Natural or Artificial Opening **8** Via Natural or Artificial Opening Endoscopic	**Z** No Device	**Z** No Qualifier
W Upper Tooth **X** Lower Tooth	**X** External	**Z** No Device	**0** Single **1** Multiple **2** All

Non-OR   0CD[W,X]XZ[0,1,2]

0 **Medical and Surgical**
C **Mouth and Throat**
F **Fragmentation**   Breaking solid matter in a body part into pieces

Body Part Character 4	Approach Character 5	Device Character 6	Qualifier Character 7
B Parotid Duct, Right NC **C** Parotid Duct, Left NC	**0** Open **3** Percutaneous **7** Via Natural or Artificial Opening **X** External	**Z** No Device	**Z** No Qualifier

NC   0CF[B,C]XZZ
Non-OR   For all body part, approach, device, and qualifier values

Mouth and Throat

Ø Medical and Surgical
C Mouth and Throat
H Insertion — Putting in a nonbiological appliance that monitors, assists, performs, or prevents a physiological function but does not physically take the place of a body part

Body Part Character 4	Approach Character 5	Device Character 6	Qualifier Character 7
7 Tongue	Ø Open 3 Percutaneous X External	1 Radioactive Element	Z No Qualifier
Y Mouth and Throat	7 Via Natural or Artificial Opening 8 Via Natural or Artificial Opening Endoscopic	B Intraluminal Device, Airway	Z No Qualifier

Non-OR ØCHY[7,8]BZ

Ø Medical and Surgical
C Mouth and Throat
J Inspection — Visually and/or manually exploring a body part

Body Part Character 4	Approach Character 5	Device Character 6	Qualifier Character 7
A Salivary Gland	Ø Open 3 Percutaneous X External	Z No Device	Z No Qualifier
S Larynx Y Mouth and Throat	Ø Open 3 Percutaneous 4 Percutaneous Endoscopic 7 Via Natural or Artificial Opening 8 Via Natural or Artificial Opening Endoscopic X External	Z No Device	Z No Qualifier

Non-OR ØCJA[Ø,3,X]ZZ
Non-OR ØCJ[S,Y][Ø,3,4,7,8,X]ZZ

Ø Medical and Surgical
C Mouth and Throat
L Occlusion — Completely closing an orifice or the lumen of a tubular body part

Body Part Character 4	Approach Character 5	Device Character 6	Qualifier Character 7
B Parotid Duct, Right C Parotid Duct, Left	Ø Open 3 Percutaneous 4 Percutaneous Endoscopic	C Extraluminal Device D Intraluminal Device Z No Device	Z No Qualifier
B Parotid Duct, Right C Parotid Duct, Left	7 Via Natural or Artificial Opening 8 Via Natural or Artificial Opening Endoscopic	D Intraluminal Device Z No Device	Z No Qualifier

Ø Medical and Surgical
C Mouth and Throat
M Reattachment — Putting back in or on all or a portion of a separated body part to its normal location or other suitable location

Body Part Character 4	Approach Character 5	Device Character 6	Qualifier Character 7
Ø Upper Lip 1 Lower Lip 3 Soft Palate 7 Tongue N Uvula	Ø Open	Z No Device	Z No Qualifier
W Upper Tooth X Lower Tooth	Ø Open X External	Z No Device	Ø Single 1 Multiple 2 All

Non-OR ØCM[W,X][Ø,X]Z[Ø,1,2]

Ø Medical and Surgical
C Mouth and Throat
N Release   Freeing a body part from an abnormal physical constraint

Body Part Character 4	Approach Character 5	Device Character 6	Qualifier Character 7
Ø Upper Lip 1 Lower Lip 2 Hard Palate 3 Soft Palate 4 Buccal Mucosa 5 Upper Gingiva 6 Lower Gingiva 7 Tongue N Uvula P Tonsils Q Adenoids	Ø Open 3 Percutaneous X External	Z No Device	Z No Qualifier
8 Parotid Gland, Right 9 Parotid Gland, Left B Parotid Duct, Right C Parotid Duct, Left D Sublingual Gland, Right F Sublingual Gland, Left G Submaxillary Gland, Right H Submaxillary Gland, Left J Minor Salivary Gland	Ø Open 3 Percutaneous	Z No Device	Z No Qualifier
W Upper Tooth X Lower Tooth	Ø Open X External	Z No Device	Ø Single 1 Multiple 2 All
M Pharynx R Epiglottis S Larynx T Vocal Cord, Right V Vocal Cord, Left	Ø Open 3 Percutaneous 4 Percutaneous Endoscopic 7 Via Natural or Artificial Opening 8 Via Natural or Artificial Opening Endoscopic	Z No Device	Z No Qualifier

Non-OR ØCN[Ø,1,5,6,7][Ø,3,X]ZZ
Non-OR ØCN[W,X][Ø,X]Z[Ø,1,2]

Ø Medical and Surgical
C Mouth and Throat
P Removal   Taking out or off a device from a body part

Body Part Character 4	Approach Character 5	Device Character 6	Qualifier Character 7
A Salivary Gland	Ø Open 3 Percutaneous	Ø Drainage Device C Extraluminal Device	Z No Qualifier
S Larynx	Ø Open 3 Percutaneous 7 Via Natural or Artificial Opening 8 Via Natural or Artificial Opening Endoscopic X External	Ø Drainage Device 7 Autologous Tissue Substitute D Intraluminal Device J Synthetic Substitute K Nonautologous Tissue Substitute	Z No Qualifier
Y Mouth and Throat	Ø Open 3 Percutaneous 7 Via Natural or Artificial Opening 8 Via Natural or Artificial Opening Endoscopic X External	Ø Drainage Device 1 Radioactive Element 7 Autologous Tissue Substitute D Intraluminal Device J Synthetic Substitute K Nonautologous Tissue Substitute	Z No Qualifier

Non-OR ØCPA[Ø,3][Ø,C]Z
Non-OR ØCPSX[Ø,7,D,J,K]Z
Non-OR ØCPY[7,8][Ø,D]Z
Non-OR ØCPYX[Ø,1,7,D,J,K]Z

Mouth and Throat

ØCQ–ØCR

Ø Medical and Surgical
C Mouth and Throat
Q Repair   Restoring, to the extent possible, a body part to its normal anatomic structure and function

Body Part Character 4	Approach Character 5	Device Character 6	Qualifier Character 7
Ø Upper Lip 1 Lower Lip 2 Hard Palate 3 Soft Palate 4 Buccal Mucosa 5 Upper Gingiva 6 Lower Gingiva 7 Tongue N Uvula P Tonsils Q Adenoids	Ø Open 3 Percutaneous X External	Z No Device	Z No Qualifier
8 Parotid Gland, Right 9 Parotid Gland, Left B Parotid Duct, Right C Parotid Duct, Left D Sublingual Gland, Right F Sublingual Gland, Left G Submaxillary Gland, Right H Submaxillary Gland, Left J Minor Salivary Gland	Ø Open 3 Percutaneous	Z No Device	Z No Qualifier
M Pharynx R Epiglottis S Larynx T Vocal Cord, Right V Vocal Cord, Left	Ø Open 3 Percutaneous 4 Percutaneous Endoscopic 7 Via Natural or Artificial Opening 8 Via Natural or Artificial Opening Endoscopic	Z No Device	Z No Qualifier
W Upper Tooth X Lower Tooth	Ø Open X External	Z No Device	Ø Single 1 Multiple 2 All

Non-OR   ØCQ[5,6][Ø,3,X]ZZ
Non-OR   ØCQ[W,X][Ø,X]Z[Ø,1,2]

Ø Medical and Surgical
C Mouth and Throat
R Replacement   Putting in or on biological or synthetic material that physically takes the place and/or function of all or a portion of a body part

Body Part Character 4	Approach Character 5	Device Character 6	Qualifier Character 7
Ø Upper Lip 1 Lower Lip 2 Hard Palate 3 Soft Palate 4 Buccal Mucosa 5 Upper Gingiva 6 Lower Gingiva 7 Tongue N Uvula	Ø Open 3 Percutaneous X External	7 Autologous Tissue Substitute J Synthetic Substitute K Nonautologous Tissue Substitute	Z No Qualifier
B Parotid Duct, Right C Parotid Duct, Left	Ø Open 3 Percutaneous	7 Autologous Tissue Substitute J Synthetic Substitute K Nonautologous Tissue Substitute	Z No Qualifier
M Pharynx R Epiglottis S Larynx T Vocal Cord, Right V Vocal Cord, Left	Ø Open 7 Via Natural or Artificial Opening 8 Via Natural or Artificial Opening Endoscopic	7 Autologous Tissue Substitute J Synthetic Substitute K Nonautologous Tissue Substitute	Z No Qualifier
W Upper Tooth X Lower Tooth	Ø Open X External	7 Autologous Tissue Substitute J Synthetic Substitute K Nonautologous Tissue Substitute	Ø Single 1 Multiple 2 All

Non-OR   ØCR[W,X][Ø,X][7,J,K][Ø,1,2]

Ø　Medical and Surgical
C　Mouth and Throat
S　Reposition　　　Moving to its normal location or other suitable location all or a portion of a body part

Body Part Character 4	Approach Character 5	Device Character 6	Qualifier Character 7
Ø　Upper Lip 1　Lower Lip 2　Hard Palate 3　Soft Palate 7　Tongue N　Uvula	Ø　Open X　External	Z　No Device	Z　No Qualifier
B　Parotid Duct, Right C　Parotid Duct, Left	Ø　Open 3　Percutaneous	Z　No Device	Z　No Qualifier
R　Epiglottis T　Vocal Cord, Right V　Vocal Cord, Left	Ø　Open 7　Via Natural or Artificial Opening 8　Via Natural or Artificial Opening 　　Endoscopic	Z　No Device	Z　No Qualifier
W　Upper Tooth X　Lower Tooth	Ø　Open X　External	5　External Fixation Device Z　No Device	Ø　Single 1　Multiple 2　All

Non-OR　ØCS[W,X][Ø,X][5,Z][Ø,1,2]

Ø　Medical and Surgical
C　Mouth and Throat
T　Resection　　　Cutting out or off, without replacement, all of a body part

Body Part Character 4	Approach Character 5	Device Character 6	Qualifier Character 7
Ø　Upper Lip 1　Lower Lip 2　Hard Palate 3　Soft Palate 7　Tongue N　Uvula P　Tonsils Q　Adenoids	Ø　Open X　External	Z　No Device	Z　No Qualifier
8　Parotid Gland, Right 9　Parotid Gland, Left B　Parotid Duct, Right C　Parotid Duct, Left D　Sublingual Gland, Right F　Sublingual Gland, Left G　Submaxillary Gland, Right H　Submaxillary Gland, Left J　Minor Salivary Gland	Ø　Open	Z　No Device	Z　No Qualifier
M　Pharynx R　Epiglottis S　Larynx T　Vocal Cord, Right V　Vocal Cord, Left	Ø　Open 4　Percutaneous Endoscopic 7　Via Natural or Artificial Opening 8　Via Natural or Artificial Opening 　　Endoscopic	Z　No Device	Z　No Qualifier
W　Upper Tooth X　Lower Tooth	Ø　Open	Z　No Device	Ø　Single 1　Multiple 2　All

Non-OR　ØCT[W,X]ØZ[Ø,1,2]

Mouth and Throat

Ø **Medical and Surgical**
C **Mouth and Throat**
U **Supplement**　　　Putting in or on biological or synthetic material that physically reinforces and/or augments the function of a portion of a body part

Body Part Character 4	Approach Character 5	Device Character 6	Qualifier Character 7
Ø Upper Lip 1 Lower Lip 2 Hard Palate 3 Soft Palate 4 Buccal Mucosa 5 Upper Gingiva 6 Lower Gingiva 7 Tongue N Uvula	Ø Open 3 Percutaneous X External	7 Autologous Tissue Substitute J Synthetic Substitute K Nonautologous Tissue Substitute	Z No Qualifier
M Pharynx R Epiglottis S Larynx T Vocal Cord, Right V Vocal Cord, Left	Ø Open 7 Via Natural or Artificial Opening 8 Via Natural or Artificial Opening Endoscopic	7 Autologous Tissue Substitute J Synthetic Substitute K Nonautologous Tissue Substitute	Z No Qualifier

Non-OR　ØCU2[Ø,3]JZ

Ø **Medical and Surgical**
C **Mouth and Throat**
V **Restriction**　　　Partially closing an orifice or the lumen of a tubular body part

Body Part Character 4	Approach Character 5	Device Character 6	Qualifier Character 7
B Parotid Duct, Right C Parotid Duct, Left	Ø Open 3 Percutaneous	C Extraluminal Device D Intraluminal Device Z No Device	Z No Qualifier
B Parotid Duct, Right C Parotid Duct, Left	7 Via Natural or Artificial Opening 8 Via Natural or Artificial Opening Endoscopic	D Intraluminal Device Z No Device	Z No Qualifier

Ø **Medical and Surgical**
C **Mouth and Throat**
W **Revision**　　　Correcting, to the extent possible, a portion of a malfunctioning device or the position of a displaced device

Body Part Character 4	Approach Character 5	Device Character 6	Qualifier Character 7
A Salivary Gland	Ø Open 3 Percutaneous X External	Ø Drainage Device C Extraluminal Device	Z No Qualifier
S Larynx	Ø Open 3 Percutaneous 7 Via Natural or Artificial Opening 8 Via Natural or Artificial Opening Endoscopic X External	Ø Drainage Device 7 Autologous Tissue Substitute D Intraluminal Device J Synthetic Substitute K Nonautologous Tissue Substitute	Z No Qualifier
Y Mouth and Throat	Ø Open 3 Percutaneous 7 Via Natural or Artificial Opening 8 Via Natural or Artificial Opening Endoscopic X External	Ø Drainage Device 1 Radioactive Element 7 Autologous Tissue Substitute D Intraluminal Device J Synthetic Substitute K Nonautologous Tissue Substitute	Z No Qualifier

Non-OR　ØCWA[Ø,3,X][Ø,C]Z
Non-OR　ØCWSX[Ø,7,D,J,K]Z
Non-OR　ØCWYØ7Z
Non-OR　ØCWYX[Ø,1,7,D,J,K]Z

Ø **Medical and Surgical**
C **Mouth and Throat**
X **Transfer**　　　Moving, without taking out, all or a portion of a body part to another location to take over the function of all or a portion of a body part

Body Part Character 4	Approach Character 5	Device Character 6	Qualifier Character 7
Ø Upper Lip 1 Lower Lip 3 Soft Palate 4 Buccal Mucosa 5 Upper Gingiva 6 Lower Gingiva 7 Tongue	Ø Open X External	Z No Device	Z No Qualifier

LC Limited Coverage　　　NC Noncovered　　　HAC associated procedure　　　Combination Only　　　DRG Non-OR　　　Non-OR　　　Revised Text in **GREEN**

Gastrointestinal System 0D1–0DY

0 Medical and Surgical
D Gastrointestinal System
1 Bypass   Altering the route of passage of the contents of a tubular body part

Body Part Character 4	Approach Character 5	Device Character 6	Qualifier Character 7
1 Esophagus, Upper 2 Esophagus, Middle 3 Esophagus, Lower 5 Esophagus	0 Open 4 Percutaneous Endoscopic 8 Via Natural or Artificial Opening Endoscopic	7 Autologous Tissue Substitute J Synthetic Substitute K Nonautologous Tissue Substitute Z No Device	4 Cutaneous 6 Stomach 9 Duodenum A Jejunum B Ileum
1 Esophagus, Upper 2 Esophagus, Middle 3 Esophagus, Lower 5 Esophagus 6 Stomach 9 Duodenum A Jejunum B Ileum H Cecum K Ascending Colon L Transverse Colon M Descending Colon N Sigmoid Colon	3 Percutaneous	J Synthetic Substitute	4 Cutaneous
6 Stomach 9 Duodenum	0 Open 4 Percutaneous Endoscopic 8 Via Natural or Artificial Opening Endoscopic	7 Autologous Tissue Substitute J Synthetic Substitute K Nonautologous Tissue Substitute Z No Device	4 Cutaneous 9 Duodenum A Jejunum B Ileum L Transverse Colon
A Jejunum	0 Open 4 Percutaneous Endoscopic 8 Via Natural or Artificial Opening Endoscopic	7 Autologous Tissue Substitute J Synthetic Substitute K Nonautologous Tissue Substitute Z No Device	4 Cutaneous A Jejunum B Ileum H Cecum K Ascending Colon L Transverse Colon M Descending Colon N Sigmoid Colon P Rectum Q Anus
B Ileum	0 Open 4 Percutaneous Endoscopic 8 Via Natural or Artificial Opening Endoscopic	7 Autologous Tissue Substitute J Synthetic Substitute K Nonautologous Tissue Substitute Z No Device	4 Cutaneous B Ileum H Cecum K Ascending Colon L Transverse Colon M Descending Colon N Sigmoid Colon P Rectum Q Anus
H Cecum	0 Open 4 Percutaneous Endoscopic 8 Via Natural or Artificial Opening Endoscopic	7 Autologous Tissue Substitute J Synthetic Substitute K Nonautologous Tissue Substitute Z No Device	4 Cutaneous H Cecum K Ascending Colon L Transverse Colon M Descending Colon N Sigmoid Colon P Rectum
K Ascending Colon	0 Open 4 Percutaneous Endoscopic 8 Via Natural or Artificial Opening Endoscopic	7 Autologous Tissue Substitute J Synthetic Substitute K Nonautologous Tissue Substitute Z No Device	4 Cutaneous K Ascending Colon L Transverse Colon M Descending Colon N Sigmoid Colon P Rectum
L Transverse Colon	0 Open 4 Percutaneous Endoscopic 8 Via Natural or Artificial Opening Endoscopic	7 Autologous Tissue Substitute J Synthetic Substitute K Nonautologous Tissue Substitute Z No Device	4 Cutaneous L Transverse Colon M Descending Colon N Sigmoid Colon P Rectum

0D1 Continued on next page

Non-OR	0D163J4
Non-OR	0D16[0,4,8][7,J,K,Z]4
HAC	0D16[0,4,8][7,J,K,Z] [9,A,B,L] when reported with PDx E66.01 and SDx K68.11 or K95.01 or K95.81 or T81.4XXA

LC Limited Coverage   NC Noncovered   HAC associated procedure   Combination Only   DRG Non-OR   Non-OR   Revised Text in **GREEN**

Gastrointestinal System

ØD1–ØD5

Ø **Medical and Surgical**
D **Gastrointestinal System**
1 **Bypass**   Altering the route of passage of the contents of a tubular body part

Body Part Character 4	Approach Character 5	Device Character 6	Qualifier Character 7
M Descending Colon	Ø Open 4 Percutaneous Endoscopic 8 Via Natural or Artificial Opening Endoscopic	7 Autologous Tissue Substitute J Synthetic Substitute K Nonautologous Tissue Substitute Z No Device	4 Cutaneous M Descending Colon N Sigmoid Colon P Rectum
N Sigmoid Colon	Ø Open 4 Percutaneous Endoscopic 8 Via Natural or Artificial Opening Endoscopic	7 Autologous Tissue Substitute J Synthetic Substitute K Nonautologous Tissue Substitute Z No Device	4 Cutaneous N Sigmoid Colon P Rectum

Ø **Medical and Surgical**
D **Gastrointestinal System**
2 **Change**   Taking out or off a device from a body part and putting back an identical or similar device in or on the same body part without cutting or puncturing the skin or a mucous membrane

Body Part Character 4	Approach Character 5	Device Character 6	Qualifier Character 7
Ø Upper Intestinal Tract D Lower Intestinal Tract	X External	Ø Drainage Device U Feeding Device Y Other Device	Z No Qualifier
U Omentum V Mesentery W Peritoneum	X External	Ø Drainage Device Y Other Device	Z No Qualifier

Non-OR   For all body part, approach, device, and qualifier values

Ø **Medical and Surgical**
D **Gastrointestinal System**
5 **Destruction**   Physical eradication of all or a portion of a body part by the direct use of energy, force, or a destructive agent

Body Part Character 4	Approach Character 5	Device Character 6	Qualifier Character 7
1 Esophagus, Upper 2 Esophagus, Middle 3 Esophagus, Lower 4 Esophagogastric Junction 5 Esophagus 6 Stomach 7 Stomach, Pylorus 8 Small Intestine 9 Duodenum A Jejunum B Ileum C Ileocecal Valve E Large Intestine F Large Intestine, Right G Large Intestine, Left H Cecum J Appendix K Ascending Colon L Transverse Colon M Descending Colon N Sigmoid Colon P Rectum	Ø Open 3 Percutaneous 4 Percutaneous Endoscopic 7 Via Natural or Artificial Opening 8 Via Natural or Artificial Opening Endoscopic	Z No Device	Z No Qualifier
Q Anus	Ø Open 3 Percutaneous 4 Percutaneous Endoscopic 7 Via Natural or Artificial Opening 8 Via Natural or Artificial Opening Endoscopic X External	Z No Device	Z No Qualifier
R Anal Sphincter S Greater Omentum T Lesser Omentum V Mesentery W Peritoneum	Ø Open 3 Percutaneous 4 Percutaneous Endoscopic	Z No Device	Z No Qualifier

Non-OR   ØD5[1,2,3,4,5,6,7,9,E,F,G,H,K,L,M,N][4,8]ZZ
Non-OR   ØD5P[Ø,3,4,7,8]ZZ
Non-OR   ØD5Q[4,8]ZZ
Non-OR   ØD5R4ZZ

0   Medical and Surgical
D   Gastrointestinal System
7   Dilation   Expanding an orifice or the lumen of a tubular body part

Body Part Character 4	Approach Character 5	Device Character 6	Qualifier Character 7
1 Esophagus, Upper **2** Esophagus, Middle **3** Esophagus, Lower **4** Esophagogastric Junction **5** Esophagus **6** Stomach **7** Stomach, Pylorus **8** Small Intestine **9** Duodenum **A** Jejunum **B** Ileum **C** Ileocecal Valve **E** Large Intestine **F** Large Intestine, Right **G** Large Intestine, Left **H** Cecum **K** Ascending Colon **L** Transverse Colon **M** Descending Colon **N** Sigmoid Colon **P** Rectum **Q** Anus	**0** Open **3** Percutaneous **4** Percutaneous Endoscopic **7** Via Natural or Artificial Opening **8** Via Natural or Artificial Opening Endoscopic	**D** Intraluminal Device **Z** No Device	**Z** No Qualifier

Non-OR 0D7[1,2,3,4,5,8,9,A,B,C,E,F,G,H,K,L,M,N,P,Q][7,8][D,Z]Z
Non-OR 0D77[4,8]DZ
Non-OR 0D7[8,9,A,B,C,E,F,G,H,K,L,M,N][0,3,4]DZ

0   Medical and Surgical
D   Gastrointestinal System
8   Division   Cutting into a body part without draining fluids and/or gases from the body part in order to separate or transect a body part

Body Part Character 4	Approach Character 5	Device Character 6	Qualifier Character 7
4 Esophagogastric Junction **7** Stomach, Pylorus	**0** Open **3** Percutaneous **4** Percutaneous Endoscopic **7** Via Natural or Artificial Opening **8** Via Natural or Artificial Opening Endoscopic	**Z** No Device	**Z** No Qualifier
R Anal Sphincter	**0** Open **3** Percutaneous	**Z** No Device	**Z** No Qualifier

Gastrointestinal System

Ø   **Medical and Surgical**
D   **Gastrointestinal System**
9   **Drainage**   Taking or letting out fluids and/or gases from a body part

Body Part Character 4	Approach Character 5	Device Character 6	Qualifier Character 7
1 Esophagus, Upper 2 Esophagus, Middle 3 Esophagus, Lower 4 Esophagogastric Junction 5 Esophagus 6 Stomach 7 Stomach, Pylorus 8 Small Intestine 9 Duodenum A Jejunum B Ileum C Ileocecal Valve E Large Intestine F Large Intestine, Right G Large Intestine, Left H Cecum J Appendix K Ascending Colon L Transverse Colon M Descending Colon N Sigmoid Colon P Rectum	Ø Open 3 Percutaneous 4 Percutaneous Endoscopic 7 Via Natural or Artificial Opening 8 Via Natural or Artificial Opening Endoscopic	Ø Drainage Device	Z No Qualifier
1 Esophagus, Upper 2 Esophagus, Middle 3 Esophagus, Lower 4 Esophagogastric Junction 5 Esophagus 6 Stomach 7 Stomach, Pylorus 8 Small Intestine 9 Duodenum A Jejunum B Ileum C Ileocecal Valve E Large Intestine F Large Intestine, Right G Large Intestine, Left H Cecum J Appendix K Ascending Colon L Transverse Colon M Descending Colon N Sigmoid Colon P Rectum	Ø Open 3 Percutaneous 4 Percutaneous Endoscopic 7 Via Natural or Artificial Opening 8 Via Natural or Artificial Opening Endoscopic	Z No Device	X Diagnostic Z No Qualifier
Q Anus	Ø Open 3 Percutaneous 4 Percutaneous Endoscopic 7 Via Natural or Artificial Opening 8 Via Natural or Artificial Opening Endoscopic X External	Ø Drainage Device	Z No Qualifier
Q Anus	Ø Open 3 Percutaneous 4 Percutaneous Endoscopic 7 Via Natural or Artificial Opening 8 Via Natural or Artificial Opening Endoscopic X External	Z No Device	X Diagnostic Z No Qualifier
R Anal Sphincter S Greater Omentum T Lesser Omentum V Mesentery W Peritoneum	Ø Open 3 Percutaneous 4 Percutaneous Endoscopic	Ø Drainage Device	Z No Qualifier
R Anal Sphincter S Greater Omentum T Lesser Omentum V Mesentery W Peritoneum	Ø Open 3 Percutaneous 4 Percutaneous Endoscopic	Z No Device	X Diagnostic Z No Qualifier

Non-OR ØD9[6,7,8,9,A,B,E,F,G,H,K,L,M,N,P][7,8]ØZ	**Non-OR** ØD9R[Ø,3,4]ZX
Non-OR ØD9[1,2,3,4,5,6,7,8,9,A,B,C,E,F,G,H,K,L,M,N,P][3,4,7,8]ZX	**Non-OR** ØD9[S,T,V,W][3,4]ØZ
Non-OR ØD9Q[Ø,3,4,7,8,X]ZX	**Non-OR** ØD9[S,T,V,W][3,4]ZZ

Ø Medical and Surgical
D Gastrointestinal System
B Excision   Cutting out or off, without replacement, a portion of a body part

Body Part Character 4	Approach Character 5	Device Character 6	Qualifier Character 7
1 Esophagus, Upper 2 Esophagus, Middle 3 Esophagus, Lower 4 Esophagogastric Junction 5 Esophagus 7 Stomach, Pylorus 8 Small Intestine 9 Duodenum A Jejunum B Ileum C Ileocecal Valve E Large Intestine F Large Intestine, Right G Large Intestine, Left H Cecum J Appendix K Ascending Colon L Transverse Colon M Descending Colon N Sigmoid Colon P Rectum	Ø Open 3 Percutaneous 4 Percutaneous Endoscopic 7 Via Natural or Artificial Opening 8 Via Natural or Artificial Opening Endoscopic	Z No Device	X Diagnostic Z No Qualifier
6 Stomach	Ø Open 3 Percutaneous 4 Percutaneous Endoscopic 7 Via Natural or Artificial Opening 8 Via Natural or Artificial Opening Endoscopic	Z No Device	3 Vertical X Diagnostic Z No Qualifier
Q Anus	Ø Open 3 Percutaneous 4 Percutaneous Endoscopic 7 Via Natural or Artificial Opening 8 Via Natural or Artificial Opening Endoscopic X External	Z No Device	X Diagnostic Z No Qualifier
R Anal Sphincter S Greater Omentum T Lesser Omentum V Mesentery W Peritoneum	Ø Open 3 Percutaneous 4 Percutaneous Endoscopic	Z No Device	X Diagnostic Z No Qualifier

Non-OR   ØDB[1,2,3,4,5,7,8,9,A,B,C,E,F,G,H,K,L,M,N,P][3,4,7,8]ZX
Non-OR   ØDB[1,2,3,5,7,9][4,8]ZZ
Non-OR   ØDB[4,E,F,G,H,K,L,M,N,P]8ZZ
Non-OR   ØDB6[3,4,7]ZX
Non-OR   ØDB6[4,8]ZZ
Non-OR   ØDBQ[Ø,3,4,7,8,X]ZX
Non-OR   ØDBR[Ø,3,4]ZX
Non-OR   ØDB[S,T,V,W][3,4]ZX

LC Limited Coverage   NC Noncovered   HAC associated procedure   Combination Only   DRG Non-OR   Non-OR   Revised Text in GREEN

ØDC–ØDF

Gastrointestinal System

Ø **Medical and Surgical**
D **Gastrointestinal System**
C **Extirpation**   Taking or cutting out solid matter from a body part

Body Part Character 4	Approach Character 5	Device Character 6	Qualifier Character 7
1 Esophagus, Upper 2 Esophagus, Middle 3 Esophagus, Lower 4 Esophagogastric Junction 5 Esophagus 6 Stomach 7 Stomach, Pylorus 8 Small Intestine 9 Duodenum A Jejunum B Ileum C Ileocecal Valve E Large Intestine F Large Intestine, Right G Large Intestine, Left H Cecum J Appendix K Ascending Colon L Transverse Colon M Descending Colon N Sigmoid Colon P Rectum	Ø Open 3 Percutaneous 4 Percutaneous Endoscopic 7 Via Natural or Artificial Opening 8 Via Natural or Artificial Opening Endoscopic	Z No Device	Z No Qualifier
Q Anus	Ø Open 3 Percutaneous 4 Percutaneous Endoscopic 7 Via Natural or Artificial Opening 8 Via Natural or Artificial Opening Endoscopic X External	Z No Device	Z No Qualifier
R Anal Sphincter S Greater Omentum T Lesser Omentum V Mesentery W Peritoneum	Ø Open 3 Percutaneous 4 Percutaneous Endoscopic	Z No Device	Z No Qualifier

Non-OR ØDC[1,2,3,4,5,6,7,8,9,A,B,C,E,F,G,H,K,L,M,N,P][7,8]ZZ
Non-OR ØDCQ[7,8,X]ZZ

Ø **Medical and Surgical**
D **Gastrointestinal System**
F **Fragmentation**   Breaking solid matter in a body part into pieces

Body Part Character 4	Approach Character 5	Device Character 6	Qualifier Character 7
5 Esophagus NC 6 Stomach NC 8 Small Intestine NC 9 Duodenum NC A Jejunum NC B Ileum NC E Large Intestine NC F Large Intestine, Right NC G Large Intestine, Left NC H Cecum NC J Appendix NC K Ascending Colon NC L Transverse Colon NC M Descending Colon NC N Sigmoid Colon NC P Rectum NC Q Anus NC	Ø Open 3 Percutaneous 4 Percutaneous Endoscopic 7 Via Natural or Artificial Opening 8 Via Natural or Artificial Opening Endoscopic X External	Z No Device	Z No Qualifier

NC ØDF[5,6,8,9,A,B,E,F,G,H,J,K,L,M,N,P,Q]XZZ
Non-OR ØDF[5,6,8,9,A,B,E,F,G,H,J,K,L,M,N,P,Q]XZZ

Ø   Medical and Surgical
D   Gastrointestinal System
H   Insertion   Putting in a nonbiological appliance that monitors, assists, performs, or prevents a physiological function but does not physically take the place of a body part

Body Part Character 4	Approach Character 5	Device Character 6	Qualifier Character 7
5 Esophagus	**Ø** Open **3** Percutaneous **4** Percutaneous Endoscopic	**1** Radioactive Element **2** Monitoring Device **3** Infusion Device **D** Intraluminal Device **U** Feeding Device	**Z** No Qualifier
5 Esophagus	**7** Via Natural or Artificial Opening **8** Via Natural or Artificial Opening Endoscopic	**1** Radioactive Element **2** Monitoring Device **3** Infusion Device **B** Intraluminal Device, Airway **D** Intraluminal Device **U** Feeding Device	**Z** No Qualifier
6 Stomach	**Ø** Open **3** Percutaneous **4** Percutaneous Endoscopic	**2** Monitoring Device **3** Infusion Device **D** Intraluminal Device **M** Stimulator Lead **U** Feeding Device	**Z** No Qualifier
6 Stomach	**7** Via Natural or Artificial Opening **8** Via Natural or Artificial Opening Endoscopic	**2** Monitoring Device **3** Infusion Device **D** Intraluminal Device **U** Feeding Device	**Z** No Qualifier
8 Small Intestine **9** Duodenum **A** Jejunum **B** Ileum	**Ø** Open **3** Percutaneous **4** Percutaneous Endoscopic **7** Via Natural or Artificial Opening **8** Via Natural or Artificial Opening Endoscopic	**2** Monitoring Device **3** Infusion Device **D** Intraluminal Device **U** Feeding Device	**Z** No Qualifier
E Large Intestine	**Ø** Open **3** Percutaneous **4** Percutaneous Endoscopic **7** Via Natural or Artificial Opening **8** Via Natural or Artificial Opening Endoscopic	**D** Intraluminal Device	**Z** No Qualifier
P Rectum	**Ø** Open **3** Percutaneous **4** Percutaneous Endoscopic **7** Via Natural or Artificial Opening **8** Via Natural or Artificial Opening Endoscopic	**1** Radioactive Element **D** Intraluminal Device	**Z** No Qualifier
Q Anus	**Ø** Open **3** Percutaneous **4** Percutaneous Endoscopic	**D** Intraluminal Device **L** Artificial Sphincter	**Z** No Qualifier
Q Anus	**7** Via Natural or Artificial Opening **8** Via Natural or Artificial Opening Endoscopic	**D** Intraluminal Device	**Z** No Qualifier
R Anal Sphincter	**Ø** Open **3** Percutaneous **4** Percutaneous Endoscopic	**M** Stimulator Lead	**Z** No Qualifier

Non-OR	ØDH5[Ø,3,4][D,U]Z
Non-OR	ØDH5[7,8][B,D,U]Z
Non-OR	ØDH6[3,4]UZ
Non-OR	ØDH[8,9,A,B][Ø,3,4,7,8][D,U]Z
Non-OR	ØDH[E,P][Ø,3,4,7,8]DZ
Non-OR	ØDHP[Ø,3,4,7,8]DZ

LC Limited Coverage   **NC** Noncovered   HAC associated procedure   Combination Only   DRG Non-OR   Non-OR   Revised Text in **GREEN**

ICD-10-PCS 2014 (Draft)   **245**

Ø **Medical and Surgical**
D **Gastrointestinal System**
J **Inspection**   Visually and/or manually exploring a body part

Body Part Character 4	Approach Character 5	Device Character 6	Qualifier Character 7
Ø Upper Intestinal Tract **6** Stomach **D** Lower Intestinal Tract	**Ø** Open **3** Percutaneous **4** Percutaneous Endoscopic **7** Via Natural or Artificial Opening **8** Via Natural or Artificial Opening Endoscopic **X** External	**Z** No Device	**Z** No Qualifier
U Omentum **V** Mesentery **W** Peritoneum	**Ø** Open **3** Percutaneous **4** Percutaneous Endoscopic **X** External	**Z** No Device	**Z** No Qualifier

Non-OR   ØDJ[Ø,6,D][3,7,8,X]ZZ
Non-OR   ØDJ[U,V,W]XZZ

Ø **Medical and Surgical**
D **Gastrointestinal System**
L **Occlusion**   Completely closing an orifice or the lumen of a tubular body part

Body Part Character 4	Approach Character 5	Device Character 6	Qualifier Character 7
1 Esophagus, Upper **2** Esophagus, Middle **3** Esophagus, Lower **4** Esophagogastric Junction **5** Esophagus **6** Stomach **7** Stomach, Pylorus **8** Small Intestine **9** Duodenum **A** Jejunum **B** Ileum **C** Ileocecal Valve **E** Large Intestine **F** Large Intestine, Right **G** Large Intestine, Left **H** Cecum **K** Ascending Colon **L** Transverse Colon **M** Descending Colon **N** Sigmoid Colon **P** Rectum	**Ø** Open **3** Percutaneous **4** Percutaneous Endoscopic	**C** Extraluminal Device **D** Intraluminal Device **Z** No Device	**Z** No Qualifier
1 Esophagus, Upper **2** Esophagus, Middle **3** Esophagus, Lower **4** Esophagogastric Junction **5** Esophagus **6** Stomach **7** Stomach, Pylorus **8** Small Intestine **9** Duodenum **A** Jejunum **B** Ileum **C** Ileocecal Valve **E** Large Intestine **F** Large Intestine, Right **G** Large Intestine, Left **H** Cecum **K** Ascending Colon **L** Transverse Colon **M** Descending Colon **N** Sigmoid Colon **P** Rectum **Q** Anus	**7** Via Natural or Artificial Opening **8** Via Natural or Artificial Opening Endoscopic	**D** Intraluminal Device **Z** No Device	**Z** No Qualifier
Q Anus	**Ø** Open **3** Percutaneous **4** Percutaneous Endoscopic **X** External	**C** Extraluminal Device **D** Intraluminal Device **Z** No Device	**Z** No Qualifier

Non-OR   ØDL[1,2,3,4,5][Ø,3,4][C,D,Z]Z
Non-OR   ØDL[1,2,3,4,5][7,8][D,Z]Z

LC Limited Coverage   **NC** Noncovered   HAC associated procedure   Combination Only   DRG Non-OR   Non-OR   Revised Text in **GREEN**

246   ICD-10-PCS 2014 (Draft)

Ø   Medical and Surgical
D   Gastrointestinal System
M   Reattachment   Putting back in or on all or a portion of a separated body part to its normal location or other suitable location

Body Part Character 4	Approach Character 5	Device Character 6	Qualifier Character 7
5 Esophagus 6 Stomach 8 Small Intestine 9 Duodenum A Jejunum B Ileum E Large Intestine F Large Intestine, Right G Large Intestine, Left H Cecum K Ascending Colon L Transverse Colon M Descending Colon N Sigmoid Colon P Rectum	Ø Open 4 Percutaneous Endoscopic	Z No Device	Z No Qualifier

Ø   Medical and Surgical
D   Gastrointestinal System
N   Release   Freeing a body part from an abnormal physical constraint

Body Part Character 4	Approach Character 5	Device Character 6	Qualifier Character 7
1 Esophagus, Upper 2 Esophagus, Middle 3 Esophagus, Lower 4 Esophagogastric Junction 5 Esophagus 6 Stomach 7 Stomach, Pylorus 8 Small Intestine 9 Duodenum A Jejunum B Ileum C Ileocecal Valve E Large Intestine F Large Intestine, Right G Large Intestine, Left H Cecum J Appendix K Ascending Colon L Transverse Colon M Descending Colon N Sigmoid Colon P Rectum	Ø Open 3 Percutaneous 4 Percutaneous Endoscopic 7 Via Natural or Artificial Opening 8 Via Natural or Artificial Opening Endoscopic	Z No Device	Z No Qualifier
Q Anus	Ø Open 3 Percutaneous 4 Percutaneous Endoscopic 7 Via Natural or Artificial Opening 8 Via Natural or Artificial Opening Endoscopic X External	Z No Device	Z No Qualifier
R Anal Sphincter S Greater Omentum T Lesser Omentum V Mesentery W Peritoneum	Ø Open 3 Percutaneous 4 Percutaneous Endoscopic	Z No Device	Z No Qualifier

Non-OR   ØDN[8,9,A,B,E,F,G,H,K,L,M,N][7,8]ZZ

Gastrointestinal System

ØDP–ØDP

Ø	**Medical and Surgical**
D	**Gastrointestinal System**
P	**Removal** Taking out or off a device from a body part

Body Part Character 4	Approach Character 5	Device Character 6	Qualifier Character 7
Ø Upper Intestinal Tract 6 Stomach D Lower Intestinal Tract	X External	Ø Drainage Device 2 Monitoring Device 3 Infusion Device D Intraluminal Device U Feeding Device	Z No Qualifier
Ø Upper Intestinal Tract D Lower Intestinal Tract	Ø Open 3 Percutaneous 4 Percutaneous Endoscopic 7 Via Natural or Artificial Opening 8 Via Natural or Artificial Opening Endoscopic	Ø Drainage Device 2 Monitoring Device 3 Infusion Device 7 Autologous Tissue Substitute C Extraluminal Device D Intraluminal Device J Synthetic Substitute K Nonautologous Tissue Substitute U Feeding Device	Z No Qualifier
5 Esophagus	Ø Open 3 Percutaneous 4 Percutaneous Endoscopic	1 Radioactive Element 2 Monitoring Device 3 Infusion Device U Feeding Device	Z No Qualifier
5 Esophagus	7 Via Natural or Artificial Opening 8 Via Natural or Artificial Opening Endoscopic	1 Radioactive Element D Intraluminal Device	Z No Qualifier
5 Esophagus	X External	1 Radioactive Element 2 Monitoring Device 3 Infusion Device D Intraluminal Device U Feeding Device	Z No Qualifier
6 Stomach	Ø Open 3 Percutaneous 4 Percutaneous Endoscopic	Ø Drainage Device 2 Monitoring Device 3 Infusion Device 7 Autologous Tissue Substitute C Extraluminal Device D Intraluminal Device J Synthetic Substitute K Nonautologous Tissue Substitute M Stimulator Lead U Feeding Device	Z No Qualifier
6 Stomach	7 Via Natural or Artificial Opening 8 Via Natural or Artificial Opening Endoscopic	Ø Drainage Device 2 Monitoring Device 3 Infusion Device 7 Autologous Tissue Substitute C Extraluminal Device D Intraluminal Device J Synthetic Substitute K Nonautologous Tissue Substitute U Feeding Device	Z No Qualifier
P Rectum	Ø Open 3 Percutaneous 4 Percutaneous Endoscopic 7 Via Natural or Artificial Opening 8 Via Natural or Artificial Opening Endoscopic X External	1 Radioactive Element	Z No Qualifier
Q Anus	Ø Open 3 Percutaneous 4 Percutaneous Endoscopic 7 Via Natural or Artificial Opening 8 Via Natural or Artificial Opening Endoscopic	L Artificial Sphincter	Z No Qualifier
R Anal Sphincter	Ø Open 3 Percutaneous 4 Percutaneous Endoscopic	M Stimulator Lead	Z No Qualifier
U Omentum V Mesentery W Peritoneum	Ø Open 3 Percutaneous 4 Percutaneous Endoscopic	Ø Drainage Device 1 Radioactive Element 7 Autologous Tissue Substitute J Synthetic Substitute K Nonautologous Tissue Substitute	Z No Qualifier

Non-OR   ØDP[Ø,6,D]X[Ø,2,3,D,U]Z
Non-OR   ØDP5[7,8]1Z
Non-OR   ØDP5X[1,2,3,D,U]Z

Non-OR   ØDP6[7,8]DZ
Non-OR   ØDPP[7,8,X]1Z

Ø Medical and Surgical
D Gastrointestinal System
Q Repair   Restoring, to the extent possible, a body part to its normal anatomic structure and function

Body Part Character 4	Approach Character 5	Device Character 6	Qualifier Character 7
1 Esophagus, Upper 2 Esophagus, Middle 3 Esophagus, Lower 4 Esophagogastric Junction 5 Esophagus 6 Stomach 7 Stomach, Pylorus 8 Small Intestine 9 Duodenum A Jejunum B Ileum C Ileocecal Valve E Large Intestine F Large Intestine, Right G Large Intestine, Left H Cecum J Appendix K Ascending Colon L Transverse Colon M Descending Colon N Sigmoid Colon P Rectum	Ø Open 3 Percutaneous 4 Percutaneous Endoscopic 7 Via Natural or Artificial Opening 8 Via Natural or Artificial Opening Endoscopic	Z No Device	Z No Qualifier
Q Anus	Ø Open 3 Percutaneous 4 Percutaneous Endoscopic 7 Via Natural or Artificial Opening 8 Via Natural or Artificial Opening Endoscopic X External	Z No Device	Z No Qualifier
R Anal Sphincter S Greater Omentum T Lesser Omentum V Mesentery W Peritoneum	Ø Open 3 Percutaneous 4 Percutaneous Endoscopic	Z No Device	Z No Qualifier

Non-OR   ØDQ[F,G,L,M]ØZZ

Ø Medical and Surgical
D Gastrointestinal System
R Replacement   Putting in or on biological or synthetic material that physically takes the place and/or function of all or a portion of a body part

Body Part Character 4	Approach Character 5	Device Character 6	Qualifier Character 7
5 Esophagus	Ø Open 4 Percutaneous Endoscopic 7 Via Natural or Artificial Opening 8 Via Natural or Artificial Opening Endoscopic	7 Autologous Tissue Substitute J Synthetic Substitute K Nonautologous Tissue Substitute	Z No Qualifier
R Anal Sphincter S Greater Omentum T Lesser Omentum V Mesentery W Peritoneum	Ø Open 4 Percutaneous Endoscopic	7 Autologous Tissue Substitute J Synthetic Substitute K Nonautologous Tissue Substitute	Z No Qualifier

Gastrointestinal System

Ø   **Medical and Surgical**
D   **Gastrointestinal System**
S   **Reposition**   Moving to its normal location or other suitable location all or a portion of a body part

Body Part Character 4	Approach Character 5	Device Character 6	Qualifier Character 7
5 Esophagus 6 Stomach 9 Duodenum A Jejunum B Ileum H Cecum K Ascending Colon L Transverse Colon M Descending Colon N Sigmoid Colon P Rectum Q Anus	Ø Open 4 Percutaneous Endoscopic 7 Via Natural or Artificial Opening 8 Via Natural or Artificial Opening Endoscopic X External	Z No Device	Z No Qualifier

Non-OR   ØDS[9,A,B,H,K,L,M,N,P]XZZ

Ø   **Medical and Surgical**
D   **Gastrointestinal System**
T   **Resection**   Cutting out or off, without replacement, all of a body part

Body Part Character 4	Approach Character 5	Device Character 6	Qualifier Character 7
1 Esophagus, Upper 2 Esophagus, Middle 3 Esophagus, Lower 4 Esophagogastric Junction 5 Esophagus 6 Stomach 7 Stomach, Pylorus 8 Small Intestine 9 Duodenum A Jejunum B Ileum C Ileocecal Valve E Large Intestine F Large Intestine, Right G Large Intestine, Left H Cecum J Appendix K Ascending Colon L Transverse Colon M Descending Colon N Sigmoid Colon P Rectum Q Anus	Ø Open 4 Percutaneous Endoscopic 7 Via Natural or Artificial Opening 8 Via Natural or Artificial Opening Endoscopic	Z No Device	Z No Qualifier
R Anal Sphincter S Greater Omentum T Lesser Omentum	Ø Open 4 Percutaneous Endoscopic	Z No Device	Z No Qualifier

Gastrointestinal System

Ø Medical and Surgical
D Gastrointestinal System
U Supplement   Putting in or on biological or synthetic material that physically reinforces and/or augments the function of a portion of a body part

Body Part Character 4	Approach Character 5	Device Character 6	Qualifier Character 7
1 Esophagus, Upper 2 Esophagus, Middle 3 Esophagus, Lower 4 Esophagogastric Junction 5 Esophagus 6 Stomach 7 Stomach, Pylorus 8 Small Intestine 9 Duodenum A Jejunum B Ileum C Ileocecal Valve E Large Intestine F Large Intestine, Right G Large Intestine, Left H Cecum K Ascending Colon L Transverse Colon M Descending Colon N Sigmoid Colon P Rectum	Ø Open 4 Percutaneous Endoscopic 7 Via Natural or Artificial Opening 8 Via Natural or Artificial Opening Endoscopic	7 Autologous Tissue Substitute J Synthetic Substitute K Nonautologous Tissue Substitute	Z No Qualifier
Q Anus	Ø Open 4 Percutaneous Endoscopic 7 Via Natural or Artificial Opening 8 Via Natural or Artificial Opening Endoscopic X External	7 Autologous Tissue Substitute J Synthetic Substitute K Nonautologous Tissue Substitute	Z No Qualifier
R Anal Sphincter S Greater Omentum T Lesser Omentum V Mesentery W Peritoneum	Ø Open 4 Percutaneous Endoscopic	7 Autologous Tissue Substitute J Synthetic Substitute K Nonautologous Tissue Substitute	Z No Qualifier

Ø Medical and Surgical
D Gastrointestinal System
V Restriction   Partially closing an orifice or the lumen of a tubular body part

Body Part Character 4	Approach Character 5	Device Character 6	Qualifier Character 7
1 Esophagus, Upper 2 Esophagus, Middle 3 Esophagus, Lower 4 Esophagogastric Junction 5 Esophagus 6 Stomach 7 Stomach, Pylorus 8 Small Intestine 9 Duodenum A Jejunum B Ileum C Ileocecal Valve E Large Intestine F Large Intestine, Right G Large Intestine, Left H Cecum K Ascending Colon L Transverse Colon M Descending Colon N Sigmoid Colon P Rectum	Ø Open 3 Percutaneous 4 Percutaneous Endoscopic	C Extraluminal Device D Intraluminal Device Z No Device	Z No Qualifier

ØDV Continued on next page

HAC ØDV64CZ when reported with PDx E66.Ø1 and SDx K68.11 or K95.Ø1 or K95.81 or T81.4XXA

ØDU—ØDV

Ø   Medical and Surgical   *ØDV Continued*
D   Gastrointestinal System
V   Restriction   Partially closing an orifice or the lumen of a tubular body part

Body Part Character 4	Approach Character 5	Device Character 6	Qualifier Character 7
1 Esophagus, Upper **2** Esophagus, Middle **3** Esophagus, Lower **4** Esophagogastric Junction **5** Esophagus **6** Stomach _{NC} **7** Stomach, Pylorus **8** Small Intestine **9** Duodenum **A** Jejunum **B** Ileum **C** Ileocecal Valve **E** Large Intestine **F** Large Intestine, Right **G** Large Intestine, Left **H** Cecum **K** Ascending Colon **L** Transverse Colon **M** Descending Colon **N** Sigmoid Colon **P** Rectum **Q** Anus	**7** Via Natural or Artificial Opening **8** Via Natural or Artificial Opening Endoscopic	**D** Intraluminal Device **Z** No Device	**Z** No Qualifier
Q Anus	**Ø** Open **3** Percutaneous **4** Percutaneous Endoscopic **X** External	**C** Extraluminal Device **D** Intraluminal Device **Z** No Device	**Z** No Qualifier

NC   ØDV6[7,8]DZ
Non-OR   ØDV6[7,8]DZ

Ø   Medical and Surgical
D   Gastrointestinal System
W   Revision   Correcting, to the extent possible, a portion of a malfunctioning device or the position of a displaced device

Body Part Character 4	Approach Character 5	Device Character 6	Qualifier Character 7
Ø Upper Intestinal Tract **D** Lower Intestinal Tract	**Ø** Open **3** Percutaneous **4** Percutaneous Endoscopic **7** Via Natural or Artificial Opening **8** Via Natural or Artificial Opening Endoscopic **X** External	**Ø** Drainage Device **2** Monitoring Device **3** Infusion Device **7** Autologous Tissue Substitute **C** Extraluminal Device **D** Intraluminal Device **J** Synthetic Substitute **K** Nonautologous Tissue Substitute **U** Feeding Device	**Z** No Qualifier
5 Esophagus	**7** Via Natural or Artificial Opening **8** Via Natural or Artificial Opening Endoscopic **X** External	**D** Intraluminal Device	**Z** No Qualifier
6 Stomach	**Ø** Open **3** Percutaneous **4** Percutaneous Endoscopic	**Ø** Drainage Device **2** Monitoring Device **3** Infusion Device **7** Autologous Tissue Substitute **C** Extraluminal Device **D** Intraluminal Device **J** Synthetic Substitute **K** Nonautologous Tissue Substitute **M** Stimulator Lead **U** Feeding Device	**Z** No Qualifier

ØDW Continued on next page

Non-OR   ØDW[Ø,D]X[Ø,2,3,7,C,D,J,K,U]Z
Non-OR   ØDW5XDZ

Ø　Medical and Surgical
D　Gastrointestinal System
W　Revision　　　Correcting, to the extent possible, a portion of a malfunctioning device or the position of a displaced device

Body Part Character 4	Approach Character 5	Device Character 6	Qualifier Character 7
6　Stomach	7　Via Natural or Artificial Opening 8　Via Natural or Artificial Opening 　　Endoscopic X　External	Ø　Drainage Device 2　Monitoring Device 3　Infusion Device 7　Autologous Tissue Substitute C　Extraluminal Device D　Intraluminal Device J　Synthetic Substitute K　Nonautologous Tissue Substitute U　Feeding Device	Z　No Qualifier
8　Small Intestine E　Large Intestine	Ø　Open 4　Percutaneous Endoscopic 7　Via Natural or Artificial Opening 8　Via Natural or Artificial Opening 　　Endoscopic	7　Autologous Tissue Substitute J　Synthetic Substitute K　Nonautologous Tissue Substitute	Z　No Qualifier
Q　Anus	Ø　Open 3　Percutaneous 4　Percutaneous Endoscopic 7　Via Natural or Artificial Opening 8　Via Natural or Artificial Opening 　　Endoscopic	L　Artificial Sphincter	Z　No Qualifier
R　Anal Sphincter	Ø　Open 3　Percutaneous 4　Percutaneous Endoscopic	M　Stimulator Lead	Z　No Qualifier
U　Omentum V　Mesentery W　Peritoneum	Ø　Open 3　Percutaneous 4　Percutaneous Endoscopic	Ø　Drainage Device 7　Autologous Tissue Substitute J　Synthetic Substitute K　Nonautologous Tissue Substitute	Z　No Qualifier

Non-OR　ØDW6X[Ø,2,3,7,C,D,J,K,U]Z
Non-OR　ØDW[U,V,W][Ø,3,4]ØZ

Ø　Medical and Surgical
D　Gastrointestinal System
X　Transfer　　　Moving, without taking out, all or a portion of a body part to another location to take over the function of all or a portion of a body part

Body Part Character 4	Approach Character 5	Device Character 6	Qualifier Character 7
6　Stomach 8　Small Intestine E　Large Intestine	Ø　Open 4　Percutaneous Endoscopic	Z　No Device	5　Esophagus

Ø　Medical and Surgical
D　Gastrointestinal System
Y　Transplantation　Putting in or on all or a portion of a living body part taken from another individual or animal to physically take the place and/or function of all or a portion of a similar body part

Body Part Character 4	Approach Character 5	Device Character 6	Qualifier Character 7
5　Esophagus 6　Stomach 8　Small Intestine　**LC** E　Large Intestine　**LC**	Ø　Open	Z　No Device	Ø　Allogeneic 1　Syngeneic 2　Zooplastic

LC　　　ØDY[8,E]ØZ[Ø,1,2]
Non-OR　ØDY5ØZ[Ø,1,2]

LC Limited Coverage　　　**NC** Noncovered　　　HAC associated procedure　　　Combination Only　　　DRG Non-OR　　　Non-OR　　　Revised Text in **GREEN**

ICD-10-PCS 2014 (Draft)　　　253

Hepatobiliary System and Pancreas

Hepatobiliary System and Pancreas ØF1–ØFY

Ø Medical and Surgical
F Hepatobiliary System and Pancreas
1 Bypass   Altering the route of passage of the contents of a tubular body part

Body Part Character 4	Approach Character 5	Device Character 6	Qualifier Character 7
4 Gallbladder 5 Hepatic Duct, Right 6 Hepatic Duct, Left 8 Cystic Duct 9 Common Bile Duct	Ø Open 4 Percutaneous Endoscopic	D Intraluminal Device Z No Device	3 Duodenum 4 Stomach 5 Hepatic Duct, Right 6 Hepatic Duct, Left 7 Hepatic Duct, Caudate 8 Cystic Duct 9 Common Bile Duct B Small Intestine
D Pancreatic Duct F Pancreatic Duct, Accessory G Pancreas	Ø Open 4 Percutaneous Endoscopic	D Intraluminal Device Z No Device	3 Duodenum B Small Intestine C Large Intestine

Ø Medical and Surgical
F Hepatobiliary System and Pancreas
2 Change   Taking out or off a device from a body part and putting back an identical or similar device in or on the same body part without cutting or puncturing the skin or a mucous membrane

Body Part Character 4	Approach Character 5	Device Character 6	Qualifier Character 7
Ø Liver 4 Gallbladder B Hepatobiliary Duct D Pancreatic Duct G Pancreas	X External	Ø Drainage Device Y Other Device	Z No Qualifier

Non-OR   For all body part, approach, device, and qualifier values

Ø Medical and Surgical
F Hepatobiliary System and Pancreas
5 Destruction   Physical eradication of all or a portion of a body part by the direct use of energy, force, or a destructive agent

Body Part Character 4	Approach Character 5	Device Character 6	Qualifier Character 7
Ø Liver 1 Liver, Right Lobe 2 Liver, Left Lobe 4 Gallbladder G Pancreas	Ø Open 3 Percutaneous 4 Percutaneous Endoscopic	Z No Device	Z No Qualifier
5 Hepatic Duct, Right 6 Hepatic Duct, Left 8 Cystic Duct 9 Common Bile Duct C Ampulla of Vater D Pancreatic Duct F Pancreatic Duct, Accessory	Ø Open 3 Percutaneous 4 Percutaneous Endoscopic 7 Via Natural or Artificial Opening 8 Via Natural or Artificial Opening Endoscopic	Z No Device	Z No Qualifier

Non-OR   ØF5G4ZZ
Non-OR   ØF5[5,6,8,9,C,D,F][4,8]ZZ

Ø Medical and Surgical
F Hepatobiliary System and Pancreas
7 Dilation   Expanding an orifice or the lumen of a tubular body part

Body Part Character 4	Approach Character 5	Device Character 6	Qualifier Character 7
5 Hepatic Duct, Right 6 Hepatic Duct, Left 8 Cystic Duct 9 Common Bile Duct C Ampulla of Vater D Pancreatic Duct F Pancreatic Duct, Accessory	Ø Open 3 Percutaneous 4 Percutaneous Endoscopic 7 Via Natural or Artificial Opening 8 Via Natural or Artificial Opening Endoscopic	D Intraluminal Device Z No Device	Z No Qualifier

DRG Non-OR   ØF7D7DZ
Non-OR   ØF7[5,6,8,9][3,4,8][D,Z]Z
Non-OR   ØF7[5,6,8,9]7DZ
Non-OR   ØF7C8[D,Z]Z
Non-OR   ØF7[D,F][4,8][D,Z]Z

Ø **Medical and Surgical**
F **Hepatobiliary System and Pancreas**
8 **Division** Cutting into a body part without draining fluids and/or gases from the body part in order to separate or transect a body part

Body Part Character 4	Approach Character 5	Device Character 6	Qualifier Character 7
G Pancreas	Ø Open 3 Percutaneous 4 Percutaneous Endoscopic	Z No Device	Z No Qualifier

Ø **Medical and Surgical**
F **Hepatobiliary System and Pancreas**
9 **Drainage** Taking or letting out fluids and/or gases from a body part

Body Part Character 4	Approach Character 5	Device Character 6	Qualifier Character 7
Ø Liver 1 Liver, Right Lobe 2 Liver, Left Lobe 4 Gallbladder G Pancreas	Ø Open 3 Percutaneous 4 Percutaneous Endoscopic	Ø Drainage Device	Z No Qualifier
Ø Liver 1 Liver, Right Lobe 2 Liver, Left Lobe 4 Gallbladder G Pancreas	Ø Open 3 Percutaneous 4 Percutaneous Endoscopic	Z No Device	X Diagnostic Z No Qualifier
5 Hepatic Duct, Right 6 Hepatic Duct, Left 8 Cystic Duct 9 Common Bile Duct C Ampulla of Vater D Pancreatic Duct F Pancreatic Duct, Accessory	Ø Open 3 Percutaneous 4 Percutaneous Endoscopic 7 Via Natural or Artificial Opening 8 Via Natural or Artificial Opening Endoscopic	Ø Drainage Device	Z No Qualifier
5 Hepatic Duct, Right 6 Hepatic Duct, Left 8 Cystic Duct 9 Common Bile Duct C Ampulla of Vater D Pancreatic Duct F Pancreatic Duct, Accessory	Ø Open 3 Percutaneous 4 Percutaneous Endoscopic 7 Via Natural or Artificial Opening 8 Via Natural or Artificial Opening Endoscopic	Z No Device	X Diagnostic Z No Qualifier

Non-OR ØF9[Ø,1,2][3,4]ØZ
Non-OR ØF944ØZ
Non-OR ØF9[Ø,1,2,4,G][3,4]ZX
Non-OR ØF9[Ø,1,2,4][3,4]ZZ
Non-OR ØF9C[4,8]ØZ
Non-OR ØF9[9,D,F]8ØZ
Non-OR ØF9[5,6,8,9,C,D,F][3,4,7,8]ZX
Non-OR ØF99[3,4,7,8]ZZ
Non-OR ØF9C[4,8]ZZ

Ø **Medical and Surgical**
F **Hepatobiliary System and Pancreas**
B **Excision** Cutting out or off, without replacement, a portion of a body part

Body Part Character 4	Approach Character 5	Device Character 6	Qualifier Character 7
Ø Liver 1 Liver, Right Lobe 2 Liver, Left Lobe 4 Gallbladder G Pancreas	Ø Open 3 Percutaneous 4 Percutaneous Endoscopic	Z No Device	X Diagnostic Z No Qualifier
5 Hepatic Duct, Right 6 Hepatic Duct, Left 8 Cystic Duct 9 Common Bile Duct C Ampulla of Vater D Pancreatic Duct F Pancreatic Duct, Accessory	Ø Open 3 Percutaneous 4 Percutaneous Endoscopic 7 Via Natural or Artificial Opening 8 Via Natural or Artificial Opening Endoscopic	Z No Device	X Diagnostic Z No Qualifier

Non-OR ØFB[Ø,1,2]3ZX
Non-OR ØFB[4,G][3,4]ZX
Non-OR ØFB[5,6,8,9,C,D,F][3,4,7,8]ZX
Non-OR ØFB[5,6,8,9,C,D,F][4,8]ZZ

Ø   Medical and Surgical
F   Hepatobiliary System and Pancreas
C   Extirpation   Taking or cutting out solid matter from a body part

Body Part Character 4	Approach Character 5	Device Character 6	Qualifier Character 7
Ø Liver 1 Liver, Right Lobe 2 Liver, Left Lobe 4 Gallbladder G Pancreas	Ø Open 3 Percutaneous 4 Percutaneous Endoscopic	Z No Device	Z No Qualifier
5 Hepatic Duct, Right 6 Hepatic Duct, Left 8 Cystic Duct 9 Common Bile Duct C Ampulla of Vater D Pancreatic Duct F Pancreatic Duct, Accessory	Ø Open 3 Percutaneous 4 Percutaneous Endoscopic 7 Via Natural or Artificial Opening 8 Via Natural or Artificial Opening Endoscopic	Z No Device	Z No Qualifier

Non-OR   ØFC[5,6,8,9][3,4,7,8]ZZ
Non-OR   ØFCC[4,8]ZZ
Non-OR   ØFC[D,F][3,4,8]ZZ

Ø   Medical and Surgical
F   Hepatobiliary System and Pancreas
F   Fragmentation   Breaking solid matter in a body part into pieces

Body Part Character 4	Approach Character 5	Device Character 6	Qualifier Character 7
4 Gallbladder `NC` 5 Hepatic Duct, Right `NC` 6 Hepatic Duct, Left `NC` 8 Cystic Duct `NC` 9 Common Bile Duct `NC` C Ampulla of Vater `NC` D Pancreatic Duct `NC` F Pancreatic Duct, Accessory `NC`	Ø Open 3 Percutaneous 4 Percutaneous Endoscopic 7 Via Natural or Artificial Opening 8 Via Natural or Artificial Opening Endoscopic X External	Z No Device	Z No Qualifier

NC   ØFF[4,5,6,8,9,C,D,F]XZZ
Non-OR   ØFF[4,5,6,8,9,C,D,F][8,X]ZZ
Non-OR   ØFF[D,F]XZZ

Ø   Medical and Surgical
F   Hepatobiliary System and Pancreas
H   Insertion   Putting in a nonbiological appliance that monitors, assists, performs, or prevents a physiological function but does not physically take the place of a body part

Body Part Character 4	Approach Character 5	Device Character 6	Qualifier Character 7
Ø Liver 1 Liver, Right Lobe 2 Liver, Left Lobe 4 Gallbladder G Pancreas	Ø Open 3 Percutaneous 4 Percutaneous Endoscopic	2 Monitoring Device 3 Infusion Device	Z No Qualifier
B Hepatobiliary Duct D Pancreatic Duct	Ø Open 3 Percutaneous 4 Percutaneous Endoscopic 7 Via Natural or Artificial Opening 8 Via Natural or Artificial Opening Endoscopic	1 Radioactive Element 2 Monitoring Device 3 Infusion Device D Intraluminal Device	Z No Qualifier

Non-OR   ØFH[Ø,1,2,4,G][Ø,3,4]3Z
Non-OR   ØFH[B,D][Ø,3,4,7,8][3,D]Z

`LC` Limited Coverage   `NC` Noncovered   HAC associated procedure   Combination Only   DRG Non-OR   Non-OR   Revised Text in **GREEN**

256   ICD-10-PCS 2014 (Draft)

Ø   Medical and Surgical
F   Hepatobiliary System and Pancreas
J   Inspection   Visually and/or manually exploring a body part

Body Part Character 4	Approach Character 5	Device Character 6	Qualifier Character 7
Ø Liver 4 Gallbladder G Pancreas	Ø Open 3 Percutaneous 4 Percutaneous Endoscopic X External	Z No Device	Z No Qualifier
B Hepatobiliary Duct D Pancreatic Duct	Ø Open 3 Percutaneous 4 Percutaneous Endoscopic 7 Via Natural or Artificial Opening 8 Via Natural or Artificial Opening Endoscopic	Z No Device	Z No Qualifier

Non-OR   ØFJ[Ø,4,G]XZZ

Ø   Medical and Surgical
F   Hepatobiliary System and Pancreas
L   Occlusion   Completely closing an orifice or the lumen of a tubular body part

Body Part Character 4	Approach Character 5	Device Character 6	Qualifier Character 7
5 Hepatic Duct, Right 6 Hepatic Duct, Left 8 Cystic Duct 9 Common Bile Duct C Ampulla of Vater D Pancreatic Duct F Pancreatic Duct, Accessory	Ø Open 3 Percutaneous 4 Percutaneous Endoscopic	C Extraluminal Device D Intraluminal Device Z No Device	Z No Qualifier
5 Hepatic Duct, Right 6 Hepatic Duct, Left 8 Cystic Duct 9 Common Bile Duct C Ampulla of Vater D Pancreatic Duct F Pancreatic Duct, Accessory	7 Via Natural or Artificial Opening 8 Via Natural or Artificial Opening Endoscopic	D Intraluminal Device Z No Device	Z No Qualifier

Non-OR   ØFL[5,6,8,9][3,4][C,D,Z]Z
Non-OR   ØFL[5,6,8,9][7,8][D,Z]Z

Ø   Medical and Surgical
F   Hepatobiliary System and Pancreas
M   Reattachment   Putting back in or on all or a portion of a separated body part to its normal location or other suitable location

Body Part Character 4	Approach Character 5	Device Character 6	Qualifier Character 7
Ø Liver 1 Liver, Right Lobe 2 Liver, Left Lobe 4 Gallbladder 5 Hepatic Duct, Right 6 Hepatic Duct, Left 8 Cystic Duct 9 Common Bile Duct C Ampulla of Vater D Pancreatic Duct F Pancreatic Duct, Accessory G Pancreas	Ø Open 4 Percutaneous Endoscopic	Z No Device	Z No Qualifier

Non-OR   ØFM[4,5,6,8,9]4ZZ

Ø　Medical and Surgical
F　Hepatobiliary System and Pancreas
N　Release　　　Freeing a body part from an abnormal physical constraint

Body Part Character 4	Approach Character 5	Device Character 6	Qualifier Character 7
Ø Liver **1** Liver, Right Lobe **2** Liver, Left Lobe **4** Gallbladder **G** Pancreas	**Ø** Open **3** Percutaneous **4** Percutaneous Endoscopic	**Z** No Device	**Z** No Qualifier
5 Hepatic Duct, Right **6** Hepatic Duct, Left **8** Cystic Duct **9** Common Bile Duct **C** Ampulla of Vater **D** Pancreatic Duct **F** Pancreatic Duct, Accessory	**Ø** Open **3** Percutaneous **4** Percutaneous Endoscopic **7** Via Natural or Artificial Opening **8** Via Natural or Artificial Opening Endoscopic	**Z** No Device	**Z** No Qualifier

Ø　Medical and Surgical
F　Hepatobiliary System and Pancreas
P　Removal　　　Taking out or off a device from a body part

Body Part Character 4	Approach Character 5	Device Character 6	Qualifier Character 7
Ø Liver	**Ø** Open **3** Percutaneous **4** Percutaneous Endoscopic **X** External	**Ø** Drainage Device **2** Monitoring Device **3** Infusion Device	**Z** No Qualifier
4 Gallbladder **G** Pancreas	**Ø** Open **3** Percutaneous **4** Percutaneous Endoscopic **X** External	**Ø** Drainage Device **2** Monitoring Device **3** Infusion Device **D** Intraluminal Device	**Z** No Qualifier
B Hepatobiliary Duct **D** Pancreatic Duct	**Ø** Open **3** Percutaneous **4** Percutaneous Endoscopic **7** Via Natural or Artificial Opening **8** Via Natural or Artificial Opening Endoscopic	**Ø** Drainage Device **1** Radioactive Element **2** Monitoring Device **3** Infusion Device **7** Autologous Tissue Substitute **C** Extraluminal Device **D** Intraluminal Device **J** Synthetic Substitute **K** Nonautologous Tissue Substitute	**Z** No Qualifier
B Hepatobiliary Duct **D** Pancreatic Duct	**X** External	**Ø** Drainage Device **1** Radioactive Element **2** Monitoring Device **3** Infusion Device **D** Intraluminal Device	**Z** No Qualifier

Non-OR　ØFPØX[Ø,2,3]Z
Non-OR　ØFP[4,G]X[Ø,2,3,D]Z
Non-OR　ØFP[B,D]X[Ø,1,2,3,D]Z

Ø　Medical and Surgical
F　Hepatobiliary System and Pancreas
Q　Repair　　　Restoring, to the extent possible, a body part to its normal anatomic structure and function

Body Part Character 4	Approach Character 5	Device Character 6	Qualifier Character 7
Ø Liver **1** Liver, Right Lobe **2** Liver, Left Lobe **4** Gallbladder **G** Pancreas	**Ø** Open **3** Percutaneous **4** Percutaneous Endoscopic	**Z** No Device	**Z** No Qualifier
5 Hepatic Duct, Right **6** Hepatic Duct, Left **8** Cystic Duct **9** Common Bile Duct **C** Ampulla of Vater **D** Pancreatic Duct **F** Pancreatic Duct, Accessory	**Ø** Open **3** Percutaneous **4** Percutaneous Endoscopic **7** Via Natural or Artificial Opening **8** Via Natural or Artificial Opening Endoscopic	**Z** No Device	**Z** No Qualifier

Ø **Medical and Surgical**
F **Hepatobiliary System and Pancreas**
R **Replacement**   Putting in or on biological or synthetic material that physically takes the place and/or function of all or a portion of a body part

Body Part Character 4	Approach Character 5	Device Character 6	Qualifier Character 7
5 Hepatic Duct, Right 6 Hepatic Duct, Left 8 Cystic Duct 9 Common Bile Duct C Ampulla of Vater D Pancreatic Duct F Pancreatic Duct, Accessory	Ø Open 4 Percutaneous Endoscopic	7 Autologous Tissue Substitute J Synthetic Substitute K Nonautologous Tissue Substitute	Z No Qualifier

Ø **Medical and Surgical**
F **Hepatobiliary System and Pancreas**
S **Reposition**   Moving to its normal location or other suitable location all or a portion of a body part

Body Part Character 4	Approach Character 5	Device Character 6	Qualifier Character 7
Ø Liver 4 Gallbladder 5 Hepatic Duct, Right 6 Hepatic Duct, Left 8 Cystic Duct 9 Common Bile Duct C Ampulla of Vater D Pancreatic Duct F Pancreatic Duct, Accessory G Pancreas	Ø Open 4 Percutaneous Endoscopic	Z No Device	Z No Qualifier

Ø **Medical and Surgical**
F **Hepatobiliary System and Pancreas**
T **Resection**   Cutting out or off, without replacement, all of a body part

Body Part Character 4	Approach Character 5	Device Character 6	Qualifier Character 7
Ø Liver 1 Liver, Right Lobe 2 Liver, Left Lobe 4 Gallbladder G Pancreas	Ø Open 4 Percutaneous Endoscopic	Z No Device	Z No Qualifier
5 Hepatic Duct, Right 6 Hepatic Duct, Left 8 Cystic Duct 9 Common Bile Duct C Ampulla of Vater D Pancreatic Duct F Pancreatic Duct, Accessory	Ø Open 4 Percutaneous Endoscopic 7 Via Natural or Artificial Opening 8 Via Natural or Artificial Opening Endoscopic	Z No Device	Z No Qualifier

Non-OR ØFT[D,F][4,8]ZZ

Ø **Medical and Surgical**
F **Hepatobiliary System and Pancreas**
U **Supplement**   Putting in or on biological or synthetic material that physically reinforces and/or augments the function of a portion of a body part

Body Part Character 4	Approach Character 5	Device Character 6	Qualifier Character 7
5 Hepatic Duct, Right 6 Hepatic Duct, Left 8 Cystic Duct 9 Common Bile Duct C Ampulla of Vater D Pancreatic Duct F Pancreatic Duct, Accessory	Ø Open 3 Percutaneous 4 Percutaneous Endoscopic	7 Autologous Tissue Substitute J Synthetic Substitute K Nonautologous Tissue Substitute	Z No Qualifier

---

LC Limited Coverage   NC Noncovered   HAC associated procedure   Combination Only   DRG Non-OR   Non-OR   Revised Text in **GREEN**

Hepatobiliary System and Pancreas

ØFV–ØFY

Ø   Medical and Surgical
F   Hepatobiliary System and Pancreas
V   Restriction   Partially closing an orifice or the lumen of a tubular body part

Body Part Character 4	Approach Character 5	Device Character 6	Qualifier Character 7
5 Hepatic Duct, Right 6 Hepatic Duct, Left 8 Cystic Duct 9 Common Bile Duct C Ampulla of Vater D Pancreatic Duct F Pancreatic Duct, Accessory	Ø Open 3 Percutaneous 4 Percutaneous Endoscopic	C Extraluminal Device D Intraluminal Device Z No Device	Z No Qualifier
5 Hepatic Duct, Right 6 Hepatic Duct, Left 8 Cystic Duct 9 Common Bile Duct C Ampulla of Vater D Pancreatic Duct F Pancreatic Duct, Accessory	7 Via Natural or Artificial Opening 8 Via Natural or Artificial Opening Endoscopic	D Intraluminal Device Z No Device	Z No Qualifier

Non-OR   ØFV[5,6,8,9][3,4][C,D,Z]Z
Non-OR   ØFV[5,6,8,9][7,8][D,Z]Z

Ø   Medical and Surgical
F   Hepatobiliary System and Pancreas
W   Revision   Correcting, to the extent possible, a portion of a malfunctioning device or the position of a displaced device

Body Part Character 4	Approach Character 5	Device Character 6	Qualifier Character 7
Ø Liver	Ø Open 3 Percutaneous 4 Percutaneous Endoscopic X External	Ø Drainage Device 2 Monitoring Device 3 Infusion Device	Z No Qualifier
4 Gallbladder G Pancreas	Ø Open 3 Percutaneous 4 Percutaneous Endoscopic X External	Ø Drainage Device 2 Monitoring Device 3 Infusion Device D Intraluminal Device	Z No Qualifier
B Hepatobiliary Duct D Pancreatic Duct	Ø Open 3 Percutaneous 4 Percutaneous Endoscopic 7 Via Natural or Artificial Opening 8 Via Natural or Artificial Opening Endoscopic X External	Ø Drainage Device 2 Monitoring Device 3 Infusion Device 7 Autologous Tissue Substitute C Extraluminal Device D Intraluminal Device J Synthetic Substitute K Nonautologous Tissue Substitute	Z No Qualifier

Non-OR   ØFWØX[Ø,2,3]Z
Non-OR   ØFW[4,G]X[Ø,2,3,D]Z
Non-OR   ØFW[B,D]X[Ø,2,3,7,C,D,J,K]Z

Ø   Medical and Surgical
F   Hepatobiliary System and Pancreas
Y   Transplantation   Putting in or on all or a portion of a living body part taken from another individual or animal to physically take the place and/or
                                 function of all or a portion of a similar body part

Body Part Character 4	Approach Character 5	Device Character 6	Qualifier Character 7
Ø Liver LC G Pancreas LC NC	Ø Open	Z No Device	Ø Allogeneic 1 Syngeneic 2 Zooplastic

NC ØFYGØZ2
NC ØFYGØZ[Ø,1] If reported alone without one of the following procedures ØTYØØZ[Ø,1,2], ØTY1ØZ[Ø,1,2] or with one of the following diagnoses E1Ø.1Ø-E1Ø.9, E89.1
LC ØFYØØZ[Ø,1,2], ØFYGØZ[Ø,1]

Endocrine System 0G2–0GW

0   Medical and Surgical
G   Endocrine System
2   Change   Taking out or off a device from a body part and putting back an identical or similar device in or on the same body part without cutting or puncturing the skin or a mucous membrane

Body Part Character 4	Approach Character 5	Device Character 6	Qualifier Character 7
0 Pituitary Gland 1 Pineal Body 5 Adrenal Gland K Thyroid Gland R Parathyroid Gland S Endocrine Gland	X External	0 Drainage Device Y Other Device	Z No Qualifier

Non-OR   For all body part, approach, device, and qualifier values

---

0   Medical and Surgical
G   Endocrine System
5   Destruction   Physical eradication of all or a portion of a body part by the direct use of energy, force, or a destructive agent

Body Part Character 4	Approach Character 5	Device Character 6	Qualifier Character 7
0 Pituitary Gland 1 Pineal Body 2 Adrenal Gland, Left 3 Adrenal Gland, Right 4 Adrenal Glands, Bilateral 6 Carotid Body, Left 7 Carotid Body, Right 8 Carotid Bodies, Bilateral 9 Para-aortic Body B Coccygeal Glomus C Glomus Jugulare D Aortic Body F Paraganglion Extremity G Thyroid Gland Lobe, Left H Thyroid Gland Lobe, Right K Thyroid Gland L Superior Parathyroid Gland, Right M Superior Parathyroid Gland, Left N Inferior Parathyroid Gland, Right P Inferior Parathyroid Gland, Left Q Parathyroid Glands, Multiple R Parathyroid Gland	0 Open 3 Percutaneous 4 Percutaneous Endoscopic	Z No Device	Z No Qualifier

Non-OR   0G5[6,7,8,9,B,C,D,F][0,3,4]ZZ

---

0   Medical and Surgical
G   Endocrine System
8   Division   Cutting into a body part without draining fluids and/or gases from the body part in order to separate or transect a body part

Body Part Character 4	Approach Character 5	Device Character 6	Qualifier Character 7
0 Pituitary Gland J Thyroid Gland Isthmus	0 Open 3 Percutaneous 4 Percutaneous Endoscopic	Z No Device	Z No Qualifier

---

LC Limited Coverage   **NC** Noncovered   HAC associated procedure   Combination Only   DRG Non-OR   Non-OR   Revised Text in **GREEN**

Ø   Medical and Surgical
G   Endocrine System
9   Drainage   Taking or letting out fluids and/or gases from a body part

Body Part Character 4	Approach Character 5	Device Character 6	Qualifier Character 7
Ø Pituitary Gland 1 Pineal Body 2 Adrenal Gland, Left 3 Adrenal Gland, Right 4 Adrenal Glands, Bilateral 6 Carotid Body, Left 7 Carotid Body, Right 8 Carotid Bodies, Bilateral 9 Para-aortic Body B Coccygeal Glomus C Glomus Jugulare D Aortic Body F Paraganglion Extremity G Thyroid Gland Lobe, Left H Thyroid Gland Lobe, Right K Thyroid Gland L Superior Parathyroid Gland, Right M Superior Parathyroid Gland, Left N Inferior Parathyroid Gland, Right P Inferior Parathyroid Gland, Left Q Parathyroid Glands, Multiple R Parathyroid Gland	Ø Open 3 Percutaneous 4 Percutaneous Endoscopic	Ø Drainage Device	Z No Qualifier
Ø Pituitary Gland 1 Pineal Body 2 Adrenal Gland, Left 3 Adrenal Gland, Right 4 Adrenal Glands, Bilateral 6 Carotid Body, Left 7 Carotid Body, Right 8 Carotid Bodies, Bilateral 9 Para-aortic Body B Coccygeal Glomus C Glomus Jugulare D Aortic Body F Paraganglion Extremity G Thyroid Gland Lobe, Left H Thyroid Gland Lobe, Right K Thyroid Gland L Superior Parathyroid Gland, Right M Superior Parathyroid Gland, Left N Inferior Parathyroid Gland, Right P Inferior Parathyroid Gland, Left Q Parathyroid Glands, Multiple R Parathyroid Gland	Ø Open 3 Percutaneous 4 Percutaneous Endoscopic	Z No Device	X Diagnostic Z No Qualifier

Non-OR   ØG9[2,3,4,G,H,K][3,4]ZX
Non-OR   ØG9[6,7,8,9,C,D,F][Ø,3,4]ØZ
Non-OR   ØG9[6,7,8,9,C,D,F][Ø,3,4]Z[X,Z]
Non-OR   ØG9[G,H,K,L,M,N,P,Q,R][3,4]ØZ
Non-OR   ØG9[G,H,K,L,M,N,P,Q,R][3,4]ZZ

0 **Medical and Surgical**
G **Endocrine System**
B **Excision**   Cutting out or off, without replacement, a portion of a body part

Body Part Character 4	Approach Character 5	Device Character 6	Qualifier Character 7
0 Pituitary Gland	**0** Open	**Z** No Device	**X** Diagnostic
1 Pineal Body	**3** Percutaneous		**Z** No Qualifier
2 Adrenal Gland, Left	**4** Percutaneous Endoscopic		
3 Adrenal Gland, Right			
4 Adrenal Glands, Bilateral			
6 Carotid Body, Left			
7 Carotid Body, Right			
8 Carotid Bodies, Bilateral			
9 Para-aortic Body			
B Coccygeal Glomus			
C Glomus Jugulare			
D Aortic Body			
F Paraganglion Extremity			
G Thyroid Gland Lobe, Left			
H Thyroid Gland Lobe, Right			
L Superior Parathyroid Gland, Right			
M Superior Parathyroid Gland, Left			
N Inferior Parathyroid Gland, Right			
P Inferior Parathyroid Gland, Left			
Q Parathyroid Glands, Multiple			
R Parathyroid Gland			

Non-OR 0GB[2,3,4,G,H][3,4]ZX
Non-OR 0GB[6,7,8,9,B,C,D,F][0,3,4]Z[X,Z]

0 **Medical and Surgical**
G **Endocrine System**
C **Extirpation**   Taking or cutting out solid matter from a body part

Body Part Character 4	Approach Character 5	Device Character 6	Qualifier Character 7
0 Pituitary Gland	**0** Open	**Z** No Device	**Z** No Qualifier
1 Pineal Body	**3** Percutaneous		
2 Adrenal Gland, Left	**4** Percutaneous Endoscopic		
3 Adrenal Gland, Right			
4 Adrenal Glands, Bilateral			
6 Carotid Body, Left			
7 Carotid Body, Right			
8 Carotid Bodies, Bilateral			
9 Para-aortic Body			
B Coccygeal Glomus			
C Glomus Jugulare			
D Aortic Body			
F Paraganglion Extremity			
G Thyroid Gland Lobe, Left			
H Thyroid Gland Lobe, Right			
K Thyroid Gland			
L Superior Parathyroid Gland, Right			
M Superior Parathyroid Gland, Left			
N Inferior Parathyroid Gland, Right			
P Inferior Parathyroid Gland, Left			
Q Parathyroid Glands, Multiple			
R Parathyroid Gland			

Non-OR 0GC[6,7,8,9,B,C,D,F][0,3,4]ZZ

0 **Medical and Surgical**
G **Endocrine System**
H **Insertion**   Putting in a nonbiological appliance that monitors, assists, performs, or prevents a physiological function but does not physically take the place of a body part

Body Part Character 4	Approach Character 5	Device Character 6	Qualifier Character 7
S Endocrine Gland	**0** Open	**2** Monitoring Device	**Z** No Qualifier
	3 Percutaneous	**3** Infusion Device	
	4 Percutaneous Endoscopic		

LC Limited Coverage **NC** Noncovered   HAC associated procedure   Combination Only   DRG Non-OR   Non-OR   Revised Text in **GREEN**

ICD-10-PCS 2014 (Draft)   263

Ø   Medical and Surgical
G   Endocrine System
J   Inspection   Visually and/or manually exploring a body part

Body Part Character 4	Approach Character 5	Device Character 6	Qualifier Character 7
Ø Pituitary Gland	Ø Open	Z No Device	Z No Qualifier
1 Pineal Body	3 Percutaneous		
5 Adrenal Gland	4 Percutaneous Endoscopic		
K Thyroid Gland			
R Parathyroid Gland			
S Endocrine Gland			

Ø   Medical and Surgical
G   Endocrine System
M   Reattachment   Putting back in or on all or a portion of a separated body part to its normal location or other suitable location

Body Part Character 4	Approach Character 5	Device Character 6	Qualifier Character 7
2 Adrenal Gland, Left	Ø Open	Z No Device	Z No Qualifier
3 Adrenal Gland, Right	4 Percutaneous Endoscopic		
G Thyroid Gland Lobe, Left			
H Thyroid Gland Lobe, Right			
L Superior Parathyroid Gland, Right			
M Superior Parathyroid Gland, Left			
N Inferior Parathyroid Gland, Right			
P Inferior Parathyroid Gland, Left			
Q Parathyroid Glands, Multiple			
R Parathyroid Gland			

Ø   Medical and Surgical
G   Endocrine System
N   Release   Freeing a body part from an abnormal physical constraint

Body Part Character 4	Approach Character 5	Device Character 6	Qualifier Character 7
Ø Pituitary Gland	Ø Open	Z No Device	Z No Qualifier
1 Pineal Body	3 Percutaneous		
2 Adrenal Gland, Left	4 Percutaneous Endoscopic		
3 Adrenal Gland, Right			
4 Adrenal Glands, Bilateral			
6 Carotid Body, Left			
7 Carotid Body, Right			
8 Carotid Bodies, Bilateral			
9 Para-aortic Body			
B Coccygeal Glomus			
C Glomus Jugulare			
D Aortic Body			
F Paraganglion Extremity			
G Thyroid Gland Lobe, Left			
H Thyroid Gland Lobe, Right			
K Thyroid Gland			
L Superior Parathyroid Gland, Right			
M Superior Parathyroid Gland, Left			
N Inferior Parathyroid Gland, Right			
P Inferior Parathyroid Gland, Left			
Q Parathyroid Glands, Multiple			
R Parathyroid Gland			

Non-OR   ØGN[6,7,8,9,B,C,D,F][Ø,3,4]ZZ

Ø   Medical and Surgical
G   Endocrine System
P   Removal   Taking out or off a device from a body part

Body Part Character 4	Approach Character 5	Device Character 6	Qualifier Character 7
Ø Pituitary Gland	Ø Open	Ø Drainage Device	Z No Qualifier
1 Pineal Body	3 Percutaneous		
5 Adrenal Gland	4 Percutaneous Endoscopic		
K Thyroid Gland	X External		
R Parathyroid Gland			
S Endocrine Gland	Ø Open	Ø Drainage Device	Z No Qualifier
	3 Percutaneous	2 Monitoring Device	
	4 Percutaneous Endoscopic	3 Infusion Device	
	X External		

Non-OR   ØGP[Ø,1,5,K,R]XØZ
Non-OR   ØGPS[Ø,3,4,X][Ø,2,3]Z

LC Limited Coverage   NC Noncovered   HAC associated procedure   Combination Only   DRG Non-OR   Non-OR   Revised Text in **GREEN**

Ø   **Medical and Surgical**
G   **Endocrine System**
Q   **Repair**   Restoring, to the extent possible, a body part to its normal anatomic structure and function

Body Part Character 4	Approach Character 5	Device Character 6	Qualifier Character 7
Ø Pituitary Gland 1 Pineal Body 2 Adrenal Gland, Left 3 Adrenal Gland, Right 4 Adrenal Glands, Bilateral 6 Carotid Body, Left 7 Carotid Body, Right 8 Carotid Bodies, Bilateral 9 Para-aortic Body B Coccygeal Glomus C Glomus Jugulare D Aortic Body F Paraganglion Extremity G Thyroid Gland Lobe, Left H Thyroid Gland Lobe, Right J Thyroid Gland Isthmus K Thyroid Gland L Superior Parathyroid Gland, Right M Superior Parathyroid Gland, Left N Inferior Parathyroid Gland, Right P Inferior Parathyroid Gland, Left Q Parathyroid Glands, Multiple R Parathyroid Gland	Ø Open 3 Percutaneous 4 Percutaneous Endoscopic	Z No Device	Z No Qualifier

Non-OR   ØGQ[6,7,8,9,B,C,D,F][Ø,3,4]ZZ

Ø   **Medical and Surgical**
G   **Endocrine System**
S   **Reposition**   Moving to its normal location or other suitable location all or a portion of a body part

Body Part Character 4	Approach Character 5	Device Character 6	Qualifier Character 7
2 Adrenal Gland, Left 3 Adrenal Gland, Right G Thyroid Gland Lobe, Left H Thyroid Gland Lobe, Right L Superior Parathyroid Gland, Right M Superior Parathyroid Gland, Left N Inferior Parathyroid Gland, Right P Inferior Parathyroid Gland, Left Q Parathyroid Glands, Multiple R Parathyroid Gland	Ø Open 4 Percutaneous Endoscopic	Z No Device	Z No Qualifier

Ø   **Medical and Surgical**
G   **Endocrine System**
T   **Resection**   Cutting out or off, without replacement, all of a body part

Body Part Character 4	Approach Character 5	Device Character 6	Qualifier Character 7
Ø Pituitary Gland 1 Pineal Body 2 Adrenal Gland, Left 3 Adrenal Gland, Right 4 Adrenal Glands, Bilateral 6 Carotid Body, Left 7 Carotid Body, Right 8 Carotid Bodies, Bilateral 9 Para-aortic Body B Coccygeal Glomus C Glomus Jugulare D Aortic Body F Paraganglion Extremity G Thyroid Gland Lobe, Left H Thyroid Gland Lobe, Right K Thyroid Gland L Superior Parathyroid Gland, Right M Superior Parathyroid Gland, Left N Inferior Parathyroid Gland, Right P Inferior Parathyroid Gland, Left Q Parathyroid Glands, Multiple R Parathyroid Gland	Ø Open 4 Percutaneous Endoscopic	Z No Device	Z No Qualifier

Non-OR   ØGT[6,7,8,9,B,C,D,F][Ø,4]ZZ

Ø   Medical and Surgical
G   Endocrine System
W   Revision   Correcting, to the extent possible, a portion of a malfunctioning device or the position of a displaced device

Body Part Character 4	Approach Character 5	Device Character 6	Qualifier Character 7
Ø Pituitary Gland 1 Pineal Body 5 Adrenal Gland K Thyroid Gland R Parathyroid Gland	Ø Open 3 Percutaneous 4 Percutaneous Endoscopic X External	Ø Drainage Device	Z No Qualifier
S Endocrine Gland	Ø Open 3 Percutaneous 4 Percutaneous Endoscopic X External	Ø Drainage Device 2 Monitoring Device 3 Infusion Device	Z No Qualifier

Non-OR   ØGW[Ø,1,5,K,R,S]XØZ
Non-OR   ØGWS[Ø,3,4,X][Ø,2,3]Z

Skin and Breast ØHØ–ØHX

Ø Medical and Surgical
H Skin and Breast
Ø Alteration　　　　Modifying the anatomic structure of a body part without affecting the function of the body part

Body Part Character 4	Approach Character 5	Device Character 6	Qualifier Character 7
T Breast, Right U Breast, Left V Breast, Bilateral	Ø Open 3 Percutaneous X External	7 Autologous Tissue Substitute J Synthetic Substitute K Nonautologous Tissue Substitute Z No Device	Z No Qualifier

Ø Medical and Surgical
H Skin and Breast
2 Change　　　　Taking out or off a device from a body part and putting back an identical or similar device in or on the same body part without cutting or puncturing the skin or a mucous membrane

Body Part Character 4	Approach Character 5	Device Character 6	Qualifier Character 7
P Skin T Breast, Right U Breast, Left	X External	Ø Drainage Device Y Other Device	Z No Qualifier

Non-OR　For all body part, approach, device, and qualifier values

Ø Medical and Surgical
H Skin and Breast
5 Destruction　　　　Physical eradication of all or a portion of a body part by the direct use of energy, force, or a destructive agent

Body Part Character 4	Approach Character 5	Device Character 6	Qualifier Character 7
Ø Skin, Scalp 1 Skin, Face 2 Skin, Right Ear 3 Skin, Left Ear 4 Skin, Neck 5 Skin, Chest 6 Skin, Back 7 Skin, Abdomen 8 Skin, Buttock 9 Skin, Perineum A Skin, Genitalia B Skin, Right Upper Arm C Skin, Left Upper Arm D Skin, Right Lower Arm E Skin, Left Lower Arm F Skin, Right Hand G Skin, Left Hand H Skin, Right Upper Leg J Skin, Left Upper Leg K Skin, Right Lower Leg L Skin, Left Lower Leg M Skin, Right Foot N Skin, Left Foot	X External	Z No Device	D Multiple Z No Qualifier
Q Finger Nail R Toe Nail	X External	Z No Device	Z No Qualifier
T Breast, Right U Breast, Left V Breast, Bilateral W Nipple, Right X Nipple, Left	Ø Open 3 Percutaneous 7 Via Natural or Artificial Opening 8 Via Natural or Artificial Opening Endoscopic X External	Z No Device	Z No Qualifier

DRG Non-OR　ØH5[Ø,1,4,5,6,7,8,9,A,B,C,D,E,F,G,H,J,K,L,M,N]XZ[D,Z]
DRG Non-OR　ØH5[Q,R]XZZ
Non-OR　ØH5[2,3]XZ[D,Z]

Skin and Breast

Ø   **Medical and Surgical**
H   **Skin and Breast**
8   **Division**   Cutting into a body part without draining fluids and/or gases from the body part in order to separate or transect a body part

Body Part Character 4	Approach Character 5	Device Character 6	Qualifier Character 7
Ø Skin, Scalp	**X** External	**Z** No Device	**Z** No Qualifier
1 Skin, Face			
2 Skin, Right Ear			
3 Skin, Left Ear			
4 Skin, Neck			
5 Skin, Chest			
6 Skin, Back			
7 Skin, Abdomen			
8 Skin, Buttock			
9 Skin, Perineum			
A Skin, Genitalia			
B Skin, Right Upper Arm			
C Skin, Left Upper Arm			
D Skin, Right Lower Arm			
E Skin, Left Lower Arm			
F Skin, Right Hand			
G Skin, Left Hand			
H Skin, Right Upper Leg			
J Skin, Left Upper Leg			
K Skin, Right Lower Leg			
L Skin, Left Lower Leg			
M Skin, Right Foot			
N Skin, Left Foot			

Non-OR   ØH8[2,3]XZZ

Ø   **Medical and Surgical**
H   **Skin and Breast**
9   **Drainage**   Taking or letting out fluids and/or gases from a body part

Body Part Character 4	Approach Character 5	Device Character 6	Qualifier Character 7
Ø Skin, Scalp	**X** External	**Ø** Drainage Device	**Z** No Qualifier
1 Skin, Face			
2 Skin, Right Ear			
3 Skin, Left Ear			
4 Skin, Neck			
5 Skin, Chest			
6 Skin, Back			
7 Skin, Abdomen			
8 Skin, Buttock			
9 Skin, Perineum			
A Skin, Genitalia			
B Skin, Right Upper Arm			
C Skin, Left Upper Arm			
D Skin, Right Lower Arm			
E Skin, Left Lower Arm			
F Skin, Right Hand			
G Skin, Left Hand			
H Skin, Right Upper Leg			
J Skin, Left Upper Leg			
K Skin, Right Lower Leg			
L Skin, Left Lower Leg			
M Skin, Right Foot			
N Skin, Left Foot			
Q Finger Nail			
R Toe Nail			

ØH9 Continued on next page

Non-OR   For all body part, approach, device, and qualifier values

LC Limited Coverage   **NC** Noncovered   HAC associated procedure   Combination Only   DRG Non-OR   Non-OR   Revised Text in **GREEN**

268   ICD-10-PCS 2014 (Draft)

Ø **Medical and Surgical** *ØH9 Continued*
H **Skin and Breast**
9 **Drainage** Taking or letting out fluids and/or gases from a body part

Body Part Character 4	Approach Character 5	Device Character 6	Qualifier Character 7
Ø Skin, Scalp	**X** External	**Z** No Device	**X** Diagnostic
1 Skin, Face			**Z** No Qualifier
2 Skin, Right Ear			
3 Skin, Left Ear			
4 Skin, Neck			
5 Skin, Chest			
6 Skin, Back			
7 Skin, Abdomen			
8 Skin, Buttock			
9 Skin, Perineum			
A Skin, Genitalia			
B Skin, Right Upper Arm			
C Skin, Left Upper Arm			
D Skin, Right Lower Arm			
E Skin, Left Lower Arm			
F Skin, Right Hand			
G Skin, Left Hand			
H Skin, Right Upper Leg			
J Skin, Left Upper Leg			
K Skin, Right Lower Leg			
L Skin, Left Lower Leg			
M Skin, Right Foot			
N Skin, Left Foot			
Q Finger Nail			
R Toe Nail			
T Breast, Right	**Ø** Open	**Ø** Drainage Device	**Z** No Qualifier
U Breast, Left	**3** Percutaneous		
V Breast, Bilateral	**7** Via Natural or Artificial Opening		
W Nipple, Right	**8** Via Natural or Artificial Opening Endoscopic		
X Nipple, Left	**X** External		
T Breast, Right	**Ø** Open	**Z** No Device	**X** Diagnostic
U Breast, Left	**3** Percutaneous		**Z** No Qualifier
V Breast, Bilateral	**7** Via Natural or Artificial Opening		
W Nipple, Right	**8** Via Natural or Artificial Opening Endoscopic		
X Nipple, Left	**X** External		

Non-OR For all body part, approach, device, and qualifier values

Ø Medical and Surgical
H Skin and Breast
B Excision   Cutting out or off, without replacement, a portion of a body part

Body Part Character 4	Approach Character 5	Device Character 6	Qualifier Character 7
Ø Skin, Scalp 1 Skin, Face 2 Skin, Right Ear 3 Skin, Left Ear 4 Skin, Neck 5 Skin, Chest 6 Skin, Back 7 Skin, Abdomen 8 Skin, Buttock 9 Skin, Perineum A Skin, Genitalia B Skin, Right Upper Arm C Skin, Left Upper Arm D Skin, Right Lower Arm E Skin, Left Lower Arm F Skin, Right Hand G Skin, Left Hand H Skin, Right Upper Leg J Skin, Left Upper Leg K Skin, Right Lower Leg L Skin, Left Lower Leg M Skin, Right Foot N Skin, Left Foot Q Finger Nail R Toe Nail	X External	Z No Device	X Diagnostic Z No Qualifier
T Breast, Right U Breast, Left V Breast, Bilateral W Nipple, Right X Nipple, Left Y Supernumerary Breast	Ø Open 3 Percutaneous 7 Via Natural or Artificial Opening 8 Via Natural or Artificial Opening Endoscopic X External	Z No Device	X Diagnostic Z No Qualifier

DRG Non-OR	ØHB9XZZ
Non-OR	ØHB[Ø,1,2,3,4,5,6,7,8,9,A,B,C,D,E,F,G,H,J,K,L,M,N,Q,R]XZ[X,Z]
Non-OR	ØHB[T,U,V,W,X,Y][3,7,8,X]ZX

Ø Medical and Surgical
H Skin and Breast
C Extirpation   Taking or cutting out solid matter from a body part

Body Part Character 4	Approach Character 5	Device Character 6	Qualifier Character 7
Ø Skin, Scalp 1 Skin, Face 2 Skin, Right Ear 3 Skin, Left Ear 4 Skin, Neck 5 Skin, Chest 6 Skin, Back 7 Skin, Abdomen 8 Skin, Buttock 9 Skin, Perineum A Skin, Genitalia B Skin, Right Upper Arm C Skin, Left Upper Arm D Skin, Right Lower Arm E Skin, Left Lower Arm F Skin, Right Hand G Skin, Left Hand H Skin, Right Upper Leg J Skin, Left Upper Leg K Skin, Right Lower Leg L Skin, Left Lower Leg M Skin, Right Foot N Skin, Left Foot Q Finger Nail R Toe Nail	X External	Z No Device	Z No Qualifier

ØHC Continued on next page

Non-OR	ØHC[Ø,1,2,3,4,5,6,7,8,9,A,B,C,D,E,F,G,H,J,K,L,M,N,Q,R]XZZ

LC Limited Coverage   **NC** Noncovered   HAC associated procedure   Combination Only   DRG Non-OR   Non-OR   Revised Text in **GREEN**

Ø **Medical and Surgical**
H **Skin and Breast**
C **Extirpation** Taking or cutting out solid matter from a body part

ØHC Continued

Body Part Character 4	Approach Character 5	Device Character 6	Qualifier Character 7
T Breast, Right U Breast, Left V Breast, Bilateral W Nipple, Right X Nipple, Left	Ø Open 3 Percutaneousv 7 Via Natural or Artificial Opening 8 Via Natural or Artificial Opening Endoscopic X External	Z No Device	Z No Qualifier

Non-OR ØHC[T,U,V,W,X][Ø,3,7,8,X]ZZ

Ø **Medical and Surgical**
H **Skin and Breast**
D **Extraction** Pulling or stripping out or off all or a portion of a body part by the use of force

Body Part Character 4	Approach Character 5	Device Character 6	Qualifier Character 7
Ø Skin, Scalp 1 Skin, Face 2 Skin, Right Ear 3 Skin, Left Ear 4 Skin, Neck 5 Skin, Chest 6 Skin, Back 7 Skin, Abdomen 8 Skin, Buttock 9 Skin, Perineum A Skin, Genitalia B Skin, Right Upper Arm C Skin, Left Upper Arm D Skin, Right Lower Arm E Skin, Left Lower Arm F Skin, Right Hand G Skin, Left Hand H Skin, Right Upper Leg J Skin, Left Upper Leg K Skin, Right Lower Leg L Skin, Left Lower Leg M Skin, Right Foot N Skin, Left Foot Q Finger Nail R Toe Nail S Hair	X External	Z No Device	Z No Qualifier

Non-OR For all body part, approach, device, and qualifier values

---

Ø **Medical and Surgical**
H **Skin and Breast**
H **Insertion** Putting in a nonbiological appliance that monitors, assists, performs, or prevents a physiological function but does not physically take the place of a body part

Body Part Character 4	Approach Character 5	Device Character 6	Qualifier Character 7
T Breast, Right U Breast, Left V Breast, Bilateral W Nipple, Right X Nipple, Left	Ø Open 3 Percutaneous 7 Via Natural or Artificial Opening 8 Via Natural or Artificial Opening Endoscopic	1 Radioactive Element N Tissue Expander	Z No Qualifier
T Breast, Right U Breast, Left V Breast, Bilateral W Nipple, Right X Nipple, Left	X External	1 Radioactive Element	Z No Qualifier

LC Limited Coverage **NC** Noncovered HAC associated procedure Combination Only DRG Non-OR Non-OR Revised Text in **GREEN**
ICD-10-PCS 2014 (Draft) 271

ØHC—ØHH

Skin and Breast

ØHJ–ØHM

Ø **Medical and Surgical**
H **Skin and Breast**
J **Inspection**   Visually and/or manually exploring a body part

Body Part Character 4	Approach Character 5	Device Character 6	Qualifier Character 7
P Skin Q Finger Nail R Toe Nail	X External	Z No Device	Z No Qualifier
T Breast, Right U Breast, Left	Ø Open 3 Percutaneous 7 Via Natural or Artificial Opening 8 Via Natural or Artificial Opening Endoscopic X External	Z No Device	Z No Qualifier

Non-OR   For all body part, approach, device, and qualifier values

Ø **Medical and Surgical**
H **Skin and Breast**
M **Reattachment**   Putting back in or on all or a portion of a separated body part to its normal location or other suitable location

Body Part Character 4	Approach Character 5	Device Character 6	Qualifier Character 7
Ø Skin, Scalp 1 Skin, Face 2 Skin, Right Ear 3 Skin, Left Ear 4 Skin, Neck 5 Skin, Chest 6 Skin, Back 7 Skin, Abdomen 8 Skin, Buttock 9 Skin, Perineum A Skin, Genitalia B Skin, Right Upper Arm C Skin, Left Upper Arm D Skin, Right Lower Arm E Skin, Left Lower Arm F Skin, Right Hand G Skin, Left Hand H Skin, Right Upper Leg J Skin, Left Upper Leg K Skin, Right Lower Leg L Skin, Left Lower Leg M Skin, Right Foot N Skin, Left Foot T Breast, Right U Breast, Left V Breast, Bilateral W Nipple, Right X Nipple, Left	X External	Z No Device	Z No Qualifier

Non-OR   ØHMØXZZ

Ø Medical and Surgical
H Skin and Breast
N Release   Freeing a body part from an abnormal physical constraint

Body Part Character 4	Approach Character 5	Device Character 6	Qualifier Character 7
Ø Skin, Scalp **1** Skin, Face **2** Skin, Right Ear **3** Skin, Left Ear **4** Skin, Neck **5** Skin, Chest **6** Skin, Back **7** Skin, Abdomen **8** Skin, Buttock **9** Skin, Perineum **A** Skin, Genitalia **B** Skin, Right Upper Arm **C** Skin, Left Upper Arm **D** Skin, Right Lower Arm **E** Skin, Left Lower Arm **F** Skin, Right Hand **G** Skin, Left Hand **H** Skin, Right Upper Leg **J** Skin, Left Upper Leg **K** Skin, Right Lower Leg **L** Skin, Left Lower Leg **M** Skin, Right Foot **N** Skin, Left Foot **Q** Finger Nail **R** Toe Nail	**X** External	**Z** No Device	**Z** No Qualifier
T Breast, Right **U** Breast, Left **V** Breast, Bilateral **W** Nipple, Right **X** Nipple, Left	**Ø** Open **3** Percutaneous **7** Via Natural or Artificial Opening **8** Via Natural or Artificial Opening Endoscopic **X** External	**Z** No Device	**Z** No Qualifier

Ø Medical and Surgical
H Skin and Breast
P Removal   Taking out or off a device from a body part

Body Part Character 4	Approach Character 5	Device Character 6	Qualifier Character 7
P Skin **Q** Finger Nail **R** Toe Nail	**X** External	**Ø** Drainage Device **7** Autologous Tissue Substitute **J** Synthetic Substitute **K** Nonautologous Tissue Substitute	**Z** No Qualifier
S Hair	**X** External	**7** Autologous Tissue Substitute **J** Synthetic Substitute **K** Nonautologous Tissue Substitute	**Z** No Qualifier
T Breast, Right **U** Breast, Left	**Ø** Open **3** Percutaneous **7** Via Natural or Artificial Opening **8** Via Natural or Artificial Opening Endoscopic	**Ø** Drainage Device **1** Radioactive Element **7** Autologous Tissue Substitute **J** Synthetic Substitute **K** Nonautologous Tissue Substitute **N** Tissue Expander	**Z** No Qualifier
T Breast, Right **U** Breast, Left	**X** External	**Ø** Drainage Device **1** Radioactive Element **7** Autologous Tissue Substitute **J** Synthetic Substitute **K** Nonautologous Tissue Substitute	**Z** No Qualifier

Non-OR ØHP[P,Q,R]X[Ø,7,J,K]Z
Non-OR ØHSX[7,J,K]Z
Non-OR ØHP[T,U][Ø,3][Ø,1,7,J,K]Z
Non-OR ØHP[T,U][7,8][Ø,1,7,J,K,N]Z
Non-OR ØHP[T,U]X[Ø,1,7,J,K]Z

Skin and Breast

ØHQ–ØHR

Ø   Medical and Surgical
H   Skin and Breast
Q   Repair   Restoring, to the extent possible, a body part to its normal anatomic structure and function

Body Part Character 4	Approach Character 5	Device Character 6	Qualifier Character 7
Ø Skin, Scalp **1** Skin, Face **2** Skin, Right Ear **3** Skin, Left Ear **4** Skin, Neck **5** Skin, Chest **6** Skin, Back **7** Skin, Abdomen **8** Skin, Buttock **9** Skin, Perineum **A** Skin, Genitalia **B** Skin, Right Upper Arm **C** Skin, Left Upper Arm **D** Skin, Right Lower Arm **E** Skin, Left Lower Arm **F** Skin, Right Hand **G** Skin, Left Hand **H** Skin, Right Upper Leg **J** Skin, Left Upper Leg **K** Skin, Right Lower Leg **L** Skin, Left Lower Leg **M** Skin, Right Foot **N** Skin, Left Foot **Q** Finger Nail **R** Toe Nail	**X** External	**Z** No Device	**Z** No Qualifier
T Breast, Right **U** Breast, Left **V** Breast, Bilateral **W** Nipple, Right **X** Nipple, Left **Y** Supernumerary Breast	**Ø** Open **3** Percutaneous **7** Via Natural or Artificial Opening **8** Via Natural or Artificial Opening Endoscopic **X** External	**Z** No Device	**Z** No Qualifier

DRG Non-OR   ØHQ9XZZ
Non-OR   ØHQ[Ø,1,2,3,4,5,6,7,8,A,B,C,D,E,F,G,H,J,K,L,M,N]XZZ
Non-OR   ØHQ[T,U,V,Y]XZZ

Ø   Medical and Surgical
H   Skin and Breast
R   Replacement   Putting in or on biological or synthetic material that physically takes the place and/or function of all or a portion of a body part

Body Part Character 4	Approach Character 5	Device Character 6	Qualifier Character 7
Ø Skin, Scalp **1** Skin, Face **2** Skin, Right Ear **3** Skin, Left Ear **4** Skin, Neck **5** Skin, Chest **6** Skin, Back **7** Skin, Abdomen **8** Skin, Buttock **9** Skin, Perineum **A** Skin, Genitalia **B** Skin, Right Upper Arm **C** Skin, Left Upper Arm **D** Skin, Right Lower Arm **E** Skin, Left Lower Arm **F** Skin, Right Hand **G** Skin, Left Hand **H** Skin, Right Upper Leg **J** Skin, Left Upper Leg **K** Skin, Right Lower Leg **L** Skin, Left Lower Leg **M** Skin, Right Foot **N** Skin, Left Foot	**X** External	**7** Autologous Tissue Substitute **K** Nonautologous Tissue Substitute	**3** Full Thickness **4** Partial Thickness

ØHR Continued on next page

LC Limited Coverage   **NC** Noncovered   HAC associated procedure   Combination Only   DRG Non-OR   Non-OR   Revised Text in **GREEN**

274   ICD-10-PCS 2014 (Draft)

Ø   Medical and Surgical   *ØHR Continued*
H   Skin and Breast
R   Replacement   Putting in or on biological or synthetic material that physically takes the place and/or function of all or a portion of a body part

Body Part Character 4	Approach Character 5	Device Character 6	Qualifier Character 7
Ø Skin, Scalp 1 Skin, Face 2 Skin, Right Ear 3 Skin, Left Ear 4 Skin, Neck 5 Skin, Chest 6 Skin, Back 7 Skin, Abdomen 8 Skin, Buttock 9 Skin, Perineum A Skin, Genitalia B Skin, Right Upper Arm C Skin, Left Upper Arm D Skin, Right Lower Arm E Skin, Left Lower Arm F Skin, Right Hand G Skin, Left Hand H Skin, Right Upper Leg J Skin, Left Upper Leg K Skin, Right Lower Leg L Skin, Left Lower Leg M Skin, Right Foot N Skin, Left Foot	X External	J Synthetic Substitute	3 Full Thickness 4 Partial Thickness Z No Qualifier
Q Finger Nail R Toe Nail S Hair	X External	7 Autologous Tissue Substitute J Synthetic Substitute K Nonautologous Tissue Substitute	Z No Qualifier
T Breast, Right U Breast, Left V Breast, Bilateral	Ø Open	7 Autologous Tissue Substitute	5 Latissimus Dorsi Myocutaneous Flap 6 Transverse Rectus Abdominis Myocutaneous Flap 7 Deep Inferior Epigastric Artery Perforator Flap 8 Superficial Inferior Epigastric Artery Flap 9 Gluteal Artery Perforator Flap Z No Qualifier
T Breast, Right U Breast, Left V Breast, Bilateral	Ø Open	J Synthetic Substitute K Nonautologous Tissue Substitute	Z No Qualifier
T Breast, Right U Breast, Left V Breast, Bilateral	3 Percutaneous X External	7 Autologous Tissue Substitute J Synthetic Substitute K Nonautologous Tissue Substitute	Z No Qualifier
W Nipple, Right X Nipple, Left	Ø Open 3 Percutaneous X External	7 Autologous Tissue Substitute J Synthetic Substitute K Nonautologous Tissue Substitute	Z No Qualifier

Non-OR   ØHRSX7Z

Ø   Medical and Surgical
H   Skin and Breast
S   Reposition   Moving to its normal location or other suitable location all or a portion of a body part

Body Part Character 4	Approach Character 5	Device Character 6	Qualifier Character 7
S Hair W Nipple, Right X Nipple, Left	X External	Z No Device	Z No Qualifier
T Breast, Right U Breast, Left V Breast, Bilateral	Ø Open	Z No Device	Z No Qualifier

Non-OR   ØHSSXZZ

Ø **Medical and Surgical**
H **Skin and Breast**
T **Resection**   Cutting out or off, without replacement, all of a body part

Body Part Character 4	Approach Character 5	Device Character 6	Qualifier Character 7
Q Finger Nail R Toe Nail W Nipple, Right X Nipple, Left	X External	Z No Device	Z No Qualifier
T Breast, Right U Breast, Left V Breast, Bilateral Y Supernumerary Breast	Ø Open	Z No Device	Z No Qualifier

Non-OR ØHT[Q,R]XZZ

Ø **Medical and Surgical**
H **Skin and Breast**
U **Supplement**   Putting in or on biological or synthetic material that physically reinforces and/or augments the function of a portion of a body part

Body Part Character 4	Approach Character 5	Device Character 6	Qualifier Character 7
T Breast, Right U Breast, Left V Breast, Bilateral W Nipple, Right X Nipple, Left	Ø Open 3 Percutaneous 7 Via Natural or Artificial Opening 8 Via Natural or Artificial Opening Endoscopic X External	7 Autologous Tissue Substitute J Synthetic Substitute K Nonautologous Tissue Substitute	Z No Qualifier

Ø **Medical and Surgical**
H **Skin and Breast**
W **Revision**   Correcting, to the extent possible, a portion of a malfunctioning device or the position of a displaced device

Body Part Character 4	Approach Character 5	Device Character 6	Qualifier Character 7
P Skin Q Finger Nail R Toe Nail T Breast, Right U Breast, Left	X External	Ø Drainage Device 7 Autologous Tissue Substitute J Synthetic Substitute K Nonautologous Tissue Substitute	Z No Qualifier
S Hair	X External	7 Autologous Tissue Substitute J Synthetic Substitute K Nonautologous Tissue Substitute	Z No Qualifier
T Breast, Right U Breast, Left	Ø Open 3 Percutaneous 7 Via Natural or Artificial Opening 8 Via Natural or Artificial Opening Endoscopic	Ø Drainage Device 7 Autologous Tissue Substitute J Synthetic Substitute K Nonautologous Tissue Substitute N Tissue Expander	Z No Qualifier

Non-OR For all body part, approach, device, and qualifier values

Ø Medical and Surgical
H Skin and Breast
X Transfer   Moving, without taking out, all or a portion of a body part to another location to take over the function of all or a portion of a body part

Body Part Character 4	Approach Character 5	Device Character 6	Qualifier Character 7
Ø Skin, Scalp	**X** External	**Z** No Device	**Z** No Qualifier
1 Skin, Face			
2 Skin, Right Ear			
3 Skin, Left Ear			
4 Skin, Neck			
5 Skin, Chest			
6 Skin, Back			
7 Skin, Abdomen			
8 Skin, Buttock			
9 Skin, Perineum			
A Skin, Genitalia			
B Skin, Right Upper Arm			
C Skin, Left Upper Arm			
D Skin, Right Lower Arm			
E Skin, Left Lower Arm			
F Skin, Right Hand			
G Skin, Left Hand			
H Skin, Right Upper Leg			
J Skin, Left Upper Leg			
K Skin, Right Lower Leg			
L Skin, Left Lower Leg			
M Skin, Right Foot			
N Skin, Left Foot			

Subcutaneous Tissue and Fascia ØJØ-ØJX

Ø   **Medical and Surgical**
J   **Subcutaneous Tissue and Fascia**
Ø   **Alteration**   Modifying the anatomic structure of a body part without affecting the function of the body part

Body Part Character 4	Approach Character 5	Device Character 6	Qualifier Character 7
1 Subcutaneous Tissue and Fascia, Face **4** Subcutaneous Tissue and Fascia, Anterior Neck **5** Subcutaneous Tissue and Fascia, Posterior Neck **6** Subcutaneous Tissue and Fascia, Chest **7** Subcutaneous Tissue and Fascia, Back **8** Subcutaneous Tissue and Fascia, Abdomen **9** Subcutaneous Tissue and Fascia, Buttock **D** Subcutaneous Tissue and Fascia, Right Upper Arm **F** Subcutaneous Tissue and Fascia, Left Upper Arm **G** Subcutaneous Tissue and Fascia, Right Lower Arm **H** Subcutaneous Tissue and Fascia, Left Lower Arm **L** Subcutaneous Tissue and Fascia, Right Upper Leg **M** Subcutaneous Tissue and Fascia, Left Upper Leg **N** Subcutaneous Tissue and Fascia, Right Lower Leg **P** Subcutaneous Tissue and Fascia, Left Lower Leg	**Ø** Open **3** Percutaneous	**Z** No Device	**Z** No Qualifier

Ø   **Medical and Surgical**
J   **Subcutaneous Tissue and Fascia**
2   **Change**   Taking out or off a device from a body part and putting back an identical or similar device in or on the same body part without cutting or puncturing the skin or a mucous membrane

Body Part Character 4	Approach Character 5	Device Character 6	Qualifier Character 7
S Subcutaneous Tissue and Fascia, Head and Neck **T** Subcutaneous Tissue and Fascia, Trunk **V** Subcutaneous Tissue and Fascia, Upper Extremity **W** Subcutaneous Tissue and Fascia, Lower Extremity	**X** External	**Ø** Drainage Device **Y** Other Device	**Z** No Qualifier

Non-OR   For all body part, approach, device, and qualifier values

Ø   **Medical and Surgical**
J   **Subcutaneous Tissue and Fascia**
5   **Destruction**   Physical eradication of all or a portion of a body part by the direct use of energy, force, or a destructive agent

Body Part Character 4	Approach Character 5	Device Character 6	Qualifier Character 7
Ø Subcutaneous Tissue and Fascia, Scalp **1** Subcutaneous Tissue and Fascia, Face **4** Subcutaneous Tissue and Fascia, Anterior Neck **5** Subcutaneous Tissue and Fascia, Posterior Neck **6** Subcutaneous Tissue and Fascia, Chest **7** Subcutaneous Tissue and Fascia, Back **8** Subcutaneous Tissue and Fascia, Abdomen **9** Subcutaneous Tissue and Fascia, Buttock **B** Subcutaneous Tissue and Fascia, Perineum **C** Subcutaneous Tissue and Fascia, Pelvic Region **D** Subcutaneous Tissue and Fascia, Right Upper Arm **F** Subcutaneous Tissue and Fascia, Left Upper Arm **G** Subcutaneous Tissue and Fascia, Right Lower Arm **H** Subcutaneous Tissue and Fascia, Left Lower Arm **J** Subcutaneous Tissue and Fascia, Right Hand **K** Subcutaneous Tissue and Fascia, Left Hand **L** Subcutaneous Tissue and Fascia, Right Upper Leg **M** Subcutaneous Tissue and Fascia, Left Upper Leg **N** Subcutaneous Tissue and Fascia, Right Lower Leg **P** Subcutaneous Tissue and Fascia, Left Lower Leg **Q** Subcutaneous Tissue and Fascia, Right Foot **R** Subcutaneous Tissue and Fascia, Left Foot	**Ø** Open **3** Percutaneous	**Z** No Device	**Z** No Qualifier

DRG Non-OR   For all body part, approach, device, and qualifier values

---

LC Limited Coverage   **NC** Noncovered   HAC associated procedure   Combination Only   DRG Non-OR   Non-OR   Revised Text in **GREEN**

278   ICD-10-PCS 2014 (Draft)

0   **Medical and Surgical**
J   **Subcutaneous Tissue and Fascia**
8   **Division**   Cutting into a body part without draining fluids and/or gases from the body part in order to separate or transect a body part

Body Part Character 4	Approach Character 5	Device Character 6	Qualifier Character 7
0 Subcutaneous Tissue and Fascia, Scalp	0 Open	Z No Device	Z No Qualifier
1 Subcutaneous Tissue and Fascia, Face	3 Percutaneous		
4 Subcutaneous Tissue and Fascia, Anterior Neck			
5 Subcutaneous Tissue and Fascia, Posterior Neck			
6 Subcutaneous Tissue and Fascia, Chest			
7 Subcutaneous Tissue and Fascia, Back			
8 Subcutaneous Tissue and Fascia, Abdomen			
9 Subcutaneous Tissue and Fascia, Buttock			
B Subcutaneous Tissue and Fascia, Perineum			
C Subcutaneous Tissue and Fascia, Pelvic Region			
D Subcutaneous Tissue and Fascia, Right Upper Arm			
F Subcutaneous Tissue and Fascia, Left Upper Arm			
G Subcutaneous Tissue and Fascia, Right Lower Arm			
H Subcutaneous Tissue and Fascia, Left Lower Arm			
J Subcutaneous Tissue and Fascia, Right Hand			
K Subcutaneous Tissue and Fascia, Left Hand			
L Subcutaneous Tissue and Fascia, Right Upper Leg			
M Subcutaneous Tissue and Fascia, Left Upper Leg			
N Subcutaneous Tissue and Fascia, Right Lower Leg			
P Subcutaneous Tissue and Fascia, Left Lower Leg			
Q Subcutaneous Tissue and Fascia, Right Foot			
R Subcutaneous Tissue and Fascia, Left Foot			
S Subcutaneous Tissue and Fascia, Head and Neck			
T Subcutaneous Tissue and Fascia, Trunk			
V Subcutaneous Tissue and Fascia, Upper Extremity			
W Subcutaneous Tissue and Fascia, Lower Extremity			

0   **Medical and Surgical**
J   **Subcutaneous Tissue and Fascia**
9   **Drainage**   Taking or letting out fluids and/or gases from a body part

Body Part Character 4	Approach Character 5	Device Character 6	Qualifier Character 7
0 Subcutaneous Tissue and Fascia, Scalp	0 Open	0 Drainage Device	Z No Qualifier
1 Subcutaneous Tissue and Fascia, Face	3 Percutaneous		
4 Subcutaneous Tissue and Fascia, Anterior Neck			
5 Subcutaneous Tissue and Fascia, Posterior Neck			
6 Subcutaneous Tissue and Fascia, Chest			
7 Subcutaneous Tissue and Fascia, Back			
8 Subcutaneous Tissue and Fascia, Abdomen			
9 Subcutaneous Tissue and Fascia, Buttock			
B Subcutaneous Tissue and Fascia, Perineum			
C Subcutaneous Tissue and Fascia, Pelvic Region			
D Subcutaneous Tissue and Fascia, Right Upper Arm			
F Subcutaneous Tissue and Fascia, Left Upper Arm			
G Subcutaneous Tissue and Fascia, Right Lower Arm			
H Subcutaneous Tissue and Fascia, Left Lower Arm			
J Subcutaneous Tissue and Fascia, Right Hand			
K Subcutaneous Tissue and Fascia, Left Hand			
L Subcutaneous Tissue and Fascia, Right Upper Leg			
M Subcutaneous Tissue and Fascia, Left Upper Leg			
N Subcutaneous Tissue and Fascia, Right Lower Leg			
P Subcutaneous Tissue and Fascia, Left Lower Leg			
Q Subcutaneous Tissue and Fascia, Right Foot			
R Subcutaneous Tissue and Fascia, Left Foot			

0J9 Continued on next page

Non-OR   0J9[0,4,5,6,7,8,9,B,C,D,F,G,H,L,M,N,P,Q,R][0,3]0Z

Ø   Medical and Surgical   *ØJ9 Continued*
J   Subcutaneous Tissue and Fascia
9   Drainage   Taking or letting out fluids and/or gases from a body part

Body Part Character 4	Approach Character 5	Device Character 6	Qualifier Character 7
Ø Subcutaneous Tissue and Fascia, Scalp 1 Subcutaneous Tissue and Fascia, Face 4 Subcutaneous Tissue and Fascia, Anterior Neck 5 Subcutaneous Tissue and Fascia, Posterior Neck 6 Subcutaneous Tissue and Fascia, Chest 7 Subcutaneous Tissue and Fascia, Back 8 Subcutaneous Tissue and Fascia, Abdomen 9 Subcutaneous Tissue and Fascia, Buttock B Subcutaneous Tissue and Fascia, Perineum C Subcutaneous Tissue and Fascia, Pelvic Region D Subcutaneous Tissue and Fascia, Right Upper Arm F Subcutaneous Tissue and Fascia, Left Upper Arm G Subcutaneous Tissue and Fascia, Right Lower Arm H Subcutaneous Tissue and Fascia, Left Lower Arm J Subcutaneous Tissue and Fascia, Right Hand K Subcutaneous Tissue and Fascia, Left Hand L Subcutaneous Tissue and Fascia, Right Upper Leg M Subcutaneous Tissue and Fascia, Left Upper Leg N Subcutaneous Tissue and Fascia, Right Lower Leg P Subcutaneous Tissue and Fascia, Left Lower Leg Q Subcutaneous Tissue and Fascia, Right Foot R Subcutaneous Tissue and Fascia, Left Foot	Ø Open 3 Percutaneous	Z No Device	X Diagnostic Z No Qualifier

Non-OR   ØJ9[Ø,1,4,5,6,7,8,9,B,C,D,F,G,H,J,K,L,M,N,P,Q,R][Ø,3]ZX
Non-OR   ØJ9[Ø,1,4,5,6,7,8,9,B,C,D,F,G,H,J,L,M,N,P,Q,R]3ZZ

Ø   Medical and Surgical
J   Subcutaneous Tissue and Fascia
B   Excision   Cutting out or off, without replacement, a portion of a body part

Body Part Character 4	Approach Character 5	Device Character 6	Qualifier Character 7
Ø Subcutaneous Tissue and Fascia, Scalp 1 Subcutaneous Tissue and Fascia, Face 4 Subcutaneous Tissue and Fascia, Anterior Neck 5 Subcutaneous Tissue and Fascia, Posterior Neck 6 Subcutaneous Tissue and Fascia, Chest 7 Subcutaneous Tissue and Fascia, Back 8 Subcutaneous Tissue and Fascia, Abdomen 9 Subcutaneous Tissue and Fascia, Buttock B Subcutaneous Tissue and Fascia, Perineum C Subcutaneous Tissue and Fascia, Pelvic Region D Subcutaneous Tissue and Fascia, Right Upper Arm F Subcutaneous Tissue and Fascia, Left Upper Arm G Subcutaneous Tissue and Fascia, Right Lower Arm H Subcutaneous Tissue and Fascia, Left Lower Arm J Subcutaneous Tissue and Fascia, Right Hand K Subcutaneous Tissue and Fascia, Left Hand L Subcutaneous Tissue and Fascia, Right Upper Leg M Subcutaneous Tissue and Fascia, Left Upper Leg N Subcutaneous Tissue and Fascia, Right Lower Leg P Subcutaneous Tissue and Fascia, Left Lower Leg Q Subcutaneous Tissue and Fascia, Right Foot R Subcutaneous Tissue and Fascia, Left Foot	Ø Open 3 Percutaneous	Z No Device	X Diagnostic Z No Qualifier

Non-OR   ØJB[Ø,1,4,5,6,7,8,9,B,C,D,F,G,H,J,K,L,M,N,P,Q,R][Ø,3]ZX
Non-OR   ØJB[Ø,4,5,6,7,8,9,B,C,D,F,G,H,L,M,N,P,Q,R]3ZZ

Ø **Medical and Surgical**
J **Subcutaneous Tissue and Fascia**
C **Extirpation**   Taking or cutting out solid matter from a body part

Body Part Character 4	Approach Character 5	Device Character 6	Qualifier Character 7
Ø Subcutaneous Tissue and Fascia, Scalp	Ø Open	Z No Device	Z No Qualifier
1 Subcutaneous Tissue and Fascia, Face	3 Percutaneous		
4 Subcutaneous Tissue and Fascia, Anterior Neck			
5 Subcutaneous Tissue and Fascia, Posterior Neck			
6 Subcutaneous Tissue and Fascia, Chest			
7 Subcutaneous Tissue and Fascia, Back			
8 Subcutaneous Tissue and Fascia, Abdomen			
9 Subcutaneous Tissue and Fascia, Buttock			
B Subcutaneous Tissue and Fascia, Perineum			
C Subcutaneous Tissue and Fascia, Pelvic Region			
D Subcutaneous Tissue and Fascia, Right Upper Arm			
F Subcutaneous Tissue and Fascia, Left Upper Arm			
G Subcutaneous Tissue and Fascia, Right Lower Arm			
H Subcutaneous Tissue and Fascia, Left Lower Arm			
J Subcutaneous Tissue and Fascia, Right Hand			
K Subcutaneous Tissue and Fascia, Left Hand			
L Subcutaneous Tissue and Fascia, Right Upper Leg			
M Subcutaneous Tissue and Fascia, Left Upper Leg			
N Subcutaneous Tissue and Fascia, Right Lower Leg			
P Subcutaneous Tissue and Fascia, Left Lower Leg			
Q Subcutaneous Tissue and Fascia, Right Foot			
R Subcutaneous Tissue and Fascia, Left Foot			

Non-OR For all body part, approach, device, and qualifier values

Ø **Medical and Surgical**
J **Subcutaneous Tissue and Fascia**
D **Extraction**   Pulling or stripping out or off all or a portion of a body part by the use of force

Body Part Character 4	Approach Character 5	Device Character 6	Qualifier Character 7
Ø Subcutaneous Tissue and Fascia, Scalp	Ø Open	Z No Device	Z No Qualifier
1 Subcutaneous Tissue and Fascia, Face	3 Percutaneous		
4 Subcutaneous Tissue and Fascia, Anterior Neck			
5 Subcutaneous Tissue and Fascia, Posterior Neck			
6 Subcutaneous Tissue and Fascia, Chest			
7 Subcutaneous Tissue and Fascia, Back			
8 Subcutaneous Tissue and Fascia, Abdomen			
9 Subcutaneous Tissue and Fascia, Buttock			
B Subcutaneous Tissue and Fascia, Perineum			
C Subcutaneous Tissue and Fascia, Pelvic Region			
D Subcutaneous Tissue and Fascia, Right Upper Arm			
F Subcutaneous Tissue and Fascia, Left Upper Arm			
G Subcutaneous Tissue and Fascia, Right Lower Arm			
H Subcutaneous Tissue and Fascia, Left Lower Arm			
J Subcutaneous Tissue and Fascia, Right Hand			
K Subcutaneous Tissue and Fascia, Left Hand			
L Subcutaneous Tissue and Fascia, Right Upper Leg			
M Subcutaneous Tissue and Fascia, Left Upper Leg			
N Subcutaneous Tissue and Fascia, Right Lower Leg			
P Subcutaneous Tissue and Fascia, Left Lower Leg			
Q Subcutaneous Tissue and Fascia, Right Foot			
R Subcutaneous Tissue and Fascia, Left Foot			

Subcutaneous Tissue and Fascia

Ø   **Medical and Surgical**
J   **Subcutaneous Tissue and Fascia**
H   **Insertion**   Putting in a nonbiological appliance that monitors, assists, performs, or prevents a physiological function but does not physically take the place of a body part

Body Part Character 4	Approach Character 5	Device Character 6	Qualifier Character 7
Ø Subcutaneous Tissue and Fascia, Scalp **1** Subcutaneous Tissue and Fascia, Face **4** Subcutaneous Tissue and Fascia, Anterior Neck **5** Subcutaneous Tissue and Fascia, Posterior Neck **9** Subcutaneous Tissue and Fascia, Buttock **B** Subcutaneous Tissue and Fascia, Perineum **C** Subcutaneous Tissue and Fascia, Pelvic Region **J** Subcutaneous Tissue and Fascia, Right Hand **K** Subcutaneous Tissue and Fascia, Left Hand **Q** Subcutaneous Tissue and Fascia, Right Foot **R** Subcutaneous Tissue and Fascia, Left Foot	**Ø** Open **3** Percutaneous	**N** Tissue Expander	**Z** No Qualifier
6 Subcutaneous Tissue and Fascia, Chest **8** Subcutaneous Tissue and Fascia, Abdomen NC	**Ø** Open **3** Percutaneous	**Ø** Monitoring Device, Hemodynamic **2** Monitoring Device **4** Pacemaker, Single Chamber **5** Pacemaker, Single Chamber Rate Responsive **6** Pacemaker, Dual Chamber **7** Cardiac Resynchronization Pacemaker Pulse Generator **8** Defibrillator Generator **9** Cardiac Resynchronization Defibrillator Pulse Generator **A** Contractility Modulation Device **B** Stimulator Generator, Single Array **C** Stimulator Generator, Single Array Rechargeable **D** Stimulator Generator, Multiple Array **E** Stimulator Generator, Multiple Array Rechargeable **H** Contraceptive Device **M** Stimulator Generator **N** Tissue Expander **P** Cardiac Rhythm Related Device **V** Infusion Device, Pump **W** Vascular Access Device, Reservoir **X** Vascular Access Device	**Z** No Qualifier

ØJH Continued on next page

NC   ØJH8[Ø,3]MZ
Non-OR   ØJH[6,8][Ø,3][4,5,6]Z
DRG Non-OR ØJH[6,8][2,H,W,X]Z

Combination Only
Pacemaker Lead/Device
One of ØJH[6,8][Ø,3][4,5,6]Z with one of Ø2H[4,6,7][Ø,4][J,M]Z with one of ØJPT[Ø,3]PZ
Or
One of ØJH[6,8][Ø,3][4,5,6]Z with one of Ø2H[6,7]3JZ with one of ØJPT[Ø,3]PZ
Or
One of ØJH[6,8][Ø,3][4,5,6]Z with one of Ø2H[K,L][Ø,3,4][J,M]Z with one of ØJPT[Ø,3]PZ
Or
One of ØJH[6,8][Ø,3][4,5,6]Z with one of Ø2H[6,7]3JZ with one of ØJPT[Ø,3]PZ
Or
One of ØJH[6,8][Ø,3][4,5,6]Z with one of Ø2H7[Ø,4][J,M]Z with one of ØJPT[Ø,3]PZ
Or
One of ØJH[6,8][Ø,3][4,5,6]Z with one of Ø2H64[J,M]Z with one of ØJPT[Ø,3]PZ
Or
One of ØJH[6,8][Ø,3][4,5,6]Z with one of Ø2H[K,L][Ø,3,4][J,M]Z with one of ØJPT[Ø,3]PZ
Or
One of ØJH[6,8][Ø,3][4,5,6]Z with one of Ø2PA[Ø,3,4,X]MZ with one of Ø2H[6,7,K,L]3JZ with one of ØJPT[Ø,3]PZ
Or
One of ØJH[6,8][Ø,3][4,5,6]Z with one of Ø2HK[3,4][J,M]Z or Ø2HL[Ø,3,4][J,M]Z with one of ØJPT[Ø,3]PZ
Or
One of ØJH[6,8][Ø,3][4,5,6,P]Z with one of Ø2HN[Ø,3,4][J,M]Z
Or
One of ØJH[6,8][Ø,3][4,5,6]Z with one of Ø2H[6,7]3MZ with one of ØJPT[Ø,3]PZ
Or
One of ØJH[6,8][Ø,3][4,5,6]Z with one of Ø2HN[Ø,3,4][J,M]Z with one of ØJPT[Ø,3]PZ

Or
One of ØJH[6,8][Ø,3][6,7,P]Z with one of Ø2H[4,6,7][Ø,4][J,M]Z or Ø2H[6,7]3JZ or Ø2H[K,L][Ø,3,4][J,M]Z
Or
One of ØJH[6,8][Ø,3][6,7,P]Z with one of Ø2H[K,L]3JZ
Or
One of ØJH[6,8][Ø,3][7,P]Z with one of Ø2PA[Ø,3,4,X]MZ with one of Ø2H[6,7,K,L]3JZ
Or
One of ØJH[6,8][Ø,3][7,P]Z with one of Ø2H[6,7]3MZ
Or
One of ØJH[6,8][Ø,3]7Z with one of Ø2H[4,6,7][Ø,3][J,M]Z or Ø2H[4,6,7]3JZ or Ø2H[K,L][Ø,3,4][J,M]Z or Ø2H43KZ

Cardioverter Defibrillator Lead/Generator
One of ØJH[6,8][Ø,3]8Z with one of Ø2H4[Ø,4]KZ or Ø2H[6,7,K,L][Ø,3,4]KZ or Ø2HN[Ø,3,4][J,K,M]Z
Or
One of ØJH[6,8][Ø,3]8Z with one of Ø2H[6,7,K,L][Ø,3,4]KZ
Or
One of ØJH[6,8]9Z with one of Ø2H4[Ø,4][J,K]Z or Ø2H43[J,K,M]Z or Ø2H[6,7,K,L][Ø,3,4]KZ or Ø2HN[Ø,3,4][J,K,M]Z
Or
One of ØJH[6,8][Ø,3]9Z with one of Ø2H[K,L][Ø,3,4]Z
Or
One of ØJH[6,8][Ø,3]AZ with one of Ø2HL[Ø,3,4]MZ

Major Brain Implant
One of ØJH[6,7,8][Ø,3][D,E]Z with one of ØØH[Ø,6][Ø,3,4]MZ

Neurotransmitter/Neurostimulator
One of ØJH[6,7,8][Ø,3][B,C,D,E] Z with one of ØØHE[Ø,3,4]MZ or Ø1HY[Ø,3,4]MZ or ØDH6[Ø,3,4]MZ
Or
One of ØJH[6,7,8][Ø,3][B,C,D,E]Z with one of ØØH[U,V][Ø,3,4]MZ

LC Limited Coverage   **NC** Noncovered   HAC associated procedure   Combination Only   DRG Non-OR   Non-OR   Revised Text in **GREEN**

ØJH Continued

Ø **Medical and Surgical**
J **Subcutaneous Tissue and Fascia**
H **Insertion**   Putting in a nonbiological appliance that monitors, assists, performs, or prevents a physiological function but does not physically take the place of a body part

Body Part Character 4	Approach Character 5	Device Character 6	Qualifier Character 7
7 Subcutaneous Tissue and Fascia, Back **NC**	**Ø** Open **3** Percutaneous	**B** Stimulator Generator, Single Array **C** Stimulator Generator, Single Array Rechargeable **D** Stimulator Generator, Multiple Array **E** Stimulator Generator, Multiple Array Rechargeable **M** Stimulator Generator **N** Tissue Expander **V** Infusion Device, Pump	**Z** No Qualifier
D Subcutaneous Tissue and Fascia, Right Upper Arm **F** Subcutaneous Tissue and Fascia, Left Upper Arm **G** Subcutaneous Tissue and Fascia, Right Lower Arm **H** Subcutaneous Tissue and Fascia, Left Lower Arm **L** Subcutaneous Tissue and Fascia, Right Upper Leg **M** Subcutaneous Tissue and Fascia, Left Upper Leg **N** Subcutaneous Tissue and Fascia, Right Lower Leg **P** Subcutaneous Tissue and Fascia, Left Lower Leg	**Ø** Open **3** Percutaneous	**H** Contraceptive Device **N** Tissue Expander **V** Infusion Pump **W** Reservoir **X** Vascular Access Device	**Z** No Qualifier
S Subcutaneous Tissue and Fascia, Head and Neck **V** Subcutaneous Tissue and Fascia, Upper Extremity **W** Subcutaneous Tissue and Fascia, Lower Extremity	**Ø** Open **3** Percutaneous	**1** Radioactive Element **3** Infusion Device	**Z** No Qualifier
T Subcutaneous Tissue and Fascia, Trunk	**Ø** Open **3** Percutaneous	**1** Radioactive Element **3** Infusion Device **V** Infusion Pump	**Z** No Qualifier

NC	ØJH7[Ø,3]MZ
DRG Non-OR	ØJH[D,F,G,H,L,M][Ø,3][W,X]
DRG Non-OR	ØJHNØ[W,X]Z
DRG Non-OR	ØJHN3[H,W,X]Z
DRG Non-OR	ØJHP[Ø,3][H,W,X]Z
Non-OR	ØJH[D,F,G,H,L,M][Ø,3][H,V]Z
Non-OR	ØJHNØ[H,V]Z
Non-OR	ØJHN3VZ
Non-OR	ØJHP[Ø,3]VZ
Non-OR	ØJH[S,V,W][Ø,3]3Z
Non-OR	ØJHT[Ø,3]3Z

Ø **Medical and Surgical**
J **Subcutaneous Tissue and Fascia**
J **Inspection**   Visually and/or manually exploring a body part

Body Part Character 4	Approach Character 5	Device Character 6	Qualifier Character 7
S Subcutaneous Tissue and Fascia, Head and Neck **T** Subcutaneous Tissue and Fascia, Trunk **V** Subcutaneous Tissue and Fascia, Upper Extremity **W** Subcutaneous Tissue and Fascia, Lower Extremity	**Ø** Open **3** Percutaneous **X** External	**Z** No Device	**Z** No Qualifier

Non-OR   For all body part, approach, device, and qualifier values

LC Limited Coverage   **NC** Noncovered   HAC associated procedure   Combination Only   DRG Non-OR   Non-OR   Revised Text in **GREEN**

ICD-10-PCS 2014 (Draft)   283

ØJH—ØJJ

Ø Medical and Surgical
J Subcutaneous Tissue and Fascia
N Release   Freeing a body part from an abnormal physical constraint

Body Part Character 4	Approach Character 5	Device Character 6	Qualifier Character 7
Ø Subcutaneous Tissue and Fascia, Scalp	Ø Open	Z No Device	Z No Qualifier
1 Subcutaneous Tissue and Fascia, Face	3 Percutaneous		
4 Subcutaneous Tissue and Fascia, Anterior Neck	X External		
5 Subcutaneous Tissue and Fascia, Posterior Neck			
6 Subcutaneous Tissue and Fascia, Chest			
7 Subcutaneous Tissue and Fascia, Back			
8 Subcutaneous Tissue and Fascia, Abdomen			
9 Subcutaneous Tissue and Fascia, Buttock			
B Subcutaneous Tissue and Fascia, Perineum			
C Subcutaneous Tissue and Fascia, Pelvic Region			
D Subcutaneous Tissue and Fascia, Right Upper Arm			
F Subcutaneous Tissue and Fascia, Left Upper Arm			
G Subcutaneous Tissue and Fascia, Right Lower Arm			
H Subcutaneous Tissue and Fascia, Left Lower Arm			
J Subcutaneous Tissue and Fascia, Right Hand			
K Subcutaneous Tissue and Fascia, Left Hand			
L Subcutaneous Tissue and Fascia, Right Upper Leg			
M Subcutaneous Tissue and Fascia, Left Upper Leg			
N Subcutaneous Tissue and Fascia, Right Lower Leg			
P Subcutaneous Tissue and Fascia, Left Lower Leg			
Q Subcutaneous Tissue and Fascia, Right Foot			
R Subcutaneous Tissue and Fascia, Left Foot			

Non-OR   ØJN[Ø,1,4,5,6,7,8,9,B,C,D,F,G,H,J,K,L,M,N,P,Q,R]XZZ

Ø Medical and Surgical
J Subcutaneous Tissue and Fascia
P Removal   Taking out or off a device from a body part

Body Part Character 4	Approach Character 5	Device Character 6	Qualifier Character 7
S Subcutaneous Tissue and Fascia, Head and Neck	Ø Open 3 Percutaneous	Ø Drainage Device 1 Radioactive Element 3 Infusion Device 7 Autologous Tissue Substitute J Synthetic Substitute K Nonautologous Tissue Substitute N Tissue Expander	Z No Qualifier
S Subcutaneous Tissue and Fascia, Head and Neck	X External	Ø Drainage Device 1 Radioactive Element 3 Infusion Device	Z No Qualifier
T Subcutaneous Tissue and Fascia, Trunk	Ø Open 3 Percutaneous	Ø Drainage Device 1 Radioactive Element 2 Monitoring Device 3 Infusion Device 7 Autologous Tissue Substitute H Contraceptive Device J Synthetic Substitute K Nonautologous Tissue Substitute M Stimulator Generator N Tissue Expander P Cardiac Rhythm Related Device V Infusion Pump W Reservoir X Vascular Access Device	Z No Qualifier

ØJP Continued on next page

Non-OR   ØJPS[Ø,3][Ø,1,3,7,J,K,N]Z
Non-OR   ØJPSX[Ø,1,3]Z
Non-OR   ØJPT[Ø,3][Ø,1,2,3,7,H,J,K,M,N,V,W,X]Z

Ø Medical and Surgical
J Subcutaneous Tissue and Fascia
P Removal Taking out or off a device from a body part

ØJP Continued

Body Part Character 4	Approach Character 5	Device Character 6	Qualifier Character 7
T Subcutaneous Tissue and Fascia, Trunk	**X** External	**Ø** Drainage Device **1** Radioactive Element **2** Monitoring Device **3** Infusion Device **H** Contraceptive Device **V** Infusion Pump **X** Vascular Access Device	**Z** No Qualifier
V Subcutaneous Tissue and Fascia, Upper Extremity **W** Subcutaneous Tissue and Fascia, Lower Extremity	**Ø** Open **3** Percutaneous	**Ø** Drainage Device **1** Radioactive Element **3** Infusion Device **7** Autologous Tissue Substitute **H** Contraceptive Device **J** Synthetic Substitute **K** Nonautologous Tissue Substitute **N** Tissue Expander **V** Infusion Pump **W** Reservoir **X** Vascular Access Device	**Z** No Qualifier
V Subcutaneous Tissue and Fascia, Upper Extremity **W** Subcutaneous Tissue and Fascia, Lower Extremity	**X** External	**Ø** Drainage Device **1** Radioactive Element **3** Infusion Device **H** Contraceptive Device **V** Infusion Pump **X** Vascular Access Device	**Z** No Qualifier

Non-OR ØJPTX[Ø,1,2,3,H,V,X]Z
Non-OR ØJP[V,W][Ø,3][Ø,1,3,7,H,J,K,N,V,W,X]Z
Non-OR ØJP[V,W]X[Ø,1,3,H,V,X]Z

Ø Medical and Surgical
J Subcutaneous Tissue and Fascia
Q Repair Restoring, to the extent possible, a body part to its normal anatomic structure and function

Body Part Character 4	Approach Character 5	Device Character 6	Qualifier Character 7
Ø Subcutaneous Tissue and Fascia, Scalp **1** Subcutaneous Tissue and Fascia, Face **4** Subcutaneous Tissue and Fascia, Anterior Neck **5** Subcutaneous Tissue and Fascia, Posterior Neck **6** Subcutaneous Tissue and Fascia, Chest **7** Subcutaneous Tissue and Fascia, Back **8** Subcutaneous Tissue and Fascia, Abdomen **9** Subcutaneous Tissue and Fascia, Buttock **B** Subcutaneous Tissue and Fascia, Perineum **C** Subcutaneous Tissue and Fascia, Pelvic Region **D** Subcutaneous Tissue and Fascia, Right Upper Arm **F** Subcutaneous Tissue and Fascia, Left Upper Arm **G** Subcutaneous Tissue and Fascia, Right Lower Arm **H** Subcutaneous Tissue and Fascia, Left Lower Arm **J** Subcutaneous Tissue and Fascia, Right Hand **K** Subcutaneous Tissue and Fascia, Left Hand **L** Subcutaneous Tissue and Fascia, Right Upper Leg **M** Subcutaneous Tissue and Fascia, Left Upper Leg **N** Subcutaneous Tissue and Fascia, Right Lower Leg **P** Subcutaneous Tissue and Fascia, Left Lower Leg **Q** Subcutaneous Tissue and Fascia, Right Foot **R** Subcutaneous Tissue and Fascia, Left Foot	**Ø** Open **3** Percutaneous	**Z** No Device	**Z** No Qualifier

LC Limited Coverage   **NC** Noncovered   HAC associated procedure   Combination Only   DRG Non-OR   Non-OR   Revised Text in **GREEN**

ICD-10-PCS 2014 (Draft)   285

Subcutaneous Tissue and Fascia

ØJP—ØJQ

Ø   Medical and Surgical
J   Subcutaneous Tissue and Fascia
R   Replacement   Putting in or on biological or synthetic material that physically takes the place and/or function of all or a portion of a body part

Body Part Character 4	Approach Character 5	Device Character 6	Qualifier Character 7
Ø Subcutaneous Tissue and Fascia, Scalp	**Ø** Open	**7** Autologous Tissue Substitute	**Z** No Qualifier
1 Subcutaneous Tissue and Fascia, Face	**3** Percutaneous	**J** Synthetic Substitute	
4 Subcutaneous Tissue and Fascia, Anterior Neck		**K** Nonautologous Tissue	
5 Subcutaneous Tissue and Fascia, Posterior Neck		Substitute	
6 Subcutaneous Tissue and Fascia, Chest			
7 Subcutaneous Tissue and Fascia, Back			
8 Subcutaneous Tissue and Fascia, Abdomen			
9 Subcutaneous Tissue and Fascia, Buttock			
B Subcutaneous Tissue and Fascia, Perineum			
C Subcutaneous Tissue and Fascia, Pelvic Region			
D Subcutaneous Tissue and Fascia, Right Upper Arm			
F Subcutaneous Tissue and Fascia, Left Upper Arm			
G Subcutaneous Tissue and Fascia, Right Lower Arm			
H Subcutaneous Tissue and Fascia, Left Lower Arm			
J Subcutaneous Tissue and Fascia, Right Hand			
K Subcutaneous Tissue and Fascia, Left Hand			
L Subcutaneous Tissue and Fascia, Right Upper Leg			
M Subcutaneous Tissue and Fascia, Left Upper Leg			
N Subcutaneous Tissue and Fascia, Right Lower Leg			
P Subcutaneous Tissue and Fascia, Left Lower Leg			
Q Subcutaneous Tissue and Fascia, Right Foot			
R Subcutaneous Tissue and Fascia, Left Foot			

Ø   Medical and Surgical
J   Subcutaneous Tissue and Fascia
U   Supplement: Putting in or on biological or synthetic material that physically reinforces and/or augments the function of a portion of a body part

Body Part Character 4	Approach Character 5	Device Character 6	Qualifier Character 7
Ø Subcutaneous Tissue and Fascia, Scalp	**Ø** Open	**7** Autologous Tissue Substitute	**Z** No Qualifier
1 Subcutaneous Tissue and Fascia, Face	**3** Percutaneous	**J** Synthetic Substitute	
4 Subcutaneous Tissue and Fascia, Anterior Neck		**K** Nonautologous Tissue	
5 Subcutaneous Tissue and Fascia, Posterior Neck		Substitute	
6 Subcutaneous Tissue and Fascia, Chest			
7 Subcutaneous Tissue and Fascia, Back			
8 Subcutaneous Tissue and Fascia, Abdomen			
9 Subcutaneous Tissue and Fascia, Buttock			
B Subcutaneous Tissue and Fascia, Perineum			
C Subcutaneous Tissue and Fascia, Pelvic Region			
D Subcutaneous Tissue and Fascia, Right Upper Arm			
F Subcutaneous Tissue and Fascia, Left Upper Arm			
G Subcutaneous Tissue and Fascia, Right Lower Arm			
H Subcutaneous Tissue and Fascia, Left Lower Arm			
J Subcutaneous Tissue and Fascia, Right Hand			
K Subcutaneous Tissue and Fascia, Left Hand			
L Subcutaneous Tissue and Fascia, Right Upper Leg			
M Subcutaneous Tissue and Fascia, Left Upper Leg			
N Subcutaneous Tissue and Fascia, Right Lower Leg			
P Subcutaneous Tissue and Fascia, Left Lower Leg			
Q Subcutaneous Tissue and Fascia, Right Foot			
R Subcutaneous Tissue and Fascia, Left Foot			

LC Limited Coverage   **NC** Noncovered   HAC associated procedure   Combination Only   DRG Non-OR   Non-OR   Revised Text in **GREEN**

286   ICD-1Ø-PCS 2Ø14 (Draft)

Ø **Medical and Surgical**
J **Subcutaneous Tissue and Fascia**
W **Revision**　　　Correcting, to the extent possible, a portion of a malfunctioning device or the position of a displaced device

Body Part Character 4	Approach Character 5	Device Character 6	Qualifier Character 7
S Subcutaneous Tissue and Fascia, Head and Neck	**Ø** Open **3** Percutaneous **X** External	**Ø** Drainage Device **3** Infusion Device **7** Autologous Tissue Substitute **J** Synthetic Substitute **K** Nonautologous Tissue Substitute **N** Tissue Expander	**Z** No Qualifier
T Subcutaneous Tissue and Fascia, Trunk	**Ø** Open **3** Percutaneous **X** External	**Ø** Drainage Device **2** Monitoring Device **3** Infusion Device **7** Autologous Tissue Substitute **H** Contraceptive Device **J** Synthetic Substitute **K** Nonautologous Tissue Substitute **M** Stimulator Generator **N** Tissue Expander **P** Cardiac Rhythm Related Device **V** Infusion Pump **W** Reservoir **X** Vascular Access Device	**Z** No Qualifier
V Subcutaneous Tissue and Fascia, Upper Extremity **W** Subcutaneous Tissue and Fascia, Lower Extremity	**Ø** Open **3** Percutaneous **X** External	**Ø** Drainage Device **3** Infusion Device **7** Autologous Tissue Substitute **H** Contraceptive Device **J** Synthetic Substitute **K** Nonautologous Tissue Substitute **N** Tissue Expander **V** Infusion Pump **W** Reservoir **X** Vascular Access Device	**Z** No Qualifier

DRG Non-OR	ØJWS[Ø,3][Ø,3,7,J,K,N]Z
DRG Non-OR	ØJWT[Ø,3][Ø,2,3,7,H,J,K,N,V,W,X]Z
DRG Non-OR	ØJW[V,W][Ø,3][Ø,3,7,H,J,K,N,V,W,X]Z
Non-OR	ØJWSX[Ø,3,7,J,K,N]Z
Non-OR	ØJWTX[Ø,2,3,7,H,J,K,N,P,V,W,X]Z
Non-OR	ØJW[V,W]X[Ø,3,7,H,J,K,N,V,W,X]Z

Ø **Medical and Surgical**
J **Subcutaneous Tissue and Fascia**
X **Transfer**　　　Moving, without taking out, all or a portion of a body part to another location to take over the function of all or a portion of a body part

Body Part Character 4	Approach Character 5	Device Character 6	Qualifier Character 7
Ø Subcutaneous Tissue and Fascia, Scalp **1** Subcutaneous Tissue and Fascia, Face **4** Subcutaneous Tissue and Fascia, Anterior Neck **5** Subcutaneous Tissue and Fascia, Posterior Neck **6** Subcutaneous Tissue and Fascia, Chest **7** Subcutaneous Tissue and Fascia, Back **8** Subcutaneous Tissue and Fascia, Abdomen **9** Subcutaneous Tissue and Fascia, Buttock **B** Subcutaneous Tissue and Fascia, Perineum **C** Subcutaneous Tissue and Fascia, Pelvic Region **D** Subcutaneous Tissue and Fascia, Right Upper Arm **F** Subcutaneous Tissue and Fascia, Left Upper Arm **G** Subcutaneous Tissue and Fascia, Right Lower Arm **H** Subcutaneous Tissue and Fascia, Left Lower Arm **J** Subcutaneous Tissue and Fascia, Right Hand **K** Subcutaneous Tissue and Fascia, Left Hand **L** Subcutaneous Tissue and Fascia, Right Upper Leg **M** Subcutaneous Tissue and Fascia, Left Upper Leg **N** Subcutaneous Tissue and Fascia, Right Lower Leg **P** Subcutaneous Tissue and Fascia, Left Lower Leg **Q** Subcutaneous Tissue and Fascia, Right Foot **R** Subcutaneous Tissue and Fascia, Left Foot	**Ø** Open **3** Percutaneous	**Z** No Device	**B** Skin and Subcutaneous Tissue **C** Skin, Subcutaneous Tissue and Fascia **Z** No Qualifier

LC Limited Coverage　　　**NC** Noncovered　　　HAC associated procedure　　　Combination Only　　　DRG Non-OR　　　Non-OR　　　Revised Text in **GREEN**

ICD-10-PCS 2014 (Draft)　　　　　　　　　　　　　　　　　　　　　　　　　　　　　　　　　　**287**

Muscles ØK2–ØKX

Ø   Medical and Surgical
K   Muscles
2   Change   Taking out or off a device from a body part and putting back an identical or similar device in or on the same body part without cutting or puncturing the skin or a mucous membrane

Body Part Character 4	Approach Character 5	Device Character 6	Qualifier Character 7
X Upper Muscle **Y** Lower Muscle	**X** External	**Ø** Drainage Device **Y** Other Device	**Z** No Qualifier

Non-OR For all body part, approach, device, and qualifier values

Ø   Medical and Surgical
K   Muscles
5   Destruction   Physical eradication of all or a portion of a body part by the direct use of energy, force, or a destructive agent

Body Part Character 4	Approach Character 5	Device Character 6	Qualifier Character 7
Ø Head Muscle **1** Facial Muscle **2** Neck Muscle, Right **3** Neck Muscle, Left **4** Tongue, Palate, Pharynx Muscle **5** Shoulder Muscle, Right **6** Shoulder Muscle, Left **7** Upper Arm Muscle, Right **8** Upper Arm Muscle, Left **9** Lower Arm and Wrist Muscle, Right **B** Lower Arm and Wrist Muscle, Left **C** Hand Muscle, Right **D** Hand Muscle, Left **F** Trunk Muscle, Right **G** Trunk Muscle, Left **H** Thorax Muscle, Right **J** Thorax Muscle, Left **K** Abdomen Muscle, Right **L** Abdomen Muscle, Left **M** Perineum Muscle **N** Hip Muscle, Right **P** Hip Muscle, Left **Q** Upper Leg Muscle, Right **R** Upper Leg Muscle, Left **S** Lower Leg Muscle, Right **T** Lower Leg Muscle, Left **V** Foot Muscle, Right **W** Foot Muscle, Left	**Ø** Open **3** Percutaneous **4** Percutaneous Endoscopic	**Z** No Device	**Z** No Qualifier

LC Limited Coverage   **NC** Noncovered   HAC associated procedure   Combination Only   DRG Non-OR   Non-OR   Revised Text in **GREEN**

288   ICD-10-PCS 2014 (Draft)

Ø　Medical and Surgical
K　Muscles
8　Division　　Cutting into a body part without draining fluids and/or gases from the body part in order to separate or transect a body part

Body Part Character 4	Approach Character 5	Device Character 6	Qualifier Character 7
Ø Head Muscle	Ø Open	Z No Device	Z No Qualifier
1 Facial Muscle	3 Percutaneous		
2 Neck Muscle, Right	4 Percutaneous Endoscopic		
3 Neck Muscle, Left			
4 Tongue, Palate, Pharynx Muscle			
5 Shoulder Muscle, Right			
6 Shoulder Muscle, Left			
7 Upper Arm Muscle, Right			
8 Upper Arm Muscle, Left			
9 Lower Arm and Wrist Muscle, Right			
B Lower Arm and Wrist Muscle, Left			
C Hand Muscle, Right			
D Hand Muscle, Left			
F Trunk Muscle, Right			
G Trunk Muscle, Left			
H Thorax Muscle, Right			
J Thorax Muscle, Left			
K Abdomen Muscle, Right			
L Abdomen Muscle, Left			
M Perineum Muscle			
N Hip Muscle, Right			
P Hip Muscle, Left			
Q Upper Leg Muscle, Right			
R Upper Leg Muscle, Left			
S Lower Leg Muscle, Right			
T Lower Leg Muscle, Left			
V Foot Muscle, Right			
W Foot Muscle, Left			

Ø　Medical and Surgical
K　Muscles
9　Drainage　　Taking or letting out fluids and/or gases from a body part

Body Part Character 4	Approach Character 5	Device Character 6	Qualifier Character 7
Ø Head Muscle	Ø Open	Ø Drainage Device	Z No Qualifier
1 Facial Muscle	3 Percutaneous		
2 Neck Muscle, Right	4 Percutaneous Endoscopic		
3 Neck Muscle, Left			
4 Tongue, Palate, Pharynx Muscle			
5 Shoulder Muscle, Right			
6 Shoulder Muscle, Left			
7 Upper Arm Muscle, Right			
8 Upper Arm Muscle, Left			
9 Lower Arm and Wrist Muscle, Right			
B Lower Arm and Wrist Muscle, Left			
C Hand Muscle, Right			
D Hand Muscle, Left			
F Trunk Muscle, Right			
G Trunk Muscle, Left			
H Thorax Muscle, Right			
J Thorax Muscle, Left			
K Abdomen Muscle, Right			
L Abdomen Muscle, Left			
M Perineum Muscle			
N Hip Muscle, Right			
P Hip Muscle, Left			
Q Upper Leg Muscle, Right			
R Upper Leg Muscle, Left			
S Lower Leg Muscle, Right			
T Lower Leg Muscle, Left			
V Foot Muscle, Right			
W Foot Muscle, Left			

ØK9 Continued on next page

ØK8—ØK9

Muscles

ØK9–ØKB

Ø   **Medical and Surgical**
K   **Muscles**
9   **Drainage**   Taking or letting out fluids and/or gases from a body part

Body Part Character 4	Approach Character 5	Device Character 6	Qualifier Character 7
Ø Head Muscle **1** Facial Muscle **2** Neck Muscle, Right **3** Neck Muscle, Left **4** Tongue, Palate, Pharynx Muscle **5** Shoulder Muscle, Right **6** Shoulder Muscle, Left **7** Upper Arm Muscle, Right **8** Upper Arm Muscle, Left **9** Lower Arm and Wrist Muscle, Right **B** Lower Arm and Wrist Muscle, Left **C** Hand Muscle, Right **D** Hand Muscle, Left **F** Trunk Muscle, Right **G** Trunk Muscle, Left **H** Thorax Muscle, Right **J** Thorax Muscle, Left **K** Abdomen Muscle, Right **L** Abdomen Muscle, Left **M** Perineum Muscle **N** Hip Muscle, Right **P** Hip Muscle, Left **Q** Upper Leg Muscle, Right **R** Upper Leg Muscle, Left **S** Lower Leg Muscle, Right **T** Lower Leg Muscle, Left **V** Foot Muscle, Right **W** Foot Muscle, Left	**Ø** Open **3** Percutaneous **4** Percutaneous Endoscopic	**Z** No Device	**X** Diagnostic **Z** No Qualifier

Non-OR   ØK9[Ø,1,2,3,4,5,6,7,8,9,B,F,G,H,J,K,L,M,N,P,Q,R,S,T,V,W]3ZZ
Non-OR   ØK9[C,D][3,4]ZZ

Ø   **Medical and Surgical**
K   **Muscles**
B   **Excision**   Cutting out or off, without replacement, a portion of a body part

Body Part Character 4	Approach Character 5	Device Character 6	Qualifier Character 7
Ø Head Muscle **1** Facial Muscle **2** Neck Muscle, Right **3** Neck Muscle, Left **4** Tongue, Palate, Pharynx Muscle **5** Shoulder Muscle, Right **6** Shoulder Muscle, Left **7** Upper Arm Muscle, Right **8** Upper Arm Muscle, Left **9** Lower Arm and Wrist Muscle, Right **B** Lower Arm and Wrist Muscle, Left **C** Hand Muscle, Right **D** Hand Muscle, Left **F** Trunk Muscle, Right **G** Trunk Muscle, Left **H** Thorax Muscle, Right **J** Thorax Muscle, Left **K** Abdomen Muscle, Right **L** Abdomen Muscle, Left **M** Perineum Muscle **N** Hip Muscle, Right **P** Hip Muscle, Left **Q** Upper Leg Muscle, Right **R** Upper Leg Muscle, Left **S** Lower Leg Muscle, Right **T** Lower Leg Muscle, Left **V** Foot Muscle, Right **W** Foot Muscle, Left	**Ø** Open **3** Percutaneous **4** Percutaneous Endoscopic	**Z** No Device	**X** Diagnostic **Z** No Qualifier

Ø   Medical and Surgical
K   Muscles
C   Extirpation   Taking or cutting out solid matter from a body part

Body Part Character 4	Approach Character 5	Device Character 6	Qualifier Character 7
Ø Head Muscle **1** Facial Muscle **2** Neck Muscle, Right **3** Neck Muscle, Left **4** Tongue, Palate, Pharynx Muscle **5** Shoulder Muscle, Right **6** Shoulder Muscle, Left **7** Upper Arm Muscle, Right **8** Upper Arm Muscle, Left **9** Lower Arm and Wrist Muscle, Right **B** Lower Arm and Wrist Muscle, Left **C** Hand Muscle, Right **D** Hand Muscle, Left **F** Trunk Muscle, Right **G** Trunk Muscle, Left **H** Thorax Muscle, Right **J** Thorax Muscle, Left **K** Abdomen Muscle, Right **L** Abdomen Muscle, Left **M** Perineum Muscle **N** Hip Muscle, Right **P** Hip Muscle, Left **Q** Upper Leg Muscle, Right **R** Upper Leg Muscle, Left **S** Lower Leg Muscle, Right **T** Lower Leg Muscle, Left **V** Foot Muscle, Right **W** Foot Muscle, Left	**Ø** Open **3** Percutaneous **4** Percutaneous Endoscopic	**Z** No Device	**Z** No Qualifier

Ø   Medical and Surgical
K   Muscles
H   Insertion   Putting in a nonbiological appliance that monitors, assists, performs, or prevents a physiological function but does not physically take the place of a body part

Body Part Character 4	Approach Character 5	Device Character 6	Qualifier Character 7
X Upper Muscle **Y** Lower Muscle	**Ø** Open **3** Percutaneous **4** Percutaneous Endoscopic	**M** Stimulator Lead	**Z** No Qualifier

Ø   Medical and Surgical
K   Muscles
J   Inspection   Visually and/or manually exploring a body part

Body Part Character 4	Approach Character 5	Device Character 6	Qualifier Character 7
X Upper Muscle **Y** Lower Muscle	**Ø** Open **3** Percutaneous **4** Percutaneous Endoscopic **X** External	**Z** No Device	**Z** No Qualifier

Non-OR   ØKJ[X,Y]XZZ

Ø   Medical and Surgical
K   Muscles
M   Reattachment   Putting back in or on all or a portion of a separated body part to its normal location or other suitable location

Body Part Character 4	Approach Character 5	Device Character 6	Qualifier Character 7
Ø Head Muscle	Ø Open	Z No Device	Z No Qualifier
1 Facial Muscle	4 Percutaneous Endoscopic		
2 Neck Muscle, Right			
3 Neck Muscle, Left			
4 Tongue, Palate, Pharynx Muscle			
5 Shoulder Muscle, Right			
6 Shoulder Muscle, Left			
7 Upper Arm Muscle, Right			
8 Upper Arm Muscle, Left			
9 Lower Arm and Wrist Muscle, Right			
B Lower Arm and Wrist Muscle, Left			
C Hand Muscle, Right			
D Hand Muscle, Left			
F Trunk Muscle, Right			
G Trunk Muscle, Left			
H Thorax Muscle, Right			
J Thorax Muscle, Left			
K Abdomen Muscle, Right			
L Abdomen Muscle, Left			
M Perineum Muscle			
N Hip Muscle, Right			
P Hip Muscle, Left			
Q Upper Leg Muscle, Right			
R Upper Leg Muscle, Left			
S Lower Leg Muscle, Right			
T Lower Leg Muscle, Left			
V Foot Muscle, Right			
W Foot Muscle, Left			

Ø   Medical and Surgical
K   Muscles
N   Release   Freeing a body part from an abnormal physical constraint

Body Part Character 4	Approach Character 5	Device Character 6	Qualifier Character 7
Ø Head Muscle	Ø Open	Z No Device	Z No Qualifier
1 Facial Muscle	3 Percutaneous		
2 Neck Muscle, Right	4 Percutaneous Endoscopic		
3 Neck Muscle, Left	X External		
4 Tongue, Palate, Pharynx Muscle			
5 Shoulder Muscle, Right			
6 Shoulder Muscle, Left			
7 Upper Arm Muscle, Right			
8 Upper Arm Muscle, Left			
9 Lower Arm and Wrist Muscle, Right			
B Lower Arm and Wrist Muscle, Left			
C Hand Muscle, Right			
D Hand Muscle, Left			
F Trunk Muscle, Right			
G Trunk Muscle, Left			
H Thorax Muscle, Right			
J Thorax Muscle, Left			
K Abdomen Muscle, Right			
L Abdomen Muscle, Left			
M Perineum Muscle			
N Hip Muscle, Right			
P Hip Muscle, Left			
Q Upper Leg Muscle, Right			
R Upper Leg Muscle, Left			
S Lower Leg Muscle, Right			
T Lower Leg Muscle, Left			
V Foot Muscle, Right			
W Foot Muscle, Left			

Non-OR   ØKN[Ø,1,2,3,4,5,6,7,8,9,B,C,D,F,G,H,J,K,L,M,N,P,Q,R,S,T,V,W]XZZ

Ø   **Medical and Surgical**
K   **Muscles**
P   **Removal**   Taking out or off a device from a body part

Body Part Character 4	Approach Character 5	Device Character 6	Qualifier Character 7
X Upper Muscle **Y** Lower Muscle	**Ø** Open **3** Percutaneous **4** Percutaneous Endoscopic	**Ø** Drainage Device **7** Autologous Tissue Substitute **J** Synthetic Substitute **K** Nonautologous Tissue Substitute **M** Stimulator Lead	**Z** No Qualifier
X Upper Muscle **Y** Lower Muscle	**X** External	**Ø** Drainage Device **M** Stimulator Lead	**Z** No Qualifier

Non-OR   ØKP[X,Y]X[Ø,M]Z

Ø   **Medical and Surgical**
K   **Muscles**
Q   **Repair**   Restoring, to the extent possible, a body part to its normal anatomic structure and function

Body Part Character 4	Approach Character 5	Device Character 6	Qualifier Character 7
Ø Head Muscle **1** Facial Muscle **2** Neck Muscle, Right **3** Neck Muscle, Left **4** Tongue, Palate, Pharynx Muscle **5** Shoulder Muscle, Right **6** Shoulder Muscle, Left **7** Upper Arm Muscle, Right **8** Upper Arm Muscle, Left **9** Lower Arm and Wrist Muscle, Right **B** Lower Arm and Wrist Muscle, Left **C** Hand Muscle, Right **D** Hand Muscle, Left **F** Trunk Muscle, Right **G** Trunk Muscle, Left **H** Thorax Muscle, Right **J** Thorax Muscle, Left **K** Abdomen Muscle, Right **L** Abdomen Muscle, Left **M** Perineum Muscle **N** Hip Muscle, Right **P** Hip Muscle, Left **Q** Upper Leg Muscle, Right **R** Upper Leg Muscle, Left **S** Lower Leg Muscle, Right **T** Lower Leg Muscle, Left **V** Foot Muscle, Right **W** Foot Muscle, Left	**Ø** Open **3** Percutaneous **4** Percutaneous Endoscopic	**Z** No Device	**Z** No Qualifier

Muscles

Ø   Medical and Surgical
K   Muscles
S   Reposition   Moving to its normal location or other suitable location all or a portion of a body part

Body Part Character 4	Approach Character 5	Device Character 6	Qualifier Character 7
Ø Head Muscle	**Ø** Open	**Z** No Device	**Z** No Qualifier
1 Facial Muscle	**4** Percutaneous Endoscopic		
2 Neck Muscle, Right			
3 Neck Muscle, Left			
4 Tongue, Palate, Pharynx Muscle			
5 Shoulder Muscle, Right			
6 Shoulder Muscle, Left			
7 Upper Arm Muscle, Right			
8 Upper Arm Muscle, Left			
9 Lower Arm and Wrist Muscle, Right			
B Lower Arm and Wrist Muscle, Left			
C Hand Muscle, Right			
D Hand Muscle, Left			
F Trunk Muscle, Right			
G Trunk Muscle, Left			
H Thorax Muscle, Right			
J Thorax Muscle, Left			
K Abdomen Muscle, Right			
L Abdomen Muscle, Left			
M Perineum Muscle			
N Hip Muscle, Right			
P Hip Muscle, Left			
Q Upper Leg Muscle, Right			
R Upper Leg Muscle, Left			
S Lower Leg Muscle, Right			
T Lower Leg Muscle, Left			
V Foot Muscle, Right			
W Foot Muscle, Left			

Ø   Medical and Surgical
K   Muscles
T   Resection   Cutting out or off, without replacement, all of a body part

Body Part Character 4	Approach Character 5	Device Character 6	Qualifier Character 7
Ø Head Muscle	**Ø** Open	**Z** No Device	**Z** No Qualifier
1 Facial Muscle	**4** Percutaneous Endoscopic		
2 Neck Muscle, Right			
3 Neck Muscle, Left			
4 Tongue, Palate, Pharynx Muscle			
5 Shoulder Muscle, Right			
6 Shoulder Muscle, Left			
7 Upper Arm Muscle, Right			
8 Upper Arm Muscle, Left			
9 Lower Arm and Wrist Muscle, Right			
B Lower Arm and Wrist Muscle, Left			
C Hand Muscle, Right			
D Hand Muscle, Left			
F Trunk Muscle, Right			
G Trunk Muscle, Left			
H Thorax Muscle, Right			
J Thorax Muscle, Left			
K Abdomen Muscle, Right			
L Abdomen Muscle, Left			
M Perineum Muscle			
N Hip Muscle, Right			
P Hip Muscle, Left			
Q Upper Leg Muscle, Right			
R Upper Leg Muscle, Left			
S Lower Leg Muscle, Right			
T Lower Leg Muscle, Left			
V Foot Muscle, Right			
W Foot Muscle, Left			

Ø   **Medical and Surgical**
K   **Muscles**
U   **Supplement**   Putting in or on biological or synthetic material that physically reinforces and/or augments the function of a portion of a body part

Body Part Character 4	Approach Character 5	Device Character 6	Qualifier Character 7
Ø Head Muscle **1** Facial Muscle **2** Neck Muscle, Right **3** Neck Muscle, Left **4** Tongue, Palate, Pharynx Muscle **5** Shoulder Muscle, Right **6** Shoulder Muscle, Left **7** Upper Arm Muscle, Right **8** Upper Arm Muscle, Left **9** Lower Arm and Wrist Muscle, Right **B** Lower Arm and Wrist Muscle, Left **C** Hand Muscle, Right **D** Hand Muscle, Left **F** Trunk Muscle, Right **G** Trunk Muscle, Left **H** Thorax Muscle, Right **J** Thorax Muscle, Left **K** Abdomen Muscle, Right **L** Abdomen Muscle, Left **M** Perineum Muscle **N** Hip Muscle, Right **P** Hip Muscle, Left **Q** Upper Leg Muscle, Right **R** Upper Leg Muscle, Left **S** Lower Leg Muscle, Right **T** Lower Leg Muscle, Left **V** Foot Muscle, Right **W** Foot Muscle, Left	**Ø** Open **4** Percutaneous Endoscopic	**7** Autologous Tissue Substitute **J** Synthetic Substitute **K** Nonautologous Tissue Substitute	**Z** No Qualifier

Ø   **Medical and Surgical**
K   **Muscles**
W   **Revision**   Correcting, to the extent possible, a portion of a malfunctioning device or the position of a displaced device

Body Part Character 4	Approach Character 5	Device Character 6	Qualifier Character 7
X Upper Muscle **Y** Lower Muscle	**Ø** Open **3** Percutaneous **4** Percutaneous Endoscopic **X** External	**Ø** Drainage Device **7** Autologous Tissue Substitute **J** Synthetic Substitute **K** Nonautologous Tissue Substitute **M** Stimulator Lead	**Z** No Qualifier

Non-OR   ØKW[X,Y]X[Ø,7,J,K,M]Z

Ø　Medical and Surgical
K　Muscles
X　Transfer　　　Moving, without taking out, all or a portion of a body part to another location to take over the function of all or a portion of a body part

Body Part Character 4	Approach Character 5	Device Character 6	Qualifier Character 7
Ø　Head Muscle **1**　Facial Muscle **2**　Neck Muscle, Right **3**　Neck Muscle, Left **4**　Tongue, Palate, Pharynx Muscle **5**　Shoulder Muscle, Right **6**　Shoulder Muscle, Left **7**　Upper Arm Muscle, Right **8**　Upper Arm Muscle, Left **9**　Lower Arm and Wrist Muscle, Right **B**　Lower Arm and Wrist Muscle, Left **C**　Hand Muscle, Right **D**　Hand Muscle, Left **F**　Trunk Muscle, Right **G**　Trunk Muscle, Left **H**　Thorax Muscle, Right **J**　Thorax Muscle, Left **M**　Perineum Muscle **N**　Hip Muscle, Right **P**　Hip Muscle, Left **Q**　Upper Leg Muscle, Right **R**　Upper Leg Muscle, Left **S**　Lower Leg Muscle, Right **T**　Lower Leg Muscle, Left **V**　Foot Muscle, Right **W**　Foot Muscle, Left	**Ø**　Open **4**　Percutaneous Endoscopic	**Z**　No Device	**Ø**　Skin **1**　Subcutaneous Tissue **2**　Skin and Subcutaneous Tissue **Z**　No Qualifier
K　Abdomen Muscle, Right **L**　Abdomen Muscle, Left	**Ø**　Open **4**　Percutaneous Endoscopic	**Z**　No Device	**Ø**　Skin **1**　Subcutaneous Tissue **2**　Skin and Subcutaneous Tissue **6**　Transverse Rectus Abdominis 　　Myocutaneous Flap **Z**　No Qualifier

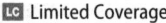 Limited Coverage　　　**NC** Noncovered　　　HAC associated procedure　　　Combination Only　　　DRG Non-OR　　　Non-OR　　　Revised Text in **GREEN**

296　　ICD-10-PCS 2014 (Draft)

Tendons 0L2–0LX

0   **Medical and Surgical**
L   **Tendons**
2   **Change**   Taking out or off a device from a body part and putting back an identical or similar device in or on the same body part without cutting or puncturing the skin or a mucous membrane

Body Part Character 4	Approach Character 5	Device Character 6	Qualifier Character 7
X Upper Tendon **Y** Lower Tendon	**X** External	**0** Drainage Device **Y** Other Device	**Z** No Qualifier

Non-OR   For all body part, approach, device, and qualifier values

0   **Medical and Surgical**
L   **Tendons**
5   **Destruction**   Physical eradication of all or a portion of a body part by the direct use of energy, force, or a destructive agent

Body Part Character 4	Approach Character 5	Device Character 6	Qualifier Character 7
0 Head and Neck Tendon **1** Shoulder Tendon, Right **2** Shoulder Tendon, Left **3** Upper Arm Tendon, Right **4** Upper Arm Tendon, Left **5** Lower Arm and Wrist Tendon, Right **6** Lower Arm and Wrist Tendon, Left **7** Hand Tendon, Right **8** Hand Tendon, Left **9** Trunk Tendon, Right **B** Trunk Tendon, Left **C** Thorax Tendon, Right **D** Thorax Tendon, Left **F** Abdomen Tendon, Right **G** Abdomen Tendon, Left **H** Perineum Tendon **J** Hip Tendon, Right **K** Hip Tendon, Left **L** Upper Leg Tendon, Right **M** Upper Leg Tendon, Left **N** Lower Leg Tendon, Right **P** Lower Leg Tendon, Left **Q** Knee Tendon, Right **R** Knee Tendon, Left **S** Ankle Tendon, Right **T** Ankle Tendon, Left **V** Foot Tendon, Right **W** Foot Tendon, Left	**0** Open **3** Percutaneous **4** Percutaneous Endoscopic	**Z** No Device	**Z** No Qualifier

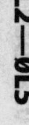

LC Limited Coverage   **NC** Noncovered   HAC associated procedure   Combination Only   DRG Non-OR   Non-OR   Revised Text in **GREEN**

Ø **Medical and Surgical**
L **Tendons**
8 **Division** — Cutting into a body part without draining fluids and/or gases from the body part in order to separate or transect a body part

Body Part Character 4	Approach Character 5	Device Character 6	Qualifier Character 7
Ø Head and Neck Tendon	**Ø** Open	**Z** No Device	**Z** No Qualifier
1 Shoulder Tendon, Right	**3** Percutaneous		
2 Shoulder Tendon, Left	**4** Percutaneous Endoscopic		
3 Upper Arm Tendon, Right			
4 Upper Arm Tendon, Left			
5 Lower Arm and Wrist Tendon, Right			
6 Lower Arm and Wrist Tendon, Left			
7 Hand Tendon, Right			
8 Hand Tendon, Left			
9 Trunk Tendon, Right			
B Trunk Tendon, Left			
C Thorax Tendon, Right			
D Thorax Tendon, Left			
F Abdomen Tendon, Right			
G Abdomen Tendon, Left			
H Perineum Tendon			
J Hip Tendon, Right			
K Hip Tendon, Left			
L Upper Leg Tendon, Right			
M Upper Leg Tendon, Left			
N Lower Leg Tendon, Right			
P Lower Leg Tendon, Left			
Q Knee Tendon, Right			
R Knee Tendon, Left			
S Ankle Tendon, Right			
T Ankle Tendon, Left			
V Foot Tendon, Right			
W Foot Tendon, Left			

Ø **Medical and Surgical**
L **Tendons**
9 **Drainage** — Taking or letting out fluids and/or gases from a body part

Body Part Character 4	Approach Character 5	Device Character 6	Qualifier Character 7
Ø Head and Neck Tendon	**Ø** Open	**Ø** Drainage Device	**Z** No Qualifier
1 Shoulder Tendon, Right	**3** Percutaneous		
2 Shoulder Tendon, Left	**4** Percutaneous Endoscopic		
3 Upper Arm Tendon, Right			
4 Upper Arm Tendon, Left			
5 Lower Arm and Wrist Tendon, Right			
6 Lower Arm and Wrist Tendon, Left			
7 Hand Tendon, Right			
8 Hand Tendon, Left			
9 Trunk Tendon, Right			
B Trunk Tendon, Left			
C Thorax Tendon, Right			
D Thorax Tendon, Left			
F Abdomen Tendon, Right			
G Abdomen Tendon, Left			
H Perineum Tendon			
J Hip Tendon, Right			
K Hip Tendon, Left			
L Upper Leg Tendon, Right			
M Upper Leg Tendon, Left			
N Lower Leg Tendon, Right			
P Lower Leg Tendon, Left			
Q Knee Tendon, Right			
R Knee Tendon, Left			
S Ankle Tendon, Right			
T Ankle Tendon, Left			
V Foot Tendon, Right			
W Foot Tendon, Left			

ØL9 Continued on next page

LC Limited Coverage　　**NC** Noncovered　　HAC associated procedure　　Combination Only　　DRG Non-OR　　Non-OR　　Revised Text in **GREEN**

298　　　　　　　　　　　　　　　　　　　　　　　　　　　　　　　　　ICD-10-PCS 2014 (Draft)

Ø   Medical and Surgical
L   Tendons
9   Drainage   Taking or letting out fluids and/or gases from a body part

Body Part Character 4	Approach Character 5	Device Character 6	Qualifier Character 7
Ø Head and Neck Tendon	Ø Open	Z No Device	X Diagnostic
1 Shoulder Tendon, Right	3 Percutaneous		Z No Qualifier
2 Shoulder Tendon, Left	4 Percutaneous Endoscopic		
3 Upper Arm Tendon, Right			
4 Upper Arm Tendon, Left			
5 Lower Arm and Wrist Tendon, Right			
6 Lower Arm and Wrist Tendon, Left			
7 Hand Tendon, Right			
8 Hand Tendon, Left			
9 Trunk Tendon, Right			
B Trunk Tendon, Left			
C Thorax Tendon, Right			
D Thorax Tendon, Left			
F Abdomen Tendon, Right			
G Abdomen Tendon, Left			
H Perineum Tendon			
J Hip Tendon, Right			
K Hip Tendon, Left			
L Upper Leg Tendon, Right			
M Upper Leg Tendon, Left			
N Lower Leg Tendon, Right			
P Lower Leg Tendon, Left			
Q Knee Tendon, Right			
R Knee Tendon, Left			
S Ankle Tendon, Right			
T Ankle Tendon, Left			
V Foot Tendon, Right			
W Foot Tendon, Left			

Non-OR   ØL9[7,8][3,4]ZZ

Ø   Medical and Surgical
L   Tendons
B   Excision   Cutting out or off, without replacement, a portion of a body part

Body Part Character 4	Approach Character 5	Device Character 6	Qualifier Character 7
Ø Head and Neck Tendon	Ø Open	Z No Device	X Diagnostic
1 Shoulder Tendon, Right	3 Percutaneous		Z No Qualifier
2 Shoulder Tendon, Left	4 Percutaneous Endoscopic		
3 Upper Arm Tendon, Right			
4 Upper Arm Tendon, Left			
5 Lower Arm and Wrist Tendon, Right			
6 Lower Arm and Wrist Tendon, Left			
7 Hand Tendon, Right			
8 Hand Tendon, Left			
9 Trunk Tendon, Right			
B Trunk Tendon, Left			
C Thorax Tendon, Right			
D Thorax Tendon, Left			
F Abdomen Tendon, Right			
G Abdomen Tendon, Left			
H Perineum Tendon			
J Hip Tendon, Right			
K Hip Tendon, Left			
L Upper Leg Tendon, Right			
M Upper Leg Tendon, Left			
N Lower Leg Tendon, Right			
P Lower Leg Tendon, Left			
Q Knee Tendon, Right			
R Knee Tendon, Left			
S Ankle Tendon, Right			
T Ankle Tendon, Left			
V Foot Tendon, Right			
W Foot Tendon, Left			

ØL9—ØLB

LC Limited Coverage   **NC** Noncovered   HAC associated procedure   Combination Only   DRG Non-OR   Non-OR   Revised Text in **GREEN**

ICD-10-PCS 2014 (Draft)   **299**

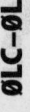

Ø   **Medical and Surgical**
L   **Tendons**
C   **Extirpation**   Taking or cutting out solid matter from a body part

Body Part Character 4	Approach Character 5	Device Character 6	Qualifier Character 7
Ø Head and Neck Tendon **1** Shoulder Tendon, Right **2** Shoulder Tendon, Left **3** Upper Arm Tendon, Right **4** Upper Arm Tendon, Left **5** Lower Arm and Wrist Tendon, Right **6** Lower Arm and Wrist Tendon, Left **7** Hand Tendon, Right **8** Hand Tendon, Left **9** Trunk Tendon, Right **B** Trunk Tendon, Left **C** Thorax Tendon, Right **D** Thorax Tendon, Left **F** Abdomen Tendon, Right **G** Abdomen Tendon, Left **H** Perineum Tendon **J** Hip Tendon, Right **K** Hip Tendon, Left **L** Upper Leg Tendon, Right **M** Upper Leg Tendon, Left **N** Lower Leg Tendon, Right **P** Lower Leg Tendon, Left **Q** Knee Tendon, Right **R** Knee Tendon, Left **S** Ankle Tendon, Right **T** Ankle Tendon, Left **V** Foot Tendon, Right **W** Foot Tendon, Left	**Ø** Open **3** Percutaneous **4** Percutaneous Endoscopic	**Z** No Device	**Z** No Qualifier

Ø   **Medical and Surgical**
L   **Tendons**
J   **Inspection**   Visually and/or manually exploring a body part

Body Part Character 4	Approach Character 5	Device Character 6	Qualifier Character 7
X Upper Tendon **Y** Lower Tendon	**Ø** Open **3** Percutaneous **4** Percutaneous Endoscopic **X** External	**Z** No Device	**Z** No Qualifier

Non-OR   ØLJ[X,Y]XZZ

LC Limited Coverage   **NC** Noncovered   HAC associated procedure   Combination Only   DRG Non-OR   Non-OR   Revised Text in **GREEN**

300   ICD-10-PCS 2014 (Draft)

Ø   **Medical and Surgical**
L   **Tendons**
M   **Reattachment**   Putting back in or on all or a portion of a separated body part to its normal location or other suitable location

Body Part Character 4	Approach Character 5	Device Character 6	Qualifier Character 7
Ø Head and Neck Tendon **1** Shoulder Tendon, Right **2** Shoulder Tendon, Left **3** Upper Arm Tendon, Right **4** Upper Arm Tendon, Left **5** Lower Arm and Wrist Tendon, Right **6** Lower Arm and Wrist Tendon, Left **7** Hand Tendon, Right **8** Hand Tendon, Left **9** Trunk Tendon, Right **B** Trunk Tendon, Left **C** Thorax Tendon, Right **D** Thorax Tendon, Left **F** Abdomen Tendon, Right **G** Abdomen Tendon, Left **H** Perineum Tendon **J** Hip Tendon, Right **K** Hip Tendon, Left **L** Upper Leg Tendon, Right **M** Upper Leg Tendon, Left **N** Lower Leg Tendon, Right **P** Lower Leg Tendon, Left **Q** Knee Tendon, Right **R** Knee Tendon, Left **S** Ankle Tendon, Right **T** Ankle Tendon, Left **V** Foot Tendon, Right **W** Foot Tendon, Left	**Ø** Open **4** Percutaneous Endoscopic	**Z** No Device	**Z** No Qualifier

Ø   **Medical and Surgical**
L   **Tendons**
N   **Release**   Freeing a body part from an abnormal physical constraint

Body Part Character 4	Approach Character 5	Device Character 6	Qualifier Character 7
Ø Head and Neck Tendon **1** Shoulder Tendon, Right **2** Shoulder Tendon, Left **3** Upper Arm Tendon, Right **4** Upper Arm Tendon, Left **5** Lower Arm and Wrist Tendon, Right **6** Lower Arm and Wrist Tendon, Left **7** Hand Tendon, Right **8** Hand Tendon, Left **9** Trunk Tendon, Right **B** Trunk Tendon, Left **C** Thorax Tendon, Right **D** Thorax Tendon, Left **F** Abdomen Tendon, Right **G** Abdomen Tendon, Left **H** Perineum Tendon **J** Hip Tendon, Right **K** Hip Tendon, Left **L** Upper Leg Tendon, Right **M** Upper Leg Tendon, Left **N** Lower Leg Tendon, Right **P** Lower Leg Tendon, Left **Q** Knee Tendon, Right **R** Knee Tendon, Left **S** Ankle Tendon, Right **T** Ankle Tendon, Left **V** Foot Tendon, Right **W** Foot Tendon, Left	**Ø** Open **3** Percutaneous **4** Percutaneous Endoscopic **X** External	**Z** No Device	**Z** No Qualifier

Non-OR   ØLN[Ø,1,2,3,4,5,6,7,8,9,B,C,D,F,G,H,J,K,L,M,N,P,Q,R,S,T,V,W]XZZ

ØLM–ØLN

LC Limited Coverage   **NC** Noncovered   HAC associated procedure   Combination Only   DRG Non-OR   Non-OR   Revised Text in **GREEN**

ICD-1Ø-PCS 2Ø14 (Draft)   **301**

Ø Medical and Surgical
L Tendons
P Removal   Taking out or off a device from a body part

Body Part Character 4	Approach Character 5	Device Character 6	Qualifier Character 7
X Upper Tendon **Y** Lower Tendon	**Ø** Open **3** Percutaneous **4** Percutaneous Endoscopic	**Ø** Drainage Device **7** Autologous Tissue Substitute **J** Synthetic Substitute **K** Nonautologous Tissue Substitute	**Z** No Qualifier
X Upper Tendon **Y** Lower Tendon	**X** External	**Ø** Drainage Device	**Z** No Qualifier

Non-OR   ØLP[X,Y]XØZ

Ø Medical and Surgical
L Tendons
Q Repair   Restoring, to the extent possible, a body part to its normal anatomic structure and function

Body Part Character 4	Approach Character 5	Device Character 6	Qualifier Character 7
Ø Head and Neck Tendon **1** Shoulder Tendon, Right **2** Shoulder Tendon, Left **3** Upper Arm Tendon, Right **4** Upper Arm Tendon, Left **5** Lower Arm and Wrist Tendon, Right **6** Lower Arm and Wrist Tendon, Left **7** Hand Tendon, Right **8** Hand Tendon, Left **9** Trunk Tendon, Right **B** Trunk Tendon, Left **C** Thorax Tendon, Right **D** Thorax Tendon, Left **F** Abdomen Tendon, Right **G** Abdomen Tendon, Left **H** Perineum Tendon **J** Hip Tendon, Right **K** Hip Tendon, Left **L** Upper Leg Tendon, Right **M** Upper Leg Tendon, Left **N** Lower Leg Tendon, Right **P** Lower Leg Tendon, Left **Q** Knee Tendon, Right **R** Knee Tendon, Left **S** Ankle Tendon, Right **T** Ankle Tendon, Left **V** Foot Tendon, Right **W** Foot Tendon, Left	**Ø** Open **3** Percutaneous **4** Percutaneous Endoscopic	**Z** No Device	**Z** No Qualifier

LC Limited Coverage   **NC** Noncovered   HAC associated procedure   Combination Only   DRG Non-OR   Non-OR   Revised Text in **GREEN**

302   ICD-10-PCS 2014 (Draft)

Ø   Medical and Surgical
L   Tendons
R   Replacement   Putting in or on biological or synthetic material that physically takes the place and/or function of all or a portion of a body part

Body Part Character 4	Approach Character 5	Device Character 6	Qualifier Character 7
Ø Head and Neck Tendon	Ø Open	7 Autologous Tissue Substitute	Z No Qualifier
1 Shoulder Tendon, Right	4 Percutaneous Endoscopic	J Synthetic Substitute	
2 Shoulder Tendon, Left		K Nonautologous Tissue Substitute	
3 Upper Arm Tendon, Right			
4 Upper Arm Tendon, Left			
5 Lower Arm and Wrist Tendon, Right			
6 Lower Arm and Wrist Tendon, Left			
7 Hand Tendon, Right			
8 Hand Tendon, Left			
9 Trunk Tendon, Right			
B Trunk Tendon, Left			
C Thorax Tendon, Right			
D Thorax Tendon, Left			
F Abdomen Tendon, Right			
G Abdomen Tendon, Left			
H Perineum Tendon			
J Hip Tendon, Right			
K Hip Tendon, Left			
L Upper Leg Tendon, Right			
M Upper Leg Tendon, Left			
N Lower Leg Tendon, Right			
P Lower Leg Tendon, Left			
Q Knee Tendon, Right			
R Knee Tendon, Left			
S Ankle Tendon, Right			
T Ankle Tendon, Left			
V Foot Tendon, Right			
W Foot Tendon, Left			

Ø   Medical and Surgical
L   Tendons
S   Reposition   Moving to its normal location or other suitable location all or a portion of a body part

Body Part Character 4	Approach Character 5	Device Character 6	Qualifier Character 7
Ø Head and Neck Tendon	Ø Open	Z No Device	Z No Qualifier
1 Shoulder Tendon, Right	4 Percutaneous Endoscopic		
2 Shoulder Tendon, Left			
3 Upper Arm Tendon, Right			
4 Upper Arm Tendon, Left			
5 Lower Arm and Wrist Tendon, Right			
6 Lower Arm and Wrist Tendon, Left			
7 Hand Tendon, Right			
8 Hand Tendon, Left			
9 Trunk Tendon, Right			
B Trunk Tendon, Left			
C Thorax Tendon, Right			
D Thorax Tendon, Left			
F Abdomen Tendon, Right			
G Abdomen Tendon, Left			
H Perineum Tendon			
J Hip Tendon, Right			
K Hip Tendon, Left			
L Upper Leg Tendon, Right			
M Upper Leg Tendon, Left			
N Lower Leg Tendon, Right			
P Lower Leg Tendon, Left			
Q Knee Tendon, Right			
R Knee Tendon, Left			
S Ankle Tendon, Right			
T Ankle Tendon, Left			
V Foot Tendon, Right			
W Foot Tendon, Left			

Ø Medical and Surgical
L Tendons
T Resection Cutting out or off, without replacement, all of a body part

Body Part Character 4	Approach Character 5	Device Character 6	Qualifier Character 7
Ø Head and Neck Tendon	Ø Open	Z No Device	Z No Qualifier
1 Shoulder Tendon, Right	4 Percutaneous Endoscopic		
2 Shoulder Tendon, Left			
3 Upper Arm Tendon, Right			
4 Upper Arm Tendon, Left			
5 Lower Arm and Wrist Tendon, Right			
6 Lower Arm and Wrist Tendon, Left			
7 Hand Tendon, Right			
8 Hand Tendon, Left			
9 Trunk Tendon, Right			
B Trunk Tendon, Left			
C Thorax Tendon, Right			
D Thorax Tendon, Left			
F Abdomen Tendon, Right			
G Abdomen Tendon, Left			
H Perineum Tendon			
J Hip Tendon, Right			
K Hip Tendon, Left			
L Upper Leg Tendon, Right			
M Upper Leg Tendon, Left			
N Lower Leg Tendon, Right			
P Lower Leg Tendon, Left			
Q Knee Tendon, Right			
R Knee Tendon, Left			
S Ankle Tendon, Right			
T Ankle Tendon, Left			
V Foot Tendon, Right			
W Foot Tendon, Left			

Ø Medical and Surgical
L Tendons
U Supplement Putting in or on biological or synthetic material that physically reinforces and/or augments the function of a portion of a body part

Body Part Character 4	Approach Character 5	Device Character 6	Qualifier Character 7
Ø Head and Neck Tendon	Ø Open	7 Autologous Tissue Substitute	Z No Qualifier
1 Shoulder Tendon, Right	4 Percutaneous Endoscopic	J Synthetic Substitute	
2 Shoulder Tendon, Left		K Nonautologous Tissue Substitute	
3 Upper Arm Tendon, Right			
4 Upper Arm Tendon, Left			
5 Lower Arm and Wrist Tendon, Right			
6 Lower Arm and Wrist Tendon, Left			
7 Hand Tendon, Right			
8 Hand Tendon, Left			
9 Trunk Tendon, Right			
B Trunk Tendon, Left			
C Thorax Tendon, Right			
D Thorax Tendon, Left			
F Abdomen Tendon, Right			
G Abdomen Tendon, Left			
H Perineum Tendon			
J Hip Tendon, Right			
K Hip Tendon, Left			
L Upper Leg Tendon, Right			
M Upper Leg Tendon, Left			
N Lower Leg Tendon, Right			
P Lower Leg Tendon, Left			
Q Knee Tendon, Right			
R Knee Tendon, Left			
S Ankle Tendon, Right			
T Ankle Tendon, Left			
V Foot Tendon, Right			
W Foot Tendon, Left			

Ø **Medical and Surgical**
L **Tendons**
W **Revision**   Correcting, to the extent possible, a portion of a malfunctioning device or the position of a displaced device

Body Part Character 4	Approach Character 5	Device Character 6	Qualifier Character 7
X Upper Tendon **Y** Lower Tendon	**Ø** Open **3** Percutaneous **4** Percutaneous Endoscopic **X** External	**Ø** Drainage Device **7** Autologous Tissue Substitute **J** Synthetic Substitute **K** Nonautologous Tissue Substitute	**Z** No Qualifier

Non-OR   ØLW[X,Y]X[Ø,7,J,K]Z

Ø **Medical and Surgical**
L **Tendons**
X **Transfer**   Moving, without taking out, all or a portion of a body part to another location to take over the function of all or a portion of a body part

Body Part Character 4	Approach Character 5	Device Character 6	Qualifier Character 7
Ø Head and Neck Tendon **1** Shoulder Tendon, Right **2** Shoulder Tendon, Left **3** Upper Arm Tendon, Right **4** Upper Arm Tendon, Left **5** Lower Arm and Wrist Tendon, Right **6** Lower Arm and Wrist Tendon, Left **7** Hand Tendon, Right **8** Hand Tendon, Left **9** Trunk Tendon, Right **B** Trunk Tendon, Left **C** Thorax Tendon, Right **D** Thorax Tendon, Left **F** Abdomen Tendon, Right **G** Abdomen Tendon, Left **H** Perineum Tendon **J** Hip Tendon, Right **K** Hip Tendon, Left **L** Upper Leg Tendon, Right **M** Upper Leg Tendon, Left **N** Lower Leg Tendon, Right **P** Lower Leg Tendon, Left **Q** Knee Tendon, Right **R** Knee Tendon, Left **S** Ankle Tendon, Right **T** Ankle Tendon, Left **V** Foot Tendon, Right **W** Foot Tendon, Left	**Ø** Open **4** Percutaneous Endoscopic	**Z** No Device	**Z** No Qualifier

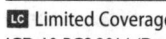

Bursae and Ligaments ØM2–ØMX

Ø   Medical and Surgical
M   Bursae and Ligaments
2   Change   Taking out or off a device from a body part and putting back an identical or similar device in or on the same body part without cutting or puncturing the skin or a mucous membrane

Body Part Character 4	Approach Character 5	Device Character 6	Qualifier Character 7
X Upper Bursa and Ligament **Y** Lower Bursa and Ligament	**X** External	**Ø** Drainage Device **Y** Other Device	**Z** No Qualifier

Non-OR   For all body part, approach, device, and qualifier values

Ø   Medical and Surgical
M   Bursae and Ligaments
5   Destruction   Physical eradication of all or a portion of a body part by the direct use of energy, force, or a destructive agent

Body Part Character 4	Approach Character 5	Device Character 6	Qualifier Character 7
Ø Head and Neck Bursa and Ligament **1** Shoulder Bursa and Ligament, Right **2** Shoulder Bursa and Ligament, Left **3** Elbow Bursa and Ligament, Right **4** Elbow Bursa and Ligament, Left **5** Wrist Bursa and Ligament, Right **6** Wrist Bursa and Ligament, Left **7** Hand Bursa and Ligament, Right **8** Hand Bursa and Ligament, Left **9** Upper Extremity Bursa and Ligament, Right **B** Upper Extremity Bursa and Ligament, Left **C** Trunk Bursa and Ligament, Right **D** Trunk Bursa and Ligament, Left **F** Thorax Bursa and Ligament, Right **G** Thorax Bursa and Ligament, Left **H** Abdomen Bursa and Ligament, Right **J** Abdomen Bursa and Ligament, Left **K** Perineum Bursa and Ligament **L** Hip Bursa and Ligament, Right **M** Hip Bursa and Ligament, Left **N** Knee Bursa and Ligament, Right **P** Knee Bursa and Ligament, Left **Q** Ankle Bursa and Ligament, Right **R** Ankle Bursa and Ligament, Left **S** Foot Bursa and Ligament, Right **T** Foot Bursa and Ligament, Left **V** Lower Extremity Bursa and Ligament, Right **W** Lower Extremity Bursa and Ligament, Left	**Ø** Open **3** Percutaneous **4** Percutaneous Endoscopic	**Z** No Device	**Z** No Qualifier

LC Limited Coverage   **NC** Noncovered   HAC associated procedure   Combination Only   DRG Non-OR   Non-OR   Revised Text in **GREEN**

306   ICD-10-PCS 2014 (Draft)

Ø   **Medical and Surgical**
M   **Bursae and Ligaments**
8   **Division**   Cutting into a body part without draining fluids and/or gases from the body part in order to separate or transect a body part

Body Part Character 4	Approach Character 5	Device Character 6	Qualifier Character 7
Ø Head and Neck Bursa and Ligament	**Ø** Open	**Z** No Device	**Z** No Qualifier
1 Shoulder Bursa and Ligament, Right	**3** Percutaneous		
2 Shoulder Bursa and Ligament, Left	**4** Percutaneous Endoscopic		
3 Elbow Bursa and Ligament, Right			
4 Elbow Bursa and Ligament, Left			
5 Wrist Bursa and Ligament, Right			
6 Wrist Bursa and Ligament, Left			
7 Hand Bursa and Ligament, Right			
8 Hand Bursa and Ligament, Left			
9 Upper Extremity Bursa and Ligament, Right			
B Upper Extremity Bursa and Ligament, Left			
C Trunk Bursa and Ligament, Right			
D Trunk Bursa and Ligament, Left			
F Thorax Bursa and Ligament, Right			
G Thorax Bursa and Ligament, Left			
H Abdomen Bursa and Ligament, Right			
J Abdomen Bursa and Ligament, Left			
K Perineum Bursa and Ligament			
L Hip Bursa and Ligament, Right			
M Hip Bursa and Ligament, Left			
N Knee Bursa and Ligament, Right			
P Knee Bursa and Ligament, Left			
Q Ankle Bursa and Ligament, Right			
R Ankle Bursa and Ligament, Left			
S Foot Bursa and Ligament, Right			
T Foot Bursa and Ligament, Left			
V Lower Extremity Bursa and Ligament, Right			
W Lower Extremity Bursa and Ligament, Left			

Non-OR   ØM8[5,6][Ø,3,4]ZZ

Ø   **Medical and Surgical**
M   **Bursae and Ligaments**
9   **Drainage**   Taking or letting out fluids and/or gases from a body part

Body Part Character 4	Approach Character 5	Device Character 6	Qualifier Character 7
Ø Head and Neck Bursa and Ligament	**Ø** Open	**Ø** Drainage Device	**Z** No Qualifier
1 Shoulder Bursa and Ligament, Right	**3** Percutaneous		
2 Shoulder Bursa and Ligament, Left	**4** Percutaneous Endoscopic		
3 Elbow Bursa and Ligament, Right			
4 Elbow Bursa and Ligament, Left			
5 Wrist Bursa and Ligament, Right			
6 Wrist Bursa and Ligament, Left			
7 Hand Bursa and Ligament, Right			
8 Hand Bursa and Ligament, Left			
9 Upper Extremity Bursa and Ligament, Right			
B Upper Extremity Bursa and Ligament, Left			
C Trunk Bursa and Ligament, Right			
D Trunk Bursa and Ligament, Left			
F Thorax Bursa and Ligament, Right			
G Thorax Bursa and Ligament, Left			
H Abdomen Bursa and Ligament, Right			
J Abdomen Bursa and Ligament, Left			
K Perineum Bursa and Ligament			
L Hip Bursa and Ligament, Right			
M Hip Bursa and Ligament, Left			
N Knee Bursa and Ligament, Right			
P Knee Bursa and Ligament, Left			
Q Ankle Bursa and Ligament, Right			
R Ankle Bursa and Ligament, Left			
S Foot Bursa and Ligament, Right			
T Foot Bursa and Ligament, Left			
V Lower Extremity Bursa and Ligament, Right			
W Lower Extremity Bursa and Ligament, Left			

ØM9 Continued on next page

Non-OR   ØM9[1,2,3,4,7,8,9,B,C,D,F,G,H,J,K,L,M,V,W][3,4]ØZ

LC Limited Coverage   **NC** Noncovered   HAC associated procedure   Combination Only   DRG Non-OR   Non-OR   Revised Text in **GREEN**

Ø   Medical and Surgical
M   Bursae and Ligaments
9   Drainage   Taking or letting out fluids and/or gases from a body part

ØM9 Continued

Body Part Character 4	Approach Character 5	Device Character 6	Qualifier Character 7
Ø Head and Neck Bursa and Ligament	**Ø** Open	**Z** No Device	**X** Diagnostic
1 Shoulder Bursa and Ligament, Right	**3** Percutaneous		**Z** No Qualifier
2 Shoulder Bursa and Ligament, Left	**4** Percutaneous Endoscopic		
3 Elbow Bursa and Ligament, Right			
4 Elbow Bursa and Ligament, Left			
5 Wrist Bursa and Ligament, Right			
6 Wrist Bursa and Ligament, Left			
7 Hand Bursa and Ligament, Right			
8 Hand Bursa and Ligament, Left			
9 Upper Extremity Bursa and Ligament, Right			
B Upper Extremity Bursa and Ligament, Left			
C Trunk Bursa and Ligament, Right			
D Trunk Bursa and Ligament, Left			
F Thorax Bursa and Ligament, Right			
G Thorax Bursa and Ligament, Left			
H Abdomen Bursa and Ligament, Right			
J Abdomen Bursa and Ligament, Left			
K Perineum Bursa and Ligament			
L Hip Bursa and Ligament, Right			
M Hip Bursa and Ligament, Left			
N Knee Bursa and Ligament, Right			
P Knee Bursa and Ligament, Left			
Q Ankle Bursa and Ligament, Right			
R Ankle Bursa and Ligament, Left			
S Foot Bursa and Ligament, Right			
T Foot Bursa and Ligament, Left			
V Lower Extremity Bursa and Ligament, Right			
W Lower Extremity Bursa and Ligament, Left			

Non-OR ØM9[Ø,1,2,3,4,5,6,7,8,C,D,F,G,L,M,N,P,Q,R,S,T][Ø,3,4]ZX   **Non-OR** ØM9[1,2,3,4,7,8,9,B,C,D,F,G,H,J,K,L,M,V,W][3,4]ØZ
Non-OR ØM9[Ø,5,6,7,8,9,B,C,D,F,G,H,J,K,N,P,Q,R,S,T,V,W][Ø,3,4]ZZ   **Non-OR** ØM9[1,2,3,4,L,M]3ZZ

Ø   Medical and Surgical
M   Bursae and Ligaments
B   Excision   Cutting out or off, without replacement, a portion of a body part

Body Part Character 4	Approach Character 5	Device Character 6	Qualifier Character 7
Ø Head and Neck Bursa and Ligament	**Ø** Open	**Z** No Device	**X** Diagnostic
1 Shoulder Bursa and Ligament, Right	**3** Percutaneous		**Z** No Qualifier
2 Shoulder Bursa and Ligament, Left	**4** Percutaneous Endoscopic		
3 Elbow Bursa and Ligament, Right			
4 Elbow Bursa and Ligament, Left			
5 Wrist Bursa and Ligament, Right			
6 Wrist Bursa and Ligament, Left			
7 Hand Bursa and Ligament, Right			
8 Hand Bursa and Ligament, Left			
9 Upper Extremity Bursa and Ligament, Right			
B Upper Extremity Bursa and Ligament, Left			
C Trunk Bursa and Ligament, Right			
D Trunk Bursa and Ligament, Left			
F Thorax Bursa and Ligament, Right			
G Thorax Bursa and Ligament, Left			
H Abdomen Bursa and Ligament, Right			
J Abdomen Bursa and Ligament, Left			
K Perineum Bursa and Ligament			
L Hip Bursa and Ligament, Right			
M Hip Bursa and Ligament, Left			
N Knee Bursa and Ligament, Right			
P Knee Bursa and Ligament, Left			
Q Ankle Bursa and Ligament, Right			
R Ankle Bursa and Ligament, Left			
S Foot Bursa and Ligament, Right			
T Foot Bursa and Ligament, Left			
V Lower Extremity Bursa and Ligament, Right			
W Lower Extremity Bursa and Ligament, Left			

Non-OR ØMB[Ø,1,2,3,4,5,6,7,8,B,C,D,F,G,L,M,N,P,Q,R,S,T][Ø,3,4]ZX   **Non-OR** ØMB94ZX

LC Limited Coverage   NC Noncovered   HAC associated procedure   Combination Only   DRG Non-OR   Non-OR   Revised Text in **GREEN**

0　**Medical and Surgical**
M　**Bursae and Ligaments**
C　**Extirpation**　　Taking or cutting out solid matter from a body part

Body Part Character 4	Approach Character 5	Device Character 6	Qualifier Character 7
0　Head and Neck Bursa and Ligament	0　Open	Z　No Device	Z　No Qualifier
1　Shoulder Bursa and Ligament, Right	3　Percutaneous		
2　Shoulder Bursa and Ligament, Left	4　Percutaneous Endoscopic		
3　Elbow Bursa and Ligament, Right			
4　Elbow Bursa and Ligament, Left			
5　Wrist Bursa and Ligament, Right			
6　Wrist Bursa and Ligament, Left			
7　Hand Bursa and Ligament, Right			
8　Hand Bursa and Ligament, Left			
9　Upper Extremity Bursa and Ligament, Right			
B　Upper Extremity Bursa and Ligament, Left			
C　Trunk Bursa and Ligament, Right			
D　Trunk Bursa and Ligament, Left			
F　Thorax Bursa and Ligament, Right			
G　Thorax Bursa and Ligament, Left			
H　Abdomen Bursa and Ligament, Right			
J　Abdomen Bursa and Ligament, Left			
K　Perineum Bursa and Ligament			
L　Hip Bursa and Ligament, Right			
M　Hip Bursa and Ligament, Left			
N　Knee Bursa and Ligament, Right			
P　Knee Bursa and Ligament, Left			
Q　Ankle Bursa and Ligament, Right			
R　Ankle Bursa and Ligament, Left			
S　Foot Bursa and Ligament, Right			
T　Foot Bursa and Ligament, Left			
V　Lower Extremity Bursa and Ligament, Right			
W　Lower Extremity Bursa and Ligament, Left			

0　**Medical and Surgical**
M　**Bursae and Ligaments**
D　**Extraction**　　Pulling or stripping out or off all or a portion of a body part by the use of force

Body Part Character 4	Approach Character 5	Device Character 6	Qualifier Character 7
0　Head and Neck Bursa and Ligament	0　Open	Z　No Device	Z　No Qualifier
1　Shoulder Bursa and Ligament, Right	3　Percutaneous		
2　Shoulder Bursa and Ligament, Left	4　Percutaneous Endoscopic		
3　Elbow Bursa and Ligament, Right			
4　Elbow Bursa and Ligament, Left			
5　Wrist Bursa and Ligament, Right			
6　Wrist Bursa and Ligament, Left			
7　Hand Bursa and Ligament, Right			
8　Hand Bursa and Ligament, Left			
9　Upper Extremity Bursa and Ligament, Right			
B　Upper Extremity Bursa and Ligament, Left			
C　Trunk Bursa and Ligament, Right			
D　Trunk Bursa and Ligament, Left			
F　Thorax Bursa and Ligament, Right			
G　Thorax Bursa and Ligament, Left			
H　Abdomen Bursa and Ligament, Right			
J　Abdomen Bursa and Ligament, Left			
K　Perineum Bursa and Ligament			
L　Hip Bursa and Ligament, Right			
M　Hip Bursa and Ligament, Left			
N　Knee Bursa and Ligament, Right			
P　Knee Bursa and Ligament, Left			
Q　Ankle Bursa and Ligament, Right			
R　Ankle Bursa and Ligament, Left			
S　Foot Bursa and Ligament, Right			
T　Foot Bursa and Ligament, Left			
V　Lower Extremity Bursa and Ligament, Right			
W　Lower Extremity Bursa and Ligament, Left			

Bursae and Ligaments

ØMJ–ØMM

Ø   **Medical and Surgical**
M   **Bursae and Ligaments**
J   **Inspection**   Visually and/or manually exploring a body part

Body Part Character 4	Approach Character 5	Device Character 6	Qualifier Character 7
X Upper Bursa and Ligament **Y** Lower Bursa and Ligament	**Ø** Open **3** Percutaneous **4** Percutaneous Endoscopic **X** External	**Z** No Device	**Z** No Qualifier

Non-OR   ØMJ[X,Y]XZZ

Ø   **Medical and Surgical**
M   **Bursae and Ligaments**
M   **Reattachment**   Putting back in or on all or a portion of a separated body part to its normal location or other suitable location

Body Part Character 4	Approach Character 5	Device Character 6	Qualifier Character 7
Ø Head and Neck Bursa and Ligament **1** Shoulder Bursa and Ligament, Rightv **2** Shoulder Bursa and Ligament, Left **3** Elbow Bursa and Ligament, Right **4** Elbow Bursa and Ligament, Left **5** Wrist Bursa and Ligament, Right **6** Wrist Bursa and Ligament, Left **7** Hand Bursa and Ligament, Right **8** Hand Bursa and Ligament, Left **9** Upper Extremity Bursa and Ligament, Right **B** Upper Extremity Bursa and Ligament, Left **C** Trunk Bursa and Ligament, Right **D** Trunk Bursa and Ligament, Left **F** Thorax Bursa and Ligament, Right **G** Thorax Bursa and Ligament, Left **H** Abdomen Bursa and Ligament, Right **J** Abdomen Bursa and Ligament, Left **K** Perineum Bursa and Ligament **L** Hip Bursa and Ligament, Right **M** Hip Bursa and Ligament, Left **N** Knee Bursa and Ligament, Right **P** Knee Bursa and Ligament, Left **Q** Ankle Bursa and Ligament, Right **R** Ankle Bursa and Ligament, Left **S** Foot Bursa and Ligament, Right **T** Foot Bursa and Ligament, Left **V** Lower Extremity Bursa and Ligament, Right **W** Lower Extremity Bursa and Ligament, Left	**Ø** Open **4** Percutaneous Endoscopic	**Z** No Device	**Z** No Qualifier

LC Limited Coverage   **NC** Noncovered   HAC associated procedure   Combination Only   DRG Non-OR   Non-OR   Revised Text in **GREEN**

310   ICD-10-PCS 2014 (Draft)

Ø   **Medical and Surgical**
M   **Bursae and Ligaments**
N   **Release**   Freeing a body part from an abnormal physical constraint

Body Part Character 4	Approach Character 5	Device Character 6	Qualifier Character 7

Ø Head and Neck Bursa and Ligament
1 Shoulder Bursa and Ligament, Right
2 Shoulder Bursa and Ligament, Left
3 Elbow Bursa and Ligament, Right
4 Elbow Bursa and Ligament, Left
5 Wrist Bursa and Ligament, Right
6 Wrist Bursa and Ligament, Left
7 Hand Bursa and Ligament, Right
8 Hand Bursa and Ligament, Left
9 Upper Extremity Bursa and Ligament,
    Right
B Upper Extremity Bursa and Ligament, Left
C Trunk Bursa and Ligament, Right
D Trunk Bursa and Ligament, Left
F Thorax Bursa and Ligament, Right
G Thorax Bursa and Ligament, Left
H Abdomen Bursa and Ligament, Right
J Abdomen Bursa and Ligament, Left
K Perineum Bursa and Ligament
L Hip Bursa and Ligament, Right
M Hip Bursa and Ligament, Left
N Knee Bursa and Ligament, Right
P Knee Bursa and Ligament, Left
Q Ankle Bursa and Ligament, Right
R Ankle Bursa and Ligament, Left
S Foot Bursa and Ligament, Right
T Foot Bursa and Ligament, Left
V Lower Extremity Bursa and Ligament,
    Right
W Lower Extremity Bursa and Ligament, Left
	Ø Open
	3 Percutaneous
	4 Percutaneous Endoscopic
	X External
		Z No Device	**Z** No Qualifier

Ø   **Medical and Surgical**
M   **Bursae and Ligaments**
P   **Removal**   Taking out or off a device from a body part

Body Part Character 4	Approach Character 5	Device Character 6	Qualifier Character 7
X Upper Bursa and Ligament **Y** Lower Bursa and Ligament	**Ø** Open **3** Percutaneous **4** Percutaneous Endoscopic	**Ø** Drainage Device **7** Autologous Tissue Substitute **J** Synthetic Substitute **K** Nonautologous Tissue Substitute	**Z** No Qualifier
X Upper Bursa and Ligament **Y** Lower Bursa and Ligament	**X** External	**Ø** Drainage Device	**Z** No Qualifier

Non-OR   ØMP[X,Y]XØZ

LC Limited Coverage   **NC** Noncovered   HAC associated procedure   Combination Only   DRG Non-OR   Non-OR   Revised Text in **GREEN**

ICD-10-PCS 2014 (Draft)   **311**

Bursae and Ligaments

ØMQ–ØMS

Ø   **Medical and Surgical**
M   **Bursae and Ligaments**
Q   **Repair**   Restoring, to the extent possible, a body part to its normal anatomic structure and function

Body Part Character 4	Approach Character 5	Device Character 6	Qualifier Character 7
Ø Head and Neck Bursa and Ligament 1 Shoulder Bursa and Ligament, Right 2 Shoulder Bursa and Ligament, Left 3 Elbow Bursa and Ligament, Right 4 Elbow Bursa and Ligament, Left 5 Wrist Bursa and Ligament, Right 6 Wrist Bursa and Ligament, Left 7 Hand Bursa and Ligament, Right 8 Hand Bursa and Ligament, Left 9 Upper Extremity Bursa and Ligament, Right B Upper Extremity Bursa and Ligament, Left C Trunk Bursa and Ligament, Right D Trunk Bursa and Ligament, Left F Thorax Bursa and Ligament, Right G Thorax Bursa and Ligament, Left H Abdomen Bursa and Ligament, Right J Abdomen Bursa and Ligament, Left K Perineum Bursa and Ligament L Hip Bursa and Ligament, Right M Hip Bursa and Ligament, Left N Knee Bursa and Ligament, Right P Knee Bursa and Ligament, Left Q Ankle Bursa and Ligament, Right R Ankle Bursa and Ligament, Left S Foot Bursa and Ligament, Right T Foot Bursa and Ligament, Left V Lower Extremity Bursa and Ligament, Right W Lower Extremity Bursa and Ligament, Left	Ø Open 3 Percutaneous 4 Percutaneous Endoscopic	Z No Device	Z No Qualifier

Ø   **Medical and Surgical**
M   **Bursae and Ligaments**
S   **Reposition**   Moving to its normal location or other suitable location all or a portion of a body part

Body Part Character 4	Approach Character 5	Device Character 6	Qualifier Character 7
Ø Head and Neck Bursa and Ligament 1 Shoulder Bursa and Ligament, Right 2 Shoulder Bursa and Ligament, Left 3 Elbow Bursa and Ligament, Right 4 Elbow Bursa and Ligament, Left 5 Wrist Bursa and Ligament, Right 6 Wrist Bursa and Ligament, Left 7 Hand Bursa and Ligament, Right 8 Hand Bursa and Ligament, Left 9 Upper Extremity Bursa and Ligament, Right B Upper Extremity Bursa and Ligament, Left C Trunk Bursa and Ligament, Right D Trunk Bursa and Ligament, Left F Thorax Bursa and Ligament, Right G Thorax Bursa and Ligament, Left H Abdomen Bursa and Ligament, Right J Abdomen Bursa and Ligament, Left K Perineum Bursa and Ligament L Hip Bursa and Ligament, Right M Hip Bursa and Ligament, Left N Knee Bursa and Ligament, Right P Knee Bursa and Ligament, Left Q Ankle Bursa and Ligament, Right R Ankle Bursa and Ligament, Left S Foot Bursa and Ligament, Right T Foot Bursa and Ligament, Left V Lower Extremity Bursa and Ligament, Right W Lower Extremity Bursa and Ligament, Left	Ø Open 4 Percutaneous Endoscopic	Z No Device	Z No Qualifier

LC Limited Coverage   **NC** Noncovered   HAC associated procedure   Combination Only   DRG Non-OR   Non-OR   Revised Text in **GREEN**

312   ICD-10-PCS 2014 (Draft)

Ø   **Medical and Surgical**
M   **Bursae and Ligaments**
T   **Resection**   Cutting out or off, without replacement, all of a body part

Body Part Character 4	Approach Character 5	Device Character 6	Qualifier Character 7
Ø Head and Neck Bursa and Ligament **1** Shoulder Bursa and Ligament, Right **2** Shoulder Bursa and Ligament, Left **3** Elbow Bursa and Ligament, Right **4** Elbow Bursa and Ligament, Left **5** Wrist Bursa and Ligament, Right **6** Wrist Bursa and Ligament, Left **7** Hand Bursa and Ligament, Right **8** Hand Bursa and Ligament, Left **9** Upper Extremity Bursa and Ligament, Right **B** Upper Extremity Bursa and Ligament, Left **C** Trunk Bursa and Ligament, Right **D** Trunk Bursa and Ligament, Left **F** Thorax Bursa and Ligament, Right **G** Thorax Bursa and Ligament, Left **H** Abdomen Bursa and Ligament, Right **J** Abdomen Bursa and Ligament, Left **K** Perineum Bursa and Ligament **L** Hip Bursa and Ligament, Right **M** Hip Bursa and Ligament, Left **N** Knee Bursa and Ligament, Right **P** Knee Bursa and Ligament, Left **Q** Ankle Bursa and Ligament, Right **R** Ankle Bursa and Ligament, Left **S** Foot Bursa and Ligament, Right **T** Foot Bursa and Ligament, Left **V** Lower Extremity Bursa and Ligament, Right **W** Lower Extremity Bursa and Ligament, Left	**Ø** Open **4** Percutaneous Endoscopic	**Z** No Device	**Z** No Qualifier

Ø   **Medical and Surgical**
M   **Bursae and Ligaments**
U   **Supplement**   Putting in or on biological or synthetic material that physically reinforces and/or augments the function of a portion of a body part

Body Part Character 4	Approach Character 5	Device Character 6	Qualifier Character 7
Ø Head and Neck Bursa and Ligament **1** Shoulder Bursa and Ligament, Right **2** Shoulder Bursa and Ligament, Left **3** Elbow Bursa and Ligament, Right **4** Elbow Bursa and Ligament, Left **5** Wrist Bursa and Ligament, Right **6** Wrist Bursa and Ligament, Left **7** Hand Bursa and Ligament, Right **8** Hand Bursa and Ligament, Left **9** Upper Extremity Bursa and Ligament, Right **B** Upper Extremity Bursa and Ligament, Left **C** Trunk Bursa and Ligament, Right **D** Trunk Bursa and Ligament, Left **F** Thorax Bursa and Ligament, Right **G** Thorax Bursa and Ligament, Left **H** Abdomen Bursa and Ligament, Right **J** Abdomen Bursa and Ligament, Left **K** Perineum Bursa and Ligament **L** Hip Bursa and Ligament, Right **M** Hip Bursa and Ligament, Left **N** Knee Bursa and Ligament, Right **P** Knee Bursa and Ligament, Left **Q** Ankle Bursa and Ligament, Right **R** Ankle Bursa and Ligament, Left **S** Foot Bursa and Ligament, Right **T** Foot Bursa and Ligament, Left **V** Lower Extremity Bursa and Ligament, Right **W** Lower Extremity Bursa and Ligament, Left	**Ø** Open **4** Percutaneous Endoscopic	**7** Autologous Tissue Substitute **J** Synthetic Substitute **K** Nonautologous Tissue Substitute	**Z** No Qualifier

LC Limited Coverage   **NC** Noncovered   HAC associated procedure   Combination Only   DRG Non-OR   Non-OR   Revised Text in **GREEN**

ICD-10-PCS 2014 (Draft)   **313**

Bursae and Ligaments

ØMW–ØMX

Ø   Medical and Surgical
M   Bursae and Ligaments
W   Revision   Correcting, to the extent possible, a portion of a malfunctioning device or the position of a displaced device

Body Part Character 4	Approach Character 5	Device Character 6	Qualifier Character 7
X Upper Bursa and Ligament Y Lower Bursa and Ligament	Ø Open 3 Percutaneous 4 Percutaneous Endoscopic X External	Ø Drainage Device 7 Autologous Tissue Substitute J Synthetic Substitute K Nonautologous Tissue Substitute	Z No Qualifier

Non-OR   ØMW[X,Y]X[Ø,7,J,K]Z

Ø   Medical and Surgical
M   Bursae and Ligaments
X   Transfer   Moving, without taking out, all or a portion of a body part to another location to take over the function of all or a portion of a body part

Body Part Character 4	Approach Character 5	Device Character 6	Qualifier Character 7
Ø Head and Neck Bursa and Ligament 1 Shoulder Bursa and Ligament, Right 2 Shoulder Bursa and Ligament, Left 3 Elbow Bursa and Ligament, Right 4 Elbow Bursa and Ligament, Left 5 Wrist Bursa and Ligament, Right 6 Wrist Bursa and Ligament, Left 7 Hand Bursa and Ligament, Right 8 Hand Bursa and Ligament, Left 9 Upper Extremity Bursa and Ligament, Right B Upper Extremity Bursa and Ligament, Left C Trunk Bursa and Ligament, Right D Trunk Bursa and Ligament, Left F Thorax Bursa and Ligament, Right G Thorax Bursa and Ligament, Left H Abdomen Bursa and Ligament, Right J Abdomen Bursa and Ligament, Left K Perineum Bursa and Ligament L Hip Bursa and Ligament, Right M Hip Bursa and Ligament, Left N Knee Bursa and Ligament, Right P Knee Bursa and Ligament, Left Q Ankle Bursa and Ligament, Right R Ankle Bursa and Ligament, Left S Foot Bursa and Ligament, Right T Foot Bursa and Ligament, Left V Lower Extremity Bursa and Ligament, Right W Lower Extremity Bursa and Ligament, Left	Ø Open 4 Percutaneous Endoscopic	Z No Device	Z No Qualifier

Head and Facial Bones ØN2–ØNW

Ø **Medical and Surgical**
N **Head and Facial Bones**
2 **Change**   Taking out or off a device from a body part and putting back an identical or similar device in or on the same body part without cutting or puncturing the skin or a mucous membrane

Body Part Character 4	Approach Character 5	Device Character 6	Qualifier Character 7
Ø Skull B Nasal Bone W Facial Bone	X External	Ø Drainage Device Y Other Device	Z No Qualifier

Non-OR	For all body part, approach, device, and qualifier values

Ø **Medical and Surgical**
N **Head and Facial Bones**
5 **Destruction**   Physical eradication of all or a portion of a body part by the direct use of energy, force, or a destructive agent

Body Part Character 4	Approach Character 5	Device Character 6	Qualifier Character 7
Ø Skull 1 Frontal Bone, Right 2 Frontal Bone, Left 3 Parietal Bone, Right 4 Parietal Bone, Left 5 Temporal Bone, Right 6 Temporal Bone, Left 7 Occipital Bone, Right 8 Occipital Bone, Left B Nasal Bone C Sphenoid Bone, Right D Sphenoid Bone, Left F Ethmoid Bone, Right G Ethmoid Bone, Left H Lacrimal Bone, Right J Lacrimal Bone, Left K Palatine Bone, Right L Palatine Bone, Left M Zygomatic Bone, Right N Zygomatic Bone, Left P Orbit, Right Q Orbit, Left R Maxilla, Right S Maxilla, Left T Mandible, Right V Mandible, Left X Hyoid Bone	Ø Open 3 Percutaneous 4 Percutaneous Endoscopic	Z No Device	Z No Qualifier

Head and Facial Bones

Ø   Medical and Surgical
N   Head and Facial Bones
8   Division   Cutting into a body part without draining fluids and/or gases from the body part in order to separate or transect a body part

Body Part Character 4	Approach Character 5	Device Character 6	Qualifier Character 7
Ø Skull	**Ø** Open	**Z** No Device	**Z** No Qualifier
1 Frontal Bone, Right	**3** Percutaneous		
2 Frontal Bone, Left	**4** Percutaneous Endoscopic		
3 Parietal Bone, Right			
4 Parietal Bone, Left			
5 Temporal Bone, Right			
6 Temporal Bone, Left			
7 Occipital Bone, Right			
8 Occipital Bone, Left			
B Nasal Bone			
C Sphenoid Bone, Right			
D Sphenoid Bone, Left			
F Ethmoid Bone, Right			
G Ethmoid Bone, Left			
H Lacrimal Bone, Right			
J Lacrimal Bone, Left			
K Palatine Bone, Right			
L Palatine Bone, Left			
M Zygomatic Bone, Right			
N Zygomatic Bone, Left			
P Orbit, Right			
Q Orbit, Left			
R Maxilla, Right			
S Maxilla, Left			
T Mandible, Right			
V Mandible, Left			
X Hyoid Bone			

Non-OR   ØN8B[Ø,3,4]ZZ

Ø   Medical and Surgical
N   Head and Facial Bones
9   Drainage   Taking or letting out fluids and/or gases from a body part

Body Part Character 4	Approach Character 5	Device Character 6	Qualifier Character 7
Ø Skull	**Ø** Open	**Ø** Drainage Device	**Z** No Qualifier
1 Frontal Bone, Right	**3** Percutaneous		
2 Frontal Bone, Left	**4** Percutaneous Endoscopic		
3 Parietal Bone, Right			
4 Parietal Bone, Left			
5 Temporal Bone, Right			
6 Temporal Bone, Left			
7 Occipital Bone, Right			
8 Occipital Bone, Left			
B Nasal Bone			
C Sphenoid Bone, Right			
D Sphenoid Bone, Left			
F Ethmoid Bone, Right			
G Ethmoid Bone, Left			
H Lacrimal Bone, Right			
J Lacrimal Bone, Left			
K Palatine Bone, Right			
L Palatine Bone, Left			
M Zygomatic Bone, Right			
N Zygomatic Bone, Left			
P Orbit, Right			
Q Orbit, Left			
R Maxilla, Right			
S Maxilla, Left			
T Mandible, Right			
V Mandible, Left			
X Hyoid Bone			

ØN9 Continued on next page

Non-OR   ØN9[B,R,S,T,V][Ø,3,4]ØZ

Ø Medical and Surgical
N Head and Facial Bones   *ØN9 Continued*
9 Drainage   Taking or letting out fluids and/or gases from a body part

Body Part Character 4	Approach Character 5	Device Character 6	Qualifier Character 7
Ø Skull	Ø Open	Z No Device	X Diagnostic
1 Frontal Bone, Right	3 Percutaneous		Z No Qualifier
2 Frontal Bone, Left	4 Percutaneous Endoscopic		
3 Parietal Bone, Right			
4 Parietal Bone, Left			
5 Temporal Bone, Right			
6 Temporal Bone, Left			
7 Occipital Bone, Right			
8 Occipital Bone, Left			
B Nasal Bone			
C Sphenoid Bone, Right			
D Sphenoid Bone, Left			
F Ethmoid Bone, Right			
G Ethmoid Bone, Left			
H Lacrimal Bone, Right			
J Lacrimal Bone, Left			
K Palatine Bone, Right			
L Palatine Bone, Left			
M Zygomatic Bone, Right			
N Zygomatic Bone, Left			
P Orbit, Right			
Q Orbit, Left			
R Maxilla, Right			
S Maxilla, Left			
T Mandible, Right			
V Mandible, Left			
X Hyoid Bone			

Non-OR   ØN9B[Ø,3,4]ZX
Non-OR   ØN9[B,R,S,T,V][Ø,3,4]ZZ

Ø Medical and Surgical
N Head and Facial Bones
B Excision   Cutting out or off, without replacement, a portion of a body part

Body Part Character 4	Approach Character 5	Device Character 6	Qualifier Character 7
Ø Skull	Ø Open	Z No Device	X Diagnostic
1 Frontal Bone, Right	3 Percutaneous		Z No Qualifier
2 Frontal Bone, Left	4 Percutaneous Endoscopic		
3 Parietal Bone, Right			
4 Parietal Bone, Left			
5 Temporal Bone, Right			
6 Temporal Bone, Left			
7 Occipital Bone, Right			
8 Occipital Bone, Left			
B Nasal Bone			
C Sphenoid Bone, Right			
D Sphenoid Bone, Left			
F Ethmoid Bone, Right			
G Ethmoid Bone, Left			
H Lacrimal Bone, Right			
J Lacrimal Bone, Left			
K Palatine Bone, Right			
L Palatine Bone, Left			
M Zygomatic Bone, Right			
N Zygomatic Bone, Left			
P Orbit, Right			
Q Orbit, Left			
R Maxilla, Right			
S Maxilla, Left			
T Mandible, Right			
V Mandible, Left			
X Hyoid Bone			

Non-OR   ØNB[B,R,S,T,V][Ø,3,4]ZX

Ø   Medical and Surgical
N   Head and Facial Bones
C   Extirpation   Taking or cutting out solid matter from a body part

Body Part Character 4	Approach Character 5	Device Character 6	Qualifier Character 7
1 Frontal Bone, Right 2 Frontal Bone, Left 3 Parietal Bone, Right 4 Parietal Bone, Left 5 Temporal Bone, Right 6 Temporal Bone, Left 7 Occipital Bone, Right 8 Occipital Bone, Left B Nasal Bone C Sphenoid Bone, Right D Sphenoid Bone, Left F Ethmoid Bone, Right G Ethmoid Bone, Left H Lacrimal Bone, Right J Lacrimal Bone, Left K Palatine Bone, Right L Palatine Bone, Left M Zygomatic Bone, Right N Zygomatic Bone, Left P Orbit, Right Q Orbit, Left R Maxilla, Right S Maxilla, Left T Mandible, Right V Mandible, Left X Hyoid Bone	Ø Open 3 Percutaneous 4 Percutaneous Endoscopic	Z No Device	Z No Qualifier

Non-OR   ØNC[B,R,S,T,V][Ø,3,4]ZZ

Ø   Medical and Surgical
N   Head and Facial Bones
H   Insertion   Putting in a nonbiological appliance that monitors, assists, performs, or prevents a physiological function but does not physically take the place of a body part

Body Part Character 4	Approach Character 5	Device Character 6	Qualifier Character 7
Ø Skull	Ø Open	4 Internal Fixation Device 5 External Fixation Device M Bone Growth Stimulator N Neurostimulator Generator	Z No Qualifier
Ø Skull	3 Percutaneous 4 Percutaneous Endoscopic	4 Internal Fixation Device 5 External Fixation Device M Bone Growth Stimulator	Z No Qualifier
1 Frontal Bone, Right 2 Frontal Bone, Left 3 Parietal Bone, Right 4 Parietal Bone, Left 7 Occipital Bone, Right 8 Occipital Bone, Left C Sphenoid Bone, Right D Sphenoid Bone, Left F Ethmoid Bone, Right G Ethmoid Bone, Left H Lacrimal Bone, Right J Lacrimal Bone, Left K Palatine Bone, Right L Palatine Bone, Left M Zygomatic Bone, Right N Zygomatic Bone, Left P Orbit, Right Q Orbit, Left X Hyoid Bone	Ø Open 3 Percutaneous 4 Percutaneous Endoscopic	4 Internal Fixation Device	Z No Qualifier

ØNH Continued on next page

Combinations Only
Major Brain Implant
One of ØNHØØNZ and one of ØØH[Ø,6][Ø,3,4]MZ

Non-OR   ØNHØØ5Z
Non-OR   ØNHØ[3,4]5Z

Head and Facial Bones

0 **Medical and Surgical**
N **Head and Facial Bones**
H **Insertion**   Putting in a nonbiological appliance that monitors, assists, performs, or prevents a physiological function but does not physically take the place of a body part

0NH Continued

Body Part Character 4	Approach Character 5	Device Character 6	Qualifier Character 7
5 Temporal Bone, Right 6 Temporal Bone, Left	0 Open 3 Percutaneous 4 Percutaneous Endoscopic	4 Internal Fixation Device S Hearing Device	Z No Qualifier
B Nasal Bone	0 Open 3 Percutaneous 4 Percutaneous Endoscopic	4 Internal Fixation Device M Bone Growth Stimulator	Z No Qualifier
R Maxilla, Right S Maxilla, Left T Mandible, Right V Mandible, Left	0 Open 3 Percutaneous 4 Percutaneous Endoscopic	4 Internal Fixation Device 5 External Fixation Device	Z No Qualifier
W Facial Bone	0 Open 3 Percutaneous 4 Percutaneous Endoscopic	M Bone Growth Stimulator	Z No Qualifier

Non-OR   0NHB[0,3,4][4,M]Z

0 **Medical and Surgical**
N **Head and Facial Bones**
J **Inspection**   Visually and/or manually exploring a body part

Body Part Character 4	Approach Character 5	Device Character 6	Qualifier Character 7
0 Skull B Nasal Bone W Facial Bone	0 Open 3 Percutaneous 4 Percutaneous Endoscopic X External	Z No Device	Z No Qualifier

Non-OR   0NJ[0,B,W]XZZ

0 **Medical and Surgical**
N **Head and Facial Bones**
N **Release**   Freeing a body part from an abnormal physical constraint

Body Part Character 4	Approach Character 5	Device Character 6	Qualifier Character 7
1 Frontal Bone, Right 2 Frontal Bone, Left 3 Parietal Bone, Right 4 Parietal Bone, Left 5 Temporal Bone, Right 6 Temporal Bone, Left 7 Occipital Bone, Right 8 Occipital Bone, Left B Nasal Bone C Sphenoid Bone, Right D Sphenoid Bone, Left F Ethmoid Bone, Right G Ethmoid Bone, Left H Lacrimal Bone, Right J Lacrimal Bone, Left K Palatine Bone, Right L Palatine Bone, Left M Zygomatic Bone, Right N Zygomatic Bone, Left P Orbit, Right Q Orbit, Left R Maxilla, Right S Maxilla, Left T Mandible, Right V Mandible, Left X Hyoid Bone	0 Open 3 Percutaneous 4 Percutaneous Endoscopic	Z No Device	Z No Qualifier

Non-OR   0NNB[0,3,4]ZZ

LC Limited Coverage   NC Noncovered   HAC associated procedure   Combination Only   DRG Non-OR   Non-OR   Revised Text in **GREEN**

Head and Facial Bones

ØNP–ØNQ

Ø   **Medical and Surgical**
N   **Head and Facial Bones**
P   **Removal**   Taking out or off a device from a body part

Body Part Character 4	Approach Character 5	Device Character 6	Qualifier Character 7
Ø Skull	Ø Open	Ø Drainage Device 4 Internal Fixation Device 5 External Fixation Device 7 Autologous Tissue Substitute J Synthetic Substitute K Nonautologous Tissue Substitute M Bone Growth Stimulator N Neurostimulator Generator S Hearing Device	Z No Qualifier
Ø Skull	3 Percutaneous 4 Percutaneous Endoscopic	Ø Drainage Device 4 Internal Fixation Device 5 External Fixation Device 7 Autologous Tissue Substitute J Synthetic Substitute K Nonautologous Tissue Substitute M Bone Growth Stimulator S Hearing Device	Z No Qualifier
Ø Skull	X External	Ø Drainage Device 4 Internal Fixation Device 5 External Fixation Device M Bone Growth Stimulator S Hearing Device	Z No Qualifier
B Nasal Bone W Facial Bone	Ø Open 3 Percutaneous 4 Percutaneous Endoscopic	Ø Drainage Device 4 Internal Fixation Device 7 Autologous Tissue Substitute J Synthetic Substitute K Nonautologous Tissue Substitute M Bone Growth Stimulator	Z No Qualifier
B Nasal Bone W Facial Bone	X External	Ø Drainage Device 4 Internal Fixation Device M Bone Growth Stimulator	Z No Qualifier

Non-OR   ØNPØ[3,4]5Z
Non-OR   ØNPØX[Ø,5]Z
Non-OR   ØNPB[Ø,3,4][Ø,4,7,J,K,M]Z
Non-OR   ØNP[B,W]X[Ø,4,M]Z

Ø   **Medical and Surgical**
N   **Head and Facial Bones**
Q   **Repair**   Restoring, to the extent possible, a body part to its normal anatomic structure and function

Body Part Character 4	Approach Character 5	Device Character 6	Qualifier Character 7
Ø Skull 1 Frontal Bone, Right 2 Frontal Bone, Left 3 Parietal Bone, Right 4 Parietal Bone, Left 5 Temporal Bone, Right 6 Temporal Bone, Left 7 Occipital Bone, Right 8 Occipital Bone, Left B Nasal Bone C Sphenoid Bone, Right D Sphenoid Bone, Left F Ethmoid Bone, Right G Ethmoid Bone, Left H Lacrimal Bone, Right J Lacrimal Bone, Left K Palatine Bone, Right L Palatine Bone, Left M Zygomatic Bone, Right N Zygomatic Bone, Left P Orbit, Right Q Orbit, Left R Maxilla, Right S Maxilla, Left T Mandible, Right V Mandible, Left X Hyoid Bone	Ø Open 3 Percutaneous 4 Percutaneous Endoscopic X External	Z No Device	Z No Qualifier

Ø   **Medical and Surgical**
N   **Head and Facial Bones**
R   **Replacement**   Putting in or on biological or synthetic material that physically takes the place and/or function of all or a portion of a body part

Body Part Character 4	Approach Character 5	Device Character 6	Qualifier Character 7
Ø Skull	**Ø** Open	**7** Autologous Tissue Substitute	**Z** No Qualifier
1 Frontal Bone, Right	**3** Percutaneous	**J** Synthetic Substitute	
2 Frontal Bone, Left	**4** Percutaneous Endoscopic	**K** Nonautologous Tissue Substitute	
3 Parietal Bone, Right			
4 Parietal Bone, Left			
5 Temporal Bone, Right			
6 Temporal Bone, Left			
7 Occipital Bone, Right			
8 Occipital Bone, Left			
B Nasal Bone			
C Sphenoid Bone, Right			
D Sphenoid Bone, Left			
F Ethmoid Bone, Right			
G Ethmoid Bone, Left			
H Lacrimal Bone, Right			
J Lacrimal Bone, Left			
K Palatine Bone, Right			
L Palatine Bone, Left			
M Zygomatic Bone, Right			
N Zygomatic Bone, Left			
P Orbit, Right			
Q Orbit, Left			
R Maxilla, Right			
S Maxilla, Left			
T Mandible, Right			
V Mandible, Left			
X Hyoid Bone			

Ø   **Medical and Surgical**
N   **Head and Facial Bones**
S   **Reposition**   Moving to its normal location or other suitable location all or a portion of a body part

Body Part Character 4	Approach Character 5	Device Character 6	Qualifier Character 7
Ø Skull	**X** External	**Z** No Device	**Z** No Qualifier
1 Frontal Bone, Right			
2 Frontal Bone, Left			
3 Parietal Bone, Right			
4 Parietal Bone, Left			
5 Temporal Bone, Right			
6 Temporal Bone, Left			
7 Occipital Bone, Right			
8 Occipital Bone, Left			
B Nasal Bone			
C Sphenoid Bone, Right			
D Sphenoid Bone, Left			
F Ethmoid Bone, Right			
G Ethmoid Bone, Left			
H Lacrimal Bone, Right			
J Lacrimal Bone, Left			
K Palatine Bone, Right			
L Palatine Bone, Left			
M Zygomatic Bone, Right			
N Zygomatic Bone, Left			
P Orbit, Right			
Q Orbit, Left			
R Maxilla, Right			
S Maxilla, Left			
T Mandible, Right			
V Mandible, Left			
X Hyoid Bone			
Ø Skull	**Ø** Open	**4** Internal Fixation Device	**Z** No Qualifier
R Maxilla, Right	**3** Percutaneous	**5** External Fixation Device	
S Maxilla, Left	**4** Percutaneous Endoscopic	**Z** No Device	
T Mandible, Right			
V Mandible, Left			

ØNS Continued on next page

Non-OR   ØNS[B,C,D,F,G,H,J,K,L,M,N,P,Q,R,S,T,V,X]XZZ
Non-OR   ØNS[R,S,T,V][3,4][4,5,Z]Z

LC Limited Coverage   **NC** Noncovered   HAC associated procedure   Combination Only   DRG Non-OR   Non-OR   Revised Text in **GREEN**

Head and Facial Bones

ØNS–ØNT

ØNS Continued

Ø   Medical and Surgical
N   Head and Facial Bones
S   Reposition   Moving to its normal location or other suitable location all or a portion of a body part

Body Part Character 4	Approach Character 5	Device Character 6	Qualifier Character 7
Ø Skull R Maxilla, Right S Maxilla, Left T Mandible, Right V Mandible, Left	X External	Z No Device	Z No Qualifier
1 Frontal Bone, Right 2 Frontal Bone, Left 3 Parietal Bone, Right 4 Parietal Bone, Left 5 Temporal Bone, Right 6 Temporal Bone, Left 7 Occipital Bone, Right 8 Occipital Bone, Left B Nasal Bone C Sphenoid Bone, Right D Sphenoid Bone, Left F Ethmoid Bone, Right G Ethmoid Bone, Left H Lacrimal Bone, Right J Lacrimal Bone, Left K Palatine Bone, Right L Palatine Bone, Left M Zygomatic Bone, Right N Zygomatic Bone, Left P Orbit, Right Q Orbit, Left X Hyoid Bone	Ø Open 3 Percutaneous 4 Percutaneous Endoscopic	4 Internal Fixation Device Z No Device	Z No Qualifier

Non-OR   ØNS[R,S,T,V]XZZ
Non-OR   ØNS[B,C,D,F,G,H,J,K,L,M,N,P,Q,X][3,4][4,Z]Z

Ø   Medical and Surgical
N   Head and Facial Bones
T   Resection   Cutting out or off, without replacement, all of a body part

Body Part Character 4	Approach Character 5	Device Character 6	Qualifier Character 7
1 Frontal Bone, Right 2 Frontal Bone, Left 3 Parietal Bone, Right 4 Parietal Bone, Left 5 Temporal Bone, Right 6 Temporal Bone, Left 7 Occipital Bone, Right 8 Occipital Bone, Left B Nasal Bone C Sphenoid Bone, Right D Sphenoid Bone, Left F Ethmoid Bone, Right G Ethmoid Bone, Left H Lacrimal Bone, Right J Lacrimal Bone, Left K Palatine Bone, Right L Palatine Bone, Left M Zygomatic Bone, Right N Zygomatic Bone, Left P Orbit, Right Q Orbit, Left R Maxilla, Right S Maxilla, Left T Mandible, Right V Mandible, Left X Hyoid Bone	Ø Open	Z No Device	Z No Qualifier

Ø **Medical and Surgical**
N **Head and Facial Bones**
U **Supplement** Putting in or on biological or synthetic material that physically reinforces and/or augments the function of a portion of a body part

Body Part — Character 4	Approach — Character 5	Device — Character 6	Qualifier — Character 7
Ø Skull 1 Frontal Bone, Right 2 Frontal Bone, Left 3 Parietal Bone, Right 4 Parietal Bone, Left 5 Temporal Bone, Right 6 Temporal Bone, Left 7 Occipital Bone, Right 8 Occipital Bone, Left B Nasal Bone C Sphenoid Bone, Right D Sphenoid Bone, Left F Ethmoid Bone, Right G Ethmoid Bone, Left H Lacrimal Bone, Right J Lacrimal Bone, Left K Palatine Bone, Right L Palatine Bone, Left M Zygomatic Bone, Right N Zygomatic Bone, Left P Orbit, Right Q Orbit, Left R Maxilla, Right S Maxilla, Left T Mandible, Right V Mandible, Left X Hyoid Bone	Ø Open 3 Percutaneous 4 Percutaneous Endoscopic	7 Autologous Tissue Substitute J Synthetic Substitute K Nonautologous Tissue Substitute	Z No Qualifier

Ø **Medical and Surgical**
N **Head and Facial Bones**
W **Revision** Correcting, to the extent possible, a portion of a malfunctioning device or the position of a displaced device

Body Part — Character 4	Approach — Character 5	Device — Character 6	Qualifier — Character 7
Ø Skull	Ø Open	Ø Drainage Device 4 Internal Fixation Device 5 External Fixation Device 7 Autologous Tissue Substitute J Synthetic Substitute K Nonautologous Tissue Substitute M Bone Growth Stimulator N Neurostimulator Generator S Hearing Device	Z No Qualifier
Ø Skull	3 Percutaneous 4 Percutaneous Endoscopic X External	Ø Drainage Device 4 Internal Fixation Device 5 External Fixation Device 7 Autologous Tissue Substitute J Synthetic Substitute K Nonautologous Tissue Substitute M Bone Growth Stimulator S Hearing Device	Z No Qualifier
B Nasal Bone W Facial Bone	Ø Open 3 Percutaneous 4 Percutaneous Endoscopic X External	Ø Drainage Device 4 Internal Fixation Device 7 Autologous Tissue Substitute J Synthetic Substitute K Nonautologous Tissue Substitute M Bone Growth Stimulator	Z No Qualifier

Non-OR ØNWØX[Ø,4,5,7,J,K,M,S]Z
Non-OR ØNW[B,W][Ø,3,4,X][Ø,4,J,K,M]Z

Upper Bones ØP2–ØPW

Ø Medical and Surgical
P Upper Bones
2 Change Taking out or off a device from a body part and putting back an identical or similar device in or on the same body part without cutting or puncturing the skin or a mucous membrane

Body Part Character 4	Approach Character 5	Device Character 6	Qualifier Character 7
Y Upper Bone	X External	Ø Drainage Device Y Other Device	Z No Qualifier

Non-OR For all body part, approach, device, and qualifier values

Ø Medical and Surgical
P Upper Bones
5 Destruction Physical eradication of all or a portion of a body part by the direct use of energy, force, or a destructive agent

Body Part Character 4	Approach Character 5	Device Character 6	Qualifier Character 7
Ø Sternum 1 Rib, Right 2 Rib, Left 3 Cervical Vertebra 4 Thoracic Vertebra 5 Scapula, Right 6 Scapula, Left 7 Glenoid Cavity, Right 8 Glenoid Cavity, Left 9 Clavicle, Right B Clavicle, Left C Humeral Head, Right D Humeral Head, Left F Humeral Shaft, Right G Humeral Shaft, Left H Radius, Right J Radius, Left K Ulna, Right L Ulna, Left M Carpal, Right N Carpal, Left P Metacarpal, Right Q Metacarpal, Left R Thumb Phalanx, Right S Thumb Phalanx, Left T Finger Phalanx, Right V Finger Phalanx, Left	Ø Open 3 Percutaneous 4 Percutaneous Endoscopic	Z No Device	Z No Qualifier

Ø Medical and Surgical
P Upper Bones
8 Division Cutting into a body part without draining fluids and/or gases from the body part in order to separate or transect a body part

Body Part Character 4	Approach Character 5	Device Character 6	Qualifier Character 7
Ø Sternum 1 Rib, Right 2 Rib, Left 3 Cervical Vertebra 4 Thoracic Vertebra 5 Scapula, Right 6 Scapula, Left 7 Glenoid Cavity, Right 8 Glenoid Cavity, Left 9 Clavicle, Right B Clavicle, Left C Humeral Head, Right D Humeral Head, Left F Humeral Shaft, Right G Humeral Shaft, Left H Radius, Right J Radius, Left K Ulna, Right L Ulna, Left M Carpal, Right N Carpal, Left P Metacarpal, Right Q Metacarpal, Left R Thumb Phalanx, Right S Thumb Phalanx, Left T Finger Phalanx, Right V Finger Phalanx, Left	Ø Open 3 Percutaneous 4 Percutaneous Endoscopic	Z No Device	Z No Qualifier

0   **Medical and Surgical**
P   **Upper Bones**
9   **Drainage**   Taking or letting out fluids and/or gases from a body part

Body Part Character 4	Approach Character 5	Device Character 6	Qualifier Character 7
0 Sternum	**0** Open	**0** Drainage Device	**Z** No Qualifier
1 Rib, Right	**3** Percutaneous		
2 Rib, Left	**4** Percutaneous Endoscopic		
3 Cervical Vertebra			
4 Thoracic Vertebra			
5 Scapula, Right			
6 Scapula, Left			
7 Glenoid Cavity, Right			
8 Glenoid Cavity, Left			
9 Clavicle, Right			
B Clavicle, Left			
C Humeral Head, Right			
D Humeral Head, Left			
F Humeral Shaft, Right			
G Humeral Shaft, Left			
H Radius, Right			
J Radius, Left			
K Ulna, Right			
L Ulna, Left			
M Carpal, Right			
N Carpal, Left			
P Metacarpal, Right			
Q Metacarpal, Left			
R Thumb Phalanx, Right			
S Thumb Phalanx, Left			
T Finger Phalanx, Right			
V Finger Phalanx, Left			
0 Sternum	**0** Open	**Z** No Device	**X** Diagnostic
1 Rib, Right	**3** Percutaneous		**Z** No Qualifier
2 Rib, Left	**4** Percutaneous Endoscopic		
3 Cervical Vertebra			
4 Thoracic Vertebra			
5 Scapula, Right			
6 Scapula, Left			
7 Glenoid Cavity, Right			
8 Glenoid Cavity, Left			
9 Clavicle, Right			
B Clavicle, Left			
C Humeral Head, Right			
D Humeral Head, Left			
F Humeral Shaft, Right			
G Humeral Shaft, Left			
H Radius, Right			
J Radius, Left			
K Ulna, Right			
L Ulna, Left			
M Carpal, Right			
N Carpal, Left			
P Metacarpal, Right			
Q Metacarpal, Left			
R Thumb Phalanx, Right			
S Thumb Phalanx, Left			
T Finger Phalanx, Right			
V Finger Phalanx, Left			

LC Limited Coverage   **NC** Noncovered   HAC associated procedure   Combination Only   DRG Non-OR   Non-OR   Revised Text in **GREEN**

ICD-10-PCS 2014 (Draft)   **325**

Upper Bones

ØPB–ØPC

Ø   Medical and Surgical
P   Upper Bones
B   Excision   Cutting out or off, without replacement, a portion of a body part

Body Part Character 4	Approach Character 5	Device Character 6	Qualifier Character 7
Ø Sternum	Ø Open	Z No Device	X Diagnostic
1 Rib, Right	3 Percutaneous		Z No Qualifier
2 Rib, Left	4 Percutaneous Endoscopic		
3 Cervical Vertebra			
4 Thoracic Vertebra			
5 Scapula, Right			
6 Scapula, Left			
7 Glenoid Cavity, Right			
8 Glenoid Cavity, Left			
9 Clavicle, Right			
B Clavicle, Left			
C Humeral Head, Right			
D Humeral Head, Left			
F Humeral Shaft, Right			
G Humeral Shaft, Left			
H Radius, Right			
J Radius, Left			
K Ulna, Right			
L Ulna, Left			
M Carpal, Right			
N Carpal, Left			
P Metacarpal, Right			
Q Metacarpal, Left			
R Thumb Phalanx, Right			
S Thumb Phalanx, Left			
T Finger Phalanx, Right			
V Finger Phalanx, Left			

Ø   Medical and Surgical
P   Upper Bones
C   Extirpation   Taking or cutting out solid matter from a body part

Body Part Character 4	Approach Character 5	Device Character 6	Qualifier Character 7
Ø Sternum	Ø Open	Z No Device	Z No Qualifier
1 Rib, Right	3 Percutaneous		
2 Rib, Left	4 Percutaneous Endoscopic		
3 Cervical Vertebra			
4 Thoracic Vertebra			
5 Scapula, Right			
6 Scapula, Left			
7 Glenoid Cavity, Right			
8 Glenoid Cavity, Left			
9 Clavicle, Right			
B Clavicle, Left			
C Humeral Head, Right			
D Humeral Head, Left			
F Humeral Shaft, Right			
G Humeral Shaft, Left			
H Radius, Right			
J Radius, Left			
K Ulna, Right			
L Ulna, Left			
M Carpal, Right			
N Carpal, Left			
P Metacarpal, Right			
Q Metacarpal, Left			
R Thumb Phalanx, Right			
S Thumb Phalanx, Left			
T Finger Phalanx, Right			
V Finger Phalanx, Left			

Ø   **Medical and Surgical**
P   **Upper Bones**
H   **Insertion**   Putting in a nonbiological appliance that monitors, assists, performs, or prevents a physiological function but does not physically take the place of a body part

Body Part Character 4	Approach Character 5	Device Character 6	Qualifier Character 7
Ø Sternum	**Ø** Open **3** Percutaneous **4** Percutaneous Endoscopic	**Ø** Internal Fixation Device, Rigid Plate **4** Internal Fixation Device	**Z** No Qualifier
1 Rib, Right **2** Rib, Left **3** Cervical Vertebra **4** Thoracic Vertebra **5** Scapula, Right **6** Scapula, Left **7** Glenoid Cavity, Right **8** Glenoid Cavity, Left **9** Clavicle, Right **B** Clavicle, Left	**Ø** Open **3** Percutaneous **4** Percutaneous Endoscopic	**4** Internal Fixation Device	**Z** No Qualifier

C Humeral Head, Right
D Humeral Head, Left
F Humeral Shaft, Right
G Humeral Shaft, Left
H Radius, Right
J Radius, Left
K Ulna, Right
L Ulna, Left
	Ø Open
	3 Percutaneous
	4 Percutaneous Endoscopic
		4 Internal Fixation Device
		5 External Fixation Device
		6 Internal Fixation Device,
		    Intramedullary
		8 External Fixation Device, Limb
		    Lengthening
		B External Fixation Device,
		    Monoplanar
		C External Fixation Device, Ring
		D External Fixation Device, Hybrid
			Z No Qualifier

M Carpal, Right **N** Carpal, Left **P** Metacarpal, Right **Q** Metacarpal, Left **R** Thumb Phalanx, Right **S** Thumb Phalanx, Left **T** Finger Phalanx, Right **V** Finger Phalanx, Left	**Ø** Open **3** Percutaneous **4** Percutaneous Endoscopic	**4** Internal Fixation Device **5** External Fixation Device	**Z** No Qualifier
Y Upper Bone	**Ø** Open **3** Percutaneous **4** Percutaneous Endoscopic	**M** Bone Growth Stimulator	**Z** No Qualifier

Non-OR   ØPH[C,D,F,G,H,J,K,L][Ø,3,4]8Z

Ø   **Medical and Surgical**
P   **Upper Bones**
J   **Inspection**   Visually and/or manually exploring a body part

Body Part Character 4	Approach Character 5	Device Character 6	Qualifier Character 7
Y Upper Bone	**Ø** Open **3** Percutaneous **4** Percutaneous Endoscopic **X** External	**Z** No Device	**Z** No Qualifier

Non-OR   ØPJYXZZ

LC Limited Coverage   **NC** Noncovered   HAC associated procedure   Combination Only   DRG Non-OR   Non-OR   Revised Text in **GREEN**

ICD-10-PCS 2014 (Draft)   327

Ø Medical and Surgical
P Upper Bones
N Release   Freeing a body part from an abnormal physical constraint

Body Part Character 4	Approach Character 5	Device Character 6	Qualifier Character 7
Ø Sternum	Ø Open	Z No Device	Z No Qualifier
1 Rib, Right	3 Percutaneous		
2 Rib, Left	4 Percutaneous Endoscopic		
3 Cervical Vertebra			
4 Thoracic Vertebra			
5 Scapula, Right			
6 Scapula, Left			
7 Glenoid Cavity, Right			
8 Glenoid Cavity, Left			
9 Clavicle, Right			
B Clavicle, Left			
C Humeral Head, Right			
D Humeral Head, Left			
F Humeral Shaft, Right			
G Humeral Shaft, Left			
H Radius, Right			
J Radius, Left			
K Ulna, Right			
L Ulna, Left			
M Carpal, Right			
N Carpal, Left			
P Metacarpal, Right			
Q Metacarpal, Left			
R Thumb Phalanx, Right			
S Thumb Phalanx, Left			
T Finger Phalanx, Right			
V Finger Phalanx, Left			

Ø Medical and Surgical
P Upper Bones
P Removal   Taking out or off a device from a body part

Body Part Character 4	Approach Character 5	Device Character 6	Qualifier Character 7
Ø Sternum	Ø Open	4 Internal Fixation Device	Z No Qualifier
1 Rib, Right	3 Percutaneous	7 Autologous Tissue Substitute	
2 Rib, Left	4 Percutaneous Endoscopic	J Synthetic Substitute	
3 Cervical Vertebra		K Nonautologous Tissue Substitute	
4 Thoracic Vertebra			
5 Scapula, Right			
6 Scapula, Left			
7 Glenoid Cavity, Right			
8 Glenoid Cavity, Left			
9 Clavicle, Right			
B Clavicle, Left			
Ø Sternum	X External	4 Internal Fixation Device	Z No Qualifier
1 Rib, Right			
2 Rib, Left			
3 Cervical Vertebra			
4 Thoracic Vertebra			
5 Scapula, Right			
6 Scapula, Left			
7 Glenoid Cavity, Right			
8 Glenoid Cavity, Left			
9 Clavicle, Right			
B Clavicle, Left			

ØPP Continued on next page

Non-OR	ØPP[Ø,1,2,3,4,5,6,7,8,9,B]X4Z

Ø Medical and Surgical
P Upper Bones
P Removal   Taking out or off a device from a body part

Body Part Character 4	Approach Character 5	Device Character 6	Qualifier Character 7
C Humeral Head, Right D Humeral Head, Left F Humeral Shaft, Right G Humeral Shaft, Left H Radius, Right J Radius, Left K Ulna, Right L Ulna, Left M Carpal, Right N Carpal, Left P Metacarpal, Right Q Metacarpal, Left R Thumb Phalanx, Right S Thumb Phalanx, Left T Finger Phalanx, Right V Finger Phalanx, Left	Ø Open 3 Percutaneous 4 Percutaneous Endoscopic	4 Internal Fixation Device 5 External Fixation Device 7 Autologous Tissue Substitute J Synthetic Substitute K Nonautologous Tissue Substitute	Z No Qualifier
C Humeral Head, Right D Humeral Head, Left F Humeral Shaft, Right G Humeral Shaft, Left H Radius, Right J Radius, Left K Ulna, Right L Ulna, Left M Carpal, Right N Carpal, Left P Metacarpal, Right Q Metacarpal, Left R Thumb Phalanx, Right S Thumb Phalanx, Left T Finger Phalanx, Right V Finger Phalanx, Left	X External	4 Internal Fixation Device 5 External Fixation Device	Z No Qualifier
Y Upper Bone	Ø Open 3 Percutaneous 4 Percutaneous Endoscopic X External	Ø Drainage Device M Bone Growth Stimulator	Z No Qualifier

Non-OR   ØPP[C,D,F,G,H,J,K,L,M,N,P,Q,R,S,T,V]X[4,5]Z
Non-OR   ØPPYX[Ø,M]Z

Ø Medical and Surgical
P Upper Bones
Q Repair   Restoring, to the extent possible, a body part to its normal anatomic structure and function

Body Part Character 4	Approach Character 5	Device Character 6	Qualifier Character 7
Ø Sternum 1 Rib, Right 2 Rib, Left 3 Cervical Vertebra 4 Thoracic Vertebra 5 Scapula, Right 6 Scapula, Left 7 Glenoid Cavity, Right 8 Glenoid Cavity, Left 9 Clavicle, Right B Clavicle, Left C Humeral Head, Right D Humeral Head, Left F Humeral Shaft, Right G Humeral Shaft, Left H Radius, Right J Radius, Left K Ulna, Right L Ulna, Left M Carpal, Right N Carpal, Left P Metacarpal, Right Q Metacarpal, Left R Thumb Phalanx, Right S Thumb Phalanx, Left T Finger Phalanx, Right V Finger Phalanx, Left	Ø Open 3 Percutaneous 4 Percutaneous Endoscopic X External	Z No Device	Z No Qualifier

Ø　Medical and Surgical
P　Upper Bones
R　Replacement　Putting in or on biological or synthetic material that physically takes the place and/or function of all or a portion of a body part

Body Part Character 4	Approach Character 5	Device Character 6	Qualifier Character 7
Ø Sternum 1 Rib, Right 2 Rib, Left 3 Cervical Vertebra 4 Thoracic Vertebra 5 Scapula, Right 6 Scapula, Left 7 Glenoid Cavity, Right 8 Glenoid Cavity, Left 9 Clavicle, Right B Clavicle, Left C Humeral Head, Right D Humeral Head, Left F Humeral Shaft, Right G Humeral Shaft, Left H Radius, Right J Radius, Left K Ulna, Right L Ulna, Left M Carpal, Right N Carpal, Left P Metacarpal, Right Q Metacarpal, Left R Thumb Phalanx, Right S Thumb Phalanx, Left T Finger Phalanx, Right V Finger Phalanx, Left	Ø Open 3 Percutaneous 4 Percutaneous Endoscopic	7 Autologous Tissue Substitute J Synthetic Substitute K Nonautologous Tissue Substitute	Z No Qualifier

Non-OR　ØPR[C,D]ØJZ

Ø　Medical and Surgical
P　Upper Bones
S　Reposition　Moving to its normal location or other suitable location all or a portion of a body part

Body Part Character 4	Approach Character 5	Device Character 6	Qualifier Character 7
Ø Sternum	Ø Open 3 Percutaneous 4 Percutaneous Endoscopic	Ø Internal Fixation Device, Rigid Plate 4 Internal Fixation Device Z No Device	Z No Qualifier
1 Rib, Right 2 Rib, Left 3 Cervical Vertebra 4 Thoracic Vertebra 5 Scapula, Right 6 Scapula, Left 7 Glenoid Cavity, Right 8 Glenoid Cavity, Left 9 Clavicle, Right B Clavicle, Left	Ø Open 3 Percutaneous 4 Percutaneous Endoscopic	4 Internal Fixation Device Z No Device	Z No Qualifier
Ø Sternum 1 Rib, Right 2 Rib, Left 3 Cervical Vertebra 4 Thoracic Vertebra 5 Scapula, Right 6 Scapula, Left 7 Glenoid Cavity, Right 8 Glenoid Cavity, Left 9 Clavicle, Right B Clavicle, Left	X External	Z No Device	Z No Qualifier

ØPS Continued on next page

Non-OR　ØPSØ[3,4]ZZ
Non-OR　ØPS[1,2,5,6,7,8,9,B][3,4]ZZ
Non-OR　ØPS[Ø,1,2,5,6,7,8,9,B]XZZ

Ø   Medical and Surgical   *ØPS Continued*
P   Upper Bones
S   Reposition   Moving to its normal location or other suitable location all or a portion of a body part

Body Part Character 4	Approach Character 5	Device Character 6	Qualifier Character 7

C Humeral Head, Right
D Humeral Head, Left
F Humeral Shaft, Right
G Humeral Shaft, Left
H Radius, Right
J Radius, Left
K Ulna, Right
L Ulna, Left
	Ø Open
	3 Percutaneous
	4 Percutaneous Endoscopic
		4 Internal Fixation Device
		5 External Fixation Device
		6 Internal Fixation Device,
		    Intramedullary
		B External Fixation Device,
		    Monoplanar
		C External Fixation Device, Ring
		D External Fixation Device, Hybrid
		Z No Device
			Z No Qualifier

C Humeral Head, Right **D** Humeral Head, Left **F** Humeral Shaft, Right **G** Humeral Shaft, Left **H** Radius, Right **J** Radius, Left **K** Ulna, Right **L** Ulna, Left	**X** External	**Z** No Device	**Z** No Qualifier
M Carpal, Right **N** Carpal, Left **P** Metacarpal, Right **Q** Metacarpal, Left **R** Thumb Phalanx, Right **S** Thumb Phalanx, Left **T** Finger Phalanx, Right **V** Finger Phalanx, Left	**Ø** Open **3** Percutaneous **4** Percutaneous Endoscopic	**4** Internal Fixation Device **5** External Fixation Device **Z** No Device	**Z** No Qualifier
M Carpal, Right **N** Carpal, Left **P** Metacarpal, Right **Q** Metacarpal, Left **R** Thumb Phalanx, Right **S** Thumb Phalanx, Left **T** Finger Phalanx, Right **V** Finger Phalanx, Left	**X** External	**Z** No Device	**Z** No Qualifier

Non-OR   ØPS[C,D,F,G,H,J,K,L][3,4]ZZ
Non-OR   ØPS[C,D,F,G,H,J,K,L]XZZ
Non-OR   ØPS[M,N,P,Q,R,S,T,V][3,4]ZZ
Non-OR   ØPS[M,N,P,Q,R,S,T,V]XZZ

Ø   Medical and Surgical
P   Upper Bones
T   Resection   Cutting out or off, without replacement, all of a body part

Body Part Character 4	Approach Character 5	Device Character 6	Qualifier Character 7
Ø Sternum **1** Rib, Right **2** Rib, Left **5** Scapula, Right **6** Scapula, Left **7** Glenoid Cavity, Right **8** Glenoid Cavity, Left **9** Clavicle, Right **B** Clavicle, Left **C** Humeral Head, Right **D** Humeral Head, Left **F** Humeral Shaft, Right **G** Humeral Shaft, Left **H** Radius, Right **J** Radius, Left **K** Ulna, Right **L** Ulna, Left **M** Carpal, Right **N** Carpal, Left **P** Metacarpal, Right **Q** Metacarpal, Left **R** Thumb Phalanx, Right **S** Thumb Phalanx, Left **T** Finger Phalanx, Right **V** Finger Phalanx, Left	**Ø** Open	**Z** No Device	**Z** No Qualifier

Ø   Medical and Surgical
P   Upper Bones
U   Supplement   Putting in or on biological or synthetic material that physically reinforces and/or augments the function of a portion of a body part

Body Part Character 4	Approach Character 5	Device Character 6	Qualifier Character 7
Ø Sternum 1 Rib, Right 2 Rib, Left 3 Cervical Vertebra 4 Thoracic Vertebra 5 Scapula, Right 6 Scapula, Left 7 Glenoid Cavity, Right 8 Glenoid Cavity, Left 9 Clavicle, Right B Clavicle, Left C Humeral Head, Right D Humeral Head, Left F Humeral Shaft, Right G Humeral Shaft, Left H Radius, Right J Radius, Left K Ulna, Right L Ulna, Left M Carpal, Right N Carpal, Left P Metacarpal, Right Q Metacarpal, Left R Thumb Phalanx, Right S Thumb Phalanx, Left T Finger Phalanx, Right V Finger Phalanx, Left	Ø Open 3 Percutaneous 4 Percutaneous Endoscopic	7 Autologous Tissue Substitute J Synthetic Substitute K Nonautologous Tissue Substitute	Z No Qualifier

Ø   Medical and Surgical
P   Upper Bones
W   Revision   Correcting, to the extent possible, a portion of a malfunctioning device or the position of a displaced device

Body Part Character 4	Approach Character 5	Device Character 6	Qualifier Character 7
Ø Sternum 1 Rib, Right 2 Rib, Left 3 Cervical Vertebra 4 Thoracic Vertebra 5 Scapula, Right 6 Scapula, Left 7 Glenoid Cavity, Right 8 Glenoid Cavity, Left 9 Clavicle, Right B Clavicle, Left	Ø Open 3 Percutaneous 4 Percutaneous Endoscopic X External	4 Internal Fixation Device 7 Autologous Tissue Substitute J Synthetic Substitute K Nonautologous Tissue Substitute	Z No Qualifier
C Humeral Head, Right D Humeral Head, Left F Humeral Shaft, Right G Humeral Shaft, Left H Radius, Right J Radius, Left K Ulna, Right L Ulna, Left M Carpal, Right N Carpal, Left P Metacarpal, Right Q Metacarpal, Left R Thumb Phalanx, Right S Thumb Phalanx, Left T Finger Phalanx, Right V Finger Phalanx, Left	Ø Open 3 Percutaneous 4 Percutaneous Endoscopic X External	4 Internal Fixation Device 5 External Fixation Device 7 Autologous Tissue Substitute J Synthetic Substitute K Nonautologous Tissue Substitute	Z No Qualifier
Y Upper Bone	Ø Open 3 Percutaneous 4 Percutaneous Endoscopic X External	Ø Drainage Device M Bone Growth Stimulator	Z No Qualifier

Non-OR   ØPW[Ø,1,2,3,4,5,6,7,8,9,B]X[4,7,J,K]Z
Non-OR   ØPW[C,D,F,G,H,J,K,L,M,N,P,Q,R,S,T,V]X[4,5,7,J,K]Z
Non-OR   ØPWYX[Ø,M]Z

Lower Bones 0Q2–0QW

0　**Medical and Surgical**
Q　**Lower Bones**
2　**Change**　　Taking out or off a device from a body part and putting back an identical or similar device in or on the same body part without cutting or puncturing the skin or a mucous membrane

Body Part Character 4	Approach Character 5	Device Character 6	Qualifier Character 7
Y Lower Bone	**X** External	**0** Drainage Device **Y** Other Device	**Z** No Qualifier

Non-OR	For all body part, approach, device, and qualifier values

0　**Medical and Surgical**
Q　**Lower Bones**
5　**Destruction**　　Physical eradication of all or a portion of a body part by the direct use of energy, force, or a destructive agent

Body Part Character 4	Approach Character 5	Device Character 6	Qualifier Character 7
0 Lumbar Vertebra **1** Sacrum **2** Pelvic Bone, Right **3** Pelvic Bone, Left **4** Acetabulum, Right **5** Acetabulum, Left **6** Upper Femur, Right **7** Upper Femur, Left **8** Femoral Shaft, Right **9** Femoral Shaft, Left **B** Lower Femur, Right **C** Lower Femur, Left **D** Patella, Right **F** Patella, Left **G** Tibia, Right **H** Tibia, Left **J** Fibula, Right **K** Fibula, Left **L** Tarsal, Right **M** Tarsal, Left **N** Metatarsal, Right **P** Metatarsal, Left **Q** Toe Phalanx, Right **R** Toe Phalanx, Left **S** Coccyx	**0** Open **3** Percutaneous **4** Percutaneous Endoscopic	**Z** No Device	**Z** No Qualifier

0　**Medical and Surgical**
Q　**Lower Bones**
8　**Division**　　Cutting into a body part without draining fluids and/or gases from the body part in order to separate or transect a body part

Body Part Character 4	Approach Character 5	Device Character 6	Qualifier Character 7
0 Lumbar Vertebra **1** Sacrum **2** Pelvic Bone, Right **3** Pelvic Bone, Left **4** Acetabulum, Right **5** Acetabulum, Left **6** Upper Femur, Right **7** Upper Femur, Left **8** Femoral Shaft, Right **9** Femoral Shaft, Left **B** Lower Femur, Right **C** Lower Femur, Left **D** Patella, Right **F** Patella, Left **G** Tibia, Right **H** Tibia, Left **J** Fibula, Right **K** Fibula, Left **L** Tarsal, Right **M** Tarsal, Left **N** Metatarsal, Right **P** Metatarsal, Left **Q** Toe Phalanx, Right **R** Toe Phalanx, Left **S** Coccyx	**0** Open **3** Percutaneous **4** Percutaneous Endoscopic	**Z** No Device	**Z** No Qualifier

LC Limited Coverage　　**NC** Noncovered　　HAC associated procedure　　Combination Only　　DRG Non-OR　　Non-OR　　Revised Text in **GREEN**

ICD-10-PCS 2014 (Draft)　　　　　　　　　　　　　　　　　　　　　　　　　　　　　　　　　　**333**

0   **Medical and Surgical**
Q   **Lower Bones**
9   **Drainage**   Taking or letting out fluids and/or gases from a body part

Body Part Character 4	Approach Character 5	Device Character 6	Qualifier Character 7
0 Lumbar Vertebra	**0** Open	**0** Drainage Device	**Z** No Qualifier
1 Sacrum	**3** Percutaneous		
2 Pelvic Bone, Right	**4** Percutaneous Endoscopic		
3 Pelvic Bone, Left			
4 Acetabulum, Right			
5 Acetabulum, Left			
6 Upper Femur, Right			
7 Upper Femur, Left			
8 Femoral Shaft, Right			
9 Femoral Shaft, Left			
B Lower Femur, Right			
C Lower Femur, Left			
D Patella, Right			
F Patella, Left			
G Tibia, Right			
H Tibia, Left			
J Fibula, Right			
K Fibula, Left			
L Tarsal, Right			
M Tarsal, Left			
N Metatarsal, Right			
P Metatarsal, Left			
Q Toe Phalanx, Right			
R Toe Phalanx, Left			
S Coccyx			
0 Lumbar Vertebra	**0** Open	**Z** No Device	**X** Diagnostic
1 Sacrum	**3** Percutaneous		**Z** No Qualifier
2 Pelvic Bone, Right	**4** Percutaneous Endoscopic		
3 Pelvic Bone, Left			
4 Acetabulum, Right			
5 Acetabulum, Left			
6 Upper Femur, Right			
7 Upper Femur, Left			
8 Femoral Shaft, Right			
9 Femoral Shaft, Left			
B Lower Femur, Right			
C Lower Femur, Left			
D Patella, Right			
F Patella, Left			
G Tibia, Right			
H Tibia, Left			
J Fibula, Right			
K Fibula, Left			
L Tarsal, Right			
M Tarsal, Left			
N Metatarsal, Right			
P Metatarsal, Left			
Q Toe Phalanx, Right			
R Toe Phalanx, Left			
S Coccyx			

LC Limited Coverage   **NC** Noncovered   HAC associated procedure   Combination Only   DRG Non-OR   Non-OR   Revised Text in **GREEN**

334   ICD-10-PCS 2014 (Draft)

0 **Medical and Surgical**
Q **Lower Bones**
B **Excision**   Cutting out or off, without replacement, a portion of a body part

Body Part Character 4	Approach Character 5	Device Character 6	Qualifier Character 7
0 Lumbar Vertebra	0 Open	Z No Device	X Diagnostic
1 Sacrum	3 Percutaneous		Z No Qualifier
2 Pelvic Bone, Right	4 Percutaneous Endoscopic		
3 Pelvic Bone, Left			
4 Acetabulum, Right			
5 Acetabulum, Left			
6 Upper Femur, Right			
7 Upper Femur, Left			
8 Femoral Shaft, Right			
9 Femoral Shaft, Left			
B Lower Femur, Right			
C Lower Femur, Left			
D Patella, Right			
F Patella, Left			
G Tibia, Right			
H Tibia, Left			
J Fibula, Right			
K Fibula, Left			
L Tarsal, Right			
M Tarsal, Left			
N Metatarsal, Right			
P Metatarsal, Left			
Q Toe Phalanx, Right			
R Toe Phalanx, Left			
S Coccyx			

0 **Medical and Surgical**
Q **Lower Bones**
C **Extirpation**   Taking or cutting out solid matter from a body part

Body Part Character 4	Approach Character 5	Device Character 6	Qualifier Character 7
0 Lumbar Vertebra	0 Open	Z No Device	Z No Qualifier
1 Sacrum	3 Percutaneous		
2 Pelvic Bone, Right	4 Percutaneous Endoscopic		
3 Pelvic Bone, Left			
4 Acetabulum, Right			
5 Acetabulum, Left			
6 Upper Femur, Right			
7 Upper Femur, Left			
8 Femoral Shaft, Right			
9 Femoral Shaft, Left			
B Lower Femur, Right			
C Lower Femur, Left			
D Patella, Right			
F Patella, Left			
G Tibia, Right			
H Tibia, Left			
J Fibula, Right			
K Fibula, Left			
L Tarsal, Right			
M Tarsal, Left			
N Metatarsal, Right			
P Metatarsal, Left			
Q Toe Phalanx, Right			
R Toe Phalanx, Left			
S Coccyx			

Ø   Medical and Surgical
Q   Lower Bones
H   Insertion   Putting in a nonbiological appliance that monitors, assists, performs, or prevents a physiological function but does not physically take the place of a body part

Body Part Character 4	Approach Character 5	Device Character 6	Qualifier Character 7
Ø Lumbar Vertebra 1 Sacrum 2 Pelvic Bone, Right 3 Pelvic Bone, Left 4 Acetabulum, Right 5 Acetabulum, Left D Patella, Right F Patella, Left L Tarsal, Right M Tarsal, Left N Metatarsal, Right P Metatarsal, Left Q Toe Phalanx, Right R Toe Phalanx, Left S Coccyx	Ø Open 3 Percutaneous 4 Percutaneous Endoscopic	4 Internal Fixation Device 5 External Fixation Device	Z No Qualifier
6 Upper Femur, Right 7 Upper Femur, Left 8 Femoral Shaft, Right 9 Femoral Shaft, Left B Lower Femur, Right C Lower Femur, Left G Tibia, Right H Tibia, Left J Fibula, Right K Fibula, Left	Ø Open 3 Percutaneous 4 Percutaneous Endoscopic	4 Internal Fixation Device 5 External Fixation Device 6 Internal Fixation Device, Intramedullary 8 External Fixation Device, Limb Lengthening B External Fixation Device, Monoplanar C External Fixation Device, Ring D External Fixation Device, Hybrid	Z No Qualifier
Y Lower Bone	Ø Open 3 Percutaneous 4 Percutaneous Endoscopic	M Bone Growth Stimulator	Z No Qualifier

Non-OR   ØQH[6,7,8,9,B,C,G,H,J,K][Ø,3,4]8Z

Ø   Medical and Surgical
Q   Lower Bones
J   Inspection   Visually and/or manually exploring a body part

Body Part Character 4	Approach Character 5	Device Character 6	Qualifier Character 7
Y Lower Bone	Ø Open 3 Percutaneous 4 Percutaneous Endoscopic X External	Z No Device	Z No Qualifier

Non-OR   ØQJYXZZ

Ø　Medical and Surgical
Q　Lower Bones
N　Release　　Freeing a body part from an abnormal physical constraint

Body Part Character 4	Approach Character 5	Device Character 6	Qualifier Character 7
Ø　Lumbar Vertebra	Ø　Open	Z　No Device	Z　No Qualifier
1　Sacrum	3　Percutaneous		
2　Pelvic Bone, Right	4　Percutaneous Endoscopic		
3　Pelvic Bone, Left			
4　Acetabulum, Right			
5　Acetabulum, Left			
6　Upper Femur, Right			
7　Upper Femur, Left			
8　Femoral Shaft, Right			
9　Femoral Shaft, Left			
B　Lower Femur, Right			
C　Lower Femur, Left			
D　Patella, Right			
F　Patella, Left			
G　Tibia, Right			
H　Tibia, Left			
J　Fibula, Right			
K　Fibula, Left			
L　Tarsal, Right			
M　Tarsal, Left			
N　Metatarsal, Right			
P　Metatarsal, Left			
Q　Toe Phalanx, Right			
R　Toe Phalanx, Left			
S　Coccyx			

Ø　Medical and Surgical
Q　Lower Bones
P　Removal　　Taking out or off a device from a body part

Body Part Character 4	Approach Character 5	Device Character 6	Qualifier Character 7
Ø　Lumbar Vertebra	Ø　Open	4　Internal Fixation Device	Z　No Qualifier
1　Sacrum	3　Percutaneous	7　Autologous Tissue Substitute	
4　Acetabulum, Right	4　Percutaneous Endoscopic	J　Synthetic Substitute	
5　Acetabulum, Left		K　Nonautologous Tissue Substitute	
S　Coccyx			
Ø　Lumbar Vertebra	X　External	4　Internal Fixation Device	Z　No Qualifier
1　Sacrum			
4　Acetabulum, Right			
5　Acetabulum, Left			
S　Coccyx			
2　Pelvic Bone, Right	X　External	4　Internal Fixation Device	Z　No Qualifier
3　Pelvic Bone, Left		5　External Fixation Device	
6　Upper Femur, Right			
7　Upper Femur, Left			
8　Femoral Shaft, Right			
9　Femoral Shaft, Left			
B　Lower Femur, Right			
C　Lower Femur, Left			
D　Patella, Right			
F　Patella, Left			
G　Tibia, Right			
H　Tibia, Left			
J　Fibula, Right			
K　Fibula, Left			
L　Tarsal, Right			
M　Tarsal, Left			
N　Metatarsal, Right			
P　Metatarsal, Left			
Q　Toe Phalanx, Right			
R　Toe Phalanx, Left			

ØQP Continued on next page

Non-OR　ØQP[Ø,1,4,5,S]X4Z
Non-OR　ØQP[2,3,6,7,8,9,B,C,D,F,G,H,J,K,L,M,N,P,Q,R]X[4,5]Z

Ø   Medical and Surgical   ***ØQP Continued***
Q   Lower Bones
P   Removal   Taking out or off a device from a body part

Body Part Character 4	Approach Character 5	Device Character 6	Qualifier Character 7
2 Pelvic Bone, Right 3 Pelvic Bone, Left 6 Upper Femur, Right 7 Upper Femur, Left 8 Femoral Shaft, Right 9 Femoral Shaft, Left B Lower Femur, Right C Lower Femur, Left D Patella, Right F Patella, Left G Tibia, Right H Tibia, Left J Fibula, Right K Fibula, Left L Tarsal, Right M Tarsal, Left N Metatarsal, Right P Metatarsal, Left Q Toe Phalanx, Right R Toe Phalanx, Left	Ø Open 3 Percutaneous 4 Percutaneous Endoscopic	4 Internal Fixation Device 5 External Fixation Device 7 Autologous Tissue Substitute J Synthetic Substitute K Nonautologous Tissue Substitute	Z No Qualifier
Y Lower Bone	Ø Open 3 Percutaneous 4 Percutaneous Endoscopic X External	Ø Drainage Device M Bone Growth Stimulator	Z No Qualifier

Non-OR   ØQPYX[Ø,M]Z

Ø   Medical and Surgical
Q   Lower Bones
Q   Repair   Restoring, to the extent possible, a body part to its normal anatomic structure and function

Body Part Character 4	Approach Character 5	Device Character 6	Qualifier Character 7
Ø Lumbar Vertebra 1 Sacrum 2 Pelvic Bone, Right 3 Pelvic Bone, Left 4 Acetabulum, Right 5 Acetabulum, Left 6 Upper Femur, Right 7 Upper Femur, Left 8 Femoral Shaft, Right 9 Femoral Shaft, Left B Lower Femur, Right C Lower Femur, Left D Patella, Right F Patella, Left G Tibia, Right H Tibia, Left J Fibula, Right K Fibula, Left L Tarsal, Right M Tarsal, Left N Metatarsal, Right P Metatarsal, Left Q Toe Phalanx, Right R Toe Phalanx, Left S Coccyx	Ø Open 3 Percutaneous 4 Percutaneous Endoscopic X External	Z No Device	Z No Qualifier

---

0   **Medical and Surgical**
Q   **Lower Bones**
R   **Replacement**   Putting in or on biological or synthetic material that physically takes the place and/or function of all or a portion of a body part

Body Part Character 4	Approach Character 5	Device Character 6	Qualifier Character 7
0 Lumbar Vertebra	**0** Open	**7** Autologous Tissue Substitute	**Z** No Qualifier
1 Sacrum	**3** Percutaneous	**J** Synthetic Substitute	
2 Pelvic Bone, Right	**4** Percutaneous Endoscopic	**K** Nonautologous Tissue Substitute	
3 Pelvic Bone, Left			
4 Acetabulum, Right			
5 Acetabulum, Left			
6 Upper Femur, Right			
7 Upper Femur, Left			
8 Femoral Shaft, Right			
9 Femoral Shaft, Left			
B Lower Femur, Right			
C Lower Femur, Left			
D Patella, Right			
F Patella, Left			
G Tibia, Right			
H Tibia, Left			
J Fibula, Right			
K Fibula, Left			
L Tarsal, Right			
M Tarsal, Left			
N Metatarsal, Right			
P Metatarsal, Left			
Q Toe Phalanx, Right			
R Toe Phalanx, Left			
S Coccyx			

0   **Medical and Surgical**
Q   **Lower Bones**
S   **Reposition**   Moving to its normal location or other suitable location all or a portion of a body part

Body Part Character 4	Approach Character 5	Device Character 6	Qualifier Character 7
0 Lumbar Vertebra	**0** Open	**4** Internal Fixation Device	**Z** No Qualifier
1 Sacrum	**3** Percutaneous	**Z** No Device	
4 Acetabulum, Right	**4** Percutaneous Endoscopic		
5 Acetabulum, Left			
S Coccyx			
0 Lumbar Vertebra	**X** External	**Z** No Device	**Z** No Qualifier
1 Sacrum			
4 Acetabulum, Right			
5 Acetabulum, Left			
S Coccyx			
2 Pelvic Bone, Right	**0** Open	**4** Internal Fixation Device	**Z** No Qualifier
3 Pelvic Bone, Left	**3** Percutaneous	**5** External Fixation Device	
D Patella, Right	**4** Percutaneous Endoscopic	**Z** No Device	
F Patella, Left			
L Tarsal, Right			
M Tarsal, Left			
N Metatarsal, Right			
P Metatarsal, Left			
Q Toe Phalanx, Right			
R Toe Phalanx, Left			
2 Pelvic Bone, Right	**X** External	**Z** No Device	**Z** No Qualifier
3 Pelvic Bone, Left			
D Patella, Right			
F Patella, Left			
L Tarsal, Right			
M Tarsal, Left			
N Metatarsal, Right			
P Metatarsal, Left			
Q Toe Phalanx, Right			
R Toe Phalanx, Left			

0QS Continued on next page

Non-OR	0QS[0,1]3ZZ
Non-OR	0QS[4,5]XZZ
Non-OR	0QS[2,3,D,F,L,M,N,P,Q,R][3,4]ZZ
Non-OR	0QS[2,3,D,F,L,M,N,P,Q,R]XZZ

LC Limited Coverage   **NC** Noncovered   HAC associated procedure   Combination Only   DRG Non-OR   Non-OR   Revised Text in **GREEN**

ICD-10-PCS 2014 (Draft)   **339**

0   Medical and Surgical   *0QS Continued*
Q   Lower Bones
S   Reposition   Moving to its normal location or other suitable location all or a portion of a body part

Body Part Character 4	Approach Character 5	Device Character 6	Qualifier Character 7

6 Upper Femur, Right
7 Upper Femur, Left
8 Femoral Shaft, Right
9 Femoral Shaft, Left
B Lower Femur, Right
C Lower Femur, Left
G Tibia, Right
H Tibia, Left
J Fibula, Right
K Fibula, Left
	0 Open
	3 Percutaneous
	4 Percutaneous Endoscopic
		4 Internal Fixation Device
		5 External Fixation Device
		6 Internal Fixation Device,
		   Intramedullary
		B External Fixation Device,
		   Monoplanar
		C External Fixation Device, Ring
		D External Fixation Device, Hybrid
		Z No Device
			Z No Qualifier

6 Upper Femur, Right 7 Upper Femur, Left 8 Femoral Shaft, Right 9 Femoral Shaft, Left B Lower Femur, Right C Lower Femur, Left G Tibia, Right H Tibia, Left J Fibula, Right K Fibula, Left	X External	Z No Device	Z No Qualifier

Non-OR   0QS[6,7,8,9,B,C,G,H,J,K][3,4]ZZ
Non-OR   0QS[6,7,8,9,B,C,G,H,J,K]XZZ

0   Medical and Surgical
Q   Lower Bones
T   Resection   Cutting out or off, without replacement, all of a body part

Body Part Character 4	Approach Character 5	Device Character 6	Qualifier Character 7
2 Pelvic Bone, Right 3 Pelvic Bone, Left 4 Acetabulum, Right 5 Acetabulum, Left 6 Upper Femur, Right 7 Upper Femur, Left 8 Femoral Shaft, Right 9 Femoral Shaft, Left B Lower Femur, Right C Lower Femur, Left D Patella, Right F Patella, Left G Tibia, Right H Tibia, Left J Fibula, Right K Fibula, Left L Tarsal, Right M Tarsal, Left N Metatarsal, Right P Metatarsal, Left Q Toe Phalanx, Right R Toe Phalanx, Left S Coccyx	0 Open	Z No Device	Z No Qualifier

0   **Medical and Surgical**
Q   **Lower Bones**
U   **Supplement**   Putting in or on biological or synthetic material that physically reinforces and/or augments the function of a portion of a body part

Body Part Character 4	Approach Character 5	Device Character 6	Qualifier Character 7
0 Lumbar Vertebra **1** Sacrum **2** Pelvic Bone, Right **3** Pelvic Bone, Left **4** Acetabulum, Right **5** Acetabulum, Left **6** Upper Femur, Right **7** Upper Femur, Left **8** Femoral Shaft, Right **9** Femoral Shaft, Left **B** Lower Femur, Right **C** Lower Femur, Left **D** Patella, Right **F** Patella, Left **G** Tibia, Right **H** Tibia, Left **J** Fibula, Right **K** Fibula, Left **L** Tarsal, Right **M** Tarsal, Left **N** Metatarsal, Right **P** Metatarsal, Left **Q** Toe Phalanx, Right **R** Toe Phalanx, Left **S** Coccyx	**0** Open **3** Percutaneous **4** Percutaneous Endoscopic	**7** Autologous Tissue Substitute **J** Synthetic Substitute **K** Nonautologous Tissue Substitute	**Z** No Qualifier

0   **Medical and Surgical**
Q   **Lower Bones**
W   **Revision**   Correcting, to the extent possible, a portion of a malfunctioning device or the position of a displaced device

Body Part Character 4	Approach Character 5	Device Character 6	Qualifier Character 7
0 Lumbar Vertebra **1** Sacrum **4** Acetabulum, Right **5** Acetabulum, Left **S** Coccyx	**0** Open **3** Percutaneous **4** Percutaneous Endoscopic **X** External	**4** Internal Fixation Device **7** Autologous Tissue Substitute **J** Synthetic Substitute **K** Nonautologous Tissue Substitute	**Z** No Qualifier
2 Pelvic Bone, Right **3** Pelvic Bone, Left **6** Upper Femur, Right **7** Upper Femur, Left **8** Femoral Shaft, Right **9** Femoral Shaft, Left **B** Lower Femur, Right **C** Lower Femur, Left **D** Patella, Right **F** Patella, Left **G** Tibia, Right **H** Tibia, Left **J** Fibula, Right **K** Fibula, Left **L** Tarsal, Right **M** Tarsal, Left **N** Metatarsal, Right **P** Metatarsal, Left **Q** Toe Phalanx, Right **R** Toe Phalanx, Left	**0** Open **3** Percutaneous **4** Percutaneous Endoscopic **X** External	**4** Internal Fixation Device **5** External Fixation Device **7** Autologous Tissue Substitute **J** Synthetic Substitute **K** Nonautologous Tissue Substitute	**Z** No Qualifier
Y Lower Bone	**0** Open **3** Percutaneous **4** Percutaneous Endoscopic **X** External	**0** Drainage Device **M** Bone Growth Stimulator	**Z** No Qualifier

Non-OR   0QW[0,1,4,5,S]X[4,7,J,K]Z
Non-OR   0QW[2,3,6,7,8,9,B,C,D,F,G,H,J,K,L,M,N,P,Q,R]X[4,5,7,J,K]Z
Non-OR   0QWYX[0,M]Z

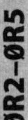

Upper Joints

Upper Joints ØR2–ØRW

Ø **Medical and Surgical**
R **Upper Joints**
2 **Change** Taking out or off a device from a body part and putting back an identical or similar device in or on the same body part without cutting or puncturing the skin or a mucous membrane

Body Part Character 4	Approach Character 5	Device Character 6	Qualifier Character 7
Y Upper Joint	X External	Ø Drainage Device Y Other Device	Z No Qualifier

Non-OR For all body part, approach, device, and qualifier values

Ø **Medical and Surgical**
R **Upper Joints**
5 **Destruction** Physical eradication of all or a portion of a body part by the direct use of energy, force, or a destructive agent

Body Part Character 4	Approach Character 5	Device Character 6	Qualifier Character 7
Ø Occipital-cervical Joint 1 Cervical Vertebral Joint 3 Cervical Vertebral Disc 4 Cervicothoracic Vertebral Joint 5 Cervicothoracic Vertebral Disc 6 Thoracic Vertebral Joint 9 Thoracic Vertebral Disc A Thoracolumbar Vertebral Joint B Thoracolumbar Vertebral Disc C Temporomandibular Joint, Right D Temporomandibular Joint, Left E Sternoclavicular Joint, Right F Sternoclavicular Joint, Left G Acromioclavicular Joint, Right H Acromioclavicular Joint, Left J Shoulder Joint, Right K Shoulder Joint, Left L Elbow Joint, Right M Elbow Joint, Left N Wrist Joint, Right P Wrist Joint, Left Q Carpal Joint, Right R Carpal Joint, Left S Metacarpocarpal Joint, Right T Metacarpocarpal Joint, Left U Metacarpophalangeal Joint, Right V Metacarpophalangeal Joint, Left W Finger Phalangeal Joint, Right X Finger Phalangeal Joint, Left	Ø Open 3 Percutaneous 4 Percutaneous Endoscopic	Z No Device	Z No Qualifier

Non-OR ØR5[3,5,9,B][3,4]ZZ

ØR2–ØR5

Upper Joints

0R9–0R9

0   **Medical and Surgical**
R   **Upper Joints**
9   **Drainage**   Taking or letting out fluids and/or gases from a body part

Body Part Character 4	Approach Character 5	Device Character 6	Qualifier Character 7
0 Occipital-cervical Joint	0 Open	0 Drainage Device	Z No Qualifier
1 Cervical Vertebral Joint	3 Percutaneous		
3 Cervical Vertebral Disc	4 Percutaneous Endoscopic		
4 Cervicothoracic Vertebral Joint			
5 Cervicothoracic Vertebral Disc			
6 Thoracic Vertebral Joint			
9 Thoracic Vertebral Disc			
A Thoracolumbar Vertebral Joint			
B Thoracolumbar Vertebral Disc			
C Temporomandibular Joint, Right			
D Temporomandibular Joint, Left			
E Sternoclavicular Joint, Right			
F Sternoclavicular Joint, Left			
G Acromioclavicular Joint, Right			
H Acromioclavicular Joint, Left			
J Shoulder Joint, Right			
K Shoulder Joint, Left			
L Elbow Joint, Right			
M Elbow Joint, Left			
N Wrist Joint, Right			
P Wrist Joint, Left			
Q Carpal Joint, Right			
R Carpal Joint, Left			
S Metacarpocarpal Joint, Right			
T Metacarpocarpal Joint, Left			
U Metacarpophalangeal Joint, Right			
V Metacarpophalangeal Joint, Left			
W Finger Phalangeal Joint, Right			
X Finger Phalangeal Joint, Left			
0 Occipital-cervical Joint	0 Open	Z No Device	X Diagnostic
1 Cervical Vertebral Joint	3 Percutaneous		Z No Qualifier
3 Cervical Vertebral Disc	4 Percutaneous Endoscopic		
4 Cervicothoracic Vertebral Joint			
5 Cervicothoracic Vertebral Disc			
6 Thoracic Vertebral Joint			
9 Thoracic Vertebral Disc			
A Thoracolumbar Vertebral Joint			
B Thoracolumbar Vertebral Disc			
C Temporomandibular Joint, Right			
D Temporomandibular Joint, Left			
E Sternoclavicular Joint, Right			
F Sternoclavicular Joint, Left			
G Acromioclavicular Joint, Right			
H Acromioclavicular Joint, Left			
J Shoulder Joint, Right			
K Shoulder Joint, Left			
L Elbow Joint, Right			
M Elbow Joint, Left			
N Wrist Joint, Right			
P Wrist Joint, Left			
Q Carpal Joint, Right			
R Carpal Joint, Left			
S Metacarpocarpal Joint, Right			
T Metacarpocarpal Joint, Left			
U Metacarpophalangeal Joint, Right			
V Metacarpophalangeal Joint, Left			
W Finger Phalangeal Joint, Right			
X Finger Phalangeal Joint, Left			

Non-OR   0R9[0,1,3,4,5,6,9,A,B,E,F,G,H,J,K,L,M,N,P,Q,R,S,T,U,V,W,X][3,4]0Z
Non-OR   0R9[0,1,3,4,5,6,9,A,B,E,F,G,H,J,K,L,M,N,P,Q,R,S,T,U,V,W,X][0,3,4]ZX

Upper Joints

Ø   Medical and Surgical
R   Upper Joints
B   Excision   Cutting out or off, without replacement, a portion of a body part

Body Part Character 4	Approach Character 5	Device Character 6	Qualifier Character 7
Ø Occipital-cervical Joint	Ø Open	Z No Device	X Diagnostic
1 Cervical Vertebral Joint	3 Percutaneous		Z No Qualifier
3 Cervical Vertebral Disc	4 Percutaneous Endoscopic		
4 Cervicothoracic Vertebral Joint			
5 Cervicothoracic Vertebral Disc			
6 Thoracic Vertebral Joint			
9 Thoracic Vertebral Disc			
A Thoracolumbar Vertebral Joint			
B Thoracolumbar Vertebral Disc			
C Temporomandibular Joint, Right			
D Temporomandibular Joint, Left			
E Sternoclavicular Joint, Right			
F Sternoclavicular Joint, Left			
G Acromioclavicular Joint, Right			
H Acromioclavicular Joint, Left			
J Shoulder Joint, Right			
K Shoulder Joint, Left			
L Elbow Joint, Right			
M Elbow Joint, Left			
N Wrist Joint, Right			
P Wrist Joint, Left			
Q Carpal Joint, Right			
R Carpal Joint, Left			
S Metacarpocarpal Joint, Right			
T Metacarpocarpal Joint, Left			
U Metacarpophalangeal Joint, Right			
V Metacarpophalangeal Joint, Left			
W Finger Phalangeal Joint, Right			
X Finger Phalangeal Joint, Left			

Non-OR   ØRB[Ø,1,3,4,5,6,9,A,B,E,F,G,H,J,K,L,M,N,P,Q,R,S,T,U,V,W,X][Ø,3,4]ZX

Ø   Medical and Surgical
R   Upper Joints
C   Extirpation   Taking or cutting out solid matter from a body part

Body Part Character 4	Approach Character 5	Device Character 6	Qualifier Character 7
Ø Occipital-cervical Joint	Ø Open	Z No Device	Z No Qualifier
1 Cervical Vertebral Joint	3 Percutaneous		
3 Cervical Vertebral Disc	4 Percutaneous Endoscopic		
4 Cervicothoracic Vertebral Joint			
5 Cervicothoracic Vertebral Disc			
6 Thoracic Vertebral Joint			
9 Thoracic Vertebral Disc			
A Thoracolumbar Vertebral Joint			
B Thoracolumbar Vertebral Disc			
C Temporomandibular Joint, Right			
D Temporomandibular Joint, Left			
E Sternoclavicular Joint, Right			
F Sternoclavicular Joint, Left			
G Acromioclavicular Joint, Right			
H Acromioclavicular Joint, Left			
J Shoulder Joint, Right			
K Shoulder Joint, Left			
L Elbow Joint, Right			
M Elbow Joint, Left			
N Wrist Joint, Right			
P Wrist Joint, Left			
Q Carpal Joint, Right			
R Carpal Joint, Left			
S Metacarpocarpal Joint, Right			
T Metacarpocarpal Joint, Left			
U Metacarpophalangeal Joint, Right			
V Metacarpophalangeal Joint, Left			
W Finger Phalangeal Joint, Right			
X Finger Phalangeal Joint, Left			

Ø **Medical and Surgical**
R **Upper Joints**
G **Fusion**　　Joining together portions of an articular body part rendering the articular body part immobile

Body Part Character 4	Approach Character 5	Device Character 6	Qualifier Character 7
Ø Occipital-cervical Joint **1** Cervical Vertebral Joint **2** Cervical Vertebral Joints, 2 or more **4** Cervicothoracic Vertebral Joint **6** Thoracic Vertebral Joint **7** Thoracic Vertebral Joints, 2 to 7 **8** Thoracic Vertebral Joints, 8 or more **A** Thoracolumbar Vertebral Joint	**Ø** Open **3** Percutaneous **4** Percutaneous Endoscopic	**7** Autologous Tissue Substitute **A** Interbody Fusion Device **J** Synthetic Substitute **K** Nonautologous Tissue Substitute **Z** No Device	**Ø** Anterior Approach, Anterior Column **1** Posterior Approach, Posterior Column **J** Posterior Approach, Anterior Column
C Temporomandibular Joint, Right **D** Temporomandibular Joint, Left **E** Sternoclavicular Joint, Right **F** Sternoclavicular Joint, Left **G** Acromioclavicular Joint, Right **H** Acromioclavicular Joint, Left **J** Shoulder Joint, Right **K** Shoulder Joint, Left	**Ø** Open **3** Percutaneous **4** Percutaneous Endoscopic	**4** Internal Fixation Device **7** Autologous Tissue Substitute **J** Synthetic Substitute **K** Nonautologous Tissue Substitute **Z** No Device	**Z** No Qualifier
L Elbow Joint, Right **M** Elbow Joint, Left **N** Wrist Joint, Right **P** Wrist Joint, Left **Q** Carpal Joint, Right **R** Carpal Joint, Left **S** Metacarpocarpal Joint, Right **T** Metacarpocarpal Joint, Left **U** Metacarpophalangeal Joint, Right **V** Metacarpophalangeal Joint, Left **W** Finger Phalangeal Joint, Right **X** Finger Phalangeal Joint, Left	**Ø** Open **3** Percutaneous **4** Percutaneous Endoscopic	**4** Internal Fixation Device **5** External Fixation Device **7** Autologous Tissue Substitute **J** Synthetic Substitute **K** Nonautologous Tissue Substitute **Z** No Device	**Z** No Qualifier

HAC ØRG[Ø,1,2,4,6,7,8,A][Ø,3,4][7,A,J,K,Z][Ø,1,J] when reported with SDx K68.11 or T81.4XXA or T81.6Ø-T84.7 with 7th character A
HAC ØRG[E,F,G,H,J,K][Ø,3,4][4,7,J,K,Z]Z when reported with SDx K68.11 or T81.4XXA or T81.6Ø-T84.7 with 7th character A
HAC ØRG[L,M][Ø,3,4][4,5,7,J,K,Z]Z when reported with SDx K68.11 or T81.4XXA or T81.6Ø-T84.7 with 7th character A

Ø **Medical and Surgical**
R **Upper Joints**
H **Insertion**　　Putting in a nonbiological appliance that monitors, assists, performs, or prevents a physiological function but does not physically take the place of a body part

Body Part Character 4	Approach Character 5	Device Character 6	Qualifier Character 7
Ø Occipital-cervical Joint **1** Cervical Vertebral Joint **4** Cervicothoracic Vertebral Joint **6** Thoracic Vertebral Joint **A** Thoracolumbar Vertebral Joint	**Ø** Open **3** Percutaneous **4** Percutaneous Endoscopic	**3** Infusion Device **4** Internal Fixation Device **8** Spacer **B** Spinal Stabilization Device, Interspinous Process **C** Spinal Stabilization Device, Pedicle-Based **D** Spinal Stabilization Device, Facet Replacement	**Z** No Qualifier
3 Cervical Vertebral Disc **5** Cervicothoracic Vertebral Disc **9** Thoracic Vertebral Disc **B** Thoracolumbar Vertebral Disc	**Ø** Open **3** Percutaneous **4** Percutaneous Endoscopic	**3** Infusion Device	**Z** No Qualifier
C Temporomandibular Joint, Right **D** Temporomandibular Joint, Left **E** Sternoclavicular Joint, Right **F** Sternoclavicular Joint, Left **G** Acromioclavicular Joint, Right **H** Acromioclavicular Joint, Left **J** Shoulder Joint, Right **K** Shoulder Joint, Left	**Ø** Open **3** Percutaneous **4** Percutaneous Endoscopic	**3** Infusion Device **4** Internal Fixation Device **8** Spacer	**Z** No Qualifier

ØRH Continued on next page

Non-OR ØRH[Ø,1,4,5,6,A][Ø,3,4][3,8]Z
Non-OR ØRH[3,5,9,B][Ø,3,4]3Z
Non-OR ØRH[E,F,G,H,J,K][Ø,3,4][3,8]Z
Non-OR ØRH[C,D][Ø,3,4]8Z

Upper Joints

ØRH Continued

Ø **Medical and Surgical**
R **Upper Joints**
H **Insertion**   Putting in a nonbiological appliance that monitors, assists, performs, or prevents a physiological function but does not physically take the place of a body part

Body Part Character 4	Approach Character 5	Device Character 6	Qualifier Character 7
L Elbow Joint, Right M Elbow Joint, Left N Wrist Joint, Right P Wrist Joint, Left Q Carpal Joint, Right R Carpal Joint, Left S Metacarpocarpal Joint, Right T Metacarpocarpal Joint, Left U Metacarpophalangeal Joint, Right V Metacarpophalangeal Joint, Left W Finger Phalangeal Joint, Right X Finger Phalangeal Joint, Left	Ø Open 3 Percutaneous 4 Percutaneous Endoscopic	3 Infusion Device 4 Internal Fixation Device 5 External Fixation Device 8 Spacer	Z No Qualifier

Non-OR   ØRH[L,M,N,P,Q,R,S,T,U,V,W,X][Ø,3,4][3,8]Z

Ø **Medical and Surgical**
R **Upper Joints**
J **Inspection**   Visually and/or manually exploring a body part

Body Part Character 4	Approach Character 5	Device Character 6	Qualifier Character 7
Ø Occipital-cervical Joint 1 Cervical Vertebral Joint 3 Cervical Vertebral Disc 4 Cervicothoracic Vertebral Joint 5 Cervicothoracic Vertebral Disc 6 Thoracic Vertebral Joint 9 Thoracic Vertebral Disc A Thoracolumbar Vertebral Joint B Thoracolumbar Vertebral Disc C Temporomandibular Joint, Right D Temporomandibular Joint, Left E Sternoclavicular Joint, Right F Sternoclavicular Joint, Left G Acromioclavicular Joint, Right H Acromioclavicular Joint, Left J Shoulder Joint, Right K Shoulder Joint, Left L Elbow Joint, Right M Elbow Joint, Left N Wrist Joint, Right P Wrist Joint, Left Q Carpal Joint, Right R Carpal Joint, Left S Metacarpocarpal Joint, Right T Metacarpocarpal Joint, Left U Metacarpophalangeal Joint, Right V Metacarpophalangeal Joint, Left W Finger Phalangeal Joint, Right X Finger Phalangeal Joint, Left	Ø Open 3 Percutaneous 4 Percutaneous Endoscopic X External	Z No Device	Z No Qualifier

Non-OR   ØRJ[Ø,1,3,4,5,6,9,A,B,C,D,E,F,G,H,J,K,L,M,N,P,Q,R,S,T,U,V,W,X]XZZ

Ø Medical and Surgical
R Upper Joints
N Release   Freeing a body part from an abnormal physical constraint

Body Part Character 4	Approach Character 5	Device Character 6	Qualifier Character 7
Ø Occipital-cervical Joint	**Ø** Open	**Z** No Device	**Z** No Qualifier
1 Cervical Vertebral Joint	**3** Percutaneous		
3 Cervical Vertebral Disc	**4** Percutaneous Endoscopic		
4 Cervicothoracic Vertebral Joint	**X** External		
5 Cervicothoracic Vertebral Disc			
6 Thoracic Vertebral Joint			
9 Thoracic Vertebral Disc			
A Thoracolumbar Vertebral Joint			
B Thoracolumbar Vertebral Disc			
C Temporomandibular Joint, Right			
D Temporomandibular Joint, Left			
E Sternoclavicular Joint, Right			
F Sternoclavicular Joint, Left			
G Acromioclavicular Joint, Right			
H Acromioclavicular Joint, Left			
J Shoulder Joint, Right			
K Shoulder Joint, Left			
L Elbow Joint, Right			
M Elbow Joint, Left			
N Wrist Joint, Right			
P Wrist Joint, Left			
Q Carpal Joint, Right			
R Carpal Joint, Left			
S Metacarpocarpal Joint, Right			
T Metacarpocarpal Joint, Left			
U Metacarpophalangeal Joint, Right			
V Metacarpophalangeal Joint, Left			
W Finger Phalangeal Joint, Right			
X Finger Phalangeal Joint, Left			

Non-OR ØRN[Ø,1,3,4,5,6,9,A,B,C,D,E,F,G,H,J,K,L,M,N,P,Q,R,S,T,U,V,W,X]XZZ

Ø Medical and Surgical
R Upper Joints
P Removal   Taking out or off a device from a body part

Body Part Character 4	Approach Character 5	Device Character 6	Qualifier Character 7
Ø Occipital-cervical Joint	**Ø** Open	**Ø** Drainage Device	**Z** No Qualifier
1 Cervical Vertebral Joint	**3** Percutaneous	**3** Infusion Device	
4 Cervicothoracic Vertebral Joint	**4** Percutaneous Endoscopic	**4** Internal Fixation Device	
6 Thoracic Vertebral Joint		**7** Autologous Tissue Substitute	
A Thoracolumbar Vertebral Joint		**8** Spacer	
C Temporomandibular Joint, Right		**A** Interbody Fusion Device	
D Temporomandibular Joint, Left		**J** Synthetic Substitute	
E Sternoclavicular Joint, Right		**K** Nonautologous Tissue Substitute	
F Sternoclavicular Joint, Left			
G Acromioclavicular Joint, Right			
H Acromioclavicular Joint, Left			
J Shoulder Joint, Right			
K Shoulder Joint, Left			
Ø Occipital-cervical Joint	**X** External	**Ø** Drainage Device	**Z** No Qualifier
1 Cervical Vertebral Joint		**3** Infusion Device	
4 Cervicothoracic Vertebral Joint		**4** Internal Fixation Device	
6 Thoracic Vertebral Joint			
A Thoracolumbar Vertebral Joint			
C Temporomandibular Joint, Right			
D Temporomandibular Joint, Left			
E Sternoclavicular Joint, Right			
F Sternoclavicular Joint, Left			
G Acromioclavicular Joint, Right			
H Acromioclavicular Joint, Left			
J Shoulder Joint, Right			
K Shoulder Joint, Left			

ØRP Continued on next page

Non-OR ØRP[Ø,1,4,6,A,C,D,E,F,G,H,J,K][Ø,3,4]8Z
Non-OR ØRP[Ø,1,4,6,A,C,D,E,F,G,H,J,K]X[Ø,3,4]Z

ØRN—ØRP

LC Limited Coverage   NC Noncovered   HAC associated procedure   Combination Only   DRG Non-OR   Non-OR   Revised Text in **GREEN**

Ø Medical and Surgical
R Upper Joints
P Removal — Taking out or off a device from a body part

ØRP Continued

Body Part Character 4	Approach Character 5	Device Character 6	Qualifier Character 7
3 Cervical Vertebral Disc **5** Cervicothoracic Vertebral Disc **9** Thoracic Vertebral Disc **B** Thoracolumbar Vertebral Disc	**Ø** Open **3** Percutaneous **4** Percutaneous Endoscopic	**Ø** Drainage Device **3** Infusion Device **7** Autologous Tissue Substitute **J** Synthetic Substitute **K** Nonautologous Tissue Substitute	**Z** No Qualifier
3 Cervical Vertebral Disc **5** Cervicothoracic Vertebral Disc **9** Thoracic Vertebral Disc **B** Thoracolumbar Vertebral Disc	**X** External	**Ø** Drainage Device **3** Infusion Device	**Z** No Qualifier
L Elbow Joint, Right **M** Elbow Joint, Left **N** Wrist Joint, Right **P** Wrist Joint, Left **Q** Carpal Joint, Right **R** Carpal Joint, Left **S** Metacarpocarpal Joint, Right **T** Metacarpocarpal Joint, Left **U** Metacarpophalangeal Joint, Right **V** Metacarpophalangeal Joint, Left **W** Finger Phalangeal Joint, Right **X** Finger Phalangeal Joint, Left	**Ø** Open **3** Percutaneous **4** Percutaneous Endoscopic	**Ø** Drainage Device **3** Infusion Device **4** Internal Fixation Device **5** External Fixation Device **7** Autologous Tissue Substitute **8** Spacer **J** Synthetic Substitute **K** Nonautologous Tissue Substitute	**Z** No Qualifier
L Elbow Joint, Right **M** Elbow Joint, Left **N** Wrist Joint, Right **P** Wrist Joint, Left **Q** Carpal Joint, Right **R** Carpal Joint, Left **S** Metacarpocarpal Joint, Right **T** Metacarpocarpal Joint, Left **U** Metacarpophalangeal Joint, Right **V** Metacarpophalangeal Joint, Left **W** Finger Phalangeal Joint, Right **X** Finger Phalangeal Joint, Left	**X** External	**Ø** Drainage Device **3** Infusion Device **4** Internal Fixation Device **5** External Fixation Device	**Z** No Qualifier

Non-OR ØRP[3,5,9,B]X[Ø,3]Z
Non-OR ØRP[L,M,N,P,Q,R,S,T,U,V,W,X][Ø,3,4]8Z
Non-OR ØRP[L,M,N,P,Q,R,S,T,U,V,W,X]X[Ø,3,4,5]Z

Ø Medical and Surgical
R Upper Joints
Q Repair — Restoring, to the extent possible, a body part to its normal anatomic structure and function

Body Part Character 4	Approach Character 5	Device Character 6	Qualifier Character 7
Ø Occipital-cervical Joint **1** Cervical Vertebral Joint **3** Cervical Vertebral Disc **4** Cervicothoracic Vertebral Joint **5** Cervicothoracic Vertebral Disc **6** Thoracic Vertebral Joint **9** Thoracic Vertebral Disc **A** Thoracolumbar Vertebral Joint **B** Thoracolumbar Vertebral Disc **C** Temporomandibular Joint, Right **D** Temporomandibular Joint, Left **E** Sternoclavicular Joint, Right **F** Sternoclavicular Joint, Left **G** Acromioclavicular Joint, Right **H** Acromioclavicular Joint, Left **J** Shoulder Joint, Right **K** Shoulder Joint, Left **L** Elbow Joint, Right **M** Elbow Joint, Left **N** Wrist Joint, Right **P** Wrist Joint, Left **Q** Carpal Joint, Right **R** Carpal Joint, Left **S** Metacarpocarpal Joint, Right **T** Metacarpocarpal Joint, Left **U** Metacarpophalangeal Joint, Right **V** Metacarpophalangeal Joint, Left **W** Finger Phalangeal Joint, Right **X** Finger Phalangeal Joint, Left	**Ø** Open **3** Percutaneous **4** Percutaneous Endoscopic **X** External	**Z** No Device	**Z** No Qualifier

Non-OR ØRQ[C,D]XZZ
HAC ØRQ[E,F,G,H,J,K,L,M][Ø,3,4,X]ZZ when reported with SDx K68.11 or T81.4XXA or T81.6Ø-T84.7 with 7th character A

LC Limited Coverage   NC Noncovered   HAC associated procedure   Combination Only   DRG Non-OR   Non-OR   Revised Text in **GREEN**

ICD-1Ø-PCS 2Ø14 (Draft)

Ø   **Medical and Surgical**
R   **Upper Joints**
R   **Replacement**   Putting in or on biological or synthetic material that physically takes the place and/or function of all or a portion of a body part

Body Part Character 4	Approach Character 5	Device Character 6	Qualifier Character 7
Ø Occipital-cervical Joint **1** Cervical Vertebral Joint **3** Cervical Vertebral Disc **4** Cervicothoracic Vertebral Joint **5** Cervicothoracic Vertebral Disc **6** Thoracic Vertebral Joint **9** Thoracic Vertebral Disc **A** Thoracolumbar Vertebral Joint **B** Thoracolumbar Vertebral Disc **C** Temporomandibular Joint, Right **D** Temporomandibular Joint, Left **E** Sternoclavicular Joint, Right **F** Sternoclavicular Joint, Left **G** Acromioclavicular Joint, Right **H** Acromioclavicular Joint, Left **L** Elbow Joint, Right **M** Elbow Joint, Left **N** Wrist Joint, Right **P** Wrist Joint, Left **Q** Carpal Joint, Right **R** Carpal Joint, Left **S** Metacarpocarpal Joint, Right **T** Metacarpocarpal Joint, Left **U** Metacarpophalangeal Joint, Right **V** Metacarpophalangeal Joint, Left **W** Finger Phalangeal Joint, Right **X** Finger Phalangeal Joint, Left	**Ø** Open	**7** Autologous Tissue Substitute **J** Synthetic Substitute **K** Nonautologous Tissue Substitute	**Z** No Qualifier
J Shoulder Joint, Right **K** Shoulder Joint, Left	**Ø** Open	**Ø** Synthetic Substitute, Reverse Ball and Socket **7** Autologous Tissue Substitute **K** Nonautologous Tissue Substitute	**Z** No Qualifier
J Shoulder Joint, Right **K** Shoulder Joint, Left	**Ø** Open	**J** Synthetic Substitute	**6** Humeral Surface **7** Glenoid Surface **Z** No Qualifier

Ø   **Medical and Surgical**
R   **Upper Joints**
S   **Reposition**   Moving to its normal location or other suitable location all or a portion of a body part

Body Part Character 4	Approach Character 5	Device Character 6	Qualifier Character 7
Ø Occipital-cervical Joint **1** Cervical Vertebral Joint **4** Cervicothoracic Vertebral Joint **6** Thoracic Vertebral Joint **A** Thoracolumbar Vertebral Joint **C** Temporomandibular Joint, Right **D** Temporomandibular Joint, Left **E** Sternoclavicular Joint, Right **F** Sternoclavicular Joint, Left **G** Acromioclavicular Joint, Right **H** Acromioclavicular Joint, Left **J** Shoulder Joint, Right **K** Shoulder Joint, Left	**Ø** Open **3** Percutaneous **4** Percutaneous Endoscopic **X** External	**4** Internal Fixation Device **Z** No Device	**Z** No Qualifier
L Elbow Joint, Right **M** Elbow Joint, Left **N** Wrist Joint, Right **P** Wrist Joint, Left **Q** Carpal Joint, Right **R** Carpal Joint, Left **S** Metacarpocarpal Joint, Right **T** Metacarpocarpal Joint, Left **U** Metacarpophalangeal Joint, Right **V** Metacarpophalangeal Joint, Left **W** Finger Phalangeal Joint, Right **X** Finger Phalangeal Joint, Left	**Ø** Open **3** Percutaneous **4** Percutaneous Endoscopic **X** External	**4** Internal Fixation Device **5** External Fixation Device **Z** No Device	**Z** No Qualifier

Non-OR   ØRS[Ø,1,4,6,A,C,D,E,F,G,H,J,K][3,4,X][4,Z]Z
Non-OR   ØRS[L,M,N,P,Q,R,S,T,U,V,W,X][3,4,X][4,5,Z]Z

LC Limited Coverage   NC Noncovered   HAC associated procedure   Combination Only   DRG Non-OR   Non-OR   Revised Text in GREEN
ICD-10-PCS 2014 (Draft)   349

ØRR—ØRS

Ø   **Medical and Surgical**
R   **Upper Joints**
T   **Resection**   Cutting out or off, without replacement, all of a body part

Body Part Character 4	Approach Character 5	Device Character 6	Qualifier Character 7
3 Cervical Vertebral Disc	**Ø** Open	**Z** No Device	**Z** No Qualifier
4 Cervicothoracic Vertebral Joint			
5 Cervicothoracic Vertebral Disc			
9 Thoracic Vertebral Disc			
B Thoracolumbar Vertebral Disc			
C Temporomandibular Joint, Right			
D Temporomandibular Joint, Left			
E Sternoclavicular Joint, Right			
F Sternoclavicular Joint, Left			
G Acromioclavicular Joint, Right			
H Acromioclavicular Joint, Left			
J Shoulder Joint, Right			
K Shoulder Joint, Left			
L Elbow Joint, Right			
M Elbow Joint, Left			
N Wrist Joint, Right			
P Wrist Joint, Left			
Q Carpal Joint, Right			
R Carpal Joint, Left			
S Metacarpocarpal Joint, Right			
T Metacarpocarpal Joint, Left			
U Metacarpophalangeal Joint, Right			
V Metacarpophalangeal Joint, Left			
W Finger Phalangeal Joint, Right			
X Finger Phalangeal Joint, Left			

Ø   **Medical and Surgical**
R   **Upper Joints**
U   **Supplement**   Putting in or on biological or synthetic material that physically reinforces and/or augments the function of a portion of a body part

Body Part Character 4	Approach Character 5	Device Character 6	Qualifier Character 7
Ø Occipital-cervical Joint	**Ø** Open	**7** Autologous Tissue Substitute	**Z** No Qualifier
1 Cervical Vertebral Joint	**3** Percutaneous	**J** Synthetic Substitute	
3 Cervical Vertebral Disc	**4** Percutaneous Endoscopic	**K** Nonautologous Tissue Substitute	
4 Cervicothoracic Vertebral Joint			
5 Cervicothoracic Vertebral Disc			
6 Thoracic Vertebral Joint			
9 Thoracic Vertebral Disc			
A Thoracolumbar Vertebral Joint			
B Thoracolumbar Vertebral Disc			
C Temporomandibular Joint, Right			
D Temporomandibular Joint, Left			
E Sternoclavicular Joint, Right			
F Sternoclavicular Joint, Left			
G Acromioclavicular Joint, Right			
H Acromioclavicular Joint, Left			
J Shoulder Joint, Right			
K Shoulder Joint, Left			
L Elbow Joint, Right			
M Elbow Joint, Left			
N Wrist Joint, Right			
P Wrist Joint, Left			
Q Carpal Joint, Right			
R Carpal Joint, Left			
S Metacarpocarpal Joint, Right			
T Metacarpocarpal Joint, Left			
U Metacarpophalangeal Joint, Right			
V Metacarpophalangeal Joint, Left			
W Finger Phalangeal			
X Finger Phalangeal Joint, Left			

HAC   ØRU[E,F,G,H,J,K,L,M][Ø,3,4][7,J,K]Z when reported with SDx K68.11 or T81.4XXA or T81.6Ø-T84.7 with 7th character A

LC Limited Coverage   **NC** Noncovered   HAC associated procedure   Combination Only   DRG Non-OR   Non-OR   Revised Text in **GREEN**

350   ICD-10-PCS 2014 (Draft)

Ø   **Medical and Surgical**
R   **Upper Joints**
W   **Revision**   Correcting, to the extent possible, a portion of a malfunctioning device or the position of a displaced device

Body Part Character 4	Approach Character 5	Device Character 6	Qualifier Character 7
Ø Occipital-cervical Joint **1** Cervical Vertebral Joint **4** Cervicothoracic Vertebral Joint **6** Thoracic Vertebral Joint **A** Thoracolumbar Vertebral Joint	**Ø** Open **3** Percutaneous **4** Percutaneous Endoscopic **X** External	**Ø** Drainage Device **3** Infusion Device **4** Internal Fixation Device **7** Autologous Tissue Substitute **8** Spacer **A** Interbody Fusion Device **J** Synthetic Substitute **K** Nonautologous Tissue Substitute	**Z** No Qualifier
3 Cervical Vertebral Disc **5** Cervicothoracic Vertebral Disc **9** Thoracic Vertebral Disc **B** Thoracolumbar Vertebral Disc	**Ø** Open **3** Percutaneous **4** Percutaneous Endoscopic **X** External	**Ø** Drainage Device **3** Infusion Device **7** Autologous Tissue Substitute **J** Synthetic Substitute **K** Nonautologous Tissue Substitute	**Z** No Qualifier
C Temporomandibular Joint, Right **D** Temporomandibular Joint, Left **E** Sternoclavicular Joint, Right **F** Sternoclavicular Joint, Left **G** Acromioclavicular Joint, Right **H** Acromioclavicular Joint, Left **J** Shoulder Joint, Right **K** Shoulder Joint, Left	**Ø** Open **3** Percutaneous **4** Percutaneous Endoscopic **X** External	**Ø** Drainage Device **3** Infusion Device **4** Internal Fixation Device **5** External Fixation Device **7** Autologous Tissue Substitute **8** Spacer **J** Synthetic Substitute **K** Nonautologous Tissue Substitute	**Z** No Qualifier
L Elbow Joint, Right **M** Elbow Joint, Left **N** Wrist Joint, Right **P** Wrist Joint, Left **Q** Carpal Joint, Right **R** Carpal Joint, Left **S** Metacarpocarpal Joint, Right **T** Metacarpocarpal Joint, Left **U** Metacarpophalangeal Joint, Right **V** Metacarpophalangeal Joint, Left **W** Finger Phalangeal Joint, Right **X** Finger Phalangeal Joint, Left	**Ø** Open **3** Percutaneous **4** Percutaneous Endoscopic **X** External	**Ø** Drainage Device **3** Infusion Device **4** Internal Fixation Device **5** External Fixation Device **7** Autologous Tissue Substitute **8** Spacer **J** Synthetic Substitute **K** Nonautologous Tissue Substitute	**Z** No Qualifier

Non-OR   ØRW[Ø,1,4,6,A]X[Ø,3,4,7,8,A,J,K]Z
Non-OR   ØRW[3,5,9,B]X[Ø,3,7,J,K]Z
Non-OR   ØRW[C,D,E,F,G,H,J,K]X[Ø,3,4,5,7,8,J,K]Z
Non-OR   ØRW[L,M,N,P,Q,R,S,T,U,V,W,X]X[Ø,3,4,5,7,8,J,K]Z

Lower Joints ØS2–ØSW

Ø   **Medical and Surgical**
S   **Lower Joints**
2   **Change**   Taking out or off a device from a body part and putting back an identical or similar device in or on the same body part without cutting or puncturing the skin or a mucous membrane

Body Part Character 4	Approach Character 5	Device Character 6	Qualifier Character 7
Y Lower Joint	X External	Ø Drainage Device Y Other Device	Z No Qualifier

Non-OR   For all body part, approach, device, and qualifier values

Ø   **Medical and Surgical**
S   **Lower Joints**
5   **Destruction**   Physical eradication of all or a portion of a body part by the direct use of energy, force, or a destructive agent

Body Part Character 4	Approach Character 5	Device Character 6	Qualifier Character 7
Ø Lumbar Vertebral Joint 2 Lumbar Vertebral Disc 3 Lumbosacral Joint 4 Lumbosacral Disc 5 Sacrococcygeal Joint 6 Coccygeal Joint 7 Sacroiliac Joint, Right 8 Sacroiliac Joint, Left 9 Hip Joint, Right B Hip Joint, Left C Knee Joint, Right D Knee Joint, Left F Ankle Joint, Right G Ankle Joint, Left H Tarsal Joint, Right J Tarsal Joint, Left K Metatarsal-Tarsal Joint, Right L Metatarsal-Tarsal Joint, Left M Metatarsal-Phalangeal Joint, Right N Metatarsal-Phalangeal Joint, Left P Toe Phalangeal Joint, Right Q Toe Phalangeal Joint, Left	Ø Open 3 Percutaneous 4 Percutaneous Endoscopic	Z No Device	Z No Qualifier

Ø   **Medical and Surgical**
S   **Lower Joints**
9   **Drainage**   Taking or letting out fluids and/or gases from a body part

Body Part Character 4	Approach Character 5	Device Character 6	Qualifier Character 7
Ø Lumbar Vertebral Joint 2 Lumbar Vertebral Disc 3 Lumbosacral Joint 4 Lumbosacral Disc 5 Sacrococcygeal Joint 6 Coccygeal Joint 7 Sacroiliac Joint, Right 8 Sacroiliac Joint, Left 9 Hip Joint, Right B Hip Joint, Left C Knee Joint, Right D Knee Joint, Left F Ankle Joint, Right G Ankle Joint, Left H Tarsal Joint, Right J Tarsal Joint, Left K Metatarsal-Tarsal Joint, Right L Metatarsal-Tarsal Joint, Left M Metatarsal-Phalangeal Joint, Right N Metatarsal-Phalangeal Joint, Left P Toe Phalangeal Joint, Right Q Toe Phalangeal Joint, Left	Ø Open 3 Percutaneous 4 Percutaneous Endoscopic	Ø Drainage Device	Z No Qualifier

ØS9 Continued on next page

Non-OR   ØS9[Ø,2,3,4,5,6,7,8,9,B,C,D,F,G,H,J,K,L,M,N,P,Q][3,4]ØZ

0S9 Continued

0   **Medical and Surgical**
S   **Lower Joints**
9   **Drainage**   Taking or letting out fluids and/or gases from a body part

Body Part Character 4	Approach Character 5	Device Character 6	Qualifier Character 7
0 Lumbar Vertebral Joint **2** Lumbar Vertebral Disc **3** Lumbosacral Joint **4** Lumbosacral Disc **5** Sacrococcygeal Joint **6** Coccygeal Joint **7** Sacroiliac Joint, Right **8** Sacroiliac Joint, Left **9** Hip Joint, Right **B** Hip Joint, Left **C** Knee Joint, Right **D** Knee Joint, Left **F** Ankle Joint, Right **G** Ankle Joint, Left **H** Tarsal Joint, Right **J** Tarsal Joint, Left **K** Metatarsal-Tarsal Joint, Right **L** Metatarsal-Tarsal Joint, Left **M** Metatarsal-Phalangeal Joint, Right **N** Metatarsal-Phalangeal Joint, Left **P** Toe Phalangeal Joint, Right **Q** Toe Phalangeal Joint, Left	**0** Open **3** Percutaneous **4** Percutaneous Endoscopic	**Z** No Device	**X** Diagnostic **Z** No Qualifier

Non-OR   0S9[0,2,3,4,5,6,7,8,9,B,C,D,F,G,H,J,K,L,M,N,P,Q][0,3,4]Z[X,Z]

0   **Medical and Surgical**
S   **Lower Joints**
B   **Excision**   Cutting out or off, without replacement, a portion of a body part

Body Part Character 4	Approach Character 5	Device Character 6	Qualifier Character 7
0 Lumbar Vertebral Joint **2** Lumbar Vertebral Disc **3** Lumbosacral Joint **4** Lumbosacral Disc **5** Sacrococcygeal Joint **6** Coccygeal Joint **7** Sacroiliac Joint, Right **8** Sacroiliac Joint, Left **9** Hip Joint, Right **B** Hip Joint, Left **C** Knee Joint, Right **D** Knee Joint, Left **F** Ankle Joint, Right **G** Ankle Joint, Left **H** Tarsal Joint, Right **J** Tarsal Joint, Left **K** Metatarsal-Tarsal Joint, Right **L** Metatarsal-Tarsal Joint, Left **M** Metatarsal-Phalangeal Joint, Right **N** Metatarsal-Phalangeal Joint, Left **P** Toe Phalangeal Joint, Right **Q** Toe Phalangeal Joint, Left	**0** Open **3** Percutaneous **4** Percutaneous Endoscopic	**Z** No Device	**X** Diagnostic **Z** No Qualifier

Non-OR   0SB[0,2,3,4,5,6,7,8,9,B,C,D,F,G,H,J,K,L,M,N,P,Q][0,3,4]ZX

LC Limited Coverage   **NC** Noncovered   HAC associated procedure   Combination Only   DRG Non-OR   Non-OR   Revised Text in **GREEN**

ICD-10-PCS 2014 (Draft)   **353**

0S9—0SB

Ø   Medical and Surgical
S   Lower Joints
C   Extirpation   Taking or cutting out solid matter from a body part

Body Part Character 4	Approach Character 5	Device Character 6	Qualifier Character 7
Ø Lumbar Vertebral Joint 2 Lumbar Vertebral Disc 3 Lumbosacral Joint 4 Lumbosacral Disc 5 Sacrococcygeal Joint 6 Coccygeal Joint 7 Sacroiliac Joint, Right 8 Sacroiliac Joint, Left 9 Hip Joint, Right B Hip Joint, Left C Knee Joint, Right D Knee Joint, Left F Ankle Joint, Right G Ankle Joint, Left H Tarsal Joint, Right J Tarsal Joint, Left K Metatarsal-Tarsal Joint, Right L Metatarsal-Tarsal Joint, Left M Metatarsal-Phalangeal Joint, Right N Metatarsal-Phalangeal Joint, Left P Toe Phalangeal Joint, Right Q Toe Phalangeal Joint, Left	Ø Open 3 Percutaneous 4 Percutaneous Endoscopic	Z No Device	Z No Qualifier

Ø   Medical and Surgical
S   Lower Joints
G   Fusion   Joining together portions of an articular body part rendering the articular body part immobile

Body Part Character 4	Approach Character 5	Device Character 6	Qualifier Character 7
Ø Lumbar Vertebral Joint 1 Lumbar Vertebral Joints, 2 or more 3 Lumbosacral Joint	Ø Open 3 Percutaneous 4 Percutaneous Endoscopic	7 Autologous Tissue Substitute A Interbody Fusion Device J Synthetic Substitute K Nonautologous Tissue Substitute Z No Device	Ø Anterior Approach, Anterior Column 1 Posterior Approach, Posterior Column J Posterior Approach, Anterior Column
5 Sacrococcygeal Joint 6 Coccygeal Joint 7 Sacroiliac Joint, Right 8 Sacroiliac Joint, Left	Ø Open 3 Percutaneous 4 Percutaneous Endoscopic	4 Internal Fixation Device 7 Autologous Tissue Substitute J Synthetic Substitute K Nonautologous Tissue Substitute Z No Device	Z No Qualifier
9 Hip Joint, Right B Hip Joint, Left C Knee Joint, Right D Knee Joint, Left F Ankle Joint, Right G Ankle Joint, Left H Tarsal Joint, Right J Tarsal Joint, Left K Metatarsal-Tarsal Joint, Right L Metatarsal-Tarsal Joint, Left M Metatarsal-Phalangeal Joint, Right N Metatarsal-Phalangeal Joint, Left P Toe Phalangeal Joint, Right Q Toe Phalangeal Joint, Left	Ø Open 3 Percutaneous 4 Percutaneous Endoscopic	4 Internal Fixation Device 5 External Fixation Device 7 Autologous Tissue Substitute J Synthetic Substitute K Nonautologous Tissue Substitute Z No Device	Z No Qualifier

HAC   ØSG[Ø,1,3][Ø,3,4][7,A,J,K,Z][Ø,1,J] when reported with SDx K68.11 or T81.4XXA or T81.6Ø-T84.7 with 7th character A

[LC] Limited Coverage   [NC] Noncovered   HAC associated procedure   Combination Only   DRG Non-OR   Non-OR   Revised Text in **GREEN**

354   ICD-10-PCS 2014 (Draft)

Ø   **Medical and Surgical**
S   **Lower Joints**
H   **Insertion**   Putting in a nonbiological appliance that monitors, assists, performs, or prevents a physiological function but does not physically take the place of a body part

Body Part Character 4	Approach Character 5	Device Character 6	Qualifier Character 7
Ø Lumbar Vertebral Joint **3** Lumbosacral Joint	**Ø** Open **3** Percutaneous **4** Percutaneous Endoscopic	**3** Infusion Device **4** Internal Fixation Device **8** Spacer **B** Spinal Stabilization Device, Interspinous Process **C** Spinal Stabilization Device, Pedicle-Based **D** Spinal Stabilization Device, Facet Replacement	**Z** No Qualifier
2 Lumbar Vertebral Disc **4** Lumbosacral Disc	**Ø** Open **3** Percutaneous **4** Percutaneous Endoscopic	**3** Infusion Device **8** Spacer	**Z** No Qualifier
5 Sacrococcygeal Joint **6** Coccygeal Joint **7** Sacroiliac Joint, Right **8** Sacroiliac Joint, Left	**Ø** Open **3** Percutaneous **4** Percutaneous Endoscopic	**3** Infusion Device **4** Internal Fixation Device **8** Spacer	**Z** No Qualifier
9 Hip Joint, Right **B** Hip Joint, Left **C** Knee Joint, Right **D** Knee Joint, Left **F** Ankle Joint, Right **G** Ankle Joint, Left **H** Tarsal Joint, Right **J** Tarsal Joint, Left **K** Metatarsal-Tarsal Joint, Right **L** Metatarsal-Tarsal Joint, Left **M** Metatarsal-Phalangeal Joint, Right **N** Metatarsal-Phalangeal Joint, Left **P** Toe Phalangeal Joint, Right **Q** Toe Phalangeal Joint, Left	**Ø** Open **3** Percutaneous **4** Percutaneous Endoscopic	**3** Infusion Device **4** Internal Fixation Device **5** External Fixation Device **8** Spacer	**Z** No Qualifier

Non-OR   ØSH[Ø,3][Ø,3,4][3,8]Z
Non-OR   ØSH[2,4][Ø,3,4][3,8]Z
Non-OR   ØSH[5,6,7,8][Ø,3,4][3,8]Z
Non-OR   ØSH[9,B,C,D,F,G,H,J,K,L,M,N,P,Q][Ø,3,4][3,8]Z

Ø   **Medical and Surgical**
S   **Lower Joints**
J   **Inspection**   Visually and/or manually exploring a body part

Body Part Character 4	Approach Character 5	Device Character 6	Qualifier Character 7
Ø Lumbar Vertebral Joint **2** Lumbar Vertebral Disc **3** Lumbosacral Joint **4** Lumbosacral Disc **5** Sacrococcygeal Joint **6** Coccygeal Joint **7** Sacroiliac Joint, Right **8** Sacroiliac Joint, Left **9** Hip Joint, Right **B** Hip Joint, Left **C** Knee Joint, Right **D** Knee Joint, Left **F** Ankle Joint, Right **G** Ankle Joint, Left **H** Tarsal Joint, Right **J** Tarsal Joint, Left **K** Metatarsal-Tarsal Joint, Right **L** Metatarsal-Tarsal Joint, Left **M** Metatarsal-Phalangeal Joint, Right **N** Metatarsal-Phalangeal Joint, Left **P** Toe Phalangeal Joint, Right **Q** Toe Phalangeal Joint, Left	**Ø** Open **3** Percutaneous **4** Percutaneous Endoscopic **X** External	**Z** No Device	**Z** No Qualifier

Non-OR   ØSJ[Ø,2,3,4,5,6,7,8,9,B,C,D,F,G,H,J,K,L,M,N,P,Q]XZZ

Ø Medical and Surgical
S Lower Joints
N Release Freeing a body part from an abnormal physical constraint

Body Part Character 4	Approach Character 5	Device Character 6	Qualifier Character 7
Ø Lumbar Vertebral Joint **2** Lumbar Vertebral Disc **3** Lumbosacral Joint **4** Lumbosacral Disc **5** Sacrococcygeal Joint **6** Coccygeal Joint **7** Sacroiliac Joint, Right **8** Sacroiliac Joint, Left **9** Hip Joint, Right **B** Hip Joint, Left **C** Knee Joint, Right **D** Knee Joint, Left **F** Ankle Joint, Right **G** Ankle Joint, Left **H** Tarsal Joint, Right **J** Tarsal Joint, Left **K** Metatarsal-Tarsal Joint, Right **L** Metatarsal-Tarsal Joint, Left **M** Metatarsal-Phalangeal Joint, Right **N** Metatarsal-Phalangeal Joint, Left **P** Toe Phalangeal Joint, Right **Q** Toe Phalangeal Joint, Left	**Ø** Open **3** Percutaneous **4** Percutaneous Endoscopic **X** External	**Z** No Device	**Z** No Qualifier

Non-OR ØSN[Ø,2,3,4,5,6,7,8,9,B,C,D,F,G,H,J,K,L,M,N,P,Q]XZZ

Ø Medical and Surgical
S Lower Joints
P Removal Taking out or off a device from a body part

Body Part Character 4	Approach Character 5	Device Character 6	Qualifier Character 7
Ø Lumbar Vertebral Joint **3** Lumbosacral Joint	**Ø** Open **3** Percutaneous **4** Percutaneous Endoscopic	**Ø** Drainage Device **3** Infusion Device **4** Internal Fixation Device **7** Autologous Tissue Substitute **8** Spacer **A** Interbody Fusion Device **J** Synthetic Substitute **K** Nonautologous Tissue Substitute	**Z** No Qualifier
Ø Lumbar Vertebral Joint **3** Lumbosacral Joint	**X** External	**Ø** Drainage Device **3** Infusion Device **4** Internal Fixation Device	**Z** No Qualifier
5 Sacrococcygeal Joint **6** Coccygeal Joint **7** Sacroiliac Joint, Right **8** Sacroiliac Joint, Left	**Ø** Open **3** Percutaneous **4** Percutaneous Endoscopic	**Ø** Drainage Device **3** Infusion Device **4** Internal Fixation Device **7** Autologous Tissue Substitute **8** Spacer **J** Synthetic Substitute **K** Nonautologous Tissue Substitute	**Z** No Qualifier
5 Sacrococcygeal Joint **6** Coccygeal Joint **7** Sacroiliac Joint, Right **8** Sacroiliac Joint, Left	**X** External	**Ø** Drainage Device **3** Infusion Device **4** Internal Fixation Device	**Z** No Qualifier
2 Lumbar Vertebral Disc **4** Lumbosacral Disc	**Ø** Open **3** Percutaneous **4** Percutaneous Endoscopic	**Ø** Drainage Device **3** Infusion Device **7** Autologous Tissue Substitute **J** Synthetic Substitute **K** Nonautologous Tissue Substitute	**Z** No Qualifier
2 Lumbar Vertebral Disc **4** Lumbosacral Disc	**X** External	**Ø** Drainage Device **3** Infusion Device	**Z** No Qualifier

ØSP Continued on next page

Non-OR ØSP[Ø,3][Ø,3,4][Ø,3,4]8Z
Non-OR ØSP[Ø,3]X[Ø,3,4]Z
Non-OR ØSP[5,6,7,8][Ø,3,4]8Z
Non-OR ØSP[5,6,7,8]X[Ø,3,4]Z
Non-OR ØSP[2,4]X[Ø,3]Z

Ø　**Medical and Surgical**
S　**Lower Joints**
P　**Removal**　　　Taking out or off a device from a body part

Body Part Character 4	Approach Character 5	Device Character 6	Qualifier Character 7
9　Hip Joint, Right B　Hip Joint, Left	Ø　Open	Ø　Drainage Device 3　Infusion Device 4　Internal Fixation Device 5　External Fixation Device 7　Autologous Tissue Substitute 8　Spacer 9　Liner B　Resurfacing Device J　Synthetic Substitute K　Nonautologous Tissue Substitute	Z　No Qualifier
9　Hip Joint, Right B　Hip Joint, Left C　Knee Joint, Right D　Knee Joint, Left	3　Percutaneous 4　Percutaneous Endoscopic	Ø　Drainage Device 3　Infusion Device 4　Internal Fixation Device 5　External Fixation Device 7　Autologous Tissue Substitute 8　Spacer J　Synthetic Substitute K　Nonautologous Tissue Substitute	Z　No Qualifier
9　Hip Joint, Right B　Hip Joint, Left C　Knee Joint, Right D　Knee Joint, Left F　Ankle Joint, Right G　Ankle Joint, Left H　Tarsal Joint, Right J　Tarsal Joint, Left K　Metatarsal-Tarsal Joint, Right L　Metatarsal-Tarsal Joint, Left M　Metatarsal-Phalangeal Joint, Right N　Metatarsal-Phalangeal Joint, Left P　Toe Phalangeal Joint, Right Q　Toe Phalangeal Joint, Left	X　External	Ø　Drainage Device 3　Infusion Device 4　Internal Fixation Device 5　External Fixation Device	Z　No Qualifier
C　Knee Joint, Right D　Knee Joint, Left	Ø　Open	Ø　Drainage Device 3　Infusion Device 4　Internal Fixation Device 5　External Fixation Device 7　Autologous Tissue Substitute 8　Spacer 9　Liner J　Synthetic Substitute K　Nonautologous Tissue Substitute	Z　No Qualifier
F　Ankle Joint, Right G　Ankle Joint, Left H　Tarsal Joint, Right J　Tarsal Joint, Left K　Metatarsal-Tarsal Joint, Right L　Metatarsal-Tarsal Joint, Left M　Metatarsal-Phalangeal Joint, Right N　Metatarsal-Phalangeal Joint, Left P　Toe Phalangeal Joint, Right Q　Toe Phalangeal Joint, Left	Ø　Open 3　Percutaneous 4　Percutaneous Endoscopic	Ø　Drainage Device 3　Infusion Device 4　Internal Fixation Device 5　External Fixation Device 7　Autologous Tissue Substitute 8　Spacer J　Synthetic Substitute K　Nonautologous Tissue Substitute	Z　No Qualifier

Non-OR　ØSP[9,B]Ø8Z
Non-OR　ØSP[9,B,C,D][3,4]8Z
Non-OR　ØSP[9,B,C,D,F,G,H,J,K,L,M,N,P,Q]X[Ø,3,4,5]Z
Non-OR　ØSP[C,D]Ø8Z
Non-OR　ØSP[F,G,H,J,K,L,M,N,P,Q][Ø,3,4]8Z

Ø   Medical and Surgical
S   Lower Joints
Q   Repair   Restoring, to the extent possible, a body part to its normal anatomic structure and function

Body Part Character 4	Approach Character 5	Device Character 6	Qualifier Character 7
Ø Lumbar Vertebral Joint	Ø Open	Z No Device	Z No Qualifier
2 Lumbar Vertebral Disc	3 Percutaneous		
3 Lumbosacral Joint	4 Percutaneous Endoscopic		
4 Lumbosacral Disc	X External		
5 Sacrococcygeal Joint			
6 Coccygeal Joint			
7 Sacroiliac Joint, Right			
8 Sacroiliac Joint, Left			
9 Hip Joint, Right			
B Hip Joint, Left			
C Knee Joint, Right			
D Knee Joint, Left			
F Ankle Joint, Right			
G Ankle Joint, Left			
H Tarsal Joint, Right			
J Tarsal Joint, Left			
K Metatarsal-Tarsal Joint, Right			
L Metatarsal-Tarsal Joint, Left			
M Metatarsal-Phalangeal Joint, Right			
N Metatarsal-Phalangeal Joint, Left			
P Toe Phalangeal Joint, Right			
Q Toe Phalangeal Joint, Left			

Ø   Medical and Surgical
S   Lower Joints
R   Replacement   Putting in or on biological or synthetic material that physically takes the place and/or function of all or a portion of a body part

Body Part Character 4	Approach Character 5	Device Character 6	Qualifier Character 7
Ø Lumbar Vertebral Joint	Ø Open	7 Autologous Tissue Substitute	Z No Qualifier
2 Lumbar Vertebral Disc NC		J Synthetic Substitute	
3 Lumbosacral Joint		K Nonautologous Tissue Substitute	
4 Lumbosacral Disc NC			
5 Sacrococcygeal Joint			
6 Coccygeal Joint			
7 Sacroiliac Joint, Right			
8 Sacroiliac Joint, Left			
H Tarsal Joint, Right			
J Tarsal Joint, Left			
K Metatarsal-Tarsal Joint, Right			
L Metatarsal-Tarsal Joint, Left			
M Metatarsal-Phalangeal Joint, Right			
N Metatarsal-Phalangeal Joint, Left			
P Toe Phalangeal Joint, Right			
Q Toe Phalangeal Joint, Left			
9 Hip Joint, Right	Ø Open	1 Synthetic Substitute, Metal	9 Cemented
B Hip Joint, Left		2 Synthetic Substitute, Metal on Polyethylene	A Uncemented
		3 Synthetic Substitute, Ceramic	Z No Qualifier
		4 Synthetic Substitute, Ceramic on Polyethylene	
		J Synthetic Substitute	
9 Hip Joint, Right	Ø Open	7 Autologous Tissue Substitute	Z No Qualifier
B Hip Joint, Left		K Nonautologous Tissue Substitute	
A Hip Joint, Acetabular Surface, Right	Ø Open	Ø Synthetic Substitute, Polyethylene	9 Cemented
E Hip Joint, Acetabular Surface, Left		1 Synthetic Substitute, Metal	A Uncemented
		3 Synthetic Substitute, Ceramic	Z No Qualifier
		J Synthetic Substitute	
A Hip Joint, Acetabular Surface, Right	Ø Open	7 Autologous Tissue Substitute	Z No Qualifier
E Hip Joint, Acetabular Surface, Left		K Nonautologous Tissue Substitute	

ØSR Continued on next page

NC   ØSR[2,4] ØJZ when beneficiary age is over 6Ø
HAC   ØSR[9,B]Ø[1,2,3,4,J][9,A,Z] when reported with SDx from I26.Ø2-I26.Ø9, I26.92-I26.99, or I82.4Ø1-I82.4Z9
HAC   ØSR[9,B]Ø[7,K]Z when reported with SDx from I26.Ø2-I26.Ø9, I26.92-I26.99, or I82.4Ø1-I82.4Z9
HAC   ØSR [A,E]Ø[Ø,1,3,J][9,A,Z] when reported with SDx from I26.Ø2-I26.Ø9, I26.92-I26.99, or I82.4Ø1-I82.4Z9
HAC   ØSR [A,E]Ø[7,K]Z when reported with SDx from I26.Ø2-I26.Ø9, I26.92-I26.99, or I82.4Ø1-I82.4Z9

Ø Medical and Surgical
S Lower Joints
R Replacement

ØSR Continued

Putting in or on biological or synthetic material that physically takes the place and/or function of all or a portion of a body part

Body Part Character 4	Approach Character 5	Device Character 6	Qualifier Character 7
C Knee Joint, Right D Knee Joint, Left F Ankle Joint, Right G Ankle Joint, Left T Knee Joint, Femoral Surface, Right U Knee Joint, Femoral Surface, Left V Knee Joint, Tibial Surface, Right W Knee Joint, Tibial Surface, Left	Ø Open	7 Autologous Tissue Substitute K Nonautologous Tissue Substitute	Z No Qualifier
C Knee Joint, Right D Knee Joint, Left F Ankle Joint, Right G Ankle Joint, Left T Knee Joint, Femoral Surface, Right U Knee Joint, Femoral Surface, Left V Knee Joint, Tibial Surface, Right W Knee Joint, Tibial Surface, Left	Ø Open	J Synthetic Substitute	9 Cemented A Uncemented Z No Qualifier
R Hip Joint, Femoral Surface, Right S Hip Joint, Femoral Surface, Left	Ø Open	1 Synthetic Substitute, Metal 3 Synthetic Substitute, Ceramic J Synthetic Substitute	9 Cemented A Uncemented Z No Qualifier
R Hip Joint, Femoral Surface, Right S Hip Joint, Femoral Surface, Left	Ø Open	7 Autologous Tissue Substitute K Nonautologous Tissue Substitute	Z No Qualifier

HAC　ØSR[C,D, T,U,V,W]Ø[7,K]Z when reported with SDx from I26.02-I26.09, I26.92-I26.99, or I82.401-I82.4Z9
HAC　ØSR[C,D,T,U,V,W]ØJ[9,A,Z] when reported with SDx from I26.02-I26.09, I26.92-I26.99, or I82.401-I82.4Z9
HAC　ØSR[R,S]Ø[1,3,J][9,A,Z] when reported with SDx from I26.02-I26.09, I26.92-I26.99, or I82.401-I82.4Z9
HAC　ØSR[R,S]Ø[7,K]Z when reported with SDx from I26.02-I26.09, I26.92-I26.99, or I82.401-I82.4Z9

Ø Medical and Surgical
S Lower Joints
S Reposition

Moving to its normal location or other suitable location all or a portion of a body part

Body Part Character 4	Approach Character 5	Device Character 6	Qualifier Character 7
Ø Lumbar Vertebral Joint 3 Lumbosacral Joint 5 Sacrococcygeal Joint 6 Coccygeal Joint 7 Sacroiliac Joint, Right 8 Sacroiliac Joint, Left	Ø Open 3 Percutaneous 4 Percutaneous Endoscopic X External	4 Internal Fixation Device Z No Device	Z No Qualifier
9 Hip Joint, Right B Hip Joint, Left C Knee Joint, Right D Knee Joint, Left F Ankle Joint, Right G Ankle Joint, Left H Tarsal Joint, Right J Tarsal Joint, Left K Metatarsal-Tarsal Joint, Right L Metatarsal-Tarsal Joint, Left M Metatarsal-Phalangeal Joint, Right N Metatarsal-Phalangeal Joint, Left P Toe Phalangeal Joint, Right Q Toe Phalangeal Joint, Left	Ø Open 3 Percutaneous 4 Percutaneous Endoscopic X External	4 Internal Fixation Device 5 External Fixation Device Z No Device	Z No Qualifier

Non-OR　ØSS[Ø,3,5,6,7,8][3,4,X][4,Z]Z
Non-OR　ØSS[9,B,C,D,F,G,H,J,K,L,M,N,P,Q][3,4,X][4,5,Z]Z

Lower Joints

ØST–ØSU

Ø   **Medical and Surgical**
S   **Lower Joints**
T   **Resection**   Cutting out or off, without replacement, all of a body part

Body Part Character 4	Approach Character 5	Device Character 6	Qualifier Character 7
2 Lumbar Vertebral Disc **4** Lumbosacral Disc **5** Sacrococcygeal Joint **6** Coccygeal Joint **7** Sacroiliac Joint, Right **8** Sacroiliac Joint, Left **9** Hip Joint, Right **B** Hip Joint, Left **C** Knee Joint, Right **D** Knee Joint, Left **F** Ankle Joint, Right **G** Ankle Joint, Left **H** Tarsal Joint, Right **J** Tarsal Joint, Left **K** Metatarsal-Tarsal Joint, Right **L** Metatarsal-Tarsal Joint, Left **M** Metatarsal-Phalangeal Joint, Right **N** Metatarsal-Phalangeal Joint, Left **P** Toe Phalangeal Joint, Right **Q** Toe Phalangeal Joint, Left	**Ø** Open	**Z** No Device	**Z** No Qualifier

Ø   **Medical and Surgical**
S   **Lower Joints**
U   **Supplement**   Putting in or on biological or synthetic material that physically reinforces and/or augments the function of a portion of a body part

Body Part Character 4	Approach Character 5	Device Character 6	Qualifier Character 7
Ø Lumbar Vertebral Joint **2** Lumbar Vertebral Disc **3** Lumbosacral Joint **4** Lumbosacral Disc **5** Sacrococcygeal Joint **6** Coccygeal Joint **7** Sacroiliac Joint, Right **8** Sacroiliac Joint, Left **F** Ankle Joint, Right **G** Ankle Joint, Left **H** Tarsal Joint, Right J Tarsal Joint, Left **K** Metatarsal-Tarsal Joint, Right **L** Metatarsal-Tarsal Joint, Left **M** Metatarsal-Phalangeal Joint, Right **N** Metatarsal-Phalangeal Joint, Left **P** Toe Phalangeal Joint, Right **Q** Toe Phalangeal Joint, Left	**Ø** Open **3** Percutaneous **4** Percutaneous Endoscopic	**7** Autologous Tissue Substitute **J** Synthetic Substitute **K** Nonautologous Tissue Substitute	**Z** No Qualifier
9 Hip Joint, Right **B** Hip Joint, Left	**Ø** Open	**7** Autologous Tissue Substitute **9** Liner **B** Resurfacing Device **J** Synthetic Substitute **K** Nonautologous Tissue Substitute	**Z** No Qualifier
9 Hip Joint, Right **B** Hip Joint, Left	**3** Percutaneous **4** Percutaneous Endoscopic	**7** Autologous Tissue Substitute **J** Synthetic Substitute **K** Nonautologous Tissue Substitute	**Z** No Qualifier
A Hip Joint, Acetabular Surface, Right **E** Hip Joint, Acetabular Surface, Left **R** Hip Joint, Femoral Surface, Right **S** Hip Joint, Femoral Surface, Left	**Ø** Open	**9** Liner **B** Resurfacing Device	**Z** No Qualifier
C Knee Joint, Right **D** Knee Joint, Left	**Ø** Open	**7** Autologous Tissue Substitute **J** Synthetic Substitute **K** Nonautologous Tissue Substitute	**Z** No Qualifier
C Knee Joint, Right **D** Knee Joint, Left	**Ø** Open	**9** Liner	**C** Patellar Surface **Z** No Qualifier
T Knee Joint, Femoral Surface, Right **U** Knee Joint, Femoral Surface, Left **V** Knee Joint, Tibial Surface, Right **W** Knee Joint, Tibial Surface, Left	**Ø** Open	**9** Liner	**Z** No Qualifier

HAC   ØSU[9,B]ØBZ when reported with SDx from I26.Ø2-I26.Ø9, I26.92-I26.99, or I82.4Ø1-I82.4Z9
HAC   ØSU[A,E,R,S]ØBZ when reported with SDx from I26.Ø2-I26.Ø9, I26.92-I26.99, or I82.4Ø1-I82.4Z9

0 **Medical and Surgical**
S **Lower Joints**
W **Revision** Correcting, to the extent possible, a portion of a malfunctioning device or the position of a displaced device

Body Part Character 4	Approach Character 5	Device Character 6	Qualifier Character 7
0 Lumbar Vertebral Joint **3** Lumbosacral Joint	**0** Open **3** Percutaneous **4** Percutaneous Endoscopic **X** External	**0** Drainage Device **3** Infusion Device **4** Internal Fixation Device **7** Autologous Tissue Substitute **8** Spacer **A** Interbody Fusion Device **J** Synthetic Substitute **K** Nonautologous Tissue Substitute	**Z** No Qualifier
2 Lumbar Vertebral Disc **4** Lumbosacral Disc	**0** Open **3** Percutaneous **4** Percutaneous Endoscopic **X** External	**0** Drainage Device **3** Infusion Device **7** Autologous Tissue Substitute **J** Synthetic Substitute **K** Nonautologous Tissue Substitute	**Z** No Qualifier
5 Sacrococcygeal Joint **6** Coccygeal Joint **7** Sacroiliac Joint, Right **8** Sacroiliac Joint, Left	**0** Open **3** Percutaneous **4** Percutaneous Endoscopic **X** External	**0** Drainage Device **3** Infusion Device **4** Internal Fixation Device **7** Autologous Tissue Substitute **8** Spacer **J** Synthetic Substitute **K** Nonautologous Tissue Substitute	**Z** No Qualifier
9 Hip Joint, Right **B** Hip Joint, Left	**0** Open	**0** Drainage Device **3** Infusion Device **4** Internal Fixation Device **5** External Fixation Device **7** Autologous Tissue Substitute **8** Spacer **9** Liner **B** Resurfacing Device **J** Synthetic Substitute **K** Nonautologous Tissue Substitute	**Z** No Qualifier
9 Hip Joint, Right **B** Hip Joint, Left **C** Knee Joint, Right **D** Knee Joint, Left	**3** Percutaneous **4** Percutaneous Endoscopic **X** External	**0** Drainage Device **3** Infusion Device **4** Internal Fixation Device **5** External Fixation Device **7** Autologous Tissue Substitute **8** Spacer **J** Synthetic Substitute **K** Nonautologous Tissue Substitute	**Z** No Qualifier
C Knee Joint, Right **D** Knee Joint, Left	**0** Open	**0** Drainage Device **3** Infusion Device **4** Internal Fixation Device **5** External Fixation Device **7** Autologous Tissue Substitute **8** Spacer **9** Liner **J** Synthetic Substitute **K** Nonautologous Tissue Substitute	**Z** No Qualifier
F Ankle Joint, Right **G** Ankle Joint, Left **H** Tarsal Joint, Right **J** Tarsal Joint, Left **K** Metatarsal-Tarsal Joint, Right **L** Metatarsal-Tarsal Joint, Left **M** Metatarsal-Phalangeal Joint, Right **N** Metatarsal-Phalangeal Joint, Left **P** Toe Phalangeal Joint, Right **Q** Toe Phalangeal Joint, Left	**0** Open **3** Percutaneous **4** Percutaneous Endoscopic **X** External	**0** Drainage Device **3** Infusion Device **4** Internal Fixation Device **5** External Fixation Device **7** Autologous Tissue Substitute **8** Spacer **J** Synthetic Substitute **K** Nonautologous Tissue Substitute	**Z** No Qualifier

Non-OR 0SW[0,3]X[0,3,4,7,8,A,J,K]Z
Non-OR 0SW[2,4]X[0,3,7,J,K]Z
Non-OR 0SW[5,6,7,8]X[0,3,4,7,8,J,K]Z
Non-OR 0SW[9,B,C,D]X[0,3,4,5,7,8,J,K]Z
Non-OR 0SW[F,G,H,J,K,L,M,N,P,Q]X[0,3,4,5,7,8,J,K]Z

LC Limited Coverage **NC** Noncovered HAC associated procedure Combination Only DRG Non-OR Non-OR Revised Text in **GREEN**
ICD-10-PCS 2014 (Draft) **361**

0SW—0SW

Urinary System ØT1–ØTY

Ø Medical and Surgical
T Urinary System
1 Bypass   Altering the route of passage of the contents of a tubular body part

Body Part Character 4	Approach Character 5	Device Character 6	Qualifier Character 7
3 Kidney Pelvis, Right **4** Kidney Pelvis, Left	**Ø** Open **4** Percutaneous Endoscopic	**7** Autologous Tissue Substitute **J** Synthetic Substitute **K** Nonautologous Tissue Substitute **Z** No Device	**3** Kidney Pelvis, Right **4** Kidney Pelvis, Left **6** Ureter, Right **7** Ureter, Left **8** Colon **9** Colocutaneous **A** Ileum **B** Bladder **C** Ileocutaneous **D** Cutaneous
3 Kidney Pelvis, Right **4** Kidney Pelvis, Left **6** Ureter, Right **7** Ureter, Left **8** Ureters, Bilateral **B** Bladder	**3** Percutaneous	**J** Synthetic Substitute	**D** Cutaneous
6 Ureter, Right **7** Ureter, Left **8** Ureters, Bilateral	**Ø** Open **4** Percutaneous Endoscopic	**7** Autologous Tissue Substitute **J** Synthetic Substitute **K** Nonautologous Tissue Substitute **Z** No Device	**6** Ureter, Right **7** Ureter, Left **8** Colon **9** Colocutaneous **A** Ileum **B** Bladder **C** Ileocutaneous **D** Cutaneous
B Bladder	**Ø** Open **4** Percutaneous Endoscopic	**7** Autologous Tissue Substitute **J** Synthetic Substitute **K** Nonautologous Tissue Substitute **Z** No Device	**9** Colocutaneous **C** Ileocutaneous **D** Cutaneous

Ø Medical and Surgical
T Urinary System
2 Change   Taking out or off a device from a body part and putting back an identical or similar device in or on the same body part without cutting or puncturing the skin or a mucous membrane

Body Part Character 4	Approach Character 5	Device Character 6	Qualifier Character 7
5 Kidney **9** Ureter **B** Bladder **D** Urethra	**X** External	**Ø** Drainage Device **Y** Other Device	**Z** No Qualifier

Non-OR   For all body part, approach, device, and qualifier values

Ø Medical and Surgical
T Urinary System
5 Destruction   Physical eradication of all or a portion of a body part by the direct use of energy, force, or a destructive agent

Body Part Character 4	Approach Character 5	Device Character 6	Qualifier Character 7
Ø Kidney, Right **1** Kidney, Left **3** Kidney Pelvis, Right **4** Kidney Pelvis, Left **6** Ureter, Right **7** Ureter, Left **B** Bladder **C** Bladder Neck	**Ø** Open **3** Percutaneous **4** Percutaneous Endoscopic **7** Via Natural or Artificial Opening **8** Via Natural or Artificial Opening Endoscopic	**Z** No Device	**Z** No Qualifier
D Urethra	**Ø** Open **3** Percutaneous **4** Percutaneous Endoscopic **7** Via Natural or Artificial Opening **8** Via Natural or Artificial Opening Endoscopic **X** External	**Z** No Device	**Z** No Qualifier

Non-OR   ØT5D[Ø,3,4,7,8,X]ZZ

0   **Medical and Surgical**
T   **Urinary System**
7   **Dilation**   Expanding an orifice or the lumen of a tubular body part

Body Part Character 4	Approach Character 5	Device Character 6	Qualifier Character 7
3 Kidney Pelvis, Right **4** Kidney Pelvis, Left **6** Ureter, Right **7** Ureter, Left **8** Ureters, Bilateral **B** Bladder **C** Bladder Neck **D** Urethra	**0** Open **3** Percutaneous **4** Percutaneous Endoscopic **7** Via Natural or Artificial Opening **8** Via Natural or Artificial Opening Endoscopic	**D** Intraluminal Device **Z** No Device	**Z** No Qualifier

Non-OR	0T7[6,7][0,3,4,7,8]DZ
Non-OR	0T7[8,D][0,3,4]DZ
Non-OR	0T7[8,D][7,8][D,Z]Z
Non-OR	0T7C[0,3,4,7,8][D,Z]Z

0   **Medical and Surgical**
T   **Urinary System**
8   **Division**   Cutting into a body part without draining fluids and/or gases from the body part in order to separate or transect a body part

Body Part Character 4	Approach Character 5	Device Character 6	Qualifier Character 7
2 Kidneys, Bilateral **C** Bladder Neck	**0** Open **3** Percutaneous **4** Percutaneous Endoscopic	**Z** No Device	**Z** No Qualifier

0   **Medical and Surgical**
T   **Urinary System**
9   **Drainage**   Taking or letting out fluids and/or gases from a body part

Body Part Character 4	Approach Character 5	Device Character 6	Qualifier Character 7
0 Kidney, Right **1** Kidney, Left **3** Kidney Pelvis, Right **4** Kidney Pelvis, Left **6** Ureter, Right **7** Ureter, Left **8** Ureters, Bilateral **B** Bladder **C** Bladder Neck	**0** Open **3** Percutaneous **4** Percutaneous Endoscopic **7** Via Natural or Artificial Opening **8** Via Natural or Artificial Opening Endoscopic	**0** Drainage Device	**Z** No Qualifier
0 Kidney, Right **1** Kidney, Left **3** Kidney Pelvis, Right **4** Kidney Pelvis, Left **6** Ureter, Right **7** Ureter, Left **8** Ureters, Bilateral **B** Bladder **C** Bladder Neck	**0** Open **3** Percutaneous **4** Percutaneous Endoscopic **7** Via Natural or Artificial Opening **8** Via Natural or Artificial Opening Endoscopic	**Z** No Device	**X** Diagnostic **Z** No Qualifier
D Urethra	**0** Open **3** Percutaneous **4** Percutaneous Endoscopic **7** Via Natural or Artificial Opening **8** Via Natural or Artificial Opening Endoscopic **X** External	**0** Drainage Device	**Z** No Qualifier
D Urethra	**0** Open **3** Percutaneous **4** Percutaneous Endoscopic **7** Via Natural or Artificial Opening **8** Via Natural or Artificial Opening Endoscopic **X** External	**Z** No Device	**X** Diagnostic **Z** No Qualifier

Non-OR	0T9[6,7,8][0,3,4,7,8]0Z
Non-OR	0T9[B,C][3,4,7,8]0Z
Non-OR	0T9[B,C][3,4,7,8]ZZ
Non-OR	0T9[0,1,3,4,6,7,8][3,4,7,8]ZX
Non-OR	0T9[0,1,3,4][3,4]ZZ
Non-OR	0T9D[0,3,4,7,8,X]ZX

LC Limited Coverage   **NC** Noncovered   HAC associated procedure   Combination Only   DRG Non-OR   Non-OR   Revised Text in **GREEN**
ICD-10-PCS 2014 (Draft)   **363**

0T7—0T9

Urinary System *(side tab)*

ØTB–ØTF *(side tab)*

Ø   **Medical and Surgical**
T   **Urinary System**
B   **Excision**   Cutting out or off, without replacement, a portion of a body part

Body Part Character 4	Approach Character 5	Device Character 6	Qualifier Character 7
Ø Kidney, Right 1 Kidney, Left 3 Kidney Pelvis, Right 4 Kidney Pelvis, Left 6 Ureter, Right 7 Ureter, Left B Bladder C Bladder Neck	Ø Open 3 Percutaneous 4 Percutaneous Endoscopic 7 Via Natural or Artificial Opening 8 Via Natural or Artificial Opening Endoscopic	Z No Device	X Diagnostic Z No Qualifier
D Urethra	Ø Open 3 Percutaneous 4 Percutaneous Endoscopic 7 Via Natural or Artificial Opening 8 Via Natural or Artificial Opening Endoscopic X External	Z No Device	X Diagnostic Z No Qualifier

Non-OR   ØTB[Ø,1,3,4,6,7][3,4,7,8]ZX
Non-OR   ØTBD[Ø,3,4,7,8,X]ZX

Ø   **Medical and Surgical**
T   **Urinary System**
C   **Extirpation**   Taking or cutting out solid matter from a body part

Body Part Character 4	Approach Character 5	Device Character 6	Qualifier Character 7
Ø Kidney, Right 1 Kidney, Left 3 Kidney Pelvis, Right 4 Kidney Pelvis, Left 6 Ureter, Right 7 Ureter, Left B Bladder C Bladder Neck	Ø Open 3 Percutaneous 4 Percutaneous Endoscopic 7 Via Natural or Artificial Opening 8 Via Natural or Artificial Opening Endoscopic	Z No Device	Z No Qualifier
D Urethra	Ø Open 3 Percutaneous 4 Percutaneous Endoscopic 7 Via Natural or Artificial Opening 8 Via Natural or Artificial Opening Endoscopic X External	Z No Device	Z No Qualifier

Non-OR   ØTC[B,C][7,8]ZZ
Non-OR   ØTCD[7,8,X]ZZ

Ø   **Medical and Surgical**
T   **Urinary System**
D   **Extraction**   Pulling or stripping out or off all or a portion of a body part by the use of force

Body Part Character 4	Approach Character 5	Device Character 6	Qualifier Character 7
Ø Kidney, Right 1 Kidney, Left	Ø Open 3 Percutaneous 4 Percutaneous Endoscopic	Z No Device	Z No Qualifier

---

Ø   **Medical and Surgical**
T   **Urinary System**
F   **Fragmentation**   Breaking solid matter in a body part into pieces

Body Part Character 4	Approach Character 5	Device Character 6	Qualifier Character 7
3 Kidney Pelvis, Right 4 Kidney Pelvis, Left 6 Ureter, Right 7 Ureter, Left B Bladder C Bladder Neck D Urethra NC	Ø Open 3 Percutaneous 4 Percutaneous Endoscopic 7 Via Natural or Artificial Opening 8 Via Natural or Artificial Opening Endoscopic X External	Z No Device	Z No Qualifier

NC   ØTFDXZZ
DRG Non-OR   ØTF[3,4,6,7,B,C]XZZ
Non-OR   ØTF[3,4][Ø,7,8]ZZ
Non-OR   ØTFD[Ø,3,4,7,8,X]ZZ
Non-OR   ØTF[6,7,B,C][Ø,3,4,7,8]ZZ

LC Limited Coverage   NC Noncovered   HAC associated procedure   Combination Only   DRG Non-OR   Non-OR   Revised Text in GREEN

ICD-10-PCS 2014 (Draft)

Ø   Medical and Surgical
T   Urinary System
H   Insertion   Putting in a nonbiological appliance that monitors, assists, performs, or prevents a physiological function but does not physically take the place of a body part

Body Part Character 4	Approach Character 5	Device Character 6	Qualifier Character 7
5 Kidney	**Ø** Open **3** Percutaneous **4** Percutaneous Endoscopic **7** Via Natural or Artificial Opening **8** Via Natural or Artificial Opening Endoscopic	**2** Monitoring Device **3** Infusion Device	**Z** No Qualifier
9 Ureter	**Ø** Open **3** Percutaneous **4** Percutaneous Endoscopic **7** Via Natural or Artificial Opening **8** Via Natural or Artificial Opening Endoscopic	**2** Monitoring Device **3** Infusion Device **M** Stimulator Lead	**Z** No Qualifier
B Bladder NC	**Ø** Open **3** Percutaneous **4** Percutaneous Endoscopic **7** Via Natural or Artificial Opening **8** Via Natural or Artificial Opening Endoscopic	**2** Monitoring Device **3** Infusion Device **L** Artificial Sphincter **M** Stimulator Lead	**Z** No Qualifier
C Bladder Neck	**Ø** Open **3** Percutaneous **4** Percutaneous Endoscopic **7** Via Natural or Artificial Opening **8** Via Natural or Artificial Opening Endoscopic	**L** Artificial Sphincter	**Z** No Qualifier
D Urethra	**Ø** Open **3** Percutaneous **4** Percutaneous Endoscopic **7** Via Natural or Artificial Opening **8** Via Natural or Artificial Opening Endoscopic **X** External	**2** Monitoring Device **3** Infusion Device **L** Artificial Sphincter	**Z** No Qualifier

NC	ØTHB[Ø,3,4,7,8]MZ
Non-OR	ØTH5[Ø,3,4,7,8]3Z
Non-OR	ØTH9[Ø,3,4,7,8]3Z
Non-OR	ØTHB[Ø,3,4,7,8]3Z
Non-OR	ØTHD[Ø,3,4,7,8,X]3Z

Ø   Medical and Surgical
T   Urinary System
J   Inspection   Visually and/or manually exploring a body part

Body Part Character 4	Approach Character 5	Device Character 6	Qualifier Character 7
5 Kidney **9** Ureter **B** Bladder **D** Urethra	**Ø** Open **3** Percutaneous **4** Percutaneous Endoscopic **7** Via Natural or Artificial Opening **8** Via Natural or Artificial Opening Endoscopic **X** External	**Z** No Device	**Z** No Qualifier

Non-OR	ØTJ[5,9][4,8,X]ZZ
Non-OR	ØTJB[8,X]ZZ
Non-OR	ØTJD[3,4,7,8,X]ZZ

Ø   **Medical and Surgical**
T   **Urinary System**
L   **Occlusion**   Completely closing an orifice or the lumen of a tubular body part

Body Part Character 4	Approach Character 5	Device Character 6	Qualifier Character 7
3 Kidney Pelvis, Right 4 Kidney Pelvis, Left 6 Ureter, Right 7 Ureter, Left B Bladder C Bladder Neck	Ø Open 3 Percutaneous 4 Percutaneous Endoscopic	C Extraluminal Device D Intraluminal Device Z No Device	Z No Qualifier
3 Kidney Pelvis, Right 4 Kidney Pelvis, Left 6 Ureter, Right 7 Ureter, Left B Bladder C Bladder Neck D Urethra	7 Via Natural or Artificial Opening 8 Via Natural or Artificial Opening Endoscopic	D Intraluminal Device Z No Device	Z No Qualifier
D Urethra	Ø Open 3 Percutaneous 4 Percutaneous Endoscopic X External	C Extraluminal Device D Intraluminal Device Z No Device	Z No Qualifier

Ø   **Medical and Surgical**
T   **Urinary System**
M   **Reattachment**   Putting back in or on all or a portion of a separated body part to its normal location or other suitable location

Body Part Character 4	Approach Character 5	Device Character 6	Qualifier Character 7
Ø Kidney, Right 1 Kidney, Left 2 Kidneys, Bilateral 3 Kidney Pelvis, Right 4 Kidney Pelvis, Left 6 Ureter, Right 7 Ureter, Left 8 Ureters, Bilateral B Bladder C Bladder Neck D Urethra	Ø Open 4 Percutaneous Endoscopic	Z No Device	Z No Qualifier

Ø   **Medical and Surgical**
T   **Urinary System**
N   **Release**   Freeing a body part from an abnormal physical constraint

Body Part Character 4	Approach Character 5	Device Character 6	Qualifier Character 7
Ø Kidney, Right 1 Kidney, Left 3 Kidney Pelvis, Right 4 Kidney Pelvis, Left 6 Ureter, Right 7 Ureter, Left B Bladder C Bladder Neck	Ø Open 3 Percutaneous 4 Percutaneous Endoscopic 7 Via Natural or Artificial Opening 8 Via Natural or Artificial Opening Endoscopic	Z No Device	Z No Qualifier
D Urethra	Ø Open 3 Percutaneous 4 Percutaneous Endoscopic 7 Via Natural or Artificial Opening 8 Via Natural or Artificial Opening Endoscopic X External	Z No Device	Z No Qualifier

Ø   Medical and Surgical
T   Urinary System
P   Removal   Taking out or off a device from a body part

Body Part Character 4	Approach Character 5	Device Character 6	Qualifier Character 7
5 Kidney	**Ø** Open **3** Percutaneous **4** Percutaneous Endoscopic **7** Via Natural or Artificial Opening **8** Via Natural or Artificial Opening Endoscopic	**Ø** Drainage Device **2** Monitoring Device **3** Infusion Device **7** Autologous Tissue Substitute **C** Extraluminal Device **D** Intraluminal Device **J** Synthetic Substitute **K** Nonautologous Tissue Substitute	**Z** No Qualifier
5 Kidney	**X** External	**Ø** Drainage Device **2** Monitoring Device **3** Infusion Device **D** Intraluminal Device	**Z** No Qualifier
9 Ureter	**Ø** Open **3** Percutaneous **4** Percutaneous Endoscopic **7** Via Natural or Artificial Opening **8** Via Natural or Artificial Opening Endoscopic	**Ø** Drainage Device **2** Monitoring Device **3** Infusion Device **7** Autologous Tissue Substitute **C** Extraluminal Device **D** Intraluminal Device **J** Synthetic Substitute **K** Nonautologous Tissue Substitute **M** Stimulator Lead	**Z** No Qualifier
9 Ureter	**X** External	**Ø** Drainage Device **2** Monitoring Device **3** Infusion Device **D** Intraluminal Device **M** Stimulator Lead	**Z** No Qualifier
B Bladder **NC**	**Ø** Open **3** Percutaneous **4** Percutaneous Endoscopic **7** Via Natural or Artificial Opening **8** Via Natural or Artificial Opening Endoscopic	**Ø** Drainage Device **2** Monitoring Device **3** Infusion Device **7** Autologous Tissue Substitute **C** Extraluminal Device **D** Intraluminal Device **J** Synthetic Substitute **K** Nonautologous Tissue Substitute **L** Artificial Sphincter **M** Stimulator Lead	**Z** No Qualifier
B Bladder	**X** External	**Ø** Drainage Device **2** Monitoring Device **3** Infusion Device **D** Intraluminal Device **L** Artificial Sphincter **M** Stimulator Lead	**Z** No Qualifier
D Urethra	**Ø** Open **3** Percutaneous **4** Percutaneous Endoscopic **7** Via Natural or Artificial Opening **8** Via Natural or Artificial Opening Endoscopic	**Ø** Drainage Device **2** Monitoring Device **3** Infusion Device **7** Autologous Tissue Substitute **C** Extraluminal Device **D** Intraluminal Device **J** Synthetic Substitute **K** Nonautologous Tissue Substitute **L** Artificial Sphincter	**Z** No Qualifier
D Urethra	**X** External	**Ø** Drainage Device **2** Monitoring Device **3** Infusion Device **D** Intraluminal Device **L** Artificial Sphincter	**Z** No Qualifier

NC   ØTPB[Ø,3,4,7,8]MZ
Non-OR   ØTP5X[Ø,2,3,D]Z
Non-OR   ØTP9X[Ø,2,3,D]Z
Non-OR   ØTPBX[Ø,2,3,D,L]Z
Non-OR   ØTPDX[Ø,2,3,D]Z

Ø Medical and Surgical
T Urinary System
Q Repair   Restoring, to the extent possible, a body part to its normal anatomic structure and function

Body Part Character 4	Approach Character 5	Device Character 6	Qualifier Character 7
Ø Kidney, Right **1** Kidney, Left **3** Kidney Pelvis, Right **4** Kidney Pelvis, Left **6** Ureter, Right **7** Ureter, Left **B** Bladder **C** Bladder Neck	**Ø** Open **3** Percutaneous **4** Percutaneous Endoscopic **7** Via Natural or Artificial Opening **8** Via Natural or Artificial Opening Endoscopic	**Z** No Device	**Z** No Qualifier
D Urethra	**Ø** Open **3** Percutaneous **4** Percutaneous Endoscopic **7** Via Natural or Artificial Opening **8** Via Natural or Artificial Opening Endoscopic **X** External	**Z** No Device	**Z** No Qualifier

Non-OR   ØTQC[Ø,3,4,7,8]ZZ

Ø Medical and Surgical
T Urinary System
R Replacement   Putting in or on biological or synthetic material that physically takes the place and/or function of all or a portion of a body part

Body Part Character 4	Approach Character 5	Device Character 6	Qualifier Character 7
3 Kidney Pelvis, Right **4** Kidney Pelvis, Left **6** Ureter, Right **7** Ureter, Left **B** Bladder **C** Bladder Neck	**Ø** Open **4** Percutaneous Endoscopic **7** Via Natural or Artificial Opening **8** Via Natural or Artificial Opening Endoscopic	**7** Autologous Tissue Substitute **J** Synthetic Substitute **K** Nonautologous Tissue Substitute	**Z** No Qualifier
D Urethra	**Ø** Open **4** Percutaneous Endoscopic **7** Via Natural or Artificial Opening **8** Via Natural or Artificial Opening Endoscopic **X** External	**7** Autologous Tissue Substitute **J** Synthetic Substitute **K** Nonautologous Tissue Substitute	**Z** No Qualifier

---

Ø Medical and Surgical
T Urinary System
S Reposition   Moving to its normal location or other suitable location all or a portion of a body part

Body Part Character 4	Approach Character 5	Device Character 6	Qualifier Character 7
Ø Kidney, Right **1** Kidney, Left **2** Kidneys, Bilateral **3** Kidney Pelvis, Right **4** Kidney Pelvis, Left **6** Ureter, Right **7** Ureter, Left **8** Ureters, Bilateral **B** Bladder **C** Bladder Neck **D** Urethra	**Ø** Open **4** Percutaneous Endoscopic	**Z** No Device	**Z** No Qualifier

LC Limited Coverage   **NC** Noncovered   HAC associated procedure   Combination Only   DRG Non-OR   Non-OR   Revised Text in **GREEN**

368   ICD-1Ø-PCS 2Ø14 (Draft)

Ø   Medical and Surgical
T   Urinary System
T   Resection   Cutting out or off, without replacement, all of a body part

Body Part Character 4	Approach Character 5	Device Character 6	Qualifier Character 7
Ø Kidney, Right **1** Kidney, Left **2** Kidneys, Bilateral	**Ø** Open **4** Percutaneous Endoscopic	**Z** No Device	**Z** No Qualifier
3 Kidney Pelvis, Right **4** Kidney Pelvis, Left **6** Ureter, Right **7** Ureter, Left **B** Bladder **C** Bladder Neck **D** Urethra	**Ø** Open **4** Percutaneous Endoscopic **7** Via Natural or Artificial Opening **8** Via Natural or Artificial Opening Endoscopic	**Z** No Device	**Z** No Qualifier

Non-OR   ØTTD[Ø,4,7,8]ZZ

Ø   Medical and Surgical
T   Urinary System
U   Supplement   Putting in or on biological or synthetic material that physically reinforces and/or augments the function of a portion of a body part

Body Part Character 4	Approach Character 5	Device Character 6	Qualifier Character 7
3 Kidney Pelvis, Right **4** Kidney Pelvis, Left **6** Ureter, Right **7** Ureter, Left **B** Bladder **C** Bladder Neck	**Ø** Open **4** Percutaneous Endoscopic **7** Via Natural or Artificial Opening **8** Via Natural or Artificial Opening Endoscopic	**7** Autologous Tissue Substitute **J** Synthetic Substitute **K** Nonautologous Tissue Substitute	**Z** No Qualifier
D Urethra	**Ø** Open **4** Percutaneous Endoscopic **7** Via Natural or Artificial Opening **8** Via Natural or Artificial Opening Endoscopic **X** External	**7** Autologous Tissue Substitute **J** Synthetic Substitute **K** Nonautologous Tissue Substitute	**Z** No Qualifier

Ø   Medical and Surgical
T   Urinary System
V   Restriction   Partially closing an orifice or the lumen of a tubular body part

Body Part Character 4	Approach Character 5	Device Character 6	Qualifier Character 7
3 Kidney Pelvis, Right **4** Kidney Pelvis, Left **6** Ureter, Right **7** Ureter, Left **B** Bladder **C** Bladder Neck **D** Urethra	**Ø** Open **3** Percutaneous **4** Percutaneous Endoscopic	**C** Extraluminal Device **D** Intraluminal Device **Z** No Device	**Z** No Qualifier
3 Kidney Pelvis, Right **4** Kidney Pelvis, Left **6** Ureter, Right **7** Ureter, Left **B** Bladder **C** Bladder Neck **D** Urethra	**7** Via Natural or Artificial Opening **8** Via Natural or Artificial Opening Endoscopic	**D** Intraluminal Device **Z** No Device	**Z** No Qualifier
D Urethra	**X** External	**Z** No Device	**Z** No Qualifier

Urinary System

ØTW–ØTY

Ø Medical and Surgical
T Urinary System
W Revision   Correcting, to the extent possible, a portion of a malfunctioning device or the position of a displaced device

Body Part Character 4	Approach Character 5	Device Character 6	Qualifier Character 7
5 Kidney	**Ø** Open **3** Percutaneous **4** Percutaneous Endoscopic **7** Via Natural or Artificial Opening **8** Via Natural or Artificial Opening Endoscopic **X** External	**Ø** Drainage Device **2** Monitoring Device **3** Infusion Device **7** Autologous Tissue Substitute **C** Extraluminal Device **D** Intraluminal Device **J** Synthetic Substitute **K** Nonautologous Tissue Substitute	**Z** No Qualifier
9 Ureter	**Ø** Open **3** Percutaneous **4** Percutaneous Endoscopic **7** Via Natural or Artificial Opening **8** Via Natural or Artificial Opening Endoscopic **X** External	**Ø** Drainage Device **2** Monitoring Device **3** Infusion Device **7** Autologous Tissue Substitute **C** Extraluminal Device **D** Intraluminal Device **J** Synthetic Substitute **K** Nonautologous Tissue Substitute **M** Stimulator Lead	**Z** No Qualifier
B Bladder	**Ø** Open **3** Percutaneous **4** Percutaneous Endoscopic **7** Via Natural or Artificial Opening **8** Via Natural or Artificial Opening Endoscopic **X** External	**Ø** Drainage Device **2** Monitoring Device **3** Infusion Device **7** Autologous Tissue Substitute **C** Extraluminal Device **D** Intraluminal Device **J** Synthetic Substitute **K** Nonautologous Tissue Substitute **L** Artificial Sphincter **M** Stimulator Lead	**Z** No Qualifier
D Urethra	**Ø** Open **3** Percutaneous **4** Percutaneous Endoscopic **7** Via Natural or Artificial Opening **8** Via Natural or Artificial Opening Endoscopic **X** External	**Ø** Drainage Device **2** Monitoring Device **3** Infusion Device **7** Autologous Tissue Substitute **C** Extraluminal Device **D** Intraluminal Device **J** Synthetic Substitute **K** Nonautologous Tissue Substitute **L** Artificial Sphincter	**Z** No Qualifier

Non-OR   ØTW5X[Ø,2,3,7,C,D,J,K]Z
Non-OR   ØTW9X[Ø,2,3,7,C,D,J,K,M]Z
Non-OR   ØTWBX[Ø,2,3,7,C,D,J,K,L,M]Z
Non-OR   ØTWDX[Ø,2,3,7,C,D,J,K,L]Z

Ø Medical and Surgical
T Urinary System
Y Transplantation   Putting in or on all or a portion of a living body part taken from another individual or animal to physically take the place and/or function of all or a portion of a similar body part

Body Part Character 4	Approach Character 5	Device Character 6	Qualifier Character 7
Ø Kidney, Right LC **1** Kidney, Left LC	**Ø** Open	**Z** No Device	**Ø** Allogeneic **1** Syngeneic **2** Zooplastic

Combinations Only
Kidney/Pancreas Transplant
One of ØTY[Ø,1]ØZ[Ø,1,2] and ØFYGØZ[Ø,1,2]

LC   ØTY[Ø,1]ØZ[Ø,1,2]

Female Reproductive System ØU1–ØUY

Ø **Medical and Surgical**
U **Female Reproductive System**
1 **Bypass**   Altering the route of passage of the contents of a tubular body part

Body Part Character 4		Approach Character 5	Device Character 6	Qualifier Character 7
5 Fallopian Tube, Right ♀	**Ø** Open	**7** Autologous Tissue Substitute	**5** Fallopian Tube, Right
6 Fallopian Tube, Left ♀	**4** Percutaneous Endoscopic	**J** Synthetic Substitute	**6** Fallopian Tube, Left
		K Nonautologous Tissue Substitute	**9** Uterus
		Z No Device	

Ø **Medical and Surgical**
U **Female Reproductive System**
2 **Change**   Taking out or off a device from a body part and putting back an identical or similar device in or on the same body part without cutting or puncturing the skin or a mucous membrane

Body Part Character 4		Approach Character 5	Device Character 6	Qualifier Character 7
3 Ovary ♀	**X** External	**Ø** Drainage Device	**Z** No Qualifier
8 Fallopian Tube ♀		**Y** Other Device	
M Vulva ♀			
D Uterus and Cervix ♀	**X** External	**Ø** Drainage Device	**Z** No Qualifier
		H Contraceptive Device	
		Y Other Device	
H Vagina and Cul-de-sac ♀	**X** External	**Ø** Drainage Device	**Z** No Qualifier
		G Pessary	
		Y Other Device	

Non-OR   For all body part, approach, device, and qualifier values

Ø **Medical and Surgical**
U **Female Reproductive System**
5 **Destruction**   Physical eradication of all or a portion of a body part by the direct use of energy, force, or a destructive agent

Body Part Character 4		Approach Character 5	Device Character 6	Qualifier Character 7
Ø Ovary, Right ♀	**Ø** Open	**Z** No Device	**Z** No Qualifier
1 Ovary, Left ♀	**3** Percutaneous		
2 Ovaries, Bilateral ♀	**4** Percutaneous Endoscopic		
4 Uterine Supporting Structure ♀			
5 Fallopian Tube, Right ♀	**Ø** Open	**Z** No Device	**Z** No Qualifier
6 Fallopian Tube, Left ♀	**3** Percutaneous		
7 Fallopian Tubes, Bilateral NC ♀	**4** Percutaneous Endoscopic		
9 Uterus ♀	**7** Via Natural or Artificial Opening		
B Endometrium ♀	**8** Via Natural or Artificial Opening Endoscopic		
C Cervix ♀			
F Cul-de-sac ♀			
G Vagina ♀	**Ø** Open	**Z** No Device	**Z** No Qualifier
K Hymen ♀	**3** Percutaneous		
	4 Percutaneous Endoscopic		
	7 Via Natural or Artificial Opening		
	8 Via Natural or Artificial Opening Endoscopic		
	X External		
J Clitoris ♀	**Ø** Open	**Z** No Device	**Z** No Qualifier
L Vestibular Gland ♀	**X** External		
M Vulva ♀			

NC ØU57[Ø,3,4,7,8]ZZ

LC Limited Coverage   **NC** Noncovered   HAC associated procedure   Combination Only   DRG Non-OR   Non-OR   Revised Text in **GREEN**

ICD-10-PCS 2014 (Draft)   **371**

Female Reproductive System

ØU7–ØU9

Ø   Medical and Surgical
U   Female Reproductive System
7   Dilation   Expanding an orifice or lumen of a tabular body part

Body Part Character 4	Approach Character 5	Device Character 6	Qualifier Character 7
5 Fallopian Tube, Right ♀ 6 Fallopian Tube, Left ♀ 7 Fallopian Tubes, Bilateral ♀ 9 Uterus ♀ C Cervix ♀ G Vagina ♀	Ø Open 3 Percutaneous 4 Percutaneous Endoscopic 7 Via Natural or Artificial Opening 8 Via Natural or Artificial Opening Endoscopic	D Intraluminal Device Z No Device	Z No Qualifier
K Hymen ♀	Ø Open 3 Percutaneous 4 Percutaneous Endoscopic 7 Via Natural or Artificial Opening 8 Via Natural or Artificial Opening Endoscopic X External	D Intraluminal Device Z No Device	Z No Qualifier

Non-OR   ØU7C[Ø,3,4,7,8][D,Z]Z
Non-OR   ØU7G[7,8][D,Z]Z

Ø   Medical and Surgical
U   Female Reproductive System
8   Division   Cutting into a body part without draining fluids and/or gases from the body part in order to separate or transect a body part

Body Part Character 4	Approach Character 5	Device Character 6	Qualifier Character 7
Ø Ovary, Right ♀ 1 Ovary, Left ♀ 2 Ovaries, Bilateral ♀ 4 Uterine Supporting Structure ♀	Ø Open 3 Percutaneous 4 Percutaneous Endoscopic	Z No Device	Z No Qualifier
K Hymen ♀	7 Via Natural or Artificial Opening 8 Via Natural or Artificial Opening Endoscopic X External	Z No Device	Z No Qualifier

Non-OR   ØU8K[7,8,X]ZZ

Ø   Medical and Surgical
U   Female Reproductive System
9   Drainage   Taking or letting out fluids and/or gases from a body part

Body Part Character 4	Approach Character 5	Device Character 6	Qualifier Character 7
Ø Ovary, Right ♀ 1 Ovary, Left ♀ 2 Ovaries, Bilateral ♀	X External	Z No Device	Z No Qualifier
Ø Ovary, Right ♀ 1 Ovary, Left ♀ 2 Ovaries, Bilateral ♀ 4 Uterine Supporting Structure ♀	Ø Open 3 Percutaneous 4 Percutaneous Endoscopic	Ø Drainage Device	Z No Qualifier
Ø Ovary, Right ♀ 1 Ovary, Left ♀ 2 Ovaries, Bilateral ♀ 4 Uterine Supporting Structure ♀	Ø Open 3 Percutaneous 4 Percutaneous Endoscopic	Z No Device	X Diagnostic Z No Qualifier
5 Fallopian Tube, Right ♀ 6 Fallopian Tube, Left ♀ 7 Fallopian Tubes, Bilateral ♀ 9 Uterus ♀ C Cervix ♀ F Cul-de-sac ♀	Ø Open 3 Percutaneous 4 Percutaneous Endoscopic 7 Via Natural or Artificial Opening 8 Via Natural or Artificial Opening Endoscopic	Ø Drainage Device	Z No Qualifier
5 Fallopian Tube, Right ♀ 6 Fallopian Tube, Left ♀ 7 Fallopian Tubes, Bilateral ♀ 9 Uterus ♀ C Cervix ♀ F Cul-de-sac ♀	Ø Open 3 Percutaneous 4 Percutaneous Endoscopic 7 Via Natural or Artificial Opening 8 Via Natural or Artificial Opening Endoscopic	Z No Device	X Diagnostic Z No Qualifier

ØU9 Continued on next page

Non-OR   ØU9[5,6,7][3,4,7,8]ZZ
Non-OR   ØU9F[3,4][Ø,Z]Z

0U9 Continued

0   **Medical and Surgical**
U   **Female Reproductive System**
9   **Drainage**   Taking or letting out fluids and/or gases from a body part

Body Part Character 4		Approach Character 5	Device Character 6	Qualifier Character 7
G Vagina ♀ **K** Hymen ♀		**0** Open **3** Percutaneous **4** Percutaneous Endoscopic **7** Via Natural or Artificial Opening **8** Via Natural or Artificial Opening Endoscopic **X** External	**0** Drainage Device	**Z** No Qualifier
G Vagina ♀ **K** Hymen ♀		**0** Open **3** Percutaneous **4** Percutaneous Endoscopic **7** Via Natural or Artificial Opening **8** Via Natural or Artificial Opening Endoscopic **X** External	**Z** No Device	**X** Diagnostic **Z** No Qualifier
J Clitoris ♀ **L** Vestibular Gland ♀ **M** Vulva ♀		**0** Open **X** External	**0** Drainage Device	**Z** No Qualifier
J Clitoris ♀ **L** Vestibular Gland ♀ **M** Vulva ♀		**0** Open **X** External	**Z** No Device	**X** Diagnostic **Z** No Qualifier

Non-OR   0U9K[0,3,4,7,8,X]0Z
Non-OR   0U9K[0,3,4,7,8,X]ZZ
Non-OR   0U9L [0,X]0Z
Non-OR   0U9L [0,X]ZZ

0   **Medical and Surgical**
U   **Female Reproductive System**
B   **Excision**   Cutting out or off, without replacement, a portion of a body part

Body Part Character 4		Approach Character 5	Device Character 6	Qualifier Character 7
0 Ovary, Right ♀ **1** Ovary, Left ♀ **2** Ovaries, Bilateral ♀ **4** Uterine Supporting Structure ♀ **5** Fallopian Tube, Right ♀ **6** Fallopian Tube, Left ♀ **7** Fallopian Tubes, Bilateral ♀ **9** Uterus ♀ **C** Cervix ♀ **F** Cul-de-sac ♀		**0** Open **3** Percutaneous **4** Percutaneous Endoscopic **7** Via Natural or Artificial Opening **8** Via Natural or Artificial Opening Endoscopic	**Z** No Device	**X** Diagnostic **Z** No Qualifier
G Vagina ♀ **K** Hymen ♀		**0** Open **3** Percutaneous **4** Percutaneous Endoscopic **7** Via Natural or Artificial Opening **8** Via Natural or Artificial Opening Endoscopic **X** External	**Z** No Device	**X** Diagnostic **Z** No Qualifier
J Clitoris ♀ **L** Vestibular Gland ♀ **M** Vulva ♀		**0** Open **X** External	**Z** No Device	**X** Diagnostic **Z** No Qualifier

Female Reproductive System

ØUC–ØUF

Ø   **Medical and Surgical**
U   **Female Reproductive System**
C   **Extirpation**   Taking or cutting out solid matter from a body part

Body Part Character 4		Approach Character 5	Device Character 6	Qualifier Character 7
Ø Ovary, Right ♀ **1** Ovary, Left ♀ **2** Ovaries, Bilateral ♀ **4** Uterine Supporting Structure ♀		**Ø** Open **3** Percutaneous **4** Percutaneous Endoscopic	**Z** No Device	**Z** No Qualifier
5 Fallopian Tube, Right ♀ **6** Fallopian Tube, Left ♀ **7** Fallopian Tubes, Bilateral ♀ **9** Uterus ♀ **B** Endometrium ♀ **C** Cervix ♀ **F** Cul-de-sac ♀		**Ø** Open **3** Percutaneous **4** Percutaneous Endoscopic **7** Via Natural or Artificial Opening **8** Via Natural or Artificial Opening Endoscopic	**Z** No Device	**Z** No Qualifier
G Vagina ♀ **K** Hymen ♀		**Ø** Open **3** Percutaneous **4** Percutaneous Endoscopic **7** Via Natural or Artificial Opening **8** Via Natural or Artificial Opening Endoscopic **X** External	**Z** No Device	**Z** No Qualifier
J Clitoris ♀ **L** Vestibular Gland ♀ **M** Vulva ♀		**Ø** Open **X** External	**Z** No Device	**Z** No Qualifier

Non-OR   ØUC9[7,8]ZZ
Non-OR   ØUC[G,K][7,8,X]ZZ
Non-OR   ØUCK[Ø,3,4]ZZ
Non-OR   ØUCMXZZ

Ø   **Medical and Surgical**
U   **Female Reproductive System**
D   **Extraction**   Pulling or stripping out or off all or a portion of a body part by the use of force

Body Part Character 4		Approach Character 5	Device Character 6	Qualifier Character 7
B Endometrium ♀		**7** Via Natural or Artificial Opening **8** Via Natural or Artificial Opening Endoscopic	**Z** No Device	**X** Diagnostic **Z** No Qualifier
N Ova ♀		**Ø** Open **3** Percutaneous **4** Percutaneous Endoscopic	**Z** No Device	**Z** No Qualifier

Ø   **Medical and Surgical**
U   **Female Reproductive System**
F   **Fragmentation**   Breaking solid matter in a body part into pieces

Body Part Character 4		Approach Character 5	Device Character 6	Qualifier Character 7
5 Fallopian Tube, Right ⓃⒸ ♀ **6** Fallopian Tube, Left ⓃⒸ ♀ **7** Fallopian Tubes, Bilateral ⓃⒸ ♀ **9** Uterus ⓃⒸ ♀		**Ø** Open **3** Percutaneous **4** Percutaneous Endoscopic **7** Via Natural or Artificial Opening **8** Via Natural or Artificial Opening Endoscopic **X** External	**Z** No Device	**Z** No Qualifier

ⓃⒸ   ØUF[5,6,7,9]XZZ
Non-OR   ØUF[5,6,7,9]XZZ

0 Medical and Surgical
U Female Reproductive System
H Insertion   Putting in a nonbiological appliance that monitors, assists, performs, or prevents a physiological function but does not physically take the place of a body part

Body Part Character 4	Approach Character 5	Device Character 6	Qualifier Character 7
3 Ovary ♀	**0** Open **3** Percutaneous **4** Percutaneous Endoscopic	**3** Infusion Device	**Z** No Qualifier
8 Fallopian Tube ♀ **D** Uterus and Cervix ♀ **H** Vagina and Cul-de-sac ♀	**0** Open **3** Percutaneous **4** Percutaneous Endoscopic **7** Via Natural or Artificial Opening **8** Via Natural or Artificial Opening Endoscopic	**3** Infusion Device	**Z** No Qualifier
9 Uterus ♀ **C** Cervix ♀	**7** Via Natural or Artificial Opening **8** Via Natural or Artificial Opening Endoscopic	**H** Contraceptive Device	**Z** No Qualifier
C Cervix ♀	**0** Open **3** Percutaneous **4** Percutaneous Endoscopic **7** Via Natural or Artificial Opening **8** Via Natural or Artificial Opening Endoscopic	**1** Radioactive Element	**Z** No Qualifier
F Cul-de-sac ♀	**7** Via Natural or Artificial Opening **8** Via Natural or Artificial Opening Endoscopic	**G** Intraluminal Device, Pessary	**Z** No Qualifier
G Vagina ♀	**0** Open **3** Percutaneous **4** Percutaneous Endoscopic **X** External	**1** Radioactive Element	**Z** No Qualifier
G Vagina ♀	**7** Via Natural or Artificial Opening **8** Via Natural or Artificial Opening Endoscopic	**1** Radioactive Element **G** Intraluminal Device, Pessary	**Z** No Qualifier

Non-OR 0UH3[0,3,4]3Z
Non-OR 0UH[8,D][0,3,4,7,8]3Z
Non-OR 0UH[9,C][7,8]HZ
Non-OR 0UHF[7,8]GZ
Non-OR 0UHG[7,8]GZ

0 Medical and Surgical
U Female Reproductive System
J Inspection   Visually and/or manually exploring a body part

Body Part Character 4	Approach Character 5	Device Character 6	Qualifier Character 7
3 Ovary ♀	**0** Open **3** Percutaneous **4** Percutaneous Endoscopic **X** External	**Z** No Device	**Z** No Qualifier
8 Fallopian Tube ♀ **D** Uterus and Cervix ♀ **H** Vagina and Cul-de-sac ♀	**0** Open **3** Percutaneous **4** Percutaneous Endoscopic **7** Via Natural or Artificial Opening **8** Via Natural or Artificial Opening Endoscopic **X** External	**Z** No Device	**Z** No Qualifier
M Vulva ♀	**0** Open **X** External	**Z** No Device	**Z** No Qualifier

Non-OR 0UJ3XZZ
Non-OR 0UJD7ZZ
Non-OR 0UJ8XZZ
Non-OR 0UJ[D,H][8,X]ZZ
Non-OR 0UJMXZZ

Female Reproductive System

ØUL–ØUN

Ø   **Medical and Surgical**
U   **Female Reproductive System**
L   **Occlusion**   Completely closing an orifice or the lumen of a tubular body part

Body Part Character 4		Approach Character 5	Device Character 6	Qualifier Character 7
5 Fallopian Tube, Right ♀ **6** Fallopian Tube, Left ♀ **7** Fallopian Tubes, Bilateral NC ♀	**Ø** Open **3** Percutaneous **4** Percutaneous Endoscopic	**C** Extraluminal Device **D** Intraluminal Device **Z** No Device	**Z** No Qualifier
5 Fallopian Tube, Right ♀ **6** Fallopian Tube, Left ♀ **7** Fallopian Tubes, Bilateral NC ♀ **F** Cul-de-sac ♀ **G** Vagina ♀	**7** Via Natural or Artificial Opening **8** Via Natural or Artificial Opening Endoscopic	**D** Intraluminal Device **Z** No Device	**Z** No Qualifier

NC   ØUL7[Ø,3,4][C,D,Z]Z
NC   ØUL7[7,8]ZZ

Ø   **Medical and Surgical**
U   **Female Reproductive System**
M   **Reattachment**   Putting back in or on all or a portion of a separated body part to its normal location or other suitable location

Body Part Character 4		Approach Character 5	Device Character 6	Qualifier Character 7
Ø Ovary, Right ♀ **1** Ovary, Left ♀ **2** Ovaries, Bilateral ♀ **4** Uterine Supporting Structure ♀ **5** Fallopian Tube, Right ♀ **6** Fallopian Tube, Left ♀ **7** Fallopian Tubes, Bilateral ♀ **9** Uterus ♀ **C** Cervix ♀ **F** Cul-de-sac ♀ **G** Vagina ♀ **K** Hymen ♀	**Ø** Open **4** Percutaneous Endoscopic	**Z** No Device	**Z** No Qualifier
J Clitoris ♀ **M** Vulva ♀	**X** External	**Z** No Device	**Z** No Qualifier
K Hymen ♀	**Ø** Open **4** Percutaneous Endoscopic **X** External	**Z** No Device	**Z** No Qualifier

Ø   **Medical and Surgical**
U   **Female Reproductive System**
N   **Release**   Freeing a body part from an abnormal physical constraint

Body Part Character 4		Approach Character 5	Device Character 6	Qualifier Character 7
Ø Ovary, Right ♀ **1** Ovary, Left ♀ **2** Ovaries, Bilateral ♀ **4** Uterine Supporting Structure ♀	**Ø** Open **3** Percutaneous **4** Percutaneous Endoscopic	**Z** No Device	**Z** No Qualifier
5 Fallopian Tube, Right ♀ **6** Fallopian Tube, Left ♀ **7** Fallopian Tubes, Bilateral ♀ **9** Uterus ♀ **C** Cervix ♀ **F** Cul-de-sac ♀	**Ø** Open **3** Percutaneous **4** Percutaneous Endoscopic **7** Via Natural or Artificial Opening **8** Via Natural or Artificial Opening Endoscopic	**Z** No Device	**Z** No Qualifier
G Vagina ♀ **K** Hymen ♀	**Ø** Open **3** Percutaneous **4** Percutaneous Endoscopic **7** Via Natural or Artificial Opening **8** Via Natural or Artificial Opening Endoscopic **X** External	**Z** No Device	**Z** No Qualifier
J Clitoris ♀ **L** Vestibular Gland ♀ **M** Vulva ♀	**Ø** Open **X** External	**Z** No Device	**Z** No Qualifier

0   **Medical and Surgical**
U   **Female Reproductive System**
P   **Removal**   Taking out or off a device from a body part

Body Part Character 4	Approach Character 5	Device Character 6	Qualifier Character 7
3 Ovary ♀	**0** Open **3** Percutaneous **4** Percutaneous Endoscopic **X** External	**0** Drainage Device **3** Infusion Device	**Z** No Qualifier
8 Fallopian Tube ♀	**0** Open **3** Percutaneous **4** Percutaneous Endoscopic **7** Via Natural or Artificial Opening **8** Via Natural or Artificial Opening Endoscopic	**0** Drainage Device **3** Infusion Device **7** Autologous Tissue Substitute **C** Extraluminal Device **D** Intraluminal Device **J** Synthetic Substitute **K** Nonautologous Tissue Substitute	**Z** No Qualifier
8 Fallopian Tube ♀	**X** External	**0** Drainage Device **3** Infusion Device **D** Intraluminal Device	**Z** No Qualifier
D Uterus and Cervix ♀	**0** Open **3** Percutaneous **4** Percutaneous Endoscopic **7** Via Natural or Artificial Opening **8** Via Natural or Artificial Opening Endoscopic	**0** Drainage Device **1** Radioactive Element **3** Infusion Device **7** Autologous Tissue Substitute **C** Extraluminal Device **D** Intraluminal Device **H** Contraceptive Device **J** Synthetic Substitute **K** Nonautologous Tissue Substitute	**Z** No Qualifier
D Uterus and Cervix ♀	**X** External	**0** Drainage Device **3** Infusion Device **D** Intraluminal Device **H** Contraceptive Device	**Z** No Qualifier
H Vagina and Cul-de-sac ♀	**0** Open **3** Percutaneous **4** Percutaneous Endoscopic **7** Via Natural or Artificial Opening **8** Via Natural or Artificial Opening Endoscopic	**0** Drainage Device **1** Radioactive Element **3** Infusion Device **7** Autologous Tissue Substitute **D** Intraluminal Device **J** Synthetic Substitute **K** Nonautologous Tissue Substitute	**Z** No Qualifier
H Vagina and Cul-de-sac ♀	**X** External	**0** Drainage Device **1** Radioactive Element **3** Infusion Device **D** Intraluminal Device	**Z** No Qualifier
M Vulva ♀	**0** Open	**0** Drainage Device **7** Autologous Tissue Substitute **J** Synthetic Substitute **K** Nonautologous Tissue Substitute	**Z** No Qualifier
M Vulva ♀	**X** External	**0** Drainage Device	**Z** No Qualifier

Non-OR   0UP3X[0,3]Z
Non-OR   0UP8X[0,3,D]Z
Non-OR   0UPD[3,4,7,8][C,H]Z
Non-OR   0UPDX[0,3,D,H]Z
Non-OR   0UPHX[0,1,3,D]Z
Non-OR   0UPMX0Z

Female Reproductive System (side tab)

ØUQ–ØUT (side tab)

Ø **Medical and Surgical**
U **Female Reproductive System**
Q **Repair**   Restoring, to the extent possible, a body part to its normal anatomic structure and function

Body Part Character 4	Approach Character 5	Device Character 6	Qualifier Character 7
Ø Ovary, Right ♀ 1 Ovary, Left ♀ 2 Ovaries, Bilateral ♀ 4 Uterine Supporting Structure ♀	Ø Open 3 Percutaneous 4 Percutaneous Endoscopic	Z No Device	Z No Qualifier
5 Fallopian Tube, Right ♀ 6 Fallopian Tube, Left ♀ 7 Fallopian Tubes, Bilateral ♀ 9 Uterus ♀ C Cervix ♀ F Cul-de-sac ♀	Ø Open 3 Percutaneous 4 Percutaneous Endoscopic 7 Via Natural or Artificial Opening 8 Via Natural or Artificial Opening Endoscopic	Z No Device	Z No Qualifier
G Vagina ♀ K Hymen ♀	Ø Open 3 Percutaneous 4 Percutaneous Endoscopic 7 Via Natural or Artificial Opening 8 Via Natural or Artificial Opening Endoscopic X External	Z No Device	Z No Qualifier
J Clitoris ♀ L Vestibular Gland ♀ M Vulva ♀	Ø Open X External	Z No Device	Z No Qualifier

DRG Non-OR   ØUQG[7,8,X]ZZ
DRG Non-OR   ØUQM[Ø,X]ZZ

Ø **Medical and Surgical**
U **Female Reproductive System**
S **Reposition**   Moving to its normal location or other suitable location all or a portion of a body part

Body Part Character 4	Approach Character 5	Device Character 6	Qualifier Character 7
Ø Ovary, Right ♀ 1 Ovary, Left ♀ 2 Ovaries, Bilateral ♀ 4 Uterine Supporting Structure ♀ 5 Fallopian Tube, Right ♀ 6 Fallopian Tube, Left ♀ 7 Fallopian Tubes, Bilateral ♀ C Cervix ♀ F Cul-de-sac ♀	Ø Open 4 Percutaneous Endoscopic	Z No Device	Z No Qualifier
9 Uterus ♀ G Vagina ♀	Ø Open 4 Percutaneous Endoscopic X External	Z No Device	Z No Qualifier

Non-OR   ØUS9XZZ

Ø **Medical and Surgical**
U **Female Reproductive System**
T **Resection**   Cutting out or off, without replacement, all of a body part

Body Part Character 4	Approach Character 5	Device Character 6	Qualifier Character 7
Ø Ovary, Right ♀ 1 Ovary, Left ♀ 2 Ovaries, Bilateral ♀ 5 Fallopian Tube, Right ♀ 6 Fallopian Tube, Left ♀ 7 Fallopian Tubes, Bilateral ♀ 9 Uterus ♀	Ø Open 4 Percutaneous Endoscopic 7 Via Natural or Artificial Opening 8 Via Natural or Artificial Opening Endoscopic F Via Natural or Artificial Opening With Percutaneous Endoscopic Assistance	Z No Device	Z No Qualifier
4 Uterine Supporting Structure ♀ C Cervix ♀ F Cul-de-sac ♀ G Vagina ♀ K Hymen ♀	Ø Open 4 Percutaneous Endoscopic 7 Via Natural or Artificial Opening 8 Via Natural or Artificial Opening Endoscopic	Z No Device	Z No Qualifier
J Clitoris ♀ L Vestibular Gland ♀ M Vulva ♀	Ø Open X External	Z No Device	Z No Qualifier
K Hymen ♀	Ø Open 4 Percutaneous Endoscopic 7 Via Natural or Artificial Opening 8 Via Natural or Artificial Opening Endoscopic X External	Z No Device	Z No Device

Ø Medical and Surgical
U Female Reproductive System
U Supplement Putting in or on biological or synthetic material that physically reinforces and/or augments the function of a portion of a body part

Body Part Character 4	Approach Character 5	Device Character 6	Qualifier Character 7
4 Uterine Supporting Structure ♀	Ø Open 4 Percutaneous Endoscopic	7 Autologous Tissue Substitute J Synthetic Substitute K Nonautologous Tissue Substitute	Z No Qualifier
5 Fallopian Tube, Right ♀ 6 Fallopian Tube, Left ♀ 7 Fallopian Tubes, Bilateral ♀ F Cul-de-sac ♀	Ø Open 4 Percutaneous Endoscopic 7 Via Natural or Artificial Opening 8 Via Natural or Artificial Opening Endoscopic	7 Autologous Tissue Substitute J Synthetic Substitute K Nonautologous Tissue Substitute	Z No Qualifier
G Vagina ♀ K Hymen ♀	Ø Open 4 Percutaneous Endoscopic 7 Via Natural or Artificial Opening 8 Via Natural or Artificial Opening Endoscopic X External	7 Autologous Tissue Substitute J Synthetic Substitute K Nonautologous Tissue Substitute	Z No Qualifier
J Clitoris ♀ M Vulva ♀	Ø Open X External	7 Autologous Tissue Substitute J Synthetic Substitute K Nonautologous Tissue Substitute	Z No Qualifier

Ø Medical and Surgical
U Female Reproductive System
V Restriction Partially closing an orifice or the lumen of a tubular body part

Body Part Character 4	Approach Character 5	Device Character 6	Qualifier Character 7
C Cervix ♀	Ø Open 3 Percutaneous 4 Percutaneous Endoscopic	C Extraluminal Device D Intraluminal Device Z No Device	Z No Qualifier
C Cervix ♀	7 Via Natural or Artificial Opening 8 Via Natural or Artificial Opening Endoscopic	D Intraluminal Device Z No Device	Z No Qualifier

Ø Medical and Surgical
U Female Reproductive System
W Revision Correcting, to the extent possible, a portion of a malfunctioning device or the position of a displaced device

Body Part Character 4	Approach Character 5	Device Character 6	Qualifier Character 7
3 Ovary ♀	Ø Open 3 Percutaneous 4 Percutaneous Endoscopic X External	Ø Drainage Device 3 Infusion Device	Z No Qualifier
8 Fallopian Tube ♀	Ø Open 3 Percutaneous 4 Percutaneous Endoscopic 7 Via Natural or Artificial Opening 8 Via Natural or Artificial Opening Endoscopic X External	Ø Drainage Device 3 Infusion Device 7 Autologous Tissue Substitute C Extraluminal Device D Intraluminal Device J Synthetic Substitute K Nonautologous Tissue Substitute	Z No Qualifier
D Uterus and Cervix ♀	Ø Open 3 Percutaneous 4 Percutaneous Endoscopic 7 Via Natural or Artificial Opening 8 Via Natural or Artificial Opening Endoscopic X External	Ø Drainage Device 1 Radioactive Element 3 Infusion Device 7 Autologous Tissue Substitute C Extraluminal Device D Intraluminal Device H Contraceptive Device J Synthetic Substitute K Nonautologous Tissue Substitute	Z No Qualifier
H Vagina and Cul-de-sac ♀	Ø Open 3 Percutaneous 4 Percutaneous Endoscopic 7 Via Natural or Artificial Opening 8 Via Natural or Artificial Opening Endoscopic X External	Ø Drainage Device 1 Radioactive Element 3 Infusion Device 7 Autologous Tissue Substitute D Intraluminal Device J Synthetic Substitute K Nonautologous Tissue Substitute	Z No Qualifier

ØUW Continued on next page

Non-OR ØUW3X[Ø,3]Z
Non-OR ØUW8X[Ø,3,7,C,D,J,K]Z
Non-OR ØUWDX[Ø,3,7,C,D,H,J,K]Z
Non-OR ØUWHX[Ø,3,7,C,D,J,K]Z

LC Limited Coverage   NC Noncovered   HAC associated procedure   Combination Only   DRG Non-OR   Non-OR   Revised Text in GREEN

ØUW Continued

Ø Medical and Surgical
U Female Reproductive System
W Revision Correcting, to the extent possible, a portion of a malfunctioning device or the position of a displaced device

Body Part Character 4	Approach Character 5	Device Character 6	Qualifier Character 7
M Vulva ♀	Ø Open X External	Ø Drainage Device 7 Autologous Tissue Substitute J Synthetic Substitute K Nonautologous Tissue Substitute	Z No Qualifier

Non-OR ØUWMX[Ø,7,J,K]Z

Ø Medical and Surgical
U Female Reproductive System
Y Transplantation Putting in or on all or a portion of a living body part taken from another individual or animal to physically take the place and/or function of all or a portion of a similar body part

Body Part Character 4	Approach Character 5	Device Character 6	Qualifier Character 7
Ø Ovary, Right ♀ 1 Ovary, Left ♀	Ø Open	Z No Device	Ø Allogeneic 1 Syngeneic 2 Zooplastic

Male Reproductive System 0V1–0VW

0   Medical and Surgical
V   Male Reproductive System
1   Bypass   Altering the route of passage of the contents of a tubular body part

Body Part Character 4		Approach Character 5	Device Character 6	Qualifier Character 7
N Vas Deferens, Right ♂ P Vas Deferens, Left ♂ Q Vas Deferens, Bilateral ♂		0 Open 4 Percutaneous Endoscopic	7 Autologous Tissue Substitute J Synthetic Substitute K Nonautologous Tissue Substitute Z No Device	J Epididymis, Right K Epididymis, Left N Vas Deferens, Right P Vas Deferens, Left

0   Medical and Surgical
V   Male Reproductive System
2   Change   Taking out or off a device from a body part and putting back an identical or similar device in or on the same body part without cutting or puncturing the skin or a mucous membrane

Body Part Character 4		Approach Character 5	Device Character 6	Qualifier Character 7
4 Prostate and Seminal Vesicles ♂ 8 Scrotum and Tunica Vaginalis ♂ D Testis ♂ M Epididymis and Spermatic Cord ♂ R Vas Deferens ♂ S Penis ♂		X External	0 Drainage Device Y Other Device	Z No Qualifier

Non-OR   For all body part, approach, device, and qualifier values

0   Medical and Surgical
V   Male Reproductive System
5   Destruction   Physical eradication of all or a portion of a body part by the direct use of energy, force, or a destructive agent

Body Part Character 4		Approach Character 5	Device Character 6	Qualifier Character 7
0 Prostate ♂		0 Open 3 Percutaneous 4 Percutaneous Endoscopic 7 Via Natural or Artificial Opening 8 Via Natural or Artificial Opening Endoscopic	Z No Device	Z No Qualifier
1 Seminal Vesicle, Right ♂ 2 Seminal Vesicle, Left ♂ 3 Seminal Vesicles, Bilateral ♂ 6 Tunica Vaginalis, Right ♂ 7 Tunica Vaginalis, Left ♂ 9 Testis, Right ♂ B Testis, Left ♂ C Testes, Bilateral ♂ F Spermatic Cord, Right ♂ G Spermatic Cord, Left ♂ H Spermatic Cords, Bilateral ♂ J Epididymis, Right ♂ K Epididymis, Left ♂ L Epididymis, Bilateral ♂ N Vas Deferens, Right NC ♂ P Vas Deferens, Left NC ♂ Q Vas Deferens, Bilateral NC ♂		0 Open 3 Percutaneous 4 Percutaneous Endoscopic	Z No Device	Z No Qualifier
5 Scrotum ♂ S Penis ♂ T Prepuce ♂		0 Open 3 Percutaneous 4 Percutaneous Endoscopic X External	Z No Device	Z No Qualifier

NC   0V5N[0,3,4]ZZ
NC   0V5P[0,3,4]ZZ
NC   0V5Q[0,3,4]ZZ
Non-OR   0V5[N,P,Q][0,3,4]ZZ
Non-OR   0V55[0,3,4,X]ZZ

Male Reproductive System

0V7–0V9

0 **Medical and Surgical**
V **Male Reproductive System**
7 **Dilation**   Expanding an orifice or the lumen of a tubular body part

Body Part Character 4		Approach Character 5	Device Character 6	Qualifier Character 7
N Vas Deferens, Right	♂	**0** Open	**D** Intraluminal Device	**Z** No Qualifier
P Vas Deferens, Left	♂	**3** Percutaneous	**Z** No Device	
Q Vas Deferens, Bilateral	♂	**4** Percutaneous Endoscopic		

0 **Medical and Surgical**
V **Male Reproductive System**
9 **Drainage**   Taking or letting out fluids and/or gases from a body part

Body Part Character 4		Approach Character 5	Device Character 6	Qualifier Character 7
0 Prostate	♂	**0** Open **3** Percutaneous **4** Percutaneous Endoscopic **7** Via Natural or Artificial Opening **8** Via Natural or Artificial Opening Endoscopic	**0** Drainage Device	**Z** No Qualifier
0 Prostate	♂	**0** Open **3** Percutaneous **4** Percutaneous Endoscopic **7** Via Natural or Artificial Opening **8** Via Natural or Artificial Opening Endoscopic	**Z** No Device	**X** Diagnostic **Z** No Qualifier
1 Seminal Vesicle, Right **2** Seminal Vesicle, Left **3** Seminal Vesicles, Bilateral **6** Tunica Vaginalis, Right **7** Tunica Vaginalis, Left **9** Testis, Right **B** Testis, Left **C** Testes, Bilateral **F** Spermatic Cord, Right **G** Spermatic Cord, Left **H** Spermatic Cords, Bilateral **J** Epididymis, Right **K** Epididymis, Left **L** Epididymis, Bilateral **N** Vas Deferens, Right **P** Vas Deferens, Left **Q** Vas Deferens, Bilateral	♂ ♂ ♂ ♂ ♂ ♂ ♂ ♂ ♂ ♂ ♂ ♂ ♂ ♂ ♂ ♂ ♂	**0** Open **3** Percutaneous **4** Percutaneous Endoscopic	**0** Drainage Device	**Z** No Qualifier
1 Seminal Vesicle, Right **2** Seminal Vesicle, Left **3** Seminal Vesicles, Bilateral **6** Tunica Vaginalis, Right **7** Tunica Vaginalis, Left **9** Testis, Right **B** Testis, Left **C** Testes, Bilateral **F** Spermatic Cord, Right **G** Spermatic Cord, Left **H** Spermatic Cords, Bilateral **J** Epididymis, Right **K** Epididymis, Left **L** Epididymis, Bilateral **N** Vas Deferens, Right **P** Vas Deferens, Left **Q** Vas Deferens, Bilateral	♂ ♂ ♂ ♂ ♂ ♂ ♂ ♂ ♂ ♂ ♂ ♂ ♂ ♂ ♂ ♂ ♂	**0** Open **3** Percutaneous **4** Percutaneous Endoscopic	**Z** No Device	**X** Diagnostic **Z** No Qualifier
5 Scrotum **S** Penis **T** Prepuce	♂ ♂ ♂	**0** Open **3** Percutaneous **4** Percutaneous Endoscopic **X** External	**0** Drainage Device	**Z** No Qualifier
5 Scrotum **S** Penis **T** Prepuce	♂ ♂ ♂	**0** Open **3** Percutaneous **4** Percutaneous Endoscopic **X** External	**Z** No Device	**X** Diagnostic **Z** No Qualifier

Non-OR 0V90[3,4]0Z	**Non-OR** 0V9[1,2,3,9,B,C][3,4]Z[X,Z]
Non-OR 0V90[3,4]ZZ	**Non-OR** 0V9[6,7,F,G,H,J,K,L,N,P,Q][0,3,4]ZX
Non-OR 0V90[3,4,7,8]ZX	**Non-OR** 0V9[6,7,F,G,H,N,P,Q][0,3,4]ZZ
Non-OR 0V9[1,2,3,9,B,C][3,4]0Z	**Non-OR** 0V95[0,3,4,X]0Z
Non-OR 0V9[6,7,F,G,H,N,P,Q][0,3,4]0Z	**Non-OR** 0V95[0,3,4,X]Z[X,Z]

Ø **Medical and Surgical**
V **Male Reproductive System**
B **Excision**   Cutting out or off, without replacement, a portion of a body part

Body Part Character 4		Approach Character 5	Device Character 6	Qualifier Character 7
Ø Prostate ♂		**Ø** Open **3** Percutaneous **4** Percutaneous Endoscopic **7** Via Natural or Artificial Opening **8** Via Natural or Artificial Opening Endoscopic	**Z** No Device	**X** Diagnostic **Z** No Qualifier
1 Seminal Vesicle, Right ♂ **2** Seminal Vesicle, Left ♂ **3** Seminal Vesicles, Bilateral ♂ **6** Tunica Vaginalis, Right ♂ **7** Tunica Vaginalis, Left ♂ **9** Testis, Right ♂ **B** Testis, Left ♂ **C** Testes, Bilateral ♂ **F** Spermatic Cord, Right ♂ **G** Spermatic Cord, Left ♂ **H** Spermatic Cords, Bilateral ♂ **J** Epididymis, Right ♂ **K** Epididymis, Left ♂ **L** Epididymis, Bilateral ♂ **N** Vas Deferens, Right ᴺᶜ ♂ **P** Vas Deferens, Left ᴺᶜ ♂ **Q** Vas Deferens, Bilateral ᴺᶜ ♂		**Ø** Open **3** Percutaneous **4** Percutaneous Endoscopic	**Z** No Device	**X** Diagnostic **Z** No Qualifier
5 Scrotum ♂ **S** Penis ♂ **T** Prepuce ♂		**Ø** Open **3** Percutaneous **4** Percutaneous Endoscopic **X** External	**Z** No Device	**X** Diagnostic **Z** No Qualifier

ᴺᶜ	ØVBN[Ø,3,4]ZZ		**Non-OR**	ØVBØ[3,4,7,8]ZX
ᴺᶜ	ØVBP[Ø,3,4]ZZ		**Non-OR**	ØVB[1,3,9,B,C][3,4]ZX
ᴺᶜ	ØVBQ[Ø,3,4]ZZ		**Non-OR**	ØVB[6,7,F,G,H,J,K,L][Ø,3,4]ZX
			Non-OR	ØVB[N,P,Q][Ø,3,4]Z[X,Z]
			Non-OR	ØVB5[Ø,3,4,X]Z[X,Z]

Ø **Medical and Surgical**
V **Male Reproductive System**
C **Extirpation**   Taking or cutting out solid matter from a body part

Body Part Character 4		Approach Character 5	Device Character 6	Qualifier Character 7
Ø Prostate ♂		**Ø** Open **3** Percutaneous **4** Percutaneous Endoscopic **7** Via Natural or Artificial Opening **8** Via Natural or Artificial Opening Endoscopic	**Z** No Device	**Z** No Qualifier
1 Seminal Vesicle, Right ♂ **2** Seminal Vesicle, Left ♂ **3** Seminal Vesicles, Bilateral ♂ **6** Tunica Vaginalis, Right ♂ **7** Tunica Vaginalis, Left ♂ **9** Testis, Right ♂ **B** Testis, Left ♂ **C** Testes, Bilateral ♂ **F** Spermatic Cord, Right ♂ **G** Spermatic Cord, Left ♂ **H** Spermatic Cords, Bilateral ♂ **J** Epididymis, Right ♂ **K** Epididymis, Left ♂ **L** Epididymis, Bilateral ♂ **N** Vas Deferens, Right ♂ **P** Vas Deferens, Left ♂ **Q** Vas Deferens, Bilateral ♂		**Ø** Open **3** Percutaneous **4** Percutaneous Endoscopic	**Z** No Device	**Z** No Qualifier
5 Scrotum ♂ **S** Penis ♂ **T** Prepuce ♂		**Ø** Open **3** Percutaneous **4** Percutaneous Endoscopic **X** External	**Z** No Device	**Z** No Qualifier

Non-OR	ØVC[6,7,N,P,Q][Ø,3,4]ZZ		**Non-OR**	ØVC[5,S][Ø,3,4,X]ZZ
Non-OR	ØVC[5,Q][Ø,3,4]ZZ		**Non-OR**	ØVC[5,S][Ø,3,4,X]ZZ
Non-OR	ØVC[5,S]XZZ			

ᴸᶜ Limited Coverage   ᴺᶜ Noncovered   HAC associated procedure   Combination Only   DRG Non-OR   Non-OR   Revised Text in **GREEN**

Ø   **Medical and Surgical**
V   **Male Reproductive System**
H   **Insertion**   Putting in a nonbiological appliance that monitors, assists, performs, or prevents a physiological function but does not physically take the place of a body part

Body Part Character 4	Approach Character 5	Device Character 6	Qualifier Character 7
Ø Prostate ♂	**Ø** Open **3** Percutaneous **4** Percutaneous Endoscopic **7** Via Natural or Artificial Opening **8** Via Natural or Artificial Opening Endoscopic	**1** Radioactive Element	**Z** No Qualifier
4 Prostate and Seminal Vesicles ♂ **8** Scrotum and Tunica Vaginalis ♂ **D** Testis ♂ **M** Epididymis and Spermatic Cord ♂ **R** Vas Deferens ♂	**Ø** Open **3** Percutaneous **4** Percutaneous Endoscopic **7** Via Natural or Artificial Opening **8** Via Natural or Artificial Opening Endoscopic	**3** Infusion Device	**Z** No Qualifier
S Penis ♂	**Ø** Open **3** Percutaneous **4** Percutaneous Endoscopic **X** External	**3** Infusion Device	**Z** No Qualifier

Non-OR   ØVH[4,8,D,M,R][Ø,3,4,7,8]3Z
Non-OR   ØVHS[Ø,3,4,X]3Z

Ø   **Medical and Surgical**
V   **Male Reproductive System**
J   **Inspection**   Visually and/or manually exploring a body part

Body Part Character 4	Approach Character 5	Device Character 6	Qualifier Character 7
4 Prostate and Seminal Vesicles ♂ **8** Scrotum and Tunica Vaginalis ♂ **D** Testis ♂ **M** Epididymis and Spermatic Cord ♂ **R** Vas Deferens ♂ **S** Penis ♂	**Ø** Open **3** Percutaneous **4** Percutaneous Endoscopic **X** External	**Z** No Device	**Z** No Qualifier

Non-OR   ØVJ[4,D,M,R]XZZ
Non-OR   ØVJ[8,S][Ø,3,4,X]ZZ

Ø   **Medical and Surgical**
V   **Male Reproductive System**
L   **Occlusion**   Completely closing an orifice or the lumen of a tubular body part

Body Part Character 4	Approach Character 5	Device Character 6	Qualifier Character 7
F Spermatic Cord, Right NC ♂ **G** Spermatic Cord, Left NC ♂ **H** Spermatic Cords, Bilateral NC ♂ **N** Vas Deferens, Right NC ♂ **P** Vas Deferens, Left NC ♂ **Q** Vas Deferens, Bilateral NC ♂	**Ø** Open **3** Percutaneous **4** Percutaneous Endoscopic	**C** Extraluminal Device **D** Intraluminal Device **Z** No Device	**Z** No Qualifier

NC ØVLF[Ø,3,4][C,D,Z]Z	**Non-OR** ØVL[F,G,H][Ø,3,4][C,D,Z]Z	
NC ØVLG[Ø,3,4][C,D,Z]Z	**Non-OR** ØVL[N,P,Q][Ø,3,4][C,Z]Z	
NC ØVLH[Ø,3,4][C,D,Z]Z		
NC ØVLN[Ø,3,4][C,Z]Z		
NC ØVLP[Ø,3,4][C,Z]Z		
NC ØVLQ[Ø,3,4][C,Z]Z		

Ø   **Medical and Surgical**
V   **Male Reproductive System**
M   **Reattachment**   Putting back in or on all or a portion of a separated body part to its normal location or other suitable location

Body Part Character 4	Approach Character 5	Device Character 6	Qualifier Character 7
5 Scrotum ♂ **S** Penis ♂	**X** External	**Z** No Device	**Z** No Qualifier
6 Tunica Vaginalis, Right ♂ **7** Tunica Vaginalis, Left ♂ **9** Testis, Right ♂ **B** Testis, Left ♂ **C** Testes, Bilateral ♂ **F** Spermatic Cord, Right ♂ **G** Spermatic Cord, Left ♂ **H** Spermatic Cords, Bilateral ♂	**Ø** Open **4** Percutaneous Endoscopic	**Z** No Device	**Z** No Qualifier

LC Limited Coverage   **NC** Noncovered   HAC associated procedure   Combination Only   DRG Non-OR   Non-OR   Revised Text in **GREEN**

384   ICD-10-PCS 2014 (Draft)

Ø Medical and Surgical
V Male Reproductive System
N Release Freeing a body part from an abnormal physical constraint

Body Part Character 4		Approach Character 5	Device Character 6	Qualifier Character 7
Ø Prostate	♂	**Ø** Open **3** Percutaneous **4** Percutaneous Endoscopic **7** Via Natural or Artificial Opening **8** Via Natural or Artificial Opening Endoscopic	**Z** No Device	**Z** No Qualifier
1 Seminal Vesicle, Right **2** Seminal Vesicle, Left **3** Seminal Vesicles, Bilateral **6** Tunica Vaginalis, Right **7** Tunica Vaginalis, Left **9** Testis, Right **B** Testis, Left **C** Testes, Bilateral **F** Spermatic Cord, Right **G** Spermatic Cord, Left **H** Spermatic Cords, Bilateral **J** Epididymis, Right **K** Epididymis, Left **L** Epididymis, Bilateral **N** Vas Deferens, Right **P** Vas Deferens, Left **Q** Vas Deferens, Bilateral	♂ ♂ ♂ ♂ ♂ ♂ ♂ ♂ ♂ ♂ ♂ ♂ ♂ ♂ ♂ ♂ ♂	**Ø** Open **3** Percutaneous **4** Percutaneous Endoscopic	**Z** No Device	**Z** No Qualifier
5 Scrotum **S** Penis **T** Prepuce	♂ ♂ ♂	**Ø** Open **3** Percutaneous **4** Percutaneous Endoscopic **X** External	**Z** No Device	**Z** No Qualifier

Non-OR ØVN[9,B,C][Ø,3,4]ZZ
Non-OR ØVNT[Ø,3,4,X]ZZ

Ø Medical and Surgical
V Male Reproductive System
P Removal Taking out or off a device from a body part

Body Part Character 4		Approach Character 5	Device Character 6	Qualifier Character 7
4 Prostate and Seminal Vesicles	♂	**Ø** Open **3** Percutaneous **4** Percutaneous Endoscopic **7** Via Natural or Artificial Opening **8** Via Natural or Artificial Opening Endoscopic	**Ø** Drainage Device **1** Radioactive Element **3** Infusion Device **7** Autologous Tissue Substitute **J** Synthetic Substitute **K** Nonautologous Tissue Substitute	**Z** No Qualifier
4 Prostate and Seminal Vesicles	♂	**X** External	**Ø** Drainage Device **1** Radioactive Element **3** Infusion Device	**Z** No Qualifier
8 Scrotum and Tunica Vaginalis **D** Testis **M** Epididymis and Spermatic Cord **S** Penis	♂ ♂ ♂ ♂	**X** External	**Ø** Drainage Device **3** Infusion Device	**Z** No Qualifier
8 Scrotum and Tunica Vaginalis **D** Testis **S** Penis	♂ ♂ ♂	**Ø** Open **3** Percutaneous **4** Percutaneous Endoscopic **7** Via Natural or Artificial Opening **8** Via Natural or Artificial Opening Endoscopic	**Ø** Drainage Device **3** Infusion Device **7** Autologous Tissue Substitute **J** Synthetic Substitute **K** Nonautologous Tissue Substitute	**Z** No Qualifier
M Epididymis and Spermatic Cord	♂	**Ø** Open **3** Percutaneous **4** Percutaneous Endoscopic **7** Via Natural or Artificial Opening **8** Via Natural or Artificial Opening Endoscopic	**Ø** Drainage Device **3** Infusion Device **7** Autologous Tissue Substitute **C** Extraluminal Device **J** Synthetic Substitute **K** Nonautologous Tissue Substitute	**Z** No Qualifier

ØVP Continued on next page

Non-OR ØVP4X[Ø,1,3]Z
Non-OR ØVP[8,D,M,S]X[Ø,3]Z

Male Reproductive System

ØVP Continued

Ø   Medical and Surgical
V   Male Reproductive System
P   Removal   Taking out or off a device from a body part

Body Part Character 4	Approach Character 5	Device Character 6	Qualifier Character 7
R Vas Deferens ♂	Ø Open 3 Percutaneous 4 Percutaneous Endoscopic 7 Via Natural or Artificial Opening 8 Via Natural or Artificial Opening Endoscopic	Ø Drainage Device 3 Infusion Device 7 Autologous Tissue Substitute C Extraluminal Device D Intraluminal Device J Synthetic Substitute K Nonautologous Tissue Substitute	Z No Qualifier
R Vas Deferens ♂	X External	Ø Drainage Device 3 Infusion Device D Intraluminal Device	Z No Qualifier

Non-OR   ØVP[8,D,S][Ø,3,4,7,8][Ø,3,7,J,K]Z
Non-OR   ØVPR[Ø,3,4,7,8][Ø,3,7,C,J,K]Z
Non-OR   ØVPRX[Ø,3,D]Z

Ø   Medical and Surgical
V   Male Reproductive System
Q   Repair   Restoring, to the extent possible, a body part to its normal anatomic structure and function

Body Part Character 4	Approach Character 5	Device Character 6	Qualifier Character 7
Ø Prostate ♂	Ø Open 3 Percutaneous 4 Percutaneous Endoscopic 7 Via Natural or Artificial Opening 8 Via Natural or Artificial Opening Endoscopic	Z No Device	Z No Qualifier
1 Seminal Vesicle, Right ♂ 2 Seminal Vesicle, Left ♂ 3 Seminal Vesicles, Bilateral ♂ 6 Tunica Vaginalis, Right ♂ 7 Tunica Vaginalis, Left ♂ 9 Testis, Right ♂ B Testis, Left ♂ C Testes, Bilateral ♂ F Spermatic Cord, Right ♂ G Spermatic Cord, Left ♂ H Spermatic Cords, Bilateral ♂ J Epididymis, Right ♂ K Epididymis, Left ♂ L Epididymis, Bilateral ♂ N Vas Deferens, Right ♂ P Vas Deferens, Left ♂ Q Vas Deferens, Bilateral ♂	Ø Open 3 Percutaneous 4 Percutaneous Endoscopic	Z No Device	Z No Qualifier
5 Scrotum ♂ S Penis ♂ T Prepuce ♂	Ø Open 3 Percutaneous 4 Percutaneous Endoscopic X External	Z No Device	Z No Qualifier

Non-OR   ØVQ[6,7][Ø,3,4]ZZ
Non-OR   ØVQ5[Ø,3,4,X]ZZ

Ø   Medical and Surgical
V   Male Reproductive System
R   Replacement   Putting in or on biological or synthetic material that physically takes the place and/or function of all or a portion of a body part

Body Part Character 4	Approach Character 5	Device Character 6	Qualifier Character 7
9 Testis, Right ♂ B Testis, Left ♂ C Testes, Bilateral ♂	Ø Open	J Synthetic Substitute	Z No Qualifier

LC Limited Coverage   **NC** Noncovered   HAC associated procedure   Combination Only   DRG Non-OR   Non-OR   Revised Text in **GREEN**

386   ICD-10-PCS 2014 (Draft)

Ø   Medical and Surgical
V   Male Reproductive System
S   Reposition   Moving to its normal location or other suitable location all or a portion of a body part

Body Part Character 4		Approach Character 5	Device Character 6	Qualifier Character 7
9 Testis, Right ♂ **B** Testis, Left ♂ **C** Testes, Bilateral ♂ **F** Spermatic Cord, Right ♂ **G** Spermatic Cord, Left ♂ **H** Spermatic Cords, Bilateral ♂		**Ø** Open **3** Percutaneous **4** Percutaneous Endoscopic	**Z** No Device	**Z** No Qualifier

Ø   Medical and Surgical
V   Male Reproductive System
T   Resection   Cutting out or off, without replacement, all of a body part

Body Part Character 4		Approach Character 5	Device Character 6	Qualifier Character 7
Ø Prostate ♂		**Ø** Open **4** Percutaneous Endoscopic **7** Via Natural or Artificial Opening **8** Via Natural or Artificial Opening Endoscopic	**Z** No Device	**Z** No Qualifier
1 Seminal Vesicle, Right ♂ **2** Seminal Vesicle, Left ♂ **3** Seminal Vesicles, Bilateral ♂ **6** Tunica Vaginalis, Right ♂ **7** Tunica Vaginalis, Left ♂ **9** Testis, Right ♂ **B** Testis, Left ♂ **C** Testes, Bilateral ♂ **F** Spermatic Cord, Right ♂ **G** Spermatic Cord, Left ♂ **H** Spermatic Cords, Bilateral ♂ **J** Epididymis, Right ♂ **K** Epididymis, Left ♂ **L** Epididymis, Bilateral ♂ **N** Vas Deferens, Right NC ♂ **P** Vas Deferens, Left NC ♂ **Q** Vas Deferens, Bilateral NC ♂		**Ø** Open **4** Percutaneous Endoscopic	**Z** No Device	**Z** No Qualifier
5 Scrotum ♂ **S** Penis ♂ **T** Prepuce ♂		**Ø** Open **4** Percutaneous Endoscopic **X** External	**Z** No Device	**Z** No Qualifier

     NC   ØVTN[Ø,4]ZZ
     NC   ØVTP[Ø,4]ZZ
     NC   ØVTQ[Ø,4]ZZ
     Non-OR   ØVT[N,P,Q][Ø,4]ZZ
     Non-OR   ØVT[5,T][Ø,4,X]ZZ

Ø   Medical and Surgical
V   Male Reproductive System
U   Supplement   Putting in or on biological or synthetic material that physically reinforces and/or augments the function of a portion of a body part

Body Part Character 4		Approach Character 5	Device Character 6	Qualifier Character 7
1 Seminal Vesicle, Right ♂ **2** Seminal Vesicle, Left ♂ **3** Seminal Vesicles, Bilateral ♂ **6** Tunica Vaginalis, Right ♂ **7** Tunica Vaginalis, Left ♂ **F** Spermatic Cord, Right ♂ **G** Spermatic Cord, Left ♂ **H** Spermatic Cords, Bilateral ♂ **J** Epididymis, Right ♂ **K** Epididymis, Left ♂ **L** Epididymis, Bilateral ♂ **N** Vas Deferens, Right ♂ **P** Vas Deferens, Left ♂ **Q** Vas Deferens, Bilateral ♂		**Ø** Open **4** Percutaneous Endoscopic	**7** Autologous Tissue Substitute **J** Synthetic Substitute **K** Nonautologous Tissue Substitute	**Z** No Qualifier
5 Scrotum ♂ **S** Penis ♂ **T** Prepuce ♂		**Ø** Open **4** Percutaneous Endoscopic **X** External	**7** Autologous Tissue Substitute **J** Synthetic Substitute **K** Nonautologous Tissue Substitute	**Z** No Qualifier
9 Testis, Right ♂ **B** Testis, Left ♂ **C** Testes, Bilateral ♂		**Ø** Open	**7** Autologous Tissue Substitute **J** Synthetic Substitute **K** Nonautologous Tissue Substitute	**Z** No Qualifier

     Non-OR   ØVUSX[7,J,K]Z

LC Limited Coverage   **NC** Noncovered   HAC associated procedure   Combination Only   DRG Non-OR   Non-OR   Revised Text in GREEN

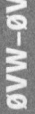

Male Reproductive System

Ø Medical and Surgical
V Male Reproductive System
W Revision   Correcting, to the extent possible, a portion of a malfunctioning device or the position of a displaced device

Body Part Character 4	Approach Character 5	Device Character 6	Qualifier Character 7
4 Prostate and Seminal Vesicles ♂ **8** Scrotum and Tunica Vaginalis ♂ **D** Testis ♂ **S** Penis ♂	**Ø** Open **3** Percutaneous **4** Percutaneous Endoscopic **7** Via Natural or Artificial Opening **8** Via Natural or Artificial Opening Endoscopic **X** External	**Ø** Drainage Device **3** Infusion Device **7** Autologous Tissue Substitute **J** Synthetic Substitute **K** Nonautologous Tissue Substitute	**Z** No Qualifier
M Epididymis and Spermatic Cord ♂	**Ø** Open **3** Percutaneous **4** Percutaneous Endoscopic **7** Via Natural or Artificial Opening **8** Via Natural or Artificial Opening Endoscopic **X** External	**Ø** Drainage Device **3** Infusion Device **7** Autologous Tissue Substitute **C** Extraluminal Device **J** Synthetic Substitute **K** Nonautologous Tissue Substitute	**Z** No Qualifier
R Vas Deferens ♂	**Ø** Open **3** Percutaneous **4** Percutaneous Endoscopic **7** Via Natural or Artificial Opening **8** Via Natural or Artificial Opening Endoscopic **X** External	**Ø** Drainage Device **3** Infusion Device **7** Autologous Tissue Substitute **C** Extraluminal Device **D** Intraluminal Device **J** Synthetic Substitute **K** Nonautologous Tissue Substitute	**Z** No Qualifier

Non-OR   ØVW[4,8,D,S][Ø,3,4,7,8,X][Ø,3,7,J,K]Z
Non-OR   ØVWMX[Ø,3,7,C,J,K]Z
Non-OR   ØVWR[Ø,3,4,7,8,X][Ø,3,7,C,D,J,K]Z

Anatomical Regions, General ØWØ–ØWW

Ø **Medical and Surgical**
W **Anatomical Regions, General**
Ø **Alteration**　　Modifying the anatomic structure of a body part without affecting the function of the body part

Body Part Character 4	Approach Character 5	Device Character 6	Qualifier Character 7
Ø Head **2** Face **4** Upper Jaw **5** Lower Jaw **6** Neck **8** Chest Wall **F** Abdominal Wall **K** Upper Back **L** Lower Back **M** Perineum, Male　　♂ **N** Perineum, Female　　♀	**Ø** Open **3** Percutaneous **4** Percutaneous Endoscopic	**7** Autologous Tissue Substitute **J** Synthetic Substitute **K** Nonautologous Tissue Substitute **Z** No Device	**Z** No Qualifier

Ø **Medical and Surgical**
W **Anatomical Regions, General**
1 **Bypass**　　Altering the route of passage of the contents of a tubular body part

Body Part Character 4	Approach Character 5	Device Character 6	Qualifier Character 7
1 Cranial Cavity	**Ø** Open	**J** Synthetic Substitute	**9** Pleural Cavity, Right **B** Pleural Cavity, Left **G** Peritoneal Cavity **J** Pelvic Cavity
9 Pleural Cavity, Right **B** Pleural Cavity, Left **G** Peritoneal Cavity **J** Pelvic Cavity　　♀	**Ø** Open **4** Percutaneous Endoscopic	**J** Synthetic Substitute	**4** Cutaneous **9** Pleural Cavity, Right **B** Pleural Cavity, Left **G** Peritoneal Cavity **J** Pelvic Cavity **Y** Lower Vein
9 Pleural Cavity, Right **B** Pleural Cavity, Left **G** Peritoneal Cavity **J** Pelvic Cavity　　♀	**3** Percutaneous	**J** Synthetic Substitute	**4** Cutaneous

　Non-OR　ØW1[9,B,G,J][Ø,4]J[4,9,B,G,J,Y]
　Non-OR　ØW1[9,B,J]3J4

Ø **Medical and Surgical**
W **Anatomical Regions, General**
2 **Change**　　Taking out or off a device from a body part and putting back an identical or similar device in or on the same body part without cutting or puncturing the skin or a mucous membrane

Body Part Character 4	Approach Character 5	Device Character 6	Qualifier Character 7
Ø Head **1** Cranial Cavity **2** Face **4** Upper Jaw **5** Lower Jaw **6** Neck **8** Chest Wall **9** Pleural Cavity, Right **B** Pleural Cavity, Left **C** Mediastinum **D** Pericardial Cavity **F** Abdominal Wall **G** Peritoneal Cavity **H** Retroperitoneum **J** Pelvic Cavity **K** Upper Back **L** Lower Back **M** Perineum, Male **N** Perineum, Female	**X** External	**Ø** Drainage Device **Y** Other Device	**Z** No Qualifier

　Non-OR　For all body part, approach, device, and qualifier values

Anatomical Regions, General

ØW3-ØW8

Ø   Medical and Surgical
W   Anatomical Regions, General
3   Control   Stopping, or attempting to stop, postprocedural bleeding

Body Part Character 4	Approach Character 5	Device Character 6	Qualifier Character 7
Ø Head 1 Cranial Cavity 2 Face 4 Upper Jaw 5 Lower Jaw 6 Neck 8 Chest Wall 9 Pleural Cavity, Right B Pleural Cavity, Left C Mediastinum D Pericardial Cavity F Abdominal Wall G Peritoneal Cavity H Retroperitoneum J Pelvic Cavity K Upper Back L Lower Back M Perineum, Male ♂ N Perineum, Female ♀	Ø Open 3 Percutaneous 4 Percutaneous Endoscopic	Z No Device	Z No Qualifier
3 Oral Cavity and Throat	Ø Open 3 Percutaneous 4 Percutaneous Endoscopic 7 Via Natural or Artificial Opening 8 Via Natural or Artificial Opening Endoscopic X External	Z No Device	Z No Qualifier
P Gastrointestinal Tract Q Respiratory Tract R Genitourinary Tract	Ø Open 3 Percutaneous 4 Percutaneous Endoscopic 7 Via Natural or Artificial Opening 8 Via Natural or Artificial Opening Endoscopic	Z No Device	Z No Qualifier

Non-OR   ØW3GØZZ
Non-OR   ØW3P8ZZ

Ø   Medical and Surgical
W   Anatomical Regions, General
4   Creation   Making a new genital structure that does not take over the function of a body part

Body Part Character 4	Approach Character 5	Device Character 6	Qualifier Character 7
M Perineum, Male ♂ NC	Ø Open	7 Autologous Tissue Substitute J Synthetic Substitute K Nonautologous Tissue Substitute Z No Device	Ø Vagina
N Perineum, Female ♀ NC	Ø Open	7 Autologous Tissue Substitute J Synthetic Substitute K Nonautologous Tissue Substitute Z No Device	1 Penis

NC   ØW4MØ[7,J,K,Z]Ø
NC   ØW4NØ[7,J,K,Z]1

Ø   Medical and Surgical
W   Anatomical Regions, General
8   Division   Cutting into a body part without draining fluids and/or gases from the body part in order to separate or transect a body part

Body Part Character 4	Approach Character 5	Device Character 6	Qualifier Character 7
N Perineum, Female ♀	X External	Z No Device	Z No Qualifier

Non-OR   ØW8NXZZ

Ø Medical and Surgical
W Anatomical Regions, General
9 Drainage   Taking or letting out fluids and/or gases from a body part

Body Part Character 4	Approach Character 5	Device Character 6	Qualifier Character 7
Ø Head **1** Cranial Cavity **2** Face **3** Oral Cavity and Throat **4** Upper Jaw **5** Lower Jaw **6** Neck **8** Chest Wall **9** Pleural Cavity, Right **B** Pleural Cavity, Left **C** Mediastinum **D** Pericardial Cavity **F** Abdominal Wall **G** Peritoneal Cavity **H** Retroperitoneum **J** Pelvic Cavity **K** Upper Back **L** Lower Back **M** Perineum, Male ♂ **N** Perineum, Female ♀	**Ø** Open **3** Percutaneous **4** Percutaneous Endoscopic	**Ø** Drainage Device	**Z** No Qualifier
Ø Head **1** Cranial Cavity **2** Face **3** Oral Cavity and Throat **4** Upper Jaw **5** Lower Jaw **6** Neck **8** Chest Wall **9** Pleural Cavity, Right **B** Pleural Cavity, Left **C** Mediastinum **D** Pericardial Cavity **F** Abdominal Wall **G** Peritoneal Cavity **H** Retroperitoneum **J** Pelvic Cavity **K** Upper Back **L** Lower Back **M** Perineum, Male ♂ **N** Perineum, Female ♀	**Ø** Open **3** Percutaneous **4** Percutaneous Endoscopic	**Z** No Device	**X** Diagnostic **Z** No Qualifier

Non-OR ØW9[Ø,8,9,B,K,L,M][Ø,3,4]ØZ	**Non-OR** ØW9[Ø,8,9,B,K,L,M][Ø,3,4]ZZ
Non-OR ØW9[1,D,F,G][3,4]ØZ	**Non-OR** ØW9[1,C,D][3,4]ZX
Non-OR ØW9J3ØZ	**Non-OR** ØW9[1,D,F,G][3,4]ZZ
Non-OR ØW9[Ø,2,3,4,5,6,8,9,B,K,L,M,N][Ø,3,4]ZX	**Non-OR** ØW9J3ZZ

Ø Medical and Surgical
W Anatomical Regions, General
B Excision   Cutting out or off, without replacement, a portion of a body part

Body Part Character 4	Approach Character 5	Device Character 6	Qualifier Character 7
Ø Head **2** Face **4** Upper Jaw **5** Lower Jaw **8** Chest Wall **K** Upper Back **L** Lower Back **M** Perineum, Male ♂ **N** Perineum, Female ♀	**Ø** Open **3** Percutaneous **4** Percutaneous Endoscopic **X** External	**Z** No Device	**X** Diagnostic **Z** No Qualifier
6 Neck **C** Mediastinum **F** Abdominal Wall **H** Retroperitoneum	**Ø** Open **3** Percutaneous **4** Percutaneous Endoscopic	**Z** No Device	**X** Diagnostic **Z** No Qualifier
6 Neck **F** Abdominal Wall	**X** External	**Z** No Device	**2** Stoma **X** Diagnostic **Z** No Qualifier

Non-OR   ØWB[Ø,2,4,5,K,L,M][Ø,3,4,X]ZX
Non-OR   ØWB6[Ø,3,4]ZX
Non-OR   ØWB[C,H][3,4]ZX

LC Limited Coverage   **NC** Noncovered   HAC associated procedure   Combination Only   DRG Non-OR   Non-OR   Revised Text in **GREEN**

ICD-10-PCS 2014 (Draft)   **391**

Anatomical Regions, General

Ø   **Medical and Surgical**
W   **Anatomical Regions, General**
C   **Extirpation**   Taking or cutting out solid matter from a body part

Body Part Character 4	Approach Character 5	Device Character 6	Qualifier Character 7
1 Cranial Cavity **3** Oral Cavity and Throat **9** Pleural Cavity, Right **B** Pleural Cavity, Left **C** Mediastinum **D** Pericardial Cavity **G** Peritoneal Cavity **J** Pelvic Cavity	**Ø** Open **3** Percutaneous **4** Percutaneous Endoscopic **X** External	**Z** No Device	**Z** No Qualifier
P Gastrointestinal Tract **Q** Respiratory Tract **R** Genitourinary Tract	**Ø** Open **3** Percutaneous **4** Percutaneous Endoscopic **7** Via Natural or Artificial Opening **8** Via Natural or Artificial Opening Endoscopic **X** External	**Z** No Device	**Z** No Qualifier

Non-OR	ØWC[1,3]XZZ
Non-OR	ØWC[9,B][Ø,3,4,X]ZZ
Non-OR	ØWC[C,D,G,J]XZZ
Non-OR	ØWCP[7,8,X]ZZ
Non-OR	ØWCQ[Ø,3,4,X]ZZ
Non-OR	ØWCR[7,8,X]ZZ

Ø   **Medical and Surgical**
W   **Anatomical Regions, General**
F   **Fragmentation**   Breaking solid matter in a body part into pieces

Body Part Character 4	Approach Character 5	Device Character 6	Qualifier Character 7
1 Cranial Cavity NC **3** Oral Cavity and Throat NC **9** Pleural Cavity, Right NC **B** Pleural Cavity, Left NC **C** Mediastinum NC **D** Pericardial Cavity **G** Peritoneal Cavity NC **J** Pelvic Cavity NC	**Ø** Open **3** Percutaneous **4** Percutaneous Endoscopic **X** External	**Z** No Device	**Z** No Qualifier
P Gastrointestinal Tract NC **Q** Respiratory Tract NC **R** Genitourinary Tract	**Ø** Open **3** Percutaneous **4** Percutaneous Endoscopic **7** Via Natural or Artificial Opening **8** Via Natural or Artificial Opening Endoscopic **X** External	**Z** No Device	**Z** No Qualifier

NC	ØWF[1,3,9,B,C,G,J]XZZ
NC	ØWF[P,Q]XZZ
DRG Non-OR	ØWFRXZZ
Non-OR	ØWF[1,3,9,B,C,G]XZZ
Non-OR	ØWFJ[Ø,3,4,X]ZZ
Non-OR	ØWFP[Ø,3,4,7,8,X]ZZ
Non-OR	ØWFQXZZ
Non-OR	ØWFR[Ø,3,4,7,8]ZZ

Ø   Medical and Surgical
W   Anatomical Regions, General
H   Insertion   Putting in a nonbiological appliance that monitors, assists, performs, or prevents a physiological function but does not physically take the place of a body part

Body Part Character 4	Approach Character 5	Device Character 6	Qualifier Character 7
Ø Head 1 Cranial Cavity 2 Face 3 Oral Cavity and Throat 4 Upper Jaw 5 Lower Jaw 6 Neck 8 Chest Wall 9 Pleural Cavity, Right B Pleural Cavity, Left C Mediastinum D Pericardial Cavity F Abdominal Wall G Peritoneal Cavity H Retroperitoneum J Pelvic Cavity K Upper Back L Lower Back M Perineum, Male N Perineum, Female ♀	Ø Open 3 Percutaneous 4 Percutaneous Endoscopic	1 Radioactive Element 3 Infusion Device Y Other Device	Z No Qualifier
P Gastrointestinal Tract Q Respiratory Tract R Genitourinary Tract	Ø Open 3 Percutaneous 4 Percutaneous Endoscopic 7 Via Natural or Artificial Opening 8 Via Natural or Artificial Opening Endoscopic	1 Radioactive Element 3 Infusion Device Y Other Device	Z No Qualifier

DRG Non-OR	ØWH[Ø,2,4,5,6,K,L,M][Ø,3,4][3,Y]Z	**Non-OR**	ØWHP[3,4,7,8][3,Y]Z
Non-OR	ØWH1[Ø,3,4]3Z	**Non-OR**	ØWHQ[Ø,7,8][3,Y]Z
Non-OR	ØWH[8,9,B][Ø,3,4][3,Y]Z	**Non-OR**	ØWHR[Ø,3,4,7,8][3,Y]Z
Non-OR	ØWHPØYZ		

Ø   Medical and Surgical
W   Anatomical Regions, General
J   Inspection   Visually and/or manually exploring a body part

Body Part Character 4	Approach Character 5	Device Character 6	Qualifier Character 7
Ø Head 2 Face 3 Oral Cavity and Throat 4 Upper Jaw 5 Lower Jaw 6 Neck 8 Chest Wall F Abdominal Wall K Upper Back L Lower Back M Perineum, Male ♂ N Perineum, Female ♀	Ø Open 3 Percutaneous 4 Percutaneous Endoscopic X External	Z No Device	Z No Qualifier
1 Cranial Cavity 9 Pleural Cavity, Right B Pleural Cavity, Left C Mediastinum D Pericardial Cavity G Peritoneal Cavity H Retroperitoneum J Pelvic Cavity	Ø Open 3 Percutaneous 4 Percutaneous Endoscopic	Z No Device	Z No Qualifier
P Gastrointestinal Tract Q Respiratory Tract R Genitourinary Tract	Ø Open 3 Percutaneous 4 Percutaneous Endoscopic 7 Via Natural or Artificial Opening 8 Via Natural or Artificial Opening Endoscopic	Z No Device	Z No Qualifier

DRG Non-OR	ØWJ[Ø,2,4,5,K,L]ØZZ
DRG Non-OR	ØWJM[Ø,4]ZZ
Non-OR	ØWJ[Ø,2,4,5,K,L,M,N][Ø,3,4,X]ZZ
Non-OR	ØWJD[Ø,3]ZZ

LC Limited Coverage   NC Noncovered   HAC associated procedure   Combination Only   DRG Non-OR   Non-OR   Revised Text in GREEN

0   **Medical and Surgical**
W   **Anatomical Regions, General**
M   **Reattachment**   Putting back in or on all or a portion of a separated body part to its normal location or other suitable location

Body Part Character 4	Approach Character 5	Device Character 6	Qualifier Character 7
2 Face **4** Upper Jaw **5** Lower Jaw **6** Neck **8** Chest Wall **F** Abdominal Wall **K** Upper Back **L** Lower Back **M** Perineum, Male ♂ **N** Perineum, Female ♀	**0** Open	**Z** No Device	**Z** No Qualifier

0   **Medical and Surgical**
W   **Anatomical Regions, General**
P   **Removal**   Taking out or off a device from a body part

Body Part Character 4	Approach Character 5	Device Character 6	Qualifier Character 7
0 Head **2** Face **4** Upper Jaw **5** Lower Jaw **6** Neck **8** Chest Wall **C** Mediastinum **F** Abdominal Wall **K** Upper Back **L** Lower Back **M** Perineum, Male ♂ **N** Perineum, Female ♀	**0** Open **3** Percutaneous **4** Percutaneous Endoscopic **X** External	**0** Drainage Device **1** Radioactive Element **3** Infusion Device **7** Autologous Tissue Substitute **J** Synthetic Substitute **K** Nonautologous Tissue Substitute **Y** Other Device	**Z** No Qualifier
1 Cranial Cavity **9** Pleural Cavity, Right **B** Pleural Cavity, Left **D** Pericardial Cavity **G** Peritoneal Cavity **H** Retroperitoneum **J** Pelvic Cavity	**X** External	**0** Drainage Device **1** Radioactive Element **3** Infusion Device	**Z** No Qualifier
1 Cranial Cavity **9** Pleural Cavity, Right **B** Pleural Cavity, Left **G** Peritoneal Cavity **J** Pelvic Cavity	**0** Open **3** Percutaneous **4** Percutaneous Endoscopic	**0** Drainage Device **1** Radioactive Element **3** Infusion Device **J** Synthetic Substitute **Y** Other Device	**Z** No Qualifier
D Pericardial Cavity **H** Retroperitoneum	**0** Open **3** Percutaneous **4** Percutaneous Endoscopic	**0** Drainage Device **1** Radioactive Element **3** Infusion Device **Y** Other Device	**Z** No Qualifier
P Gastrointestinal Tract **Q** Respiratory Tract **R** Genitourinary Tract	**0** Open **3** Percutaneous **4** Percutaneous Endoscopic **7** Via Natural or Artificial Opening **8** Via Natural or Artificial Opening Endoscopic **X** External	**1** Radioactive Element **3** Infusion Device **Y** Other Device	**Z** No Qualifier

Non-OR   For all body part, approach, device, and qualifier values

Ø **Medical and Surgical**
W **Anatomical Regions, General**
Q **Repair** Restoring, to the extent possible, a body part to its normal anatomic structure and function

Body Part Character 4	Approach Character 5	Device Character 6	Qualifier Character 7
Ø Head 2 Face 4 Upper Jaw 5 Lower Jaw 8 Chest Wall K Upper Back L Lower Back M Perineum, Male N Perineum, Female ♀	Ø Open 3 Percutaneous 4 Percutaneous Endoscopic X External	Z No Device	Z No Qualifier
6 Neck C Mediastinum F Abdominal Wall	Ø Open 3 Percutaneous 4 Percutaneous Endoscopic	Z No Device	Z No Qualifier
6 Neck F Abdominal Wall	X External	Z No Device	2 Stoma Z No Qualifier

Non-OR ØWQNXZZ

Ø **Medical and Surgical**
W **Anatomical Regions, General**
U **Supplement** Putting in or on biological or synthetic material that physically reinforces and/or augments the function of a portion of a body part

Body Part Character 4	Approach Character 5	Device Character 6	Qualifier Character 7
Ø Head 2 Face 4 Upper Jaw 5 Lower Jaw 6 Neck 8 Chest Wall C Mediastinum F Abdominal Wall K Upper Back L Lower Back M Perineum, Male ♂ N Perineum, Female ♀	Ø Open 4 Percutaneous Endoscopic	7 Autologous Tissue Substitute J Synthetic Substitute K Nonautologous Tissue Substitute	Z No Qualifier

Ø **Medical and Surgical**
W **Anatomical Regions, General**
W **Revision** Correcting, to the extent possible, a portion of a malfunctioning device or the position of a displaced device

Body Part Character 4	Approach Character 5	Device Character 6	Qualifier Character 7
Ø Head 2 Face 4 Upper Jaw 5 Lower Jaw 6 Neck 8 Chest Wall C Mediastinum F Abdominal Wall K Upper Back L Lower Back M Perineum, Male ♂ N Perineum, Female ♀	Ø Open 3 Percutaneous 4 Percutaneous Endoscopic X External	Ø Drainage Device 1 Radioactive Element 3 Infusion Device 7 Autologous Tissue Substitute J Synthetic Substitute K Nonautologous Tissue Substitute Y Other Device	Z No Qualifier
1 Cranial Cavity 9 Pleural Cavity, Right B Pleural Cavity, Left G Peritoneal Cavity J Pelvic Cavity	Ø Open 3 Percutaneous 4 Percutaneous Endoscopic X External	Ø Drainage Device 1 Radioactive Element 3 Infusion Device J Synthetic Substitute Y Other Device	Z No Qualifier
D Pericardial Cavity H Retroperitoneum	Ø Open 3 Percutaneous 4 Percutaneous Endoscopic X External	Ø Drainage Device 1 Radioactive Element 3 Infusion Device Y Other Device	Z No Qualifier

ØWW Continued on next page

DRG Non-OR ØWW[Ø,2,4,5,6,K,L][Ø,3,4][Ø,1,3,7,J,K,Y]Z	**Non-OR** ØWW[1,G,J]X[Ø,1,3,J,Y]Z
DRG Non-OR ØWWM[Ø,3,4][Ø,1,3,J,Y]Z	**Non-OR** ØWW[9,B][Ø,3,4,X][Ø,1,3,J,Y]Z
Non-OR ØWW[Ø,2,4,5,6,C,F,K,L,M,N]X[Ø,1,3,7,J,K,Y]Z	**Non-OR** ØWW[D,H]X[Ø,1,3,Y]Z
Non-OR ØWW8[Ø,3,4,X][Ø,1,3,7,J,K,Y]Z	

Anatomical Regions, General

ØWW–ØWW

Ø   Medical and Surgical   *ØWW Continued*
W   Anatomical Regions, General
W   Revision   Correcting, to the extent possible, a portion of a malfunctioning device or the position of a displaced device

Body Part Character 4	Approach Character 5	Device Character 6	Qualifier Character 7
P Gastrointestinal Tract **Q** Respiratory Tract **R** Genitourinary Tract	**Ø** Open **3** Percutaneous **4** Percutaneous Endoscopic **7** Via Natural or Artificial Opening **8** Via Natural or Artificial Opening 　　Endoscopic **X** External	**1** Radioactive Element **3** Infusion Device **Y** Other Device	**Z** No Qualifier

Non-OR	ØWWP[3,4,7,8,X][1,3,Y]Z
Non-OR	ØWWQ[Ø,X][1,3,Y]Z
Non-OR	ØWWR[Ø,3,4,7,8,X][1,3,Y]Z

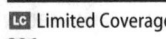 Limited Coverage   **NC** Noncovered   HAC associated procedure   Combination Only   DRG Non-OR   Non-OR   Revised Text in **GREEN**

396   ICD-10-PCS 2014 (Draft)

Anatomical Regions, Upper Extremities 0X0–0XX

0   **Medical and Surgical**
X   **Anatomical Regions, Upper Extremities**
0   **Alteration**   Modifying the anatomic structure of a body part without affecting the function of the body part

Body Part Character 4	Approach Character 5	Device Character 6	Qualifier Character 7
2 Shoulder Region, Right **3** Shoulder Region, Left **4** Axilla, Right **5** Axilla, Left **6** Upper Extremity, Right **7** Upper Extremity, Left **8** Upper Arm, Right **9** Upper Arm, Left **B** Elbow Region, Right **C** Elbow Region, Left **D** Lower Arm, Right **F** Lower Arm, Left **G** Wrist Region, Right **H** Wrist Region, Left	**0** Open **3** Percutaneous **4** Percutaneous Endoscopic	**7** Autologous Tissue Substitute **J** Synthetic Substitute **K** Nonautologous Tissue Substitute **Z** No Device	**Z** No Qualifier

0   **Medical and Surgical**
X   **Anatomical Regions, Upper Extremities**
2   **Change**   Taking out or off a device from a body part and putting back an identical or similar device in or on the same body part without cutting or puncturing the skin or a mucous membrane

Body Part Character 4	Approach Character 5	Device Character 6	Qualifier Character 7
6 Upper Extremity, Right **7** Upper Extremity, Left	**X** External	**0** Drainage Device **Y** Other Device	**Z** No Qualifier

> **Non-OR**   For all body part, approach, device, and qualifier values

0   **Medical and Surgical**
X   **Anatomical Regions, Upper Extremities**
3   **Control**   Stopping, or attempting to stop, postprocedural bleeding

Body Part Character 4	Approach Character 5	Device Character 6	Qualifier Character 7
2 Shoulder Region, Right **3** Shoulder Region, Left **4** Axilla, Right **5** Axilla, Left **6** Upper Extremity, Right **7** Upper Extremity, Left **8** Upper Arm, Right **9** Upper Arm, Left **B** Elbow Region, Right **C** Elbow Region, Left **D** Lower Arm, Right **F** Lower Arm, Left **G** Wrist Region, Right **H** Wrist Region, Left **J** Hand, Right **K** Hand, Left	**0** Open **3** Percutaneous **4** Percutaneous Endoscopic	**Z** No Device	**Z** No Qualifier

0   **Medical and Surgical**
X   **Anatomical Regions, Upper Extremities**
6   **Detachment**   Cutting off all or a portion of the upper or lower extremities

Body Part Character 4	Approach Character 5	Device Character 6	Qualifier Character 7
0 Forequarter, Right **1** Forequarter, Left **2** Shoulder Region, Right **3** Shoulder Region, Left **B** Elbow Region, Right **C** Elbow Region, Left	**0** Open	**Z** No Device	**Z** No Qualifier
8 Upper Arm, Right **9** Upper Arm, Left **D** Lower Arm, Right **F** Lower Arm, Left	**0** Open	**Z** No Device	**1** High **2** Mid **3** Low

0X6 Continued on next page

Anatomical Regions, Upper Extremities *(left margin)*

ØX6–ØX9 *(left margin)*

Ø   **Medical and Surgical**   *ØX6 Continued*
X   **Anatomical Regions, Upper Extremities**
6   **Detachment**   Cutting off all or a portion of the upper or lower extremities

Body Part Character 4	Approach Character 5	Device Character 6	Qualifier Character 7
J Hand, Right K Hand, Left	Ø Open	Z No Device	Ø Complete 4 Complete 1st Ray 5 Complete 2nd Ray 6 Complete 3rd Ray 7 Complete 4th Ray 8 Complete 5th Ray 9 Partial 1st Ray B Partial 2nd Ray C Partial 3rd Ray D Partial 4th Ray F Partial 5th Ray
L Thumb, Right M Thumb, Left N Index Finger, Right P Index Finger, Left Q Middle Finger, Right R Middle Finger, Left S Ring Finger, Right T Ring Finger, Left V Little Finger, Right W Little Finger, Left	Ø Open	Z No Device	Ø Complete 1 High 2 Mid 3 Low

Ø   **Medical and Surgical**
X   **Anatomical Regions, Upper Extremities**
9   **Drainage**   Taking or letting out fluids and/or gases from a body part

Body Part Character 4	Approach Character 5	Device Character 6	Qualifier Character 7
2 Shoulder Region, Right 3 Shoulder Region, Left 4 Axilla, Right 5 Axilla, Left 6 Upper Extremity, Right 7 Upper Extremity, Left 8 Upper Arm, Right 9 Upper Arm, Left B Elbow Region, Right C Elbow Region, Left D Lower Arm, Right F Lower Arm, Left G Wrist Region, Right H Wrist Region, Left J Hand, Right K Hand, Left	Ø Open 3 Percutaneous 4 Percutaneous Endoscopic	Ø Drainage Device	Z No Qualifier
2 Shoulder Region, Right 3 Shoulder Region, Left 4 Axilla, Right 5 Axilla, Left 6 Upper Extremity, Right 7 Upper Extremity, Left 8 Upper Arm, Right 9 Upper Arm, Left B Elbow Region, Right C Elbow Region, Left D Lower Arm, Right F Lower Arm, Left G Wrist Region, Right H Wrist Region, Left J Hand, Right K Hand, Left	Ø Open 3 Percutaneous 4 Percutaneous Endoscopic	Z No Device	X Diagnostic Z No Qualifier

Non-OR   For all body part, approach, device, and qualifier values

---

Ø   Medical and Surgical
X   Anatomical Regions, Upper Extremities
B   Excision   Cutting out or off, without replacement, a portion of a body part

Body Part Character 4	Approach Character 5	Device Character 6	Qualifier Character 7
2 Shoulder Region, Right	Ø Open	Z No Device	X Diagnostic
3 Shoulder Region, Left	3 Percutaneous		Z No Qualifier
4 Axilla, Right	4 Percutaneous Endoscopic		
5 Axilla, Left			
6 Upper Extremity, Right			
7 Upper Extremity, Left			
8 Upper Arm, Right			
9 Upper Arm, Left			
B Elbow Region, Right			
C Elbow Region, Left			
D Lower Arm, Right			
F Lower Arm, Left			
G Wrist Region, Right			
H Wrist Region, Left			
J Hand, Right			
K Hand, Left			

Non-OR   ØXB[2,3,4,5,6,7,8,9,B,C,D,F,G,H,J,K][Ø,3,4]ZX

Ø   Medical and Surgical
X   Anatomical Regions, Upper Extremities
H   Insertion   Putting in a nonbiological appliance that monitors, assists, performs, or prevents a physiological function but does not physically take the place of a body part

Body Part Character 4	Approach Character 5	Device Character 6	Qualifier Character 7
2 Shoulder Region, Right	Ø Open	1 Radioactive Element	Z No Qualifier
3 Shoulder Region, Left	3 Percutaneous	3 Infusion Device	
4 Axilla, Right	4 Percutaneous Endoscopic	Y Other Device	
5 Axilla, Left			
6 Upper Extremity, Right			
7 Upper Extremity, Left			
8 Upper Arm, Right			
9 Upper Arm, Left			
B Elbow Region, Right			
C Elbow Region, Left			
D Lower Arm, Right			
F Lower Arm, Left			
G Wrist Region, Right			
H Wrist Region, Left			
J Hand, Right			
K Hand, Left			

DRG Non-OR   ØXH[2,3,4,5,6,7,8,9,B,C,D,F,G,H,J,K][Ø,3,4][3,Y]Z

Ø   Medical and Surgical
X   Anatomical Regions, Upper Extremities
J   Inspection   Visually and/or manually exploring a body part

Body Part Character 4	Approach Character 5	Device Character 6	Qualifier Character 7
2 Shoulder Region, Right	Ø Open	Z No Device	Z No Qualifier
3 Shoulder Region, Left	3 Percutaneous		
4 Axilla, Right	4 Percutaneous Endoscopic		
5 Axilla, Left	X External		
6 Upper Extremity, Right			
7 Upper Extremity, Left			
8 Upper Arm, Right			
9 Upper Arm, Left			
B Elbow Region, Right			
C Elbow Region, Left			
D Lower Arm, Right			
F Lower Arm, Left			
G Wrist Region, Right			
H Wrist Region, Left			
J Hand, Right			
K Hand, Left			

DRG Non-OR   ØXJ[2,3,4,5,6,7,8,9,B,C,D,F,G,H,J,K]ØZZ
Non-OR   ØXJ[2,3,4,5,6,7,8,9,B,C,D,F,G,H][3,4,X]ZZ
Non-OR   ØXJ[J,K]XZZ

LC Limited Coverage   NC Noncovered   HAC associated procedure   Combination Only   DRG Non-OR   Non-OR   Revised Text in GREEN

Anatomical Regions, Upper Extremities

ØXM–ØXP

Ø   Medical and Surgical
X   Anatomical Regions, Upper Extremities
M   Reattachment   Putting back in or on all or a portion of a separated body part to its normal location or other suitable location

Body Part Character 4	Approach Character 5	Device Character 6	Qualifier Character 7
Ø Forequarter, Right	Ø Open	Z No Device	Z No Qualifier
1 Forequarter, Left			
2 Shoulder Region, Right			
3 Shoulder Region, Left			
4 Axilla, Right			
5 Axilla, Left			
6 Upper Extremity, Right			
7 Upper Extremity, Left			
8 Upper Arm, Right			
9 Upper Arm, Left			
B Elbow Region, Right			
C Elbow Region, Left			
D Lower Arm, Right			
F Lower Arm, Left			
G Wrist Region, Right			
H Wrist Region, Left			
J Hand, Right			
K Hand, Left			
L Thumb, Right			
M Thumb, Left			
N Index Finger, Right			
P Index Finger, Left			
Q Middle Finger, Right			
R Middle Finger, Left			
S Ring Finger, Right			
T Ring Finger, Left			
V Little Finger, Right			
W Little Finger, Left			

Ø   Medical and Surgical
X   Anatomical Regions, Upper Extremities
P   Removal   Taking out or off a device from a body part

Body Part Character 4	Approach Character 5	Device Character 6	Qualifier Character 7
6 Upper Extremity, Right	Ø Open	Ø Drainage Device	Z No Qualifier
7 Upper Extremity, Left	3 Percutaneous	1 Radioactive Element	
	4 Percutaneous Endoscopic	3 Infusion Device	
	X External	7 Autologous Tissue Substitute	
		J Synthetic Substitute	
		K Nonautologous Tissue Substitute	
		Y Other Device	

Non-OR   For all body part, approach, device, and qualifier values

Ø   **Medical and Surgical**
X   **Anatomical Regions, Upper Extremities**
Q   **Repair**   Restoring, to the extent possible, a body part to its normal anatomic structure and function

Body Part Character 4	Approach Character 5	Device Character 6	Qualifier Character 7
2 Shoulder Region, Right	**Ø** Open	**Z** No Device	**Z** No Qualifier
3 Shoulder Region, Left	**3** Percutaneous		
4 Axilla, Right	**4** Percutaneous Endoscopic		
5 Axilla, Left	**X** External		
6 Upper Extremity, Right			
7 Upper Extremity, Left			
8 Upper Arm, Right			
9 Upper Arm, Left			
B Elbow Region, Right			
C Elbow Region, Left			
D Lower Arm, Right			
F Lower Arm, Left			
G Wrist Region, Right			
H Wrist Region, Left			
J Hand, Right			
K Hand, Left			
L Thumb, Right			
M Thumb, Left			
N Index Finger, Right			
P Index Finger, Left			
Q Middle Finger, Right			
R Middle Finger, Left			
S Ring Finger, Right			
T Ring Finger, Left			
V Little Finger, Right			
W Little Finger, Left			

Ø   **Medical and Surgical**
X   **Anatomical Regions, Upper Extremities**
R   **Replacement**   Putting in or on biological or synthetic material that physically takes the place and/or function of all or a portion of a body part

Body Part Character 4	Approach Character 5	Device Character 6	Qualifier Character 7
L Thumb, Right	**Ø** Open	**7** Autologous Tissue Substitute	**N** Toe, Right
M Thumb, Left	**4** Percutaneous Endoscopic		**P** Toe, Left

Ø   **Medical and Surgical**
X   **Anatomical Regions, Upper Extremities**
U   **Supplement**   Putting in or on biological or synthetic material that physically reinforces and/or augments the function of a portion of a body part

Body Part Character 4	Approach Character 5	Device Character 6	Qualifier Character 7
2 Shoulder Region, Right	**Ø** Open	**7** Autologous Tissue Substitute	**Z** No Qualifier
3 Shoulder Region, Left	**4** Percutaneous Endoscopic	**J** Synthetic Substitute	
4 Axilla, Right		**K** Nonautologous Tissue Substitute	
5 Axilla, Left			
6 Upper Extremity, Right			
7 Upper Extremity, Left			
8 Upper Arm, Right			
9 Upper Arm, Left			
B Elbow Region, Right			
C Elbow Region, Left			
D Lower Arm, Right			
F Lower Arm, Left			
G Wrist Region, Right			
H Wrist Region, Left			
J Hand, Right			
K Hand, Left			
L Thumb, Right			
M Thumb, Left			
N Index Finger, Right			
P Index Finger, Left			
Q Middle Finger, Right			
R Middle Finger, Left			
S Ring Finger, Right			
T Ring Finger, Left			
V Little Finger, Right			
W Little Finger, Left			

Ø　Medical and Surgical
X　Anatomical Regions, Upper Extremities
W　Revision　　　　Correcting, to the extent possible, a portion of a malfunctioning device or the position of a displaced device

Body Part Character 4	Approach Character 5	Device Character 6	Qualifier Character 7
6 Upper Extremity, Right **7** Upper Extremity, Left	**Ø** Open **3** Percutaneous **4** Percutaneous Endoscopic **X** External	**Ø** Drainage Device **3** Infusion Device **7** Autologous Tissue Substitute **J** Synthetic Substitute **K** Nonautologous Tissue Substitute **Y** Other Device	**Z** No Qualifier

Non-OR　ØXW[6,7]X[Ø,3,7,J,K,Y]Z

Ø　Medical and Surgical
X　Anatomical Regions, Upper Extremities
X　Transfer　　　　Moving, without taking out, all or a portion of a body part to another location to take over the function of all or a portion of a body part

Body Part Character 4	Approach Character 5	Device Character 6	Qualifier Character 7
N Index Finger, Right	**Ø** Open	**Z** No Device	**L** Thumb, Right
P Index Finger, Left	**Ø** Open	**Z** No Device	**M** Thumb, Left

Anatomical Regions, Lower Extremities ØYØ–ØYW

Ø   Medical and Surgical
Y   Anatomical Regions, Lower Extremities
Ø   Alteration   Modifying the anatomic structure of a body part without affecting the function of the body part

Body Part Character 4	Approach Character 5	Device Character 6	Qualifier Character 7
Ø Buttock, Right **1** Buttock, Left **9** Lower Extremity, Right **B** Lower Extremity, Left **C** Upper Leg, Right **D** Upper Leg, Left **F** Knee Region, Right **G** Knee Region, Left **H** Lower Leg, Right **J** Lower Leg, Left **K** Ankle Region, Right **L** Ankle Region, Left	**Ø** Open **3** Percutaneous **4** Percutaneous Endoscopic	**7** Autologous Tissue Substitute **J** Synthetic Substitute **K** Nonautologous Tissue Substitute **Z** No Device	**Z** No Qualifier

Ø   Medical and Surgical
Y   Anatomical Regions, Lower Extremities
2   Change   Taking out or off a device from a body part and putting back an identical or similar device in or on the same body part without cutting or puncturing the skin or a mucous membrane

Body Part Character 4	Approach Character 5	Device Character 6	Qualifier Character 7
9 Lower Extremity, Right **B** Lower Extremity, Left	**X** External	**Ø** Drainage Device **Y** Other Device	**Z** No Qualifier

Non-OR   For all body part, approach, device, and qualifier values

Ø   Medical and Surgical
Y   Anatomical Regions, Lower Extremities
3   Control   Stopping, or attempting to stop, postprocedural bleeding

Body Part Character 4	Approach Character 5	Device Character 6	Qualifier Character 7
Ø Buttock, Right **1** Buttock, Left **5** Inguinal Region, Right **6** Inguinal Region, Left **7** Femoral Region, Right **8** Femoral Region, Left **9** Lower Extremity, Right **B** Lower Extremity, Left **C** Upper Leg, Right **D** Upper Leg, Left **F** Knee Region, Right **G** Knee Region, Left **H** Lower Leg, Right **J** Lower Leg, Left **K** Ankle Region, Right **L** Ankle Region, Left **M** Foot, Right **N** Foot, Left	**Ø** Open **3** Percutaneous **4** Percutaneous Endoscopic	**Z** No Device	**Z** No Qualifier

Ø   Medical and Surgical
Y   Anatomical Regions, Lower Extremities
6   Detachment   Cutting off all or a portion of the upper or lower extremities

Body Part Character 4	Approach Character 5	Device Character 6	Qualifier Character 7
2 Hindquarter, Right **3** Hindquarter, Left **4** Hindquarter, Bilateral **7** Femoral Region, Right **8** Femoral Region, Left **F** Knee Region, Right **G** Knee Region, Left	**Ø** Open	**Z** No Device	**Z** No Qualifier
C Upper Leg, Right **D** Upper Leg, Left **H** Lower Leg, Right **J** Lower Leg, Left	**Ø** Open	**Z** No Device	**1** High **2** Mid **3** Low

ØY6 Continued on next page

LC Limited Coverage   **NC** Noncovered   HAC associated procedure   Combination Only   DRG Non-OR   Non-OR   Revised Text in **GREEN**

ICD-10-PCS 2014 (Draft)   403

Anatomical Regions, Lower Extremities *(side margin)*

ØY6–ØY9 *(side margin)*

ØY6 Continued

Ø   **Medical and Surgical**
Y   **Anatomical Regions, Lower Extremities**
6   **Detachment**   Cutting off all or a portion of the upper or lower extremities

Body Part Character 4	Approach Character 5	Device Character 6	Qualifier Character 7
M Foot, Right N Foot, Left	Ø Open	Z No Device	Ø Complete 4 Complete 1st Ray 5 Complete 2nd Ray 6 Complete 3rd Ray 7 Complete 4th Ray 8 Complete 5th Ray 9 Partial 1st Ray B Partial 2nd Ray C Partial 3rd Ray D Partial 4th Ray F Partial 5th Ray
P 1st Toe, Right Q 1st Toe, Left R 2nd Toe, Right S 2nd Toe, Left T 3rd Toe, Right U 3rd Toe, Left V 4th Toe, Right W 4th Toe, Left X 5th Toe, Right Y 5th Toe, Left	Ø Open	Z No Device	Ø Complete 1 High 2 Mid 3 Low

Ø   **Medical and Surgical**
Y   **Anatomical Regions, Lower Extremities**
9   **Drainage**   Taking or letting out fluids and/or gases from a body part

Body Part Character 4	Approach Character 5	Device Character 6	Qualifier Character 7
Ø Buttock, Right 1 Buttock, Left 5 Inguinal Region, Right 6 Inguinal Region, Left 7 Femoral Region, Right 8 Femoral Region, Left 9 Lower Extremity, Right B Lower Extremity, Left C Upper Leg, Right D Upper Leg, Left F Knee Region, Right G Knee Region, Left H Lower Leg, Right J Lower Leg, Left K Ankle Region, Right L Ankle Region, Left M Foot, Right N Foot, Left	Ø Open 3 Percutaneous 4 Percutaneous Endoscopic	Ø Drainage Device	Z No Qualifier
Ø Buttock, Right 1 Buttock, Left 5 Inguinal Region, Right 6 Inguinal Region, Left 7 Femoral Region, Right 8 Femoral Region, Left 9 Lower Extremity, Right B Lower Extremity, Left C Upper Leg, Right D Upper Leg, Left F Knee Region, Right G Knee Region, Left H Lower Leg, Right J Lower Leg, Left K Ankle Region, Right L Ankle Region, Left M Foot, Right N Foot, Left	Ø Open 3 Percutaneous 4 Percutaneous Endoscopic	Z No Device	X Diagnostic Z No Qualifier

Non-OR   ØY9[Ø,1,7,8,9,B,C,D,F,G,H,J,K,L,M,N][Ø,3,4]ØZ
Non-OR   ØY9[Ø,1,7,8,9,B,C,D,F,G,H,J,K,L,M,N][Ø,3,4]Z[X,Z]

Ø   **Medical and Surgical**
Y   **Anatomical Regions, Lower Extremities**
B   **Excision**   Cutting out or off, without replacement, a portion of a body part

Body Part Character 4	Approach Character 5	Device Character 6	Qualifier Character 7
Ø Buttock, Right	**Ø** Open	**Z** No Device	**X** Diagnostic
1 Buttock, Left	**3** Percutaneous		**Z** No Qualifier
5 Inguinal Region, Right	**4** Percutaneous Endoscopic		
6 Inguinal Region, Left			
7 Femoral Region, Right			
8 Femoral Region, Left			
9 Lower Extremity, Right			
B Lower Extremity, Left			
C Upper Leg, Right			
D Upper Leg, Left			
F Knee Region, Right			
G Knee Region, Left			
H Lower Leg, Right			
J Lower Leg, Left			
K Ankle Region, Right			
L Ankle Region, Left			
M Foot, Right			
N Foot, Left			

Non-OR   ØYB[Ø,1,9,B,C,D,F,G,H,J,K,L,M,N][Ø,3,4]ZX

Ø   **Medical and Surgical**
Y   **Anatomical Regions, Lower Extremities**
H   **Insertion**   Putting in a nonbiological appliance that monitors, assists, performs, or prevents a physiological function but does not physically take the place of a body part

Body Part Character 4	Approach Character 5	Device Character 6	Qualifier Character 7
Ø Buttock, Right	**Ø** Open	**1** Radioactive Element	**Z** No Qualifier
1 Buttock, Left	**3** Percutaneous	**3** Infusion Device	
5 Inguinal Region, Right	**4** Percutaneous Endoscopic	**Y** Other Device	
6 Inguinal Region, Left			
7 Femoral Region, Right			
8 Femoral Region, Left			
9 Lower Extremity, Right			
B Lower Extremity, Left			
C Upper Leg, Right			
D Upper Leg, Left			
F Knee Region, Right			
G Knee Region, Left			
H Lower Leg, Right			
J Lower Leg, Left			
K Ankle Region, Right			
L Ankle Region, Left			
M Foot, Right			
N Foot, Left			

DRG Non-OR   ØYH[Ø,1,5,6,7,8,9,B,C,D,F,G,H,J,K,L,M,N][Ø,3,4][3,Y]Z

Ø   Medical and Surgical
Y   Anatomical Regions, Lower Extremities
J   Inspection   Visually and/or manually exploring a body part

Body Part Character 4	Approach Character 5	Device Character 6	Qualifier Character 7
Ø Buttock, Right	Ø Open	Z No Device	Z No Qualifier
1 Buttock, Left	3 Percutaneous		
5 Inguinal Region, Right	4 Percutaneous Endoscopic		
6 Inguinal Region, Left	X External		
7 Femoral Region, Right			
8 Femoral Region, Left			
9 Lower Extremity, Right			
A Inguinal Region, Bilateral			
B Lower Extremity, Left			
C Upper Leg, Right			
D Upper Leg, Left			
E Femoral Region, Bilateral			
F Knee Region, Right			
G Knee Region, Left			
H Lower Leg, Right			
J Lower Leg, Left			
K Ankle Region, Right			
L Ankle Region, Left			
M Foot, Right			
N Foot, Left			

DRG Non-OR   ØYJ[Ø,1,8,9,B,C,D,E,F,G,H,J,K,L,M,N]ØZZ
Non-OR   ØYJ[Ø,1,5,6,8,9,A,B,C,D,E,F,G,H,J,K,L,M,N][3,4,X]ZZ

Ø   Medical and Surgical
Y   Anatomical Regions, Lower Extremities
M   Reattachment   Putting back in or on all or a portion of a separated body part to its normal location or other suitable location

Body Part Character 4	Approach Character 5	Device Character 6	Qualifier Character 7
Ø Buttock, Right	Ø Open	Z No Device	Z No Qualifier
1 Buttock, Left			
2 Hindquarter, Right			
3 Hindquarter, Left			
4 Hindquarter, Bilateral			
5 Inguinal Region, Right			
6 Inguinal Region, Left			
7 Femoral Region, Right			
8 Femoral Region, Left			
9 Lower Extremity, Right			
B Lower Extremity, Left			
C Upper Leg, Right			
D Upper Leg, Left			
F Knee Region, Right			
G Knee Region, Left			
H Lower Leg, Right			
J Lower Leg, Left			
K Ankle Region, Right			
L Ankle Region, Left			
M Foot, Right			
N Foot, Left			
P 1st Toe, Right			
Q 1st Toe, Left			
R 2nd Toe, Right			
S 2nd Toe, Left			
T 3rd Toe, Right			
U 3rd Toe, Left			
V 4th Toe, Right			
W 4th Toe, Left			
X 5th Toe, Right			
Y 5th Toe, Left			

Ø   **Medical and Surgical**
Y   **Anatomical Regions, Lower Extremities**
P   **Removal**   Taking out or off a device from a body part

Body Part Character 4	Approach Character 5	Device Character 6	Qualifier Character 7
9 Lower Extremity, Right B Lower Extremity, Left	Ø Open 3 Percutaneous 4 Percutaneous Endoscopic X External	Ø Drainage Device 1 Radioactive Element 3 Infusion Device 7 Autologous Tissue Substitute J Synthetic Substitute K Nonautologous Tissue Substitute Y Other Device	Z No Qualifier

Non-OR   For all body part, approach, device, and qualifier values

Ø   **Medical and Surgical**
Y   **Anatomical Regions, Lower Extremities**
Q   **Repair**   Restoring, to the extent possible, a body part to its normal anatomic structure and function

Body Part Character 4	Approach Character 5	Device Character 6	Qualifier Character 7
Ø Buttock, Right 1 Buttock, Left 5 Inguinal Region, Right 6 Inguinal Region, Left 7 Femoral Region, Right 8 Femoral Region, Left 9 Lower Extremity, Right A Inguinal Region, Bilateral B Lower Extremity, Left C Upper Leg, Right D Upper Leg, Left E Femoral Region, Bilateral F Knee Region, Right G Knee Region, Left H Lower Leg, Right J Lower Leg, Left K Ankle Region, Right L Ankle Region, Left M Foot, Right N Foot, Left P 1st Toe, Right Q 1st Toe, Left R 2nd Toe, Right S 2nd Toe, Left T 3rd Toe, Right U 3rd Toe, Left V 4th Toe, Right W 4th Toe, Left X 5th Toe, Right Y 5th Toe, Left	Ø Open 3 Percutaneous 4 Percutaneous Endoscopic X External	Z No Device	Z No Qualifier

Non-OR   ØYQ[5,6,7,8,A,E]XZZ

LC Limited Coverage   **NC** Noncovered   HAC associated procedure   Combination Only   DRG Non-OR   Non-OR   Revised Text in **GREEN**

ICD-10-PCS 2014 (Draft)   **407**

Ø   **Medical and Surgical**
Y   **Anatomical Regions, Lower Extremities**
U   **Supplement**   Putting in or on biological or synthetic material that physically reinforces and/or augments the function of a portion of a body part

Body Part Character 4	Approach Character 5	Device Character 6	Qualifier Character 7
Ø Buttock, Right	**Ø** Open	**7** Autologous Tissue Substitute	**Z** No Qualifier
1 Buttock, Left	**4** Percutaneous Endoscopic	**J** Synthetic Substitute	
5 Inguinal Region, Right		**K** Nonautologous Tissue Substitute	
6 Inguinal Region, Left			
7 Femoral Region, Right			
8 Femoral Region, Left			
9 Lower Extremity, Right			
A Inguinal Region, Bilateral			
B Lower Extremity, Left			
C Upper Leg, Right			
D Upper Leg, Left			
E Femoral Region, Bilateral			
F Knee Region, Right			
G Knee Region, Left			
H Lower Leg, Right			
J Lower Leg, Left			
K Ankle Region, Right			
L Ankle Region, Left			
M Foot, Right			
N Foot, Left			
P 1st Toe, Right			
Q 1st Toe, Left			
R 2nd Toe, Right			
S 2nd Toe, Left			
T 3rd Toe, Right			
U 3rd Toe, Left			
V 4th Toe, Right			
W 4th Toe, Left			
X 5th Toe, Right			
Y 5th Toe, Left			

Ø   **Medical and Surgical**
Y   **Anatomical Regions, Lower Extremities**
W   **Revision**   Correcting, to the extent possible, a portion of a malfunctioning device or the position of a displaced device

Body Part Character 4	Approach Character 5	Device Character 6	Qualifier Character 7
9 Lower Extremity, Right	**Ø** Open	**Ø** Drainage Device	**Z** No Qualifier
B Lower Extremity, Left	**3** Percutaneous	**3** Infusion Device	
	4 Percutaneous Endoscopic	**7** Autologous Tissue Substitute	
	X External	**J** Synthetic Substitute	
		K Nonautologous Tissue Substitute	
		Y Other Device	

DRG Non-OR	ØYW[9,B][Ø,3,4][Ø,3,7,J,K,Y]Z
Non-OR	ØYW[9,B]X[Ø,3,7,J,K,Y]Z

Obstetrics 1Ø2–1ØY

1   Obstetrics
Ø   Pregnancy
2   Change   Taking out or off a device from a body part and putting back an identical or similar device in or on the same body part without cutting or puncturing the skin or a mucous membrane

Body Part Character 4		Approach Character 5	Device Character 6	Qualifier Character 7
Ø Products of Conception	♀	**7** Via Natural or Artificial Opening	**3** Monitoring Electrode **Y** Other Device	**Z** No Qualifier

Non-OR   For all body part, approach, device, and qualifier values

1   Obstetrics
Ø   Pregnancy
9   Drainage   Taking or letting out fluids and/or gases from a body part

Body Part Character 4		Approach Character 5	Device Character 6	Qualifier Character 7
Ø Products of Conception	♀	**Ø** Open **3** Percutaneous **4** Percutaneous Endoscopic **7** Via Natural or Artificial Opening **8** Via Natural or Artificial Opening Endoscopic	**Z** No Device	**9** Fetal Blood **A** Fetal Cerebrospinal Fluid **B** Fetal Fluid, Other **C** Amniotic Fluid, Therapeutic **D** Fluid, Other **U** Amniotic Fluid, Diagnostic

Non-OR   For all body part, approach, device, and qualifier values

1   Obstetrics
Ø   Pregnancy
A   Abortion   Artificially terminating a pregnancy

Body Part Character 4		Approach Character 5	Device Character 6	Qualifier Character 7
Ø Products of Conception	♀	**Ø** Open **3** Percutaneous **4** Percutaneous Endoscopic **8** Via Natural or Artificial Opening Endoscopic	**Z** No Device	**Z** No Qualifier
Ø Products of Conception	♀	**7** Via Natural or Artificial Opening	**Z** No Device	**6** Vacuum **W** Laminaria **X** Abortifacient **Z** No Qualifier

Non-OR   1ØAØ7Z[6,W,X]

1   Obstetrics
Ø   Pregnancy
D   Extraction   Pulling or stripping out or off all or a portion of a body part

Body Part Character 4		Approach Character 5	Device Character 6	Qualifier Character 7
Ø Products of Conception	♀	**Ø** Open	**Z** No Device	**Ø** Classical **1** Low Cervical **2** Extraperitoneal
Ø Products of Conception	♀	**7** Via Natural or Artificial Opening	**Z** No Device	**3** Low Forceps **4** Mid Forceps **5** High Forceps **6** Vacuum **7** Internal Version **8** Other
1 Products of Conception, Retained **2** Products of Conception, Ectopic	♀ ♀	**7** Via Natural or Artificial Opening **8** Via Natural or Artificial Opening Endoscopic	**Z** No Device	**Z** No Qualifier

DRG Non-OR   1ØDØ7Z[3,4,5,6,7,8]

1   Obstetrics
Ø   Pregnancy
E   Delivery   Assisting the passage of the products of conception from the genital canal

Body Part Character 4		Approach Character 5	Device Character 6	Qualifier Character 7
Ø Products of Conception	♀	**X** External	**Z** No Device	**Z** No Qualifier

DRG Non-OR   1ØEØXZZ

LC Limited Coverage   **NC** Noncovered   HAC associated procedure   Combination Only   DRG Non-OR   Non-OR   Revised Text in **GREEN**

1 Obstetrics
0 Pregnancy
H Insertion   Putting in a nonbiological appliance that monitors, assists, performs, or prevents a physiological function but does not physically take the place of a body part

Body Part Character 4	Approach Character 5	Device Character 6	Qualifier Character 7
0 Products of Conception ♀	0 Open 7 Via Natural or Artificial Opening	3 Monitoring Electrode Y Other Device	Z No Qualifier

Non-OR   For all body part, approach, device, and qualifier values

1 Obstetrics
0 Pregnancy
J Inspection   Visually and/or manually exploring a body part

Body Part Character 4	Approach Character 5	Device Character 6	Qualifier Character 7
0 Products of Conception ♀ 1 Products of Conception, Retained ♀ 2 Products of Conception, Ectopic ♀	0 Open 3 Percutaneous 4 Percutaneous Endoscopic 7 Via Natural or Artificial Opening 8 Via Natural or Artificial Opening Endoscopic X External	Z No Device	Z No Qualifier

Non-OR   For all body part, approach, device, and qualifier values

1 Obstetrics
0 Pregnancy
P Removal   Taking out or off a device from a body part, region or orifice

Body Part Character 4	Approach Character 5	Device Character 6	Qualifier Character 7
0 Products of Conception ♀	0 Open 7 Via Natural or Artificial Opening	3 Monitoring Electrode Y Other Device	Z No Qualifier

1 Obstetrics
0 Pregnancy
Q Repair   Restoring, to the extent possible, a body part to its normal anatomic structure and function

Body Part Character 4	Approach Character 5	Device Character 6	Qualifier Character 7
0 Products of Conception ♀	0 Open 3 Percutaneous 4 Percutaneous Endoscopic 7 Via Natural or Artificial Opening 8 Via Natural or Artificial Opening Endoscopic	Y Other Device Z No Device	E Nervous System F Cardiovascular System G Lymphatics and Hemic H Eye J Ear, Nose and Sinus K Respiratory System L Mouth and Throat M Gastrointestinal System N Hepatobiliary and Pancreas P Endocrine System Q Skin R Musculoskeletal System S Urinary System T Female Reproductive System V Male Reproductive System Y Other Body System

Non-OR   For all body part, approach, device, and qualifier values

1 Obstetrics
0 Pregnancy
S Reposition   Moving to its normal location or other suitable location all or a portion of a body part

Body Part Character 4	Approach Character 5	Device Character 6	Qualifier Character 7
0 Products of Conception ♀	7 Via Natural or Artificial Opening X External	Z No Device	Z No Qualifier
2 Products of Conception, Ectopic ♀	0 Open 3 Percutaneous 4 Percutaneous Endoscopic 7 Via Natural or Artificial Opening 8 Via Natural or Artificial Opening Endoscopic	Z No Device	Z No Qualifier

DRG Non-OR   10S07ZZ
Non-OR   10S0XZZ

LC Limited Coverage   **NC** Noncovered   HAC associated procedure   Combination Only   DRG Non-OR   Non-OR   Revised Text in **GREEN**

410   ICD-10-PCS 2014 (Draft)

1　Obstetrics
0　Pregnancy
T　Resection　　Cutting out or off, without replacement, all of a body part

Body Part Character 4	Approach Character 5	Device Character 6	Qualifier Character 7
2　Products of Conception, Ectopic　♀	0　Open 3　Percutaneous 4　Percutaneous Endoscopic 7　Via Natural or Artificial Opening 8　Via Natural or Artificial Opening Endoscopic	Z　No Device	Z　No Qualifier

1　Obstetrics
0　Pregnancy
Y　Transplantation　　Putting in or on all or a portion of a living body part taken from another individual or animal to physically take the place and/or function of all or a portion of a similar body part

Body Part Character 4	Approach Character 5	Device Character 6	Qualifier Character 7
0　Products of Conception　♀	3　Percutaneous 4　Percutaneous Endoscopic 7　Via Natural or Artificial Opening	Z　No Device	E　Nervous System F　Cardiovascular System G　Lymphatics and Hemic H　Eye J　Ear, Nose and Sinus K　Respiratory System L　Mouth and Throat M　Gastrointestinal System N　Hepatobiliary and Pancreas P　Endocrine System Q　Skin R　Musculoskeletal System S　Urinary System T　Female Reproductive System V　Male Reproductive System Y　Other Body System

Non-OR　　For all body part, approach, device, and qualifier values

Placement—Anatomical Regions 2W0–2W6

2   **Placement**
W   **Anatomical Regions**
0   **Change**   Taking out or off a device from a body part and putting back an identical or similar device in or on the same body part without cutting or puncturing the skin or a mucous membrane

Body Region Character 4	Approach Character 5	Device Character 6	Qualifier Character 7
0 Head	**X** External	**0** Traction Apparatus	**Z** No Qualifier
1 Face		**1** Splint	
2 Neck		**2** Cast	
3 Abdominal Wall		**3** Brace	
4 Chest Wall		**4** Bandage	
5 Back		**5** Packing Material	
6 Inguinal Region, Right		**6** Pressure Dressing	
7 Inguinal Region, Left		**7** Intermittent Pressure Device	
8 Upper Extremity, Right		**Y** Other Device	
9 Upper Extremity, Left			
A Upper Arm, Right			
B Upper Arm, Left			
C Lower Arm, Right			
D Lower Arm, Left			
E Hand, Right			
F Hand, Left			
G Thumb, Right			
H Thumb, Left			
J Finger, Right			
K Finger, Left			
L Lower Extremity, Right			
M Lower Extremity, Left			
N Upper Leg, Right			
P Upper Leg, Left			
Q Lower Leg, Right			
R Lower Leg, Left			
S Foot, Right			
T Foot, Left			
U Toe, Right			
V Toe, Left			
1 Face	**X** External	**0** Traction Apparatus	**Z** No Qualifier
		1 Splint	
		2 Cast	
		3 Brace	
		4 Bandage	
		5 Packing Material	
		6 Pressure Dressing	
		7 Intermittent Pressure Device	
		9 Wire	
		Y Other Device	

2 Placement
W Anatomical Regions
1 Compression   Putting pressure on a body region

Body Region Character 4	Approach Character 5	Device Character 6	Qualifier Character 7
0 Head	X External	6 Pressure Dressing	Z No Qualifier
1 Face		7 Intermittent Pressure Device	
2 Neck			
3 Abdominal Wall			
4 Chest Wall			
5 Back			
6 Inguinal Region, Right			
7 Inguinal Region, Left			
8 Upper Extremity, Right			
9 Upper Extremity, Left			
A Upper Arm, Right			
B Upper Arm, Left			
C Lower Arm, Right			
D Lower Arm, Left			
E Hand, Right			
F Hand, Left			
G Thumb, Right			
H Thumb, Left			
J Finger, Right			
K Finger, Left			
L Lower Extremity, Right			
M Lower Extremity, Left			
N Upper Leg, Right			
P Upper Leg, Left			
Q Lower Leg, Right			
R Lower Leg, Left			
S Foot, Right			
T Foot, Left			
U Toe, Right			
V Toe, Left			

2 Placement
W Anatomical Regions
2 Dressing   Putting material on a body region for protection

Body Region Character 4	Approach Character 5	Device Character 6	Qualifier Character 7
0 Head	X External	4 Bandage	Z No Qualifier
1 Face			
2 Neck			
3 Abdominal Wall			
4 Chest Wall			
5 Back			
6 Inguinal Region, Right			
7 Inguinal Region, Left			
8 Upper Extremity, Right			
9 Upper Extremity, Left			
A Upper Arm, Right			
B Upper Arm, Left			
C Lower Arm, Right			
D Lower Arm, Left			
E Hand, Right			
F Hand, Left			
G Thumb, Right			
H Thumb, Left			
J Finger, Right			
K Finger, Left			
L Lower Extremity, Right			
M Lower Extremity, Left			
N Upper Leg, Right			
P Upper Leg, Left			
Q Lower Leg, Right			
R Lower Leg, Left			
S Foot, Right			
T Foot, Left			
U Toe, Right			
V Toe, Left			

Placement—Anatomical Regions   2W1—2W2

2   Placement
W   Anatomical Regions
3   Immobilization   Limiting or preventing motion of a body region

Body Region Character 4	Approach Character 5	Device Character 6	Qualifier Character 7
Ø Head	X External	1 Splint	Z No Qualifier
2 Neck		2 Cast	
3 Abdominal Wall		3 Brace	
4 Chest Wall		Y Other Device	
5 Back			
6 Inguinal Region, Right			
7 Inguinal Region, Left			
8 Upper Extremity, Right			
9 Upper Extremity, Left			
A Upper Arm, Right			
B Upper Arm, Left			
C Lower Arm, Right			
D Lower Arm, Left			
E Hand, Right			
F Hand, Left			
G Thumb, Right			
H Thumb, Left			
J Finger, Right			
K Finger, Left			
L Lower Extremity, Right			
M Lower Extremity, Left			
N Upper Leg, Right			
P Upper Leg, Left			
Q Lower Leg, Right			
R Lower Leg, Left			
S Foot, Right			
T Foot, Left			
U Toe, Right			
V Toe, Left			
1 Face	X External	1 Splint	Z No Qualifier
		2 Cast	
		3 Brace	
		9 Wire	
		Y Other Device	

2   Placement
W   Anatomical Regions
4   Packing   Putting material in a body region or orifice

Body Region Character 4	Approach Character 5	Device Character 6	Qualifier Character 7
Ø Head	X External	5 Packing Material	Z No Qualifier
1 Face			
2 Neck			
3 Abdominal Wall			
4 Chest Wall			
5 Back			
6 Inguinal Region, Right			
7 Inguinal Region, Left			
8 Upper Extremity, Right			
9 Upper Extremity, Left			
A Upper Arm, Right			
B Upper Arm, Left			
C Lower Arm, Right			
D Lower Arm, Left			
E Hand, Right			
F Hand, Left			
G Thumb, Right			
H Thumb, Left			
J Finger, Right			
K Finger, Left			
L Lower Extremity, Right			
M Lower Extremity, Left			
N Upper Leg, Right			
P Upper Leg, Left			
Q Lower Leg, Right			
R Lower Leg, Left			
S Foot, Right			
T Foot, Left			
U Toe, Right			
V Toe, Left			

2   **Placement**
W   **Anatomical Regions**
5   **Removal**   Taking out or off a device from a body part

Body Region Character 4	Approach Character 5	Device Character 6	Qualifier Character 7
Ø Head **2** Neck **3** Abdominal Wall **4** Chest Wall **5** Back **6** Inguinal Region, Right **7** Inguinal Region, Left **8** Upper Extremity, Right **9** Upper Extremity, Left **A** Upper Arm, Right **B** Upper Arm, Left **C** Lower Arm, Right **D** Lower Arm, Left **E** Hand, Right **F** Hand, Left **G** Thumb, Right **H** Thumb, Left **J** Finger, Right **K** Finger, Left **L** Lower Extremity, Right **M** Lower Extremity, Left **N** Upper Leg, Right **P** Upper Leg, Left **Q** Lower Leg, Right **R** Lower Leg, Left **S** Foot, Right **T** Foot, Left **U** Toe, Right **V** Toe, Left	**X** External	**Ø** Traction Apparatus **1** Splint **2** Cast **3** Brace **4** Bandage **5** Packing Material **6** Pressure Dressing **7** Intermittent Pressure Device **Y** Other Device	**Z** No Qualifier
1 Face	**X** External	**Ø** Traction Apparatus **1** Splint **2** Cast **3** Brace **4** Bandage **5** Packing Material **6** Pressure Dressing **7** Intermittent Pressure Device **9** Wire **Y** Other Device	**Z** No Qualifier

LC Limited Coverage   **NC** Noncovered   HAC associated procedure   Combination Only   DRG Non-OR   Non-OR   Revised Text in **GREEN**

ICD-10-PCS 2014 (Draft)   **415**

2 **Placement**
W **Anatomical Regions**
6 **Traction**　　　　Exerting a pulling force on a body region in a distal direction

Body Region Character 4	Approach Character 5	Device Character 6	Qualifier Character 7
0 Head	**X** External	**0** Traction Apparatus	**Z** No Qualifier
1 Face		**Z** No Device	
2 Neck			
3 Abdominal Wall			
4 Chest Wall			
5 Back			
6 Inguinal Region, Right			
7 Inguinal Region, Left			
8 Upper Extremity, Right			
9 Upper Extremity, Left			
A Upper Arm, Right			
B Upper Arm, Left			
C Lower Arm, Right			
D Lower Arm, Left			
E Hand, Right			
F Hand, Left			
G Thumb, Right			
H Thumb, Left			
J Finger, Right			
K Finger, Left			
L Lower Extremity, Right			
M Lower Extremity, Left			
N Upper Leg, Right			
P Upper Leg, Left			
Q Lower Leg, Right			
R Lower Leg, Left			
S Foot, Right			
T Foot, Left			
U Toe, Right			
V Toe, Left			

Placement—Anatomical Orifices 2Y0–2Y5

2   **Placement**
Y   **Anatomical Orifices**
0   **Change**   Taking out or off a device from a body part and putting back an identical or similar device in or on the same body part without cutting or puncturing the skin or a mucous membrane

Body Region Character 4	Approach Character 5	Device Character 6	Qualifier Character 7
0 Mouth and Pharynx **1** Nasal **2** Ear **3** Anorectal **4** Female Genital Tract ♀ **5** Urethra	**X** External	**5** Packing Material	**Z** No Qualifier

2   **Placement**
Y   **Anatomical Orifices**
4   **Packing**   Putting material in a body region or orifice

Body Region Character 4	Approach Character 5	Device Character 6	Qualifier Character 7
0 Mouth and Pharynx **1** Nasal **2** Ear **3** Anorectal **4** Female Genital Tract ♀ **5** Urethra	**X** External	**5** Packing Material	**Z** No Qualifier

2   **Placement**
Y   **Anatomical Orifices**
5   **Removal**   Taking out or off a device from a body part

Body Region Character 4	Approach Character 5	Device Character 6	Qualifier Character 7
0 Mouth and Pharynx **1** Nasal **2** Ear **3** Anorectal **4** Female Genital Tract ♀ **5** Urethra	**X** External	**5** Packing Material	**Z** No Qualifier

LC Limited Coverage   **NC** Noncovered   HAC associated procedure   Combination Only   DRG Non-OR   Non-OR   Revised Text in **GREEN**

ICD-10-PCS 2014 (Draft)   **417**

Administration 302–3E1

3   **Administration**
0   **Circulatory**
2   **Transfusion**   Putting in blood or blood products

Body System/Region Character 4		Approach Character 5		Substance Character 6		Qualifier Character 7	
3 Peripheral Vein	NC	**0** Open		**A** Stem Cells, Embryonic		**Z** No Qualifier	
4 Central Vein	NC	**3** Percutaneous					
3 Peripheral Vein	NC	**0** Open		**G** Bone Marrow		**0** Autologous	
4 Central Vein	NC	**3** Percutaneous		**H** Whole Blood		**1** Nonautologous	
5 Peripheral Artery	NC			**J** Serum Albumin			
6 Central Artery	NC			**K** Frozen Plasma			
				L Fresh Plasma			
				M Plasma Cryoprecipitate			
				N Red Blood Cells			
				P Frozen Red Cells			
				Q White Cells			
				R Platelets			
				S Globulin			
				T Fibrinogen			
				V Antihemophilic Factors			
				W Factor IX			
				X Stem Cells, Cord Blood			
				Y Stem Cells, Hematopoietic			
7 Products of Conception, Circulatory	♀	**3** Percutaneous		**H** Whole Blood		**1** Nonautologous	
		7 Via Natural or Artificial Opening		**J** Serum Albumin			
				K Frozen Plasma			
				L Fresh Plasma			
				M Plasma Cryoprecipitate			
				N Red Blood Cells			
				P Frozen Red Cells			
				Q White Cells			
				R Platelets			
				S Globulin			
				T Fibrinogen			
				V Antihemophilic Factors			
				W Factor IX			
8 Vein		**0** Open		**B** 4-Factor Prothrombin Complex Concentrate		**1** Nonautologous	
		3 Percutaneous					

NC 3023[0,3]AZ Only when reported with PDx or SDx of C91.00, C92.00, C92.10, C92.11, C92.40, C92.50, C92.60, C92.A0, C93.00, C94.00, C95.00
NC 3024[0,3]0Z Only when reported with PDx or SDx of C91.00, C92.00, C92.10, C92.11, C92.40, C92.50, C92.60, C92.A0, C93.00, C94.00, C95.00
NC 3023[0,3][G,Y]0 Only when reported with PDx or SDx of C91.00, C92.00, C92.10, C92.11, C92.40, C92.50, C92.60, C92.A0, C93.00, C94.00, C95.00
NC 3023[0,3][G,Y]1 Only when reported with PDx or SDx of C90.00, C90.01
NC 3024[0,3][G,Y]0 Only when reported with PDx or SDx of C91.00, C92.00, C92.10, C92.11, C92.40, C92.50, C92.60, C92.A0, C93.00, C94.00, C95.00
NC 3024[0,3][G,Y]1 Only when reported with PDx or SDx of C90.00, C90.01
NC 3025[0,3][G,Y]0 Only when reported with PDx or SDx of C91.00, C92.00, C92.10, C92.11, C92.40, C92.50, C92.60, C92.A0, C93.00, C94.00, C95.00
NC 3025[0,3][G,Y]1 Only when reported with PDx or SDx of C90.00, C90.01
NC 3026[0,3][G,Y]0 Only when reported with PDx or SDx of C91.00, C92.00, C92.10, C92.11, C92.40, C92.50, C92.60, C92.A0, C93.00, C94.00, C95.00
NC 3026[0,3][G,Y]1 Only when reported with PDx or SDx of C90.00, C90.01

3   **Administration**
C   **Indwelling Device**
1   **Irrigation**   Putting in or on a cleansing substance

Body System/Region Character 4	Approach Character 5	Substance Character 6	Qualifier Character 7
Z None	**X** External	**8** Irrigating Substance	**Z** No Qualifier

3 Administration
E Physiological Systems and Anatomical Regions
0 Introduction Putting in or on a therapeutic, diagnostic, nutritional, physiological, or prophylactic substance except blood or blood products

Body System/Region Character 4	Approach Character 5	Substance Character 6	Qualifier Character 7
0 Skin and Mucous Membranes	X External	0 Antineoplastic	5 Other Antineoplastic M Monoclonal Antibody
0 Skin and Mucous Membranes	X External	2 Anti-infective	8 Oxazolidinones 9 Other Anti-infective
0 Skin and Mucous Membranes	X External	3 Anti-inflammatory 4 Serum, Toxoid and Vaccine B Local Anesthetic K Other Diagnostic Substance M Pigment N Analgesics, Hypnotics, Sedatives T Destructive Agent	Z No Qualifier
0 Skin and Mucous Membranes	X External	G Other Therapeutic Substance	C Other Substance
1 Subcutaneous Tissue	0 Open	2 Anti-infective	A Anti-infective Envelope
1 Subcutaneous Tissue	3 Percutaneous	V Hormone	G Insulin J Other Hormone
1 Subcutaneous Tissue	3 Percutaneous	2 Anti-infective	8 Oxazolidinones 9 Other Anti-infective A Anti-infective Envelope
1 Subcutaneous Tissue 2 Muscle	3 Percutaneous	3 Anti-inflammatory 4 Serum, Toxoid and Vaccine 6 Nutritional Substance 7 Electrolytic and Water Balance Substance B Local Anesthetic H Radioactive Substance K Other Diagnostic Substance N Analgesics, Hypnotics, Sedatives T Destructive Agent	Z No Qualifier
1 Subcutaneous Tissue 2 Muscle A Bone Marrow F Respiratory Tract L Pleural Cavity M Peritoneal Cavity Q Cranial Cavity and Brain R Spinal Canal S Epidural Space T Peripheral Nerves and Plexi W Lymphatics X Cranial Nerves Y Pericardial Cavity	3 Percutaneous	G Other Therapeutic Substance	C Other Substance
1 Subcutaneous Tissue 2 Muscle A Bone Marrow V Bones W Lymphatics	3 Percutaneous	0 Antineoplastic	5 Other Antineoplastic M Monoclonal Antibody
2 Muscle F Respiratory Tract L Pleural Cavity M Peritoneal Cavity Q Cranial Cavity and Brain R Spinal Canal S Epidural Space U Joints V Bones W Lymphatics Y Pericardial Cavity	3 Percutaneous	2 Anti-infective	8 Oxazolidinones 9 Other Anti-infective
3 Peripheral Vein	0 Open 3 Percutaneous	U Pancreatic Islet Cells	0 Autologous 1 Nonautologous

3E0 Continued on next page

3E0 Continued on next page

DRG Non-OR	3E03[0,3]U[0,1]

Administration

3E0 Continued

3   **Administration**
E   **Physiological Systems and Anatomical Regions**
0   **Introduction**   Putting in or on a therapeutic, diagnostic, nutritional, physiological, or prophylactic substance except blood or blood products

Body System/Region Character 4		Approach Character 5		Substance Character 6		Qualifier Character 7	
3 4 5 6	Peripheral Vein Central Vein Peripheral Artery Central Artery	0 3	Open Percutaneous	0	Antineoplastic	2 3 5 M P	High-dose Interleukin-2 Low-dose Interleukin-2 Other Antineoplastic Monoclonal Antibody Clofarabine
3 4 5 6	Peripheral Vein Central Vein Peripheral Artery Central Artery	0 3	Open Percutaneous	2	Anti-infective	8 9	Oxazolidinones Other Anti-infective
3 4 5 6	Peripheral Vein Central Vein Peripheral Artery Central Artery	0 3	Open Percutaneous	3 4 6 7 F H K N P R T X	Anti-inflammatory Serum, Toxoid and Vaccine Nutritional Substance Electrolytic and Water Balance Substance Intracirculatory Anesthetic Radioactive Substance Other Diagnostic Substance Analgesics, Hypnotics, Sedatives Platelet Inhibitor Antiarrhythmic Destructive Agent Vasopressor	Z	No Qualifier
5 6	Peripheral Artery Central Artery	0 3	Open Percutaneous	G	Other Therapeutic Substance	C N	Other Substance Blood Brain Barrier Disruption
3 4 5 6	Peripheral Vein Central Vein Peripheral Artery Central Artery	0 3	Open Percutaneous	V	Hormone	G H J	Insulin Human B-type Natriuretic Peptide Other Hormone
3 4	Peripheral Vein Central Vein	0	Open	G	Other Therapeutic Substance	C N Q	Other Substance Blood Brain Barrier Disruption Glucarpidase
3 4	Peripheral Vein Central Vein	3	Percutaneous Substance	G	Other Therapeutic Substance	C N Q	Other Substance Blood Brain Barrier Disruption Glucarpidase
3 4 5 6	Peripheral Vein Central Vein Peripheral Artery Central Artery	0 3	Open Percutaneous	W	Immunotherapeutic	K L	Immunostimulator Immunosuppressive
3 4 5 6 7 8	Peripheral Vein Central Vein Peripheral Artery Central Artery Coronary Artery Heart	0 3	Open Percutaneous	1	Thrombolytic	6 7	Recombinant Human-activated Protein C Other Thrombolytic
7 8	Coronary Artery Heart	0 3	Open Percutaneous	G	Other Therapeutic Substance	C	Other Substance
7 8	Coronary Artery Heart	0 3	Open Percutaneous	K P	Other Diagnostic Substance Platelet Inhibitor	Z	No Qualifier
9	Nose	3 7 X	Percutaneous Via Natural or Artificial Opening External	0	Antineoplastic	5 M	Other Antineoplastic Monoclonal Antibody
9	Nose	3 7 X	Percutaneous Via Natural or Artificial Opening External	3 4 B H K N T	Anti-inflammatory Serum, Toxoid and Vaccine Local Anesthetic Radioactive Substance Other Diagnostic Substance Analgesics, Hypnotics, Sedatives Destructive Agent	Z	No Qualifier

3E0 Continued on next page

DRG Non-OR 3E03[0,3]02	**DRG Non-OR** 3E04[0,3]17
DRG Non-OR 3E043[0,3]02	**DRG Non-OR** 3E05[0,3]17
DRG Non-OR 3E05[0,3]02	**DRG Non-OR** 3E06[0,3]17
DRG Non-OR 3E06[0,3]02	**DRG Non-OR** 3E08[0,3]17
DRG Non-OR 3E03[0,3]17	

3 **Administration**
E **Physiological Systems and Anatomical Regions**
0 **Introduction**   Putting in or on a therapeutic, diagnostic, nutritional, physiological, or prophylactic substance except blood or blood products

3E0 Continued

Body System/Region Character 4	Approach Character 5	Substance Character 6	Qualifier Character 7
9 Nose **B** Ear **C** Eye **D** Mouth and Pharynx	**3** Percutaneous **7** Via Natural or Artificial Opening **X** External	**2** Anti-infective	**8** Oxazolidinones **9** Other Anti-infective
9 Nose **B** Ear **C** Eye **D** Mouth and Pharynx	**3** Percutaneous **7** Via Natural or Artificial Opening **X** External	**G** Other Therapeutic Substance	**C** Other Substance
B Ear	**3** Percutaneous **7** Via Natural or Artificial Opening **X** External	**3** Anti-inflammatory **B** Local Anesthetic **H** Radioactive Substance **K** Other Diagnostic Substance **N** Analgesics, Hypnotics, Sedatives **T** Destructive Agent	**Z** No Qualifier
B Ear **C** Eye **D** Mouth and Pharynx	**3** Percutaneous **7** Via Natural or Artificial Opening **X** External	**0** Antineoplastic	**4** Liquid Brachytherapy Radioisotope **5** Other Antineoplastic **M** Monoclonal Antibody
C Eye	**3** Percutaneous **7** Via Natural or Artificial Opening **X** External	**3** Anti-inflammatory **B** Local Anesthetic **H** Radioactive Substance **K** Other Diagnostic Substance **M** Pigment **N** Analgesics, Hypnotics, Sedatives **T** Destructive Agent	**Z** No Qualifier
C Eye	**3** Percutaneous **7** Via Natural or Artificial Opening **X** External	**S** Gas	**F** Other Gas
D Mouth and Pharynx	**3** Percutaneous **7** Via Natural or Artificial Opening **X** External	**3** Anti-inflammatory **4** Serum, Toxoid and Vaccine **6** Nutritional Substance **7** Electrolytic and Water Balance Substance **B** Local Anesthetic **H** Radioactive Substance **K** Other Diagnostic Substance **N** Analgesics, Hypnotics, Sedatives **R** Antiarrhythmic **T** Destructive Agent	**Z** No Qualifier
E Products of Conception ♀ **F** Respiratory Tract **G** Upper GI **H** Lower GI **J** Biliary and Pancreatic Tract **K** Genitourinary Tract **N** Male Reproductive ♂ **P** Female Reproductive ♀	**3** Percutaneous **7** Via Natural or Artificial Opening **8** Via Natural or Artificial Opening Endoscopic	**0** Antineoplastic	**4** Liquid Brachytherapy Radioisotope **5** Other Antineoplastic **M** Monoclonal Antibody
E Products of Conception ♀ **F** Respiratory Tract **G** Upper GI **H** Lower GI **J** Biliary and Pancreatic Tract **K** Genitourinary Tract **N** Male Reproductive ♂ **P** Female Reproductive ♀	**3** Percutaneous **7** Via Natural or Artificial Opening **8** Via Natural or Artificial Opening Endoscopic	**2** Anti-infective	**8** Oxazolidinones **9** Other Anti-infective
E Products of Conception ♀ **F** Respiratory Tract **G** Upper GI **H** Lower GI **J** Biliary and Pancreatic Tract **K** Genitourinary Tract **N** Male Reproductive ♂ **P** Female Reproductive ♀	**3** Percutaneous **7** Via Natural or Artificial Opening **8** Via Natural or Artificial Opening Endoscopic	**G** Other Therapeutic Substance	**C** Other Substance

3E0 Continued on next page

LC Limited Coverage   **NC** Noncovered   HAC associated procedure   Combination Only   DRG Non-OR   Non-OR   Revised Text in **GREEN**

ICD-10-PCS 2014 (Draft)   **421**

3E0 Continued

3   **Administration**
E   **Physiological Systems and Anatomical Regions**
0   **Introduction**   Putting in or on a therapeutic, diagnostic, nutritional, physiological, or prophylactic substance except blood or blood products

Body System/Region Character 4	Approach Character 5	Substance Character 6	Qualifier Character 7
E Products of Conception ♀ **G** Upper GI **H** Lower GI **J** Biliary and Pancreatic Tract **K** Genitourinary Tract **N** Male Reproductive ♂	**3** Percutaneous **7** Via Natural or Artificial Opening **8** Via Natural or Artificial Opening Endoscopic	**3** Anti-inflammatory **6** Nutritional Substance **7** Electrolytic and Water Balance Substance **B** Local Anesthetic **H** Radioactive Substance **K** Other Diagnostic Substance **N** Analgesics, Hypnotics, Sedatives **T** Destructive Agent	**Z** No Qualifier
E Products of Conception ♀ **G** Upper GI **H** Lower GI **J** Biliary and Pancreatic Tract **K** Genitourinary Tract **N** Male Reproductive ♂ **P** Female Reproductive ♀	**3** Percutaneous **7** Via Natural or Artificial Opening **8** Via Natural or Artificial Opening Endoscopic	**S** Gas	**F** Other Gas
F Respiratory Tract	**3** Percutaneous **7** Via Natural or Artificial Opening **8** Via Natural or Artificial Opening Endoscopic	**S** Gas	**D** Nitric Oxide **F** Other Gas
F Respiratory Tract	**7** Via Natural or Artificial Opening **8** Via Natural or Artificial Opening Endoscopic	**3** Anti-inflammatory **6** Nutritional Substance **7** Electrolytic and Water Balance Substance **B** Local Anesthetic **D** Inhalation Anesthetic **H** Radioactive Substance **K** Other Diagnostic Substance **N** Analgesics, Hypnotics, Sedatives **T** Destructive Agent	**Z** No Qualifier
F Respiratory Tract **L** Pleural Cavity **M** Peritoneal Cavity **W** Lymphatics **Y** Pericardial Cavity	**3** Percutaneous	**3** Anti-inflammatory **6** Nutritional Substance **7** Electrolytic and Water Balance Substance **B** Local Anesthetic **H** Radioactive Substance **K** Other Diagnostic Substance **N** Analgesics, Hypnotics, Sedatives **T** Destructive Agent	**Z** No Qualifier
J Biliary and Pancreatic Tract	**3** Percutaneous **7** Via Natural or Artificial Opening **8** Via Natural or Artificial Opening Endoscopic	**U** Pancreatic Islet Cells	**0** Autologous **1** Nonautologous
L Pleural Cavity **M** Peritoneal Cavity **P** Female Reproductive ♀	**0** Open	**5** Adhesion Barrier	**Z** No Qualifier
L Pleural Cavity **M** Peritoneal Cavity **Q** Cranial Cavity and Brain **R** Spinal Canal **S** Epidural Space **Y** Pericardial Cavity	**3** Percutaneous **7** Via Natural or Artificial Opening	**S** Gas	**F** Other Gas
L Pleural Cavity **M** Peritoneal Cavity **Q** Cranial Cavity and Brain **Y** Pericardial Cavity	**3** Percutaneous **7** Via Natural or Artificial Opening	**0** Antineoplastic	**4** Liquid Brachytherapy Radioisotope **5** Other Antineoplastic **M** Monoclonal Antibody

3E0 Continued on next page

DRG Non-OR 3E0J[3,7,8]U[0,1]
DRG Non-OR 3E0Q[3,7]05

LC Limited Coverage   **NC** Noncovered   HAC associated procedure   Combination Only   DRG Non-OR   Non-OR   Revised Text in **GREEN**

422   ICD-10-PCS 2014 (Draft)

3E0 Continued

3   **Administration**
E   **Physiological Systems and Anatomical Regions**
0   **Introduction**   Putting in or on a therapeutic, diagnostic, nutritional, physiological, or prophylactic substance except blood or blood products

Body System/Region Character 4	Approach Character 5	Substance Character 6	Qualifier Character 7
P Female Reproductive ♀	**3** Percutaneous **7** Via Natural or Artificial Opening	**3** Anti-inflammatory **6** Nutritional Substance **7** Electrolytic and Water Balance Substance **B** Local Anesthetic **H** Radioactive Substance **K** Other Diagnostic Substance **L** Sperm **N** Analgesics, Hypnotics, Sedatives **T** Destructive Agent	**Z** No Qualifier
P Female Reproductive ♀	**3** Percutaneous **7** Via Natural or Artificial Opening	**Q** Fertilized Ovum	**0** Autologous **1** Nonautologous
P Female Reproductive ♀	**8** Via Natural or Artificial Opening Endoscopic	**3** Anti-inflammatory **6** Nutritional Substance **7** Electrolytic and Water Balance Substance **B** Local Anesthetic **H** Radioactive Substance **K** Other Diagnostic Substance **N** Analgesics, Hypnotics, Sedatives **T** Destructive Agent	**Z** No Qualifier
Q Cranial Cavity and Brain	**3** Percutaneous	**3** Anti-inflammatory **6** Nutritional Substance **7** Electrolytic and Water Balance Substance **A** Stem Cells, Embryonic **B** Local Anesthetic **H** Radioactive Substance **K** Other Diagnostic Substance **N** Analgesics, Hypnotics, Sedatives **T** Destructive Agent	**Z** No Qualifier
Q Cranial Cavity and Brain **R** Spinal Canal	**0** Open	**A** Stem Cells, Embryonic	**Z** No Qualifier
Q Cranial Cavity and Brain **R** Spinal Canal	**0** Open **3** Percutaneous	**E** Stem Cells, Somatic	**0** Autologous **1** Nonautologous
R Spinal Canal	**3** Percutaneous	**3** Anti-inflammatory **6** Nutritional Substance **7** Electrolytic and Water Balance Substance **A** Stem Cells, Embryonic **B** Local Anesthetic **C** Regional Anesthetic **H** Radioactive Substance **K** Other Diagnostic Substance **N** Analgesics, Hypnotics, Sedatives **T** Destructive Agent	**Z** No Qualifier
R Spinal Canal **S** Epidural Space	**3** Percutaneous	**0** Antineoplastic	**2** High-dose Interleukin-2 **3** Low-dose Interleukin-2 **4** Liquid Brachytherapy Radioisotope **5** Other Antineoplastic **M** Monoclonal Antibody
S Epidural Space	**3** Percutaneous	**3** Anti-inflammatory **6** Nutritional Substance **7** Electrolytic and Water Balance Substance **B** Local Anesthetic **C** Regional Anesthetic **H** Radioactive Substance **K** Other Diagnostic Substance **N** Analgesics, Hypnotics, Sedatives **T** Destructive Agent	**Z** No Qualifier
T Peripheral Nerves and Plexi **X** Cranial Nerves	**3** Percutaneous	**3** Anti-inflammatory **C** Regional Anesthetic **T** Destructive Agent	**Z** No Qualifier

3E0 Continued on next page

DRG Non-OR   3E0[R,S]302

Administration

3   **Administration**
E   **Physiological Systems and Anatomical Regions**
0   **Introduction**   Putting in or on a therapeutic, diagnostic, nutritional, physiological, or prophylactic substance except blood or blood products

Body System/Region Character 4	Approach Character 5	Substance Character 6	Qualifier Character 7
U Joints V Bones	0 Open	G Other Therapeutic Substance	B Recombinant Bone Morphogenetic Protein
U Joints	0 Open	2 Anti-infective	8 Oxazolidinones 9 Other Anti-infective
U Joints	3 Percutaneous	0 Antineoplastic	4 Liquid Brachytherapy Radioisotope 5 Other Antineoplastic M Monoclonal Antibody
U Joints	3 Percutaneous	2 Anti-infective	8 Oxazolidinones 9 Other Anti-infective
U Joints	3 Percutaneous	S Gas	F Other Gas
U Joints V Bones	3 Percutaneous	3 Anti-inflammatory 6 Nutritional Substance 7 Electrolytic and Water Balance Substance B Local Anesthetic H Radioactive Substance K Other Diagnostic Substance N Analgesics, Hypnotics, Sedatives T Destructive Agent	Z No Qualifier
V Bones	3 Percutaneous	0 Antineoplastic	5 Other Antineoplastic M Monoclonal Antibody
V Bones	3 Percutaneous	2 Anti-infective	8 Oxazolidinones 9 Other Anti-infective
U Joints V Bones	3 Percutaneous	G Other Therapeutic Substance	B Recombinant Bone Morphogenetic Protein C Other Substance

3   **Administration**
E   **Physiological Systems and Anatomical Regions**
1   **Irrigation**   Putting in or on a cleansing substance

Body System/Region Character 4	Approach Character 5	Substance Character 6	Qualifier Character 7
0 Skin and Mucous Membranes C Eye	3 Percutaneous X External	8 Irrigating Substance	X Diagnostic Z No Qualifier
9 Nose B Ear F Respiratory Tract G Upper GI H Lower GI J Biliary and Pancreatic Tract K Genitourinary Tract N Male Reproductive ♂ P Female Reproductive ♀	3 Percutaneous 7 Via Natural or Artificial Opening 8 Via Natural or Artificial Opening Endoscopic	8 Irrigating Substance	X Diagnostic Z No Qualifier
L Pleural Cavity M Peritoneal Cavity Q Cranial Cavity and Brain R Spinal Canal S Epidural Space U Joints Y Pericardial Cavity	3 Percutaneous	8 Irrigating Substance	X Diagnostic Z No Qualifier
M Peritoneal Cavity	3 Percutaneous	9 Dialysate	Z No Qualifier

LC Limited Coverage   **NC** Noncovered   HAC associated procedure   Combination Only   DRG Non-OR   Non-OR   Revised Text in **GREEN**

424   ICD-10-PCS 2014 (Draft)

Measurement and Monitoring 4AØ–4BØ

4　Measurement and Monitoring
A　Physiological Systems
Ø　Measurement　Determining the level of a physiological or physical function at a point in time

Body System Character 4	Approach Character 5	Function/Device Character 6	Qualifier Character 7
Ø Central Nervous	Ø Open	2 Conductivity 4 Electrical Activity B Pressure	Z No Qualifier
Ø Central Nervous	3 Percutaneous	4 Electrical Activity	Z No Qualifier
Ø Central Nervous	3 Percutaneous 7 Via Natural or Artificial Opening	B Pressure K Temperature R Saturation	D Intracranial
Ø Central Nervous	X External	2 Conductivity 4 Electrical Activity	Z No Qualifier
1 Peripheral Nervous	Ø Open 3 Percutaneous X External	2 Conductivity	9 Sensory B Motor
1 Peripheral Nervous	Ø Open 3 Percutaneous X External	4 Electrical Activity	Z No Qualifier
2 Cardiac	Ø Open 3 Percutaneous	N Sampling and Pressure	6 Right Heart 7 Left Heart 8 Bilateral
2 Cardiac	Ø Open 3 Percutaneous	4 Electrical Activity 9 Output C Rate F Rhythm H Sound P Action Currents	Z No Qualifier
2 Cardiac	X External	9 Output C Rate F Rhythm H Sound P Action Currents	Z No Qualifier
2 Cardiac	X External	M Total Activity	4 Stress
2 Cardiac	X External	4 Electrical Activity	A Guidance Z No Qualifier
3 Arterial	Ø Open 3 Percutaneous	5 Flow J Pulse	1 Peripheral 3 Pulmonary C Coronary
3 Arterial	Ø Open 3 Percutaneous	B Pressure	1 Peripheral 3 Pulmonary C Coronary F Other Thoracic
3 Arterial	Ø Open 3 Percutaneous	H Sound R Saturation	1 Peripheral
3 Arterial	X External	5 Flow B Pressure H Sound J Pulse R Saturation	1 Peripheral
4 Venous	Ø Open 3 Percutaneous	5 Flow B Pressure J Pulse	Ø Central 1 Peripheral 2 Portal 3 Pulmonary
4 Venous	Ø Open 3 Percutaneous	R Saturation	1 Peripheral
4 Venous	X External	5 Flow B Pressure J Pulse R Saturation	1 Peripheral
5 Circulatory	X External	L Volume	Z No Qualifier
6 Lymphatic	Ø Open 3 Percutaneous	5 Flow B Pressure	Z No Qualifier

4AØ Continued on next page

DRG Non-OR　4AØ2[Ø,3]N[6,7,8]
DRG Non-OR　4AØ23FZ

Measurement and Monitoring (side margin)

4A0 Continued

4   Measurement and Monitoring
A   Physiological Systems
0   Measurement   Determining the level of a physiological or physical function at a point in time

Body System Character 4	Approach Character 5	Function/Device Character 6	Qualifier Character 7
7 Visual	X External	0 Acuity 7 Mobility B Pressure	Z No Qualifier
8 Olfactory	X External	0 Acuity	Z No Qualifier
9 Respiratory	7 Via Natural or Artificial Opening 8 Via Natural or Artificial Opening Endoscopic X External	1 Capacity 5 Flow C Rate D Resistance L Volume M Total Activity	Z No Qualifier
B Gastrointestinal	7 Via Natural or Artificial Opening 8 Via Natural or Artificial Opening Endoscopic	8 Motility B Pressure G Secretion	Z No Qualifier
C Biliary	3 Percutaneous 4 Percutaneous Endoscopic 7 Via Natural or Artificial Opening 8 Via Natural or Artificial Opening Endoscopic	5 Flow B Pressure	Z No Qualifier
D Urinary	7 Via Natural or Artificial Opening	3 Contractility 5 Flow B Pressure D Resistance L Volume	Z No Qualifier
F Musculoskeletal	3 Percutaneous X External	3 Contractility	Z No Qualifier
H Products of Conception, Cardiac ♀	7 Via Natural or Artificial Opening 8 Via Natural or Artificial Opening Endoscopic X External	4 Electrical Activity C Rate F Rhythm H Sound	Z No Qualifier
J Products of Conception, Nervous ♀	7 Via Natural or Artificial Opening 8 Via Natural or Artificial Opening Endoscopic X External	2 Conductivity 4 Electrical Activity B Pressure	Z No Qualifier
Z None	7 Via Natural or Artificial Opening	6 Metabolism K Temperature	Z No Qualifier
Z None	X External	6 Metabolism K Temperature Q Sleep	Z No Qualifier

4   Measurement and Monitoring
A   Physiological Systems
1   Monitoring   Determining the level of a physiological or physical function at a point in time

Body System Character 4	Approach Character 5	Function/Device Character 6	Qualifier Character 7
0 Central Nervous	0 Open	2 Conductivity B Pressure	Z No Qualifier
0 Central Nervous	0 Open X External	4 Electrical Activity	G Intraoperative Z No Qualifier
0 Central Nervous	3 Percutaneous 7 Via Natural or Artificial Opening	B Pressure K Temperature R Saturation	D Intracranial
0 Central Nervous	3 Percutaneous	4 Electrical Activity	G Intraoperative Z No Qualifier
0 Central Nervous	X External	2 Conductivity	Z No Qualifier
1 Peripheral Nervous	0 Open 3 Percutaneous X External	2 Conductivity	9 Sensory B Motor
1 Peripheral Nervous	0 Open 3 Percutaneous X External	4 Electrical Activity	G Intraoperative Z No Qualifier

4A1 Continued on next page

4　Measurement and Monitoring
A　Physiological Systems
1　Monitoring　　Determining the level of a physiological or physical function repetitively over a period of time

Body System Character 4	Approach Character 5	Function/Device Character 6	Qualifier Character 7
2 Cardiac	**Ø** Open **3** Percutaneous	**4** Electrical Activity **9** Output **C** Rate **F** Rhythm **H** Sound	**Z** No Qualifier
2 Cardiac	**X** External	**4** Electrical Activity	**5** Ambulatory **Z** No Qualifier
2 Cardiac	**X** External	**9** Output **C** Rate **F** Rhythm **H** Sound	**Z** No Qualifier
2 Cardiac	**X** External	**M** Total Activity	**4** Stress
3 Arterial	**Ø** Open **3** Percutaneous	**5** Flow **B** Pressure **J** Pulse	**1** Peripheral **3** Pulmonary **C** Coronary
3 Arterial	**Ø** Open **3** Percutaneous	**H** Sound **R** Saturation	**1** Peripheral
3 Arterial	**X** External	**5** Flow **B** Pressure **H** Sound **J** Pulse **R** Saturation	**1** Peripheral
4 Venous	**Ø** Open **3** Percutaneous	**5** Flow **B** Pressure **J** Pulse	**Ø** Central **1** Peripheral **2** Portal **3** Pulmonary
4 Venous	**Ø** Open **3** Percutaneous	**R** Saturation	**Ø** Central **2** Portal **3** Pulmonary
4 Venous	**X** External	**5** Flow **B** Pressure **J** Pulse	**1** Peripheral
6 Lymphatic	**Ø** Open **3** Percutaneous	**5** Flow **B** Pressure	**Z** No Qualifier
9 Respiratory	**7** Via Natural or Artificial Opening **X** External	**1** Capacity **5** Flow **C** Rate **D** Resistance **L** Volume	**Z** No Qualifier
B Gastrointestinal	**7** Via Natural or Artificial Opening **8** Via Natural or Artificial Opening Endoscopic	**8** Motility **B** Pressure **G** Secretion	**Z** No Qualifier
D Urinary	**7** Via Natural or Artificial Opening	**3** Contractility **5** Flow **B** Pressure **D** Resistance **L** Volume	**Z** No Qualifier
H Products of Conception, Cardiac ♀	**7** Via Natural or Artificial Opening **8** Via Natural or Artificial Opening Endoscopic **X** External	**4** Electrical Activity **C** Rate **F** Rhythm **H** Sound	**Z** No Qualifier
J Products of Conception, Nervous ♀	**7** Via Natural or Artificial Opening **8** Via Natural or Artificial Opening Endoscopic **X** External	**2** Conductivity **4** Electrical Activity **B** Pressure	**Z** No Qualifier
Z None	**7** Via Natural or Artificial Opening	**K** Temperature	**Z** No Qualifier
Z None	**X** External	**K** Temperature **Q** Sleep	**Z** No Qualifier

Measurement and Monitoring

4B0–4B0

4   Measurement and Monitoring
B   Physiological Devices
0   Measurement   Determining the level of a physiological or physical function at a point in time

Body System Character 4	Approach Character 5	Function/Device Character 6	Qualifier Character 7
0 Central Nervous **1** Peripheral Nervous **F** Musculoskeletal	**X** External	**V** Stimulator	**Z** No Qualifier
2 Cardiac	**X** External	**S** Pacemaker **T** Defibrillator	**Z** No Qualifier
9 Respiratory	**X** External	**S** Pacemaker	**Z** No Qualifier

LC Limited Coverage   **NC** Noncovered   HAC associated procedure   Combination Only   DRG Non-OR   Non-OR   Revised Text in **GREEN**

428   ICD-10-PCS 2014 (Draft)

Extracorporeal Assistance and Performance 5A0–5A2

5 **Extracorporeal Assistance and Performance**
A **Physiological Systems**
0 **Assistance**   Taking over a portion of a physiological function by extracorporeal means

Body System Character 4	Duration Character 5	Function Character 6	Qualifier Character 7
2 Cardiac	**1** Intermittent **2** Continuous	**1** Output	**0** Balloon Pump **5** Pulsatile Compression **6** Other Pump **D** Impeller Pump
5 Circulatory	**1** Intermittent **2** Continuous	**2** Oxygenation	**1** Hyperbaric **C** Supersaturated
9 Respiratory	**3** Less than 24 Consecutive Hours **4** 24-96 Consecutive Hours **5** Greater than 96 Consecutive Hours	**5** Ventilation	**7** Continuous Positive Airway Pressure **8** Intermittent Positive Airway Pressure **9** Continuous Negative Airway Pressure **B** Intermittent Negative Airway Pressure **Z** No Qualifier

5 **Extracorporeal Assistance and Performance**
A **Physiological Systems**
1 **Performance**   Completely taking over a physiological function by extracorporeal means

Body System Character 4	Duration Character 5	Function Character 6	Qualifier Character 7
2 Cardiac	**0** Single	**1** Output	**2** Manual
2 Cardiac	**1** Intermittent	**3** Pacing	**Z** No Qualifier
2 Cardiac	**2** Continuous	**1** Output **3** Pacing	**Z** No Qualifier
5 Circulatory	**2** Continuous	**2** Oxygenation	**3** Membrane
9 Respiratory	**0** Single	**5** Ventilation	**4** Nonmechanical
9 Respiratory	**3** Less than 24 Consecutive Hours **4** 24-96 Consecutive Hours **5** Greater than 96 Consecutive Hours	**5** Ventilation	**Z** No Qualifier
C Biliary **D** Urinary	**0** Single **6** Multiple	**0** Filtration	**Z** No Qualifier

DRG Non-OR 5A19[3,4,5]5Z
Note: For code 5A1955Z, length of stay must be >= 4 days.

5 **Extracorporeal Assistance and Performance**
A **Physiological Systems**
2 **Restoration**   Returning, or attempting to return, a physiological function to its original state by extracorporeal means.

Body System Character 4	Duration Character 5	Function Character 6	Qualifier Character 7
2 Cardiac	**0** Single	**4** Rhythm	**Z** No Qualifier

Extracorporeal Therapies

Extracorporeal Therapies 6A0–6A9

6   **Extracorporeal Therapies**
A   **Physiological Systems**
0   **Atmospheric Control**   Extracorporeal control of atmospheric pressure and composition

Body System Character 4	Duration Character 5	Qualifier Character 6	Qualifier Character 7
Z None	0 Single 1 Multiple	Z No Qualifier	Z No Qualifier

6   **Extracorporeal Therapies**
A   **Physiological Systems**
1   **Decompression**   Extracorporeal elimination of undissolved gas from body fluids

Body System Character 4	Duration Character 5	Qualifier Character 6	Qualifier Character 7
5 Circulatory	0 Single 1 Multiple	Z No Qualifier	Z No Qualifier

6   **Extracorporeal Therapies**
A   **Physiological Systems**
2   **Electromagnetic Therapy**   Extracorporeal treatment by electromagnetic rays

Body System Character 4	Duration Character 5	Qualifier Character 6	Qualifier Character 7
1 Urinary 2 Central Nervous	0 Single 1 Multiple	Z No Qualifier	Z No Qualifier

6   **Extracorporeal Therapies**
A   **Physiological Systems**
3   **Hyperthermia**   Extracorporeal raising of body temperature

Body System Character 4	Duration Character 5	Qualifier Character 6	Qualifier Character 7
Z None	0 Single 1 Multiple	Z No Qualifier	Z No Qualifier

6   **Extracorporeal Therapies**
A   **Physiological Systems**
4   **Hypothermia**   Extracorporeal lowering of body temperature

Body System Character 4	Duration Character 5	Qualifier Character 6	Qualifier Character 7
Z None	0 Single 1 Multiple	Z No Qualifier	Z No Qualifier

6   **Extracorporeal Therapies**
A   **Physiological Systems**
5   **Pheresis**   Extracorporeal separation of blood products

Body System Character 4	Duration Character 5	Qualifier Character 6	Qualifier Character 7
5 Circulatory	0 Single 1 Multiple	Z No Qualifier	0 Erythrocytes 1 Leukocytes 2 Platelets 3 Plasma T Stem Cells, Cord Blood V Stem Cells, Hematopoietic

6   **Extracorporeal Therapies**
A   **Physiological Systems**
6   **Phototherapy**   Extracorporeal treatment by light rays

Body System Character 4	Duration Character 5	Qualifier Character 6	Qualifier Character 7
0 Skin 5 Circulatory	0 Single 1 Multiple	Z No Qualifier	Z No Qualifier

6   **Extracorporeal Therapies**
A   **Physiological Systems**
7   **Ultrasound Therapy**   Extracorporeal treatment by ultrasound

Body System Character 4	Duration Character 5	Qualifier Character 6	Qualifier Character 7
5 Circulatory	**Ø** Single **1** Multiple	**Z** No Qualifier	**4** Head and Neck Vessels **5** Heart **6** Peripheral Vessels **7** Other Vessels **Z** No Qualifier

6   **Extracorporeal Therapies**
A   **Physiological Systems**
8   **Ultraviolet Light Therapy**   Extracorporeal treatment by ultraviolet light

Body System Character 4	Duration Character 5	Qualifier Character 6	Qualifier Character 7
Ø Skin	**Ø** Single **1** Multiple	**Z** No Qualifier	**Z** No Qualifier

6   **Extracorporeal Therapies**
A   **Physiological Systems**
9   **Shock Wave Therapy**   Extracorporeal treatment by shock waves

Body System Character 4	Duration Character 5	Qualifier Character 6	Qualifier Character 7
3 Musculoskeletal	**Ø** Single **1** Multiple	**Z** No Qualifier	**Z** No Qualifier

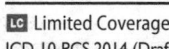

Osteopathic 7WØ

7   **Osteopathic**
W   **Anatomical Regions**
Ø   **Treatment**   Manual treatment to eliminate or alleviate somatic dysfunction and related disorders

Body Region Character 4	Approach Character 5	Method Character 6	Qualifier Character 7
Ø Head	**X** External	**Ø** Articulatory-Raising	**Z** None
1 Cervical		**1** Fascial Release	
2 Thoracic		**2** General Mobilization	
3 Lumbar		**3** High Velocity-Low Amplitude	
4 Sacrum		**4** Indirect	
5 Pelvis		**5** Low Velocity-High Amplitude	
6 Lower Extremities		**6** Lymphatic Pump	
7 Upper Extremities		**7** Muscle Energy-Isometric	
8 Rib Cage		**8** Muscle Energy-Isotonic	
9 Abdomen		**9** Other Method	

Other Procedures 8C0–8E0

8   **Other Procedures**
C   **Indwelling Device**
0   **Other Procedures**   Methodologies which attempt to remediate or cure a disorder or disease

Body Region Character 4	Approach Character 5	Method Character 6	Qualifier Character 7
1 Nervous System	**X** External	**6** Collection	**J** Cerebrospinal Fluid **L** Other Fluid
2 Circulatory System	**X** External	**6** Collection	**K** Blood **L** Other Fluid

8   **Other Procedures**
E   **Physiological Systems and Anatomical Regions**
0   **Other Procedures**   Methodologies which attempt to remediate or cure a disorder or disease

Body Region Character 4	Approach Character 5	Method Character 6	Qualifier Character 7
1 Nervous System **K** Musculoskeletal System **U** Female Reproductive System ♀	**X** External	**Y** Other Method	**7** Examination
2 Circulatory System	**3** Percutaneous	**D** Near Infrared Spectroscopy	**Z** No Qualifier
9 Head and Neck Region **W** Trunk Region	**0** Open **3** Percutaneous **4** Percutaneous Endoscopic **7** Via Natural or Artificial Opening **8** Via Natural or Artificial Opening Endoscopic **X** External	**C** Robotic Assisted Procedure	**Z** No Qualifier
9 Head and Neck Region **W** Trunk Region **X** Upper Extremity **Y** Lower Extremity	**X** External	**B** Computer Assisted Procedure	**F** With Fluoroscopy **G** With Computerized Tomography **H** With Magnetic Resonance Imaging **Z** No Qualifier
9 Head and Neck Region **W** Trunk Region **X** Upper Extremity **Y** Lower Extremity	**X** External	**Y** Other Method	**8** Suture Removal
H Integumentary System and Breast	**3** Percutaneous	**0** Acupuncture	**0** Anesthesia **Z** No Qualifier
H Integumentary System and Breast ♀	**X** External	**6** Collection	**2** Breast Milk
H Integumentary System and Breast	**X** External	**Y** Other Method	**9** Piercing
K Musculoskeletal System	**X** External	**1** Therapeutic Massage	**Z** No Qualifier
V Male Reproductive System ♂	**X** External	**1** Therapeutic Massage	**C** Prostate **D** Rectum
V Male Reproductive System ♂	**X** External	**6** Collection	**3** Sperm
X Upper Extremity **Y** Lower Extremity	**0** Open **3** Percutaneous **4** Percutaneous Endoscopic **X** External	**C** Robotic Assisted Procedure	**Z** No Qualifier
Z None	**X** External	**Y** Other Method	**1** In Vitro Fertilization **4** Yoga Therapy **5** Meditation **6** Isolation

LC Limited Coverage   **NC** Noncovered   HAC associated procedure   Combination Only   DRG Non-OR   Non-OR   Revised Text in **GREEN**

ICD-10-PCS 2014 (Draft)   **433**

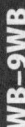

Chiropractic 9WB

9　Chiropractic
W　Anatomical Regions
B　Manipulation　　Manual procedure that involves a directed thrust to move a joint past the physiological range of motion, without exceeding the anatomical limit

Body Region Character 4	Approach Character 5	Method Character 6	Qualifier Character 7
0　Head 1　Cervical 2　Thoracic 3　Lumbar 4　Sacrum 5　Pelvis 6　Lower Extremities 7　Upper Extremities 8　Rib Cage 9　Abdomen	X　External	B　Non-Manual C　Indirect Visceral D　Extra-Articular F　Direct Visceral G　Long Lever Specific Contact H　Short Lever Specific Contact J　Long and Short Lever Specific 　　Contact K　Mechanically Assisted L　Other Method	Z　None

Imaging B00–BY4

B　**Imaging**
0　**Central Nervous System**
0　**Plain Radiography**　Planar display of an image developed from the capture of external ionizing radiation on photographic or photoconductive plate

Body Part Character 4	Contrast Character 5	Qualifier Character 6	Qualifier Character 7
B Spinal Cord	**0** High Osmolar **1** Low Osmolar **Y** Other Contrast **Z** None	**Z** None	**Z** None

B　**Imaging**
0　**Central Nervous System**
1　**Fluoroscopy**　Single plane or bi-plane real time display of an image developed from the capture of external ionizing radioation on a fluorescent screen. The image may also be stored by either digital or analog means

Body Part Character 4	Contrast Character 5	Qualifier Character 6	Qualifier Character 7
B Spinal Cord	**0** High Osmolar **1** Low Osmolar **Y** Other Contrast **Z** None	**Z** None	**Z** None

B　**Imaging**
0　**Central Nervous System**
2　**Computerized Tomography (CT Scan)**　Computer reformatted digital display of multiplanar images developed from the capture of multiple exposures of external ionizing radiation

Body Part Character 4	Contrast Character 5	Qualifier Character 6	Qualifier Character 7
0 Brain **7** Cisterna **8** Cerebral Ventricle(s) **9** Sella Turcica/Pituitary Gland **B** Spinal Cord	**0** High Osmolar **1** Low Osmolar **Y** Other Contrast	**0** Unenhanced and Enhanced **Z** None	**Z** None
0 Brain **7** Cisterna **8** Cerebral Ventricle(s) **9** Sella Turcica/Pituitary Gland **B** Spinal Cord	**Z** None	**Z** None	**Z** None

B　**Imaging**
0　**Central Nervous System**
3　**Magnetic Resonance Imaging (MRI)**　Computer reformatted digital display of multiplanar images developed from the capture of radio-frequency signals emitted by nuclei in a body site excited within a magnetic field

Body Part Character 4	Contrast Character 5	Qualifier Character 6	Qualifier Character 7
0 Brain **9** Sella Turcica/Pituitary Gland **B** Spinal Cord **C** Acoustic Nerves	**Y** Other Contrast	**0** Unenhanced and Enhanced **Z** None	**Z** None
0 Brain **9** Sella Turcica/Pituitary Gland **B** Spinal Cord **C** Acoustic Nerves	**Z** None	**Z** None	**Z** None

B　**Imaging**
0　**Central Nervous System**
4　**Ultrasonography**　Real time display of images of anatomy or flow information developed from the capture of relected and attenuated high frequency sound waves

Body Part Character 4	Contrast Character 5	Qualifier Character 6	Qualifier Character 7
0 Brain **B** Spinal Cord	**Z** None	**Z** None	**Z** None

LC Limited Coverage　　**NC** Noncovered　　HAC associated procedure　　Combination Only　　DRG Non-OR　　Non-OR　　Revised Text in **GREEN**

ICD-10-PCS 2014 (Draft)　　　　**435**

Imaging

B   **Imaging**
2   **Heart**
Ø   **Plain Radiography**   Planar display of an image developed from the capture of external ionizing radiation on photographic or photoconductive plate

Body Part Character 4	Contrast Character 5	Qualifier Character 6	Qualifier Character 7
Ø Coronary Artery, Single **1** Coronary Arteries, Multiple **2** Coronary Artery Bypass Graft, Single **3** Coronary Artery Bypass Grafts, Multiple **4** Heart, Right **5** Heart, Left **6** Heart, Right and Left **7** Internal Mammary Bypass Graft, Right **8** Internal Mammary Bypass Graft, Left **F** Bypass Graft, Other	**Ø** High Osmolar **1** Low Osmolar **Y** Other Contrast	**Z** None	**Z** None

DRG Non-OR   For all body part, approach, device, and qualifier values

---

B   **Imaging**
2   **Heart**
1   **Fluoroscopy**   Single plane or bi-plane real time display of an image developed from the capture of external ionizing radioation on a fluorescent screen. The image may also be stored by either digital or analog means

Body Part Character 4	Contrast Character 5	Qualifier Character 6	Qualifier Character 7
Ø Coronary Artery, Single **1** Coronary Arteries, Multiple **2** Coronary Artery Bypass Graft, Single **3** Coronary Artery Bypass Grafts, Multiple	**Ø** High Osmolar **1** Low Osmolar **Y** Other Contrast	**1** Laser	**Ø** Intraoperative
Ø Coronary Artery, Single **1** Coronary Arteries, Multiple **2** Coronary Artery Bypass Graft, Single **3** Coronary Artery Bypass Grafts, Multiple **4** Heart, Right **5** Heart, Left **6** Heart, Right and Left **7** Internal Mammary Bypass Graft, Right **8** Internal Mammary Bypass Graft, Left **F** Bypass Graft, Other	**Ø** High Osmolar **1** Low Osmolar **Y** Other Contrast	**Z** None	**Z** None

DRG Non-OR   All body part values, all contrast values, with qualifier values of NONE

B   **Imaging**
2   **Heart**
2   **Computerized Tomography (CT Scan)**   Computer reformatted digital display of multiplanar images developed from the capture of multiple exposures of external ionizing radiation

Body Part Character 4	Contrast Character 5	Qualifier Character 6	Qualifier Character 7
1 Coronary Arteries, Multiple **3** Coronary Artery Bypass Grafts, Multiple **6** Heart, Right and Left	**Ø** High Osmolar **1** Low Osmolar **Y** Other Contrast	**Ø** Unenhanced and Enhanced **Z** None	**Z** None
1 Coronary Arteries, Multiple **3** Coronary Artery Bypass Grafts, Multiple **6** Heart, Right and Left	**Z** None	**2** Intravascular Optical Coherence **Z** None	**Z** None

B **Imaging**
2 **Heart**
3 **Magnetic Resonance Imaging (MRI)** Computer reformatted digital display of multiplanar images developed from the capture of radio-frequency signals emitted by nuclei in a body site excited within a magnetic field

Body Part Character 4	Contrast Character 5	Qualifier Character 6	Qualifier Character 7
1 Coronary Arteries, Multiple 3 Coronary Artery Bypass Grafts, Multiple 6 Heart, Right and Left	Y Other Contrast	Ø Unenhanced and Enhanced Z None	Z None
1 Coronary Arteries, Multiple 3 Coronary Artery Bypass Grafts, Multiple 6 Heart, Right and Left	Z None	Z None	Z None

B **Imaging**
2 **Heart**
4 **Ultrasonography** Real time display of images of anatomy or flow information developed from the capture of relected and attenuated high frequency sound waves

Body Part Character 4	Contrast Character 5	Qualifier Character 6	Qualifier Character 7
Ø Coronary Artery, Single 1 Coronary Arteries, Multiple 4 Heart, Right 5 Heart, Left 6 Heart, Right and Left B Heart with Aorta C Pericardium D Pediatric Heart	Y Other Contrast	Z None	Z None
Ø Coronary Artery, Single 1 Coronary Arteries, Multiple 4 Heart, Right 5 Heart, Left 6 Heart, Right and Left B Heart with Aorta C Pericardium D Pediatric Heart	Z None	Z None	3 Intravascular 4 Transesophageal Z None

B **Imaging**
3 **Upper Arteries**
Ø **Plain Radiography** Planar display of an image developed from the capture of external ionizing radiation on photographic or photoconductive plate

Body Part Character 4	Contrast Character 5	Qualifier Character 6	Qualifier Character 7
Ø Thoracic Aorta 1 Brachiocephalic-Subclavian Artery, Right 2 Subclavian Artery, Left 3 Common Carotid Artery, Right 4 Common Carotid Artery, Left 5 Common Carotid Arteries, Bilateral 6 Internal Carotid Artery, Right 7 Internal Carotid Artery, Left 8 Internal Carotid Arteries, Bilateral 9 External Carotid Artery, Right B External Carotid Artery, Left C External Carotid Arteries, Bilateral D Vertebral Artery, Right F Vertebral Artery, Left G Vertebral Arteries, Bilateral H Upper Extremity Arteries, Right J Upper Extremity Arteries, Left K Upper Extremity Arteries, Bilateral L Intercostal and Bronchial Arteries M Spinal Arteries N Upper Arteries, Other P Thoraco-Abdominal Aorta Q Cervico-Cerebral Arch R Intracranial Arteries S Pulmonary Artery, Right T Pulmonary Artery, Left	Ø High Osmolar 1 Low Osmolar Y Other Contrast Z None	Z None	Z None

B Imaging
3 Upper Arteries
1 Fluoroscopy Fluoroscopy: Single plane or bi-plane real time display of an image developed from the capture of external ionizing radiation on a fluorescent screen. The image may also be stored by either digital or analog means

Body Part Character 4	Contrast Character 5	Qualifier Character 6	Qualifier Character 7
0 Thoracic Aorta	**0** High Osmolar	**1** Laser	**0** Intraoperative
1 Brachiocephalic-Subclavian Artery, Right	**1** Low Osmolar		
2 Subclavian Artery, Left	**Y** Other Contrast		
3 Common Carotid Artery, Right			
4 Common Carotid Artery, Left			
5 Common Carotid Arteries, Bilateral			
6 Internal Carotid Artery, Right			
7 Internal Carotid Artery, Left			
8 Internal Carotid Arteries, Bilateral			
9 External Carotid Artery, Right			
B External Carotid Artery, Left			
C External Carotid Arteries, Bilateral			
D Vertebral Artery, Right			
F Vertebral Artery, Left			
G Vertebral Arteries, Bilateral			
H Upper Extremity Arteries, Right			
J Upper Extremity Arteries, Left			
K Upper Extremity Arteries, Bilateral			
L Intercostal and Bronchial Arteries			
M Spinal Arteries			
N Upper Arteries, Other			
P Thoraco-Abdominal Aorta			
Q Cervico-Cerebral Arch			
R Intracranial Arteries			
S Pulmonary Artery, Right			
T Pulmonary Artery, Left			
0 Thoracic Aorta	**0** High Osmolar	**Z** None	**Z** None
1 Brachiocephalic-Subclavian Artery, Right	**1** Low Osmolar		
2 Subclavian Artery, Left	**Y** Other Contrast		
3 Common Carotid Artery, Right			
4 Common Carotid Artery, Left			
5 Common Carotid Arteries, Bilateral			
6 Internal Carotid Artery, Right			
7 Internal Carotid Artery, Left			
8 Internal Carotid Arteries, Bilateral			
9 External Carotid Artery, Right			
B External Carotid Artery, Left			
C External Carotid Arteries, Bilateral			
D Vertebral Artery, Right			
F Vertebral Artery, Left			
G Vertebral Arteries, Bilateral			
H Upper Extremity Arteries, Right			
J Upper Extremity Arteries, Left			
K Upper Extremity Arteries, Bilateral			
L Intercostal and Bronchial Arteries			
M Spinal Arteries			
N Upper Arteries, Other			
P Thoraco-Abdominal Aorta			
Q Cervico-Cerebral Arch			
R Intracranial Arteries			
S Pulmonary Artery, Right			
T Pulmonary Artery, Left			

B31 Continued on next page

LC Limited Coverage   **NC** Noncovered   HAC associated procedure   Combination Only   DRG Non-OR   Non-OR   Revised Text in **GREEN**

B   **Imaging**
3   **Upper Arteries**

1   **Fluoroscopy**   Fluoroscopy: Single plane or bi-plane real time display of an image developed from the capture of external ionizing radiation on a fluorescent screen. The image may also be stored by either digital or analog means

Body Part Character 4	Contrast Character 5	Qualifier Character 6	Qualifier Character 7
Ø Thoracic Aorta **1** Brachiocephalic-Subclavian Artery, Right **2** Subclavian Artery, Left **3** Common Carotid Artery, Right **4** Common Carotid Artery, Left **5** Common Carotid Arteries, Bilateral **6** Internal Carotid Artery, Right **7** Internal Carotid Artery, Left **8** Internal Carotid Arteries, Bilateral **9** External Carotid Artery, Right **B** External Carotid Artery, Left **C** External Carotid Arteries, Bilateral **D** Vertebral Artery, Right **F** Vertebral Artery, Left **G** Vertebral Arteries, Bilateral **H** Upper Extremity Arteries, Right **J** Upper Extremity Arteries, Left **K** Upper Extremity Arteries, Bilateral **L** Intercostal and Bronchial Arteries **M** Spinal Arteries **N** Upper Arteries, Other **P** Thoraco-Abdominal Aorta **Q** Cervico-Cerebral Arch **R** Intracranial Arteries **S** Pulmonary Artery, Right **T** Pulmonary Artery, Left	**Z** None	**Z** None	**Z** None

B   **Imaging**
3   **Upper Arteries**
2   **Computerized Tomography (CT Scan)**   Computer reformatted digital display of multiplanar images developed from the capture of multiple exposures of external ionizing radiation

Body Part Character 4	Contrast Character 5	Qualifier Character 6	Qualifier Character 7
Ø Thoracic Aorta **5** Common Carotid Arteries, Bilateral **8** Internal Carotid Arteries, Bilateral **G** Vertebral Arteries, Bilateral **R** Intracranial Arteries **S** Pulmonary Artery, Right **T** Pulmonary Artery, Left	**Ø** High Osmolar **1** Low Osmolar **Y** Other Contrast	**Z** None	**Z** None
Ø Thoracic Aorta **5** Common Carotid Arteries, Bilateral **8** Internal Carotid Arteries, Bilateral **G** Vertebral Arteries, Bilateral **R** Intracranial Arteries **S** Pulmonary Artery, Right **T** Pulmonary Artery, Left	**Z** None	**2** Intravascular Optical Coherence **Z** None	**Z** None

[LC] Limited Coverage   [NC] Noncovered   HAC associated procedure   Combination Only   DRG Non-OR   Non-OR   Revised Text in **GREEN**

ICD-10-PCS 2014 (Draft)   **439**

B31—B32

B **Imaging**
3 **Upper Arteries**
3 **Magnetic Resonance Imaging (MRI)** Computer reformatted digital display of multiplanar images developed from the capture of radio-frequency signals emitted by nuclei in a body site excited within a magnetic field

Body Part Character 4	Contrast Character 5	Qualifier Character 6	Qualifier Character 7
Ø Thoracic Aorta **5** Common Carotid Arteries, Bilateral **8** Internal Carotid Arteries, Bilateral **G** Vertebral Arteries, Bilateral **H** Upper Extremity Arteries, Right **J** Upper Extremity Arteries, Left **K** Upper Extremity Arteries, Bilateral **M** Spinal Arteries **Q** Cervico-Cerebral Arch **R** Intracranial Arteries	**Y** Other Contrast	**Ø** Unenhanced and Enhanced **Z** None	**Z** None
Ø Thoracic Aorta **5** Common Carotid Arteries, Bilateral **8** Internal Carotid Arteries, Bilateral **G** Vertebral Arteries, Bilateral **H** Upper Extremity Arteries, Right **J** Upper Extremity Arteries, Left **K** Upper Extremity Arteries, Bilateral **M** Spinal Arteries **Q** Cervico-Cerebral Arch **R** Intracranial Arteries	**Z** None	**Z** None	**Z** None

B **Imaging**
3 **Upper Arteries**
4 **Ultrasonography** Real time display of images of anatomy or flow information developed from the capture of relected and attenuated high frequency sound waves

Body Part Character 4	Contrast Character 5	Qualifier Character 6	Qualifier Character 7
Ø Thoracic Aorta **1** Brachiocephalic-Subclavian Artery, Right **2** Subclavian Artery, Left **3** Common Carotid Artery, Right **4** Common Carotid Artery, Left **5** Common Carotid Arteries, Bilateral **6** Internal Carotid Artery, Right **7** Internal Carotid Artery, Left **8** Internal Carotid Arteries, Bilateral **H** Upper Extremity Arteries, Right **J** Upper Extremity Arteries, Left **K** Upper Extremity Arteries, Bilateral **R** Intracranial Arteries **S** Pulmonary Artery, Right **T** Pulmonary Artery, Left **V** Ophthalmic Arteries	**Z** None	**Z** None	**3** Intravascular **Z** None

B **Imaging**
4 **Lower Arteries**
Ø **Plain Radiography** Planar display of an image developed from the capture of external ionizing radiation on photographic or photoconductive plate

Body Part Character 4	Contrast Character 5	Qualifier Character 6	Qualifier Character 7
Ø Abdominal Aorta **2** Hepatic Artery **3** Splenic Arteries **4** Superior Mesenteric Artery **5** Inferior Mesenteric Artery **6** Renal Artery, Right **7** Renal Artery, Left **8** Renal Arteries, Bilateral **9** Lumbar Arteries **B** Intra-Abdominal Arteries, Other **C** Pelvic Arteries **D** Aorta and Bilateral Lower Extremity Arteries **F** Lower Extremity Arteries, Right **G** Lower Extremity Arteries, Left **J** Lower Arteries, Other **M** Renal Artery Transplant	**Ø** High Osmolar **1** Low Osmolar **Y** Other Contrast	**Z** None	**Z** None

LC Limited Coverage   **NC** Noncovered   HAC associated procedure   Combination Only   DRG Non-OR   Non-OR   Revised Text in **GREEN**

440   ICD-10-PCS 2014 (Draft)

B33–B40

B **Imaging**
4 **Lower Arteries**
1 **Fluoroscopy**   Single plane or bi-plane real time display of an image developed from the capture of external ionizing radiation on a fluorescent screen. The image may also be stored by either digital or analog means

Body Part Character 4	Contrast Character 5	Qualifier Character 6	Qualifier Character 7
Ø Abdominal Aorta **2** Hepatic Artery **3** Splenic Arteries **4** Superior Mesenteric Artery **5** Inferior Mesenteric Artery **6** Renal Artery, Right **7** Renal Artery, Left **8** Renal Arteries, Bilateral **9** Lumbar Arteries **B** Intra-Abdominal Arteries, Other **C** Pelvic Arteries **D** Aorta and Bilateral Lower Extremity Arteries **F** Lower Extremity Arteries, Right **G** Lower Extremity Arteries, Left **J** Lower Arteries, Other	**Ø** High Osmolar **1** Low Osmolar **Y** Other Contrast	**1** Laser	**Ø** Intraoperative
Ø Abdominal Aorta **2** Hepatic Artery **3** Splenic Arteries **4** Superior Mesenteric Artery **5** Inferior Mesenteric Artery **6** Renal Artery, Right **7** Renal Artery, Left **8** Renal Arteries, Bilateral **9** Lumbar Arteries **B** Intra-Abdominal Arteries, Other **C** Pelvic Arteries **D** Aorta and Bilateral Lower Extremity Arteries **F** Lower Extremity Arteries, Right **G** Lower Extremity Arteries, Left **J** Lower Arteries, Other	**Ø** High Osmolar **1** Low Osmolar **Y** Other Contrast	**Z** None	**Z** None
Ø Abdominal Aorta **2** Hepatic Artery **3** Splenic Arteries **4** Superior Mesenteric Artery **5** Inferior Mesenteric Artery **6** Renal Artery, Right **7** Renal Artery, Left **8** Renal Arteries, Bilateral **9** Lumbar Arteries **B** Intra-Abdominal Arteries, Other **C** Pelvic Arteries **D** Aorta and Bilateral Lower Extremity Arteries **F** Lower Extremity Arteries, Right **G** Lower Extremity Arteries, Left **J** Lower Arteries, Other	**Z** None	**Z** None	**Z** None

LC Limited Coverage   **NC** Noncovered   HAC associated procedure   Combination Only   DRG Non-OR   Non-OR   Revised Text in **GREEN**

ICD-10-PCS 2014 (Draft)   **441**

B41—B41

B   Imaging
4   Lower Arteries
2   Computerized Tomography (CT Scan) Computer reformatted digital display of multiplanar images developed from the capture of multiple exposures of external ionizing radiation

Body Part Character 4	Contrast Character 5	Qualifier Character 6	Qualifier Character 7
Ø Abdominal Aorta **1** Celiac Artery **4** Superior Mesenteric Artery **8** Renal Arteries, Bilateral **C** Pelvic Arteries **F** Lower Extremity Arteries, Right **G** Lower Extremity Arteries, Left **H** Lower Extremity Arteries, Bilateral **M** Renal Artery Transplant	**Ø** High Osmolar **1** Low Osmolar **Y** Other Contrast	**Z** None	**Z** None
Ø Abdominal Aorta **1** Celiac Artery **4** Superior Mesenteric Artery **8** Renal Arteries, Bilateral **C** Pelvic Arteries **F** Lower Extremity Arteries, Right **G** Lower Extremity Arteries, Left **H** Lower Extremity Arteries, Bilateral **M** Renal Artery Transplant	**Z** None	**2** Intravascular Optical Coherence **Z** None	**Z** None

B   Imaging
4   Lower Arteries
3   Magnetic Resonance Imaging (MRI) Computer reformatted digital display of multiplanar images developed from the capture of radio-frequency signals emitted by nuclei in a body site excited within a magnetic field

Body Part Character 4	Contrast Character 5	Qualifier Character 6	Qualifier Character 7
Ø Abdominal Aorta **1** Celiac Artery **4** Superior Mesenteric Artery **8** Renal Arteries, Bilateral **C** Pelvic Arteries **F** Lower Extremity Arteries, Right **G** Lower Extremity Arteries, Left **H** Lower Extremity Arteries, Bilateral	**Y** Other Contrast	**Ø** Unenhanced and Enhanced **Z** None	**Z** None
Ø Abdominal Aorta **1** Celiac Artery **4** Superior Mesenteric Artery **8** Renal Arteries, Bilateral **C** Pelvic Arteries **F** Lower Extremity Arteries, Right **G** Lower Extremity Arteries, Left **H** Lower Extremity Arteries, Bilateral	**Z** None	**Z** None	**Z** None

B   Imaging
4   Lower Arteries
4   Ultrasonography Real time display of images of anatomy or flow information developed from the capture of relected and attenuated high frequency sound waves

Body Part Character 4	Contrast Character 5	Qualifier Character 6	Qualifier Character 7
Ø Abdominal Aorta **4** Superior Mesenteric Artery **5** Inferior Mesenteric Artery **6** Renal Artery, Right **7** Renal Artery, Left **8** Renal Arteries, Bilateral **B** Intra-Abdominal Arteries, Other **F** Lower Extremity Arteries, Right **G** Lower Extremity Arteries, Left **H** Lower Extremity Arteries, Bilateral **K** Celiac and Mesenteric Arteries **L** Femoral Artery **N** Penile Arteries	**Z** None	**Z** None	**3** Intravascular **Z** None

LC Limited Coverage   **NC** Noncovered   HAC associated procedure   Combination Only   DRG Non-OR   Non-OR   Revised Text in **GREEN**

442   ICD-10-PCS 2014 (Draft)

B   Imaging
5   Veins
0   Plain Radiography   Planar display of an image developed from the capture of external ionizing radiation on photographic or photoconductive plate

Body Part Character 4	Contrast Character 5	Qualifier Character 6	Qualifier Character 7
0 Epidural Veins	0 High Osmolar	Z None	Z None
1 Cerebral and Cerebellar Veins	1 Low Osmolar		
2 Intracranial Sinuses	Y Other Contrast		
3 Jugular Veins, Right			
4 Jugular Veins, Left			
5 Jugular Veins, Bilateral			
6 Subclavian Vein, Right			
7 Subclavian Vein, Left			
8 Superior Vena Cava			
9 Inferior Vena Cava			
B Lower Extremity Veins, Right			
C Lower Extremity Veins, Left			
D Lower Extremity Veins, Bilateral			
F Pelvic (Iliac) Veins, Right			
G Pelvic (Iliac) Veins, Left			
H Pelvic (Iliac) Veins, Bilateral			
J Renal Vein, Right			
K Renal Vein, Left			
L Renal Veins, Bilateral			
M Upper Extremity Veins, Right			
N Upper Extremity Veins, Left			
P Upper Extremity Veins, Bilateral			
Q Pulmonary Vein, Right			
R Pulmonary Vein, Left			
S Pulmonary Veins, Bilateral			
T Portal and Splanchnic Veins			
V Veins, Other			
W Dialysis Shunt/Fistula			

B   Imaging
5   Veins
1   Fluoroscopy   Single plane or bi-plane real time display of an image developed from the capture of external ionizing radioation on a fluorescent screen. The image may also be stored by either digital or analog means

Body Part Character 4	Contrast Character 5	Qualifier Character 6	Qualifier Character 7
0 Epidural Veins	0 High Osmolar	Z None	A Guidance
1 Cerebral and Cerebellar Veins	1 Low Osmolar		Z None
2 Intracranial Sinuses	Y Other Contrast		
3 Jugular Veins, Right	Z None		
4 Jugular Veins, Left			
5 Jugular Veins, Bilateral			
6 Subclavian Vein, Right			
7 Subclavian Vein, Left			
8 Superior Vena Cava			
9 Inferior Vena Cava			
B Lower Extremity Veins, Right			
C Lower Extremity Veins, Left			
D Lower Extremity Veins, Bilateral			
F Pelvic (Iliac) Veins, Right			
G Pelvic (Iliac) Veins, Left			
H Pelvic (Iliac) Veins, Bilateral			
J Renal Vein, Right			
K Renal Vein, Left			
L Renal Veins, Bilateral			
M Upper Extremity Veins, Right			
N Upper Extremity Veins, Left			
P Upper Extremity Veins, Bilateral			
Q Pulmonary Vein, Right			
R Pulmonary Vein, Left			
S Pulmonary Veins, Bilateral			
T Portal and Splanchnic Veins			
V Veins, Other			
W Dialysis Shunt/Fistula			

B   **Imaging**
5   **Veins**
2   **Computerized Tomography (CT Scan)** Computer reformatted digital display of multiplanar images developed from the capture of multiple exposures of external ionizing radiation

Body Part Character 4	Contrast Character 5	Qualifier Character 6	Qualifier Character 7
2 Intracranial Sinuses **8** Superior Vena Cava **9** Inferior Vena Cava **F** Pelvic (Iliac) Veins, Right **G** Pelvic (Iliac) Veins, Left **H** Pelvic (Iliac) Veins, Bilateral **J** Renal Vein, Right **K** Renal Vein, Left **L** Renal Veins, Bilateral **Q** Pulmonary Vein, Right **R** Pulmonary Vein, Left **S** Pulmonary Veins, Bilateral **T** Portal and Splanchnic Veins	**Ø** High Osmolar **1** Low Osmolar **Y** Other Contrast	**Ø** Unenhanced and Enhanced **Z** None	**Z** None
2 Intracranial Sinuses **8** Superior Vena Cava **9** Inferior Vena Cava **F** Pelvic (Iliac) Veins, Right **G** Pelvic (Iliac) Veins, Left **H** Pelvic (Iliac) Veins, Bilateral **J** Renal Vein, Right **K** Renal Vein, Left **L** Renal Veins, Bilateral **Q** Pulmonary Vein, Right **R** Pulmonary Vein, Left **S** Pulmonary Veins, Bilateral **T** Portal and Splanchnic Veins	**Z** None	**2** Intravascular Optical Coherence **Z** None	**Z** None

B   **Imaging**
5   **Veins**
3   **Magnetic Resonance Imaging (MRI)** Computer reformatted digital display of multiplanar images developed from the capture of radio-frequency signals emitted by nuclei in a body site excited within a magnetic field

Body Part Character 4	Contrast Character 5	Qualifier Character 6	Qualifier Character 7
1 Cerebral and Cerebellar Veins **2** Intracranial Sinuses **5** Jugular Veins, Bilateral **8** Superior Vena Cava **9** Inferior Vena Cava **B** Lower Extremity Veins, Right **C** Lower Extremity Veins, Left **D** Lower Extremity Veins, Bilateral **H** Pelvic (Iliac) Veins, Bilateral **L** Renal Veins, Bilateral **M** Upper Extremity Veins, Right **N** Upper Extremity Veins, Left **P** Upper Extremity Veins, Bilateral **S** Pulmonary Veins, Bilateral **T** Portal and Splanchnic Veins **V** Veins, Other	**Y** Other Contrast	**Ø** Unenhanced and Enhanced **Z** None	**Z** None
1 Cerebral and Cerebellar Veins **2** Intracranial Sinuses **5** Jugular Veins, Bilateral **8** Superior Vena Cava **9** Inferior Vena Cava **B** Lower Extremity Veins, Right **C** Lower Extremity Veins, Left **D** Lower Extremity Veins, Bilateral **H** Pelvic (Iliac) Veins, Bilateral **L** Renal Veins, Bilateral **M** Upper Extremity Veins, Right **N** Upper Extremity Veins, Left **P** Upper Extremity Veins, Bilateral **S** Pulmonary Veins, Bilateral **T** Portal and Splanchnic Veins **V** Veins, Other	**Z** None	**Z** None	**Z** None

LC Limited Coverage   **NC** Noncovered   HAC associated procedure   Combination Only   DRG Non-OR   Non-OR   Revised Text in **GREEN**

444   ICD-10-PCS 2014 (Draft)

B Imaging
5 Veins
4 Ultrasonography — Real time display of images of anatomy or flow information developed from the capture of relected and attenuated high frequency sound waves

Body Part Character 4	Contrast Character 5	Qualifier Character 6	Qualifier Character 7
3 Jugular Veins, Right 4 Jugular Veins, Left 6 Subclavian Vein, Right 7 Subclavian Vein, Left 9 Inferior Vena Cava B Lower Extremity Veins, Right C Lower Extremity Veins, Left D Lower Extremity Veins, Bilateral J Renal Vein, Right K Renal Vein, Left L Renal Veins, Bilateral M Upper Extremity Veins, Right N Upper Extremity Veins, Left P Upper Extremity Veins, Bilateral T Portal and Splanchnic Veins	Z None	Z None	3 Intravascular A Guidance Z None

B Imaging
7 Lymphatic System
0 Plain Radiography — Planar display of an image developed from the capture of external ionizing radiation on photographic or photoconductive plate

Body Part Character 4	Contrast Character 5	Qualifier Character 6	Qualifier Character 7
0 Abdominal/Retroperitoneal Lymphatics, Unilateral 1 Abdominal/Retroperitoneal Lymphatics, Bilateral 4 Lymphatics, Head and Neck 5 Upper Extremity Lymphatics, Right 6 Upper Extremity Lymphatics, Left 7 Upper Extremity Lymphatics, Bilateral 8 Lower Extremity Lymphatics, Right 9 Lower Extremity Lymphatics, Left B Lower Extremity Lymphatics, Bilateral C Lymphatics, Pelvic	0 High Osmolar 1 Low Osmolar Y Other Contrast	Z None	Z None

B Imaging
8 Eye
0 Plain Radiography — Planar display of an image developed from the capture of external ionizing radiation on photographic or photoconductive plate

Body Part Character 4	Contrast Character 5	Qualifier Character 6	Qualifier Character 7
0 Lacrimal Duct, Right 1 Lacrimal Duct, Left 2 Lacrimal Ducts, Bilateral	0 High Osmolar 1 Low Osmolar Y Other Contrast	Z None	Z None
3 Optic Foramina, Right 4 Optic Foramina, Left 5 Eye, Right 6 Eye, Left 7 Eyes, Bilateral	Z None	Z None	Z None

B Imaging
8 Eye
2 Computerized Tomography (CT Scan) — Computer reformatted digital display of multiplanar images developed from the capture of multiple exposures of external ionizing radiation

Body Part Character 4	Contrast Character 5	Qualifier Character 6	Qualifier Character 7
5 Eye, Right 6 Eye, Left 7 Eyes, Bilateral	0 High Osmolar 1 Low Osmolar Y Other Contrast	0 Unenhanced and Enhanced Z None	Z None
5 Eye, Right 6 Eye, Left 7 Eyes, Bilateral	Z None	Z None	Z None

B   Imaging
8   Eye
3   Magnetic Resonance Imaging (MRI)   Computer reformatted digital display of multiplanar images developed from the capture of radio-frequency signals emitted by nuclei in a body site excited within a magnetic field

Body Part Character 4	Contrast Character 5	Qualifier Character 6	Qualifier Character 7
5 Eye, Right **6** Eye, Left **7** Eyes, Bilateral	**Y** Other Contrast	**Ø** Unenhanced and Enhanced **Z** None	**Z** None
5 Eye, Right **6** Eye, Left **7** Eyes, Bilateral	**Z** None	**Z** None	**Z** None

B   Imaging
8   Eye
4   Ultrasonography   Real time display of images of anatomy or flow information developed from the capture of relected and attenuated high frequency sound waves

Body Part Character 4	Contrast Character 5	Qualifier Character 6	Qualifier Character 7
5 Eye, Right **6** Eye, Left **7** Eyes, Bilateral	**Z** None	**Z** None	**Z** None

B   Imaging
9   Ear, Nose, Mouth and Throat
Ø   Plain Radiography   Planar display of an image developed from the capture of external ionizing radiation on photographic or photoconductive plate

Body Part Character 4	Contrast Character 5	Qualifier Character 6	Qualifier Character 7
2 Paranasal Sinuses **F** Nasopharynx/Oropharynx **H** Mastoids	**Z** None	**Z** None	**Z** None
4 Parotid Gland, Right **5** Parotid Gland, Left **6** Parotid Glands, Bilateral **7** Submandibular Gland, Right **8** Submandibular Gland, Left **9** Submandibular Glands, Bilateral **B** Salivary Gland, Right **C** Salivary Gland, Left **D** Salivary Glands, Bilateral	**Ø** High Osmolar **1** Low Osmolar **Y** Other Contrast	**Z** None	**Z** None

B   Imaging
9   Ear, Nose, Mouth and Throat
1   Fluoroscopy   Single plane or bi-plane real time display of an image developed from the capture of external ionizing radioation on a fluorescent screen. The image may also be stored by either digital or analog means

Body Part Character 4	Contrast Character 5	Qualifier Character 6	Qualifier Character 7
G Pharynx and Epiglottis **J** Larynx	**Y** Other Contrast **Z** None	**Z** None	**Z** None

B   Imaging
9   Ear, Nose, Mouth and Throat
2   Computerized Tomography (CT Scan)   Computer reformatted digital display of multiplanar images developed from the capture of multiple exposures of external ionizing radiation

Body Part Character 4	Contrast Character 5	Qualifier Character 6	Qualifier Character 7
Ø Ear **2** Paranasal Sinuses **6** Parotid Glands, Bilateral **9** Submandibular Glands, Bilateral **D** Salivary Glands, Bilateral **F** Nasopharynx/Oropharynx **J** Larynx	**Ø** High Osmolar **1** Low Osmolar **Y** Other Contrast	**Ø** Unenhanced and Enhanced **Z** None	**Z** None
Ø Ear **2** Paranasal Sinuses **6** Parotid Glands, Bilateral **9** Submandibular Glands, Bilateral **D** Salivary Glands, Bilateral **F** Nasopharynx/Oropharynx **J** Larynx	**Z** None	**Z** None	**Z** None

B　Imaging
9　Ear, Nose, Mouth and Throat
3　Magnetic Resonance Imaging (MRI)　Computer reformatted digital display of multiplanar images developed from the capture of radio-frequency signals emitted by nuclei in a body site excited within a magnetic field

Body Part Character 4	Contrast Character 5	Qualifier Character 6	Qualifier Character 7
Ø　Ear 2　Paranasal Sinuses 6　Parotid Glands, Bilateral 9　Submandibular Glands, Bilateral D　Salivary Glands, Bilateral F　Nasopharynx/Oropharynx J　Larynx	Y　Other Contrast	Ø　Unenhanced and Enhanced Z　None	Z　None
Ø　Ear 2　Paranasal Sinuses 6　Parotid Glands, Bilateral 9　Submandibular Glands, Bilateral D　Salivary Glands, Bilateral F　Nasopharynx/Oropharynx J　Larynx	Z　None	Z　None	Z　None

B　Imaging
B　Respiratory System
Ø　Plain Radiography　Planar display of an image developed from the capture of external ionizing radiation on photographic or photoconductive plate

Body Part Character 4	Contrast Character 5	Qualifier Character 6	Qualifier Character 7
7　Tracheobronchial Tree, Right 8　Tracheobronchial Tree, Left 9　Tracheobronchial Trees, Bilateral	Y　Other Contrast	Z　None	Z　None
D　Upper Airways	Z　None	Z　None	Z　None

B　Imaging
B　Respiratory System
1　Fluoroscopy　Single plane or bi-plane real time display of an image developed from the capture of external ionizing radioation on a fluorescent screen. The image may also be stored by either digital or analog means

Body Part Character 4	Contrast Character 5	Qualifier Character 6	Qualifier Character 7
2　Lung, Right 3　Lung, Left 4　Lungs, Bilateral 6　Diaphragm C　Mediastinum D　Upper Airways	Z　None	Z　None	Z　None
7　Tracheobronchial Tree, Right 8　Tracheobronchial Tree, Left 9　Tracheobronchial Trees, Bilateral	Y　Other Contrast	Z　None	Z　None

B　Imaging
B　Respiratory System
2　Computerized Tomography (CT Scan)　Computer reformatted digital display of multiplanar images developed from the capture of multiple exposures of external ionizing radiation

Body Part Character 4	Contrast Character 5	Qualifier Character 6	Qualifier Character 7
4　Lungs, Bilateral 7　Tracheobronchial Tree, Right 8　Tracheobronchial Tree, Left 9　Tracheobronchial Trees, Bilateral F　Trachea/Airways	Ø　High Osmolar 1　Low Osmolar Y　Other Contrast	Ø　Unenhanced and Enhanced Z　None	Z　None
4　Lungs, Bilateral 7　Tracheobronchial Tree, Right 8　Tracheobronchial Tree, Left 9　Tracheobronchial Trees, Bilateral F　Trachea/Airways	Z　None	Z　None	Z　None

LC Limited Coverage　　　NC Noncovered　　　HAC associated procedure　　　Combination Only　　　DRG Non-OR　　　Non-OR　　　Revised Text in **GREEN**
ICD-10-PCS 2014 (Draft)　　　　　　　　　　　　　　　　　　　　　　　　　　　　447

B93—BB2

B **Imaging**
B **Respiratory System**
3 **Magnetic Resonance Imaging (MRI)**   Computer reformatted digital display of multiplanar images developed from the capture of radio-frequency signals emitted by nuclei in a body site excited within a magnetic field

Body Part Character 4	Contrast Character 5	Qualifier Character 6	Qualifier Character 7
G Lung Apices	**Y** Other Contrast	**Ø** Unenhanced and Enhanced **Z** None	**Z** None
G Lung Apices	**Z** None	**Z** None	**Z** None

B **Imaging**
B **Respiratory System**
4 **Ultrasonography**   Real time display of images of anatomy or flow information developed from the capture of relected and attenuated high frequency sound waves

Body Part Character 4	Contrast Character 5	Qualifier Character 6	Qualifier Character 7
B Pleura **C** Mediastinum	**Z** None	**Z** None	**Z** None

B **Imaging**
D **Gastrointestinal System**
1 **Fluoroscopy**   Single plane or bi-plane real time display of an image developed from the capture of external ionizing radioation on a fluorescent screen. The image may also be stored by either digital or analog means

Body Part Character 4	Contrast Character 5	Qualifier Character 6	Qualifier Character 7
1 Esophagus **2** Stomach **3** Small Bowel **4** Colon **5** Upper GI **6** Upper GI and Small Bowel **9** Duodenum **B** Mouth/Oropharynx	**Y** Other Contrast **Z** None	**Z** None	**Z** None

B **Imaging**
D **Gastrointestinal System**
2 **Computerized Tomography (CT Scan)**   Computer reformatted digital display of multiplanar images developed from the capture of multiple exposures of external ionizing radiation

Body Part Character 4	Contrast Character 5	Qualifier Character 6	Qualifier Character 7
4 Colon	**Ø** High Osmolar **1** Low Osmolar **Y** Other Contrast	**Ø** Unenhanced and Enhanced **Z** None	**Z** None
4 Colon	**Z** None	**Z** None	**Z** None

B **Imaging**
D **Gastrointestinal System**
4 **Ultrasonography**   Real time display of images of anatomy or flow information developed from the capture of relected and attenuated high frequency sound waves

Body Part Character 4	Contrast Character 5	Qualifier Character 6	Qualifier Character 7
1 Esophagus **2** Stomach **7** Gastrointestinal Tract **8** Appendix **9** Duodenum **C** Rectum	**Z** None	**Z** None	**Z** None

B **Imaging**
F **Hepatobiliary System and Pancreas**
Ø **Plain Radiography**   Planar display of an image developed from the capture of external ionizing radiation on photographic or photoconductive plate

Body Part Character 4	Contrast Character 5	Qualifier Character 6	Qualifier Character 7
Ø Bile Ducts **3** Gallbladder and Bile Ducts **C** Hepatobiliary System, All	**Ø** High Osmolar **1** Low Osmolar **Y** Other Contrast	**Z** None	**Z** None

LC Limited Coverage   **NC** Noncovered   HAC associated procedure   Combination Only   DRG Non-OR   Non-OR   Revised Text in **GREEN**

448   ICD-10-PCS 2014 (Draft)

B   **Imaging**
F   **Hepatobiliary System and Pancreas**
1   **Fluoroscopy**   Single plane or bi-plane real time display of an image developed from the capture of external ionizing radiation on a fluorescent screen. The image may also be stored by either digital or analog means

Body Part Character 4	Contrast Character 5	Qualifier Character 6	Qualifier Character 7
Ø Bile Ducts **1** Biliary and Pancreatic Ducts **2** Gallbladder **3** Gallbladder and Bile Ducts **4** Gallbladder, Bile Ducts and Pancreatic Ducts **8** Pancreatic Ducts	**Ø** High Osmolar **1** Low Osmolar **Y** Other Contrast	**Z** None	**Z** None

B   **Imaging**
F   **Hepatobiliary System and Pancreas**
2   **Computerized Tomography (CT Scan)**   Computer reformatted digital display of multiplanar images developed from the capture of multiple exposures of external ionizing radiation

Body Part Character 4	Contrast Character 5	Qualifier Character 6	Qualifier Character 7
5 Liver **6** Liver and Spleen **7** Pancreas **C** Hepatobiliary System, All	**Ø** High Osmolar **1** Low Osmolar **Y** Other Contrast	**Ø** Unenhanced and Enhanced **Z** None	**Z** None
5 Liver **6** Liver and Spleen **7** Pancreas **C** Hepatobiliary System, All	**Z** None	**Z** None	**Z** None

B   **Imaging**
F   **Hepatobiliary System and Pancreas**
3   **Magnetic Resonance Imaging (MRI)**   Computer reformatted digital display of multiplanar images developed from the capture of radio-frequency signals emitted by nuclei in a body site excited within a magnetic field

Body Part Character 4	Contrast Character 5	Qualifier Character 6	Qualifier Character 7
5 Liver **6** Liver and Spleen **7** Pancreas	**Y** Other Contrast	**Ø** Unenhanced and Enhanced **Z** None	**Z** None
5 Liver **6** Liver and Spleen **7** Pancreas	**Z** None	**Z** None	**Z** None

B   **Imaging**
F   **Hepatobiliary System and Pancreas**
4   **Ultrasonography**   Real time display of images of anatomy or flow information developed from the capture of relected and attenuated high frequency sound waves

Body Part Character 4	Contrast Character 5	Qualifier Character 6	Qualifier Character 7
Ø Bile Ducts **2** Gallbladder **3** Gallbladder and Bile Ducts **5** Liver **6** Liver and Spleen **7** Pancreas **C** Hepatobiliary System, All	**Z** None	**Z** None	**Z** None

B   **Imaging**
G   **Endocrine System**
2   **Computerized Tomography (CT Scan)**   Computer reformatted digital display of multiplanar images developed from the capture of multiple exposures of external ionizing radiation

Body Part Character 4	Contrast Character 5	Qualifier Character 6	Qualifier Character 7
2 Adrenal Glands, Bilateral **3** Parathyroid Glands **4** Thyroid Gland	**Ø** High Osmolar **1** Low Osmolar **Y** Other Contrast	**Ø** Unenhanced and Enhanced **Z** None	**Z** None
2 Adrenal Glands, Bilateral **3** Parathyroid Glands **4** Thyroid Gland	**Z** None	**Z** None	**Z** None

B **Imaging**
G **Endocrine System**
3 **Magnetic Resonance Imaging (MRI)** Computer reformatted digital display of multiplanar images developed from the capture of radio-frequency signals emitted by nuclei in a body site excited within a magnetic field

Body Part Character 4	Contrast Character 5	Qualifier Character 6	Qualifier Character 7
2 Adrenal Glands, Bilateral 3 Parathyroid Glands 4 Thyroid Gland	Y Other Contrast	Ø Unenhanced and Enhanced Z None	Z None
2 Adrenal Glands, Bilateral 3 Parathyroid Glands 4 Thyroid Gland	Z None	Z None	Z None

B **Imaging**
G **Endocrine System**
4 **Ultrasonography** Real time display of images of anatomy or flow information developed from the capture of relected and attenuated high frequency sound waves

Body Part Character 4	Contrast Character 5	Qualifier Character 6	Qualifier Character 7
Ø Adrenal Gland, Right 1 Adrenal Gland, Left 2 Adrenal Glands, Bilateral 3 Parathyroid Glands 4 Thyroid Gland	Z None	Z None	Z None

B **Imaging**
H **Skin, Subcutaneous Tissue and Breast**
Ø **Plain Radiography** Planar display of an image developed from the capture of external ionizing radiation on photographic or photoconductive plate

Body Part Character 4	Contrast Character 5	Qualifier Character 6	Qualifier Character 7
Ø Breast, Right 1 Breast, Left 2 Breasts, Bilateral	Z None	Z None	Z None
3 Single Mammary Duct, Right 4 Single Mammary Duct, Left 5 Multiple Mammary Ducts, Right 6 Multiple Mammary Ducts, Left	Ø High Osmolar 1 Low Osmolar Y Other Contrast Z None	Z None	Z None

B **Imaging**
H **Skin, Subcutaneous Tissue and Breast**
3 **Magnetic Resonance Imaging (MRI)** Computer reformatted digital display of multiplanar images developed from the capture of radio-frequency signals emitted by nuclei in a body site excited within a magnetic field

Body Part Character 4	Contrast Character 5	Qualifier Character 6	Qualifier Character 7
Ø Breast, Right 1 Breast, Left 2 Breasts, Bilateral D Subcutaneous Tissue, Head/Neck F Subcutaneous Tissue, Upper Extremity G Subcutaneous Tissue, Thorax H Subcutaneous Tissue, Abdomen and Pelvis J Subcutaneous Tissue, Lower Extremity	Y Other Contrast	Ø Unenhanced and Enhanced Z None	Z None
Ø Breast, Right 1 Breast, Left 2 Breasts, Bilateral D Subcutaneous Tissue, Head/Neck F Subcutaneous Tissue, Upper Extremity G Subcutaneous Tissue, Thorax H Subcutaneous Tissue, Abdomen and Pelvis J Subcutaneous Tissue, Lower Extremity	Z None	Z None	Z None

B   **Imaging**
H   **Skin, Subcutaneous Tissue and Breast**
4   **Ultrasonography**   Real time display of images of anatomy or flow information developed from the capture of relected and attenuated high frequency sound waves

Body Part Character 4	Contrast Character 5	Qualifier Character 6	Qualifier Character 7
0 Breast, Right **1** Breast, Left **2** Breasts, Bilateral **7** Extremity, Upper **8** Extremity, Lower **9** Abdominal Wall **B** Chest Wall **C** Head and Neck	**Z** None	**Z** None	**Z** None

B   **Imaging**
L   **Connective Tissue**
3   **Magnetic Resonance Imaging (MRI)**   Computer reformatted digital display of multiplanar images developed from the capture of radio-frequency signals emitted by nuclei in a body site excited within a magnetic field

Body Part Character 4	Contrast Character 5	Qualifier Character 6	Qualifier Character 7
0 Connective Tissue, Upper Extremity **1** Connective Tissue, Lower Extremity **2** Tendons, Upper Extremity **3** Tendons, Lower Extremity	**Y** Other Contrast	**0** Unenhanced and Enhanced **Z** None	**Z** None
0 Connective Tissue, Upper Extremity **1** Connective Tissue, Lower Extremity **2** Tendons, Upper Extremity **3** Tendons, Lower Extremity	**Z** None	**Z** None	**Z** None

B   **Imaging**
L   **Connective Tissue**
4   **Ultrasonography**   Real time display of images of anatomy or flow information developed from the capture of relected and attenuated high frequency sound waves

Body Part Character 4	Contrast Character 5	Qualifier Character 6	Qualifier Character 7
0 Connective Tissue, Upper Extremity **1** Connective Tissue, Lower Extremity **2** Tendons, Upper Extremity **3** Tendons, Lower Extremity	**Z** None	**Z** None	**Z** None

B   **Imaging**
N   **Skull and Facial Bones**
0   **Plain Radiography**   Planar display of an image developed from the capture of external ionizing radiation on photographic or photoconductive plate

Body Part Character 4	Contrast Character 5	Qualifier Character 6	Qualifier Character 7
0 Skull **1** Orbit, Right **2** Orbit, Left **3** Orbits, Bilateral **4** Nasal Bones **5** Facial Bones **6** Mandible **B** Zygomatic Arch, Right **C** Zygomatic Arch, Left **D** Zygomatic Arches, Bilateral **G** Tooth, Single **H** Teeth, Multiple **J** Teeth, All	**Z** None	**Z** None	**Z** None
7 Temporomandibular Joint, Right **8** Temporomandibular Joint, Left **9** Temporomandibular Joints, Bilateral	**0** High Osmolar **1** Low Osmolar **Y** Other Contrast **Z** None	**Z** None	**Z** None

LC Limited Coverage   **NC** Noncovered   HAC associated procedure   Combination Only   DRG Non-OR   Non-OR   Revised Text in **GREEN**

ICD-10-PCS 2014 (Draft)   451

BH4—BN0

B   Imaging
N   Skull and Facial Bones
1   Fluoroscopy   Single plane or bi-plane real time display of an image developed from the capture of external ionizing radioation on a fluorescent screen. The image may also be stored by either digital or analog means

Body Part Character 4	Contrast Character 5	Qualifier Character 6	Qualifier Character 7
7 Temporomandibular Joint, Right 8 Temporomandibular Joint, Left 9 Temporomandibular Joints, Bilateral	Ø High Osmolar 1 Low Osmolar Y Other Contrast Z None	Z None	Z None

B   Imaging
N   Skull and Facial Bones
2   Computerized Tomography (CT Scan)   Computer reformatted digital display of multiplanar images developed from the capture of multiple exposures of external ionizing radiation

Body Part Character 4	Contrast Character 5	Qualifier Character 6	Qualifier Character 7
Ø Skull 3 Orbits, Bilateral 5 Facial Bones 6 Mandible 9 Temporomandibular Joints, Bilateral F Temporal Bones	Ø High Osmolar 1 Low Osmolar Y Other Contrast Z None	Z None	Z None

B   Imaging
N   Skull and Facial Bones
3   Magnetic Resonance Imaging (MRI)   Computer reformatted digital display of multiplanar images developed from the capture of radio-frequency signals emitted by nuclei in a body site excited within a magnetic field

Body Part Character 4	Contrast Character 5	Qualifier Character 6	Qualifier Character 7
9 Temporomandibular Joints, Bilateral	Y Other Contrast Z None	Z None	Z None

B   Imaging
P   Non-Axial Upper Bones
Ø   Plain Radiography   Planar display of an image developed from the capture of external ionizing radiation on photographic or photoconductive plate

Body Part Character 4	Contrast Character 5	Qualifier Character 6	Qualifier Character 7
Ø Sternoclavicular Joint, Right 1 Sternoclavicular Joint, Left 2 Sternoclavicular Joints, Bilateral 3 Acromioclavicular Joints, Bilateral 4 Clavicle, Right 5 Clavicle, Left 6 Scapula, Right 7 Scapula, Left A Humerus, Right B Humerus, Left E Upper Arm, Right F Upper Arm, Left J Forearm, Right K Forearm, Left N Hand, Right P Hand, Left R Finger(s), Right S Finger(s), Left X Ribs, Right Y Ribs, Left	Z None	Z None	Z None
8 Shoulder, Right 9 Shoulder, Left C Hand/Finger Joint, Right D Hand/Finger Joint, Left G Elbow, Right H Elbow, Left L Wrist, Right M Wrist, Left	Ø High Osmolar 1 Low Osmolar Y Other Contrast Z None	Z None	Z None

B   **Imaging**
P   **Non-Axial Upper Bones**
1   **Fluoroscopy**   Single plane or bi-plane real time display of an image developed from the capture of external ionizing radioation on a fluorescent screen. The image may also be stored by either digital or analog means

Body Part Character 4	Contrast Character 5	Qualifier Character 6	Qualifier Character 7
Ø Sternoclavicular Joint, Right **1** Sternoclavicular Joint, Left **2** Sternoclavicular Joints, Bilateral **3** Acromioclavicular Joints, Bilateral **4** Clavicle, Right **5** Clavicle, Left **6** Scapula, Right **7** Scapula, Left **A** Humerus, Right **B** Humerus, Left **E** Upper Arm, Right **F** Upper Arm, Left **J** Forearm, Right **K** Forearm, Left **N** Hand, Right **P** Hand, Left **R** Finger(s), Right **S** Finger(s), Left **X** Ribs, Right **Y** Ribs, Left	**Z** None	**Z** None	**Z** None
8 Shoulder, Right **9** Shoulder, Left **L** Wrist, Right **M** Wrist, Left	**Ø** High Osmolar **1** Low Osmolar **Y** Other Contrast **Z** None	**Z** None	**Z** None
C Hand/Finger Joint, Right **D** Hand/Finger Joint, Left **G** Elbow, Right **H** Elbow, Left	**Ø** High Osmolar **1** Low Osmolar **Y** Other Contrast	**Z** None	**Z** None

B   **Imaging**
P   **Non-Axial Upper Bones**
2   **Computerized Tomography (CT Scan)**   Computer reformatted digital display of multiplanar images developed from the capture of multiple exposures of external ionizing radiation

Body Part Character 4	Contrast Character 5	Qualifier Character 6	Qualifier Character 7
Ø Sternoclavicular Joint, Right **1** Sternoclavicular Joint, Left **W** Thorax	**Ø** High Osmolar **1** Low Osmolar **Y** Other Contrast	**Z** None	**Z** None
2 Sternoclavicular Joints, Bilateral **3** Acromioclavicular Joints, Bilateral **4** Clavicle, Right **5** Clavicle, Left **6** Scapula, Right **7** Scapula, Left **8** Shoulder, Right **9** Shoulder, Left **A** Humerus, Right **B** Humerus, Left **E** Upper Arm, Right **F** Upper Arm, Left **G** Elbow, Right **H** Elbow, Left **J** Forearm, Right **K** Forearm, Left **L** Wrist, Right **M** Wrist, Left **N** Hand, Right **P** Hand, Left **Q** Hands and Wrists, Bilateral **R** Finger(s), Right **S** Finger(s), Left **T** Upper Extremity, Right **U** Upper Extremity, Left **V** Upper Extremities, Bilateral **X** Ribs, Right **Y** Ribs, Left	**Ø** High Osmolar **1** Low Osmolar **Y** Other Contrast **Z** None	**Z** None	**Z** None
C Hand/Finger Joint, Right **D** Hand/Finger Joint, Left	**Z** None	**Z** None	**Z** None

---

LC Limited Coverage   **NC** Noncovered   HAC associated procedure   Combination Only   DRG Non-OR   Non-OR   Revised Text in **GREEN**

B   **Imaging**
P   **Non-Axial Upper Bones**
3   **Magnetic Resonance Imaging (MRI)**   Computer reformatted digital display of multiplanar images developed from the capture of radio-frequency signals emitted by nuclei in a body site excited within a magnetic field

Body Part Character 4	Contrast Character 5	Qualifier Character 6	Qualifier Character 7
8 Shoulder, Right **9** Shoulder, Left **C** Hand/Finger Joint, Right **D** Hand/Finger Joint, Left **E** Upper Arm, Right **F** Upper Arm, Left **G** Elbow, Right **H** Elbow, Left **J** Forearm, Right **K** Forearm, Left **L** Wrist, Right **M** Wrist, Left	**Y** Other Contrast	**Ø** Unenhanced and Enhanced **Z** None	**Z** None
8 Shoulder, Right **9** Shoulder, Left **C** Hand/Finger Joint, Right **D** Hand/Finger Joint, Left **E** Upper Arm, Right **F** Upper Arm, Left **G** Elbow, Right **H** Elbow, Left **J** Forearm, Right **K** Forearm, Left **L** Wrist, Right **M** Wrist, Left	**Z** None	**Z** None	**Z** None

B   **Imaging**
P   **Non-Axial Upper Bones**
4   **Ultrasonography**   Real time display of images of anatomy or flow information developed from the capture of reflected and attenuated high frequency sound waves

Body Part Character 4	Contrast Character 5	Qualifier Character 6	Qualifier Character 7
8 Shoulder, Right **9** Shoulder, Left **G** Elbow, Right **H** Elbow, Left **L** Wrist, Right **M** Wrist, Left **N** Hand, Right **P** Hand, Left	**Z** None	**Z** None	**1** Densitometry **Z** None

B   **Imaging**
Q   **Non-Axial Lower Bones**
Ø   **Plain Radiography**   Planar display of an image developed from the capture of external ionizing radiation on photographic or photoconductive plate

Body Part Character 4	Contrast Character 5	Qualifier Character 6	Qualifier Character 7
Ø Hip, Right **1** Hip, Left **3** Femur, Right **4** Femur, Left	**Z** None	**Z** None	**1** Densitometry **Z** None
Ø Hip, Right **1** Hip, Left **X** Foot/Toe Joint, Right **Y** Foot/Toe Joint, Left	**Ø** High Osmolar **1** Low Osmolar **Y** Other Contrast	**Z** None	**Z** None
7 Knee, Right **8** Knee, Left **G** Ankle, Right **H** Ankle, Left	**Ø** High Osmolar **1** Low Osmolar **Y** Other Contrast **Z** None	**Z** None	**Z** None
D Lower Leg, Right **F** Lower Leg, Left **J** Calcaneus, Right **K** Calcaneus, Left **L** Foot, Right **M** Foot, Left **P** Toe(s), Right **Q** Toe(s), Left **V** Patella, Right **W** Patella, Left	**Z** None	**Z** None	**Z** None

LC Limited Coverage   **NC** Noncovered   HAC associated procedure   Combination Only   DRG Non-OR   Non-OR   Revised Text in **GREEN**

454   ICD-10-PCS 2014 (Draft)

B   **Imaging**
Q   **Non-Axial Lower Bones**
1   **Fluoroscopy**   Single plane or bi-plane real time display of an image developed from the capture of external ionizing radioation on a fluorescent screen. The image may also be stored by either digital or analog means

Body Part Character 4	Contrast Character 5	Qualifier Character 6	Qualifier Character 7
0 Hip, Right **1** Hip, Left **7** Knee, Right **8** Knee, Left **G** Ankle, Right **H** Ankle, Left **X** Foot/Toe Joint, Right **Y** Foot/Toe Joint, Left	**0** High Osmolar **1** Low Osmolar **Y** Other Contrast **Z** None	**Z** None	**Z** None
3 Femur, Right **4** Femur, Left **D** Lower Leg, Right **F** Lower Leg, Left **J** Calcaneus, Right **K** Calcaneus, Left **L** Foot, Right **M** Foot, Left **P** Toe(s), Right **Q** Toe(s), Left **V** Patella, Right **W** Patella, Left	**Z** None	**Z** None	**Z** None

B   **Imaging**
Q   **Non-Axial Lower Bones**
2   **Computerized Tomography (CT Scan)**   Computer reformatted digital display of multiplanar images developed from the capture of multiple exposures of external ionizing radiation

Body Part Character 4	Contrast Character 5	Qualifier Character 6	Qualifier Character 7
0 Hip, Right **1** Hip, Left **3** Femur, Right **4** Femur, Left **7** Knee, Right **8** Knee, Left **D** Lower Leg, Right **F** Lower Leg, Left **G** Ankle, Right **H** Ankle, Left **J** Calcaneus, Right **K** Calcaneus, Left **L** Foot, Right **M** Foot, Left **P** Toe(s), Right **Q** Toe(s), Left **R** Lower Extremity, Right **S** Lower Extremity, Left **V** Patella, Right **W** Patella, Left **X** Foot/Toe Joint, Right **Y** Foot/Toe Joint, Left	**0** High Osmolar **1** Low Osmolar **Y** Other Contrast **Z** None	**Z** None	**Z** None
B Tibia/Fibula, Right **C** Tibia/Fibula, Left	**0** High Osmolar **1** Low Osmolar **Y** Other Contrast	**Z** None	**Z** None

LC Limited Coverage   **NC** Noncovered   HAC associated procedure   Combination Only   DRG Non-OR   Non-OR   Revised Text in **GREEN**

ICD-10-PCS 2014 (Draft)   455

B   **Imaging**
Q   **Non-Axial Lower Bones**
3   **Magnetic Resonance Imaging (MRI)**   Computer reformatted digital display of multiplanar images developed from the capture of radio-frequency signals emitted by nuclei in a body site excited within a magnetic field

Body Part Character 4	Contrast Character 5	Qualifier Character 6	Qualifier Character 7
Ø Hip, Right 1 Hip, Left 3 Femur, Right 4 Femur, Left 7 Knee, Right 8 Knee, Left D Lower Leg, Right F Lower Leg, Left G Ankle, Right H Ankle, Left J Calcaneus, Right K Calcaneus, Left L Foot, Right M Foot, Left P Toe(s), Right Q Toe(s), Left V Patella, Right W Patella, Left	Y Other Contrast	Ø Unenhanced and Enhanced Z None	Z None
Ø Hip, Right 1 Hip, Left 3 Femur, Right 4 Femur, Left 7 Knee, Right 8 Knee, Left D Lower Leg, Right F Lower Leg, Left G Ankle, Right H Ankle, Left J Calcaneus, Right K Calcaneus, Left L Foot, Right M Foot, Left P Toe(s), Right Q Toe(s), Left V Patella, Right W Patella, Left	Z None	Z None	Z None

B   **Imaging**
Q   **Non-Axial Lower Bones**
4   **Ultrasonography**   Real time display of images of anatomy or flow information developed from the capture of relected and attenuated high frequency sound waves

Body Part Character 4	Contrast Character 5	Qualifier Character 6	Qualifier Character 7
Ø Hip, Right 1 Hip, Left 2 Hips, Bilateral 7 Knee, Right 8 Knee, Left 9 Knees, Bilateral	Z None	Z None	Z None

LC Limited Coverage   **NC** Noncovered   HAC associated procedure   Combination Only   DRG Non-OR   Non-OR   Revised Text in **GREEN**

456   ICD-10-PCS 2014 (Draft)

B　Imaging
R　Axial Skeleton, Except Skull and Facial Bones
0　Plain Radiography　Planar display of an image developed from the capture of external ionizing radiation on photographic or photoconductive plate

Body Part Character 4	Contrast Character 5	Qualifier Character 6	Qualifier Character 7
0　Cervical Spine 7　Thoracic Spine 9　Lumbar Spine G　Whole Spine	Z　None	Z　None	1　Densitometry Z　None
1　Cervical Disc(s) 2　Thoracic Disc(s) 3　Lumbar Disc(s) 4　Cervical Facet Joint(s) 5　Thoracic Facet Joint(s) 6　Lumbar Facet Joint(s) D　Sacroiliac Joints	0　High Osmolar 1　Low Osmolar Y　Other Contrast Z　None	Z　None	Z　None
8　Thoracolumbar Joint B　Lumbosacral Joint C　Pelvis F　Sacrum and Coccyx H　Sternum	Z　None	Z　None	Z　None

B　Imaging
R　Axial Skeleton, Except Skull and Facial Bones
1　Fluoroscopy　Single plane or bi-plane real time display of an image developed from the capture of external ionizing radioation on a fluorescent screen. The image may also be stored by either digital or analog means

Body Part Character 4	Contrast Character 5	Qualifier Character 6	Qualifier Character 7
0　Cervical Spine 1　Cervical Disc(s) 2　Thoracic Disc(s) 3　Lumbar Disc(s) 4　Cervical Facet Joint(s) 5　Thoracic Facet Joint(s) 6　Lumbar Facet Joint(s) 7　Thoracic Spine 8　Thoracolumbar Joint 9　Lumbar Spine B　Lumbosacral Joint C　Pelvis D　Sacroiliac Joints F　Sacrum and Coccyx G　Whole Spine H　Sternum	0　High Osmolar 1　Low Osmolar Y　Other Contrast Z　None	Z　None	Z　None

B　Imaging
R　Axial Skeleton, Except Skull and Facial Bones
2　Computerized Tomography (CT Scan)　Computer reformatted digital display of multiplanar images developed from the capture of multiple exposures of external ionizing radiation

Body Part Character 4	Contrast Character 5	Qualifier Character 6	Qualifier Character 7
0　Cervical Spine 7　Thoracic Spine 9　Lumbar Spine C　Pelvis D　Sacroiliac Joints F　Sacrum and Coccyx	0　High Osmolar 1　Low Osmolar Y　Other Contrast Z　None	Z　None	Z　None

LC Limited Coverage　　NC Noncovered　　HAC associated procedure　　Combination Only　　DRG Non-OR　　Non-OR　　Revised Text in GREEN

B   **Imaging**
R   **Axial Skeleton, Except Skull and Facial Bones**
3   **Magnetic Resonance Imaging (MRI)**   Computer reformatted digital display of multiplanar images developed from the capture of radio-frequency signals emitted by nuclei in a body site excited within a magnetic field

Body Part Character 4	Contrast Character 5	Qualifier Character 6	Qualifier Character 7
Ø Cervical Spine **1** Cervical Disc(s) **2** Thoracic Disc(s) **3** Lumbar Disc(s) **7** Thoracic Spine **9** Lumbar Spine **C** Pelvis **F** Sacrum and Coccyx	**Y** Other Contrast	**Ø** Unenhanced and Enhanced **Z** None	**Z** None
Ø Cervical Spine **1** Cervical Disc(s) **2** Thoracic Disc(s) **3** Lumbar Disc(s) **7** Thoracic Spine **9** Lumbar Spine **C** Pelvis **F** Sacrum and Coccyx	**Z** None	**Z** None	**Z** None

B   **Imaging**
R   **Axial Skeleton, Except Skull and Facial Bones**
4   **Ultrasonography**   Real time display of images of anatomy or flow information developed from the capture of relected and attenuated high frequency sound waves

Body Part Character 4	Contrast Character 5	Qualifier Character 6	Qualifier Character 7
Ø Cervical Spine **7** Thoracic Spine **9** Lumbar Spine **F** Sacrum and Coccyx	**Z** None	**Z** None	**Z** None

B   **Imaging**
T   **Urinary System**
Ø   **Plain Radiography**   Planar display of an image developed from the capture of external ionizing radiation on photographic or photoconductive plate

Body Part Character 4	Contrast Character 5	Qualifier Character 6	Qualifier Character 7
Ø Bladder **1** Kidney, Right **2** Kidney, Left **3** Kidneys, Bilateral **4** Kidneys, Ureters and Bladder **5** Urethra **6** Ureter, Right **7** Ureter, Left **8** Ureters, Bilateral **B** Bladder and Urethra **C** Ileal Diversion Loop	**Ø** High Osmolar **1** Low Osmolar **Y** Other Contrast **Z** None	**Z** None	**Z** None

B   **Imaging**
T   **Urinary System**
1   **Fluoroscopy**   Single plane or bi-plane real time display of an image developed from the capture of external ionizing radioation on a fluorescent screen. The image may also be stored by either digital or analog means

Body Part Character 4	Contrast Character 5	Qualifier Character 6	Qualifier Character 7
Ø Bladder **1** Kidney, Right **2** Kidney, Left **3** Kidneys, Bilateral **4** Kidneys, Ureters and Bladder **5** Urethra **6** Ureter, Right **7** Ureter, Left **B** Bladder and Urethra **C** Ileal Diversion Loop **D** Kidney, Ureter and Bladder, Right **F** Kidney, Ureter and Bladder, Left **G** Ileal Loop, Ureters and Kidneys	**Ø** High Osmolar **1** Low Osmolar **Y** Other Contrast **Z** None	**Z** None	**Z** None

B   **Imaging**
T   **Urinary System**
2   **Computerized Tomography (CT Scan)**   Computer reformatted digital display of multiplanar images developed from the capture of multiple exposures of external ionizing radiation

Body Part Character 4	Contrast Character 5	Qualifier Character 6	Qualifier Character 7
0 Bladder 1 Kidney, Right 2 Kidney, Left 3 Kidneys, Bilateral 9 Kidney Transplant	0 High Osmolar 1 Low Osmolar Y Other Contrast	0 Unenhanced and Enhanced Z None	Z None
0 Bladder 1 Kidney, Right 2 Kidney, Left 3 Kidneys, Bilateral 9 Kidney Transplant	Z None	Z None	Z None

B   **Imaging**
T   **Urinary System**
3   **Magnetic Resonance Imaging (MRI)**   Computer reformatted digital display of multiplanar images developed from the capture of radio-frequency signals emitted by nuclei in a body site excited within a magnetic field

Body Part Character 4	Contrast Character 5	Qualifier Character 6	Qualifier Character 7
0 Bladder 1 Kidney, Right 2 Kidney, Left 3 Kidneys, Bilateral 9 Kidney Transplant	Y Other Contrast	0 Unenhanced and Enhanced Z None	Z None
0 Bladder 1 Kidney, Right 2 Kidney, Left 3 Kidneys, Bilateral 9 Kidney Transplant	Z None	Z None	Z None

B   **Imaging**
T   **Urinary System**
4   **Ultrasonography**   Real time display of images of anatomy or flow information developed from the capture of relected and attenuated high frequency sound waves

Body Part Character 4	Contrast Character 5	Qualifier Character 6	Qualifier Character 7
0 Bladder 1 Kidney, Right 2 Kidney, Left 3 Kidneys, Bilateral 5 Urethra 6 Ureter, Right 7 Ureter, Left 8 Ureters, Bilateral 9 Kidney Transplant J Kidneys and Bladder	Z None	Z None	Z None

B   **Imaging**
U   **Female Reproductive System**
0   **Plain Radiography**   Planar display of an image developed from the capture of external ionizing radiation on photographic or photoconductive plate

Body Part Character 4	Contrast Character 5	Qualifier Character 6	Qualifier Character 7
0 Fallopian Tube, Right ♀ 1 Fallopian Tube, Left ♀ 2 Fallopian Tubes, Bilateral ♀ 6 Uterus ♀ 8 Uterus and Fallopian Tubes ♀ 9 Vagina ♀	0 High Osmolar 1 Low Osmolar Y Other Contrast	Z None	Z None

B   **Imaging**
U   **Female Reproductive System**
1   **Fluoroscopy**   Single plane or bi-plane real time display of an image developed from the capture of external ionizing radioation on a fluorescent screen. The image may also be stored by either digital or analog means

Body Part Character 4		Contrast Character 5	Qualifier Character 6	Qualifier Character 7
Ø Fallopian Tube, Right	♀	**Ø** High Osmolar	**Z** None	**Z** None
1 Fallopian Tube, Left	♀	**1** Low Osmolar		
2 Fallopian Tubes, Bilateral	♀	**Y** Other Contrast		
6 Uterus	♀	**Z** None		
8 Uterus and Fallopian Tubes	♀			
9 Vagina	♀			

B   **Imaging**
U   **Female Reproductive System**
3   **Magnetic Resonance Imaging (MRI)**   Computer reformatted digital display of multiplanar images developed from the capture of radio-frequency signals emitted by nuclei in a body site excited within a magnetic field

Body Part Character 4		Contrast Character 5	Qualifier Character 6	Qualifier Character 7
3 Ovary, Right	♀	**Y** Other Contrast	**Ø** Unenhanced and Enhanced	**Z** None
4 Ovary, Left	♀		**Z** None	
5 Ovaries, Bilateral	♀			
6 Uterus	♀			
9 Vagina	♀			
B Pregnant Uterus	♀			
C Uterus and Ovaries	♀			
3 Ovary, Right	♀	**Z** None	**Z** None	**Z** None
4 Ovary, Left	♀			
5 Ovaries, Bilateral	♀			
6 Uterus	♀			
9 Vagina	♀			
B Pregnant Uterus	♀			
C Uterus and Ovaries	♀			

B   **Imaging**
U   **Female Reproductive System**
4   **Ultrasonography**   Real time display of images of anatomy or flow information developed from the capture of relected and attenuated high frequency sound waves

Body Part Character 4		Contrast Character 5	Qualifier Character 6	Qualifier Character 7
Ø Fallopian Tube, Right	♀	**Y** Other Contrast	**Z** None	**Z** None
1 Fallopian Tube, Left	♀	**Z** None		
2 Fallopian Tubes, Bilateral	♀			
3 Ovary, Right	♀			
4 Ovary, Left	♀			
5 Ovaries, Bilateral	♀			
6 Uterus	♀			
C Uterus and Ovaries	♀			

B   **Imaging**
V   **Male Reproductive System**
Ø   **Plain Radiography**   Planar display of an image developed from the capture of external ionizing radiation on photographic or photoconductive plate

Body Part Character 4		Contrast Character 5	Qualifier Character 6	Qualifier Character 7
Ø Corpora Cavernosa	♂	**Ø** High Osmolar	**Z** None	**Z** None
1 Epididymis, Right	♂	**1** Low Osmolar		
2 Epididymis, Left	♂	**Y** Other Contrast		
3 Prostate	♂			
5 Testicle, Right	♂			
6 Testicle, Left	♂			
8 Vasa Vasorum	♂			

B   **Imaging**
V   **Male Reproductive System**
1   **Fluoroscopy**   Single plane or bi-plane real time display of an image developed from the capture of external ionizing radioation on a fluorescent screen. The image may also be stored by either digital or analog means

Body Part Character 4		Contrast Character 5	Qualifier Character 6	Qualifier Character 7
Ø Corpora Cavernosa	♂	**Ø** High Osmolar	**Z** None	**Z** None
8 Vasa Vasorum	♂	**1** Low Osmolar		
		Y Other Contrast		
		Z None		

LC Limited Coverage   **NC** Noncovered   HAC associated procedure   Combination Only   DRG Non-OR   Non-OR   Revised Text in **GREEN**

460   ICD-10-PCS 2014 (Draft)

B   Imaging
V   Male Reproductive System
2   Computerized Tomography (CT Scan) Computer reformatted digital display of multiplanar images developed from the capture of multiple exposures of external ionizing radiation

Body Part Character 4		Contrast Character 5	Qualifier Character 6	Qualifier Character 7
3 Prostate	♂	**Ø** High Osmolar **1** Low Osmolar **Y** Other Contrast	**Ø** Unenhanced and Enhanced **Z** None	**Z** None
3 Prostate	♂	**Z** None	**Z** None	**Z** None

B   Imaging
V   Male Reproductive System
3   Magnetic Resonance Imaging (MRI) Computer reformatted digital display of multiplanar images developed from the capture of radio-frequency signals emitted by nuclei in a body site excited within a magnetic field

Body Part Character 4		Contrast Character 5	Qualifier Character 6	Qualifier Character 7
Ø Corpora Cavernosa **3** Prostate **4** Scrotum **5** Testicle, Right **6** Testicle, Left **7** Testicles, Bilateral	♂ ♂ ♂ ♂ ♂ ♂	**Y** Other Contrast	**Ø** Unenhanced and Enhanced **Z** None	**Z** None
Ø Corpora Cavernosa **3** Prostate **4** Scrotum **5** Testicle, Right **6** Testicle, Left **7** Testicles, Bilateral	♂ ♂ ♂ ♂ ♂ ♂	**Z** None	**Z** None	**Z** None

B   Imaging
V   Male Reproductive System
4   Ultrasonography Real time display of images of anatomy or flow information developed from the capture of relected and attenuated high frequency sound waves

Body Part Character 4		Contrast Character 5	Qualifier Character 6	Qualifier Character 7
4 Scrotum **9** Prostate and Seminal Vesicles **B** Penis	♂ ♂ ♂	**Z** None	**Z** None	**Z** None

B   Imaging
W   Anatomical Regions
Ø   Plain Radiography Planar display of an image developed from the capture of external ionizing radiation on photographic or photoconductive plate

Body Part Character 4	Contrast Character 5	Qualifier Character 6	Qualifier Character 7
Ø Abdomen **1** Abdomen and Pelvis **3** Chest **B** Long Bones, All **C** Lower Extremity **J** Upper Extremity **K** Whole Body **L** Whole Skeleton **M** Whole Body, Infant	**Z** None	**Z** None	**Z** None

B   Imaging
W   Anatomical Regions
1   Fluoroscopy Single plane or bi-plane real time display of an image developed from the capture of external ionizing radioation on a fluorescent screen. The image may also be stored by either digital or analog means

Body Part Character 4	Contrast Character 5	Qualifier Character 6	Qualifier Character 7
1 Abdomen and Pelvis **9** Head and Neck **C** Lower Extremity **J** Upper Extremity	**Ø** High Osmolar **1** Low Osmolar **Y** Other Contrast **Z** None	**Z** None	**Z** None

B   **Imaging**
W   **Anatomical Regions**
2   **Computerized Tomography (CT Scan)** Computer reformatted digital display of multiplanar images developed from the capture of multiple exposures of external ionizing radiation

Body Part Character 4	Contrast Character 5	Qualifier Character 6	Qualifier Character 7
0 Abdomen **1** Abdomen and Pelvis **4** Chest and Abdomen **5** Chest, Abdomen and Pelvis **8** Head **9** Head and Neck **F** Neck **G** Pelvic Region	**0** High Osmolar **1** Low Osmolar **Y** Other Contrast	**0** Unenhanced and Enhanced **Z** None	**Z** None
0 Abdomen **1** Abdomen and Pelvis **4** Chest and Abdomen **5** Chest, Abdomen and Pelvis **8** Head **9** Head and Neck **F** Neck **G** Pelvic Region	**Z** None	**Z** None	**Z** None

B   **Imaging**
W   **Anatomical Regions**
3   **Magnetic Resonance Imaging (MRI)** Computer reformatted digital display of multiplanar images developed from the capture of radio-frequency signals emitted by nuclei in a body site excited within a magnetic field

Body Part Character 4	Contrast Character 5	Qualifier Character 6	Qualifier Character 7
0 Abdomen **3** Chest **8** Head **F** Neck **G** Pelvic Region **H** Retroperitoneum **P** Brachial Plexus	**Y** Other Contrast	**0** Unenhanced and Enhanced **Z** None	**Z** None
0 Abdomen **8** Head **F** Neck **G** Pelvic Region **H** Retroperitoneum **P** Brachial Plexus	**Z** None	**Z** None	**Z** None

B   **Imaging**
W   **Anatomical Regions**
4   **Ultrasonography** Real time display of images of anatomy or flow information developed from the capture of relected and attenuated high frequency sound waves

Body Part Character 4	Contrast Character 5	Qualifier Character 6	Qualifier Character 7
0 Abdomen **1** Abdomen and Pelvis **F** Neck **G** Pelvic Region	**Z** None	**Z** None	**Z** None

B   Imaging
Y   Fetus and Obstetrical
3   Magnetic Resonance Imaging (MRI)   Computer reformatted digital display of multiplanar images developed from the capture of radio-frequency signals emitted by nuclei in a body site excited within a magnetic field

Body Part Character 4		Contrast Character 5	Qualifier Character 6	Qualifier Character 7
Ø Fetal Head ♀ **1** Fetal Heart ♀ **2** Fetal Thorax ♀ **3** Fetal Abdomen ♀ **4** Fetal Spine ♀ **5** Fetal Extremities ♀ **6** Whole Fetus ♀		**Y** Other Contrast	**Ø** Unenhanced and Enhanced **Z** None	**Z** None
Ø Fetal Head ♀ **1** Fetal Heart ♀ **2** Fetal Thorax ♀ **3** Fetal Abdomen ♀ **4** Fetal Spine ♀ **5** Fetal Extremities ♀ **6** Whole Fetus ♀		**Z** None	**Z** None	**Z** None

B   Imaging
Y   Fetus and Obstetrical
4   Ultrasonography   Real time display of images of anatomy or flow information developed from the capture of relected and attenuated high frequency sound waves

Body Part Character 4		Contrast Character 5	Qualifier Character 6	Qualifier Character 7
7 Fetal Umbilical Cord ♀ **8** Placenta ♀ **9** First Trimester, Single Fetus ♀ **B** First Trimester, Multiple Gestation ♀ **C** Second Trimester, Single Fetus ♀ **D** Second Trimester, Multiple Gestation ♀ **F** Third Trimester, Single Fetus ♀ **G** Third Trimester, Multiple Gestation ♀		**Z** None	**Z** None	**Z** None

Nuclear Medicine C01–CW7

C   **Nuclear Medicine**
0   **Central Nervous System**
1   **Planar Nuclear Medicine Imaging**   Introduction of radioactive materials into the body for single plane display of images developed from the capture of radioactive emissions

Body Part Character 4	Radionuclide Character 5	Qualifier Character 6	Qualifier Character 7
0 Brain	**1** Technetium 99m (Tc-99m) **Y** Other Radionuclide	**Z** None	**Z** None
5 Cerebrospinal Fluid	**D** Indium 111 (In-111) **Y** Other Radionuclide	**Z** None	**Z** None
Y Central Nervous System	**Y** Other Radionuclide	**Z** None	**Z** None

C   **Nuclear Medicine**
0   **Central Nervous System**
2   **Tomographic (Tomo) Nuclear Medicine Imaging**   Introduction of radioactive materials into the body for three dimensional display of images developed from the capture of radioactive emissions

Body Part Character 4	Radionuclide Character 5	Qualifier Character 6	Qualifier Character 7
0 Brain	**1** Technetium 99m (Tc-99m) **F** Iodine 123 (I-123) **S** Thallium 201 (Tl-201) **Y** Other Radionuclide	**Z** None	**Z** None
5 Cerebrospinal Fluid	**D** Indium 111 (In-111) **Y** Other Radionuclide	**Z** None	**Z** None
Y Central Nervous System	**Y** Other Radionuclide	**Z** None	**Z** None

C   **Nuclear Medicine**
0   **Central Nervous System**
3   **Positron Emission Tomographic (PET) Imaging**   Introduction of radioactive materials into the body for three dimensional display of images developed from the simultaneous capture, 180 degrees apart, of radioactive emissions

Body Part Character 4	Radionuclide Character 5	Qualifier Character 6	Qualifier Character 7
0 Brain	**B** Carbon 11 (C-11) **K** Fluorine 18 (F-18) **M** Oxygen 15 (O-15) **Y** Other Radionuclide	**Z** None	**Z** None
Y Central Nervous System	**Y** Other Radionuclide	**Z** None	**Z** None

C   **Nuclear Medicine**
0   **Central Nervous System**
5   **Nonimaging Nuclear Medicine Probe**   Introduction of radioactive materials into the body for the study of distribution and fate of certain substances by the detection of radioactive emissions; or, alternatively, measurement of absorption of radioactive emissions from an external source

Body Part Character 4	Radionuclide Character 5	Qualifier Character 6	Qualifier Character 7
0 Brain	**V** Xenon 133 (Xe-133) **Y** Other Radionuclide	**Z** None	**Z** None
Y Central Nervous System	**Y** Other Radionuclide	**Z** None	**Z** None

C   **Nuclear Medicine**
2   **Heart**
1   **Planar Nuclear Medicine Imaging**   Introduction of radioactive materials into the body for single plane display of images developed from the capture of radioactive emissions

Body Part Character 4	Radionuclide Character 5	Qualifier Character 6	Qualifier Character 7
6 Heart, Right and Left	**1** Technetium 99m (Tc-99m) **Y** Other Radionuclide	**Z** None	**Z** None
G Myocardium	**1** Technetium 99m (Tc-99m) **D** Indium 111 (In-111) **S** Thallium 201 (Tl-201) **Y** Other Radionuclide **Z** None	**Z** None	**Z** None
Y Heart	**Y** Other Radionuclide	**Z** None	**Z** None

LC Limited Coverage   **NC** Noncovered   HAC associated procedure   Combination Only   DRG Non-OR   Non-OR   Revised Text in **GREEN**

464   ICD-10-PCS 2014 (Draft)

C   **Nuclear Medicine**
2   **Heart**
2   **Tomographic (Tomo) Nuclear Medicine Imaging**   Introduction of radioactive materials into the body for three dimensional display of images developed from the capture of radioactive emissions

Body Part Character 4	Radionuclide Character 5	Qualifier Character 6	Qualifier Character 7
6 Heart, Right and Left	**1** Technetium 99m (Tc-99m) **Y** Other Radionuclide	**Z** None	**Z** None
G Myocardium	**1** Technetium 99m (Tc-99m) **D** Indium 111 (In-111) **K** Fluorine 18 (F-18) **S** Thallium 201 (Tl-201) **Y** Other Radionuclide **Z** None	**Z** None	**Z** None
Y Heart	**Y** Other Radionuclide	**Z** None	**Z** None

C   **Nuclear Medicine**
2   **Heart**
3   **Positron Emission Tomographic (PET) Imaging**   Introduction of radioactive materials into the body for three dimensional display of images developed from the simultaneous capture, 180 degrees apart, of radioactive emissions

Body Part Character 4	Radionuclide Character 5	Qualifier Character 6	Qualifier Character 7
G Myocardium	**K** Fluorine 18 (F-18) **M** Oxygen 15 (O-15) **Q** Rubidium 82 (Rb-82) **R** Nitrogen 13 (N-13) **Y** Other Radionuclide	**Z** None	**Z** None
Y Heart	**Y** Other Radionuclide	**Z** None	**Z** None

C   **Nuclear Medicine**
2   **Heart**
5   **Nonimaging Nuclear Medicine Probe**   Introduction of radioactive materials into the body for the study of distribution and fate of certain substances by the detection of radioactive emissions; or, alternatively, measurement of absorption of radioactive emissions from an external source

Body Part Character 4	Radionuclide Character 5	Qualifier Character 6	Qualifier Character 7
6 Heart, Right and Left	**1** Technetium 99m (Tc-99m) **Y** Other Radionuclide	**Z** None	**Z** None
Y Heart	**Y** Other Radionuclide	**Z** None	**Z** None

C   **Nuclear Medicine**
5   **Veins**
1   **Planar Nuclear Medicine Imaging**   Introduction of radioactive materials into the body for single plane display of images developed from the capture of radioactive emissions

Body Part Character 4	Radionuclide Character 5	Qualifier Character 6	Qualifier Character 7
B Lower Extremity Veins, Right **C** Lower Extremity Veins, Left **D** Lower Extremity Veins, Bilateral **N** Upper Extremity Veins, Right **P** Upper Extremity Veins, Left **Q** Upper Extremity Veins, Bilateral **R** Central Veins	**1** Technetium 99m (Tc-99m) **Y** Other Radionuclide	**Z** None	**Z** None
Y Veins	**Y** Other Radionuclide	**Z** None	**Z** None

LC Limited Coverage   **NC** Noncovered   HAC associated procedure   Combination Only   DRG Non-OR   Non-OR   Revised Text in **GREEN**

ICD-10-PCS 2014 (Draft)   **465**

C   Nuclear Medicine
7   Lymphatic and Hematologic System
1   Planar Nuclear Medicine Imaging   Introduction of radioactive materials into the body for single plane display of images developed from the capture of radioactive emissions

Body Part Character 4	Radionuclide Character 5	Qualifier Character 6	Qualifier Character 7
0 Bone Marrow	**1** Technetium 99m (Tc-99m) **D** Indium 111 (In-111) **Y** Other Radionuclide	**Z** None	**Z** None
2 Spleen **5** Lymphatics, Head and Neck **D** Lymphatics, Pelvic **J** Lymphatics, Head **K** Lymphatics, Neck **L** Lymphatics, Upper Chest **M** Lymphatics, Trunk **N** Lymphatics, Upper Extremity **P** Lymphatics, Lower Extremity	**1** Technetium 99m (Tc-99m) **Y** Other Radionuclide	**Z** None	**Z** None
3 Blood	**D** Indium 111 (In-111) **Y** Other Radionuclide	**Z** None	**Z** None
Y Lymphatic and Hematologic System	**Y** Other Radionuclide	**Z** None	**Z** None

C   Nuclear Medicine
7   Lymphatic and Hematologic System
2   Tomographic (Tomo) Nuclear Medicine Imaging   Introduction of radioactive materials into the body for three dimensional display of images developed from the capture of radioactive emissions

Body Part Character 4	Radionuclide Character 5	Qualifier Character 6	Qualifier Character 7
2 Spleen	**1** Technetium 99m (Tc-99m) **Y** Other Radionuclide	**Z** None	**Z** None
Y Lymphatic and Hematologic System	**Y** Other Radionuclide	**Z** None	**Z** None

C   Nuclear Medicine
7   Lymphatic and Hematologic System
5   Nonimaging Nuclear Medicine Probe   Introduction of radioactive materials into the body for the study of distribution and fate of certain substances by the detection of radioactive emissions; or, alternatively, measurement of absorption of radioactive emissions from an external source

Body Part Character 4	Radionuclide Character 5	Qualifier Character 6	Qualifier Character 7
5 Lymphatics, Head and Neck **D** Lymphatics, Pelvic **J** Lymphatics, Head **K** Lymphatics, Neck **L** Lymphatics, Upper Chest **M** Lymphatics, Trunk **N** Lymphatics, Upper Extremity **P** Lymphatics, Lower Extremity	**1** Technetium 99m (Tc-99m) **Y** Other Radionuclide	**Z** None	**Z** None
Y Lymphatic and Hematologic System	**Y** Other Radionuclide	**Z** None	**Z** None

C   Nuclear Medicine
7   Lymphatic and Hematologic System
6   Nonimaging Nuclear Medicine Assay   Introduction of radioactive materials into the body for the study of body fluids and blood elements, by the detection of radioactive emissions

Body Part Character 4	Radionuclide Character 5	Qualifier Character 6	Qualifier Character 7
3 Blood	**1** Technetium 99m (Tc-99m) **7** Cobalt 58 (Co-58) **C** Cobalt 57 (Co-57) **D** Indium 111 (In-111) **H** Iodine 125 (I-125) **W** Chromium (Cr-51) **Y** Other Radionuclide	**Z** None	**Z** None
Y Lymphatic and Hematologic System	**Y** Other Radionuclide	**Z** None	**Z** None

C Nuclear Medicine
8 Eye
1 Planar Nuclear Medicine Imaging Introduction of radioactive materials into the body for single plane display of images developed from the capture of radioactive emissions

Body Part Character 4	Radionuclide Character 5	Qualifier Character 6	Qualifier Character 7
9 Lacrimal Ducts, Bilateral	**1** Technetium 99m (Tc-99m) **Y** Other Radionuclide	**Z** None	**Z** None
Y Eye	**Y** Other Radionuclide	**Z** None	**Z** None

C Nuclear Medicine
9 Ear, Nose, Mouth and Throat
1 Planar Nuclear Medicine Imaging Introduction of radioactive materials into the body for single plane display of images developed from the capture of radioactive emissions

Body Part Character 4	Radionuclide Character 5	Qualifier Character 6	Qualifier Character 7
B Salivary Glands, Bilateral	**1** Technetium 99m (Tc-99m) **Y** Other Radionuclide	**Z** None	**Z** None
Y Ear, Nose, Mouth and Throat	**Y** Other Radionuclide	**Z** None	**Z** None

C Nuclear Medicine
B Respiratory System
1 Planar Nuclear Medicine Imaging Introduction of radioactive materials into the body for single plane display of images developed from the capture of radioactive emissions

Body Part Character 4	Radionuclide Character 5	Qualifier Character 6	Qualifier Character 7
2 Lungs and Bronchi	**1** Technetium 99m (Tc-99m) **9** Krypton (Kr-81m) **T** Xenon 127 (Xe-127) **V** Xenon 133 (Xe-133) **Y** Other Radionuclide	**Z** None	**Z** None
Y Respiratory System	**Y** Other Radionuclide	**Z** None	**Z** None

C Nuclear Medicine
B Respiratory System
2 Tomographic (Tomo) Nuclear Medicine Imaging Introduction of radioactive materials into the body for three dimensional display of images developed from the capture of radioactive emissions

Body Part Character 4	Radionuclide Character 5	Qualifier Character 6	Qualifier Character 7
2 Lungs and Bronchi	**1** Technetium 99m (Tc-99m) **9** Krypton (Kr-81m) **Y** Other Radionuclide	**Z** None	**Z** None
Y Respiratory System	**Y** Other Radionuclide	**Z** None	**Z** None

C Nuclear Medicine
B Respiratory System
3 Positron Emission Tomographic (PET) Imaging Introduction of radioactive materials into the body for three dimensional display of images developed from the simultaneous capture, 180 degrees apart, of radioactive emissions

Body Part Character 4	Radionuclide Character 5	Qualifier Character 6	Qualifier Character 7
2 Lungs and Bronchi	**K** Fluorine 18 (F-18) **Y** Other Radionuclide	**Z** None	**Z** None
Y Respiratory System	**Y** Other Radionuclide	**Z** None	**Z** None

C Nuclear Medicine
D Gastrointestinal System
1 Planar Nuclear Medicine Imaging Introduction of radioactive materials into the body for single plane display of images developed from the capture of radioactive emissions

Body Part Character 4	Radionuclide Character 5	Qualifier Character 6	Qualifier Character 7
5 Upper Gastrointestinal Tract **7** Gastrointestinal Tract	**1** Technetium 99m (Tc-99m) **D** Indium 111 (In-111) **Y** Other Radionuclide	**Z** None	**Z** None
Y Digestive System	**Y** Other Radionuclide	**Z** None	**Z** None

C   **Nuclear Medicine**
D   **Gastrointestinal System**
2   **Tomographic (Tomo) Nuclear Medicine Imaging** Introduction of radioactive materials into the body for three dimensional display of images developed from the capture of radioactive emissions

Body Part Character 4	Radionuclide Character 5	Qualifier Character 6	Qualifier Character 7
7 Gastrointestinal Tract	**1** Technetium 99m (Tc-99m) **D** Indium 111 (In-111) **Y** Other Radionuclide	**Z** None	**Z** None
Y Digestive System	**Y** Other Radionuclide	**Z** None	**Z** None

C   **Nuclear Medicine**
F   **Hepatobiliary System and Pancreas**
1   **Planar Nuclear Medicine Imaging** Introduction of radioactive materials into the body for single plane display of images developed from the capture of radioactive emissions

Body Part Character 4	Radionuclide Character 5	Qualifier Character 6	Qualifier Character 7
4 Gallbladder **5** Liver **6** Liver and Spleen **C** Hepatobiliary System, All	**1** Technetium 99m (Tc-99m) **Y** Other Radionuclide	**Z** None	**Z** None
Y Hepatobiliary System and Pancreas	**Y** Other Radionuclide	**Z** None	**Z** None

C   **Nuclear Medicine**
F   **Hepatobiliary System and Pancreas**
2   **Tomographic (Tomo) Nuclear Medicine Imaging** Introduction of radioactive materials into the body for three dimensional display of images developed from the capture of radioactive emissions

Body Part Character 4	Radionuclide Character 5	Qualifier Character 6	Qualifier Character 7
4 Gallbladder **5** Liver **6** Liver and Spleen	**1** Technetium 99m (Tc-99m) **Y** Other Radionuclide	**Z** None	**Z** None
Y Hepatobiliary System and Pancreas	**Y** Other Radionuclide	**Z** None	**Z** None

C   **Nuclear Medicine**
G   **Endocrine System**
1   **Planar Nuclear Medicine Imaging** Introduction of radioactive materials into the body for single plane display of images developed from the capture of radioactive emissions

Body Part Character 4	Radionuclide Character 5	Qualifier Character 6	Qualifier Character 7
1 Parathyroid Glands	**1** Technetium 99m (Tc-99m) **S** Thallium 201 (Tl-201) **Y** Other Radionuclide	**Z** None	**Z** None
2 Thyroid Gland	**1** Technetium 99m (Tc-99m) **F** Iodine 123 (I-123) **G** Iodine 131 (I-131) **Y** Other Radionuclide	**Z** None	**Z** None
4 Adrenal Glands, Bilateral	**G** Iodine 131 (I-131) **Y** Other Radionuclide	**Z** None	**Z** None
Y Endocrine System	**Y** Other Radionuclide	**Z** None	**Z** None

C   **Nuclear Medicine**
G   **Endocrine System**
2   **Tomographic (Tomo) Nuclear Medicine Imaging** Introduction of radioactive materials into the body for three dimensional display of images developed from the capture of radioactive emissions

Body Part Character 4	Radionuclide Character 5	Qualifier Character 6	Qualifier Character 7
1 Parathyroid Glands	**1** Technetium 99m (Tc-99m) **S** Thallium 201 (Tl-201) **Y** Other Radionuclide	**Z** None	**Z** None
Y Endocrine System	**Y** Other Radionuclide	**Z** None	**Z** None

C **Nuclear Medicine**
G **Endocrine System**
4 **Nonimaging Nuclear Medicine Uptake**   Introduction of radioactive materials into the body for measurements of organ function, from the detection of radioactive emmissions

Body Part Character 4	Radionuclide Character 5	Qualifier Character 6	Qualifier Character 7
2 Thyroid Gland	**1** Technetium 99m (Tc-99m) **F** Iodine 123 (I-123) **G** Iodine 131 (I-131) **Y** Other Radionuclide	**Z** None	**Z** None
Y Endocrine System	**Y** Other Radionuclide	**Z** None	**Z** None

C **Nuclear Medicine**
H **Skin, Subcutaneous Tissue and Breast**
1 **Planar Nuclear Medicine Imaging**   Introduction of radioactive materials into the body for single plane display of images developed from the capture of radioactive emissions

Body Part Character 4	Radionuclide Character 5	Qualifier Character 6	Qualifier Character 7
Ø Breast, Right **1** Breast, Left **2** Breasts, Bilateral	**1** Technetium 99m (Tc-99m) **S** Thallium 201 (Tl-201) **Y** Other Radionuclide	**Z** None	**Z** None
Y Skin, Subcutaneous Tissue and Breast	**Y** Other Radionuclide	**Z** None	**Z** None

C **Nuclear Medicine**
H **Skin, Subcutaneous Tissue and Breast**
2 **Tomographic (Tomo) Nuclear Medicine Imaging**   Introduction of radioactive materials into the body for three dimensional display of images developed from the capture of radioactive emissions

Body Part Character 4	Radionuclide Character 5	Qualifier Character 6	Qualifier Character 7
Ø Breast, Right **1** Breast, Left **2** Breasts, Bilateral	**1** Technetium 99m (Tc-99m) **S** Thallium 201 (Tl-201) **Y** Other Radionuclide	**Z** None	**Z** None
Y Skin, Subcutaneous Tissue and Breast	**Y** Other Radionuclide	**Z** None	**Z** None

C **Nuclear Medicine**
P **Musculoskeletal System**
1 **Planar Nuclear Medicine Imaging**   Introduction of radioactive materials into the body for single plane display of images developed from the capture of radioactive emissions

Body Part Character 4	Radionuclide Character 5	Qualifier Character 6	Qualifier Character 7
1 Skull **4** Thorax **5** Spine **6** Pelvis **7** Spine and Pelvis **8** Upper Extremity, Right **9** Upper Extremity, Left **B** Upper Extremities, Bilateral **C** Lower Extremity, Right **D** Lower Extremity, Left **F** Lower Extremities, Bilateral **Z** Musculoskeletal System, All	**1** Technetium 99m (Tc-99m) **Y** Other Radionuclide	**Z** None	**Z** None
Y Musculoskeletal System, Other	**Y** Other Radionuclide	**Z** None	**Z** None

C **Nuclear Medicine**
P **Musculoskeletal System**
2 **Tomographic (Tomo) Nuclear Medicine Imaging** Introduction of radioactive materials into the body for three dimensional display of images developed from the capture of radioactive emissions

Body Part Character 4	Radionuclide Character 5	Qualifier Character 6	Qualifier Character 7
1 Skull **2** Cervical Spine **3** Skull and Cervical Spine **4** Thorax **6** Pelvis **7** Spine and Pelvis **8** Upper Extremity, Right **9** Upper Extremity, Left **B** Upper Extremities, Bilateral **C** Lower Extremity, Right **D** Lower Extremity, Left **F** Lower Extremities, Bilateral **G** Thoracic Spine **H** Lumbar Spine **J** Thoracolumbar Spine	**1** Technetium 99m (Tc-99m) **Y** Other Radionuclide	**Z** None	**Z** None
Y Musculoskeletal System, Other	**Y** Other Radionuclide	**Z** None	**Z** None

C **Nuclear Medicine**
P **Musculoskeletal System**
5 **Nonimaging Nuclear Medicine Probe** Introduction of radioactive materials into the body for the study of distribution and fate of certain substances by the detection of radioactive emissions; or, alternatively, measurement of absorption of radioactive emissions from an external source

Body Part Character 4	Radionuclide Character 5	Qualifier Character 6	Qualifier Character 7
5 Spine **N** Upper Extremities **P** Lower Extremities	**Z** None	**Z** None	**Z** None
Y Musculoskeletal System, Other	**Y** Other Radionuclide	**Z** None	**Z** None

C **Nuclear Medicine**
T **Urinary System**
1 **Planar Nuclear Medicine Imaging** Introduction of radioactive materials into the body for single plane display of images developed from the capture of radioactive emissions

Body Part Character 4	Radionuclide Character 5	Qualifier Character 6	Qualifier Character 7
3 Kidneys, Ureters and Bladder	**1** Technetium 99m (Tc-99m) **F** Iodine 123 (I-123) **G** Iodine 131 (I-131) **Y** Other Radionuclide	**Z** None	**Z** None
H Bladder and Ureters	**1** Technetium 99m (Tc-99m) **Y** Other Radionuclide	**Z** None	**Z** None
Y Urinary System	**Y** Other Radionuclide	**Z** None	**Z** None

C **Nuclear Medicine**
T **Urinary System**
2 **Tomographic (Tomo) Nuclear Medicine Imaging** Introduction of radioactive materials into the body for three dimensional display of images developed from the capture of radioactive emissions

Body Part Character 4	Radionuclide Character 5	Qualifier Character 6	Qualifier Character 7
3 Kidneys, Ureters and Bladder	**1** Technetium 99m (Tc-99m) **Y** Other Radionuclide	**Z** None	**Z** None
Y Urinary System	**Y** Other Radionuclide	**Z** None	**Z** None

C **Nuclear Medicine**
T **Urinary System**
6 **Nonimaging Nuclear Medicine Assay** Introduction of radioactive materials into the body for the study of body fluids and blood elements, by the detection of radioactive emissions

Body Part Character 4	Radionuclide Character 5	Qualifier Character 6	Qualifier Character 7
3 Kidneys, Ureters and Bladder	**1** Technetium 99m (Tc-99m) **F** Iodine 123 (I-123) **G** Iodine 131 (I-131) **H** Iodine 125 (I-125) **Y** Other Radionuclide	**Z** None	**Z** None
Y Urinary System	**Y** Other Radionuclide	**Z** None	**Z** None

C Nuclear Medicine
V Male Reproductive System
1 Planar Nuclear Medicine Imaging Introduction of radioactive materials into the body for single plane display of images developed from the capture of radioactive emissions

Body Part Character 4	Radionuclide Character 5	Qualifier Character 6	Qualifier Character 7
9 Testicles, Bilateral	**1** Technetium 99m (Tc-99m) **Y** Other Radionuclide	**Z** None	**Z** None
Y Male Reproductive System	**Y** Other Radionuclide	**Z** None	**Z** None

C Nuclear Medicine
W Anatomical Regions
1 Planar Nuclear Medicine Imaging Introduction of radioactive materials into the body for single plane display of images developed from the capture of radioactive emissions

Body Part Character 4	Radionuclide Character 5	Qualifier Character 6	Qualifier Character 7
Ø Abdomen **1** Abdomen and Pelvis **4** Chest and Abdomen **6** Chest and Neck **B** Head and Neck **D** Lower Extremity **J** Pelvic Region **M** Upper Extremity **N** Whole Body	**1** Technetium 99m (Tc-99m) **D** Indium 111 (In-111) **F** Iodine 123 (I-123) **G** Iodine 131 (I-131) **L** Gallium 67 (Ga-67) **S** Thallium 201 (Tl-201) **Y** Other Radionuclide	**Z** None	**Z** None
3 Chest	**1** Technetium 99m (Tc-99m) **D** Indium 111 (In-111) **F** Iodine 123 (I-123) **G** Iodine 131 (I-131) **K** Fluorine 18 (F-18) **L** Gallium 67 (Ga-67) **S** Thallium 201 (Tl-201) **Y** Other Radionuclide	**Z** None	**Z** None
Y Anatomical Regions, Multiple	**Y** Other Radionuclide	**Z** None	**Z** None
Z Anatomical Region, Other	**Z** None	**Z** None	**Z** None

C Nuclear Medicine
W Anatomical Regions
2 Tomographic (Tomo) Nuclear Medicine Imaging Introduction of radioactive materials into the body for three dimensional display of images developed from the capture of radioactive emissions

Body Part Character 4	Radionuclide Character 5	Qualifier Character 6	Qualifier Character 7
Ø Abdomen **1** Abdomen and Pelvis **3** Chest **4** Chest and Abdomen **6** Chest and Neck **B** Head and Neck **D** Lower Extremity **J** Pelvic Region **M** Upper Extremity	**1** Technetium 99m (Tc-99m) **D** Indium 111 (In-111) **F** Iodine 123 (I-123) **G** Iodine 131 (I-131) **K** Fluorine 18 (F-18) **L** Gallium 67 (Ga-67) **S** Thallium 201 (Tl-201) **Y** Other Radionuclide	**Z** None	**Z** None
Y Anatomical Regions, Multiple	**Y** Other Radionuclide	**Z** None	**Z** None

C Nuclear Medicine
W Anatomical Regions
3 Positron Emission Tomographic (PET) Imaging Introduction of radioactive materials into the body for three dimensional display of images developed from the simultaneous capture, 180 degrees apart, of radioactive emissions

Body Part Character 4	Radionuclide Character 5	Qualifier Character 6	Qualifier Character 7
N Whole Body	**Y** Other Radionuclide	**Z** None	**Z** None

LC Limited Coverage **NC** Noncovered HAC associated procedure Combination Only DRG Non-OR Non-OR Revised Text in **GREEN**

ICD-10-PCS 2014 (Draft) 471

Nuclear Medicine

C Nuclear Medicine
W Anatomical Regions
5 Nonimaging Nuclear Medicine Probe Introduction of radioactive materials into the body for the study of distribution and fate of certain substances by the detection of radioactive emissions; or, alternatively, measurement of absorption of radioactive emissions from an external source

Body Part Character 4	Radionuclide Character 5	Qualifier Character 6	Qualifier Character 7
Ø Abdomen **1** Abdomen and Pelvis **3** Chest **4** Chest and Abdomen **6** Chest and Neck **B** Head and Neck **D** Lower Extremity **J** Pelvic Region **M** Upper Extremity	**1** Technetium 99m (Tc-99m) **D** Indium 111 (In-111) **Y** Other Radionuclide	**Z** None	**Z** None

C Nuclear Medicine
W Anatomical Regions
7 Systemic Nuclear Medicine Therapy Introduction of radioactive materials into the body for treatment

Body Part Character 4	Radionuclide Character 5	Qualifier Character 6	Qualifier Character 7
Ø Abdomen **3** Chest	**N** Phosphorus 32 (P-32) **Y** Other Radionuclide	**Z** None	**Z** None
G Thyroid	**G** Iodine 131 (I-131) **Y** Other Radionuclide	**Z** None	**Z** None
N Whole Body	**8** Samarium 153 (Sm-153) **G** Iodine 131 (I-131) **N** Phosphorus 32 (P-32) **P** Strontium 89 (Sr-89) **Y** Other Radionuclide	**Z** None	**Z** None
Y Anatomical Regions, Multiple	**Y** Other Radionuclide	**Z** None	**Z** None

LC Limited Coverage   **NC** Noncovered   HAC associated procedure   Combination Only   DRG Non-OR   Non-OR   Revised Text in **GREEN**

472   ICD-10-PCS 2014 (Draft)

Radiation Therapy D00–DWY

D　Radiation Therapy
0　Central and Peripheral Nervous System
0　Beam Radiation

Treatment Site Character 4	Modal. Qualifier Character 5	Isotope Character 6	Qualifier Character 7
0　Brain 1　Brain Stem 6　Spinal Cord 7　Peripheral Nerve	0　Photons <1 MeV 1　Photons 1- 10 MeV 2　Photons >10 MeV 4　Heavy Particles (Protons, Ions) 5　Neutrons 6　Neutron Capture	Z　None	Z　None
0　Brain 1　Brain Stem 6　Spinal Cord 7　Peripheral Nerve	3　Electrons	Z　None	0　Intraoperative Z　None

D　Radiation Therapy
0　Central and Peripheral Nervous System
1　Brachytherapy

Treatment Site Character 4	Modal. Qualifier Character 5	Isotope Character 6	Qualifier Character 7
0　Brain 1　Brain Stem 6　Spinal Cord 7　Peripheral Nerve	9　High Dose Rate (HDR) B　Low Dose Rate (LDR)	7　Cesium 137 (Cs-137) 8　Iridium 192 (Ir-192) 9　Iodine 125 (I-125) B　Palladium 103 (Pd-103) C　Californium 252 (Cf-252) Y　Other Isotope	Z　None

D　Radiation Therapy
0　Central and Peripheral Nervous System
2　Stereotactic Radiosurgery

Treatment Site Character 4	Modal. Qualifier Character 5	Isotope Character 6	Qualifier Character 7
0　Brain 1　Brain Stem 6　Spinal Cord 7　Peripheral Nerve	D　Stereotactic Other Photon 　　Radiosurgery H　Stereotactic Particulate Radiosurgery J　Stereotactic Gamma Beam 　　Radiosurgery	Z　None	Z　None

DRG Non-OR　For all body part, approach, device, and qualifier values

D　Radiation Therapy
0　Central and Peripheral Nervous System
Y　Other Radiation

Treatment Site Character 4	Modal. Qualifier Character 5	Isotope Character 6	Qualifier Character 7
0　Brain 1　Brain Stem 6　Spinal Cord 7　Peripheral Nerve	7　Contact Radiation 8　Hyperthermia F　Plaque Radiation K　Laser Interstitial Thermal Therapy	Z　None	Z　None

Radiation Therapy

D7Ø–D7Y

D Radiation Therapy
7 Lymphatic and Hematologic System
Ø Beam Radiation

Treatment Site Character 4	Modal. Qualifier Character 5	Isotope Character 6	Qualifier Character 7
Ø Bone Marrow 1 Thymus 2 Spleen 3 Lymphatics, Neck 4 Lymphatics, Axillary 5 Lymphatics, Thorax 6 Lymphatics, Abdomen 7 Lymphatics, Pelvis 8 Lymphatics, Inguinal	Ø Photons <1 MeV 1 Photons 1- 1Ø MeV 2 Photons >1Ø MeV 4 Heavy Particles (Protons, Ions) 5 Neutrons 6 Neutron Capture	Z None	Z None
Ø Bone Marrow 1 Thymus 2 Spleen 3 Lymphatics, Neck 4 Lymphatics, Axillary 5 Lymphatics, Thorax 6 Lymphatics, Abdomen 7 Lymphatics, Pelvis 8 Lymphatics, Inguinal	3 Electrons	Z None	Ø Intraoperative Z None

D Radiation Therapy
7 Lymphatic and Hematologic System
1 Brachytherapy

Treatment Site Character 4	Modal. Qualifier Character 5	Isotope Character 6	Qualifier Character 7
Ø Bone Marrow 1 Thymus 2 Spleen 3 Lymphatics, Neck 4 Lymphatics, Axillary 5 Lymphatics, Thorax 6 Lymphatics, Abdomen 7 Lymphatics, Pelvis 8 Lymphatics, Inguinal	9 High Dose Rate (HDR) B Low Dose Rate (LDR)	7 Cesium 137 (Cs-137) 8 Iridium 192 (Ir-192) 9 Iodine 125 (I-125) B Palladium 1Ø3 (Pd-1Ø3) C Californium 252 (Cf-252) Y Other Isotope	Z None

D Radiation Therapy
7 Lymphatic and Hematologic System
2 Stereotactic Radiosurgery

Treatment Site Character 4	Modal. Qualifier Character 5	Isotope Character 6	Qualifier Character 7
Ø Bone Marrow 1 Thymus 2 Spleen 3 Lymphatics, Neck 4 Lymphatics, Axillary 5 Lymphatics, Thorax 6 Lymphatics, Abdomen 7 Lymphatics, Pelvis 8 Lymphatics, Inguinal	D Stereotactic Other Photon Radiosurgery H Stereotactic Particulate Radiosurgery J Stereotactic Gamma Beam Radiosurgery	Z None	Z None

DRG Non-OR For all body part, approach, device, and qualifier values

D Radiation Therapy
7 Lymphatic and Hematologic System
Y Other Radiation

Treatment Site Character 4	Modal. Qualifier Character 5	Isotope Character 6	Qualifier Character 7
Ø Bone Marrow 1 Thymus 2 Spleen 3 Lymphatics, Neck 4 Lymphatics, Axillary 5 Lymphatics, Thorax 6 Lymphatics, Abdomen 7 Lymphatics, Pelvis 8 Lymphatics, Inguinal	8 Hyperthermia F Plaque Radiation	Z None	Z None

D Radiation Therapy
8 Eye
Ø Beam Radiation

Treatment Site Character 4	Modal. Qualifier Character 5	Isotope Character 6	Qualifier Character 7
Ø Eye	Ø Photons <1 MeV 1 Photons 1- 1Ø MeV 2 Photons >1Ø MeV 4 Heavy Particles (Protons, Ions) 5 Neutrons 6 Neutron Capture	Z None	Z None
Ø Eye	3 Electrons	Z None	Ø Intraoperative Z None

D Radiation Therapy
8 Eye
1 Brachytherapy

Treatment Site Character 4	Modal. Qualifier Character 5	Isotope Character 6	Qualifier Character 7
Ø Eye	9 High Dose Rate (HDR) B Low Dose Rate (LDR)	7 Cesium 137 (Cs-137) 8 Iridium 192 (Ir-192) 9 Iodine 125 (I-125) B Palladium 1Ø3 (Pd-1Ø3) C Californium 252 (Cf-252) Y Other Isotope	Z None

D Radiation Therapy
8 Eye
2 Stereotactic Radiosurgery

Treatment Site Character 4	Modal. Qualifier Character 5	Isotope Character 6	Qualifier Character 7
Ø Eye	D Stereotactic Other Photon Radiosurgery H Stereotactic Particulate Radiosurgery J Stereotactic Gamma Beam Radiosurgery	Z None	Z None

DRG Non-OR For all body part, approach, device, and qualifier values

D Radiation Therapy
8 Eye
Y Other Radiation

Treatment Site Character 4	Modal. Qualifier Character 5	Isotope Character 6	Qualifier Character 7
Ø Eye	7 Contact Radiation 8 Hyperthermia F Plaque Radiation	Z None	Z None

LC Limited Coverage   **NC** Noncovered   HAC associated procedure   Combination Only   DRG Non-OR   Non-OR   Revised Text in **GREEN**

ICD-10-PCS 2014 (Draft)   **475**

Radiation Therapy

D90–D92

D   **Radiation Therapy**
9   **Ear, Nose, Mouth and Throat**
Ø   **Beam Radiation**

Treatment Site Character 4	Modal. Qualifier Character 5	Isotope Character 6	Qualifier Character 7
Ø Ear 1 Nose 3 Hypopharynx 4 Mouth 5 Tongue 6 Salivary Glands 7 Sinuses 8 Hard Palate 9 Soft Palate B Larynx D Nasopharynx F Oropharynx	Ø Photons <1 MeV 1 Photons 1- 1Ø MeV 2 Photons >1Ø MeV 4 Heavy Particles (Protons, Ions) 5 Neutrons 6 Neutron Capture	Z None	Z None
Ø Ear 1 Nose 3 Hypopharynx 4 Mouth 5 Tongue 6 Salivary Glands 7 Sinuses 8 Hard Palate 9 Soft Palate B Larynx D Nasopharynx F Oropharynx	3 Electrons	Z None	Ø Intraoperative Z None

D   **Radiation Therapy**
9   **Ear, Nose, Mouth and Throat**
1   **Brachytherapy**

Treatment Site Character 4	Modal. Qualifier Character 5	Isotope Character 6	Qualifier Character 7
Ø Ear 1 Nose 3 Hypopharynx 4 Mouth 5 Tongue 6 Salivary Glands 7 Sinuses 8 Hard Palate 9 Soft Palate B Larynx D Nasopharynx F Oropharynx	9 High Dose Rate (HDR) B Low Dose Rate (LDR)	7 Cesium 137 (Cs-137) 8 Iridium 192 (Ir-192) 9 Iodine 125 (I-125) B Palladium 1Ø3 (Pd-1Ø3) C Californium 252 (Cf-252) Y Other Isotope	Z None

D   **Radiation Therapy**
9   **Ear, Nose, Mouth and Throat**
2   **Stereotactic Radiosurgery**

Treatment Site Character 4	Modal. Qualifier Character 5	Isotope Character 6	Qualifier Character 7
Ø Ear 1 Nose 4 Mouth 5 Tongue 6 Salivary Glands 7 Sinuses 8 Hard Palate 9 Soft Palate B Larynx C Pharynx D Nasopharynx	D Stereotactic Other Photon Radiosurgery H Stereotactic Particulate Radiosurgery J Stereotactic Gamma Beam Radiosurgery	Z None	Z None

DRG Non-OR   For all body part, approach, device, and qualifier values

D   Radiation Therapy
9   Ear, Nose, Mouth and Throat
Y   Other Radiation

Treatment Site Character 4	Modal. Qualifier Character 5	Isotope Character 6	Qualifier Character 7
0 Ear **1** Nose **5** Tongue **6** Salivary Glands **7** Sinuses **8** Hard Palate **9** Soft Palate	**7** Contact Radiation **8** Hyperthermia **F** Plaque Radiation	**Z** None	**Z** None
3 Hypopharynx **F** Oropharynx	**7** Contact Radiation **8** Hyperthermia	**Z** None	**Z** None
4 Mouth **B** Larynx **D** Nasopharynx	**7** Contact Radiation **8** Hyperthermia **C** Intraoperative Radiation Therapy (IORT) **F** Plaque Radiation	**Z** None	**Z** None
C Pharynx	**C** Intraoperative Radiation Therapy (IORT) **F** Plaque Radiation	**Z** None	**Z** None

D   Radiation Therapy
B   Respiratory System
0   Beam Radiation

Treatment Site Character 4	Modal. Qualifier Character 5	Isotope Character 6	Qualifier Character 7
0 Trachea **1** Bronchus **2** Lung **5** Pleura **6** Mediastinum **7** Chest Wall **8** Diaphragm	**0** Photons <1 MeV **1** Photons 1- 10 MeV **2** Photons >10 MeV **4** Heavy Particles (Protons, Ions) **5** Neutrons **6** Neutron Capture	**Z** None	**Z** None
0 Trachea **1** Bronchus **2** Lung **5** Pleura **6** Mediastinum **7** Chest Wall **8** Diaphragm	**3** Electrons	**Z** None	**0** Intraoperative **Z** None

D   Radiation Therapy
B   Respiratory System
1   Brachytherapy

Treatment Site Character 4	Modal. Qualifier Character 5	Isotope Character 6	Qualifier Character 7
0 Trachea **1** Bronchus **2** Lung **5** Pleura **6** Mediastinum **7** Chest Wall **8** Diaphragm	**9** High Dose Rate (HDR) **B** Low Dose Rate (LDR)	**7** Cesium 137 (Cs-137) **8** Iridium 192 (Ir-192) **9** Iodine 125 (I-125) **B** Palladium 103 (Pd-103) **C** Californium 252 (Cf-252) **Y** Other Isotope	**Z** None

D   Radiation Therapy
B   Respiratory System
2   Stereotactic Radiosurgery

Treatment Site Character 4	Modal. Qualifier Character 5	Isotope Character 6	Qualifier Character 7
0 Trachea **1** Bronchus **2** Lung **5** Pleura **6** Mediastinum **7** Chest Wall **8** Diaphragm	**D** Stereotactic Other Photon Radiosurgery **H** Stereotactic Particulate Radiosurgery **J** Stereotactic Gamma Beam Radiosurgery	**Z** None	**Z** None

DRG Non-OR   For all body part, approach, device, and qualifier values

LC Limited Coverage   **NC** Noncovered   HAC associated procedure   Combination Only   DRG Non-OR   Non-OR   Revised Text in **GREEN**

ICD-10-PCS 2014 (Draft)

477

D9Y—DB2

Radiation Therapy

D   **Radiation Therapy**
B   **Respiratory System**
Y   **Other Radiation**

Treatment Site Character 4	Modal. Qualifier Character 5	Isotope Character 6	Qualifier Character 7
Ø Trachea 1 Bronchus 2 Lung 5 Pleura 6 Mediastinum 7 Chest Wall 8 Diaphragm	7 Contact Radiation 8 Hyperthermia F Plaque Radiation K Laser Interstitial Thermal Therapy	Z None	Z None

D   **Radiation Therapy**
D   **Gastrointestinal System**
Ø   **Beam Radiation**

Treatment Site Character 4	Modal. Qualifier Character 5	Isotope Character 6	Qualifier Character 7
Ø Esophagus 1 Stomach 2 Duodenum 3 Jejunum 4 Ileum 5 Colon 7 Rectum	Ø Photons <1 MeV 1 Photons 1- 1Ø MeV 2 Photons >1Ø MeV 4 Heavy Particles (Protons, Ions) 5 Neutrons 6 Neutron Capture	Z None	Z None
Ø Esophagus 1 Stomach 2 Duodenum 3 Jejunum 4 Ileum 5 Colon 7 Rectum	3 Electrons	Z None	Ø Intraoperative Z None

D   **Radiation Therapy**
D   **Gastrointestinal System**
1   **Brachytherapy**

Treatment Site Character 4	Modal. Qualifier Character 5	Isotope Character 6	Qualifier Character 7
Ø Esophagus 1 Stomach 2 Duodenum 3 Jejunum 4 Ileum 5 Colon 7 Rectum	9 High Dose Rate (HDR) B Low Dose Rate (LDR)	7 Cesium 137 (Cs-137) 8 Iridium 192 (Ir-192) 9 Iodine 125 (I-125) B Palladium 1Ø3 (Pd-1Ø3) C Californium 252 (Cf-252) Y Other Isotope	Z None

D   **Radiation Therapy**
D   **Gastrointestinal System**
2   **Stereotactic Radiosurgery**

Treatment Site Character 4	Modal. Qualifier Character 5	Isotope Character 6	Qualifier Character 7

Ø   Esophagus
1   Stomach
2   Duodenum
3   Jejunum
4   Ileum
5   Colon
7   Rectum
	D Stereotactic Other Photon
	      Radiosurgery
	H Stereotactic Particulate Radiosurgery
	J Stereotactic Gamma Beam
	      Radiosurgery
		Z None	Z None

DRG Non-OR   For all body part, approach, device, and qualifier values

D   **Radiation therapy**
D   **Gastrointestinal System**
Y   **Other Radiation**

Treatment Site Character 4	Modal. Qualifier Character 5	Isotope Character 6	Qualifier Character 7
Ø Esophagus	**7** Contact Radiation **8** Hyperthermia **F** Plaque Radiation **K** Laser Interstitial Thermal Therapy	**Z** None	**Z** None
1 Stomach **2** Duodenum **3** Jejunum **4** Ileum **5** Colon **7** Rectum	**7** Contact Radiation **8** Hyperthermia **C** Intraoperative Radiation Therapy (IORT) **F** Plaque Radiation **K** Laser Interstitial Thermal Therapy	**Z** None	**Z** None
8 Anus	**C** Intraoperative Radiation Therapy (IORT) **F** Plaque Radiation **K** Laser Interstitial Thermal Therapy	**Z** None	**Z** None

D   **Radiation Therapy**
F   **Hepatobiliary System and Pancreas**
Ø   **Beam Radiation**

Treatment Site Character 4	Modal. Qualifier Character 5	Isotope Character 6	Qualifier Character 7
Ø Liver **1** Gallbladder **2** Bile Ducts **3** Pancreas	**Ø** Photons <1 MeV **1** Photons 1- 10 MeV **2** Photons >10 MeV **4** Heavy Particles (Protons, Ions) **5** Neutrons **6** Neutron Capture	**Z** None	**Z** None
Ø Liver **1** Gallbladder **2** Bile Ducts **3** Pancreas	**3** Electrons	**Z** None	**Ø** Intraoperative **Z** None

D   **Radiation Therapy**
F   **Hepatobiliary System and Pancreas**
1   **Brachytherapy**

Treatment Site Character 4	Modal. Qualifier Character 5	Isotope Character 6	Qualifier Character 7
Ø Liver **1** Gallbladder **2** Bile Ducts **3** Pancreas	**9** High Dose Rate (HDR) **B** Low Dose Rate (LDR)	**7** Cesium 137 (Cs-137) **8** Iridium 192 (Ir-192) **9** Iodine 125 (I-125) **B** Palladium 103 (Pd-103) **C** Californium 252 (Cf-252) **Y** Other Isotope	**Z** None

D   **Radiation Therapy**
F   **Hepatobiliary System and Pancreas**
2   **Stereotactic Radiosurgery**

Treatment Site Character 4	Modal. Qualifier Character 5	Isotope Character 6	Qualifier Character 7
Ø Liver **1** Gallbladder **2** Bile Ducts **3** Pancreas	**D** Stereotactic Other Photon Radiosurgery **H** Stereotactic Particulate Radiosurgery **J** Stereotactic Gamma Beam Radiosurgery	**Z** None	**Z** None

DRG Non-OR   For all body part, approach, device, and qualifier values

D   **Radiation Therapy**
F   **Hepatobiliary System and Pancreas**
Y   **Other Radiation**

Treatment Site Character 4	Modal. Qualifier Character 5	Isotope Character 6	Qualifier Character 7
Ø Liver **1** Gallbladder **2** Bile Ducts **3** Pancreas	**7** Contact Radiation **8** Hyperthermia **C** Intraoperative Radiation Therapy (IORT) **F** Plaque Radiation **K** Laser Interstitial Thermal Therapy	**Z** None	**Z** None

LC Limited Coverage   **NC** Noncovered   HAC associated procedure   Combination Only   DRG Non-OR   Non-OR   Revised Text in **GREEN**

ICD-10-PCS 2014 (Draft)   **479**

Radiation Therapy

D **Radiation Therapy**
G **Endocrine System**
0 **Beam Radiation**

Treatment Site Character 4	Modal. Qualifier Character 5	Isotope Character 6	Qualifier Character 7
0 Pituitary Gland 1 Pineal Body 2 Adrenal Glands 4 Parathyroid Glands 5 Thyroid	0 Photons <1 MeV 1 Photons 1- 10 MeV 2 Photons >10 MeV 5 Neutrons 6 Neutron Capture	Z None	Z None
0 Pituitary Gland 1 Pineal Body 2 Adrenal Glands 4 Parathyroid Glands 5 Thyroid	3 Electrons	Z None	0 Intraoperative Z None

D **Radiation Therapy**
G **Endocrine System**
1 **Brachytherapy**

Treatment Site Character 4	Modal. Qualifier Character 5	Isotope Character 6	Qualifier Character 7
0 Pituitary Gland 1 Pineal Body 2 Adrenal Glands 4 Parathyroid Glands 5 Thyroid	9 High Dose Rate (HDR) B Low Dose Rate (LDR)	7 Cesium 137 (Cs-137) 8 Iridium 192 (Ir-192) 9 Iodine 125 (I-125) B Palladium 103 (Pd-103) C Californium 252 (Cf-252) Y Other Isotope	Z None

D **Radiation Therapy**
G **Endocrine System**
2 **Stereotactic Radiosurgery**

Treatment Site Character 4	Modal. Qualifier Character 5	Isotope Character 6	Qualifier Character 7
0 Pituitary Gland 1 Pineal Body 2 Adrenal Glands 4 Parathyroid Glands 5 Thyroid	D Stereotactic Other Photon Radiosurgery H Stereotactic Particulate Radiosurgery J Stereotactic Gamma Beam Radiosurgery	Z None	Z None

DRG Non-OR For all body part, approach, device, and qualifier values

D **Radiation therapy**
G **Endocrine System**
Y **Other Radiation**

Treatment Site Character 4	Modal. Qualifier Character 5	Isotope Character 6	Qualifier Character 7
0 Pituitary Gland 1 Pineal Body 2 Adrenal Glands 4 Parathyroid Glands 5 Thyroid	7 Contact Radiation 8 Hyperthermia F Plaque Radiation K Laser Interstitial Thermal Therapy	Z None	Z None

D **Radiation Therapy**
H **Skin**
0 **Beam Radiation**

Treatment Site Character 4	Modal. Qualifier Character 5	Isotope Character 6	Qualifier Character 7
2 Skin, Face 3 Skin, Neck 4 Skin, Arm 6 Skin, Chest 7 Skin, Back 8 Skin, Abdomen 9 Skin, Buttock B Skin, Leg	0 Photons <1 MeV 1 Photons 1- 10 MeV 2 Photons >10 MeV 4 Heavy Particles (Protons, Ions) 5 Neutrons 6 Neutron Capture	Z None	Z None
2 Skin, Face 3 Skin, Neck 4 Skin, Arm 6 Skin, Chest 7 Skin, Back 8 Skin, Abdomen 9 Skin, Buttock B Skin, Leg	3 Electrons	Z None	0 Intraoperative Z None

LC Limited Coverage   **NC** Noncovered   HAC associated procedure   Combination Only   DRG Non-OR   Non-OR   Revised Text in **GREEN**

480   ICD-10-PCS 2014 (Draft)

D　Radiation Therapy
H　Skin
Y　Other Radiation

Treatment Site Character 4	Modal. Qualifier Character 5	Isotope Character 6	Qualifier Character 7
2　Skin, Face 3　Skin, Neck 4　Skin, Arm 6　Skin, Chest 7　Skin, Back 8　Skin, Abdomen 9　Skin, Buttock B　Skin, Leg	7　Contact Radiation 8　Hyperthermia F　Plaque Radiation	Z　None	Z　None
5　Skin, Hand C　Skin, Foot	F　Plaque Radiation	Z　None	Z　None

D　Radiation Therapy
M　Breast
Ø　Beam Radiation

Treatment Site Character 4	Modal. Qualifier Character 5	Isotope Character 6	Qualifier Character 7
Ø　Breast, Left 1　Breast, Right	Ø　Photons <1 MeV 1　Photons 1- 1Ø MeV 2　Photons >1Ø MeV 4　Heavy Particles (Protons, Ions) 5　Neutrons 6　Neutron Capture	Z　None	Z　None
Ø　Breast, Left 1　Breast, Right	3　Electrons	Z　None	Ø　Intraoperative Z　None

D　Radiation Therapy
M　Breast
1　Brachytherapy

Treatment Site Character 4	Modal. Qualifier Character 5	Isotope Character 6	Qualifier Character 7
Ø　Breast, Left 1　Breast, Right	9　High Dose Rate (HDR) B　Low Dose Rate (LDR)	7　Cesium 137 (Cs-137) 8　Iridium 192 (Ir-192) 9　Iodine 125 (I-125) B　Palladium 1Ø3 (Pd-1Ø3) C　Californium 252 (Cf-252) Y　Other Isotope	Z　None

D　Radiation Therapy
M　Breast
2　Stereotactic Radiosurgery

Treatment Site Character 4	Modal. Qualifier Character 5	Isotope Character 6	Qualifier Character 7
Ø　Breast, Left 1　Breast, Right	D　Stereotactic Other Photon 　　Radiosurgery H　Stereotactic Particulate Radiosurgery J　Stereotactic Gamma Beam 　　Radiosurgery	Z　None	Z　None

DRG Non-OR　For all body part, approach, device, and qualifier values

D　Radiation Therapy
M　Breast
Y　Other Radiation

Treatment Site Character 4	Modal. Qualifier Character 5	Isotope Character 6	Qualifier Character 7
Ø　Breast, Left 1　Breast, Right	7　Contact Radiation 8　Hyperthermia F　Plaque Radiation K　Laser Interstitial Thermal Therapy	Z　None	Z　None

LC Limited Coverage　　**NC** Noncovered　　HAC associated procedure　　Combination Only　　DRG Non-OR　　Non-OR　　Revised Text in **GREEN**

ICD-10-PCS 2014 (Draft)　　　　　　　　　　　　　　　　　　　　　　　　481

DP0–DT1

D   **Radiation Therapy**
P   **Musculoskeletal System**
0   **Beam Radiation**

Treatment Site Character 4	Modal. Qualifier Character 5	Isotope Character 6	Qualifier Character 7
0 Skull 2 Maxilla 3 Mandible 4 Sternum 5 Rib(s) 6 Humerus 7 Radius/Ulna 8 Pelvic Bones 9 Femur B Tibia/Fibula C Other Bone	0 Photons <1 MeV 1 Photons 1- 10 MeV 2 Photons >10 MeV 4 Heavy Particles (Protons, Ions) 5 Neutrons 6 Neutron Capture	Z None	Z None
0 Skull 2 Maxilla 3 Mandible 4 Sternum 5 Rib(s) 6 Humerus 7 Radius/Ulna 8 Pelvic Bones 9 Femur B Tibia/Fibula C Other Bone	3 Electrons	Z None	0 Intraoperative Z None

D   **Radiation Therapy**
P   **Musculoskeletal System**
Y   **Other Radiation**

Treatment Site Character 4	Modal. Qualifier Character 5	Isotope Character 6	Qualifier Character 7
0 Skull 2 Maxilla 3 Mandible 4 Sternum 5 Rib(s) 6 Humerus 7 Radius/Ulna 8 Pelvic Bones 9 Femur B Tibia/Fibula C Other Bone	7 Contact Radiation 8 Hyperthermia F Plaque Radiation	Z None	Z None

D   **Radiation Therapy**
T   **Urinary System**
0   **Beam Radiation**

Treatment Site Character 4	Modal. Qualifier Character 5	Isotope Character 6	Qualifier Character 7
0 Kidney 1 Ureter 2 Bladder 3 Urethra	0 Photons <1 MeV 1 Photons 1- 10 MeV 2 Photons >10 MeV 4 Heavy Particles (Protons, Ions) 5 Neutrons 6 Neutron Capture	Z None	Z None
0 Kidney 1 Ureter 2 Bladder 3 Urethra	3 Electrons	Z None	0 Intraoperative Z None

D   **Radiation Therapy**
T   **Urinary System**
1   **Brachytherapy**

Treatment Site Character 4	Modal. Qualifier Character 5	Isotope Character 6	Qualifier Character 7
0 Kidney 1 Ureter 2 Bladder 3 Urethra	9 High Dose Rate (HDR) B Low Dose Rate (LDR)	7 Cesium 137 (Cs-137) 8 Iridium 192 (Ir-192) 9 Iodine 125 (I-125) B Palladium 103 (Pd-103) C Californium 252 (Cf-252) Y Other Isotope	Z None

D Radiation Therapy
T Urinary System
2 Stereotactic Radiosurgery

Treatment Site Character 4	Modal. Qualifier Character 5	Isotope Character 6	Qualifier Character 7

Ø Kidney
1 Ureter
2 Bladder
3 Urethra
	D Stereotactic Other Photon
	   Radiosurgery
	H Stereotactic Particulate Radiosurgery
	J Stereotactic Gamma Beam
	   Radiosurgery
		Z None	Z None

DRG Non-OR For all body part, approach, device, and qualifier values

D Radiation Therapy
T Urinary System
Y Other Radiation

Treatment Site Character 4	Modal. Qualifier Character 5	Isotope Character 6	Qualifier Character 7
Ø Kidney 1 Ureter 2 Bladder 3 Urethra	7 Contact Radiation 8 Hyperthermia C Intraoperative Radiation Therapy (IORT) F Plaque Radiation	Z None	Z None

D Radiation Therapy
U Female Reproductive System
Ø Beam Radiation

Treatment Site Character 4		Modal. Qualifier Character 5	Isotope Character 6	Qualifier Character 7
Ø Ovary 1 Cervix 2 Uterus	♀ ♀ ♀	Ø Photons <1 MeV 1 Photons 1- 1Ø MeV 2 Photons >1Ø MeV 4 Heavy Particles (Protons, Ions) 5 Neutrons 6 Neutron Capture	Z None	Z None
Ø Ovary 1 Cervix 2 Uterus	♀ ♀ ♀	3 Electrons	Z None	Ø Intraoperative Z None

D Radiation Therapy
U Female Reproductive System
1 Brachytherapy

Treatment Site Character 4		Modal. Qualifier Character 5	Isotope Character 6	Qualifier Character 7
Ø Ovary 1 Cervix 2 Uterus	♀ ♀ ♀	9 High Dose Rate (HDR) B Low Dose Rate (LDR)	7 Cesium 137 (Cs-137) 8 Iridium 192 (Ir-192) 9 Iodine 125 (I-125) B Palladium 1Ø3 (Pd-1Ø3) C Californium 252 (Cf-252) Y Other Isotope	Z None

D Radiation Therapy
U Female Reproductive System
2 Stereotactic Radiosurgery

Treatment Site Character 4		Modal. Qualifier Character 5	Isotope Character 6	Qualifier Character 7

Ø Ovary
1 Cervix
2 Uterus
	♀
	♀
	♀
		D Stereotactic Other Photon
		   Radiosurgery
		H Stereotactic Particulate Radiosurgery
		J Stereotactic Gamma Beam
		   Radiosurgery
			Z None	Z None

DRG Non-OR For all body part, approach, device, and qualifier values

LC Limited Coverage   **NC** Noncovered   HAC associated procedure   Combination Only   DRG Non-OR   Non-OR   Revised Text in **GREEN**

ICD-10-PCS 2014 (Draft)

483

D   **Radiation Therapy**
U   **Female Reproductive System**
Y   **Other Radiation**

Treatment Site Character 4		Modal. Qualifier Character 5	Isotope Character 6	Qualifier Character 7
0 Ovary	♀	**7** Contact Radiation	**Z** None	**Z** None
1 Cervix	♀	**8** Hyperthermia		
2 Uterus	♀	**C** Intraoperative Radiation Therapy (IORT)		
		F Plaque Radiation		

D   **Radiation Therapy**
V   **Male Reproductive System**
0   **Beam Radiation**

Treatment Site Character 4		Modal. Qualifier Character 5	Isotope Character 6	Qualifier Character 7
0 Prostate	♂	**0** Photons <1 MeV	**Z** None	**Z** None
1 Testis	♂	**1** Photons 1- 10 MeV		
		2 Photons >10 MeV		
		4 Heavy Particles (Protons, Ions)		
		5 Neutrons		
		6 Neutron Capture		
0 Prostate	♂	**3** Electrons	**Z** None	**0** Intraoperative
1 Testis	♂			**Z** None

D   **Radiation Therapy**
V   **Male Reproductive System**
1   **Brachytherapy**

Treatment Site Character 4		Modal. Qualifier Character 5	Isotope Character 6	Qualifier Character 7
0 Prostate	♂	**9** High Dose Rate (HDR)	**7** Cesium 137 (Cs-137)	**Z** None
1 Testis	♂	**B** Low Dose Rate (LDR)	**8** Iridium 192 (Ir-192)	
			9 Iodine 125 (I-125)	
			B Palladium 103 (Pd-103)	
			C Californium 252 (Cf-252)	
			Y Other Isotope	

D   **Radiation Therapy**
V   **Male Reproductive System**
2   **Stereotactic Radiosurgery**

Treatment Site Character 4		Modal. Qualifier Character 5	Isotope Character 6	Qualifier Character 7
0 Prostate	♂	**D** Stereotactic Other Photon Radiosurgery	**Z** None	**Z** None
1 Testis	♂	**H** Stereotactic Particulate Radiosurgery		
		J Stereotactic Gamma Beam Radiosurgery		

DRG Non-OR   For all body part, approach, device, and qualifier values

D   **Radiation Therapy**
V   **Male Reproductive System**
Y   **Other Radiation**

Treatment Site Character 4		Modal. Qualifier Character 5	Isotope Character 6	Qualifier Character 7
0 Prostate	♂	**7** Contact Radiation	**Z** None	**Z** None
		8 Hyperthermia		
		C Intraoperative Radiation Therapy (IORT)		
		F Plaque Radiation		
		K Laser Interstitial Thermal Therapy		
1 Testis	♂	**7** Contact Radiation	**Z** None	**Z** None
		8 Hyperthermia		
		F Plaque Radiation		

LC Limited Coverage   **NC** Noncovered   HAC associated procedure   Combination Only   DRG Non-OR   Non-OR   Revised Text in **GREEN**

484   ICD-10-PCS 2014 (Draft)

D Radiation Therapy
W Anatomical Regions
0 Beam Radiation

Treatment Site Character 4	Modal. Qualifier Character 5	Isotope Character 6	Qualifier Character 7
1 Head and Neck 2 Chest 3 Abdomen 4 Hemibody 5 Whole Body 6 Pelvic Region	0 Photons <1 MeV 1 Photons 1- 10 MeV 2 Photons >10 MeV 4 Heavy Particles (Protons, Ions) 5 Neutrons 6 Neutron Capture	Z None	Z None
1 Head and Neck 2 Chest 3 Abdomen 4 Hemibody 5 Whole Body 6 Pelvic Region	3 Electrons	Z None	0 Intraoperative Z None

D Radiation Therapy
W Anatomical Regions
1 Brachytherapy

Treatment Site Character 4	Modal. Qualifier Character 5	Isotope Character 6	Qualifier Character 7
1 Head and Neck 2 Chest 3 Abdomen 6 Pelvic Region	9 High Dose Rate (HDR) B Low Dose Rate (LDR)	7 Cesium 137 (Cs-137) 8 Iridium 192 (Ir-192) 9 Iodine 125 (I-125) B Palladium 103 (Pd-103) C Californium 252 (Cf-252) Y Other Isotope	Z None

D Radiation Therapy
W Anatomical Regions
2 Stereotactic Radiosurgery

Treatment Site Character 4	Modal. Qualifier Character 5	Isotope Character 6	Qualifier Character 7
1 Head and Neck 2 Chest 3 Abdomen 6 Pelvic Region	D Stereotactic Other Photon Radiosurgery H Stereotactic Particulate Radiosurgery J Stereotactic Gamma Beam Radiosurgery	Z None	Z None

DRG Non-OR For all body part, approach, device, and qualifier values

D Radiation Therapy
W Anatomical Regions
Y Other Radiation

Treatment Site Character 4	Modal. Qualifier Character 5	Isotope Character 6	Qualifier Character 7
1 Head and Neck 2 Chest 3 Abdomen 4 Hemibody 5 Whole Body 6 Pelvic Region	7 Contact Radiation 8 Hyperthermia F Plaque Radiation	Z None	Z None
5 Whole Body	G Isotope Administration	D Iodine 131 (I-131) F Phosphorus 32 (P-32) G Strontium 89 (Sr-89) H Strontium 90 (Sr-90) Y Other Isotope	Z None

DW0—DWY

LC Limited Coverage   **NC** Noncovered   HAC associated procedure   Combination Only   DRG Non-OR   Non-OR   Revised Text in GREEN

ICD-10-PCS 2014 (Draft)   485

Physical Rehabilitation and Diagnostic Audiology F00–F15

F **Physical Rehabilitation and Diagnostic Audiology**
0 **Rehabilitation**
0 **Speech Assessment** Measurement of speech and related functions

Body System/Region Character 4	Type Qualifier Character 5	Equipment Character 6	Qualifier Character 7
3 Neurological System - Whole Body	G Communicative/Cognitive Integration Skills	K Audiovisual M Augmentative / Alternative Communication P Computer Y Other Equipment Z None	Z None
Z None	0 Filtered Speech 3 Staggered Spondaic Word Q Performance Intensity Phonetically Balanced Speech Discrimination R Brief Tone Stimuli S Distorted Speech T Dichotic Stimuli V Temporal Ordering of Stimuli W Masking Patterns	1 Audiometer 2 Sound Field / Booth K Audiovisual Z None	Z None
Z None	1 Speech Threshold 2 Speech/Word Recognition	1 Audiometer 2 Sound Field / Booth 9 Cochlear Implant K Audiovisual Z None	Z None
Z None	4 Sensorineural Acuity Level	1 Audiometer 2 Sound Field / Booth Z None	Z None
Z None	5 Synthetic Sentence Identification	1 Audiometer 2 Sound Field / Booth 9 Cochlear Implant K Audiovisual	Z None
Z None	6 Speech and/or Language Screening 7 Nonspoken Language 8 Receptive/Expressive Language C Aphasia G Communicative/Cognitive Integration Skills L Augmentative/Alternative Communication System	K Audiovisual M Augmentative / Alternative Communication P Computer Y Other Equipment Z None	Z None
Z None	9 Articulation/Phonology	K Audiovisual P Computer Q Speech Analysis Y Other Equipment Z None	Z None
Z None	B Motor Speech	K Audiovisual N Biosensory Feedback P Computer Q Speech Analysis T Aerodynamic Function Y Other Equipment Z None	Z None
Z None	D Fluency	K Audiovisual N Biosensory Feedback P Computer Q Speech Analysis S Voice Analysis T Aerodynamic Function Y Other Equipment Z None	Z None

F00 Continued on next page

DRG Non-OR All body system/region, type qualifier, equipment, and qualifier values

---

F   **Physical Rehabilitation and Diagnostic Audiology**   *F00 Continued*
Ø   **Rehabilitation**
Ø   **Speech Assessment**   Measurement of speech and related functions

Body System/Region Character 4	Type Qualifier Character 5	Equipment Character 6	Qualifier Character 7
Z None	**F** Voice	**K** Audiovisual **N** Biosensory Feedback **P** Computer **S** Voice Analysis **T** Aerodynamic Function **Y** Other Equipment **Z** None	**Z** None
Z None	**H** Bedside Swallowing and Oral Function **P** Oral Peripheral Mechanism	**Y** Other Equipment **Z** None	**Z** None
Z None	**J** Instrumental Swallowing and Oral Function	**T** Aerodynamic Function **W** Swallowing **Y** Other Equipment	**Z** None
Z None	**K** Orofacial Myofunctional	**K** Audiovisual **P** Computer **Y** Other Equipment **Z** None	**Z** None
Z None	**M** Voice Prosthetic	**K** Audiovisual **P** Computer **S** Voice Analysis **V** Speech Prosthesis **Y** Other Equipment **Z** None	**Z** None
Z None	**N** Non-invasive Instrumental Status	**N** Biosensory Feedback **P** Computer **Q** Speech Analysis **S** Voice Analysis **T** Aerodynamic Function **Y** Other Equipment	**Z** None
Z None	**X** Other Specified Central Auditory Processing	**Z** None	**Z** None

DRG Non-OR   All body system/region, type qualifier, equipment, and qualifier values

F   **Physical Rehabilitation and Diagnostic Audiology**
Ø   **Rehabilitation**
1   **Motor and/or Nerve Function Assessment**   Measurement of motor, nerve, and related functions

Body System/Region Character 4	Type Qualifier Character 5	Equipment Character 6	Qualifier Character 7
Ø Neurological System - Head and Neck **1** Neurological System - Upper Back/Upper Extremity **2** Neurological System - Lower Back/Lower Extremity **3** Neurological System - Whole Body	**1** Integumentary Integrity **3** Coordination/Dexterity **4** Motor Function **G** Reflex Integrity	**Z** None	**Z** None
Ø Neurological System - Head and Neck **1** Neurological System - Upper Back/Upper Extremity **2** Neurological System - Lower Back/Lower Extremity **3** Neurological System - Whole Body **D** Integumentary System - Head and Neck **F** Integumentary System - Upper Back/Upper Extremity **G** Integumentary System - Lower Back/Lower Extremity **H** Integumentary System - Whole Body **J** Musculoskeletal System - Head and Neck **K** Musculoskeletal System - Upper Back/ Upper Extremity **L** Musculoskeletal System - Lower Back/ Lower Extremity **M** Musculoskeletal System - Whole Body	**5** Range of Motion and Joint Integrity **6** Sensory Awareness/Processing/Integrity	**Y** Other Equipment **Z** None	**Z** None

F01 Continued on next page

DRG Non-OR   All body system/region, type qualifier, equipment, and qualifier values

---

LC Limited Coverage   **NC** Noncovered   HAC associated procedure   Combination Only   DRG Non-OR   Non-OR   Revised Text in **GREEN**

ICD-10-PCS 2014 (Draft)   **487**

Physical Rehabilitation and Diagnostic Audiology — side tab

F   **Physical Rehabilitation and Diagnostic Audiology**
Ø   **Rehabilitation**
1   **Motor and/or Nerve Function Assessment**   Measurement of motor, nerve, and related functions

F01 Continued

Body System/Region Character 4	Type Qualifier Character 5	Equipment Character 6	Qualifier Character 7
Ø Neurological System - Head and Neck **1** Neurological System - Upper Back/ Upper Extremity **2** Neurological System - Lower Back/ Lower Extremity **3** Neurological System - Whole Body **D** Integumentary System - Head and Neck **F** Integumentary System - Upper Back/ Upper Extremity **G** Integumentary System - Lower Back/ Lower Extremity **H** Integumentary System - Whole Body **J** Musculoskeletal System - Head and Neck **K** Musculoskeletal System - Upper Back/ Upper Extremity **L** Musculoskeletal System - Lower Back/ Lower Extremity **M** Musculoskeletal System - Whole Body **N** Genitourinary System	**Ø** Muscle Performance	**E** Orthosis **F** Assistive, Adaptive, Supportive or Protective **U** Prosthesis **Y** Other Equipment **Z** None	**Z** None
D Integumentary System - Head and Neck **F** Integumentary System - Upper Back/ Upper Extremity **G** Integumentary System - Lower Back/ Lower Extremity **H** Integumentary System - Whole Body **J** Musculoskeletal System - Head and Neck **K** Musculoskeletal System - Upper Back/ Upper Extremity **L** Musculoskeletal System - Lower Back/ Lower Extremity **M** Musculoskeletal System - Whole Body	**1** Integumentary Integrity	**Z** None	**Z** None
Z None	**2** Visual Motor Integration	**K** Audiovisual **M** Augmentative / Alternative Communication **N** Biosensory Feedback **P** Computer **Q** Speech Analysis **S** Voice Analysis **Y** Other Equipment **Z** None	**Z** None
Z None	**7** Facial Nerve Function	**7** Electrophysiologic	**Z** None
Z None	**9** Somatosensory Evoked Potentials	**J** Somatosensory	**Z** None
Z None	**B** Bed Mobility **C** Transfer **F** Wheelchair Mobility	**E** Orthosis **F** Assistive, Adaptive, Supportive or Protective **U** Prosthesis **Z** None	**Z** None
Z None	**D** Gait and/or Balance	**E** Orthosis **F** Assistive, Adaptive, Supportive or Protective **U** Prosthesis **Y** Other Equipment **Z** None	**Z** None

DRG Non-OR All body system/region, type qualifier, equipment, and qualifier values

F   Physical Rehabilitation and Diagnostic Audiology
0   Rehabilitation
2   Activities of Daily Living Assessment   Measurement of functional level for activities of daily living

Body System/Region Character 4	Type Qualifier Character 5	Equipment Character 6	Qualifier Character 7
0 Neurological System - Head and Neck	**9** Cranial Nerve Integrity **D** Neuromotor Development	**Y** Other Equipment **Z** None	**Z** None
1 Neurological System - Upper Back/ Upper Extremity **2** Neurological System - Lower Back/ Lower Extremity **3** Neurological System - Whole Body	**D** Neuromotor Development	**Y** Other Equipment **Z** None	**Z** None
4 Circulatory System - Head and Neck **5** Circulatory System - Upper Back/Upper Extremity **6** Circulatory System - Lower Back/Lower Extremity **7** Circulatory System - Whole Body **8** Respiratory System - Head and Neck **9** Respiratory System - Upper Back/ Upper Extremity **B** Respiratory System - Lower Back/ Lower Extremity **C** Respiratory System - Whole Body	**G** Ventilation, Respiration and Circulation	**C** Mechanical **G** Aerobic Endurance and Conditioning **Y** Other Equipment **Z** None	**Z** None
7 Circulatory System - Whole Body **C** Respiratory System - Whole Body	**7** Aerobic Capacity and Endurance	**E** Orthosis **G** Aerobic Endurance and Conditioning **U** Prosthesis **Y** Other Equipment **Z** None	**Z** None
Z None	**0** Bathing/Showering **1** Dressing **3** Grooming/Personal Hygiene **4** Home Management	**E** Orthosis **F** Assistive, Adaptive, Supportive or Protective **U** Prosthesis **Z** None	**Z** None
Z None	**2** Feeding/Eating **8** Anthropometric Characteristics **F** Pain	**Y** Other Equipment **Z** None	**Z** None
Z None	**5** Perceptual Processing	**K** Audiovisual **M** Augmentative / Alternative Communication **N** Biosensory Feedback **P** Computer **Q** Speech Analysis **S** Voice Analysis **Y** Other Equipment **Z** None	**Z** None
Z None	**6** Psychosocial Skills	**Z** None	**Z** None
Z None	**B** Environmental, Home and Work Barriers **C** Ergonomics and Body Mechanics	**E** Orthosis **F** Assistive, Adaptive, Supportive or Protective **U** Prosthesis **Y** Other Equipment **Z** None	**Z** None
Z None	**H** Vocational Activities and Functional Community or Work Reintegration Skills	**E** Orthosis **F** Assistive, Adaptive, Supportive or Protective **G** Aerobic Endurance and Conditioning **U** Prosthesis **Y** Other Equipment **Z** None	**Z** None

DRG Non-OR   All body system/region, type qualifier, equipment, and qualifier values

F   **Physical Rehabilitation and Diagnostic Audiology**
Ø   **Rehabilitation**
6   **Speech Treatment**   Application of techniques to improve, augment, or compensate for speech and related functional impairment

Body System/Region Character 4	Type Qualifier Character 5	Equipment Character 6	Qualifier Character 7
3 Neurological System - Whole Body	**6** Communicative/Cognitive Integration Skills	**K** Audiovisual **M** Augmentative / Alternative Communication **P** Computer **Y** Other Equipment **Z** None	**Z** None
Z None	**Ø** Nonspoken Language **3** Aphasia **6** Communicative/Cognitive Integration Skills	**K** Audiovisual **M** Augmentative / Alternative Communication **P** Computer **Y** Other Equipment **Z** None	**Z** None
Z None	**1** Speech-Language Pathology and Related Disorders Counseling **2** Speech-Language Pathology and Related Disorders Prevention	**K** Audiovisual **Z** None	**Z** None
Z None	**4** Articulation/Phonology	**K** Audiovisual **P** Computer **Q** Speech Analysis **T** Aerodynamic Function **Y** Other Equipment **Z** None	**Z** None
Z None	**5** Aural Rehabilitation	**K** Audiovisual **L** Assistive Listening **M** Augmentative / Alternative Communication **N** Biosensory Feedback **P** Computer **Q** Speech Analysis **S** Voice Analysis **Y** Other Equipment **Z** None	**Z** None
Z None	**7** Fluency	**4** Electroacoustic Immitance / Acoustic Reflex **K** Audiovisual **N** Biosensory Feedback **Q** Speech Analysis **S** Voice Analysis **T** Aerodynamic Function **Y** Other Equipment **Z** None	**Z** None
Z None	**8** Motor Speech	**K** Audiovisual **N** Biosensory Feedback **P** Computer **Q** Speech Analysis **S** Voice Analysis **T** Aerodynamic Function **Y** Other Equipment **Z** None	**Z** None
Z None	**9** Orofacial Myofunctional	**K** Audiovisual **P** Computer **Y** Other Equipment **Z** None	**Z** None
Z None	**B** Receptive/Expressive Language	**K** Audiovisual **L** Assistive Listening **M** Augmentative / Alternative Communication **P** Computer **Y** Other Equipment **Z** None	**Z** None

F06 Continued on next page

DRG Non-OR   All body system/region, type qualifier, equipment, and qualifier values

LC Limited Coverage   **NC** Noncovered   HAC associated procedure   Combination Only   DRG Non-OR   Non-OR   Revised Text in **GREEN**

490   ICD-10-PCS 2014 (Draft)

F   **Physical Rehabilitation and Diagnostic Audiology**   *F06 Continued*
Ø   **Rehabilitation**
6   **Speech Treatment**   Application of techniques to improve, augment, or compensate for speech and related functional impairment

Body System/Region Character 4	Type Qualifier Character 5	Equipment Character 6	Qualifier Character 7
Z None	**C** Voice	**K** Audiovisual **N** Biosensory Feedback **P** Computer **S** Voice Analysis **T** Aerodynamic Function **V** Speech Prosthesis **Y** Other Equipment **Z** None	**Z** None
Z None	**D** Swallowing Dysfunction	**M** Augmentative / Alternative Communication **T** Aerodynamic Function **V** Speech Prosthesis **Y** Other Equipment **Z** None	**Z** None

DRG Non-OR   All body system/region, type qualifier, equipment, and qualifier values

F   **Physical Rehabilitation and Diagnostic Audiology**
Ø   **Rehabilitation**
7   **Motor Treatment**   Exercise or activities to increase or facilitate motor function

Body System/Region Character 4	Type Qualifier Character 5	Equipment Character 6	Qualifier Character 7
Ø Neurological System - Head and Neck **1** Neurological System - Upper Back/Upper Extremity **2** Neurological System - Lower Back/Lower Extremity **3** Neurological System - Whole Body **4** Circulatory System - Head and Neck **5** Circulatory System - Upper Back/Upper Extremity **6** Circulatory System - Lower Back/Lower Extremity **7** Circulatory System - Whole Body **8** Respiratory System - Head and Neck **9** Respiratory System - Upper Back/Upper Extremity **B** Respiratory System - Lower Back/Lower Extremity **C** Respiratory System - Whole Body **D** Integumentary System - Head and Neck **F** Integumentary System - Upper Back/Upper Extremity **G** Integumentary System - Lower Back/Lower Extremity **H** Integumentary System - Whole Body **J** Musculoskeletal System - Head and Neck **K** Musculoskeletal System - Upper Back/Upper Extremity **L** Musculoskeletal System - Lower Back/Lower Extremity **M** Musculoskeletal System - Whole Body **N** Genitourinary System	**6** Therapeutic Exercise	**B** Physical Agents **C** Mechanical **D** Electrotherapeutic **E** Orthosis **F** Assistive, Adaptive, Supportive or Protective **G** Aerobic Endurance and Conditioning **H** Mechanical or Electromechanical **U** Prosthesis **Y** Other Equipment **Z** None	**Z** None

F07 Continued on next page

DRG Non-OR   All body system/region, type qualifier, equipment, and qualifier values

Physical Rehabilitation and Diagnostic Audiology (side tab)

F07–F07 (side tab)

F   **Physical Rehabilitation and Diagnostic Audiology**
Ø   **Rehabilitation**
7   **Motor Treatment**   Exercise or activities to increase or facilitate motor function

F07 Continued

Body System/Region Character 4	Type Qualifier Character 5	Equipment Character 6	Qualifier Character 7
Ø Neurological System - Head and Neck 1 Neurological System - Upper Back/Upper Extremity 2 Neurological System - Lower Back/Lower Extremity 3 Neurological System - Whole Body D Integumentary System - Head and Neck F Integumentary System - Upper Back/Upper Extremity G Integumentary System - Lower Back/Lower Extremity H Integumentary System - Whole Body J Musculoskeletal System - Head and Neck K Musculoskeletal System - Upper Back/Upper Extremity L Musculoskeletal System - Lower Back/Lower Extremity M Musculoskeletal System - Whole Body	Ø Range of Motion and Joint Mobility 1 Muscle Performance 2 Coordination/Dexterity 3 Motor Function	E Orthosis F Assistive, Adaptive, Supportive or Protective U Prosthesis Y Other Equipment Z None	Z None
Ø Neurological System - Head and Neck 1 Neurological System - Upper Back/Upper Extremity 2 Neurological System - Lower Back/Lower Extremity 3 Neurological System - Whole Body D Integumentary System - Head and Neck F Integumentary System - Upper Back/Upper Extremity G Integumentary System - Lower Back/Lower Extremity H Integumentary System - Whole Body J Musculoskeletal System - Head and Neck K Musculoskeletal System - Upper Back/Upper Extremity L Musculoskeletal System - Lower Back/Lower Extremity M Musculoskeletal System - Whole Body	7 Manual Therapy Techniques	Z None	Z None
N Genitourinary System	1 Muscle Performance	E Orthosis F Assistive, Adaptive, Supportive or Protective U Prosthesis Y Other Equipment Z None	Z None
Z None	4 Wheelchair Mobility	D Electrotherapeutic E Orthosis F Assistive, Adaptive, Supportive or Protective U Prosthesis Y Other Equipment Z None	Z None
Z None	5 Bed Mobility	C Mechanical E Orthosis F Assistive, Adaptive, Supportive or Protective U Prosthesis Y Other Equipment Z None	Z None
Z None	8 Transfer Training	C Mechanical D Electrotherapeutic E Orthosis F Assistive, Adaptive, Supportive or Protective U Prosthesis Y Other Equipment Z None	Z None

DRG Non-OR   All body system/region, type qualifier, equipment, and qualifier values

---

F　Physical Rehabilitation and Diagnostic Audiology
0　Rehabilitation
7　Motor Treatment　　Exercise or activities to increase or facilitate motor function

F07 Continued

Body System/Region Character 4	Type Qualifier Character 5	Equipment Character 6	Qualifier Character 7
Z None	9 Gait Training/Functional Ambulation	C Mechanical D Electrotherapeutic E Orthosis F Assistive, Adaptive, Supportive or Protective G Aerobic Endurance and Conditioning U Prosthesis Y Other Equipment Z None	Z None

DRG Non-OR All body system/region, type qualifier, equipment, and qualifier values

F　Physical Rehabilitation and Diagnostic Audiology
0　Rehabilitation
8　Activities of Daily Living Treatment　　Exercise or activities to facilitate functional competence for activities of daily living

Body System/Region Character 4	Type Qualifier Character 5	Equipment Character 6	Qualifier Character 7
D Integumentary System - Head and Neck F Integumentary System - Upper Back/Upper Extremity G Integumentary System - Lower Back/Lower Extremity H Integumentary System - Whole Body J Musculoskeletal System - Head and Neck K Musculoskeletal System - Upper Back/Upper Extremity L Musculoskeletal System - Lower Back/Lower Extremity M Musculoskeletal System - Whole Body	5 Wound Management	B Physical Agents C Mechanical D Electrotherapeutic E Orthosis F Assistive, Adaptive, Supportive or Protective U Prosthesis Y Other Equipment Z None	Z None
Z None	0 Bathing/Showering Techniques 1 Dressing Techniques 2 Grooming/Personal Hygiene	E Orthosis F Assistive, Adaptive, Supportive or Protective U Prosthesis Y Other Equipment Z None	Z None
Z None	3 Feeding/Eating	C Mechanical D Electrotherapeutic E Orthosis F Assistive, Adaptive, Supportive or Protective U Prosthesis Y Other Equipment Z None	Z None
Z None	4 Home Management	D Electrotherapeutic E Orthosis F Assistive, Adaptive, Supportive or Protective U Prosthesis Y Other Equipment Z None	Z None
Z None	6 Psychosocial Skills	Z None	Z None
Z None	7 Vocational Activities and Functional Community or Work Reintegration Skills	B Physical Agents C Mechanical D Electrotherapeutic E Orthosis F Assistive, Adaptive, Supportive or Protective G Aerobic Endurance and Conditioning U Prosthesis Y Other Equipment Z None	Z None

DRG Non-OR All body system/region, type qualifier, equipment, and qualifier values

LC Limited Coverage　　**NC** Noncovered　　HAC associated procedure　　Combination Only　　DRG Non-OR　　Non-OR　　Revised Text in **GREEN**

ICD-10-PCS 2014 (Draft)　　　　493

Physical Rehabilitation and Diagnostic Audiology

F   **Physical Rehabilitation and Diagnostic Audiology**
0   **Rehabilitation**
9   **Hearing Treatment**   Application of techniques to improve, augment, or compensate for hearing and related functional impairment

Body System/Region Character 4	Type Qualifier Character 5	Equipment Character 6	Qualifier Character 7
Z None	0 Hearing and Related Disorders Counseling 1 Hearing and Related Disorders Prevention	K Audiovisual Z None	Z None
Z None	2 Auditory Processing	K Audiovisual L Assistive Listening P Computer Y Other Equipment Z None	Z None
Z None	3 Cerumen Management	X Cerumen Management Z None	Z None

DRG Non-OR   All body system/region, type qualifier, equipment, and qualifier values

---

F   **Physical Rehabilitation and Diagnostic Audiology**
0   **Rehabilitation**
B   **Cochlear Implant Treatment**   Application of techniques to improve the communication abilities of individuals with cochlear implant

Body System/Region Character 4	Type Qualifier Character 5	Equipment Character 6	Qualifier Character 7
Z None	0 Cochlear Implant Rehabilitation	1 Audiometer 2 Sound Field / Booth 9 Cochlear Implant K Audiovisual P Computer Y Other Equipment	Z None

DRG Non-OR   All body system/region, type qualifier, equipment, and qualifier values

---

F   **Physical Rehabilitation and Diagnostic Audiology**
0   **Rehabilitation**
C   **Vestibular Treatment**   Application of techniques to improve, augment, or compensate for vestibular and related functional impairment

Body System/Region Character 4	Type Qualifier Character 5	Equipment Character 6	Qualifier Character 7
3 Neurological System - Whole Body H Integumentary System - Whole Body M Musculoskeletal System - Whole Body	3 Postural Control	E Orthosis F Assistive, Adaptive, Supportive or Protective U Prosthesis Y Other Equipment Z None	Z None
Z None	0 Vestibular	8 Vestibular / Balance Z None	Z None
Z None	1 Perceptual Processing 2 Visual Motor Integration	K Audiovisual L Assistive Listening N Biosensory Feedback P Computer Q Speech Analysis S Voice Analysis T Aerodynamic Function Y Other Equipment Z None	Z None

DRG Non-OR   All body system/region, type qualifier, equipment, and qualifier values

F   **Physical Rehabilitation and Diagnostic Audiology**
Ø   **Rehabilitation**
D   **Device Fitting**   Fitting of a device designed to facilitate or support achievement of a higher level of function

Body System/Region Character 4	Type Qualifier Character 5	Equipment Character 6	Qualifier Character 7
Z None	Ø Tinnitus Masker	5 Hearing Aid Selection / Fitting / Test Z None	Z None
Z None	1 Monaural Hearing Aid 2 Binaural Hearing Aid 5 Assistive Listening Device	1 Audiometer 2 Sound Field / Booth 5 Hearing Aid Selection / Fitting / Test K Audiovisual L Assistive Listening Z None	Z None
Z None	3 Augmentative/Alternative Communication System	M Augmentative / Alternative Communication	Z None
Z None	4 Voice Prosthetic	S Voice Analysis V Speech Prosthesis	Z None
Z None	6 Dynamic Orthosis 7 Static Orthosis 8 Prosthesis 9 Assistive, Adaptive,Supportive or Protective Devices	E Orthosis F Assistive, Adaptive, Supportive or Protective U Prosthesis Z None	Z None

DRG Non-OR	FØDZØ[5,Ø]Z
DRG Non-OR	FØDZ[1, 2,5][1,2,5, K,L,Z]Z
DRG Non-OR	FØDZ3MZ
DRG Non-OR	FØDZ4[S,V]Z
DRG Non-OR	FØDZ[6,7][E,F,U,Z]Z
DRG Non-OR	FØDZ8[E,F,Z,U]

F   **Physical Rehabilitation and Diagnostic Audiology**
Ø   **Rehabilitation**
F   **Caregiver Training**   Training in activities to support patient's optimal level of function

Body System/Region Character 4	Type Qualifier Character 5	Equipment Character 6	Qualifier Character 7
Z None	Ø Bathing/Showering Technique 1 Dressing 2 Feeding and Eating 3 Grooming/Personal Hygiene 4 Bed Mobility 5 Transfer 6 Wheelchair Mobility 7 Therapeutic Exercise 8 Airway Clearance Techniques 9 Wound Management B Vocational Activities and Functional Community or Work Reintegration Skills C Gait Training/Functional Ambulation D Application, Proper Use and Care of Assistive, Adaptive, Supportive or Protective Devices F Application, Proper Use and Care of Orthoses G Application, Proper Use and Care of Prosthesis H Home Management	E Orthosis F Assistive, Adaptive, Supportive or Protective U Prosthesis Z None	Z None
Z None	J Communication Skills	K Audiovisual L Assistive Listening M Augmentative / Alternative Communication P Computer Z None	Z None

DRG Non-OR	All body system/region, type qualifier, equipment, and qualifier values

LC Limited Coverage   **NC** Noncovered   HAC associated procedure   Combination Only   DRG Non-OR   Non-OR   Revised Text in **GREEN**

ICD-10-PCS 2014 (Draft)   **495**

F   **Physical Rehabilitation and Diagnostic Audiology**
1   **Diagnostic Audiology**
3   **Hearing Assessment**   Measurement of hearing and related functions

Body System/Region Character 4	Type Qualifier Character 5	Equipment Character 6	Qualifier Character 7
Z None	**0** Hearing Screening	**0** Occupational Hearing **1** Audiometer **2** Sound Field / Booth **3** Tympanometer **8** Vestibular / Balance **9** Cochlear Implant **Z** None	**Z** None
Z None	**1** Pure Tone Audiometry, Air **2** Pure Tone Audiometry, Air and Bone	**0** Occupational Hearing **1** Audiometer **2** Sound Field / Booth **Z** None	**Z** None
Z None	**3** Bekesy Audiometry **6** Visual Reinforcement Audiometry **9** Short Increment Sensitivity Index **B** Stenger **C** Pure Tone Stenger	**1** Audiometer **2** Sound Field / Booth **Z** None	**Z** None
Z None	**4** Conditioned Play Audiometry **5** Select Picture Audiometry	**1** Audiometer **2** Sound Field / Booth **K** Audiovisual **Z** None	**Z** None
Z None	**7** Alternate Binaural or Monaural Loudness Balance	**1** Audiometer **K** Audiovisual **Z** None	**Z** None
Z None	**8** Tone Decay **D** Tympanometry **F** Eustachian Tube Function **G** Acoustic Reflex Patterns **H** Acoustic Reflex Threshold **J** Acoustic Reflex Decay	**3** Tympanometer **4** Electroacoustic Immitance / Acoustic Reflex **Z** None	**Z** None
Z None	**K** Electrocochleography **L** Auditory Evoked Potentials	**7** Electrophysiologic **Z** None	**Z** None
Z None	**M** Evoked Otoacoustic Emissions, Screening **N** Evoked Otoacoustic Emissions, Diagnostic	**6** Otoacoustic Emission (OAE) **Z** None	**Z** None
Z None	**P** Aural Rehabilitation Status	**1** Audiometer **2** Sound Field / Booth **4** Electroacoustic Immitance / Acoustic Reflex **9** Cochlear Implant **K** Audiovisual **L** Assistive Listening **P** Computer **Z** None	**Z** None
Z None	**Q** Auditory Processing	**K** Audiovisual **P** Computer **Y** Other Equipment **Z** None	**Z** None

F Physical Rehabilitation and Diagnostic Audiology
1 Diagnostic Audiology
4 Hearing Aid Assessment Measurement of the appropriateness and/or effectiveness of a hearing device

Body System/Region Character 4	Type Qualifier Character 5	Equipment Character 6	Qualifier Character 7
Z None	Ø Cochlear Implant	1 Audiometer 2 Sound Field / Booth 3 Tympanometer 4 Electroacoustic Immitance / Acoustic Reflex 5 Hearing Aid Selection / Fitting / Test 7 Electrophysiologic 9 Cochlear Implant K Audiovisual L Assistive Listening P Computer Y Other Equipment Z None	Z None
Z None	1 Ear Canal Probe Microphone 6 Binaural Electroacoustic Hearing Aid Check 8 Monaural Electroacoustic Hearing Aid Check	5 Hearing Aid Selection / Fitting / Test Z None	Z None
Z None	2 Monaural Hearing Aid 3 Binaural Hearing Aid	1 Audiometer 2 Sound Field / Booth 3 Tympanometer 4 Electroacoustic Immitance / Acoustic Reflex 5 Hearing Aid Selection / Fitting / Test K Audiovisual L Assistive Listening P Computer Z None	Z None
Z None	4 Assistive Listening System/Device Selection	1 Audiometer 2 Sound Field / Booth 3 Tympanometer 4 Electroacoustic Immitance / Acoustic Reflex K Audiovisual L Assistive Listening Z None	Z None
Z None	5 Sensory Aids	1 Audiometer 2 Sound Field / Booth 3 Tympanometer 4 Electroacoustic Immitance / Acoustic Reflex 5 Hearing Aid Selection / Fitting / Test K Audiovisual L Assistive Listening Z None	Z None
Z None	7 Ear Protector Attentuation	Ø Occupational Hearing Z None	Z None

F Physical Rehabilitation and Diagnostic Audiology
1 Diagnostic Audiology
5 Vestibular Assessment Measurement of the vestibular system and related functions

Body System/Region Character 4	Type Qualifier Character 5	Equipment Character 6	Qualifier Character 7
Z None	Ø Bithermal, Binaural Caloric Irrigation 1 Bithermal, Monaural Caloric Irrigation 2 Unithermal Binaural Screen 3 Oscillating Tracking 4 Sinusoidal Vertical Axis Rotational 5 Dix-Hallpike Dynamic 6 Computerized Dynamic Posturography	8 Vestibular / Balance Z None	Z None
Z None	7 Tinnitus Masker	5 Hearing Aid Selection / Fitting / Test Z None	Z None

Mental Health GZ1–GZJ

G   **Mental Health**
Z   **None**
1   **Psychological Tests**   The administration and interpretation of standardized psychological tests and measurement instruments for the assessment of psychological function

Type Qualifier Character 4	Qualifier Character 5	Qualifier Character 6	Qualifier Character 7
Ø Developmental **1** Personality and Behavioral **2** Intellectual and Psychoeducational **3** Neuropsychological **4** Neurobehavioral and Cognitive Status	**Z** None	**Z** None	**Z** None

G   **Mental Health**
Z   **None**
2   **Crisis Intervention**   Treatment of a traumatized, acutely disturbed or distressed individual for the purpose of short-term stabilization

Type Qualifier Character 4	Qualifier Character 5	Qualifier Character 6	Qualifier Character 7
Z None	**Z** None	**Z** None	**Z** None

G   **Mental Health**
Z   **None**
3   **Medication Management**   Monitoring and adjusting the use of medications for the treatment of a mental health disorder

Type Qualifier Character 4	Qualifier Character 5	Qualifier Character 6	Qualifier Character 7
Z None	**Z** None	**Z** None	**Z** None

G   **Mental Health**
Z   **None**
5   **Individual Psychotherapy**   Treatment of an individual with a mental health disorder by behavioral, cognitive, psychoanalytic, psychodynamic or psychophysiological means to improve functioning or well-being

Type Qualifier Character 4	Qualifier Character 5	Qualifier Character 6	Qualifier Character 7
Ø Interactive **1** Behavioral **2** Cognitive **3** Interpersonal **4** Psychoanalysis **5** Psychodynamic **6** Supportive **8** Cognitive-Behavioral **9** Psychophysiological	**Z** None	**Z** None	**Z** None

G   **Mental Health**
Z   **None**
6   **Counseling**   The application of psychological methods to treat an individual with normal developmental issues and psychological problems in order to increase function, improve well-being, alleviate distress, maladjustment or resolve crises

Type Qualifier Character 4	Qualifier Character 5	Qualifier Character 6	Qualifier Character 7
Ø Educational **1** Vocational **3** Other Counseling	**Z** None	**Z** None	**Z** None

G   **Mental Health**
Z   **None**
7   **Family Psychotherapy**   Treatment that includes one or more family members of an individual with a mental health disorder by behavioral, cognitive, psychoanalytic, psychodynamic or psychophysiological means to improve functioning or well-being

Type Qualifier Character 4	Qualifier Character 5	Qualifier Character 6	Qualifier Character 7
2 Other Family Psychotherapy	**Z** None	**Z** None	**Z** None

LC Limited Coverage   **NC** Noncovered   HAC associated procedure   Combination Only   DRG Non-OR   Non-OR   Revised Text in **GREEN**

498   ICD-10-PCS 2014 (Draft)

G **Mental Health**
Z **None**
B **Electroconvulsive Therapy**   The application of controlled electrical voltages to treat a mental health disorder

Type Qualifier Character 4	Qualifier Character 5	Qualifier Character 6	Qualifier Character 7
0 Unilateral-Single Seizure **1** Unilateral-Multiple Seizure **2** Bilateral-Single Seizure **3** Bilateral-Multiple Seizure **4** Other Electroconvulsive Therapy	**Z** None	**Z** None	**Z** None

G **Mental Health**
Z **None**
C **Biofeedback**   Provision of information from the monitoring and regulating of physiological processes in conjunction with cognitive-behavioral techniques to improve patient functioning or well-being

Type Qualifier Character 4	Qualifier Character 5	Qualifier Character 6	Qualifier Character 7
9 Other Biofeedback	**Z** None	**Z** None	**Z** None

G **Mental Health**
Z **None**
F **Hypnosis**   Induction of a state of heightened suggestibility by auditory, visual and tactile techniques to elicit an emotional or behavioral response

Type Qualifier Character 4	Qualifier Character 5	Qualifier Character 6	Qualifier Character 7
Z None	**Z** None	**Z** None	**Z** None

G **Mental Health**
Z **None**
G **Narcosynthesis**   Administration of intravenous barbiturates in order to release suppressed or repressed thoughts

Type Qualifier Character 4	Qualifier Character 5	Qualifier Character 6	Qualifier Character 7
Z None	**Z** None	**Z** None	**Z** None

G **Mental Health**
Z **None**
H **Group Psychotherapy**   Treatment of two or more individuals with a mental health disorder by behavioral, cognitive, psychoanalytic, psychodynamic or psychophysiological means to improve functioning or well-being

Type Qualifier Character 4	Qualifier Character 5	Qualifier Character 6	Qualifier Character 7
Z None	**Z** None	**Z** None	**Z** None

G **Mental Health**
Z **None**
J **Light Therapy**   Application of specialized light treatments to improve functioning or well-being

Type Qualifier Character 4	Qualifier Character 5	Qualifier Character 6	Qualifier Character 7
Z None	**Z** None	**Z** None	**Z** None

LC Limited Coverage   **NC** Noncovered   HAC associated procedure   Combination Only   DRG Non-OR   Non-OR   Revised Text in **GREEN**

ICD-10-PCS 2014 (Draft)   **499**

Substance Abuse Treatment *(side tab)*

HZ2–HZ5 *(side tab)*

Substance Abuse Treatment HZ2–HZ9

H   **Substance Abuse Treatment**
Z   **None**
2   **Detoxification Services**   Detoxification from alcohol and/or drugs

Type Qualifier Character 4	Qualifier Character 5	Qualifier Character 6	Qualifier Character 7
Z None	**Z** None	**Z** None	**Z** None

H   **Substance Abuse Treatment**
Z   **None**
3   **Individual Counseling**   The application of psychological methods to treat an individual with addictive behavior

Type Qualifier Character 4	Qualifier Character 5	Qualifier Character 6	Qualifier Character 7
Ø Cognitive **1** Behavioral **2** Cognitive-Behavioral **3** 12-Step **4** Interpersonal **5** Vocational **6** Psychoeducation **7** Motivational Enhancement **8** Confrontational **9** Continuing Care **B** Spiritual **C** Pre/Post-Test Infectious Disease	**Z** None	**Z** None	**Z** None

H   **Substance Abuse Treatment**
Z   **None**
4   **Group Counseling**   The application of psychological methods to treat two or more individuals with addictive behavior

Type Qualifier Character 4	Qualifier Character 5	Qualifier Character 6	Qualifier Character 7
Ø Cognitive **1** Behavioral **2** Cognitive-Behavioral **3** 12-Step **4** Interpersonal **5** Vocational **6** Psychoeducation **7** Motivational Enhancement **8** Confrontational **9** Continuing Care **B** Spiritual **C** Pre/Post-Test Infectious Disease	**Z** None	**Z** None	**Z** None

H   **Substance Abuse Treatment**
Z   **None**
5   **Individual Psychotherapy**   Treatment of an individual with addictive behavior by behavioral, cognitive, psychoanalytic, psychodynamic or psychophysiological means

Type Qualifier Character 4	Qualifier Character 5	Qualifier Character 6	Qualifier Character 7
Ø Cognitive **1** Behavioral **2** Cognitive-Behavioral **3** 12-Step **4** Interpersonal **5** Interactive **6** Psychoeducation **7** Motivational Enhancement **8** Confrontational **9** Supportive **B** Psychoanalysis **C** Psychodynamic **D** Psychophysiological	**Z** None	**Z** None	**Z** None

DRG Non-OR   For all type qualifier and qualifier values

H **Substance Abuse Treatment**
Z **None**
6 **Family Counseling**   The application of psychological methods that includes one or more family members to treat an individual with addictive behavior

Type Qualifier Character 4	Qualifier Character 5	Qualifier Character 6	Qualifier Character 7
3 Other Family Counseling	Z None	Z None	Z None

DRG Non-OR   For all type qualifier and qualifier values

H **Substance Abuse Treatment**
Z **None**
8 **Medication Management**   Monitoring or adjusting the use of replacement medications for the treatment of addiction

Type Qualifier Character 4	Qualifier Character 5	Qualifier Character 6	Qualifier Character 7
Ø Nicotine Replacement 1 Methadone Maintenance 2 Levo-alpha-acetyl-methadol (LAAM) 3 Antabuse 4 Naltrexone 5 Naloxone 6 Clonidine 7 Bupropion 8 Psychiatric Medication 9 Other Replacement Medication	Z None	Z None	Z None

DRG Non-OR   For all type qualifier and qualifier values

H **Substance Abuse Treatment**
Z **None**
9 **Pharmacotherapy**   The use of replacement medications for the treatment of addiction

Type Qualifier Character 4	Qualifier Character 5	Qualifier Character 6	Qualifier Character 7
Ø Nicotine Replacement 1 Methadone Maintenance 2 Levo-alpha-acetyl-methadol (LAAM) 3 Antabuse 4 Naltrexone 5 Naloxone 6 Clonidine 7 Bupropion 8 Psychiatric Medication 9 Other Replacement Medication	Z None	Z None	Z None

DRG Non-OR   For all type qualifier and qualifier values

Appendix A: Root Operations Definitions

Ø	Medical and Surgical		
Ø	Alteration	Definition:	Modifying the natural anatomic structure of a body part without affecting the function of the body part
		Explanation:	Principal purpose is to improve appearance
		Examples:	Face lift, breast augmentation
1	Bypass	Definition:	Altering the route of passage of the contents of a tubular body part
		Explanation:	Rerouting contents of a body part to a downstream area of the normal route, to a similar route and body part, or to an abnormal route and dissimilar body part. Includes one or more anastomoses, with or without the use of a device
		Examples:	Coronary artery bypass, colostomy formation
2	Change	Definition:	Taking out or off a device from a body part and putting back an identical or similar device in or on the same body part without cutting or puncturing the skin or a mucous membrane
		Explanation:	All CHANGE procedures are coded using the approach EXTERNAL
		Example:	Urinary catheter change, gastrostomy tube change
3	Control	Definition:	Stopping, or attempting to stop, postprocedural bleeding
		Explanation:	The site of the bleeding is coded as an anatomical region and not to a specific body part.
		Examples:	Control of post-prostatectomy hemorrhage, control of post-tonsillectomy hemorrhage
4	Creation	Definition:	Making a new genital structure that does not take over the function of a body part
		Explanation:	Used only for sex change operations
		Examples:	Creation of vagina in a male, creation of penis in a female
5	Destruction	Definition:	Physical eradication of all or a portion of a body part by the direct use of energy, force, or a destructive agent
		Explanation:	None of the body part is physically taken out.
		Examples:	Fulguration of rectal polyp, cautery of skin lesion
6	Detachment	Definition:	Cutting off all or part of the upper or lower extremities
		Explanation:	The body part value is the site of the detachment, with a qualifier if applicable to further specify the level where the extremity was detached
		Examples:	Below knee amputation, disarticulation of shoulder
7	Dilation	Definition:	Expanding an orifice or the lumen of a tubular body part
		Explanation:	The orifice can be a natural orifice or an artificially created orifice. Accomplished by stretching a tubular body part using intraluminal pressure or by cutting part of the orifice or wall of the tubular body part.
		Examples:	Percutaneous transluminal angioplasty, pyloromyotomy
8	Division	Definition:	Cutting into a body part without draining fluids and/or gases from the body part in order to separate or transect a body part
		Explanation:	All or a portion of the body part is separated into two or more portions.
		Examples:	Spinal cordotomy, osteotomy
9	Drainage	Definition:	Taking or letting out fluids and/or gases from a body part
		Explanation:	The qualifier *diagnostic* is used to identify drainage procedures that are biopsies.
		Examples:	Thoracentesis, incision and drainage
B	Excision	Definition:	Cutting out or off, without replacement, a portion of a body part
		Explanation:	The qualifier *diagnostic* is used to identify excision procedures that are biopsies.
		Examples:	Partial nephrectomy, liver biopsy
C	Extirpation	Definition:	Taking or cutting out solid matter from a body part
		Explanation:	The solid matter may be an abnormal byproduct of a biological function or a foreign body; it may be imbedded in a body part or in the lumen of a tubular body part. The solid matter may or may not have been previously broken into pieces.
		Examples:	Thrombectomy, choledocholithotomy, endarterectomy

Continued on next page

Ø	Medical and Surgical		*Continued from previous page*
D	Extraction	Definition:	Pulling or stripping out or off all or a portion of a body part by the use of force
		Explanation:	The qualifier DIAGNOSTIC is used to identify extractions that are biopsies.
		Examples:	Dilation and curettage, vein stripping
F	Fragmentation	Definition:	Breaking solid matter in a body part into pieces
		Explanation:	Physical force (e.g., manual, ultrasonic) applied directly or indirectly through intervening body parts are used to break the solid matter into pieces. The solid matter may be an abnormal byproduct of a biological function or a foreign body. The pieces of solid matter are not taken out, but are eliminated or absorbed through normal biological functions.
		Examples:	Extracorporeal shockwave lithotripsy, transurethral lithotripsy
G	Fusion	Definition:	Joining together portions of an articular body part, rendering the articular body part immobile
		Explanation:	The body part is joined together by fixation device, bone graft, or other means.
		Examples:	Spinal fusion, ankle arthrodesis
H	Insertion	Definition:	Putting in a nonbiological appliance that monitors, assists, performs, or prevents a physiological function but does not physically take the place of a body part
		Explanation:	None
		Examples:	Insertion of radioactive implant, insertion of central venous catheter
J	Inspection	Definition:	Visually and/or manually exploring a body part
		Explanation:	Visual exploration may be performed with or without optical instrumentation. Manual exploration may be performed directly or through intervening body layers.
		Examples:	Diagnostic arthroscopy, exploratory laparotomy
K	Map	Definition:	Locating the route of passage of electrical impulses and/or locating functional areas in a body part
		Explanation:	Applicable only to the cardiac conduction mechanism and the central nervous system
		Examples:	Cardiac mapping, cortical mapping
L	Occlusion	Definition:	Completely closing an orifice or lumen of a tubular body part
		Explanation:	The orifice can be a natural orifice or an artificially created orifice.
		Examples:	Fallopian tube ligation, ligation of inferior vena cava
M	Reattachment	Definition:	Putting back in or on all or a portion of a separated body part to its normal location or other suitable location
		Explanation:	Vascular circulation and nervous pathways may or may not be reestablished.
		Examples:	Reattachment of hand, reattachment of avulsed kidney
N	Release	Definition:	Freeing a body part from an abnormal physical constraint by cutting or by use of force
		Explanation:	Some of the restraining tissue may be taken out but none of the body part is taken out.
		Examples:	Adhesiolysis, carpal tunnel release
P	Removal	Definition:	Taking out or off a device from a body part
		Explanation:	If a device is taken out and a similar device put in without cutting or puncturing the skin or mucous membrane, the procedure is coded to the root operation CHANGE. Otherwise, the procedure for taking out the device is coded to the root operation REMOVAL, and the procedure for putting in the new device is coded to the root operation performed.
		Examples:	Drainage tube removal, cardiac pacemaker removal
Q	Repair	Definition:	Restoring, to the extent possible, a body part to its normal anatomic structure and function
		Explanation:	Used only when the method to accomplish the repair is not one of the other root operations
		Examples:	Colostomy takedown, herniorrhaphy, suture of laceration
R	Replacement	Definition:	Putting in or on a biological or synthetic material that physically takes the place and/or function of all or a portion of a body part
		Explanation:	The body part may have been taken out or replaced, or may be taken out, physically eradicated, or rendered nonfunctional during the REPLACEMENT procedure. A REMOVAL procedure is coded for taking out the device used in a previous replacement procedure
		Examples:	Total hip replacement, free skin graft
S	Reposition	Definition:	Moving to its normal location or other suitable location all or a portion of a body part
		Explanation:	The body part is moved to a new location from an abnormal location, or from a normal location where it is not functioning correctly. The body part may or may not be cut out or off to be moved to the new location.
		Examples:	Reposition of undescended testicle, fracture reduction

Continued on next page

Ø	**Medical and Surgical**		*Continued from previous page*
T	Resection	Definition:	Cutting out or off, without replacement, all of a body part
		Explanation:	None
		Examples:	Total nephrectomy, total lobectomy of lung
V	Restriction	Definition:	Partially closing an orifice or the lumen of a tubular body part
		Explanation:	The orifice can be a natural orifice or an artificially created orifice.
		Examples:	Esophagogastric fundoplication, cervical cerclage
W	Revision	Definition:	Correcting, to the extent possible, a portion of a malfunctioning device or the position of a displaced device
		Explanation:	Revision can include correcting a malfunctioning or displaced device by taking out or putting in components of the device such as a screw or pin.
		Examples:	Adjustment of position of pacemaker lead, recementing of hip prosthesis
U	Supplement	Definition:	Putting in or on biological or synthetic material that physically reinforces and/or augments the function of a portion of a body part
		Explanation:	The biological material is non-living, or is living and from the same individual. The body part may have been previously replaced, and the SUPPLEMENT procedure is performed to physically reinforce and/or augment the function of the replaced body part
		Examples:	Herniorrhaphy using mesh, free nerve graft, mitral valve ring annuloplasty, put a new acetabular liner in a previous hip replacement
X	Transfer	Definition:	Moving, without taking out, all or a portion of a body part to another location to take over the function of all or a portion of a body part
		Explanation:	The body part transferred remains connected to its vascular and nervous supply.
		Examples:	Tendon transfer, skin pedicle flap transfer
Y	Transplantation	Definition:	Putting in or on all or a portion of a living body part taken from another individual or animal to physically take the place and/or function of all or a portion of a similar body part
		Explanation:	The native body part may or may not be taken out, and the transplanted body part may take over all or a portion of its function.
		Examples:	Kidney transplant, heart transplant

Root Operation Definitions for Other Sections

1	**Obstetrics**		
A	Abortion	Definition:	Artificially terminating a pregnancy
		Explanation:	Subdivided according to whether an additional device such as a laminaria or abortifacient is used, or whether the abortion was performed by mechanical means
		Examples:	Transvaginal abortion using vacuum aspiration technique
E	Delivery	Definition:	Assisting the passage of the products of conception from the genital canal
		Explanation:	Applies only to manually-assisted, vaginal delivery
		Examples:	Manually-assisted delivery

2	**Placement**		
Ø	Change	Definition:	Taking out or off a device from a body region and putting back an identical or similar device in or on the same body region without cutting or puncturing the skin or a mucous membrane
		Explanation:	Procedures performed without making an incision or a puncture.
		Examples:	Change of vaginal packing
1	Compression	Definition:	Putting pressure on a body region
		Explanation:	Procedures performed without making an incision or a puncture
		Examples:	Placement of pressure dressing on abdominal wall
2	Dressing	Definition:	Putting material on a body region for protection
		Explanation:	Procedures performed without making an incision or a puncture
		Examples:	Application of sterile dressing to head wound

Continued on next page

2 Placement

Continued from previous page

3	Immobilization	Definition:	Limiting or preventing motion of a body region
		Explanation:	Procedures to fit a device, such as splints and braces, as described in FØDZ6EZ and FØDZ7EZ, apply only to the rehabilitation setting.
		Examples:	Placement of splint on left finger
4	Packing	Definition:	Putting material in a body region or orifice
		Explanation:	Procedures performed without making an incision or a puncture
		Examples:	Placement of nasal packing
5	Removal	Definition:	Taking out or off a device from a body region
		Explanation:	Procedures performed without making an incision or a puncture
		Examples:	Removal of stereotactic head frame
6	Traction	Definition:	Exerting a pulling force on a body region in a distal direction
		Explanation:	Traction in this section includes only the task performed using a mechanical traction apparatus.
		Examples:	Lumbar traction using motorized split-traction table

3 Administration

Ø	Introduction	Definition:	Putting in or on a therapeutic, diagnostic, nutritional, physiological, or prophylactic substance except blood or blood products
		Explanation:	All other substances administered, such as antineoplastic substance
		Examples:	Nerve block injection to median nerve
1	Irrigation	Definition:	Putting in or on a cleansing substance
		Explanation:	Substance given is a cleansing substance or dialysate
		Examples:	Flushing of eye
2	Transfusion	Definition:	Putting in blood or blood products
		Explanation:	Substance given is a blood product or a stem cell substance
		Examples:	Transfusion of cell saver red cells into central venous line

4 Measurement and Monitoring

Ø	Measurement	Definition:	Determining the level of a physiological or physical function at a point in time
		Explanation:	A single temperature reading is considered measurement.
		Examples:	External electrocardiogram(EKG), single reading
1	Monitoring	Definition:	Determining the level of a physiological or physical function repetitively over a period of time
		Explanation:	Temperature taken every half hour for 8 hours is considered monitoring
		Examples:	Urinary pressure monitoring

5 Extracorporeal Assistance and Performance

Ø	Assistance	Definition:	Taking over a portion of a physiological function by extracorporeal means
		Explanation:	Procedures that support a physiological function but do not take complete control of it, such as intra-aortic balloon pump to support cardiac output and hyperbaric oxygen treatment
		Examples:	Hyperbaric oxygenation of wound
1	Performance	Definition:	Completely taking over a physiological function by extracorporeal means
		Explanation:	Procedures in which complete control is exercised over a physiological function, such as total mechanical ventilation, cardiac pacing, and cardiopulmonary bypass
		Examples:	Cardiopulmonary bypass in conjunction with CABG
2	Restoration	Definition:	Returning, or attempting to return, a physiological function to its original state by extracorporeal means
		Explanation:	Only external cardioversion and defibrillation procedures. Failed cardioversion procedures are also included in the definition of restoration, and are coded the same as successful procedures
		Examples:	Attempted cardiac defibrillation, unsuccessful

6   Extracorporeal Therapies

Ø	Atmospheric Control	Definition:	Extracorporeal control of atmospheric pressure and composition
		Explanation:	None
		Examples:	Antigen-free air conditioning, series treatment
1	Decompression	Definition:	Extracorporeal elimination of undissolved gas from body fluids
		Explanation:	A single type of procedure—treatment for decompression sickness (the bends) in a hyperbaric chamber
		Examples:	Hyperbaric decompression treatment, single
2	Electromagnetic Therapy	Definition:	Extracorporeal treatment by electromagnetic rays
		Explanation:	None
		Examples:	TMS (transcranial magnetic stimulation), series treatment
3	Hyperthermia	Definition:	Extracorporeal raising of body temperature
		Explanation:	To treat temperature imbalance, and as an adjunct radiation treatment for cancer. When performed to treat temperature imbalance, the procedure is coded to this section. When performed for cancer treatment, whole-body hyperthermia is classified as a modality qualifier in section D, "Radiation Therapy."
		Examples:	None
4	Hypothermia	Definition:	Extracorporeal lowering of body temperature
		Explanation:	None
		Examples:	Whole body hypothermia treatment for temperature imbalances, series
5	Pheresis	Definition:	Extracorporeal separation of blood products
		Explanation:	Used in medical practice for two main purposes: to treat diseases where too much of a blood component is produced, such as leukemia, or to remove a blood product such as platelets from a donor, for transfusion into a patient who needs them
		Examples:	Therapeutic leukopheresis, single treatment
6	Phototherapy	Definition:	Extracorporeal treatment by light rays
		Explanation:	Phototherapy to the circulatory system means exposing the blood to light rays outside the body, using a machine that recirculates the blood and returns it to the body after phototherapy.
		Examples:	Phototherapy of circulatory system, series treatment
7	Ultrasound Therapy	Definition:	Extracorporeal treatment by ultrasound
		Explanation:	None
		Examples:	Therapeutic ultrasound of peripheral vessels, single treatment
8	Ultraviolet Light Therapy	Definition:	Extracorporeal treatment by ultraviolet light
		Explanation:	None
		Examples:	Ultraviolet light phototherapy, series treatment
9	Shock Wave Therapy	Definition:	Extracorporeal treatment by shockwaves
		Explanation:	None
		Examples:	Shockwave therapy of plantar fascia, single treatment

7   Osteopathic

Ø	Treatment	Definition:	Manual treatment to eliminate or alleviate somatic dysfunction and related disorders
		Explanation:	None
		Examples:	Fascial release of abdomen, osteopathic treatment

8   Other Procedures

Ø	Other Procedures	Definition:	Methodologies that attempt to remediate or cure a disorder or disease
		Explanation:	For nontraditional, whole-body therapies including acupuncture and meditation
		Examples:	Acupuncture

9	Chiropractic		
B	Manipulation	Definition:	Manual procedure that involves a directed thrust to move a joint past the physiological range of motion, without exceeding the anatomical limit
		Explanation:	None
		Examples:	Chiropractic treatment of cervical spine, short lever specific contact

Note: Sections B-H (Imaging through Substance Abuse Treatment) do not include root operations. Character 3 position represents type of procedure, therefore those definitions are not included in this appendix. See appendix D for definitions of the type (character 3) or type qualifiers (character 5) that provide details of the procedures performed.

Appendix B: Comparison of Medical and Surgical Root Operations

Note: the character associated with each operation appears in parentheses after its title.

Procedures That Take Out Some or All of a Body Part

Operation	Action	Target	Clarification	Example
Excision (B)	Cutting out or off	Some of a body part	Without replacing body part	Breast lumpectomy
Resection (T)	Cutting out or off	All of a body part	Without replacing body part	Total nephrectomy
Extraction (D)	Pulling out or off	All or a portion of a body part	Without replacing body part	Suction D&C
Destruction (5)	Eradicating	All or a portion of a body part	Without taking out or replacing body part	Rectal polyp fulguration
Detachment (6)	Cutting out/off	Extremity only, any level	Without replacing extremity	Below knee amputation

Procedures That Put in/Put Back or Move Some/All of a Body Part

Operation	Action	Target	Clarification	Example
Transplantation (Y)	Putting in	All or a portion of a living body part from other individual or animal	Physically takes the place and/or function of all or a portion of a body part	Heart transplant, kidney transplant
Reattachment (M)	Putting back in or on	All or a portion of a separated body part	Put in its normal or other suitable location. The vascular circulation and nervous pathways may or may not be reestablished.	Finger reattachment
Reposition (S)	Moving	All or a portion of a body part	Moving to its normal or other suitable location. Body part may or may not be cut out or off	Reposition undescended testicle
Transfer (X)	Moving to function for a similar body part	All or a portion of a body part	Without taking out body part; assumes function of similar body part and remains connected to its vascular and nervous supply	Tendon transfer, skin transfer flap

Procedures That Take Out or Eliminate Solid Matter, Fluids, or Gases From a Body Part

Operation	Action	Target	Clarification	Example
Drainage (9)	Taking or letting out	Fluids and/or gases from a body part	Without taking out any of the body part. The qualifier DIAGNOSTIC is used to identify drainage procedures that are biopsies.	Incision and drainage
Extirpation (C)	Taking or cutting out	Solid matter in a body part	Without taking out any of the body part. The solid matter may be an abnormal byproduct of a biological function or a foreign body; it may be imbedded in a body part or in the lumen of a tubular body part. The solid matter may or may not have been previously broken into pieces.	Thrombectomy
Fragmentation (F)	Breaking down	Solid matter into pieces within a body part	The physical force (e.g., manual, ultrasonic) is applied directly or indirectly, without taking out any of the body part or any solid matter. The solid matter may be an abnormal byproduct of a biological function or a foreign body. The pieces of solid matter are not taken out.	Lithotripsy

Procedures That Involve Only Examination of Body Parts and Regions

Operation	Action	Target	Clarification	Example
Inspection (J)	Visual and/or manual exploration	Some or all of a body part	Performed with or without optical instrumentation, directly or through body layers	Diagnostic arthroscopy, diagnostic cystoscopy
Map (K)	Locating	Route of passage of electrical impulses or functional areas in a body part	Applicable only to cardiac conduction mechanism and central nervous system	Cardiac mapping

Procedures That Alter the Diameter/Route of a Tubular Body Part

Operation	Action	Target	Clarification	Example
Bypass (1)	Altering the route of passage	Contents of tubular body part	May include use of living tissue, nonliving biological material or synthetic material which does not take the place of the body part. Includes one or more anastomoses, with or without the use of a device.	Gastrojejunal bypass, coronary artery bypass (CABG)
Dilation (7)	Expanding	Orifice or lumen of tubular body part	By application of intraluminal pressure or by cutting the wall of the orifice	Percutaneous transluminal angioplasty
Occlusion (L)	Completely closing	Orifice or lumen of tubular body part	Orifice may be natural or artificially created	Fallopian tube ligation
Restriction (V)	Partially closing	Orifice or lumen of tubular body part	Orifice may be natural or artificially created	Cervical cerclage, gastroesophageal fundoplication

Procedures That Always Involve Devices

Operation	Action	Target	Clarification	Example
Insertion (H)	Putting in non-biological device	Device in or on a body part	Putting in a non-biological device that monitors, performs, assists, or prevents a physical function, does not physically take the place of a body part	Pacemaker insertion, central line insertion
Replacement (R)	Putting in or on	Biological or synthetic material; living tissue taken from same individual	Physically takes the place of all or a portion of a body part. A REMOVAL procedure is assigned for taking out the device used in a previous replacement procedure.	Total hip replacement
Supplement (U)	Putting in or on	Device that reinforces or augments a body part	Biological material is nonliving or living and from the same individual	Herniorrhaphy using mesh
Removal (P)	Taking a device out or off	Device from a body part	If a new device is inserted via an incision or puncture, that procedure is coded separately	Cardiac pacemaker removal, central line removal
Change (2)	Taking a device out or off and putting back an indentical or similar device	Identical or similar device in or on a body part	Without cutting or puncturing skin or mucous membrane; all *change* procedures are coded using the *External* approach	Drainage tube change
Revision (W)	Correcting	Malfunctioning or displaced device in or on a body part	To the extent possible	Hip prosthesis adjustment, revision of pacemaker lead

Procedures Involving Cutting or Separation Only

Operation	Action	Target	Clarification	Example
Division (8)	Cutting into/Separating	A body part	Without taking out any of the body part or draining fluids and/or gases. All or a portion of the body part is separated into two or more portions.	Osteotomy, neurotomy
Release (N)	Freeing, by cutting or by the use of force	A body part	Eliminating abnormal constraint without taking out any of the body part. Some of the restraining tissue may be taken out, but none of the body part is taken out.	Peritoneal adhesiolysis

Procedures That Define Other Repairs

Operation	Action	Target	Clarification	Example
Control (3)	Stopping or attempting to stop	Postprocedural bleeding	Limited to anatomic regions not specific body parts	Control of postprostatectomy bleeding
Repair (Q)	Restoring	A body part to its natural anatomic structure and function	To the extent possible	Hernia repair, suture laceration

Procedures That Define Objectives

Operation	Action	Target	Clarification	Example
Alteration (Ø)	Modifying	Natural anatomical structure of a body part	Without affecting function of body part, performed for cosmetic purposes	Face lift
Creation (4)	Making	New genital structure	Does not physically take the place of a body part, used only for sex change operations	Artificial vagina creation
Fusion (G)	Unification and immobilization	Joint or articular body part	Stabilization of damaged joints by graft and/or fixation	Spinal fusion

Appendix C: Body Part Key

Anatomical Term	PCS Description
Abdominal aortic plexus	Abdominal Sympathetic Nerve
Abdominal esophagus	Esophagus, Lower
Abductor hallucis muscle	Foot Muscle, Right
	Foot Muscle, Left
Accessory cephalic vein	Cephalic Vein, Right
	Cephalic Vein, Left
Accessory obturator nerve	Lumbar Plexus
Accessory phrenic nerve	Phrenic nerve
Accessory spleen	Spleen
Acetabulofemoral joint	Hip Joint, Left
	Hip Joint, Right
Achilles tendon	Lower Leg Tendon, Right
	Lower Leg Tendon, Left
Acromioclavicular ligament	Shoulder Bursa and Ligament, Right
	Shoulder Bursa and Ligament, Left
Acromion (process)	Scapula, Left
	Scapula, Right
Adductor brevis muscle	Upper Leg Muscle, Right
	Upper Leg Muscle, Left
Adductor hallucis muscle	Foot Muscle, Right
	Foot Muscle, Left
Adductor longus muscle	Upper Leg Muscle, Right
	Upper Leg Muscle, Left
Adductor magnus muscle	Upper Leg Muscle, Right
	Upper Leg Muscle, Left
Adenohypophysis	Pituitary Gland
Alar ligament of axis	Head and Neck Bursa and Ligament
Alveolar process of mandible	Mandible, Left
	Mandible, Right
Alveolar process of maxilla	Maxilla, Left
	Maxilla, Right
Anal orifice	Anus
Anatomical snuffbox	Lower Arm and Wrist Tendon, Right
	Lower Arm and Wrist Tendon, Left
Angular artery	Face Artery
Angular vein	Face Vein, Left
	Face Vein, Right
Annular ligament	Elbow Bursa and Ligament, Right
	Elbow Bursa and Ligament, Left
Anorectal junction	Rectum
Ansa cervicalis	Cervical Plexus
Antebrachial fascia	Subcutaneous Tissue and Fascia, Right Lower Arm
	Subcutaneous Tissue and Fascia, Left Lower Arm
Anterior (pectoral) lymph node	Lymphatic, Left Axillary
	Lymphatic, Right Axillary

Anatomical Term	PCS Description
Anterior cerebral artery	Intracranial Artery
Anterior cerebral vein	Intracranial Vein
Anterior choroidal artery	Intracranial Artery
Anterior circumflex humeral artery	Axillary Artery, Right
	Axillary Artery, Left
Anterior communicating artery	Intracranial Artery
Anterior cruciate ligament (ACL)	Knee Bursa and Ligament, Right
	Knee Bursa and Ligament, Left
Anterior crural nerve	Femoral Nerve
Anterior facial vein	Face Vein, Left
	Face Vein, Right
Anterior intercostal artery	Internal Mammary Artery, Right
	Internal Mammary Artery, Left
Anterior interosseous nerve	Median Nerve
Anterior lateral malleolar artery	Anterior Tibial Artery, Right
	Anterior Tibial Artery, Left
Anterior lingual gland	Minor Salivary Gland
Anterior medial malleolar artery	Anterior Tibial Artery, Right
	Anterior Tibial Artery, Left
Anterior spinal artery	Vertebral Artery, Right
	Vertebral Artery, Left
Anterior tibial recurrent artery	Anterior Tibial Artery, Right
	Anterior Tibial Artery, Left
Anterior ulnar recurrent artery	Ulnar Artery, Right
	Ulnar Artery, Left
Anterior vagal trunk	Vagus Nerve
Anterior vertebral muscle	Neck Muscle, Right
	Neck Muscle, Left
Antihelix	External Ear, Right
	External Ear, Left
	External Ear, Bilateral
Antitragus	External Ear, Right
	External Ear, Left
	External Ear, Bilateral
Antrum of Highmore	Maxillary Sinus, Right
	Maxillary Sinus, Left
Aortic annulus	Aortic Valve
Aortic arch	Thoracic Aorta
Aortic intercostal artery	Thoracic Aorta
Apical (subclavicular) lymph node	Lymphatic, Left Axillary
	Lymphatic, Right Axillary
Apneustic center	Pons
Aqueduct of Sylvius	Cerebral Ventricle
Aqueous humour	Anterior Chamber, Right
	Anterior Chamber, Left

Anatomical Term	PCS Description
Arachnoid mater	Cerebral Meninges
	Spinal Meninges
Arcuate artery	Foot Artery, Right
	Foot Artery, Right
Areola	Nipple, Left
	Nipple, Right
Arterial canal (duct)	Pulmonary Artery, Left
Aryepiglottic fold	Larynx
Arytenoid cartilage	Larynx
Arytenoid muscle	Neck Muscle, Right
	Neck Muscle, Left
Ascending aorta	Thoracic Aorta
Ascending palatine artery	Face Artery
Ascending pharyngeal artery	External Carotid Artery, Right
	External Carotid Artery, Left
Atlantoaxial joint	Cervical Vertebral Joint
Atrioventricular node	Conduction Mechanism
Atrium dextrum cordis	Atrium, Right
Atrium pulmonale	Atrium, Left
Auditory tube	Eustachian Tube, Right
	Eustachian Tube, Left
Auerbach's (myenteric) plexus	Abdominal Sympathetic Nerve
Auricle	External Ear, Right
	External Ear, Left
	External Ear, Bilateral
Auricularis muscle	Head Muscle
Axillary fascia	Subcutaneous Tissue and Fascia, Right Upper Arm
	Subcutaneous Tissue and Fascia, Left Upper Arm
Axillary nerve	Brachial Plexus
Bartholin's (greater vestibular) gland	Vestibular Gland
Basal (internal) cerebral vein	Intracranial Vein
Basal nuclei	Basal Ganglia
Basilar artery	Intracranial Artery
Basis pontis	Pons
Biceps brachii muscle	Upper Arm Muscle, Right
	Upper Arm Muscle, Left
Biceps femoris muscle	Upper Leg Muscle, Right
	Upper Leg Muscle, Left
Bicipital aponeurosis	Subcutaneous Tissue and Fascia, Right Lower Arm
	Subcutaneous Tissue and Fascia, Left Lower Arm
Bicuspid valve	Mitral Valve
Body of femur	Femoral Shaft, Right
	Femoral Shaft, Left
Body of fibula	Fibula, Left
	Fibula, Right

Anatomical Term	PCS Description
Bony labyrinth	Inner Ear, Left
	Inner Ear, Right
Bony orbit	Orbit, Left
	Orbit, Right
Bony vestibule	Inner Ear, Left
	Inner Ear, Right
Botallo's duct	Pulmonary Artery, Left
Brachial (lateral) lymph node	Lymphatic, Left Axillary
	Lymphatic, Right Axillary
Brachialis muscle	Upper Arm Muscle, Right
	Upper Arm Muscle, Left
Brachiocephalic artery or trunk	Innominate Artery
	Innominate Artery
Brachiocephalic vein	Innominate Vein, Right
	Innominate Vein, Left
Brachioradialis muscle	Lower Arm and Wrist Muscle, Right
	Lower Arm and Wrist Muscle, Left
Broad ligament	Uterine Supporting Structure
Bronchial artery	Thoracic Aorta
Buccal gland	Buccal Mucosa
Buccinator lymph node	Lymphatic, Head
Buccinator muscle	Facial Muscle
Bulbospongiosus muscle	Perineum Muscle
Bulbourethral (Cowper's) gland	Urethra
Bundle of His	Conduction Mechanism
Bundle of Kent	Conduction Mechanism
Calcaneocuboid ligament	Foot Bursa and Ligament, Right
	Foot Bursa and Ligament, Left
Calcaneocuboid joint	Tarsal Joint, Right
	Tarsal Joint, Left
Calcaneofibular ligament	Ankle Bursa and Ligament, Right
	Ankle Bursa and Ligament, Left
Calcaneus	Tarsal, Left
	Tarsal, Right
Capitate bone	Carpal, Left
	Carpal, Right
Cardia	Esophagogastric Junction
Cardiac plexus	Thoracic Sympathetic Nerve
Cardioesophageal junction	Esophagogastric Junction
Caroticotympanic artery	Internal Carotid Artery, Right
	Internal Carotid Artery, Left
Carotid glomus	Carotid Bodies, Bilateral
	Carotid Body, Right
	Carotid Body, Left
Carotid sinus nerve	Glossopharyngeal Nerve
Carotid sinus	Internal Carotid Artery, Right
	Internal Carotid Artery, Left
Carpometacarpal (CMC) joint	Metacarpocarpal Joint, Right
	Metacarpocarpal Joint, Left

Anatomical Term	PCS Description
Carpometacarpal ligament	Hand Bursa and Ligament, Right
	Hand Bursa and Ligament, Left
Cauda equina	Lumbar Spinal Cord
Cavernous plexus	Head and Neck Sympathetic Nerve
Celiac ganglion	Abdominal Sympathetic Nerve
Celiac (solar) plexus	Abdominal Sympathetic Nerve
Celiac lymph node	Lymphatic, Aortic
Celiac trunk	Celiac Artery
Central axillary lymph node	Lymphatic, Left Axillary
	Lymphatic, Right Axillary
Cerebral aqueduct (Sylvius)	Cerebral Ventricle
Cerebrum	Brain
Cervical esophagus	Esophagus, Upper
Cervical facet joint	Cervical Vertebral Joints, 2 or more
	Cervical Vertebral Joint
Cervical ganglion	Head and Neck Sympathetic Nerve
Cervical intertransverse ligament	Head and Neck Bursa and Ligament
Cervical interspinous ligament	Head and Neck Bursa and Ligament
Cervical ligamentum flavum	Head and Neck Bursa and Ligament
Cervical lymph node	Lymphatic, Left Neck
	Lymphatic, Right Neck
Cervicothoracic facet joint	Cervicothoracic Vertebral Joint
Choana	Nasopharynx
Chondroglossus muscle	Tongue, Palate, Pharynx Muscle
Chorda tympani	Facial Nerve
Choroid plexus	Cerebral Ventricle
Ciliary body	Eye, Left
	Eye, Right
Ciliary ganglion	Head and Neck Sympathetic Nerve
Circle of Willis	Intracranial Artery
Circumflex illiac artery	Femoral Artery, Right
	Femoral Artery, Left
Claustrum	Basal Ganglia
Coccygeal body	Coccygeal Glomus
Coccygeus muscle	Trunk Muscle, Left
Cochlea	Inner Ear, Left
	Inner Ear, Right
Cochlear nerve	Acoustic Nerve
Columella	Nose
Common digital vein	Foot Vein, Left
	Foot Vein, Right
Common facial vein	Face Vein, Left
	Face Vein, Right
Common fibular nerve	Peroneal Nerve
Common hepatic artery	Hepatic Artery
Common iliac (subaortic) lymph node	Lymphatic, Pelvis

Anatomical Term	PCS Description
Common interosseous artery	Ulnar Artery, Right
	Ulnar Artery, Left
Common peroneal nerve	Peroneal Nerve
Condyloid process	Mandible, Left
	Mandible, Right
Conus arteriosus	Ventricle, Right
Conus medullaris	Lumbar Spinal Cord
Coracoacromial ligament	Shoulder Bursa and Ligament, Right
	Shoulder Bursa and Ligament, Left
Coracobrachialis muscle	Upper Arm Muscle, Right
	Upper Arm Muscle, Left
Coracoclavicular ligament	Shoulder Bursa and Ligament, Right
	Shoulder Bursa and Ligament, Left
Coracohumeral ligament	Shoulder Bursa and Ligament, Right
	Shoulder Bursa and Ligament, Left
Coracoid process	Scapula, Left
	Scapula, Right
Corniculate cartilage	Larynx
Corpus callosum	Brain
Corpus cavernosum	Penis
Corpus spongiosum	Penis
Corpus striatum	Basal Ganglia
Corrugator supercilii muscle	Facial Muscle
Costocervical trunk	Subclavian Artery, Right
	Subclavian Artery, Left
Costoclavicular ligament	Shoulder Bursa and Ligament, Right
	Shoulder Bursa and Ligament, Left
Costotransverse joint	Thoracic Vertebral Joints, 8 or more
	Thoracic Vertebral Joints, 2 to 7
	Thoracic Vertebral Joint
Costotransverse ligament	Thorax Bursa and Ligament, Right
	Thorax Bursa and Ligament, Left
Costovertebral joint	Thoracic Vertebral Joints, 8 or more
	Thoracic Vertebral Joints, 2 to 7
	Thoracic Vertebral Joint
Costoxiphoid ligament	Thorax Bursa and Ligament, Right
	Thorax Bursa and Ligament, Left
Cowper's (bulbourethral) gland	Urethra
Cranial dura mater	Dura Mater
Cranial epidural space	Epidural Space
Cranial subarachnoid space	Subarachnoid Space
Cranial subdural space	Subdural Space
Cremaster muscle	Perineum Muscle
Cribriform plate	Ethmoid Bone, Right
	Ethmoid Bone, Left
Cricoid cartilage	Larynx
Cricothyroid artery	Thyroid Artery, Right
	Thyroid Artery, Left

Anatomical Term	PCS Description
Cricothyroid muscle	Neck Muscle, Right
	Neck Muscle, Left
Crural fascia	Subcutaneous Tissue and Fascia, Right Upper Leg
	Subcutaneous Tissue and Fascia, Left Upper Leg
Cubital lymph node	Lymphatic, Left Upper Extremity
	Lymphatic, Right Upper Extremity
Cubital nerve	Ulnar Nerve
Cuboid bone	Tarsal, Left
	Tarsal, Right
Cuboideonavicular joint	Tarsal Joint, Right
	Tarsal Joint, Left
Culmen	Cerebellum
Cuneiform cartilage	Larynx
Cuneonavicular ligament	Foot Bursa and Ligament, Right
	Foot Bursa and Ligament, Left
Cuneonavicular joint	Tarsal Joint, Right
	Tarsal Joint, Left
Cutaneous (transverse) cervical nerve	Cervical Plexus
Deep cervical fascia	Subcutaneous Tissue and Fascia, Anterior Neck
Deep cervical vein	Vertebral Vein, Right
	Vertebral Vein, Left
Deep circumflex iliac artery	External Iliac Artery, Right
	External Iliac Artery, Left
Deep facial vein	Face Vein, Left
	Face Vein, Right
Deep femoral artery	Femoral Artery, Right
	Femoral Artery, Left
Deep femoral (profunda femoris) vein	Femoral Vein, Right
	Femoral Vein, Left
Deep palmar arch	Hand Artery, Right
	Hand Artery, Left
Deep transverse perineal muscle	Perineum Muscle
Deferential artery	Internal Iliac Artery, Right
	Internal Iliac Artery, Left
Deltoid fascia	Subcutaneous Tissue and Fascia, Right Upper Arm
	Subcutaneous Tissue and Fascia, Left Upper Arm
Deltoid ligament	Ankle Bursa and Ligament, Right
	Ankle Bursa and Ligament, Left
Deltoid muscle	Shoulder Muscle, Right
	Shoulder Muscle, Left
Deltopectoral (infraclavicular) lymph node	Lymphatic, Left Upper Extremity
	Lymphatic, Right Upper Extremity
Dentate ligament	Dura Mater
Denticulate ligament	Spinal Meninges
Depressor anguli oris muscle	Facial Muscle

Anatomical Term	PCS Description
Depressor labii inferioris muscle	Facial Muscle
Depressor septi nasi muscle	Facial Muscle
Depressor supercilii muscle	Facial Muscle
Dermis	Skin
Descending genicular artery	Femoral Artery, Right
	Femoral Artery, Left
Diaphragma sellae	Dura Mater
Distal radioulnar joint	Wrist Joint, Right
	Wrist Joint, Left
Dorsal digital nerve	Radial Nerve
Dorsal metacarpal vein	Hand Vein, Left
	Hand Vein, Right
Dorsal metatarsal artery	Foot Artery, Right
	Foot Artery, Left
Dorsal metatarsal vein	Foot Vein, Left
	Foot Vein, Right
Dorsal scapular artery	Subclavian Artery, Right
	Subclavian Artery, Left
Dorsal scapular nerve	Brachial Plexus
Dorsal venous arch	Foot Vein, Left
	Foot Vein, Right
Dorsalis pedis artery	Anterior Tibial Artery, Right
	Anterior Tibial Artery, Left
Duct of Santorini	Pancreatic Duct, Accessory
Duct of Wirsung	Pancreatic Duct
Ductus deferens	Vas Deferens, Right
	Vas Deferens, Left
	Vas Deferens, Bilateral
	Vas Deferens
Duodenal ampulla	Ampulla of Vater
Duodenojejunal flexure	Jejunum
Dural venous sinus	Intracranial Vein
Earlobe	External Ear, Right
	External Ear, Left
	External Ear, Bilateral
Eighth cranial nerve	Acoustic Nerve
Ejaculatory duct	Vas Deferens, Right
	Vas Deferens, Left
	Vas Deferens, Bilateral
	Vas Deferens
Eleventh cranial nerve	Accessory Nerve
Encephalon	Brain
Ependyma	Cerebral Ventricle
Epidermis	Skin
Epiploic foramen	Peritoneum
Epithalamus	Thalamus
Epitroclear lymph node	Lymphatic, Left Upper Extremity
	Lymphatic, Right Upper Extremity

Anatomical Term	PCS Description
Erector spinae muscle	Trunk Muscle, Right
	Trunk Muscle, Left
Esophageal artery	Thoracic Aorta
Esophageal plexus	Thoracic Sympathetic Nerve
Ethmoidal air cell	Ethmoid Sinus, Right
	Ethmoid Sinus, Left
Extensor carpi radialis muscle	Lower Arm and Wrist Muscle, Right
Extensor carpi ulnaris muscle	Lower Arm and Wrist Muscle, Right
Extensor digitorum brevis muscle	Foot Muscle, Right
	Foot Muscle, Left
Extensor digitorum longus muscle	Lower Leg Muscle, Right
	Lower Leg Muscle, Left
Extensor hallucis brevis muscle	Foot Muscle, Right
	Foot Muscle, Left
Extensor hallucis longus muscle	Lower Leg Muscle, Right
	Lower Leg Muscle, Left
External anal sphincter	Anal Sphincter
External auditory meatus	External Auditory Canal, Right
	External Auditory Canal, Left
External maxillary artery	Face Artery
External naris	Nose
External oblique aponeurosis	Subcutaneous Tissue and Fascia, Trunk
External oblique muscle	Abdomen Muscle, Right
	Abdomen Muscle, Left
External popliteal nerve	Peroneal Nerve
External pudendal artery	Femoral Artery, Right
	Femoral Artery, Left
External pudendal vein	Greater Saphenous Vein, Right
	Greater Saphenous Vein, Left
External urethral sphincter	Urethra
Extradural space	Epidural Space
Facial artery	Face Artery
False vocal cord	Larynx
Falx cerebri	Dura Mater
Fascia lata	Subcutaneous Tissue and Fascia, Right Upper Leg
	Subcutaneous Tissue and Fascia, Left Upper Leg
Femoral head	Upper Femur, Right
	Upper Femur, Left
Femoral lymph node	Lymphatic, Left Lower Extremity
	Lymphatic, Right Lower Extremity
Femoropatellar joint	Knee Joint, Right
	Knee Joint, Left
	Knee Joint, Femoral Surface, Right
	Knee Joint, Femoral Surface, Left

Anatomical Term	PCS Description
Femorotibial joint	Knee Joint, Right
	Knee Joint, Left
	Knee Joint, Tibial Surface, Right
	Knee Joint, Tibial Surface, Left
Fibular artery	Peroneal Artery, Right
	Peroneal Artery, Left
Fibularis brevis muscle	Lower Leg Muscle, Right
	Lower Leg Muscle, Left
Fibularis longus muscle	Lower Leg Muscle, Right
	Lower Leg Muscle, Left
Fifth cranial nerve	Trigeminal Nerve
First cranial nerve	Olfactory Nerve
First intercostal nerve	Brachial Plexus
Flexor carpi ulnaris muscle	Lower Arm and Wrist Muscle, Left
	Lower Arm and Wrist Muscle, Right
Flexor digitorum brevis muscle	Foot Muscle, Right
	Foot Muscle, Left
Flexor digitorum longus muscle	Lower Leg Muscle, Right
	Lower Leg Muscle, Left
Flexor hallucis brevis muscle	Foot Muscle, Right
	Foot Muscle, Left
Flexor hallucis longus muscle	Lower Leg Muscle, Right
	Lower Leg Muscle, Left
Flexor pollicis longus muscle	Lower Arm and Wrist Muscle, Right
	Lower Arm and Wrist Muscle, Left
Foramen magnum	Occipital Bone, Right
	Occipital Bone, Left
Foramen of Monro (intraventricular)	Cerebral Ventricle
Foreskin	Prepuce
Fossa of Rosenmuller	Nasopharynx
Fourth cranial nerve	Trochlear Nerve
Fourth ventricle	Cerebral Ventricle
Fovea	Retina, Left
	Retina, Right
Frenulum labii inferioris	Lower Lip
Frenulum labii superioris	Upper Lip
Frenulum linguae	Tongue
Frontal lobe	Cerebral Hemisphere
Frontal vein	Face Vein, Left
	Face Vein, Right
Fundus uteri	Uterus
Galea aponeurotica	Subcutaneous Tissue and Fascia, Scalp
Ganglion impar (ganglion of Walther)	Sacral Sympathetic Nerve
Gasserian ganglion	Trigeminal Nerve
Gastric lymph node	Lymphatic, Aortic
Gastric plexus	Abdominal Sympathetic Nerve
Gastrocnemius muscle	Lower Leg Muscle, Right
	Lower Leg Muscle, Left
Gastrocolic ligament	Greater Omentum
Gastrocolic omentum	Greater Omentum

Anatomical Term	PCS Description
Gastroduodenal artery	Hepatic Artery
Gastroesophageal (GE) junction	Esophagogastric Junction
Gastrohepatic omentum	Lesser Omentum
Gastrophrenic ligament	Greater Omentum
Gastrosplenic ligament	Greater Omentum
Gemellus muscle	Hip Muscle, Right
	Hip Muscle, Left
Geniculate ganglion	Facial Nerve
Geniculate nucleus	Thalamus
Genioglossus muscle	Tongue, Palate, Pharynx Muscle
Genitofemoral nerve	Lumbar Plexus
Glans penis	Prepuce
Glenohumeral joint	Shoulder Joint, Right
	Shoulder Joint, Left
Glenohumeral ligament	Shoulder Bursa and Ligament, Right
	Shoulder Bursa and Ligament, Left
Glenoid fossa (of scapula)	Glenoid Cavity, Right
	Glenoid Cavity, Left
Glenoid ligament (labrum)	Shoulder Bursa and Ligament, Right
	Shoulder Bursa and Ligament, Left
Globus pallidus	Basal Ganglia
Glossoepiglottic fold	Epiglottis
Glottis	Larynx
Gluteal lymph node	Lymphatic, Pelvis
Gluteal vein	Hypogastric Vein, Right
	Hypogastric Vein, Left
Gluteus maximus muscle	Hip Muscle, Right
	Hip Muscle, Left
Gluteus medius muscle	Hip Muscle, Right
	Hip Muscle, Left
Gluteus minimus muscle	Hip Muscle, Right
	Hip Muscle, Left
Gracilis muscle	Upper Leg Muscle, Right
	Upper Leg Muscle, Left
Great auricular nerve	Cervical Plexus
Great cerebral vein	Intracranial Vein
Great saphenous vein	Greater Saphenous Vein, Right
	Greater Saphenous Vein, Left
Greater alar cartilage	Nose
Greater occipital nerve	Cervical Nerve
Greater splanchnic nerve	Thoracic Sympathetic Nerve
Greater superficial petrosal nerve	Facial Nerve
Greater trochanter	Upper Femur, Right
	Upper Femur, Left
Greater tuberosity	Humeral Head, Right
	Humeral Head, Left
Greater vestibular (Bartholin's) gland	Vestibular Gland

Anatomical Term	PCS Description
Greater wing	Sphenoid Bone, Right
	Sphenoid Bone, Left
Hallux	1st Toe, Left
	1st Toe, Right
Hamate bone	Carpal, Left
	Carpal, Right
Head of fibula	Fibula, Left
	Fibula, Right
Helix	External Ear, Right
	External Ear, Left
	External Ear, Bilateral
Hepatic artery proper	Hepatic Artery
Hepatic flexure	Ascending Colon
Hepatic lymph node	Lymphatic, Aortic
Hepatic plexus	Abdominal Sympathetic Nerve
Hepatic portal vein	Portal Vein
Hepatogastric ligament	Lesser Omentum
Hepatopancreatic ampulla	Ampulla of Vater
Humeroradial joint	Elbow Joint, Right
	Elbow Joint, Left
Humeroulnar joint	Elbow Joint, Right
	Elbow Joint, Left
Humerus, distal	Humeral Shaft
Humerus, distal involving joint	Joint, Elbow
Hyoglossus muscle	Tongue, Palate, Pharynx Muscle
Hyoid artery	Thyroid Artery, Right
	Thyroid Artery, Left
Hypogastric artery	Internal Iliac Artery, Right
	Internal Iliac Artery, Left
Hypopharynx	Pharynx
Hypophysis	Pituitary Gland
Hypothenar muscle	Hand Muscle, Right
	Hand Muscle, Left
Ileal artery	Superior Mesenteric Artery
Ileocolic artery	Superior Mesenteric Artery
Ileocolic vein	Colic Vein
Iliac crest	Pelvic Bone, Right
	Pelvic Bone, Left
Iliac fascia	Subcutaneous Tissue and Fascia, Right Upper Leg
	Subcutaneous Tissue and Fascia, Left Upper Leg
Iliac lymph node	Lymphatic, Pelvis
Iliacus muscle	Hip Muscle, Right
	Hip Muscle, Left
Iliofemoral ligament	Hip Bursa and Ligament, Right
	Hip Bursa and Ligament, Left
Iliohypogastric nerve	Lumbar Plexus
Ilioinguinal nerve	Lumbar Plexus

Anatomical Term	PCS Description
Iliolumbar artery	Internal Iliac Artery, Right
	Internal Iliac Artery, Left
Iliolumbar ligament	Trunk Bursa and Ligament, Right
	Trunk Bursa and Ligament, Left
Iliotibial tract (band)	Subcutaneous Tissue and Fascia, Right Upper Leg
	Subcutaneous Tissue and Fascia, Left Upper Leg
Ilium	Pelvic Bone, Right
	Pelvic Bone, Left
Incus	Auditory Ossicle, Right
	Auditory Ossicle, Left
Inferior cardiac nerve	Thoracic Sympathetic Nerve
Inferior cerebellar vein	Intracranial Vein
Inferior cerebral vein	Intracranial Vein
Inferior epigastric artery	External Iliac Artery, Right
	External Iliac Artery, Left
Inferior epigastric lymph node	Lymphatic, Pelvis
Inferior genicular artery	Popliteal Artery, Right
	Popliteal Artery, Left
Inferior gluteal artery	Internal Iliac Artery, Right
	Internal Iliac Artery, Left
Inferior gluteal nerve	Sacral Plexus
Inferior hypogastric plexus	Abdominal Sympathetic Nerve
Inferior labial artery	Face Artery
Inferior longitudinal muscle	Tongue, Palate, Pharynx Muscle
Inferior mesenteric ganglion	Abdominal Sympathetic Nerve
Inferior mesenteric lymph node	Lymphatic, Mesenteric
Inferior mesenteric plexus	Abdominal Sympathetic Nerve
Inferior oblique muscle	Extraocular Muscle, Right
	Extraocular Muscle, Left
Inferior pancreaticoduo-denal artery	Superior Mesenteric Artery
Inferior phrenic artery	Abdominal Aorta
Inferior rectus muscle	Extraocular Muscle, Right
	Extraocular Muscle, Left
Inferior suprarenal artery	Renal Artery, Right
	Renal Artery, Left
Inferior tarsal plate	Lower Eyelid, Right
	Lower Eyelid, Left
Inferior thyroid vein	Innominate Vein, Right
	Innominate Vein, Left
Inferior tibiofibular joint	Ankle Joint, Right
	Ankle Joint, Left
Inferior turbinate	Nasal Turbinate
Inferior ulnar collateral artery	Brachial Artery, Right
	Brachial Artery, Left

Anatomical Term	PCS Description
Inferior vesical artery	Internal Iliac Artery, Right
	Internal Iliac Artery, Left
Infraauricular lymph node	Lymphatic, Head
Infraclavicular (deltopectoral) lymph node	Lymphatic, Left Upper Extremity
	Lymphatic, Right Upper Extremity
Infrahyoid muscle	Neck Muscle, Right
	Neck Muscle, Left
Infraparotid lymph node	Lymphatic, Head
Infraspinatus fascia	Subcutaneous Tissue and Fascia, Right Upper Arm
	Subcutaneous Tissue and Fascia, Left Upper Arm
Infraspinatus muscle	Shoulder Muscle, Right
	Shoulder Muscle, Left
Infundibulopelvic ligament	Uterine Supporting Structure
Inguinal canal	Inguinal Region, Right
	Inguinal Region, Left
	Inguinal Region, Bilateral
Inguinal triangle	Inguinal Region, Right
	Inguinal Region, Left
	Inguinal Region, Bilateral
Interatrial septum	Atrial Septum
Intercarpal joint	Carpal Joint, Right
	Carpal Joint, Left
Intercarpal ligament	Hand Bursa and Ligament, Right
	Hand Bursa and Ligament, Left
Interclavicular ligament	Shoulder Bursa and Ligament, Right
	Shoulder Bursa and Ligament, Left
Intercostal lymph node	Lymphatic, Thorax
Intercostal nerve	Thoracic Nerve
Intercostal muscle	Thorax Muscle, Right
	Thorax Muscle, Left
Intercostobrachial nerve	Thoracic Nerve
Intercuneiform joint	Tarsal Joint, Right
	Tarsal Joint, Left
Intermediate cuneiform bone	Tarsal, Left
	Tarsal, Right
Internal (basal) cerebral vein	Intracranial Vein
Internal anal sphincter	Anal Sphincter
Internal carotid plexus	Head and Neck Sympathetic Nerve
Internal iliac vein	Hypogastric Vein, Right
	Hypogastric Vein, Left
Internal maxillary artery	External Carotid Artery, Right
	External Carotid Artery, Left
Internal naris	Nose
Internal oblique muscle	Abdomen Muscle, Right
	Abdomen Muscle, Left
Internal pudendal artery	Internal Iliac Artery, Left
	Internal Iliac Artery, Right

Anatomical Term	PCS Description
Internal pudendal vein	Hypogastric Vein, Right
	Hypogastric Vein, Left
Internal thoracic artery	Internal Mammary Artery, Right
	Internal Mammary Artery, Left
	Subclavian Artery, Right
	Subclavian Artery, Left
Internal urethral sphincter	Urethra
Interphalangeal (IP) joint	Finger Phalangeal Joint, Right
	Finger Phalangeal Joint, Left
	Toe Phalangeal Joint, Right
	Toe Phalangeal Joint, Left
Interphalangeal ligament	Foot Bursa and Ligament, Right
	Foot Bursa and Ligament, Left
	Hand Bursa and Ligament, Right
	Hand Bursa and Ligament, Left
Interspinalis muscle	Trunk Muscle, Right
	Trunk Muscle, Left
Interspinous ligament	Trunk Bursa and Ligament, Right
	Trunk Bursa and Ligament, Left
Intertransverse ligament	Trunk Bursa and Ligament, Right
	Trunk Bursa and Ligament, Left
Intertransversarius muscle	Trunk Muscle, Right
	Trunk Muscle, Left
Interventricular foramen (Monro)	Cerebral Ventricle
Interventricular septum	Ventricular Septum
Intestinal lymphatic trunk	Cisterna Chyli
Ischiatic nerve	Sciatic Nerve
Ischiocavernosus muscle	Perineum Muscle
Ischiofemoral ligament	Hip Bursa and Ligament, Right
	Hip Bursa and Ligament, Left
Ischium	Pelvic Bone, Right
	Pelvic Bone, Left
Jejunal artery	Superior Mesenteric Artery
Jugular body	Glomus Jugulare
Jugular lymph node	Lymphatic, Left Neck
	Lymphatic, Right Neck
Labia majora	Vulva
Labia minora	Vulva
Labial gland	Upper Lip
	Lower Lip
Lacrimal canaliculus	Lacrimal Duct, Right
	Lacrimal Duct, Left
Lacrimal punctum	Lacrimal Duct, Right
	Lacrimal Duct, Left
Lacrimal sac	Lacrimal Duct, Right
	Lacrimal Duct, Left
Laryngopharynx	Pharynx
Lateral (brachial) lymph node	Lymphatic, Left Axillary
	Lymphatic, Right Axillary

Anatomical Term	PCS Description
Lateral canthus	Upper Eyelid, Right
	Upper Eyelid, Left
Lateral collateral ligament (LCL)	Knee Bursa and Ligament, Right
	Knee Bursa and Ligament, Left
Lateral condyle of femur	Lower Femur, Right
	Lower Femur, Left
Lateral condyle of tibia	Tibia, Left
	Tibia, Right
Lateral cuneiform bone	Tarsal, Left
	Tarsal, Right
Lateral epicondyle of femur	Lower Femur, Right
	Lower Femur, Left
Lateral epicondyle of humerus	Humeral Shaft, Right
	Humeral Shaft, Left
Lateral femoral cutaneous nerve	Lumbar Plexus
Lateral malleolus	Fibula, Left
	Fibula, Right
Lateral meniscus	Knee Joint, Right
	Knee Joint, Left
Lateral nasal cartilage	Nose
Lateral plantar artery	Foot Artery, Right
	Foot Artery, Left
Lateral plantar nerve	Tibial Nerve
Lateral rectus muscle	Extraocular Muscle, Right
	Extraocular Muscle, Left
Lateral sacral artery	Internal Iliac Artery, Right
	Internal Iliac Artery, Left
Lateral sacral vein	Hypogastric Vein, Right
	Hypogastric Vein, Left
Lateral sural cutaneous nerve	Peroneal Nerve
Lateral tarsal artery	Foot Artery, Right
	Foot Artery, Left
Lateral temporo-mandibular ligament	Head and Neck Bursa and Ligament
Lateral thoracic artery	Axillary Artery, Right
	Axillary Artery, Left
Latissimus dorsi muscle	Trunk Muscle, Right
	Trunk Muscle, Left
Least splanchnic nerve	Thoracic Sympathetic Nerve
Left ascending lumbar vein	Hemiazygos Vein
Left atrioventricular valve	Mitral Valve
Left auricular appendix	Atrium, Left
Left colic vein	Colic Vein
Left coronary sulcus	Heart, Left
Left gastric artery	Gastric Artery
Left gastroepiploic artery	Splenic Artery
Left gastroepiploic vein	Splenic Vein
Left inferior phrenic vein	Renal Vein, Left

Anatomical Term	PCS Description
Left inferior pulmonary vein	Pulmonary Vein, Left
Left jugular trunk	Thoracic Duct
Left lateral ventricle	Cerebral Ventricle
Left ovarian vein	Renal Vein, Left
Left second lumbar vein	Renal Vein, Left
Left subclavian trunk	Thoracic Duct
Left subcostal vein	Hemiazygos Vein
Left superior pulmonary vein	Pulmonary Vein, Left
Left suprarenal vein	Renal Vein, Left
Left testicular vein	Renal Vein, Left
Leptomeninges	Cerebral Meninges
	Spinal Meninges
Lesser alar cartilage	Nose
Lesser occipital nerve	Cervical Plexus
Lesser splanchnic nerve	Thoracic Sympathetic Nerve
Lesser trochanter	Upper Femur, Right
	Upper Femur, Left
Lesser tuberosity	Humeral Head, Right
	Humeral Head, Left
Lesser wing	Sphenoid Bone, Right
	Sphenoid Bone, Left
Levator anguli oris muscle	Facial Muscle
Levator ani muscle	Trunk Muscle, Left
Levator labii superioris alaeque nasi muscle	Facial Muscle
Levator labii superioris muscle	Facial Muscle
Levator palpebrae superioris muscle	Upper Eyelid, Right
	Upper Eyelid, Left
Levator scapulae muscle	Neck Muscle, Right
	Neck Muscle, Left
Levator veli palatini muscle	Tongue, Palate, Pharynx Muscle
Levatores costarum muscle	Thorax Muscle, Right
	Thorax Muscle, Left
Ligament of head of fibula	Knee Bursa and Ligament, Right
	Knee Bursa and Ligament, Left
Ligament of the lateral malleolus	Ankle Bursa and Ligament, Right
	Ankle Bursa and Ligament, Left
Ligamentum flavum	Trunk Bursa and Ligament, Right
	Trunk Bursa and Ligament, Left
Lingual artery	External Carotid Artery, Right
	External Carotid Artery, Left
Lingual tonsil	Tongue
Locus ceruleus	Pons
Long thoracic nerve	Brachial Plexus
Lumbar artery	Abdominal Aorta
Lumbar facet joint	Lumbar Vertebral Joints, 2 or more
	Lumbar Vertebral Joint

Anatomical Term	PCS Description
Lumbar ganglion	Lumbar Sympathetic Nerve
Lumbar lymph node	Lymphatic, Aortic
Lumbar lymphatic trunk	Cisterna Chyli
Lumbar splanchnic nerve	Lumbar Sympathetic Nerve
Lumbosacral facet joint	Lumbosacral Joint
Lumbosacral trunk	Lumbar Nerve
Lunate bone	Carpal, Left
	Carpal, Right
Lunotriquetral ligament	Hand Bursa and Ligament, Right
	Hand Bursa and Ligament, Left
Macula	Retina, Left
	Retina, Right
Malleus	Auditory Ossicle, Right
	Auditory Ossicle, Left
Mammary duct	Breast, Bilateral
	Breast, Left
	Breast, Right
Mammary gland	Breast, Bilateral
	Breast, Left
	Breast, Right
Mammillary body	Hypothalamus
Mandibular nerve	Trigeminal Nerve
Mandibular notch	Mandible, Left
	Mandible, Right
Manubrium	Sternum
Masseter muscle	Head Muscle
Masseteric fascia	Subcutaneous Tissue and Fascia, Face
Mastoid (postauricular) lymph node	Lymphatic, Left Neck
	Lymphatic, Right Neck
Mastoid air cells	Mastoid Sinus, Right
	Mastoid Sinus, Left
Mastoid process	Temporal Bone, Right
	Temporal Bone, Left
Maxillary artery	External Carotid Artery, Right
	External Carotid Artery, Left
Maxillary nerve	Trigeminal Nerve
Medial canthus	Lower Eyelid, Right
	Lower Eyelid, Left
Medial collateral ligament (MCL)	Knee Bursa and Ligament, Right
	Knee Bursa and Ligament, Left
Medial condyle of femur	Lower Femur, Right
	Lower Femur, Left
Medial condyle of tibia	Tibia, Left
	Tibia, Right
Medial cuneiform bone	Tarsal, Left
	Tarsal, Right
Medial epicondyle of femur	Lower Femur, Right
	Lower Femur, Left
Medial epicondyle of humerus	Humeral Shaft, Right
	Humeral Shaft, Left

Anatomical Term	PCS Description
Medial malleolus	Tibia, Left
	Tibia, Right
Medial meniscus	Knee Joint, Right
	Knee Joint, Left
Medial plantar artery	Foot Artery, Right
	Foot Artery, Left
Medial plantar nerve	Tibial Nerve
Medial popliteal nerve	Tibial Nerve
Medial rectus muscle	Extraocular Muscle, Right
	Extraocular Muscle, Left
Medial sural cutaneous nerve	Tibial Nerve
Median antebrachial vein	Basilic Vein, Right
	Basilic Vein, Left
Median cubital vein	Basilic Vein, Right
	Basilic Vein, Left
Median sacral artery	Abdominal Aorta
Mediastinal lymph node	Lymphatic, Thorax
Meissner's (submucous) plexus	Abdominal Sympathetic Nerve
Membranous urethra	Urethra
Mental foramen	Mandible, Left
	Mandible, Right
Mentalis muscle	Facial Muscle
Mesoappendix	Mesentery
Mesocolon	Mesentery
Metacarpal ligament	Hand Bursa and Ligament, Right
	Hand Bursa and Ligament, Left
Metacarpophalangeal ligament	Hand Bursa and Ligament, Right
	Hand Bursa and Ligament, Left
Metatarsal ligament	Foot Bursa and Ligament, Right
	Foot Bursa and Ligament, Left
Metatarsophalangeal ligament	Foot Bursa and Ligament, Right
	Foot Bursa and Ligament, Left
Metatarsophalangeal (MTP) joint	Metatarsal-Phalangeal Joint, Right
	Metatarsal-Phalangeal Joint, Left
Metathalamus	Thalamus
Midcarpal joint	Carpal Joint, Right
	Carpal Joint, Left
Middle cardiac nerve	Thoracic Sympathetic Nerve
Middle cerebral artery	Intracranial Artery
Middle cerebral vein	Intracranial Vein
Middle colic vein	Colic Vein
Middle genicular artery	Popliteal Artery, Right
	Popliteal Artery, Left
Middle hemorrhoidal vein	Hypogastric Vein, Right
	Hypogastric Vein, Left
Middle rectal artery	Internal Iliac Artery, Right
	Internal Iliac Artery, Left
Middle suprarenal artery	Abdominal Aorta
Middle temporal artery	Temporal Artery, Right
	Temporal Artery, Left

Anatomical Term	PCS Description
Middle turbinate	Nasal Turbinate
Mitral annulus	Mitral Valve
Molar gland	Buccal Mucosa
Musculocutaneous nerve	Brachial Plexus
Musculophrenic artery	Internal Mammary Artery, Right
	Internal Mammary Artery, Left
Musculospiral nerve	Radial Nerve
Myelencephalon	Medulla Oblongata
Myenteric (Auerbach's) plexus	Abdominal Sympathetic Nerve
Myometrium	Uterus
Nail bed	Finger Nail
	Toe Nail
Nail plate	Finger Nail
	Toe Nail
Nasal cavity	Nose
Nasal concha	Nasal Turbinate
Nasalis muscle	Facial Muscle
Nasolacrimal duct	Lacrimal Duct, Right
	Lacrimal Duct, Left
Navicular bone	Tarsal, Left
	Tarsal, Right
Neck of femur	Upper Femur, Right
	Upper Femur, Left
Neck of humerus (anatomical) (surgical)	Humeral Head, Right
	Humeral Head, Left
Nerve to the stapedius	Facial Nerve
Neurohypophysis	Pituitary Gland
Ninth cranial nerve	Glossopharyngeal Nerve
Nostril	Nose
Obturator artery	Internal Iliac Artery, Right
	Internal Iliac Artery, Left
Obturator lymph node	Lymphatic, Pelvis
Obturator muscle	Hip Muscle, Right
	Hip Muscle, Left
Obturator nerve	Lumbar Plexus
Obturator vein	Hypogastric Vein, Right
	Hypogastric Vein, Left
Obtuse margin	Heart, Left
Occipital artery	External Carotid Artery, Right
	External Carotid Artery, Left
Occipital lobe	Cerebral Hemisphere
Occipital lymph node	Lymphatic, Left Neck
	Lymphatic, Right Neck
Occipitofrontalis muscle	Facial Muscle
Olecranon bursa	Elbow Bursa and Ligament, Right
	Elbow Bursa and Ligament, Left
Olecranon process	Ulna, Left
	Ulna, Right
Olfactory bulb	Olfactory Nerve

Anatomical Term	PCS Description
Ophthalmic artery	Internal Carotid Artery, Right
	Internal Carotid Artery, Left
Ophthalmic nerve	Trigeminal Nerve
Ophthalmic vein	Intracranial Vein
Optic chiasma	Optic Nerve
Optic disc	Retina, Left
	Retina, Right
Optic foramen	Sphenoid Bone, Right
	Sphenoid Bone, Left
Orbicularis oculi muscle	Upper Eyelid, Right
	Upper Eyelid, Left
Orbicularis oris muscle	Facial Muscle
Orbital fascia	Subcutaneous Tissue and Fascia, Face
Orbital portion of ethmoid bone	Orbit, Left
	Orbit, Right
Orbital portion of frontal bone	Orbit, Left
	Orbit, Right
Orbital portion of lacrimal bone	Orbit, Left
	Orbit, Right
Orbital portion of maxilla	Orbit, Left
	Orbit, Right
Orbital portion of palatine bone	Orbit, Left
	Orbit, Right
Orbital portion of sphenoid bone	Orbit, Left
	Orbit, Right
Orbital portion of zygomatic bone	Orbit, Left
	Orbit, Right
Oropharynx	Pharynx
Ossicular chain	Auditory Ossicle, Right
	Auditory Ossicle, Left
Otic ganglion	Head and Neck Sympathetic Nerve
Oval window	Middle Ear, Left
	Middle Ear, Right
Ovarian artery	Abdominal Aorta
Ovarian ligament	Uterine Supporting Structure
Oviduct	Fallopian Tube, Right
	Fallopian Tube, Left
Palatine gland	Buccal Mucosa
Palatine tonsil	Tonsils
Palatine uvula	Uvula
Palatoglossal muscle	Tongue, Palate, Pharynx Muscle
Palatopharyngeal muscle	Tongue, Palate, Pharynx Muscle
Palmar (volar) metacarpal vein	Hand Vein, Right
	Hand Vein, Left
Palmar (volar) digital vein	Hand Vein, Left
	Hand Vein, Right
Palmar cutaneous nerve	Median Nerve
	Radial Nerve
Palmar fascia (aponeurosis)	Subcutaneous Tissue and Fascia, Right Hand
	Subcutaneous Tissue and Fascia, Left Hand

Anatomical Term	PCS Description
Palmar interosseous muscle	Hand Muscle, Right
	Hand Muscle, Left
Palmar ulnocarpal ligament	Wrist Bursa and Ligament, Right
	Wrist Bursa and Ligament, Left
Palmaris longus muscle	Lower Arm and Wrist Muscle, Right
	Lower Arm and Wrist Muscle, Left
Pancreatic artery	Splenic Artery
Pancreatic plexus	Abdominal Sympathetic Nerve
Pancreatic vein	Splenic Vein
Pancreaticos-plenic lymph node	Lymphatic, Aortic
Paraaortic lymph node	Lymphatic, Aortic
Pararectal lymph node	Lymphatic, Mesenteric
Parasternal lymph node	Lymphatic, Thorax
Paratracheal lymph node	Lymphatic, Thorax
Paraurethral (Skene's) gland	Vestibular Gland
Parietal lobe	Cerebral Hemisphere
Parotid lymph node	Lymphatic, Head
Parotid plexus	Facial Nerve
Pars flaccida	Tympanic Membrane, Right
	Tympanic Membrane, Left
Patellar ligament	Knee Bursa and Ligament, Right
	Knee Bursa and Ligament, Left
Patellar tendon	Knee Tendon, Right
	Knee Tendon, Left
Patellofemoral joint	Knee Joint, Right
	Knee Joint, Left
	Knee Joint, Femoral Surface, Right
	Knee Joint, Femoral Surface, Left
Pectineus muscle	Upper Leg Muscle, Right
	Upper Leg Muscle, Left
Pectoral (anterior) lymph node	Lymphatic, Left Axillary
	Lymphatic, Right Axillary
Pectoral fascia	Subcutaneous Tissue and Fascia, Chest
Pectoralis major muscle	Thorax Muscle, Left
	Thorax Muscle, Right
Pectoralis minor muscle	Thorax Muscle, Left
	Thorax Muscle, Right
Pelvic fascia	Subcutaneous Tissue and Fascia, Trunk
Pelvic splanchnic nerve	Abdominal Sympathetic Nerve
	Sacral Sympathetic Nerve
Penile urethra	Urethra
Pericardiophrenic artery	Internal Mammary Artery, Right
	Internal Mammary Artery, Left
Perimetrium	Uterus
Peroneus brevis muscle	Lower Leg Muscle, Right
	Lower Leg Muscle, Left
Peroneus longus muscle	Lower Leg Muscle, Right
	Lower Leg Muscle, Left
Petrous part of temporal bone	Temporal Bone, Right
	Temporal Bone, Left

Anatomical Term	PCS Description
Pharyngeal constrictor muscle	Tongue, Palate, Pharynx Muscle
Pharyngeal plexus	Vagus Nerve
Pharyngeal recess	Nasopharynx
Pharyngeal tonsil	Adenoids
Pharyngotym-panic tube	Eustachian Tube, Right
	Eustachian Tube, Left
Pia mater	Cerebral Meninges
	Spinal Meninges
Pinna	External Ear, Right
	External Ear, Left
	External Ear, Bilateral
Piriform recess (sinus)	Pharynx
Piriformis muscle	Hip Muscle, Right
	Hip Muscle, Left
Pisiform bone	Carpal, Left
	Carpal, Right
Pisohamate ligament	Hand Bursa and Ligament, Right
	Hand Bursa and Ligament, Left
Pisometacarpal ligament	Hand Bursa and Ligament, Right
	Hand Bursa and Ligament, Left
Plantar digital vein	Foot Vein, Left
	Foot Vein, Right
Plantar fascia (aponeurosis)	Subcutaneous Tissue and Fascia, Right Foot
	Subcutaneous Tissue and Fascia, Left Foot
Plantar metatarsal vein	Foot Vein, Left
	Foot Vein, Right
Plantar venous arch	Foot Vein, Left
	Foot Vein, Right
Platysma muscle	Neck Muscle, Right
	Neck Muscle, Left
Plica semilunaris	Conjunctiva, Right
	Conjunctiva, Left
Pneumogastric nerve	Vagus Nerve
Pneumotaxic center	Pons
Pontine tegmentum	Pons
Popliteal lymph node	Lymphatic, Left Lower Extremity
	Lymphatic, Right Lower Extremity
Popliteal ligament	Knee Bursa and Ligament, Right
	Knee Bursa and Ligament, Left
Popliteal vein	Femoral Vein, Right
	Femoral Vein, Left
Popliteus muscle	Lower Leg Muscle, Right
	Lower Leg Muscle, Left
Postauricular (mastoid) lymph node	Lymphatic, Left Neck
	Lymphatic, Right Neck
Postcava	Inferior Vena Cava
Posterior (subscapular) lymph node	Lymphatic, Left Axillary
	Lymphatic, Right Axillary

Anatomical Term	PCS Description
Posterior auricular artery	External Carotid Artery, Right
	External Carotid Artery, Left
Posterior auricular nerve	Facial Nerve
Posterior auricular vein	External Jugular Vein, Right
	External Jugular Vein, Left
Posterior cerebral artery	Intracranial Artery
Posterior chamber	Eye, Left
	Eye, Right
Posterior circumflex humeral artery	Axillary Artery, Right
	Axillary Artery, Left
Posterior communicating artery	Intracranial Artery
Posterior cruciate ligament (PCL)	Knee Bursa and Ligament, Right
	Knee Bursa and Ligament, Left
Posterior facial (retromandibular) vein	Face Vein, Left
	Face Vein, Right
Posterior femoral cutaneous nerve	Sacral Plexus
Posterior inferior cerebellar artery (PICA)	Intracranial Artery
Posterior interosseous nerve	Radial Nerve
Posterior labial nerve	Pudendal Nerve
Posterior scrotal nerve	Pudendal Nerve
Posterior spinal artery	Vertebral Artery, Right
	Vertebral Artery, Left
Posterior tibial recurrent artery	Anterior Tibial Artery, Right
	Anterior Tibial Artery, Left
Posterior ulnar recurrent artery	Ulnar Artery, Right
	Ulnar Artery, Left
Posterior vagal trunk	Vagus Nerve
Preauricular lymph node	Lymphatic, Head
Precava	Superior Vena Cava
Prepatellar bursa	Knee Bursa and Ligament, Right
	Knee Bursa and Ligament, Left
Pretracheal fascia	Subcutaneous Tissue and Fascia, Anterior Neck
Prevertebral fascia	Subcutaneous Tissue and Fascia, Posterior Neck
Princeps pollicis artery	Hand Artery, Right
	Hand Artery, Left
Procerus muscle	Facial Muscle
Profunda brachii	Brachial Artery, Right
	Brachial Artery, Left
Profunda femoris (deep femoral) vein	Femoral Vein, Right
	Femoral Vein, Left
Pronator quadratus muscle	Lower Arm and Wrist Muscle, Right
	Lower Arm and Wrist Muscle, Left
Pronator teres muscle	Lower Arm and Wrist Muscle, Right
	Lower Arm and Wrist Muscle, Left
Prostatic urethra	Urethra

Anatomical Term	PCS Description
Proximal radioulnar joint	Elbow Joint, Right
	Elbow Joint, Left
Psoas muscle	Hip Muscle, Right
	Hip Muscle, Left
Pterygoid muscle	Head Muscle
Pterygoid process	Sphenoid Bone, Right
	Sphenoid Bone, Left
Pterygopalatine (sphenopalatine) ganglion	Head and Neck Sympathetic Nerve
Pubic ligament	Trunk Bursa and Ligament, Right
	Trunk Bursa and Ligament, Left
Pubis	Pelvic Bone, Right
	Pelvic Bone, Left
Pubofemoral ligament	Hip Bursa and Ligament, Right
	Hip Bursa and Ligament, Left
Pudendal nerve	Sacral Plexus
Pulmoaortic canal	Pulmonary Artery, Left
Pulmonary annulus	Pulmonary Valve
Pulmonary plexus	Thoracic Sympathetic Nerve
	Vagus Nerve
Pulmonic valve	Pulmonary Valve
Pulvinar	Thalamus
Pyloric antrum	Stomach, Pylorus
Pyloric canal	Stomach, Pylorus
Pyloric sphincter	Stomach, Pylorus
Pyramidalis muscle	Abdomen Muscle, Right
	Abdomen Muscle, Left
Quadrangular cartilage	Nasal Septum
Quadrate lobe	Liver
Quadratus femoris muscle	Hip Muscle, Right
	Hip Muscle, Left
Quadratus lumborum muscle	Trunk Muscle, Right
	Trunk Muscle, Left
Quadratus plantae muscle	Foot Muscle, Right
	Foot Muscle, Left
Quadriceps (femoris)	Upper Leg Muscle, Right
	Upper Leg Muscle, Left
	Upper Leg Tendon, Right
	Upper Leg Tendon, Left
Radial collateral ligament	Elbow Bursa and Ligament, Right
	Elbow Bursa and Ligament, Left
Radial collateral carpal ligament	Wrist Bursa and Ligament, Right
	Wrist Bursa and Ligament, Left
Radial notch	Ulna, Left
	Ulna, Right
Radial recurrent artery	Radial Artery, Right
	Radial Artery, Left
Radial vein	Brachial Vein, Right
	Brachial Vein, Left
Radialis indicis	Hand Artery, Right
	Hand Artery, Left

Anatomical Term	PCS Description
Radiocarpal joint	Wrist Joint, Right
	Wrist Joint, Left
Radiocarpal ligament	Wrist Bursa and Ligament, Right
	Wrist Bursa and Ligament, Left
Rectosigmoid junction	Sigmoid Colon
Radioulnar ligament	Wrist Bursa and Ligament, Right
	Wrist Bursa and Ligament, Left
Rectus abdominis muscle	Abdomen Muscle, Right
	Abdomen Muscle, Left
Rectus femoris muscle	Upper Leg Muscle, Right
	Upper Leg Muscle, Left
Recurrent laryngeal nerve	Vagus Nerve
Renal calyx	Kidney
	Kidney, Left
	Kidney, Right
	Kidneys, Bilateral
Renal capsule	Kidney
	Kidney, Left
	Kidney, Right
	Kidneys, Bilateral
Renal cortex	Kidney
	Kidney, Left
	Kidney, Right
	Kidneys, Bilateral
Renal plexus	Abdominal Sympathetic Nerve
Renal segment	Kidney
	Kidney, Left
	Kidney, Right
	Kidneys, Bilateral
Renal segmental artery	Renal Artery, Right
	Renal Artery, Left
Retroperitoneal lymph node	Lymphatic, Aortic
Retroperitoneal space	Retroperitoneum
Retropharyngeal lymph node	Lymphatic, Left Neck
	Lymphatic, Right Neck
Retropubic space	Pelvic Cavity
Rhinopharynx	Nasopharynx
Rhomboid major muscle	Trunk Muscle, Right
	Trunk Muscle, Left
Rhomboid minor muscle	Trunk Muscle, Right
	Trunk Muscle, Left
Right ascending lumbar vein	Azygos Vein
Right atrioventricular valve	Tricuspid Valve
Right auricular appendix	Atrium, Right
Right colic vein	Colic Vein
Right coronary sulcus	Heart, Right
Right gastric artery	Gastric Artery
Right gastroepiploic vein	Superior Mesenteric Vein

Anatomical Term	PCS Description
Right inferior phrenic vein	Inferior Vena Cava
Right inferior pulmonary vein	Pulmonary Vein, Right
Right jugular trunk	Lymphatic, Right Neck
Right lateral ventricle	Cerebral Ventricle
Right lymphatic duct	Lymphatic, Right Neck
Right ovarian vein	Inferior Vena Cava
Right second lumbar vein	Inferior Vena Cava
Right subclavian trunk	Lymphatic, Right Neck
Right subcostal vein	Azygos Vein
Right superior pulmonary vein	Pulmonary Vein, Right
Right suprarenal vein	Inferior Vena Cava
Right testicular vein	Inferior Vena Cava
Rima glottidis	Larynx
Risorius muscle	Facial Muscle
Round ligament of uterus	Uterine Supporting Structure
Round window	Inner Ear, Left
	Inner Ear, Right
Sacral ganglion	Sacral Sympathetic Nerve
Sacral lymph node	Lymphatic, Pelvis
Sacral splanchnic nerve	Sacral Sympathetic Nerve
Sacrococcygeal ligament	Trunk Bursa and Ligament, Right
	Trunk Bursa and Ligament, Left
Sacrococcygeal symphysis	Sacrococcygeal Joint
Sacroiliac ligament	Trunk Bursa and Ligament, Right
	Trunk Bursa and Ligament, Left
Sacrospinous ligament	Trunk Bursa and Ligament, Right
	Trunk Bursa and Ligament, Left
Sacrotuberous ligament	Trunk Bursa and Ligament, Right
	Trunk Bursa and Ligament, Left
Salpingopharyngeus muscle	Tongue, Palate, Pharynx Muscle
Salpinx	Fallopian Tube, Left
	Fallopian Tube, Right
Saphenous nerve	Femoral Nerve
Sartorius muscle	Upper Leg Muscle, Right
	Upper Leg Muscle, Left
Scalene muscle	Neck Muscle, Right
	Neck Muscle, Left
Scaphoid bone	Carpal, Left
	Carpal, Right
Scapholunate ligament	Hand Bursa and Ligament, Right
	Hand Bursa and Ligament, Left
Scaphotrapezium ligament	Hand Bursa and Ligament, Right
	Hand Bursa and Ligament, Left
Scarpa's (vestibular) ganglion	Acoustic Nerve
Sebaceous gland	Skin
Second cranial nerve	Optic Nerve

Anatomical Term	PCS Description
Sella turcica	Sphenoid Bone, Right
	Sphenoid Bone, Left
Semicircular canal	Inner Ear, Left
	Inner Ear, Right
Semimembranosus muscle	Upper Leg Muscle, Right
	Upper Leg Muscle, Left
Semitendinosus muscle	Upper Leg Muscle, Right
	Upper Leg Muscle, Left
Septal cartilage	Nasal Septum
Serratus anterior muscle	Thorax Muscle, Right
	Thorax Muscle, Left
Serratus posterior muscle	Trunk Muscle, Right
	Trunk Muscle, Left
Seventh cranial nerve	Facial Nerve
Short gastric artery	Splenic Artery
Sigmoid artery	Inferior Mesenteric Artery
Sigmoid flexure	Sigmoid Colon
Sigmoid vein	Inferior Mesenteric Vein
Sinoatrial node	Conduction Mechanism
Sinus venosus	Atrium, Right
Sixth cranial nerve	Abducens Nerve
Skene's (paraurethral) gland	Vestibular Gland
Small saphenous vein	Lesser Saphenous Vein, Right
	Lesser Saphenous Vein, Left
Solar (celiac) plexus	Abdominal Sympathetic Nerve
Soleus muscle	Lower Leg Muscle, Right
	Lower Leg Muscle, Left
Sphenomandibular ligament	Head and Neck Bursa and Ligament
Sphenopalatine (pterygopalatine) ganglion	Head and Neck Sympathetic Nerve
Spinal dura mater	Dura Mater
Spinal epidural space	Epidural Space
Spinal nerve, cervical	Cervical Nerve
Spinal nerve, lumbar	Lumbar Nerve
Spinal nerve, sacral	Sacral Nerve
Spinal nerve, thoracic	Thoracic Nerve
Spinal subarachnoid space	Subarachnoid Space
Spinal subdural space	Subdural Space
Spinous process	Cervical Vertebra
	Lumbar Vertebra
	Thoracic Vertebra
Spiral ganglion	Acoustic Nerve
Splenic flexure	Transverse Colon
Splenic plexus	Abdominal Sympathetic Nerve
Splenius capitis muscle	Head Muscle
Splenius cervicis muscle	Neck Muscle, Right
	Neck Muscle, Left
Stapes	Auditory Ossicle, Right
	Auditory Ossicle, Left

Anatomical Term	PCS Description
Stellate ganglion	Head and Neck Sympathetic Nerve
Stensen's duct	Parotid Duct, Right
	Parotid Duct, Left
Sternoclavicular ligament	Shoulder Bursa and Ligament, Right
	Shoulder Bursa and Ligament, Left
Sternocleido-mastoid artery	Thyroid Artery, Right
	Thyroid Artery, Left
Sternocleido-mastoid muscle	Neck Muscle, Right
	Neck Muscle, Left
Sternocostal ligament	Thorax Bursa and Ligament, Right
	Thorax Bursa and Ligament, Left
Styloglossus muscle	Tongue, Palate, Pharynx Muscle
Stylomandibular ligament	Head and Neck Bursa and Ligament
Stylopharyngeus muscle	Tongue, Palate, Pharynx Muscle
Subacromial bursa	Shoulder Bursa and Ligament, Right
	Shoulder Bursa and Ligament, Left
Subaortic (common iliac) lymph node	Lymphatic, Pelvis
Subclavicular (apical) lymph node	Lymphatic, Left Axillary
	Lymphatic, Right Axillary
Subclavius muscle	Thorax Muscle, Right
	Thorax Muscle, Left
Subclavius nerve	Brachial Plexus
Subcostal artery	Thoracic Aorta
Subcostal muscle	Thorax Muscle, Right
	Thorax Muscle, Left
Subcostal nerve	Thoracic Nerve
Submandibular ganglion	Facial Nerve
	Head and Neck Sympathetic Nerve
Submandibular gland	Submaxillary Gland, Right
	Submaxillary Gland, Left
Submandibular lymph node	Lymphatic, Head
Submaxillary ganglion	Head and Neck Sympathetic Nerve
Submaxillary lymph node	Lymphatic, Head
Submental artery	Face Artery
Submental lymph node	Lymphatic, Head
Submucous (Meissner's) plexus	Abdominal Sympathetic Nerve
Suboccipital nerve	Cervical Nerve
Suboccipital venous plexus	Vertebral Vein, Right
	Vertebral Vein, Left
Subparotid lymph node	Lymphatic, Head
Subscapular aponeurosis	Subcutaneous Tissue and Fascia, Right Upper Arm
	Subcutaneous Tissue and Fascia, Left Upper Arm
Subscapular artery	Axillary Artery, Right
	Axillary Artery, Left
Subscapular (posterior) lymph node	Lymphatic, Left Axillary
	Lymphatic, Right Axillary

Anatomical Term	PCS Description
Subscapularis muscle	Shoulder Muscle, Right
	Shoulder Muscle, Left
Substantia nigra	Basal Ganglia
Subtalar (talocalcaneal) joint	Tarsal Joint, Right
	Tarsal Joint, Left
Subtalar ligament	Foot Bursa and Ligament, Right
	Foot Bursa and Ligament, Left
Subthalamic nucleus	Basal Ganglia
Superficial epigastric artery	Femoral Artery, Left
	Femoral Artery, Right
Superficial epigastric vein	Greater Saphenous Vein, Left
	Greater Saphenous Vein, Right
Superficial circumflex iliac vein	Greater Saphenous Vein, Left
	Greater Saphenous Vein, Right
Superficial palmar arch	Hand Artery, Right
	Hand Artery, Left
Superficial palmar venous arch	Hand Vein, Left
	Hand Vein, Right
Superficial transverse perineal muscle	Perineum Muscle
Superficial temporal artery	Temporal Artery, Right
	Temporal Artery, Left
Superior cardiac nerve	Thoracic Sympathetic Nerve
Superior cerebellar vein	Intracranial Vein
Superior cerebral vein	Intracranial Vein
Superior clunic (cluneal) nerve	Lumbar Nerve
Superior epigastric artery	Internal Mammary Artery, Right
	Internal Mammary Artery, Left
Superior genicular artery	Popliteal Artery, Right
	Popliteal Artery, Left
Superior gluteal artery	Internal Iliac Artery, Right
	Internal Iliac Artery, Left
Superior gluteal nerve	Lumbar Plexus
Superior hypogastric plexus	Abdominal Sympathetic Nerve
Superior labial artery	Face Artery
Superior laryngeal artery	Thyroid Artery, Right
	Thyroid Artery, Left
Superior laryngeal nerve	Vagus Nerve
Superior longitudinal muscle	Tongue, Palate, Pharynx Muscle
Superior mesenteric ganglion	Abdominal Sympathetic Nerve
Superior mesenteric lymph node	Lymphatic, Mesenteric
Superior mesenteric plexus	Abdominal Sympathetic Nerve
Superior oblique muscle	Extraocular Muscle, Right
	Extraocular Muscle, Left
Superior olivary nucleus	Pons
Superior rectal artery	Inferior Mesenteric Artery

Anatomical Term	PCS Description
Superior rectal muscle	Extraocular Muscle, Right
	Extraocular Muscle, Left
Superior rectal vein	Inferior Mesenteric Vein
Superior tarsal plate	Upper Eyelid, Right
	Upper Eyelid, Left
Superior thoracic artery	Axillary Artery, Right
	Axillary Artery, Left
Superior thyroid artery	External Carotid Artery, Right
	External Carotid Artery, Left
	Thyroid Artery, Right
	Thyroid Artery, Left
Superior turbinate	Nasal Turbinate
Superior ulnar collateral artery	Brachial Artery, Right
	Brachial Artery, Left
Supraclavicular nerve	Cervical Plexus
Supraclavicular (Virchow's) lymph node	Lymphatic, Left Neck
	Lymphatic, Right Neck
Suprahyoid lymph node	Lymphatic, Head
Suprahyoid muscle	Neck Muscle, Right
	Neck Muscle, Left
Suprainguinal lymph node	Lymphatic, Pelvis
Supraorbital vein	Face Vein, Left
	Face Vein, Right
Suprarenal gland	Adrenal Glands, Bilateral
	Adrenal Gland, Right
	Adrenal Gland, Left
	Adrenal Gland
Suprarenal plexus	Abdominal Sympathetic Nerve
Suprascapular nerve	Brachial Plexus
Supraspinatus fascia	Subcutaneous Tissue and Fascia, Right Upper Arm
	Subcutaneous Tissue and Fascia, Left Upper Arm
Supraspinatus muscle	Shoulder Muscle, Right
	Shoulder Muscle, Left
Supraspinous ligament	Trunk Bursa and Ligament, Right
	Trunk Bursa and Ligament, Left
Suprasternal notch	Sternum
Supratrochlear lymph node	Lymphatic, Left Upper Extremity
	Lymphatic, Right Upper Extremity
Sural artery	Popliteal Artery, Right
	Popliteal Artery, Left
Sweat gland	Skin
Talocalcaneal ligament	Foot Bursa and Ligament, Right
	Foot Bursa and Ligament, Left
Talocalcaneal (subtalar) joint	Tarsal Joint, Right
	Tarsal Joint, Left
Talocalcaneonavicular joint	Tarsal Joint, Right
	Tarsal Joint, Left
Talocalcaneonavicular ligament	Foot Bursa and Ligament, Right
	Foot Bursa and Ligament, Left

Anatomical Term	PCS Description
Talocrural joint	Ankle Joint, Right
	Ankle Joint, Left
Talofibular ligament	Ankle Bursa and Ligament, Right
	Ankle Bursa and Ligament, Left
Talus bone	Tarsal, Left
	Tarsal, Right
Tarsometatarsal joint	Metatarsal-Tarsal Joint, Right
	Metatarsal-Tarsal Joint, Left
Tarsometatarsal ligament	Foot Bursa and Ligament, Right
	Foot Bursa and Ligament, Left
Temporal lobe	Cerebral Hemisphere
Temporalis muscle	Head Muscle
Temporoparietalis muscle	Head Muscle
Tensor fasciae latae muscle	Hip Muscle, Right
	Hip Muscle, Left
Tensor veli palatini muscle	Tongue, Palate, Pharynx Muscle
Tenth cranial nerve	Vagus Nerve
Tentorium cerebelli	Dura Mater
Teres major muscle	Shoulder Muscle, Right
	Shoulder Muscle, Left
Teres minor muscle	Shoulder Muscle, Right
	Shoulder Muscle, Left
Testicular artery	Abdominal Aorta
Thenar muscle	Hand Muscle, Right
	Hand Muscle, Left
Third cranial nerve	Oculomotor Nerve
Third occipital nerve	Cervical Nerve
Third ventricle	Cerebral Ventricle
Thoracic aortic plexus	Thoracic Sympathetic Nerve
Thoracic esophagus	Esophagus, Middle
Thoracic facet joint	Thoracic Vertebral Joints, 8 or more
	Thoracic Vertebral Joints, 2 to 7
	Thoracic Vertebral Joint
Thoracic ganglion	Thoracic Sympathetic Nerve
Thoracoacromial artery	Axillary Artery, Right
	Axillary Artery, Left
Thoracolumbar facet joint	Thoracolumbar Vertebral Joint
Thymus gland	Thymus
Thyroarytenoid muscle	Neck Muscle, Right
	Neck Muscle, Left
Thyrocervical trunk	Thyroid Artery, Right
	Thyroid Artery, Left
Thyroid cartilage	Larynx
Tibialis anterior muscle	Lower Leg Muscle, Right
	Lower Leg Muscle, Left
Tibialis posterior muscle	Lower Leg Muscle, Right
	Lower Leg Muscle, Left

Anatomical Term	PCS Description
Tibiofemoral joint	Knee Joint, Right
	Knee Joint, Left
	Knee Joint, Tibial Surface, Right
	Knee Joint, Tibial Surface, Left
Tracheobronchial lymph node	Lymphatic, Thorax
Tragus	External Ear, Right
	External Ear, Left
	External Ear, Bilateral
Transversalis fascia	Subcutaneous Tissue and Fascia, Trunk
Transverse acetabular ligament	Hip Bursa and Ligament, Left
	Hip Bursa and Ligament, Right
Transverse (cutaneous) cervical nerve	Cervical Plexus
Transverse facial artery	Temporal Artery, Right
	Temporal Artery, Left
Transverse humeral ligament	Shoulder Bursa and Ligament, Right
	Shoulder Bursa and Ligament, Left
Transverse ligament of atlas	Head and Neck Bursa and Ligament
Transverse scapular ligament	Shoulder Bursa and Ligament, Right
	Shoulder Bursa and Ligament, Left
Transverse thoracis muscle	Thorax Muscle, Right
	Thorax Muscle, Left
Transversospinalis muscle	Trunk Muscle, Right
	Trunk Muscle, Left
Transversus abdominis muscle	Abdomen Muscle, Right
	Abdomen Muscle, Left
Trapezium bone	Carpal, Left
	Carpal, Right
Trapezius muscle	Trunk Muscle, Right
	Trunk Muscle, Left
Trapezoid bone	Carpal, Left
	Carpal, Right
Triceps brachii muscle	Upper Arm Muscle, Right
	Upper Arm Muscle, Left
Tricuspid annulus	Tricuspid Valve
Trifacial nerve	Trigeminal Nerve
Trigone of bladder	Bladder
Triquetral bone	Carpal, Left
	Carpal, Right
Trochanteric bursa	Hip Bursa and Ligament, Right
	Hip Bursa and Ligament, Left
Twelfth cranial nerve	Hypoglossal Nerve
Tympanic cavity	Middle Ear, Right
	Middle Ear, Left
Tympanic nerve	Glossopharyngeal Nerve
Tympanic part of temoporal bone	Temporal Bone, Right
	Temporal Bone, Left
Ulnar collateral ligament	Elbow Bursa and Ligament, Right
	Elbow Bursa and Ligament, Left

Anatomical Term	PCS Description
Ulnar collateral carpal ligament	Wrist Bursa and Ligament, Right
	Wrist Bursa and Ligament, Left
Ulnar notch	Radius, Left
	Radius, Right
Ulnar vein	Brachial Vein, Right
	Brachial Vein, Left
Umbilical artery	Internal Iliac Artery, Right
	Internal Iliac Artery, Left
Ureteral orifice	Ureter
	Ureter, Left
	Ureter, Right
	Ureters, Bilateral
Ureteropelvic junction (UPJ)	Kidney Pelvis, Right
	Kidney Pelvis, Left
Ureterovesical orifice	Ureter, Left
	Ureter, Right
Uterine artery	Internal Iliac Artery, Right
	Internal Iliac Artery, Left
Uterine cornu	Uterus
Uterine tube	Fallopian Tube, Right
	Fallopian Tube, Left
Uterine vein	Hypogastric Vein, Right
	Hypogastric Vein, Left
Vaginal artery	Internal Iliac Artery, Right
	Internal Iliac Artery, Left
Vaginal vein	Hypogastric Vein, Right
	Hypogastric Vein, Left
Vastus intermedius muscle	Upper Leg Muscle, Right
	Upper Leg Muscle, Left
Vastus lateralis muscle	Upper Leg Muscle, Right
	Upper Leg Muscle, Left
Vastus medialis muscle	Upper Leg Muscle, Right
	Upper Leg Muscle, Left
Ventricular fold	Larynx
Vermiform appendix	Appendix
Vermilion border	Lower Lip
	Upper Lip
Vertebral arch	Cervical Vertebra
	Lumbar Vertebra
	Thoracic Vertebra
Vertebral canal	Spinal Canal
Vertebral foramen	Cervical Vertebra
	Lumbar Vertebra
	Thoracic Vertebra
Vertebral lamina	Cervical Vertebra
	Lumbar Vertebra
	Thoracic Vertebra
Vertebral pedicle	Cervical Vertebra
	Lumbar Vertebra
	Thoracic Vertebra

Anatomical Term	PCS Description
Vesical vein	Hypogastric Vein, Right
	Hypogastric Vein, Left
Vestibular (Scarpa's) ganglion	Acoustic Nerve
Vestibular nerve	Acoustic Nerve
Vestibulocochlear nerve	Acoustic Nerve
Virchow's (supraclavicular) lymph node	Lymphatic, Left Neck
	Lymphatic, Right Neck
Vitreous body	Vitreous, Left
	Vitreous, Right
Vocal fold	Vocal Cord, Right
	Vocal Cord, Left
Volar (palmar) digital vein	Hand Vein, Left
	Hand Vein, Right
Volar (palmar) metacarpal vein	Hand Vein, Left
	Hand Vein, Right
Vomer bone	Nasal Septum (bone
Xiphoid process	Sternum
Zonule of Zinn	Lens, Left
	Lens, Right
Zygomatic process of frontal bone	Frontal Bone, Right
	Frontal Bone, Left
Zygomatic process of temporal bone	Temporal Bone, Right
	Temporal Bone, Left
Zygomaticus muscle	Facial Muscle

Appendix D: Device Key and Aggregation Table

Device Key

Device Term	PCS Description
3f (Aortic) Bioprosthesis valve	Zooplastic Tissue in Heart and Great Vessels
AbioCor® Total Replacement Heart	Synthetic Substitute
Acellular Hydrated Dermis	Nonautologous Tissue Substitute
Activa PC neurostimulator	Stimulator Generator, Multiple Array for Insertion in Subcutaneous Tissue and Fascia
Activa RC neurostimulator	Stimulator Generator, Multiple Array Rechargeable for Insertion in Subcutaneous Tissue and Fascia
Activa SC neurostimulator	Stimulator Generator, Single Array for Insertion in Subcutaneous Tissue and Fascia
ACUITY™ Steerable Lead	Cardiac Lead in Heart and Great Vessels
AMPLATZER® Muscular VSD Occluder	Synthetic Substitute
AMS 800® Urinary Control System	Artificial Sphincter in Urinary System
AneuRx® AAA Advantage®	Intraluminal Device
Annuloplasty ring	Synthetic Substitute
Artificial anal sphincter (AAS)	Artificial Sphincter in Gastrointestinal System
Artificial bowel sphincter (neosphincter)	Artificial Sphincter in Gastrointestinal System
Artificial urinary sphincter (AUS)	Artificial Sphincter in Urinary System
Assurant (Cobalt) stent	Intraluminal Device
Attain Ability® Lead	Cardiac Lead, Pacemaker for Insertion in Heart and Great Vessels
Attain StarFix® (OTW) Lead	Cardiac Lead in Heart and Great Vessels
Autograft	Autologous Tissue Substitute
Autologous artery graft	Autologous Arterial Tissue in Heart and Great Vessels Autologous Arterial Tissue in Upper Arteries Autologous Arterial Tissue in Lower Arteries Autologous Arterial Tissue in Upper Veins Autologous Arterial Tissue in Lower Veins

Device Term	PCS Description
Autologous vein graft	Autologous Venous Tissue in Heart and Great Vessels Autologous Venous Tissue in Upper Arteries Autologous Venous Tissue in Lower Arteries Autologous Venous Tissue in Upper Veins Autologous Venous Tissue in Lower Veins
Axial Lumbar Interbody Fusion System	Interbody Fusion Device in Lower Joints
AxiaLIF® System	Interbody Fusion Device in Lower Joints
BAK/C® Interbody Cervical Fusion System	Interbody Fusion Device in Upper Joints
Bard® Composix® (E/X)(LP) mesh	Synthetic Substitute
Bard® Composix® Kugel® patch	Synthetic Substitute
Bard® Dulex™ mesh	Synthetic Substitute
Bard® Ventralex™ Hernia Patch	Synthetic Substitute
Baroreflex Activation Therapy® (BAT®)	Stimulator Lead in Upper Arteries Cardiac Rhythm Related Device in Subcutaneous Tissue and Fascia
Berlin Heart Ventricular Assist Device	Implantable Heart Assist System in Heart and Great Vessels
Bioactive embolization coil(s)	Intraluminal Device, Bioactive in Upper Arteries
Biventricular external heart assist system	External Heart Assist System in Heart and Great Vessels
Blood glucose monitoring system	Monitoring Device
Bone anchored hearing device	Hearing Device, Bone Conduction for Insertion in Ear, Nose, Sinus Hearing Device, Bone Conduction in Head and Facial Bones
Bone bank bone graft	Nonautologous Tissue Substitute
Bone screw (interlocking)(lag)(pedicle)(recessed)	Internal Fixation Device in Head and Facial Bones Internal Fixation Device in Upper Bones Internal Fixation Device in Lower Bones
Bovine pericardial valve	Zooplastic Tissue in Heart and Great Vessels
Bovine pericardium graft	Zooplastic Tissue in Heart and Great Vessels
Brachytherapy seeds	Radioactive Element
BRYAN® Cervical Disc System	Synthetic Substitute
BVS 5000 Ventricular Assist Device	External Heart Assist System in Heart and Great Vessels

Device Term	PCS Description
Cardiac contractility modulation lead	Cardiac Lead in Heart and Great Vessels
Cardiac event recorder	Monitoring Device
Cardiac resynchronization therapy (CRT) lead	Cardiac Lead, Pacemaker for Insertion in Heart and Great Vessels Cardiac Lead, Defibrillator for Insertion in Heart and Great Vessels
CardioMEMS® pressure sensor	Monitoring Device, Pressure Sensor for Insertion in Heart and Great Vessels
Carotid (artery) sinus (baroreceptor) lead	Stimulator Lead in Upper Arteries
Carotid WALLSTENT® Monorail® Endoprosthesis	Intraluminal Device
Centrimag® Blood Pump	Intraluminal Device
Clamp and rod internal fixation system (CRIF)	Internal Fixation Device in Upper Bones Internal Fixation Device in Lower Bones
CoAxia NeuroFlo catheter	Intraluminal Device
Cobalt/chromium head and polyethylene socket	Synthetic Substitute, Metal on Polyethylene for Replacement in Lower Joints
Cobalt/chromium head and socket	Synthetic Substitute, Metal for Replacement in Lower Joints
Cochlear implant (CI), multiple channel (electrode)	Hearing Device, Multiple Channel Cochlear Prosthesis for Insertion in Ear, Nose, Sinus
Cochlear implant (CI), single channel (electrode)	Hearing Device, Single Channel Cochlear Prosthesis for Insertion in Ear, Nose, Sinus
COGNIS® CRT-D	Cardiac Resynchronization Defibrillator Pulse Generator for Insertion in Subcutaneous Tissue and Fascia
Colonic Z-Stent®	Intraluminal Device
Complete (SE) stent	Intraluminal Device
Concerto II CRT-D	Cardiac Resynchronization Defibrillator Pulse Generator for Insertion in Subcutaneous Tissue and Fascia
CONSERVE® PLUS Total Resurfacing Hip System	Resurfacing Device in Lower Joints
Consulta CRT-D	Cardiac Resynchronization Defibrillator Pulse Generator for Insertion in Subcutaneous Tissue and Fascia
Consulta CRT-P	Cardiac Resynchronization Pacemaker Pulse Generator for Insertion in Subcutaneous Tissue and Fascia
CONTAK RENEWAL® 3 RF (HE) CRT-D	Cardiac Resynchronization Defibrillator Pulse Generator for Insertion in Subcutaneous Tissue and Fascia
Contegra Pulmonary Valved Conduit	Zooplastic Tissue in Heart and Great Vessels

Device Term	PCS Description
Continuous Glucose Monitoring (CGM) device	Monitoring Device
CoreValve transcatheter aortic valve	Zooplastic Tissue in Heart and Great Vessels
Cormet Hip Resurfacing System	Resurfacing Device in Lower Joints
CoRoent® XL	Interbody Fusion Device in Lower Joints
Corox (OTW) Bipolar Lead	Cardiac Lead, Pacemaker for Insertion in Heart and Great Vessels Cardiac Lead, Defibrillator for Insertion in Heart and Great Vessels
Cortical strip neurostimulator lead	Neurostimulator Lead in Central Nervous System
Cultured epidermal cell autograft	Autologous Tissue Substitute
CYPHER® Stent	Intraluminal Device, Drug-eluting in Heart and Great Vessels
Cystostomy tube	Drainage Device
DBS lead	Neurostimulator Lead in Central Nervous System
DeBakey Left Ventricular Assist Device	Implantable Heart Assist System in Heart and Great Vessels
Deep brain neurostimulator lead	Neurostimulator Lead in Central Nervous System
Delta frame external fixator	External Fixation Device, Hybrid for Insertion in Upper Bones External Fixation Device, Hybrid for Reposition in Upper Bones External Fixation Device, Hybrid for Insertion in Lower Bones External Fixation Device, Hybrid for Reposition in Lower Bones
Delta III Reverse shoulder prosthesis	Synthetic Substitute, Reverse Ball and Socket for Replacement in Upper Joints
Diaphragmatic pacemaker generator	Stimulator Generator in Subcutaneous Tissue and Fascia
Direct Lateral Interbody Fusion (DLIF) device	Interbody Fusion Device in Lower Joints
Driver stent (RX) (OTW)	Intraluminal Device
DuraHeart Left Ventricular Assist System	Implantable Heart Assist System in Heart and Great Vessels
Durata® Defibrillation Lead	Cardiac Lead, Defibrillator for Insertion in Heart and Great Vessels
Dynesys® Dynamic Stabilization System	Spinal Stabilization Device, Pedicle-Based for Insertion in Upper Joints Spinal Stabilization Device, Pedicle-Based for Insertion in Lower Joints
E-Luminexx™ (Biliary)(Vascular) Stent	Intraluminal Device
Electrical bone growth stimulator (EBGS)	Bone Growth Stimulator in Head and Facial Bones Bone Growth Stimulator in Upper Bones Bone Growth Stimulator in Lower Bones

Device Term	PCS Description
Electrical muscle stimulation (EMS) lead	Stimulator Lead in Muscles
Electronic muscle stimulator lead	Stimulator Lead in Muscles
Embolization coil(s)	Intraluminal Device
Endeavor® (III)(IV) (Sprint) Zotarolimus-eluting Coronary Stent System	Intraluminal Device, Drug-eluting in Heart and Great Vessels
EndoSure® sensor	Monitoring Device, Pressure Sensor for Insertion in Heart and Great Vessels
ENDOTAK RELIANCE® (G) Defibrillation Lead	Cardiac Lead, Defibrillator for Insertion in Heart and Great Vessels
Endotracheal tube (cuffed)(double-lumen)	Intraluminal Device, Endotracheal Airway in Respiratory System
Endurant® Endovascular Stent Graft	Intraluminal Device
EnRhythm	Pacemaker, Dual Chamber for Insertion in Subcutaneous Tissue and Fascia
Enterra gastric neurostimulator	Stimulator Generator, Multiple Array
Epicel® cultured epidermal autograft	Autologous Tissue Substitute
Epic™ Stented Tissue Valve (aortic)	Zooplastic Tissue in Heart and Great Vessels
Epiretinal visual prosthesis	Epiretinal Visual Prosthesis in Eye
Esophageal obturator airway (EOA)	Intraluminal Device, Airway in Gastrointestinal System
Esteem® implantable hearing system	Hearing Device in Ear, Nose, Sinus
Everolimus-eluting coronary stent	Intraluminal Device, Drug-eluting in Heart and Great Vessels
Ex-PRESS™ mini glaucoma shunt	Synthetic Substitute
Express® (LD) Premounted Stent System	Intraluminal Device
Express® Biliary SD Monorail® Premounted Stent System	Intraluminal Device
Express® SD Renal Monorail® Premounted Stent System	Intraluminal Device
External fixator	External Fixation Device in Head and Facial Bones External Fixation Device in Upper Bones External Fixation Device in Lower Bones External Fixation Device in Upper Joints External Fixation Device in Lower Joints
EXtreme Lateral Interbody Fusion (XLIF) device	Interbody Fusion Device in Lower Joints
Facet replacement spinal stabilization device	Spinal Stabilization Device, Facet Replacement for Insertion in Upper Joints Spinal Stabilization Device, Facet Replacement for Insertion in Lower Joints

Device Term	PCS Description
FLAIR® Endovascular Stent Graft	Intraluminal Device
Flexible Composite Mesh	Synthetic Substitute
Foley catheter	Drainage Device
Formula™ Balloon-Expandable Renal Stent System	Intraluminal Device
Freestyle (Stentless) Aortic Root Bioprosthesis	Zooplastic Tissue in Heart and Great Vessels
Fusion screw (compression)(lag)(locking)	Internal Fixation Device in Upper Joints Internal Fixation Device in Lower Joints
Gastric electrical stimulation (GES) lead	Stimulator Lead in Gastrointestinal System
Gastric pacemaker lead	Stimulator Lead in Gastrointestinal System
GORE® DUALMESH®	Synthetic Substitute
Guedel airway	Intraluminal Device, Airway in Mouth and Throat
Hancock Bioprosthesis (aortic)(mitral) valve	Zooplastic Tissue
Hancock Bioprosthetic Valved Conduit	Zooplastic Tissue in Heart and Great Vessels
HeartMate II® Left Ventricular Assist Device (LVAD)	Implantable Heart Assist System in Heart and Great Vessels
HeartMate XVE® Left Ventricular Assist Device (LVAD)	Implantable Heart Assist System in Heart and Great Vessels
Hip (joint) liner	Liner in Lower Joints
Holter valve ventricular shunt	Synthetic Substitute
Ilizarov external fixator	External Fixation Device, Ring for Insertion in Upper Bones External Fixation Device, Ring for Reposition in Upper Bones External Fixation Device, Ring for Insertion in Lower Bones External Fixation Device, Ring for Reposition in Lower Bones
Ilizarov-Vecklich device	External Fixation Device, Limb Lengthening for Insertion in Upper Bones External Fixation Device, Limb Lengthening for Insertion in Lower Bones
Impella® (2.5)(5.0)(LD) cardiac assist device	Intraluminal Device
Implantable cardioverter-defibrillator (ICD)	Defibrillator Generator for Insertion in Subcutaneous Tissue and Fascia
Implantable gastric pacemaker generator	Stimulator Generator in Subcutaneous Tissue and Fascia
Implantable glucose monitoring device	Monitoring Device
Implantable hemodynamic monitor (IHM)	Monitoring Device, Hemodynamic for Insertion in Subcutaneous Tissue and Fascia
Implantable hemodynamic monitoring system (IHMS)	Monitoring Device, Hemodynamic for Insertion in Subcutaneous Tissue and Fascia

Device Term	PCS Description
Implantable Miniature Telescope™ (IMT)	Synthetic Substitute, Intraocular Telescope for Replacement in Eye
Implantable pain pump	Implantable Drug Infusion Pump (antispasmodic) (chemotherapy) (pain)
Implanted (venous)(access) port	Vascular Access Device, Reservoir in Subcutaneous Tissue and Fascia
InDura, intrathecal catheter (1P) (spinal)	Infusion Device
Injection reservoir, port	Vascular Access Device, Reservoir in Subcutaneous Tissue and Fascia
Injection reservoir, pump	Infusion Device, Pump in Subcutaneous Tissue and Fascia
Interbody fusion (spine) cage	Interbody Fusion Device in Upper Joints Interbody Fusion Device in Lower Joints
Interspinous process spinal stabilization device	Spinal Stabilization Device, Interspinous Process for Insertion in Upper Joints Spinal Stabilization Device, Interspinous Process for Insertion in Lower Joints
InterStim® Therapy lead	Neurostimulator Lead in Peripheral Nervous System
InterStim® Therapy neurostimulator	Stimulator Generator Single Array
Intramedullary (IM) rod (nail)	Internal Fixation Device, Intramedullary in Upper Bones Internal Fixation Device, Intramedullary in Lower Bones
Intramedullary skeletal kinetic distractor (ISKD)	Internal Fixation Device, Intramedullary in Upper Bones Internal Fixation Device, Intramedullary in Lower Bones
Intrauterine Device (IUD)	Contraceptive Device in Female Reproductive System
Itrel (3)(4) neurostimulator	Stimulator Generator, Single Array for Insertion in Subcutaneous Tissue and Fascia
Joint fixation plate	Internal Fixation Device in Upper Joints Internal Fixation Device in Lower Joints
Joint liner (insert)	Liner in Lower Joints
Joint spacer (antibiotic)	Spacer in Upper Joints Spacer in Lower Joints
Kappa	Pacemaker, Dual Chamber for Insertion in Subcutaneous Tissue and Fascia
Kinetra® neurostimulator	Stimulator Generator, Multiple Array for Insertion in Subcutaneous Tissue and Fascia

Device Term	PCS Description
Kirschner wire (K-wire)	Internal Fixation Device in Head and Facial Bones Internal Fixation Device in Upper Bones Internal Fixation Device in Lower Bones Internal Fixation Device in Upper Joints Internal Fixation Device in Lower Joints
Knee (implant) insert	Liner in Lower Joints
Kuntscher nail	Internal Fixation Device, Intramedullary in Upper Bones Internal Fixation Device, Intramedullary in Lower Bones
LAP-BAND® Adjustable Gastric Banding System	Extraluminal Device
LifeStent® (Flexstar)(XL) Vascular Stent System	Intraluminal Device
LIVIAN™ CRT-D	Cardiac Resynchronization Defibrillator Pulse Generator for Insertion in Subcutaneous Tissue and Fascia
Loop recorder, implantable	Monitoring Device
Mark IV Breathing Pacemaker System	Stimulator Generator in Subcutaneous Tissue and Fascia
Maximo II DR (VR)	Defibrillator Generator for Insertion in Subcutaneous Tissue and Fascia
Maximo II DR CRT-D	Cardiac Resynchronization Defibrillator Pulse Generator for Insertion in Subcutaneous Tissue and Fascia
Melody® transcatheter pulmonary valve	Zooplastic Tissue in Heart and Great Vessels
Micro-Driver stent (RX) (OTW)	Intraluminal Device
MicroMed HeartAssist	Implantable Heart Assist System in Heart and Great Vessels
Micrus CERECYTE Microcoil	Intraluminal Device, Bioactive in Upper Arteries
MitraClip valve repair system	Synthetic Substitute
Mitroflow® Aortic Pericardial Heart Valve	Zooplastic Tissue in Heart and Great Vessels
Nasopharyngeal airway (NPA)	Intraluminal Device, Airway in Ear, Nose, Sinus
Neuromuscular electrical stimulation (NEMS) lead	Stimulator Lead in Muscles
Neurostimulator generator, multiple channel	Stimulator Generator, Multiple Array for Insertion in Subcutaneous Tissue and Fascia
Neurostimulator generator, multiple channel rechargeable	Stimulator Generator, Multiple Array Rechargeable for Insertion in Subcutaneous Tissue and Fascia
Neurostimulator generator, single channel	Stimulator Generator, Single Array for Insertion in Subcutaneous Tissue and Fascia
Neurostimulator generator, single channel rechargeable	Stimulator Generator, Single Array Rechargeable for Insertion in Subcutaneous Tissue and Fascia

Device Term	PCS Description
Neutralization plate	Internal Fixation Device in Head and Facial Bones Internal Fixation Device in Upper Bones Internal Fixation Device in Lower Bones
Nitinol framed polymer mesh	Synthetic Substitute
Non-tunneled central venous catheter	Infusion Device
Novacor Left Ventricular Assist Device	Implantable Heart Assist System in Heart and Great Vessels
Novation® Ceramic AHS® (articulation hip system)	Synthetic Substitute, Ceramic for Replacement in Lower Joints
Optimizer™ III implantable pulse generator	Contractility Modulation Device for Insertion in Subcutaneous Tissue and Fascia
Oropharyngeal airway (OPA)	Intraluminal Device, Airway in Mouth and Throat
Ovatio™ CRT-D	Cardiac Resynchronization Defibrillator Pulse Generator for Insertion in Subcutaneous Tissue and Fascia
Oxidized zirconium ceramic hip bearing surface	Synthetic Substitute, Ceramic on Polyethylene for Replacement in Lower Joints
Paclitaxel-eluting coronary stent	Intraluminal Device, Drug-eluting in Heart and Great Vessels
Paclitaxel-eluting peripheral stent	Intraluminal Device, Drug-eluting in Upper Arteries Intraluminal Device, Drug-eluting in Lower Arteries
Partially absorbable mesh	Synthetic Substitute
Pedicle-based dynamic stabilization device	Spinal Stabilization Device, Pedicle-Based for Insertion in Upper Joints Spinal Stabilization Device, Pedicle-Based for Insertion in Lower Joints
Percutaneous endoscopic gastrojejunostomy (PEG/J) tube	Feeding Device in Gastrointestinal System
Percutaneous endoscopic gastrostomy (PEG) tube	Feeding Device in Gastrointestinal System
Percutaneous nephrostomy catheter	Drainage Device
Peripherally inserted central catheter (PICC)	Infusion Device
Pessary ring	Intraluminal Device, Pessary in Female Reproductive System
Phrenic nerve stimulator generator	Stimulator Generator in Subcutaneous Tissue and Fascia
Phrenic nerve stimulator lead	Diaphragmatic Pacemaker Lead in Respiratory System
PHYSIOMESH™ Flexible Composite Mesh	Synthetic Substitute
Pipeline™ Embolization device (PED)	Intraluminal Device
Polyethylene socket	Synthetic Substitute, Polyethylene for Replacement in Lower Joints

Device Term	PCS Description
Polymethylmethacrylate (PMMA)	Synthetic Substitute
Polypropylene mesh	Synthetic Substitute
Porcine (bioprosthetic) valve	Zooplastic Tissue in Heart and Great Vessels
PRESTIGE® Cervical Disc	Synthetic Substitute
PrimeAdvanced neurostimulator	Stimulator Generator, Multiple Array for Insertion in Subcutaneous Tissue and Fascia
PROCEED™ Ventral Patch	Synthetic Substitute
Prodisc-C	Synthetic Substitute
Prodisc-L	Synthetic Substitute
PROLENE Polypropylene Hernia System (PHS)	Synthetic Substitute
Protecta XT CRT-D	Cardiac Resynchronization Defibrillator Pulse Generator for Insertion in Subcutaneous Tissue and Fascia
Protecta XT DR (XT VR)	Defibrillator Generator for Insertion in Subcutaneous Tissue and Fascia
Protégé® RX Carotid Stent System	Intraluminal Device
Pump reservoir	Vascular Access Device, Reservoir in Subcutaneous Tissue and Fascia
REALIZE® Adjustable Gastric Band	Extraluminal Device
Rebound HRD® (Hernia Repair Device)	Synthetic Substitute
RestoreAdvanced neurostimulator	Stimulator Generator, Multiple Array Rechargeable for Insertion in Subcutaneous Tissue and Fascia
RestoreSensor neurostimulator	Stimulator Generator, Multiple Array Rechargeable for Insertion in Subcutaneous Tissue and Fascia
RestoreUltra neurostimulator	Stimulator Generator, Multiple Array Rechargeable for Insertion in Subcutaneous Tissue and Fascia
Reveal (DX)(XT)	Monitoring Device
Reverse® Shoulder Prosthesis	Synthetic Substitute, Reverse Ball and Socket for Replacement in Upper Joints
Revo MRI™ SureScan® pacemaker	Pacemaker, Dual Chamber for Insertion in Subcutaneous Tissue and Fascia
Rheos® System device	Cardiac Rhythm Related Device in Subcutaneous Tissue and Fascia
Rheos® System lead	Stimulator Lead in Upper Arteries
RNS System lead	Neurostimulator Lead in Central Nervous System
RNS system neurostimulator generator	Neurostimulator Generator in Head and Facial Bones
Sacral nerve modulation (SNM) lead	Stimulator Lead in Urinary System
Sacral neuromodulation lead	Stimulator Lead in Urinary System
SAPIEN transcatheter aortic valve	Zooplastic Tissue in Heart and Great Vessels

Device Term	PCS Description
Secura (DR) (VR)	Defibrillator Generator for Insertion in Subcutaneous Tissue and Fascia
Sheffield hybrid external fixator	External Fixation Device, Hybrid for Insertion in Upper Bones External Fixation Device, Hybrid for Reposition in Upper Bones External Fixation Device, Hybrid for Insertion in Lower Bones External Fixation Device, Hybrid for Reposition in Lower Bones
Sheffield ring external fixator	External Fixation Device, Ring for Insertion in Upper Bones External Fixation Device, Ring for Reposition in Upper Bones External Fixation Device, Ring for Insertion in Lower Bones External Fixation Device, Ring for Reposition in Lower Bones
Single lead pacemaker (atrium)(ventricle)	Pacemaker, Single Chamber for Insertion in Subcutaneous Tissue and Fascia
Single lead rate responsive pacemaker (atrium)(ventricle)	Pacemaker, Single Chamber Rate Responsive for Insertion in Subcutaneous Tissue and Fascia
Sirolimus-eluting coronary stent	Intraluminal Device, Drug-eluting in Heart and Great Vessels
SJM Biocor® Stented Valve System	Zooplastic Tissue in Heart and Great Vessels
Soletra® single-channel neurostimulator	Stimulator Generator, Single Array for Insertion in Subcutaneous Tissue and Fascia
Spinal cord neurostimulator lead	Neurostimulator Lead in Central Nervous System
Spiration IBV™ Valve System	Intraluminal Device, Endobronchial Valve in Respiratory System
Stent (angioplasty)(embolization)	Intraluminal Device
Stented tissue valve	Zooplastic Tissue in Heart and Great Vessels
Stratos LV	Cardiac Resynchronization Pacemaker Pulse Generator for Insertion in Subcutaneous Tissue and Fascia
Subcutaneous injection reservoir, port	Vascular Access Device, Reservoir in Subcutaneous Tissue and Fascia
Subcutaneous injection reservoir, pump	Infusion Device, Pump in Subcutaneous Tissue and Fascia
Subdermal progesterone implant	Contraceptive Device in Subcutaneous Tissue and Fascia
SynCardia Total Artificial Heart	Synthetic Substitute
Synchra CRT-P	Cardiac Resynchronization Pacemaker Pulse Generator for Insertion in Subcutaneous Tissue and Fascia
Talent® Abdominal Stent Graft System	Talent Abdominal Stent Graft (Abdominal) (Thoracic)
Talent® Converter	Intraluminal Device
Talent® Occluder	Intraluminal Device

Device Term	PCS Description
TandemHeart® System	External Heart Assist System in Heart and Great Vessels
TAXUS® Liberté® Paclitaxel-eluting Coronary Stent System	Intraluminal Device, Drug-eluting in Heart and Great Vessels
Therapeutic occlusion coil(s)	Intraluminal Device
Thoracostomy tube	Drainage Device
Thoratec IVAD (implantable ventricular assist device)	Implantable Heart Assist System in Heart and Great Vessels
Thoratec Paracorporeal Ventricular Assist Device	External Heart Assist System in Heart and Great Vessels
TigerPaw® system for closure of left atrial appendage	Extraluminal Device
Tissue bank graft	Nonautologous Tissue Substitute
Tissue expander (inflatable)(injectable)	Tissue Expander in Skin and Breast Tissue Expander in Subcutaneous Tissue and Fascia
Titanium Sternal Fixation System (TSFS)	Internal Fixation Device, Rigid Plate for Insertion in Upper Bones Internal Fixation Device, Rigid Plate for Reposition in Upper Bones
Total artificial (replacement) heart	Synthetic Substitute
Tracheostomy tube	Tracheostomy Device in Respiratory System
Trifecta™ Valve (aortic)	Zooplastic Tissue in Heart and Great Vessels
Tunneled central venous catheter	Vascular Access Device in Subcutaneous Tissue and Fascia
Tunneled spinal (intrathecal) catheter	Infusion Device
Two lead pacemaker	Pacemaker, Dual Chamber for Insertion in Subcutaneous Tissue and Fascia
Ultraflex™ Precision Colonic Stent System	Intraluminal Device
ULTRAPRO Hernia System (UHS)	Synthetic Substitute
ULTRAPRO Partially Absorbable Lightweight Mesh	Synthetic Substitute
ULTRAPRO Plug	Synthetic Substitute
Ultrasonic osteogenic stimulator	Bone Growth Stimulator in Head and Facial Bones Bone Growth Stimulator in Upper Bones Bone Growth Stimulator in Lower Bones
Ultrasound bone healing system	Bone Growth Stimulator in Head and Facial Bones Bone Growth Stimulator in Upper Bones Bone Growth Stimulator in Lower Bones

Device Term	PCS Description	Device Term	PCS Description
Uniplanar external fixator	External Fixation Device, Monoplanar for Insertion in Upper Bones External Fixation Device, Monoplanar for Reposition in Upper Bones External Fixation Device, Monoplanar for Insertion in Lower Bones External Fixation Device, Monoplanar for Reposition in Lower Bones	Xenograft	Zooplastic Tissue in Heart and Great Vessels
		XIENCE V Everolimus Eluting Coronary Stent System	Intraluminal Device, Drug-eluting in Heart and Great Vessels
		XLIF® System	Interbody Fusion Device in Lower Joints
Urinary incontinence stimulator lead	Stimulator Lead in Urinary System	Zenith Flex® AAA Endovascular Graft	Intraluminal Device
Vaginal pessary	Intraluminal Device, Pessary in Female Reproductive System	Zenith TX2® TAA Endovascular Graft	Intraluminal Device
Valiant Thoracic Stent Graft	Synthetic Substitute	Zenith® Renu™ AAA Ancillary Graft	Intraluminal Device
Vectra® Vascular Access Graft	Vascular Access Device in Subcutaneous Tissue and Fascia	Zilver® PTX® (paclitaxel) Drug-Eluting Peripheral Stent	Intraluminal Device, Drug-eluting in Upper Arteries Intraluminal Device, Drug-eluting in Lower Arteries
Ventrio™ Hernia Patch	Synthetic Substitute		
Versa	Pacemaker, Dual Chamber	Zimmer® NexGen® LPS Mobile Bearing Knee	Synthetic Substitute
Virtuoso (II) (DR) (VR)	Defibrillator Generator for Insertion in Subcutaneous Tissue and Fascia	Zimmer® NexGen® LPS-Flex Mobile Knee	Synthetic Substitute
WALLSTENT® Endoprosthesis	Intraluminal Device	Zotarolimus-eluting coronary stent	Intraluminal Device, Drug-eluting in Heart and Great Vessels
X-STOP® Spacer	Spinal Stabilization Device, Interspinous Process for Insertion in Upper Joints Spinal Stabilization Device, Interspinous Process for Insertion in Lower Joints		

Device Aggregation Table

This table crosswalks specific device character value definitions for specific root operations in a specific body system to the more general device character value to be used when the root operation covers a wide range of body parts and the device character represents an entire family of devices.

Specific Device	for Operation	in Body System	General Device	
Autologous Arterial Tissue (A)	All applicable	Heart and Great Vessels Lower Arteries Lower Veins Upper Arteries Upper Veins	7	Autologous Tissue Substitute
Autologous Venous Tissue (9)	All applicable	Heart and Great Vessels Lower Arteries Lower Veins Upper Arteries Upper Veins	7	Autologous Tissue Substitute
Cardiac Lead, Defibrillator (K)	Insertion	Heart and Great Vessels	M	Cardiac Lead
Cardiac Lead, Pacemaker (J)	Insertion	Heart and Great Vessels	M	Cardiac Lead
Cardiac Resynchronization Defibrillator Pulse Generator (9)	Insertion	Subcutaneous Tissue and Fascia	P	Cardiac Rhythm Related Device
Cardiac Resynchronization Pacemaker Pulse Generator (7)	Insertion	Subcutaneous Tissue and Fascia	P	Cardiac Rhythm Related Device
Contractility Modulation Device (A)	Insertion	Subcutaneous Tissue and Fascia	P	Cardiac Rhythm Related Device
Defibrillator Generator (8)	Insertion	Subcutaneous Tissue and Fascia	P	Cardiac Rhythm Related Device
Epiretinal Visual Prosthesis	All applicable	Eye	J	Synthetic Substitute
External Fixation Device, Hybrid (D)	Insertion	Lower Bones Upper Bones	5	External Fixation Device

Specific Device	for Operation	in Body System	General Device	
External Fixation Device, Hybrid (D)	Reposition	Lower Bones Upper Bones	5	External Fixation Device
External Fixation Device, Limb Lengthening (8)	Insertion	Lower Bones Upper Bones	5	External Fixation Device
External Fixation Device, Monoplanar (B)	Insertion	Lower Bones Upper Bones	5	External Fixation Device
External Fixation Device, Monoplanar (B)	Reposition	Lower Bones Upper Bones	5	External Fixation Device
External Fixation Device, Ring (C)	Insertion	Lower Bones Upper Bones	5	External Fixation Device
External Fixation Device, Ring (C)	Reposition	Lower Bones Upper Bones	5	External Fixation Device
Hearing Device, Bone Conduction (S)	All applicable	Head and Facial Bones	S	Hearing Device, Bone Conduction
Hearing Device, Bone Conduction (4)	Insertion	Ear, Nose, Sinus	S	Hearing Device
Hearing Device, Multiple Channel Cochlear Prosthesis (6)	Insertion	Ear, Nose, Sinus	S	Hearing Device
Hearing Device, Single Channel Cochlear Prosthesis (5)	Insertion	Ear, Nose, Sinus	S	Hearing Device
Internal Fixation Device, Intramedullary (6)	All applicable	Lower Bones Upper Bones	4	Internal Fixation Device
Internal Fixation Device, Rigid Plate (Ø)	Insertion	Upper Bones	4	Internal Fixation Device
Internal Fixation Device, Rigid Plate (Ø)	Reposition	Upper Bones	4	Internal Fixation Device
Intraluminal Device, Pessary (G)	All applicable	Female Reproductive System	D	Intraluminal Device
Intraluminal Device, Airway (B)	All applicable	Ear, Nose, Sinus Gastrointestinal System Mouth and Throat	D	Intraluminal Device
Intraluminal Device, Bioactive (B)	All applicable	Upper Arteries	D	Intraluminal Device
Intraluminal Device, Drug-eluting (4)	All applicable	Heart and Great Vessels Lower Arteries Upper Arteries	D	Intraluminal Device
Intraluminal Device, Endobronchial Valve (G)	All applicable	Respiratory System	D	Intraluminal Device
Intraluminal Device, Endotracheal Airway (E)	All applicable	Respiratory System	D	Intraluminal Device
Intraluminal Device, Radioactive (T)	All applicable	Heart and Great Vessels	D	Intraluminal Device
Monitoring Device, Hemodynamic (Ø)	Insertion	Subcutaneous Tissue and Fascia	2	Monitoring Device
Monitoring Device, Pressure Sensor (Ø)	Insertion	Heart and Great Vessels	2	Monitoring Device
Pacemaker, Dual Chamber (6)	Insertion	Subcutaneous Tissue and Fascia	P	Cardiac Rhythm Related Device
Pacemaker, Single Chamber (4)	Insertion	Subcutaneous Tissue and Fascia	P	Cardiac Rhythm Related Device
Pacemaker, Single Chamber Rate Responsive (5)	Insertion	Subcutaneous Tissue and Fascia	P	Cardiac Rhythm Related Device
Spinal Stabilization Device, Facet Replacement (D)	Insertion	Lower Joints Upper Joints	4	Internal Fixation Device
Spinal Stabilization Device, Interspinous Process (B)	Insertion	Lower Joints Upper Joints	4	Internal Fixation Device
Spinal Stabilization Device, Pedicle-Based (C)	Insertion	Lower Joints Upper Joints	4	Internal Fixation Device
Stimulator Generator, Multiple Array (D)	Insertion	Subcutaneous Tissue and Fascia	M	Stimulator Generator
Stimulator Generator, Multiple Array Rechargeable (E)	Insertion	Subcutaneous Tissue and Fascia	M	Stimulator Generator
Stimulator Generator, Single Array (B)	Insertion	Subcutaneous Tissue and Fascia	M	Stimulator Generator
Stimulator Generator, Single Array Rechargeable (C)	Insertion	Subcutaneous Tissue and Fascia	M	Stimulator Generator
Synthetic Substitute, Ceramic (3)	Replacement	Lower Joints	J	Synthetic Substitute
Synthetic Substitute, Ceramic on Polyethylene (4)	Replacement	Lower Joints	J	Synthetic Substitute
Synthetic Substitute, Intraocular Telescope (Ø)	Replacement	Eye	J	Synthetic Substitute
Synthetic Substitute, Metal (1)	Replacement	Lower Joints	J	Synthetic Substitute
Synthetic Substitute, Metal on Polyethylene (2)	Replacement	Lower Joints	J	Synthetic Substitute
Synthetic Substitute, Polyethylene (Ø)	Replacement	Lower Joints	J	Synthetic Substitute
Synthetic Substitute, Reverse Ball and Socket (Ø)	Replacement	Upper Joints	J	Synthetic Substitute

Appendix E: Type and Type Qualifier Definitions Sections B–H

Section B–Imaging

Type (Character 3)	Definition
Computerized Tomography (CT Scan) (2)	Computer reformatted digital display of multiplanar images developed from the capture of multiple exposures of external ionizing radiation
Fluoroscopy (1)	Single plane or bi-plane real time display of an image developed from the capture of external ionizing radiation on a fluorescent screen. The image may also be stored by either digital or analog means
Magnetic Resonance Imaging (MRI) (3)	Computer reformatted digital display of multiplanar images developed from the capture of radiofrequency signals emitted by nuclei in a body site excited within a magnetic field
Plain Radiography (Ø)	Planar display of an image developed from the capture of external ionizing radiation on photographic or photoconductive plate
Ultrasonography (4)	Real time display of images of anatomy or flow information developed from the capture of reflected and attenuated high frequency sound waves

Section C–Nuclear Medicine

Type (Character 3)	Definition
Nonimaging Nuclear Medicine Assay (6)	Introduction of radioactive materials into the body for the study of body fluids and blood elements, by the detection of radioactive emissions
Nonimaging Nuclear Medicine Probe (5)	Introduction of radioactive materials into the body for the study of distribution and fate of certain substances by the detection of radioactive emissions; or, alternatively, measurement of absorption of radioactive emissions from an external source
Nonimaging Nuclear Medicine Uptake (4)	Introduction of radioactive materials into the body for measurements of organ function, from the detection of radioactive emissions
Planar Nuclear Medicine Imaging (1)	Introduction of radioactive materials into the body for single plane display of images developed from the capture of radioactive emissions
Positron Emission Tomographic (PET) Imaging (3)	Introduction of radioactive materials into the body for three dimensional display of images developed from the simultaneous capture, 18Ø degrees apart, of radioactive emissions
Systemic Nuclear Medicine Therapy (7)	Introduction of unsealed radioactive materials into the body for treatment
Tomographic (Tomo) Nuclear Medicine Imaging (2)	Introduction of radioactive materials into the body for three dimensional display of images developed from the capture of radioactive emissions

Section F–Physical Rehabilitation and Diagnostic Audiology

Type (Character 3)	Definition
Activities of Daily Living Assessment (2)	Measurement of functional level for activities of daily living
Activities of Daily Living Treatment (8)	Exercise or activities to facilitate functional competence for activities of daily living
Caregiver Training (F)	Training in activities to support patient's optimal level of function
Cochlear Implant Treatment (B)	Application of techniques to improve the communication abilities of individuals with cochlear implant
Device Fitting (D)	Fitting of a device designed to facilitate or support achievement of a higher level of function
Hearing Aid Assessment (4)	Measurement of the appropriateness and/or effectiveness of a hearing device
Hearing Assessment (3)	Measurement of hearing and related functions

Continued on next page

Section F–Physical Rehabilitation and Diagnostic Audiology

Continued from previous page

Type (Character 3)	Definition
Hearing Treatment (9)	Application of techniques to improve, augment, or compensate for hearing and related functional impairment
Motor Function Assessment/Nerve Function Assessment (1)	Measurement of motor, nerve, and related functions
Motor Treatment (7)	Exercise or activities to increase or facilitate motor function
Speech Assessment (Ø)	Measurement of speech and related functions
Speech Treatment (6)	Application of techniques to improve, augment, or compensate for speech and related functional impairment
Vestibular Assessment (5)	Measurement of the vestibular system and related functions
Vestibular Treatment (C)	Application of techniques to improve, augment, or compensate for vestibular and related functional impairment

Section F–Physical Rehabilitation and Diagnostic Audiology

Type Qualifier (Character 5)	Definition
Acoustic Reflex Decay (J)	Measures reduction in size/strength of acoustic reflex over time Includes/Examples: Includes site of lesion test
Acoustic Reflex Patterns (G)	Defines site of lesion based upon presence/absence of acoustic reflexes with ipsilateral vs. contralateral stimulation
Acoustic Reflex Threshold (H)	Determines minimal intensity that acoustic reflex occurs with ipsilateral and/or contralateral stimulation
Aerobic Capacity and Endurance (7)	Measures autonomic responses to positional changes; perceived exertion, dyspnea or angina during activity; performance during exercise protocols; standard vital signs; and blood gas analysis or oxygen consumption
Alternate Binaural or Monaural Loudness Balance (7)	Determines auditory stimulus parameter that yields the same objective sensation Includes/Examples: Sound intensities that yield same loudness perception
Anthropometric Characteristics (B)	Measures edema, body fat composition, height, weight, length and girth
Aphasia (Assessment) (C)	Measures expressive and receptive speech and language function including reading and writing
Aphasia (Treatment) (3)	Applying techniques to improve, augment, or compensate for receptive/ expressive language impairments
Articulation/Phonology (Assessment) (9)	Measures speech production
Articulation/Phonology (Treatment) (4)	Applying techniques to correct, improve, or compensate for speech productive impairment
Assistive Listening Device (5)	Assists in use of effective and appropriate assistive listening device/system
Assistive Listening System Device Selection (4)	Measures the effectiveness and appropriateness of assistive listening systems/devices
Assistive, Adaptive,Supportive or Protective Devices (9)	Explanation: Devices to facilitate or support achievement of a higher level of function in wheelchair mobility; bed mobility; transfer or ambulation ability; bath and showering ability; dressing; grooming; personal hygiene; play or leisure
Auditory Evoked Potentials (L)	Measures electric responses produced by the VIIIth cranial nerve and brainstem following auditory stimulation
Auditory Processing (Assessment) (Q)	Evaluates ability to receive and process auditory information and comprehension of spoken language
Auditory Processing (Treatment) (2)	Applying techniques to improve the receiving and processing of auditory information and comprehension of spoken language

Continued on next page

Section F–Physical Rehabilitation and Diagnostic Audiology   *Continued from previous page*

Type Qualifier (Character 5)	Definition
Augmentative/Alternative Communication System (Assessment) (L)	Determines the appropriateness of aids, techniques, symbols, and/or strategies to augment or replace speech and enhance communication Includes/Examples: Includes the use of telephones, writing equipment, emergency equipment, and TDD
Augmentative/Alternative Communication System (Treatment) (3)	Includes/Examples: Includes augmentative communication devices and aids
Aural Rehabilitation (5)	Applying techniques to improve the communication abilities associated with hearing loss
Aural Rehabilitation Status (P)	Measures impact of a hearing loss including evaluation of receptive and expressive communication skills
Bathing/Showering (Ø)	Includes/Examples: Includes obtaining and using supplies; soaping, rinsing, and drying body parts; maintaining bathing position; and transferring to and from bathing positions
Bathing/Showering Techniques (Ø)	Activities to facilitate obtaining and using supplies, soaping, rinsing and drying body parts, maintaining bathing position, and transferring to and from bathing positions
Bed Mobility (Assessment) (B)	Transitional movement within bed
Bed Mobility (Treatment) (5)	Exercise or activities to facilitate transitional movements within bed
Bedside Swallowing and Oral Function (H)	Includes/Examples: Bedside swallowing includes assessment of sucking, masticating, coughing, and swallowing. Oral function includes assessment of musculature for controlled movements, structures, and functions to determine coordination and phonation
Bekesy Audiometry (3)	Uses an instrument that provides a choice of discrete or continuously varying pure tones; choice of pulsed or continuous signal
Binaural Electroacoustic Hearing Aid Check (6)	Determines mechanical and electroacoustic function of bilateral hearing aids using hearing aid test box
Binaural Hearing Aid (Assessment) (3)	Measures the candidacy, effectiveness, and appropriateness of a hearing aid Explanation: Measures bilateral fit
Binaural Hearing Aid (Treatment) (2)	Explanation: Assists in achieving maximum understanding and performance
Bithermal, Binaural Caloric Irrigation (Ø)	Measures the rhythmic eye movements stimulated by changing the temperature of the vestibular system
Bithermal, Monaural Caloric Irrigation (1)	Measures the rhythmic eye movements stimulated by changing the temperature of the vestibular system in one ear
Brief Tone Stimuli (R)	Measures specific central auditory process
Cerumen Management (3)	Includes examination of external auditory canal and tympanic membrane and removal of cerumen from external ear canal
Cochlear Implant (Ø)	Measures candidacy for cochlear implant
Cochlear Implant Rehabilitation (Ø)	Applying techniques to improve the communication abilities of individuals with cochlear implant; includes programming the device, providing patients/families with information
Communicative/Cognitive Integration Skills (Assessment) (G)	Measures ability to use higher cortical functions Includes/Examples: Includes orientation, recognition, attention span, initiation and termination of activity, memory, sequencing, categorizing, concept formation, spatial operations, judgment, problem solving, generalization and pragmatic communication
Communicative/Cognitive Integration Skills (Treatment) (6)	Activities to facilitate the use of higher cortical functions Includes/Examples: Includes level of arousal, orientation, recognition, attention span, initiation and termination of activity, memory sequencing, judgment and problem solving, learning and generalization, and pragmatic communication
Computerized Dynamic Posturography (6)	Measures the status of the peripheral and central vestibular system and the sensory/motor component of balance; evaluates the efficacy of vestibular rehabilitation
Conditioned Play Audiometry (4)	Behavioral measures using nonspeech and speech stimuli to obtain frequency-specific and ear-specific information on auditory status from the patient Explanation: Obtains speech reception threshold by having patient point to pictures of spondaic words

Continued on next page

Section F–Physical Rehabilitation and Diagnostic Audiology

Continued from previous page

Type Qualifier (Character 5)	Definition
Coordination/Dexterity (Assessment) (3)	Measures large and small muscle groups for controlled goal- directed movements Explanation: Dexterity includes object manipulation
Coordination/Dexterity (Treatment) (2)	Exercise or activities to facilitate gross coordination and fine coordination
Cranial Nerve Integrity (9)	Measures cranial nerve sensory and motor functions, including tastes, smell and facial expression
Dichotic Stimuli (T)	Measures specific central auditory process
Distorted Speech (S)	Measures specific central auditory process
Dix-Hallpike Dynamic (5)	Measures nystagmus following Dix-Hallpike maneuver
Dressing (1)	Includes/Examples: Includes selecting clothing and accessories, obtaining clothing from storage, dressing, fastening and adjusting clothing and shoes, and applying and removing personal devices, prosthesis or orthosis
Dressing Techniques (1)	Activities to facilitate selecting clothing and accessories, dressing and undressing, adjusting clothing and shoes, applying and removing devices, prostheses or orthoses
Dynamic Orthosis (6)	Includes/Examples: Includes customized and prefabricated splints, inhibitory casts, spinal and other braces, and protective devices; allows motion through transfer of movement from other body parts or by use of outside forces
Ear Canal Probe Microphone (1)	Real ear measures
Ear Protector Attentuation (7)	Measures ear protector fit and effectiveness
Electrocochleography (K)	Measures the VIIIth cranial nerve action potential
Environmental, Home, Work Barriers (B)	Measures current and potential barriers to optimal function, including safety hazards, access problems and home or office design
Ergonomics and Body Mechanics (C)	Ergonomic measurement of job tasks, work hardening or work conditioning needs; functional capacity; and body mechanics
Eustachian Tube Function (F)	Measures eustachian tube function and patency of eustachian tube
Evoked Otoacoustic Emissions, Diagnostic (N)	Measures auditory evoked potentials in a diagnostic format
Evoked Otoacoustic Emissions, Screening (M)	Measures auditory evoked potentials in a screening format
Facial Nerve Function (7)	Measures electrical activity of the VIIth cranial nerve (facial nerve)
Feeding/Eating (Assessment) (2)	Includes/Examples: Includes setting up food, selecting and using utensils and tableware, bringing food or drink to mouth, cleaning face, hands, and clothing, and management of alternative methods of nourishment
Feeding/Eating (Treatment) (3)	Exercise or activities to facilitate setting up food, selecting and using utensils and tableware, bringing food or drink to mouth, cleaning face, hands, and clothing, and management of alternative methods of nourishment
Filtered Speech (Ø)	Uses high or low pass filtered speech stimuli to assess central auditory processing disorders, site of lesion testing
Fluency (Assessment) (D)	Measures speech fluency or stuttering
Fluency (Treatment) (7)	Applying techniques to improve and augment fluent speech
Gait Training/Functional Ambulation (9)	Exercise or activities to facilitate ambulation on a variety of surfaces and in a variety of environments
Gait/Balance (D)	Measures biomechanical, arthrokinematic and other spatial and temporal characteristics of gait and balance

Continued on next page

Section F–Physical Rehabilitation and Diagnostic Audiology

Continued from previous page

Type Qualifier (Character 5)	Definition
Grooming/Personal Hygiene (Assessment) (3)	Includes/Examples: Includes ability to obtain and use supplies in a sequential fashion, general grooming, oral hygiene, toilet hygiene, personal care devices, including care for artificial airways
Grooming/Personal Hygiene (Treatment) (2)	Activities to facilitate obtaining and using supplies in a sequential fashion: general grooming, oral hygiene, toilet hygiene, cleaning body, and personal care devices, including artificial airways
Hearing and Related Disorders Counseling (Ø)	Provides patients/families/caregivers with information, support, referrals to facilitate recovery from a communication disorder Includes/Examples: Includes strategies for psychosocial adjustment to hearing loss for clients and families/caregivers
Hearing and Related Disorders Prevention (1)	Provides patients/families/caregivers with information and support to prevent communication disorders
Hearing Screening (Ø)	Pass/refer measures designed to identify need for further audiologic assessment
Home Management (Assessment) (4)	Obtaining and maintaining personal and household possessions and environment Includes/Examples: Includes clothing care, cleaning, meal preparation and cleanup, shopping, money management, household maintenance, safety procedures, and childcare/parenting
Home Management (Treatment) (4)	Activities to facilitate obtaining and maintaining personal household possessions and environment Includes/Examples: Includes clothing care, cleaning, meal preparation and clean-up, shopping, money management, household maintenance, safety procedures, childcare/parenting
Instrumental Swallowing and Oral Function (J)	Definition: Measures swallowing function using instrumental diagnostic procedures Explanation: Methods include videofluoroscopy, ultrasound, manometry, endoscopy
Integumentary Integrity (1)	Includes/Examples: Includes burns, skin conditions, ecchymosis, bleeding, blisters, scar tissue, wounds and other traumas, tissue mobility, turgor and texture
Manual Therapy Techniques (7)	Techniques in which the therapist uses his/her hands to administer skilled movements Includes/Examples: Includes connective tissue massage, joint mobilization and manipulation, manual lymph drainage, manual traction, soft tissue mobilization and manipulation
Masking Patterns (W)	Measures central auditory processing status
Monaural Electroacoustic Hearing Aid Check (8)	Determines mechanical and electroacoustic function of one hearing aid using hearing aid test box
Monaural Hearing Aid (Assessment) (2)	Measures the candidacy, effectiveness, and appropriateness of a hearing aid Explanation: Measures unilateral fit
Monaural Hearing Aid (Treatment) (1)	Explanation: Assists in achieving maximum understanding and performance
Motor Function (Assessment) (4)	Measures the body's functional and versatile movement patterns Includes/Examples: Includes motor assessment scales, analysis of head, trunk and limb movement, and assessment of motor learning
Motor Function (Treatment) (3)	Exercise or activities to facilitate crossing midline, laterality, bilateral integration, praxis, neuromuscular relaxation, inhibition, facilitation, motor function and motor learning
Motor Speech (Assessment) (B)	Measures neurological motor aspects of speech production
Motor Speech (Treatment) (B)	Applying techniques to improve and augment the impaired neurological motor aspects of speech production
Muscle Performance (Assessment) (Ø)	Measures muscle strength, power and endurance using manual testing, dynamometry or computer-assisted electromechanical muscle test; functional muscle strength, power and endurance; muscle pain, tone, or soreness; or pelvic-floor musculature Explanation: Muscle endurance refers to the ability to contract a muscle repeatedly over time
Muscle Performance (Treatment) (1)	Exercise or activities to increase the capacity of a muscle to do work in terms of strength, power, and/or endurance Explanation: Muscle strength is the force exerted to overcome resistance in one maximal effort. Muscle power is work produced per unit of time, or the product of strength and speed. Muscle endurance is the ability to contract a muscle repeatedly over time

Continued on next page

Section F–Physical Rehabilitation and Diagnostic Audiology

Continued from previous page

Type Qualifier (Character 5)	Definition
Neuromotor Development (D)	Measures motor development, righting and equilibrium reactions, and reflex and equilibrium reactions
Neurophysiologic Intraoperative (8)	Monitors neural status during surgery
Non-invasive Instrumental Status (N)	Instrumental measures of oral, nasal, vocal, and velopharyngeal functions as they pertain to speech production
Nonspoken Language (Assessment) (7)	Measures nonspoken language (print, sign, symbols) for communication
Nonspoken Language (Treatment) (Ø)	Applying techniques that improve, augment, or compensate spoken communication
Oral Peripheral Mechanism (P)	Structural measures of face, jaw, lips, tongue, teeth, hard and soft palate, pharynx as related to speech production
Orofacial Myofunctional (Assessment) (K)	Measures orofacial myofunctional patterns for speech and related functions
Orofacial Myofunctional (Treatment) (9)	Applying techniques to improve, alter, or augment impaired orofacial myofunctional patterns and related speech production errors
Oscillating Tracking (3)	Measures ability to visually track
Pain (F)	Measures muscle soreness, pain and soreness with joint movement, and pain perception Includes/Examples: Includes questionnaires, graphs, symptom magnification scales or visual analog scales
Perceptual Processing (Assessment) (5)	Measures stereognosis, kinesthesia, body schema, right-left discrimination, form constancy, position in space, visual closure, figure-ground, depth perception, spatial relations and topographical orientation
Perceptual Processing (Treatment) (1)	Exercise and activities to facilitate perceptual processing Explanation: Includes stereognosis, kinesthesia, body schema, right-left discrimination, form constancy, position in space, visual closure, figure-ground, depth perception, spatial relations, and topographical orientation Includes/Examples: Includes stereognosis, kinesthesia, body schema, right-left discrimination, form constancy, position in space, visual closure, figure-ground, depth perception, spatial relations, and topographical orientation
Performance Intensity Phonetically Balanced Speech Discrimination (Q)	Measures word recognition over varying intensity levels
Postural Control (3)	Exercise or activities to increase postural alignment and control
Prosthesis (8)	Explanation: Artificial substitutes for missing body parts that augment performance or function
Psychosocial Skills (Assessment) (6)	The ability to interact in society and to process emotions Includes/Examples: Includes psychological (values, interests, self-concept); social (role performance, social conduct, interpersonal skills, self expression); self-management (coping skills, time management, self-control)
Psychosocial Skills (Treatment) (6)	The ability to interact in society and to process emotions Includes/Examples: Includes psychological (values, interests, self-concept); social (role performance, social conduct, interpersonal skills, self expression); self-management (coping skills, time management, self-control)
Pure Tone Audiometry, Air (1)	Air-conduction pure tone threshold measures with appropriate masking
Pure Tone Audiometry, Air and Bone (2)	Air-conduction and bone-conduction pure tone threshold measures with appropriate masking
Pure Tone Stenger (C)	Measures unilateral nonorganic hearing loss based on simultaneous presentation of pure tones of differing volume
Range of Motion and Joint Integrity (5)	Measures quantity, quality, grade, and classification of joint movement and/or mobility Explanation: Range of Motion is the space, distance or angle through which movement occurs at a joint or series of joints. Joint integrity is the conformance of joints to expected anatomic, biomechanical and kinematic norms

Continued on next page

Section F–Physical Rehabilitation and Diagnostic Audiology

Continued from previous page

Type Qualifier (Character 5)	Definition
Range of Motion and Joint Mobility (0)	Exercise or activities to increase muscle length and joint mobility
Receptive/Expressive Language (Assessment) (8)	Measures receptive and expressive language
Receptive/Expressive Language (Treatment) (B)	Applying techniques to improve and augment receptive/expressive language
Reflex Integrity (G)	Measures the presence, absence, or exaggeration of developmentally appropriate, pathologic or normal reflexes
Select Picture Audiometry (5)	Establishes hearing threshold levels for speech using pictures
Sensorineural Acuity Level (4)	Measures sensorineural acuity masking presented via bone conduction
Sensory Aids (5)	Determines the appropriateness of a sensory prosthetic device, other than a hearing aid or assistive listening system/device
Sensory Awareness/ Processing/ Integrity (6)	Includes/Examples: Includes light touch, pressure, temperature, pain, sharp/dull, proprioception, vestibular, visual, auditory, gustatory, and olfactory
Short Increment Sensitivity Index (9)	Measures the ear's ability to detect small intensity changes; site of lesion test requiring a behavioral response
Sinusoidal Vertical Axis Rotational (4)	Measures nystagmus following rotation
Somatosensory Evoked Potentials (9)	Measures neural activity from sites throughout the body
Speech/Language Screening (6)	Identifies need for further speech and/or language evaluation
Speech Threshold (1)	Measures minimal intensity needed to repeat spondaic words
Speech/Word Recognition (2)	Measures ability to repeat/identify single syllable words; scores given as a percentage; includes word recognition/speech discrimination
Speech-Language Pathology and Related Disorders Counseling (1)	Provides patients/families with information, support, referrals to facilitate recovery from a communication disorder
Speech-Language Pathology and Related Disorders Prevention (2)	Applying techniques to avoid or minimize onset and/or development of a communication disorder
Staggered Spondaic Word (3)	Measures central auditory processing site of lesion based upon dichotic presentation of spondaic words
Static Orthosis (7)	Includes/Examples: Includes customized and prefabricated splints, inhibitory casts, spinal and other braces, and protective devices; has no moving parts, maintains joint(s) in desired position
Stenger (B)	Measures unilateral nonorganic hearing loss based on simultaneous presentation of signals of differing volume
Swallowing Dysfunction (D)	Activities to improve swallowing function in coordination with respiratory function Includes/Examples: Includes function and coordination of sucking, mastication, coughing, swallowing
Synthetic Sentence Identification (5)	Measures central auditory dysfunction using identification of third order approximations of sentences and competing messages
Temporal Ordering of Stimuli (V)	Measures specific central auditory process
Therapeutic Exercise (7)	Exercise or activities to facilitate sensory awareness, sensory processing, sensory integration, balance training, conditioning, reconditioning Includes/Examples: Includes developmental activities, breathing exercises, aerobic endurance activities, aquatic exercises, stretching and ventilatory muscle training
Tinnitus Masker (Assessment) (7)	Determines candidacy for tinnitus masker
Tinnitus Masker (Treatment) (0)	Explanation: Used to verify physical fit, acoustic appropriateness, and benefit; assists in achieving maximum benefit

Continued on next page

Section F–Physical Rehabilitation and Diagnostic Audiology

Continued from previous page

Type Qualifier (Character 5)	Definition
Tone Decay (B)	Measures decrease in hearing sensitivity to a tone; site of lesion test requiring a behavioral response
Transfer (5)	Transitional movement from one surface to another
Transfer Training (8)	Exercise or activities to facilitate movement from one surface to another
Tympanometry (D)	Measures the integrity of the middle ear; measures ease at which sound flows through the tympanic membrane while air pressure against the membrane is varied
Unithermal Binaural Screen (2)	Measures the rhythmic eye movements stimulated by changing the temperature of the vestibular system in both ears using warm water, screening format
Ventilation/Respiration/Circulation (G)	Measures ventilatory muscle strength, power and endurance, pulmonary function and ventilatory mechanics Includes/Examples: Includes ability to clear airway, activities that aggravate or relieve edema, pain, dyspnea or other symptoms, chest wall mobility, cardiopulmonary response to performance of ADL and IAD, cough and sputum, standard vital signs
Vestibular (Ø)	Applying techniques to compensate for balance disorders; includes habituation, exercise therapy, and balance retraining
Visual Motor Integration (Assessment) (2)	Coordinating the interaction of information from the eyes with body movement during activity
Visual Motor Integration (Treatment) (2)	Exercise or activities to facilitate coordinating the interaction of information from eyes with body movement during activity
Visual Reinforcement Audiometry (6)	Behavioral measures using nonspeech and speech stimuli to obtain frequency/ear-specific information on auditory status Includes/Examples: Includes a conditioned response of looking toward a visual reinforcer (e.g., lights, animated toy) every time auditory stimuli are heard
Vocational Activities and Functional Community or Work Reintegration Skills (Assessment) (H)	Measures environmental, home, work (job/school/play) barriers that keep patients from functioning optimally in their environment Includes/Examples: Includes assessment of vocational skills and interests, environment of work (job/school/play), injury potential and injury prevention or reduction, ergonomic stressors, transportation skills, and ability to access and use community resources
Vocational Activities/Functional Community Skills/Work Reintegration Skills (Treatment) (7)	Activities to facilitate vocational exploration, body mechanics training, job acquisition, and environmental or work (job/school/play) task adaptation Includes/Examples: Includes injury prevention and reduction, ergonomic stressor reduction, job coaching and simulation, work hardening and conditioning, driving training, transportation skills, and use of community resources
Voice (Assessment) (F)	Measures vocal structure, function and production
Voice (Treatment) (C)	Applying techniques to improve voice and vocal function
Voice Prosthetic (Assessment) (M)	Determines the appropriateness of voice prosthetic/adaptive device to enhance or facilitate communication
Voice Prosthetic (Treatment) (4)	Includes/Examples: Includes electrolarynx, and other assistive, adaptive, supportive devices
Wheelchair Mobility (Assessment) (F)	Measures fit and functional abilities within wheelchair in a variety of environments
Wheelchair Mobility (Treatment) (4)	Management, maintenance and controlled operation of a wheelchair, scooter or other device, in and on a variety of surfaces and environments
Wound Management (5)	Includes/Examples: Includes non-selective and selective debridement (enzymes, autolysis, sharp debridement), dressings (wound coverings, hydrogel, vacuum-assisted closure), topical agents, etc.

Section G–Mental Health

Type (Character 3)	Definition
Biofeedback (C)	Provision of information from the monitoring and regulating of physiological processes in conjunction with cognitive-behavioral techniques to improve patient functioning or well-being Includes/Examples: Includes EEG, blood pressure, skin temperature or peripheral blood flow, ECG, electrooculogram, EMG, respirometry or capnometry, GSR/EDR, perineometry to monitor/regulate bowel/bladder activity, electrogastrogram to monitor/regulate gastric motility
Counseling (6)	The application of psychological methods to treat an individual with normal developmental issues and psychological problems in order to increase function, improve well-being, alleviate distress, maladjustment or resolve crises
Crisis Intervention (2)	Treatment of a traumatized, acutely disturbed or distressed individual for the purpose of short-term stabilization Includes/Examples: Includes defusing, debriefing, counseling, psychotherapy and/or coordination of care with other providers or agencies
Electroconvulsive Therapy (B)	The application of controlled electrical voltages to treat a mental health disorder Includes/Examples: Includes appropriate sedation and other preparation of the individual
Family Psychotherapy (7)	Treatment that includes one or more family members of an individual with a mental health disorder by behavioral, cognitive, psychoanalytic, psychodynamic or psychophysiological means to improve functioning or well-being Explanation: Remediation of emotional or behavioral problems presented by one or more family members in cases where psychotherapy with more than one family member is indicated
Group Psychotherapy (H)	Treatment of two or more individuals with a mental health disorder by behavioral, cognitive, psychoanalytic, psychodynamic or psychophysiological means to improve functioning or well-being
Hypnosis (F)	Induction of a state of heightened suggestibility by auditory, visual and tactile techniques to elicit an emotional or behavioral response
Individual Psychotherapy (5)	Treatment of an individual with a mental health disorder by behavioral, cognitive, psychoanalytic, psychodynamic or psychophysiological means to improve functioning or well-being
Light Therapy (J)	Application of specialized light treatments to improve functioning or well-being
Medication Management (3)	Monitoring and adjusting the use of medications for the treatment of a mental health disorder
Narcosynthesis (G)	Administration of intravenous barbiturates in order to release suppressed or repressed thoughts
Psychological Tests (1)	The administration and interpretation of standardized psychological tests and measurement instruments for the assessment of psychological function

Section G–Mental Health

Type Qualifier (Character 4)	Definition
Behavioral (1)	Primarily to modify behavior Includes/Examples: Includes modeling and role playing, positive reinforcement of target behaviors, response cost, and training of self-management skills
Cognitive (2)	Primarily to correct cognitive distortions and errors
Cognitive-Behavioral (8)	Combining cognitive and behavioral treatment strategies to improve functioning Explanation: Maladaptive responses are examined to determine how cognitions relate to behavior patterns in response to an event. Uses learning principles and information-processing models
Developmental (Ø)	Age-normed developmental status of cognitive, social and adaptive behavior skills
Intellectual and Psychoeducational (2)	Intellectual abilities, academic achievement and learning capabilities (including behaviors and emotional factors affecting learning)

Continued on next page

Section G–Mental Health

Continued from previous page

Type Qualifier (Character 4)	Definition
Interactive (0)	Uses primarily physical aids and other forms of non-oral interaction with a patient who is physically, psychologically or developmentally unable to use ordinary language for communication Includes/Examples: Includes the use of toys in symbolic play
Interpersonal (3)	Helps an individual make changes in interpersonal behaviors to reduce psychological dysfunction Includes/Examples: Includes exploratory techniques, encouragement of affective expression, clarification of patient statements, analysis of communication patterns, use of therapy relationship and behavior change techniques
Neurobehavioral Status/Cognitive Status (4)	Includes neurobehavioral status exam, interview(s), and observation for the clinical assessment of thinking, reasoning and judgment, acquired knowledge, attention, memory, visual spatial abilities, language functions, and planning
Neuropsychological (3)	Thinking, reasoning and judgment, acquired knowledge, attention, memory, visual spatial abilities, language functions, planning
Personality and Behavioral (1)	Mood, emotion, behavior, social functioning, psychopathological conditions, personality traits and characteristics
Psychoanalysis (4)	Methods of obtaining a detailed account of past and present mental and emotional experiences to determine the source and eliminate or diminish the undesirable effects of unconscious conflicts Explanation: Accomplished by making the individual aware of their existence, origin, and inappropriate expression in emotions and behavior
Psychodynamic (5)	Exploration of past and present emotional experiences to understand motives and drives using insight-oriented techniques to reduce the undesirable effects of internal conflicts on emotions and behavior Explanation: Techniques include empathetic listening, clarifying self-defeating behavior patterns, and exploring adaptive alternatives
Psychophysiological (9)	Monitoring and alteration of physiological processes to help the individual associate physiological reactions combined with cognitive and behavioral strategies to gain improved control of these processes to help the individual cope more effectively
Supportive (6)	Formation of therapeutic relationship primarily for providing emotional support to prevent further deterioration in functioning during periods of particular stress Explanation: Often used in conjunction with other therapeutic approaches
Vocational (1)	Exploration of vocational interests, aptitudes and required adaptive behavior skills to develop and carry out a plan for achieving a successful vocational placement Includes/Examples: Includes enhancing work related adjustment and/or pursuing viable options in training education or preparation

Section H - Substance Abuse Treatment

Type (Character 3)	Definition
Detoxification Services (2)	Detoxification from alcohol and/or drugs Explanation: Not a treatment modality, but helps the patient stabilize physically and psychologically until the body becomes free of drugs and the effects of alcohol
Family Counseling (6)	The application of psychological methods that includes one or more family members to treat an individual with addictive behavior Explanation: Provides support and education for family members of addicted individuals. Family member participation is seen as a critical area of substance abuse treatment
Group Counseling (4)	The application of psychological methods to treat two or more individuals with addictive behavior Explanation: Provides structured group counseling sessions and healing power through the connection with others
Individual Counseling (3)	The application of psychological methods to treat an individual with addictive behavior Explanation: Comprised of several different techniques, which apply various strategies to address drug addiction
Individual Psychotherapy (5)	Treatment of an individual with addictive behavior by behavioral, cognitive, psychoanalytic, psychodynamic or psychophysiological means
Medication Management (8)	Monitoring and adjusting the use of replacement medications for the treatment of addiction
Pharmacotherapy (9)	The use of replacement medications for the treatment of addiction

Appendix F: Components of the Medical and Surgical Approach Definitions

Approach	Definition	Access Location	Method	Type of Instrumentation	Example
Open (Ø)	Cutting through the skin or mucous membrane and any other body layers necessary to expose the site of the procedure.	Skin or mucous membraneany other body layers	Cutting	None	Abdominal hysterectomy
Percutaneous (3)	Entry, by puncture or minor incision, of instrumentation through the skin or mucous membrane and/or any other body layers necessary to reach the site of the procedure	Skin or mucous membrane, any other body layers	Puncture or minor incision	Without visualization	Needle biopsy of liver, Liposuction
Percutaneous endoscopic (4)	Entry, by puncture or minor incision, of instrumentation through the skin or mucous membrane and/or any other body layers necessary to reach and visualize the site of the procedure	Skin or mucous membrane, any other body layers	Puncture or minor incision	With visualization	Arthroscopy, Laparoscopic cholecystectomy
Via natural or artificial opening (7)	Entry of instrumentation through a natural or artificial external opening to reach the site of the procedure	Natural or artificial external opening	Direct entry	Without visualization	Endotracheal tube insertion, Foley catheter placement
Via natural or artificial opening endoscopic (8)	Entry of instrumentation through a natural or artificial external opening to reach and visualize the site of the procedure	Natural or artificial external opening	Direct entry with puncture or minor incision for instrumentation only	With visualization	Sigmoidoscopy, EGD, ERCP
Via natural or artificial opening with percutaneous endoscopic assistance (F)	Entry of instrumentation through a natural or artificial external opening and entry, by puncture or minor incision, of instrumentation through the skin or mucous membrane and any other body layers necessary to aid in the performance of the procedure	Skin or mucous membrane, any other body layers	Cutting	With visualization	Laparoscopic-assisted vaginal hysterectomy
External (X)	Procedures performed directly on the skin or mucous membrane and procedures performed indirectly by the application of external force through the skin or mucous membrane	Skin or mucous membrane	Direct or indirect application	None	Closed fracture reduction, Resection of tonsils

Appendix G: Character Meanings

Ø: Medical and Surgical
Ø: Central Nervous System

Operation–Character 3	Body Part–Character 4	Approach–Character 5	Device–Character 6	Qualifier–Character 7
1 Bypass	Ø Brain	Ø Open	Ø Drainage Device	Ø Nasopharynx
2 Change	1 Cerebral Meninges	3 Percutaneous	2 Monitoring Device	1 Mastoid Sinus
5 Destruction	2 Dura Mater	4 Percutaneous Endoscopic	3 Infusion Device	2 Atrium
8 Division	3 Epidural Space	X External	7 Autologous Tissue Substitute	3 Blood Vessel
9 Drainage	4 Subdural Space		J Synthetic Substitute	4 Pleural Cavity
B Excision	5 Subarachnoid Space		K Nonautologous Tissue Substitute	5 Intestine
C Extirpation	6 Cerebral Ventricle		M Electrode	6 Peritoneal Cavity
D Extraction	7 Cerebral Hemisphere		Y Other Device	7 Urinary Tract
F Fragmentation	8 Basal Ganglia		Z No Device	8 Bone Marrow
H Insertion	9 Thalamus			9 Fallopian Tube
J Inspection	A Hypothalamus			B Cerebral Cisterns
K Map	B Pons			F Olfactory Nerve
N Release	C Cerebellum			G Optic Nerve
P Removal	D Medulla Oblongata			H Oculomotor Nerve
Q Repair	E Cranial Nerve			J Trochlear Nerve
S Reposition	F Olfactory Nerve			K Trigeminal Nerve
T Resection	G Optic Nerve			L Abducens Nerve
U Supplement	H Oculomotor Nerve			M Facial Nerve
W Revision	J Trochlear Nerve			N Acoustic Nerve
X Transfer	K Trigeminal Nerve			P Glossopharyngeal Nerve
	L Abducens Nerve			Q Vagus Nerve
	M Facial Nerve			R Accessory Nerve
	N Acoustic Nerve			S Hypoglossal Nerve
	P Glossopharyngeal Nerve			X Diagnostic
	Q Vagus Nerve			Z No Qualifier
	R Accessory Nerve			
	S Hypoglossal Nerve			
	T Spinal Meninges			
	U Spinal Canal			
	V Spinal Cord			
	W Cervical Spinal Cord			
	X Thoracic Spinal Cord			
	Y Lumbar Spinal Cord			

Ø: Medical and Surgical

1: Peripheral Nervous System

Operation–Character 3	Body Part–Character 4	Approach–Character 5	Device–Character 6	Qualifier–Character 7
2　Change	Ø　Cervical Plexus	Ø　Open	Ø　Drainage Device	1　Cervical Nerve
5　Destruction	1　Cervical Nerve	3　Percutaneous	2　Monitoring Device	2　Phrenic Nerve
8　Division	2　Phrenic Nerve	4　Percutaneous Endoscopic	7　Autologous Tissue Substitute	4　Ulnar Nerve
9　Drainage	3　Brachial Plexus	X　External	M　Neurostimulator Lead	5　Median Nerve
B　Excision	4　Ulnar Nerve		Y　Other Device	6　Radial Nerve
C　Extirpation	5　Median Nerve		Z　No Device	8　Thoracic Nerve
D　Extraction	6　Radial Nerve			B　Lumbar Nerve
H　Insertion	8　Thoracic Nerve			C　Perineal Nerve
J　Inspection	9　Lumbar Plexus			D　Femoral Nerve
N　Release	A　Lumbosacral Plexus			F　Sciatic Nerve
P　Removal	B　Lumbar Nerve			G　Tibial Nerve
Q　Repair	C　Pudendal Nerve			H　Peroneal Nerve
S　Reposition	D　Femoral Nerve			X　Diagnostic
U　Supplement	F　Sciatic Nerve			Z　No Qualifier
W　Revision	G　Tibial Nerve			
X　Transfer	H　Peroneal Nerve			
	K　Head and Neck Sympathetic Nerve			
	L　Thoracic Sympathetic Nerve			
	M　Abdominal Sympathetic Nerve			
	N　Lumbar Sympathetic Nerve			
	P　Sacral Sympathetic Nerve			
	Q　Sacral Plexus			
	R　Sacral Nerve			
	Y　Peripheral Nerve			

Ø: Medical and Surgical
2: Heart and Great Vessels

Operation–Character 3	Body Part–Character 4	Approach–Character 5	Device–Character 6	Qualifier–Character 7
1 Bypass	Ø Coronary Artery, One Site	Ø Open	Ø Monitoring Device, Pressure Sensor	Ø Allogeneic
5 Destruction	1 Coronary Artery, Two Sites	3 Percutaneous	2 Monitoring Device	1 Syngeneic
7 Dilation	2 Coronary Artery, Three Sites	4 Percutaneous Endoscopic	3 Infusion Device	2 Zooplastic
8 Division	3 Coronary Artery, Four or More Sites	X External	4 Intraluminal Device, Drug-eluting	3 Coronary Artery
B Excision	4 Coronary Vein		7 Autologous Tissue Substitute	4 Coronary Vein
C Extirpation	5 Atrial Septum		8 Zooplastic Tissue	5 Coronary Circulation
F Fragmentation	6 Atrium, Right		9 Autologous Venous Tissue	6 Bifurcation
H Insertion	7 Atrium, Left		A Autologous Arterial Tissue	7 Atrium, Left
J Inspection	8 Conduction Mechanism		C Extraluminal Device	8 Internal Mammary, Right
K Map	9 Chordae Tendineae		D Intraluminal Device	9 Internal Mammary, Left
L Occlusion	A Heart		J Synthetic Substitute OR Cardiac Lead, Pacemaker (for root operation INSERTION only)	A Pacemaker Lead
N Release	B Heart, Right		K Nonautologous Tissue Substitute OR Cardiac Lead, Defibrillator (for root operation INSERTION only)	B Subclavian
P Removal	C Heart, Left		M Cardiac Lead	C Thoracic Artery
Q Repair	D Papillary Muscle		Q Implantable Heart Assist System	D Carotid
R Replacement	F Aortic Valve		R External Heart Assist System	E Defibrillator Lead
S Reposition	G Mitral Valve		T Intraluminal Device, Radioactive	F Abdominal Artery
T Resection	H Pulmonary Valve		Z No Device	G Pressure Sensor
U Supplement	J Tricuspid Valve			H Transapical
V Restriction	K Ventricle, Right			J Temporary
W Revision	L Ventricle, Left			K Left Atrial Appendage
Y Transplantation	M Ventricular Septum			P Pulmonary Trunk
	N Pericardium			Q Pulmonary Artery, Right
	P Pulmonary Trunk			R Pulmonary Artery, Left
	Q Pulmonary Artery, Right			S Biventricular
	R Pulmonary Artery, Left			T Ductus Arteriosus
	S Pulmonary Vein, Right			W Aorta
	T Pulmonary Vein, Left			X Diagnostic
	V Superior Vena Cava			Z No Qualifier
	W Thoracic Aorta			
	Y Great Vessel			

Ø: Medical and Surgical

3: Upper Arteries

Operation–Character 3	Body Part–Character 4	Approach–Character 5	Device–Character 6	Qualifier–Character 7
1 Bypass	Ø Internal Mammary Artery, Right	Ø Open	Ø Drainage Device	Ø Upper Arm Artery, Right
5 Destruction	1 Internal Mammary Artery, Left	3 Percutaneous	2 Monitoring Device	1 Upper Arm Artery, Left
7 Dilation	2 Innominate Artery	4 Percutaneous Endoscopic	3 Infusion Device	2 Upper Arm Artery, Bilateral
9 Drainage	3 Subclavian Artery, Right	X External	4 Intraluminal Device, Drug-eluting	3 Lower Arm Artery, Right
B Excision	4 Subclavian Artery, Left		7 Autologous Tissue Substitute	4 Lower Arm Artery, Left
C Extirpation	5 Axillary Artery, Right		9 Autologous Venous Tissue	5 Lower Arm Artery, Bilateral
H Insertion	6 Axillary Artery, Left		A Autologous Arterial Tissue	6 Upper Leg Artery, Right
J Inspection	7 Brachial Artery, Right		B Intraluminal Device, Bioactive	7 Upper Leg Artery, Left
L Occlusion	8 Brachial Artery, Left		C Extraluminal Device	8 Upper Leg Artery, Bilateral
N Release	9 Ulnar Artery, Right		D Intraluminal Device	9 Lower Leg Artery, Right
P Removal	A Ulnar Artery, Left		J Synthetic Substitute	B Lower Leg Artery, Left
Q Repair	B Radial Artery, Right		K Nonautologous Tissue Substitute	C Lower Leg Artery, Bilateral
R Replacement	C Radial Artery, Left		M Stimulator Lead	D Upper Arm Vein
S Reposition	D Hand Artery, Right		Z No Device	F Lower Arm Vein
U Supplement	F Hand Artery, Left			G Intracranial Artery
V Restriction	G Intracranial Artery			J Extracranial Artery, Right
W Revision	H Common Carotid Artery, Right			K Extracranial Artery, Left
	J Common Carotid Artery, Left			M Pulmonary Artery, Right
	K Internal Carotid Artery, Right			N Pulmonary Artery, Left
	L Internal Carotid Artery, Left			X Diagnostic
	M External Carotid Artery, Right			Z No Qualifier
	N External Carotid Artery, Left			
	P Vertebral Artery, Right			
	Q Vertebral Artery, Left			
	R Face Artery			
	S Temporal Artery, Right			
	T Temporal Artery, Left			
	U Thyroid Artery, Right			
	V Thyroid Artery, Left			
	Y Upper Artery			

Ø: Medical and Surgical

4: Lower Arteries

Operation–Character 3	Body Part–Character 4	Approach–Character 5	Device–Character 6	Qualifier–Character 7
1 Bypass	Ø Abdominal Aorta	Ø Open	Ø Drainage Device	Ø Abdominal Aorta
5 Destruction	1 Celiac Artery	3 Percutaneous	1 Radioactive Element	1 Celiac Artery
7 Dilation	2 Gastric Artery	4 Percutaneous Endoscopic	2 Monitoring Device	2 Mesenteric Artery
9 Drainage	3 Hepatic Artery	X External	3 Infusion Device	3 Renal Artery, Right
B Excision	4 Splenic Artery		4 Intraluminal Device, Drug-eluting	4 Renal Artery, Left
C Extirpation	5 Superior Mesenteric Artery		7 Autologous Tissue Substitute	5 Renal Artery, Bilateral
H Insertion	6 Colic Artery, Right		9 Autologous Venous Tissue	6 Common Iliac Artery, Right
J Inspection	7 Colic Artery, Left		A Autologous Arterial Tissue	7 Common Iliac Artery, Left
L Occlusion	8 Colic Artery, Middle		C Extraluminal Device	8 Common Iliac Arteries, Bilateral
N Release	9 Renal Artery, Right		D Intraluminal Device	9 Internal Iliac Artery, Right
P Removal	A Renal Artery, Left		J Synthetic Substitute	B Internal Iliac Artery, Left
Q Repair	B Inferior Mesenteric Artery		K Nonautologous Tissue Substitute	C Internal Iliac Arteries, Bilateral
R Replacement	C Common Iliac Artery, Right		Z No Device	D External Iliac Artery, Right
S Reposition	D Common Iliac Artery, Left			F External Iliac Artery, Left
U Supplement	E Internal Iliac Artery, Right			G External Iliac Arteries, Bilateral
V Restriction	F Internal Iliac Artery, Left			H Femoral Artery, Right
W Revision	H External Iliac Artery, Right			J Femoral Artery, Left OR Temporary (for root operation Restriction only)
	J External Iliac Artery, Left			K Femoral Arteries, Bilateral
	K Femoral Artery, Right			L Popliteal Artery
	L Femoral Artery, Left			M Peroneal Artery
	M Popliteal Artery, Right			N Posterior Tibial Artery
	N Popliteal Artery, Left			P Foot Artery
	P Anterior Tibial Artery, Right			Q Lower Extremity Artery
	Q Anterior Tibial Artery, Left			R Lower Artery
	R Posterior Tibial Artery, Right			S Lower Extremity Vein
	S Posterior Tibial Artery, Left			T Uterine Artery, Right
	T Peroneal Artery, Right			U Uterine Artery, Left
	U Peroneal Artery, Left			X Diagnostic
	V Foot Artery, Right			Z No Qualifier
	W Foot Artery, Left			
	Y Lower Artery			

Ø: Medical and Surgical

5: Upper Veins

Operation–Character 3	Body Part–Character 4	Approach–Character 5	Device–Character 6	Qualifier–Character 7
1 Bypass	Ø Azygos Vein	Ø Open	Ø Drainage Device	X Diagnostic
5 Destruction	1 Hemiazygos Vein	3 Percutaneous	2 Monitoring Device	Y Upper Vein
7 Dilation	3 Innominate Vein, Right	4 Percutaneous Endoscopic	3 Infusion Device	Z No Qualifier
9 Drainage	4 Innominate Vein, Left	X External	7 Autologous Tissue Substitute	
B Excision	5 Subclavian Vein, Right		9 Autologous Venous Tissue	
C Extirpation	6 Subclavian Vein, Left		A Autologous Arterial Tissue	
D Extraction	7 Axillary Vein, Right		C Extraluminal Device	
H Insertion	8 Axillary Vein, Left		D Intraluminal Device	
J Inspection	9 Brachial Vein, Right		J Synthetic Substitute	
L Occlusion	A Brachial Vein, Left		K Nonautologous Tissue Substitute	
N Release	B Basilic Vein, Right		Z No Device	
P Removal	C Basilic Vein, Left			
Q Repair	D Cephalic Vein, Right			
R Replacement	F Cephalic Vein, Left			
S Reposition	G Hand Vein, Right			
U Supplement	H Hand Vein, Left			
V Restriction	L Intracranial Vein			
W Revision	M Internal Jugular Vein, Right			
	N Internal Jugular Vein, Left			
	P External Jugular Vein, Right			
	Q External Jugular Vein, Left			
	R Vertebral Vein, Right			
	S Vertebral Vein, Left			
	T Face Vein, Right			
	V Face Vein, Left			
	Y Upper Vein			

Ø: Medical and Surgical

6: Lower Veins

Operation–Character 3	Body Part–Character 4	Approach–Character 5	Device–Character 6	Qualifier–Character 7
1 Bypass	Ø Inferior Vena Cava	Ø Open	Ø Drainage Device	5 Superior Mesenteric Vein
5 Destruction	1 Splenic Vein	3 Percutaneous	2 Monitoring Device	6 Inferior Mesenteric Vein
7 Dilation	2 Gastric Vein	4 Percutaneous Endoscopic	3 Infusion Device	9 Renal Vein, Right
9 Drainage	3 Esophageal Vein	X External	7 Autologous Tissue Substitute	B Renal Vein, Left
B Excision	4 Hepatic Vein		9 Autologous Venous Tissue	C Hemorrhoidal Plexus
C Extirpation	5 Superior Mesenteric Vein		A Autologous Arterial Tissue	T Via Umbilical Vein
D Extraction	6 Inferior Mesenteric Vein		C Extraluminal Device	X Diagnostic
H Insertion	7 Colic Vein		D Intraluminal Device	Y Lower Vein
J Inspection	8 Portal Vein		J Synthetic Substitute	Z No Qualifier
L Occlusion	9 Renal Vein, Right		K Nonautologous Tissue Substitute	
N Release	B Renal Vein, Left		Z No Device	
P Removal	C Common Iliac Vein, Right			
Q Repair	D Common Iliac Vein, Left			
R Replacement	F External Iliac Vein, Right			
S Reposition	G External Iliac Vein, Left			
U Supplement	H Hypogastric Vein, Right			
V Restriction	J Hypogastric Vein, Left			
W Revision	M Femoral Vein, Right			
	N Femoral Vein, Left			
	P Greater Saphenous Vein, Right			
	Q Greater Saphenous Vein, Left			
	R Lesser Saphenous Vein, Right			
	S Lesser Saphenous Vein, Left			
	T Foot Vein, Right			
	V Foot Vein, Left			
	Y Lower Vein			

Ø: Medical and Surgical
7: Lymphatic and Hemic Systems*

Operation–Character 3	Body Part–Character 4	Approach–Character 5	Device–Character 6	Qualifier–Character 7
2 Change	Ø Lymphatic, Head	Ø Open	Ø Drainage Device	Ø Allogeneic
5 Destruction	1 Lymphatic, Right Neck	3 Percutaneous	3 Infusion Device	1 Syngeneic
9 Drainage	2 Lymphatic, Left Neck	4 Percutaneous Endoscopic	7 Autologous Tissue Substitute	2 Zooplastic
B Excision	3 Lymphatic, Right Upper Extremity	X External	C Extraluminal Device	X Diagnostic
C Extirpation	4 Lymphatic, Left Upper Extremity		D Intraluminal Device	Z No Qualifier
D Extraction	5 Lymphatic, Right Axillary		J Synthetic Substitute	
H Insertion	6 Lymphatic, Left Axillary		K Nonautologous Tissue Substitute	
J Inspection	7 Lymphatic, Thorax		Y Other Device	
L Occlusion	8 Lymphatic, Internal Mammary, Right		Z No Device	
N Release	9 Lymphatic, Internal Mammary, Left			
P Removal	B Lymphatic, Mesenteric			
Q Repair	C Lymphatic, Pelvis			
S Reposition	D Lymphatic, Aortic			
T Resection	F Lymphatic, Right Lower Extremity			
U Supplement	G Lymphatic, Left Lower Extremity			
V Restriction	H Lymphatic, Right Inguinal			
W Revision	J Lymphatic, Left Inguinal			
Y Transplantation	K Thoracic Duct			
	L Cisterna Chyli			
	M Thymus			
	N Lymphatic			
	P Spleen			
	Q Bone Marrow, Sternum			
	R Bone Marrow, Iliac			
	S Bone Marrow, Vertebral			
	T Bone Marrow			

* Includes lymph vessels and lymph nodes.

Ø: Medical and Surgical

8: Eye

Operation–Character 3	Body Part–Character 4	Approach–Character 5	Device–Character 6	Qualifier–Character 7
Ø Alteration	Ø Eye, Right	Ø Open	Ø Drainage Device OR Synthetic Substitute, Intraocular Telescope (for root operation REPLACEMENT only)	3 Nasal Cavity
1 Bypass	1 Eye, Left	3 Percutaneous	1 Radioactive Element	4 Sclera
2 Change	2 Anterior Chamber, Right	7 Via Natural or Artificial Opening	3 Infusion Device	X Diagnostic
5 Destruction	3 Anterior Chamber, Left	8 Via Natural or Artificial Opening Endoscopic	5 Epiretinal Visual Prosthesis	Z No Qualifier
7 Dilation	4 Vitreous, Right	X External	7 Autologous Tissue Substitute	
9 Drainage	5 Vitreous, Left		C Extraluminal Device	
B Excision	6 Sclera, Right		D Intraluminal Device	
C Extirpation	7 Sclera, Left		J Synthetic Substitute	
D Extraction	8 Cornea, Right		K Nonautologous Tissue Substitute	
F Fragmentation	9 Cornea, Left		Y Other Device	
H Insertion	A Choroid, Right		Z No Device	
J Inspection	B Choroid, Left			
L Occlusion	C Iris, Right			
M Reattachment	D Iris, Left			
N Release	E Retina, Right			
P Removal	F Retina, Left			
Q Repair	G Retinal Vessel, Right			
R Replacement	H Retinal Vessel, Left			
S Reposition	J Lens, Right			
T Resection	K Lens, Left			
U Supplement	L Extraocular Muscle, Right			
V Restriction	M Extraocular Muscle, Left			
W Revision	N Upper Eyelid, Right			
X Transfer	P Upper Eyelid, Left			
	Q Lower Eyelid, Right			
	R Lower Eyelid, Left			
	S Conjunctiva, Right			
	T Conjunctiva, Left			
	V Lacrimal Gland, Right			
	W Lacrimal Gland, Left			
	X Lacrimal Duct, Right			
	Y Lacrimal Duct, Left			

Ø: Medical and Surgical
9: Ear, Nose, Sinus*

Operation–Character 3	Body Part–Character 4	Approach–Character 5	Device–Character 6	Qualifier–Character 7
Ø Alteration	Ø External Ear, Right	Ø Open	Ø Drainage Device	Ø Endolymphatic
1 Bypass	1 External Ear, Left	3 Percutaneous	4 Hearing Device, Bone Conduction	X Diagnostic
2 Change	2 External Ear, Bilateral	4 Percutaneous Endoscopic	5 Hearing Device, Single Channel Cochlear Prosthesis	Z No Qualifier
5 Destruction	3 External Auditory Canal, Right	7 Via Natural or Artificial Opening	6 Hearing Device, Multiple Channel Cochlear Prosthesis	
7 Dilation	4 External Auditory Canal, Left	8 Via Natural or Artificial Opening Endoscopic	7 Autologous Tissue Substitute	
8 Division	5 Middle Ear, Right	X External	B Intraluminal Device, Airway	
9 Drainage	6 Middle Ear, Left		D Intraluminal Device	
B Excision	7 Tympanic Membrane, Right		J Synthetic Substitute	
C Extirpation	8 Tympanic Membrane, Left		K Nonautologous Tissue Substitute	
D Extraction	9 Auditory Ossicle, Right		S Hearing Device	
H Insertion	A Auditory Ossicle, Left		Y Other Device	
J Inspection	B Mastoid Sinus, Right		Z No Device	
M Reattachment	C Mastoid Sinus, Left			
N Release	D Inner Ear, Right			
P Removal	E Inner Ear, Left			
Q Repair	F Eustachian Tube, Right			
R Replacement	G Eustachian Tube, Left			
S Reposition	H Ear, Right			
T Resection	J Ear, Left			
U Supplement	K Nose			
W Revision	L Nasal Turbinate			
	M Nasal Septum			
	N Nasopharynx			
	P Accessory Sinus			
	Q Maxillary Sinus, Right			
	R Maxillary Sinus, Left			
	S Frontal Sinus, Right			
	T Frontal Sinus, Left			
	U Ethmoid Sinus, Right			
	V Ethmoid Sinus, Left			
	W Sphenoid Sinus, Right			
	X Sphenoid Sinus, Left			
	Y Sinus			

* Includes sinus ducts.

Ø: Medical and Surgical

B: Respiratory System

Operation–Character 3	Body Part–Character 4	Approach–Character 5	Device–Character 6	Qualifier–Character 7
1 Bypass	Ø Tracheobronchial Tree	Ø Open	Ø Drainage Device	Ø Allogeneic
2 Change	1 Trachea	3 Percutaneous	1 Radioactive Element	1 Syngeneic
5 Destruction	2 Carina	4 Percutaneous Endoscopic	2 Monitoring Device	2 Zooplastic
7 Dilation	3 Main Bronchus, Right	7 Via Natural or Artificial Opening	3 Infusion Device	4 Cutaneous
9 Drainage	4 Upper Lobe Bronchus, Right	8 Via Natural or Artificial Opening Endoscopic	7 Autologous Tissue Substitute	6 Esophagus
B Excision	5 Middle Lobe Bronchus, Right	X External	C Extraluminal Device	X Diagnostic
C Extirpation	6 Lower Lobe Bronchus, Right		D Intraluminal Device	Z No Qualifier
D Extraction	7 Main Bronchus, Left		E Intraluminal Device, Endotracheal Airway	
F Fragmentation	8 Upper Lobe Bronchus, Left		F Tracheostomy Device	
H Insertion	9 Lingula Bronchus		G Intraluminal Endobronchial Valve	
J Inspection	B Lower Lobe Bronchus, Left		J Synthetic Substitute	
L Occlusion	C Upper Lung Lobe, Right		K Nonautologous Tissue Substitute	
M Reattachment	D Middle Lung Lobe, Right		M Diaphragmatic Pacemaker Lead	
N Release	F Lower Lung Lobe, Right		Y Other Device	
P Removal	G Upper Lung Lobe, Left		Z No Device	
Q Repair	H Lung Lingula			
S Reposition	J Lower Lung Lobe, Left			
T Resection	K Lung, Right			
U Supplement	L Lung, Left			
V Restriction	M Lungs, Bilateral			
W Revision	N Pleura, Right			
Y Transplantation	P Pleura, Left			
	Q Pleura			
	R Diaphragm, Right			
	S Diaphragm, Left			
	T Diaphragm			

Ø: Medical and Surgical
C: Mouth and Throat

Operation–Character 3	Body Part–Character 4	Approach–Character 5	Device–Character 6	Qualifier–Character 7
Ø Alteration	Ø Upper Lip	Ø Open	Ø Drainage Device	Ø Single
2 Change	1 Lower Lip	3 Percutaneous	1 Radioactive Element	1 Multiple
5 Destruction	2 Hard Palate	4 Percutaneous Endoscopic	5 External Fixation Device	2 All
7 Dilation	3 Soft Palate	7 Via Natural or Artificial Opening	7 Autologous Tissue Substitute	X Diagnostic
9 Drainage	4 Buccal Mucosa	8 Via Natural or Artificial Opening Endoscopic	B Intraluminal Device, Airway	Z No Qualifier
B Excision	5 Upper Gingiva	X External	C Extraluminal Device	
C Extirpation	6 Lower Gingiva		D Intraluminal Device	
D Extraction	7 Tongue		J Synthetic Substitute	
F Fragmentation	8 Parotid Gland, Right		K Nonautologous Tissue Substitute	
H Insertion	9 Parotid Gland, Left		Y Other Device	
J Inspection	A Salivary Gland		Z No Device	
L Occlusion	B Parotid Duct, Right			
M Reattachment	C Parotid Duct, Left			
N Release	D Sublingual Gland, Right			
P Removal	F Sublingual Gland, Left			
Q Repair	G Submaxillary Gland, Right			
R Replacement	H Submaxillary Gland, Left			
S Reposition	J Minor Salivary Gland			
T Resection	M Pharynx			
U Supplement	N Uvula			
V Restriction	P Tonsils			
W Revision	Q Adenoids			
X Transfer	R Epiglottis			
	S Larynx			
	T Vocal Cord, Right			
	V Vocal Cord, Left			
	W Upper Tooth			
	X Lower Tooth			
	Y Mouth and Throat			

Ø: Medical and Surgical
D: Gastrointestinal System

Operation–Character 3	Body Part–Character 4	Approach–Character 5	Device–Character 6	Qualifier–Character 7
1 Bypass	Ø Upper Intestinal Tract	Ø Open	Ø Drainage Device	Ø Allogeneic
2 Change	1 Esophagus, Upper	3 Percutaneous	1 Radioactive Element	1 Syngeneic
5 Destruction	2 Esophagus, Middle	4 Percutaneous Endoscopic	2 Monitoring Device	2 Zooplastic
7 Dilation	3 Esophagus, Lower	7 Via Natural or Artificial Opening	3 Infusion Device	3 Vertical
8 Division	4 Esophagogastric Junction	8 Via Natural or Artificial Opening Endoscopic	7 Autologous Tissue Substitute	4 Cutaneous
9 Drainage	5 Esophagus	X External	B Intraluminal Device, Airway	5 Esophagus
B Excision	6 Stomach		C Extraluminal Device	6 Stomach
C Extirpation	7 Stomach, Pylorus		D Intraluminal Device	9 Duodenum
F Fragmentation	8 Small Intestine		J Synthetic Substitute	A Jejunum
H Insertion	9 Duodenum		K Nonautologous Tissue Substitute	B Ileum
J Inspection	A Jejunum		L Artificial Sphincter	H Cecum
L Occlusion	B Ileum		M Stimulator Lead	K Ascending Colon
M Reattachment	C Ileocecal Valve		U Feeding Device	L Transverse Colon
N Release	D Lower Intestinal Tract		Y Other Device	M Descending Colon
P Removal	E Large Intestine		Z No Device	N Sigmoid Colon
Q Repair	F Large Intestine, Right			P Rectum
R Replacement	G Large Intestine, Left			Q Anus
S Reposition	H Cecum			X Diagnostic
T Resection	J Appendix			Z No Qualifier
U Supplement	K Ascending Colon			
V Restriction	L Transverse Colon			
W Revision	M Descending Colon			
X Transfer	N Sigmoid Colon			
Y Transplantation	P Rectum			
	Q Anus			
	R Anal Sphincter			
	S Greater Omentum			
	T Lesser Omentum			
	U Omentum			
	V Mesentery			
	W Peritoneum			

Ø: Medical and Surgical

F: Hepatobiliary System and Pancreas

Operation–Character 3	Body Part–Character 4	Approach–Character 5	Device–Character 6	Qualifier–Character 7
1 Bypass	Ø Liver	Ø Open	Ø Drainage Device	Ø Allogeneic
2 Change	1 Liver, Right Lobe	3 Percutaneous	1 Radioactive Element	1 Syngeneic
5 Destruction	2 Liver, Left Lobe	4 Percutaneous Endoscopic	2 Monitoring Device	2 Zooplastic
7 Dilation	4 Gallbladder	7 Via Natural or Artificial Opening	3 Infusion Device	3 Duodenum
8 Division	5 Hepatic Duct, Right	8 Via Natural or Artificial Opening Endoscopic	7 Autologous Tissue Substitute	4 Stomach
9 Drainage	6 Hepatic Duct, Left	X External	C Extraluminal Device	5 Hepatic Duct, Right
B Excision	8 Cystic Duct		D Intraluminal Device	6 Hepatic Duct, Left
C Extirpation	9 Common Bile Duct		J Synthetic Substitute	7 Hepatic Duct, Caudate
F Fragmentation	B Hepatobiliary Duct		K Nonautologous Tissue Substitute	8 Cystic Duct
H Insertion	C Ampulla of Vater		Y Other Device	9 Common Bile Duct
J Inspection	D Pancreatic Duct		Z No Device	B Small Intestine
L Occlusion	F Pancreatic Duct, Accessory			C Large Intestine
M Reattachment	G Pancreas			X Diagnostic
N Release				Z No Qualifier
P Removal				
Q Repair				
R Replacement				
S Reposition				
T Resection				
U Supplement				
V Restriction				
W Revision				
Y Transplantation				

Ø: Medical and Surgical

G: Endocrine System

Operation–Character 3	Body Part–Character 4	Approach–Character 5	Device–Character 6	Qualifier–Character 7
2 Change	Ø Pituitary Gland	Ø Open	Ø Drainage Device	X Diagnostic
5 Destruction	1 Pineal Body	3 Percutaneous	2 Monitoring Device	Z No Qualifier
8 Division	2 Adrenal Gland, Left	4 Percutaneous Endoscopic	3 Infusion Device	
9 Drainage	3 Adrenal Gland, Right	X External	Y Other Device	
B Excision	4 Adrenal Glands, Bilateral		Z No Device	
C Extirpation	5 Adrenal Gland			
H Insertion	6 Carotid Body, Left			
J Inspection	7 Carotid Body, Right			
M Reattachment	8 Carotid Bodies, Bilateral			
N Release	9 Para-aortic Body			
P Removal	B Coccygeal Glomus			
Q Repair	C Glomus Jugulare			
S Reposition	D Aortic Body			
T Resection	F Paraganglion Extremity			
W Revision	G Thyroid Gland Lobe, Left			
	H Thyroid Gland Lobe, Right			
	J Thyroid Gland Isthmus			
	K Thyroid Gland			
	L Superior Parathyroid Gland, Right			
	M Superior Parathyroid Gland, Left			
	N Inferior Parathyroid Gland, Right			
	P Inferior Parathyroid Gland, Left			
	Q Parathyroid Glands, Multiple			
	R Parathyroid Gland			
	S Endocrine Gland			

Ø: Medical and Surgical

H: Skin and Breast*

Operation–Character 3	Body Part–Character 4	Approach–Character 5	Device–Character 6	Qualifier–Character 7
Ø Alteration	Ø Skin, Scalp	Ø Open	Ø Drainage Device	3 Full Thickness
2 Change	1 Skin, Face	3 Percutaneous	1 Radioactive Element	4 Partial Thickness
5 Destruction	2 Skin, Right Ear	7 Via Natural or Artificial Opening	7 Autologous Tissue Substitute	5 Latissimus Dorsi Myocutaneous Flap
8 Division	3 Skin, Left Ear	8 Via Natural or Artificial Opening Endoscopic	J Synthetic Substitute	6 Transverse Rectus Abdominis Myocutaneous Flap
9 Drainage	4 Skin, Neck	X External	K Nonautologous Tissue Substitute	7 Deep Inferior Epigastric Artery Perforator Flap
B Excision	5 Skin, Chest		N Tissue Expander	8 Superficial Inferior Epigastric Artery Flap
C Extirpation	6 Skin, Back		Y Other Device	9 Gluteal Artery Perforator Flap
D Extraction	7 Skin, Abdomen		Z No Device	D Multiple
H Insertion	8 Skin, Buttock			X Diagnostic
J Inspection	9 Skin, Perineum			Z No Qualifier
M Reattachment	A Skin, Genitalia			
N Release	B Skin, Right Upper Arm			
P Removal	C Skin, Left Upper Arm			
Q Repair	D Skin, Right Lower Arm			
R Replacement	E Skin, Left Lower Arm			
S Reposition	F Skin, Right Hand			
T Resection	G Skin, Left Hand			
U Supplement	H Skin, Right Upper Leg			
W Revision	J Skin, Left Upper Leg			
X Transfer	K Skin, Right Lower Leg			
	L Skin, Left Lower Leg			
	M Skin, Right Foot			
	N Skin, Left Foot			
	P Skin			
	Q Finger Nail			
	R Toe Nail			
	S Hair			
	T Breast, Right			
	U Breast, Left			
	V Breast, Bilateral			
	W Nipple, Right			
	X Nipple, Left			
	Y Supernumerary Breast			

* Includes skin and breast glands and ducts.

Ø: Medical and Surgical
J: Subcutaneous Tissue and Fascia

Operation–Character 3	Body Part–Character 4	Approach–Character 5	Device–Character 6	Qualifier–Character 7
Ø Alteration	Ø Subcutaneous Tissue and Fascia, Scalp	Ø Open	Ø Monitoring Device, Hemodynamic	B Skin and Subcutaneous Tissue
2 Change	1 Subcutaneous Tissue and Fascia, Face	3 Percutaneous	1 Radioactive Element	C Skin, Subcutaneous Tissue and Fascia
5 Destruction	4 Subcutaneous Tissue and Fascia, Anterior Neck	X External	2 Monitoring Device	X Diagnostic
8 Division	5 Subcutaneous Tissue and Fascia, Posterior Neck		3 Infusion Device	Z No Qualifier
9 Drainage	6 Subcutaneous Tissue and Fascia, Chest		4 Pacemaker, Single Chamber	
B Excision	7 Subcutaneous Tissue and Fascia, Back		5 Pacemaker, Single Chamber Rate Responsive	
C Extirpation	8 Subcutaneous Tissue and Fascia, Abdomen		6 Pacemaker, Dual Chamber	
D Extraction	9 Subcutaneous Tissue and Fascia, Buttock		7 Autologous Tissue Substitute OR Cardiac Resynchronization Pacemaker Pulse Generator (for root operation INSERTION only)	
H Insertion	B Subcutaneous Tissue and Fascia, Perineum		8 Defibrillator Generator	
J Inspection	C Subcutaneous Tissue and Fascia, Pelvic Region		9 Cardiac Resynchronization Defibrillator Pulse Generator	
N Release	D Subcutaneous Tissue and Fascia, Right Upper Arm		A Contractility Modulation Device	
P Removal	F Subcutaneous Tissue and Fascia, Left Upper Arm		B Stimulator Generator, Single Array	
Q Repair	G Subcutaneous Tissue and Fascia, Right Lower Arm		C Stimulator Generator, Single Array Rechargeable	
R Replacement	H Subcutaneous Tissue and Fascia, Left Lower Arm		D Stimulator Generator, Multiple Array	
U Supplement	J Subcutaneous Tissue and Fascia, Right Hand		E Stimulator Generator, Multiple Array Rechargea	
W Revision	K Subcutaneous Tissue and Fascia, Left Hand		H Contraceptive Device	
X Transfer	L Subcutaneous Tissue and Fascia, Right Upper Leg		J Synthetic Substitute	
	M Subcutaneous Tissue and Fascia, Left Upper Leg		K Nonautologous Tissue Substitute	
	N Subcutaneous Tissue and Fascia, Right Lower Leg		M Stimulator Generator	
	P Subcutaneous Tissue and Fascia, Left Lower Leg		N Tissue Expander	
	Q Subcutaneous Tissue and Fascia, Right Foot		P Cardiac Rhythm Related Device	
	R Subcutaneous Tissue and Fascia, Left Foot		V Infusion Pump	
	S Subcutaneous Tissue and Fascia, Head and Neck		W Reservoir	
	T Subcutaneous Tissue and Fascia, Trunk		X Vascular Access Device	
	V Subcutaneous Tissue and Fascia, Upper Extremity		Y Other Device	
	W Subcutaneous Tissue and Fascia, Lower Extremity		Z No Device	

Ø: Medical and Surgical

K: Muscles

Operation–Character 3	Body Part–Character 4	Approach–Character 5	Device–Character 6	Qualifier–Character 7
2 Change	Ø Head Muscle	Ø Open	Ø Drainage Device	Ø Skin
5 Destruction	1 Facial Muscle	3 Percutaneous	7 Autologous Tissue Substitute	1 Subcutaneous Tissue
8 Division	2 Neck Muscle, Right	4 Percutaneous Endoscopic	J Synthetic Substitute	2 Skin and Subcutaneous Tissue
9 Drainage	3 Neck Muscle, Left	X External	K Nonautologous Tissue Substitute	6 Transverse Rectus Abdominis Myocutaneous Flap
B Excision	4 Tongue, Palate, Pharynx Muscle		M Stimulator Lead	X Diagnostic
C Extirpation	5 Shoulder Muscle, Right		Y Other Device	Z No Qualifier
H Insertion	6 Shoulder Muscle, Left		Z No Device	
J Inspection	7 Upper Arm Muscle, Right			
M Reattachment	8 Upper Arm Muscle, Left			
N Release	9 Lower Arm and Wrist Muscle, Right			
P Removal	B Lower Arm and Wrist Muscle, Left			
Q Repair	C Hand Muscle, Right			
S Reposition	D Hand Muscle, Left			
T Resection	F Trunk Muscle, Right			
U Supplement	G Trunk Muscle, Left			
W Revision	H Thorax Muscle, Right			
X Transfer	J Thorax Muscle, Left			
	K Abdomen Muscle, Right			
	L Abdomen Muscle, Left			
	M Perineum Muscle			
	N Hip Muscle, Right			
	P Hip Muscle, Left			
	Q Upper Leg Muscle, Right			
	R Upper Leg Muscle, Left			
	S Lower Leg Muscle, Right			
	T Lower Leg Muscle, Left			
	V Foot Muscle, Right			
	W Foot Muscle, Left			
	X Upper Muscle			
	Y Lower Muscle			

Ø: Medical and Surgical
L: Tendons*

Operation–Character 3	Body Part–Character 4	Approach–Character 5	Device–Character 6	Qualifier–Character 7
2　Change	Ø　Head and Neck Tendon	Ø　Open	Ø　Drainage Device	X　Diagnostic
5　Destruction	1　Shoulder Tendon, Right	3　Percutaneous	7　Autologous Tissue Substitute	Z　No Qualifier
8　Division	2　Shoulder Tendon, Left	4　Percutaneous Endoscopic	J　Synthetic Substitute	
9　Drainage	3　Upper Arm Tendon, Right	X　External	K　Nonautologous Tissue Substitute	
B　Excision	4　Upper Arm Tendon, Left		Y　Other Device	
C　Extirpation	5　Lower Arm and Wrist Tendon, Right		Z　No Device	
J　Inspection	6　Lower Arm and Wrist Tendon, Left			
M　Reattachment	7　Hand Tendon, Right			
N　Release	8　Hand Tendon, Left			
P　Removal	9　Trunk Tendon, Right			
Q　Repair	B　Trunk Tendon, Left			
R　Replacement	C　Thorax Tendon, Right			
S　Reposition	D　Thorax Tendon, Left			
T　Resection	F　Abdomen Tendon, Right			
U　Supplement	G　Abdomen Tendon, Left			
W　Revision	H　Perineum Tendon			
X　Transfer	J　Hip Tendon, Right			
	K　Hip Tendon, Left			
	L　Upper Leg Tendon, Right			
	M　Upper Leg Tendon, Left			
	N　Lower Leg Tendon, Right			
	P　Lower Leg Tendon, Left			
	Q　Knee Tendon, Right			
	R　Knee Tendon, Left			
	S　Ankle Tendon, Right			
	T　Ankle Tendon, Left			
	V　Foot Tendon, Right			
	W　Foot Tendon, Left			
	X　Upper Tendon			
	Y　Lower Tendon			

* Includes synovial membrane.

Ø: Medical and Surgical

M: Bursae and Ligaments*

Operation–Character 3	Body Part–Character 4	Approach–Character 5	Device–Character 6	Qualifier–Character 7
2 Change	Ø Head and Neck Bursa and Ligament	Ø Open	Ø Drainage Device	X Diagnostic
5 Destruction	1 Shoulder Bursa and Ligament, Right	3 Percutaneous	7 Autologous Tissue Substitute	Z No Qualifier
8 Division	2 Shoulder Bursa and Ligament, Left	4 Percutaneous Endoscopic	J Synthetic Substitute	
9 Drainage	3 Elbow Bursa and Ligament, Right	X External	K Nonautologous Tissue Substitute	
B Excision	4 Elbow Bursa and Ligament, Left		Y Other Device	
C Extirpation	5 Wrist Bursa and Ligament, Right		Z No Device	
D Extraction	6 Wrist Bursa and Ligament, Left			
J Inspection	7 Hand Bursa and Ligament, Right			
M Reattachment	8 Hand Bursa and Ligament, Left			
N Release	9 Upper Extremity Bursa and Ligament, Right			
P Removal	B Upper Extremity Bursa and Ligament, Left			
Q Repair	C Trunk Bursa and Ligament, Right			
S Reposition	D Trunk Bursa and Ligament, Left			
T Resection	F Thorax Bursa and Ligament, Right			
U Supplement	G Thorax Bursa and Ligament, Left			
W Revision	H Abdomen Bursa and Ligament, Right			
X Transfer	J Abdomen Bursa and Ligament, Left			
	K Perineum Bursa and Ligament			
	L Hip Bursa and Ligament, Right			
	M Hip Bursa and Ligament, Left			
	N Knee Bursa and Ligament, Right			
	P Knee Bursa and Ligament, Left			
	Q Ankle Bursa and Ligament, Right			
	R Ankle Bursa and Ligament, Left			
	S Foot Bursa and Ligament, Right			
	T Foot Bursa and Ligament, Left			
	V Lower Extremity Bursa and Ligament, Right			
	W Lower Extremity Bursa and Ligament, Left			
	X Upper Bursa and Ligament			
	Y Lower Bursa and Ligament			

* Includes synovial membrane.

Ø: Medical and Surgical
N: Head and Facial Bones

Operation–Character 3	Body Part–Character 4	Approach–Character 5	Device–Character 6	Qualifier–Character 7
2 Change	Ø Skull	Ø Open	Ø Drainage Device	X Diagnostic
5 Destruction	1 Frontal Bone, Right	3 Percutaneous	4 Internal Fixation Device	Z No Qualifier
8 Division	2 Frontal Bone, Left	4 Percutaneous Endoscopic	5 External Fixation Device	
9 Drainage	3 Parietal Bone, Right	X External	7 Autologous Tissue Substitute	
B Excision	4 Parietal Bone, Left		J Synthetic Substitute	
C Extirpation	5 Temporal Bone, Right		K Nonautologous Tissue Substitute	
H Insertion	6 Temporal Bone, Left		M Bone Growth Stimulator	
J Inspection	7 Occipital Bone, Right		N Neurostimulator Generator	
N Release	8 Occipital Bone, Left		S Hearing Device	
P Removal	B Nasal Bone		Y Other Device	
Q Repair	C Sphenoid Bone, Right		Z No Device	
R Replacement	D Sphenoid Bone, Left			
S Reposition	F Ethmoid Bone, Right			
T Resection	G Ethmoid Bone, Left			
U Supplement	H Lacrimal Bone, Right			
W Revision	J Lacrimal Bone, Left			
	K Palatine Bone, Right			
	L Palatine Bone, Left			
	M Zygomatic Bone, Right			
	N Zygomatic Bone, Left			
	P Orbit, Right			
	Q Orbit, Left			
	R Maxilla, Right			
	S Maxilla, Left			
	T Mandible, Right			
	V Mandible, Left			
	W Facial Bone			
	X Hyoid Bone			

Ø: Medical and Surgical

P: Upper Bones

Operation–Character 3	Body Part–Character 4	Approach–Character 5	Device–Character 6	Qualifier–Character 7
2 Change	Ø Sternum	Ø Open	Ø Drainage Device OR Internal Fixation Device, Rigid Plate (for root operation INSERTION only)	X Diagnostic
5 Destruction	1 Rib, Right	3 Percutaneous	4 Internal Fixation Device	Z No Qualifier
8 Division	2 Rib, Left	4 Percutaneous Endoscopic	5 External Fixation Device	
9 Drainage	3 Cervical Vertebra	X External	6 Internal Fixation Device, Intramedullary	
B Excision	4 Thoracic Vertebra		7 Autologous Tissue Substitute	
C Extirpation	5 Scapula, Right		8 External Fixation Device, Limb Lengthening	
H Insertion	6 Scapula, Left		B External Fixation Device, Monoplanar	
J Inspection	7 Glenoid Cavity, Right		C External Fixation Device, Ring	
N Release	8 Glenoid Cavity, Left		D External Fixation Device, Hybrid	
P Removal	9 Clavicle, Right		J Synthetic Substitute	
Q Repair	B Clavicle, Left		K Nonautologous Tissue Substitute	
R Replacement	C Humeral Head, Right		M Bone Growth Stimulator	
S Reposition	D Humeral Head, Left		Y Other Device	
T Resection	F Humeral Shaft, Right		Z No Device	
U Supplement	G Humeral Shaft, Left			
W Revision	H Radius, Right			
	J Radius, Left			
	K Ulna, Right			
	L Ulna, Left			
	M Carpal, Right			
	N Carpal, Left			
	P Metacarpal, Right			
	Q Metacarpal, Left			
	R Thumb Phalanx, Right			
	S Thumb Phalanx, Left			
	T Finger Phalanx, Right			
	V Finger Phalanx, Left			
	Y Upper Bone			

Ø: Medical and Surgical

Q: Lower Bones

Operation–Character 3	Body Part–Character 4	Approach–Character 5	Device–Character 6	Qualifier–Character 7
2 Change	Ø Lumbar Vertebra	Ø Open	Ø Drainage Device	X Diagnostic
5 Destruction	1 Sacrum	3 Percutaneous	4 Internal Fixation Device	Z No Qualifier
8 Division	2 Pelvic Bone, Right	4 Percutaneous Endoscopic	5 External Fixation Device	
9 Drainage	3 Pelvic Bone, Left	X External	6 Internal Fixation Device, Intramedullary	
B Excision	4 Acetabulum, Right		7 Autologous Tissue Substitute	
C Extirpation	5 Acetabulum, Left		8 External Fixation Device, Limb Lengthening	
H Insertion	6 Upper Femur, Right		B External Fixation Device, Monoplanar	
J Inspection	7 Upper Femur, Left		C External Fixation Device, Ring	
N Release	8 Femoral Shaft, Right		D External Fixation Device, Hybrid	
P Removal	9 Femoral Shaft, Left		J Synthetic Substitute	
Q Repair	B Lower Femur, Right		K Nonautologous Tissue Substitute	
R Replacement	C Lower Femur, Left		M Bone Growth Stimulator	
S Reposition	D Patella, Right		Y Other Device	
T Resection	F Patella, Left		Z No Device	
U Supplement	G Tibia, Right			
W Revision	H Tibia, Left			
	J Fibula, Right			
	K Fibula, Left			
	L Tarsal, Right			
	M Tarsal, Left			
	N Metatarsal, Right			
	P Metatarsal, Left			
	Q Toe Phalanx, Right			
	R Toe Phalanx, Left			
	S Coccyx			
	Y Lower Bone			

Ø: Medical and Surgical

R: Upper Joints*

Operation–Character 3	Body Part–Character 4	Approach–Character 5	Device–Character 6	Qualifier–Character 7
2 Change	Ø Occipital-cervical Joint	Ø Open	Ø Drainage Device OR Synthetic Substitute, Reverse Ball and Socket (for root operation REPLACEMENT only)	Ø Anterior Approach, Anterior Column
5 Destruction	1 Cervical Vertebral Joint	3 Percutaneous	3 Infusion Device	1 Posterior Approach, Posterior Column
9 Drainage	2 Cervical Vertebral Joint, 2 or more	4 Percutaneous Endoscopic	4 Internal Fixation Device	6 Humeral Surface
B Excision	3 Cervical Vertebral Disc	X External	5 External Fixation Device	7 Glenoid Surface
C Extirpation	4 Cervicothoracic Vertebral Joint		7 Autologous Tissue Substitute	J Posterior Approach, Anterior Column
G Fusion	5 Cervicothoracic Vertebral Disc		8 Spacer	X Diagnostic
H Insertion	6 Thoracic Vertebral Joint		A Interbody Fusion Device	Z No Qualifier
J Inspection	7 Thoracic Vertebral Joint, 2 to 7		B Spinal Stabilization Device, Interspinous Process	
N Release	8 Thoracic Vertebral Joint, 8 or more		C Spinal Stabilization Device, Pedicle-Based	
P Removal	9 Thoracic Vertebral Disc		D Spinal Stabilization Device, Facet Replacement	
Q Repair	A Thoracolumbar Vertebral Joint		J Synthetic Substitute	
R Replacement	B Thoracolumbar Vertebral Disc		K Nonautologous Tissue Substitute	
S Reposition	C Temporomandibular Joint, Right		Y Other Device	
T Resection	D Temporomandibular Joint, Left		Z No Device	
U Supplement	E Sternoclavicular Joint, Right			
W Revision	F Sternoclavicular Joint, Left			
	G Acromioclavicular Joint, Right			
	H Acromioclavicular Joint, Left			
	J Shoulder Joint, Right			
	K Shoulder Joint, Left			
	L Elbow Joint, Right			
	M Elbow Joint, Left			
	N Wrist Joint, Right			
	P Wrist Joint, Left			
	Q Carpal Joint, Right			
	R Carpal Joint, Left			
	S Metacarpocarpal Joint, Right			
	T Metacarpocarpal Joint, Left			
	U Metacarpophalangeal Joint, Right			
	V Metacarpophalangeal Joint, Left			
	W Finger Phalangeal Joint, Right			
	X Finger Phalangeal Joint, Left			
	Y Upper Joint			

* Includes synovial membrane.

Ø: Medical and Surgical

S: Lower Joints*

Operation–Character 3	Body Part–Character 4	Approach–Character 5	Device–Character 6	Qualifier–Character 7
2 Change	Ø Lumbar Vertebral Joint	Ø Open	Ø Drainage Device OR Synthetic Substitute, Polyethylene (for root operation REPLACEMENT only)	Ø Anterior Approach, Anterior Column
5 Destruction	1 Lumbar Vertebral Joint, 2 or more	3 Percutaneous	1 Synthetic Substitute, Metal	1 Approach, Posterior Posterior Column
9 Drainage	2 Lumbar Vertebral Disc	4 Percutaneous Endoscopic	2 Synthetic Substitute, Metal on Polyethylene	9 Cemented
B Excision	3 Lumbosacral Joint	X External	3 Infusion Device OR Synthetic Substitute, Ceramic (for root operation REPLACEMENT only)	A Uncemented
C Extirpation	4 Lumbosacral Disc		4 Internal Fixation Device OR Synthetic Substitute, Ceramic on Polyethylene (for root operation REPLACEMENT only)	C Patellar Surface
G Fusion	5 Sacrococcygeal Joint		5 External Fixation Device	J Posterior Approach, Anterior Column
H Insertion	6 Coccygeal Joint		7 Autologous Tissue Substitute	X Diagnostic
J Inspection	7 Sacroiliac Joint, Right		8 Spacer	Z No Qualifier
N Release	8 Sacroiliac Joint, Left		9 Liner	
P Removal	9 Hip Joint, Right		A Interbody Fusion Device	
Q Repair	B Hip Joint, Left		B Resurfacing Device OR Spinal Stabilization Device, Interspinous Process (for root operation INSERTION only)	
R Replacement	C Knee Joint, Right		C Spinal Stabilization Device, Pedicle-Based	
S Reposition	D Knee Joint, Left		D Spinal Stabilization Device, Facet Replacement	
T Resection	F Ankle Joint, Right		J Synthetic Substitute	
U Supplement	G Ankle Joint, Left		K Nonautologous Tissue Substitute	

* Includes synovial membrane.

Operation–Character 3	Body Part–Character 4	Approach–Character 5	Device–Character 6	Qualifier–Character 7
W Revision	H Tarsal Joint, Right		Y Other Device	
	J Tarsal Joint, Left		Z No Device	
	K Metatarsal-Tarsal Joint, Right			
	L Metatarsal-Tarsal Joint, Left			
	M Metatarsal-Phalangeal Joint, Right			
	N Metatarsal-Phalangeal Joint, Left			
	P Toe Phalangeal Joint, Right			
	Q Toe Phalangeal Joint, Left			
	Y Lower Joint			

* Includes synovial membrane.

0: Medical and Surgical

T: Urinary System

Operation–Character 3	Body Part–Character 4	Approach–Character 5	Device–Character 6	Qualifier–Character 7
1 Bypass	0 Kidney, Right	0 Open	0 Drainage Device	0 Allogeneic
2 Change	1 Kidney, Left	3 Percutaneous	2 Monitoring Device	1 Syngeneic
5 Destruction	2 Kidneys, Bilateral	4 Percutaneous Endoscopic	3 Infusion Device	2 Zooplastic
7 Dilation	3 Kidney Pelvis, Right	7 Via Natural or Artificial Opening	7 Autologous Tissue Substitute	3 Kidney Pelvis, Right
8 Division	4 Kidney Pelvis, Left	8 Via Natural or Artificial Opening Endoscopic	C Extraluminal Device	4 Kidney Pelvis, Left
9 Drainage	5 Kidney	X External	D Intraluminal Device	6 Ureter, Right
B Excision	6 Ureter, Right		J Synthetic Substitute	7 Ureter, Left
C Extirpation	7 Ureter, Left		K Nonautologous Tissue Substitute	8 Colon
D Extraction	8 Ureters, Bilateral		L Artificial Sphincter	9 Colocutaneous
F Fragmentation	9 Ureter		M Stimulator Lead	A Ileum
H Insertion	B Bladder		Y Other Device	B Bladder
J Inspection	C Bladder Neck		Z No Device	C Ileocutaneous
L Occlusion	D Urethra			D Cutaneous
M Reattachment				X Diagnostic
N Release				Z No Qualifier
P Removal				
Q Repair				
R Replacement				
S Reposition				
T Resection				
U Supplement				
V Restriction				
W Revision				
X Transfer				
Y Transplantation				

Ø: Medical and Surgical

U: Female Reproductive System

Operation–Character 3	Body Part–Character 4	Approach–Character 5	Device–Character 6	Qualifier–Character 7
1 Bypass	Ø Ovary, Right	Ø Open	Ø Drainage Device	Ø Allogeneic
2 Change	1 Ovary, Left	3 Percutaneous	1 Radioactive Element	1 Syngeneic
5 Destruction	2 Ovaries, Bilateral	4 Percutaneous Endoscopic	3 Infusion Device	2 Zooplastic
7 Dilation	3 Ovary	7 Via Natural or Artificial Opening	7 Autologous Tissue Substitute	5 Fallopian Tube, Right
8 Division	4 Uterine Supporting Structure	8 Via Natural or Artificial Opening Endoscopic	C Extraluminal Device	6 Fallopian Tube, Left
9 Drainage	5 Fallopian Tube, Right	F Via Natural or Artificial Opening With Percutaneous Endoscopic Assistance	D Intraluminal Device	9 Uterus
B Excision	6 Fallopian Tube, Left	X External	G Intraluminal Device, Pessary	X Diagnostic
C Extirpation	7 Fallopian Tubes, Bilateral		H Contraceptive Device	Z No Qualifier
D Extraction	8 Fallopian Tube		J Synthetic Substitute	
F Fragmentation	9 Uterus		K Nonautologous Tissue Substitute	
H Insertion	B Endometrium		Y Other Device	
J Inspection	C Cervix		Z No Device	
L Occlusion	D Uterus and Cervix			
M Reattachment	F Cul-de-sac			
N Release	G Vagina			
P Removal	H Vagina and Cul-de-sac			
Q Repair	J Clitoris			
S Reposition	K Hymen			
T Resection	L Vestibular Gland			
U Supplement	M Vulva			
V Restriction	N Ova			
W Revision				
X Transfer				
Y Transplantation				

Ø: Medical and Surgical

V: Male Reproductive System

Operation–Character 3		Body Part–Character 4		Approach–Character 5		Device–Character 6		Qualifier–Character 7	
1	Bypass	Ø	Prostate	Ø	Open	Ø	Drainage Device	J	Epididymis, Right
2	Change	1	Seminal Vesicle, Right	3	Percutaneous	1	Radioactive Element	K	Epididymis, Left
5	Destruction	2	Seminal Vesicle, Left	4	Percutaneous Endoscopic	3	Infusion Device	N	Vas Deferens, Right
7	Dilation	3	Seminal Vesicles, Bilateral	7	Via Natural or Artificial Opening	7	Autologous Tissue Substitute	P	Vas Deferens, Left
9	Drainage	4	Prostate and Seminal Vesicles	8	Via Natural or Artificial Opening Endoscopic	C	Extraluminal Device	X	Diagnostic
B	Excision	5	Scrotum	X	External	D	Intraluminal Device	Z	No Qualifier
C	Extirpation	6	Tunica Vaginalis, Right			J	Synthetic Substitute		
H	Insertion	7	Tunica Vaginalis, Left			K	Nonautologous Tissue Substitute		
J	Inspection	8	Scrotum and Tunica Vaginalis			Y	Other Device		
L	Occlusion	9	Testis, Right			Z	No Device		
M	Reattachment	B	Testis, Left						
N	Release	C	Testes, Bilateral						
P	Removal	D	Testis						
Q	Repair	F	Spermatic Cord, Right						
R	Replacement	G	Spermatic Cord, Left						
S	Reposition	H	Spermatic Cords, Bilateral						
T	Resection	J	Epididymis, Right						
U	Supplement	K	Epididymis, Left						
W	Revision	L	Epididymis, Bilateral						
		M	Epididymis and Spermatic Cord						
		N	Vas Deferens, Right						
		P	Vas Deferens, Left						
		Q	Vas Deferens, Bilateral						
		R	Vas Deferens						
		S	Penis						
		T	Prepuce						
		V	Male External Genitalia						

0: Medical and Surgical
W: Anatomical Regions, General

Operation–Character 3	Body Region–Character 4	Approach–Character 5	Device–Character 6	Qualifier–Character 7
Ø Alteration	Ø Head	Ø Open	Ø Drainage Device	Ø Vagina
1 Bypass	1 Cranial Cavity	3 Percutaneous	1 Radioactive Element	1 Penis
2 Change	2 Face	4 Percutaneous Endoscopic	3 Infusion Device	2 Stoma
3 Control	3 Oral Cavity and Throat	7 Via Natural or Artificial Opening	7 Autologous Tissue Substitute	4 Cutaneous
4 Creation	4 Upper Jaw	8 Via Natural or Artificial Opening Endoscopic	J Synthetic Substitute	9 Pleural Cavity, Right
8 Division	5 Lower Jaw	X External	K Nonautologous Tissue Substitute	B Pleural Cavity, Left
9 Drainage	6 Neck		Y Other Device	G Peritoneal Cavity
B Excision	8 Chest Wall		Z No Device	J Pelvic Cavity
C Extirpation	9 Pleural Cavity, Right			X Diagnostic
F Fragmentation	B Pleural Cavity, Left			Y Lower Vein
H Insertion	C Mediastinum			Z No Qualifier
J Inspection	D Pericardial Cavity			
M Reattachment	F Abdominal Wall			
P Removal	G Peritoneal Cavity			
Q Repair	H Retroperitoneum			
U Supplement	J Pelvic Cavity			
W Revision	K Upper Back			
	L Lower Back			
	M Perineum, Male			
	N Perineum, Female			
	P Gastrointestinal Tract			
	Q Respiratory Tract			
	R Genitourinary Tract			

Ø: Medical and Surgical
X: Anatomical Regions, Upper Extremities

Operation–Character 3	Body Part–Character 4	Approach–Character 5	Device–Character 6	Qualifier–Character 7
Ø Alteration	Ø Forequarter, Right	Ø Open	Ø Drainage Device	Ø Complete
2 Change	1 Forequarter, Left	3 Percutaneous	1 Radioactive Element	1 High
3 Control	2 Shoulder Region, Right	4 Percutaneous Endoscopic	3 Infusion Device	2 Mid
6 Detachment	3 Shoulder Region, Left	X External	7 Autologous Tissue Substitute	3 Low
9 Drainage	4 Axilla, Right		J Synthetic Substitute	4 Complete 1st Ray
B Excision	5 Axilla, Left		K Nonautologous Tissue Substitute	5 Complete 2nd Ray
H Insertion	6 Upper Extremity, Right		Y Other Device	6 Complete 3rd Ray
J Inspection	7 Upper Extremity, Left		Z No Device	7 Complete 4th Ray
M Reattachment	8 Upper Arm, Right			8 Complete 5th Ray
P Removal	9 Upper Arm, Left			9 Partial 1st Ray
Q Repair	B Elbow Region, Right			B Partial 2nd Ray
R Replacement	C Elbow Region, Left			C Partial 3rd Ray
U Supplement	D Lower Arm, Right			D Partial 4th Ray
W Revision	F Lower Arm, Left			F Partial 5th Ray
X Transfer	G Wrist Region, Right			L Thumb, Right
	H Wrist Region, Left			M Thumb, Left
	J Hand, Right			N Toe, Right
	K Hand, Left			P Toe, Left
	L Thumb, Right			X Diagnostic
	M Thumb, Left			Z No Qualifier
	N Index Finger, Right			
	P Index Finger, Left			
	Q Middle Finger, Right			
	R Middle Finger, Left			
	S Ring Finger, Right			
	T Ring Finger, Left			
	V Little Finger, Right			
	W Little Finger, Left			

0: Medical and Surgical

Y: Anatomical Regions, Lower Extremities

Operation–Character 3	Body Part–Character 4	Approach–Character 5	Device–Character 6	Qualifier–Character 7
0 Alteration	0 Buttock, Right	0 Open	0 Drainage Device	0 Complete
2 Change	1 Buttock, Left	3 Percutaneous	1 Radioactive Element	1 High
3 Control	2 Hindquarter, Right	4 Percutaneous Endoscopic	3 Infusion Device	2 Mid
6 Detachment	3 Hindquarter, Left	X External	7 Autologous Tissue Substitute	3 Low
9 Drainage	4 Hindquarter, Bilateral		J Synthetic Substitute	4 Complete 1st Ray
B Excision	5 Inguinal Region, Right		K Nonautologous Tissue Substitute	5 Complete 2nd Ray
H Insertion	6 Inguinal Region, Left		Y Other Device	6 Complete 3rd Ray
J Inspection	7 Femoral Region, Right		Z No Device	7 Complete 4th Ray
M Reattachment	8 Femoral Region, Left			8 Complete 5th Ray
P Removal	9 Lower Extremity, Right			9 Partial 1st Ray
Q Repair	A Inguinal Region, Bilateral			B Partial 2nd Ray
U Supplement	B Lower Extremity, Left			C Partial 3rd Ray
W Revision	C Upper Leg, Right			D Partial 4th Ray
	D Upper Leg, Left			F Partial 5th Ray
	E Femoral Region, Bilateral			X Diagnostic
	F Knee Region, Right			Z No Qualifier
	G Knee Region, Left			
	H Lower Leg, Right			
	J Lower Leg, Left			
	K Ankle Region, Right			
	L Ankle Region, Left			
	M Foot, Right			
	N Foot, Left			
	P 1st Toe, Right			
	Q 1st Toe, Left			
	R 2nd Toe, Right			
	S 2nd Toe, Left			
	T 3rd Toe, Right			
	U 3rd Toe, Left			
	V 4th Toe, Right			
	W 4th Toe, Left			
	X 5th Toe, Right			
	Y 5th Toe, Left			

1: Obstetrics

0: Pregnancy

Operation–Character 3	Body Part–Character 4	Approach–Character 5	Device–Character 6	Qualifier–Character 7
2 Change	0 Products of Conception	0 Open	3 Monitoring Electrode	0 Classical
9 Drainage	1 Products of Conception, Retained	3 Percutaneous	Y Other Device	1 Low Cervical
A Abortion	2 Products of Conception, Ectopic	4 Percutaneous Endoscopic	Z No Device	2 Extraperitoneal
D Extraction		7 Via Natural or Artificial Opening		3 Low Forceps
E Delivery		8 Via Natural or Artificial Opening Endoscopic		4 Mid Forceps
H Insertion		X External		5 High Forceps
J Inspection				6 Vacuum
P Removal				7 Internal Version
Q Repair				8 Other
S Reposition				9 Fetal Blood
T Resection				A Fetal Cerebrospinal Fluid
Y Transplantation				B Fetal Fluid, Other
				C Amniotic Fluid, Therapeutic
				D Fluid, Other
				E Nervous System
				F Cardiovascular System
				G Lymphatics & Hemic
				H Eye
				J Ear, Nose & Sinus
				K Respiratory System
				L Mouth & Throat
				M Gastrointestinal System
				N Hepatobiliary & Pancreas
				P Endocrine System
				Q Skin
				R Musculoskeletal System
				S Urinary System
				T Female Reproductive System
				U Amniotic Fluid, Diagnostic
				V Male Reproductive System
				W Laminaria
				X Abortifacient
				Y Other Body Systems
				Z No Qualifier

2: Placement
W: Anatomical Regions

Operation–Character 3	Body Region Character 4	Approach–Character 5	Device–Character 6	Qualifier–Character 7
Ø Change	Ø Head	X External	Ø Traction Apparatus	Z No Qualifier
1 Compression	1 Face		1 Splint	
2 Dressing	2 Neck		2 Cast	
3 Immobilization	3 Abdominal Wall		3 Brace	
4 Packing	4 Chest Wall		4 Bandage	
5 Removal	5 Back		5 Packing Material	
6 Traction	6 Inguinal Region, Right		6 Pressure Dressing	
	7 Inguinal Region, Left		7 Intermittent Pressure Device	
	8 Upper Extremity, Right		8 Stereotatic Apparatus	
	9 Upper Extremity, Left		9 Wire	
	A Upper Arm, Right		Y Other Device	
	B Upper Arm, Left		Z No Device	
	C Lower Arm, Right			
	D Lower Arm, Left			
	E Hand, Right			
	F Hand, Left			
	G Thumb, Right			
	H Thumb, Left			
	J Finger, Right			
	K Finger, Left			
	L Lower Extremity, Right			
	M Lower Extremity, Left			
	N Upper Leg, Right			
	P Upper Leg, Left			
	Q Lower Leg, Right			
	R Lower Leg, Left			
	S Foot, Right			
	T Foot, Left			
	U Toe, Right			
	V Toe, Left			

2: Placement
Y: Anatomical Orifices

Operation–Character 3	Body Orifice–Character 4	Approach Character–5	Device Character–6	Qualifier Character–7
Ø Change	Ø Mouth and Pharynx	X External	5 Packing Material	Z No Qualifier
4 Packing	1 Nasal			
5 Removal	2 Ear			
	3 Anorectal			
	4 Female Genital Tract			
	5 Urethra			

3: Administration
0: Circulatory

Operation–Character 3	Body System/Region Character 4	Approach–Character 5	Substance–Character 6	Qualifier–Character 7
2 Transfusion	3 Peripheral Vein	0 Open	A Stem Cells, Embryonic	0 Autologous
	4 Central Vein	3 Percutaneous	B 4-Factor Prothrombin Complex Concentrate	1 Nonautologous
	5 Peripheral Artery	7 Via Natural or Artificial Opening	G Bone Marrow	Z No Qualifier
	6 Central Artery		H Whole Blood	
	7 Products of Conception, Circulatory		J Serum Albumin	
			K Frozen Plasma	
			L Fresh Plasma	
			M Plasma Cryoprecipitate	
			N Red Blood Cells	
			P Frozen Red Cells	
			Q White Cells	
			R Platelets	
			S Globulin	
			T Fibrinogen	
			V Antihemophilic Factors	
			W Factor IX	
			X Stem Cells, Cord Blood	
			Y Stem Cells, Hematopoietic	

3: Administration
C: Indwelling Device

Operation–Character 3	Body System/Region Character 4	Approach–Character 5	Substance–Character 6	Qualifier–Character 7
1 Irrigation	Z None	X External	8 Irrigating Substance	Z No Qualifier

3: Administration

E: Physiological Systems and Anatomical Regions

Operation–Character 3	Body System/Region–Character 4	Approach–Character 5	Substance–Character 6	Qualifier–Character 7
Ø Introduction	Ø Skin and Mucous Membranes	Ø Open	Ø Antineoplastic	Ø Autologous
1 Irrigation	1 Subcutaneous Tissue	3 Percutaneous	1 Thrombolytic	1 Nonautologous
	2 Muscle	7 Via Natural or Artificial Opening	2 Anti-infective	2 High-dose Interleukin-2
	3 Peripheral Vein	8 Via Natural or Artificial Opening Endoscopic	3 Anti-inflammatory	3 Low-dose Interleukin-2
	4 Central Vein	X External	4 Serum, Toxoid and Vaccine	4 Liquid Brachytherapy Radioisotope
	5 Peripheral Artery		5 Adhesion Barrier	5 Other Antineoplastic
	6 Central Artery		6 Nutritional Substance	6 Recombinant Human-activated Protein C
	7 Coronary Artery		7 Electrolytic and Water Balance Substance	7 Other Thrombolytic
	8 Heart		8 Irrigating Substance	8 Oxazolidinones
	9 Nose		9 Dialysate	9 Other Anti-infective
	A Bone Marrow		A Stem Cells, Embryonic	A Anti-infective Envelope
	B Ear		B Local Anesthetic	B Recombinant Bone Morphogenetic Protein
	C Eye		C Regional Anesthetic	C Other Substance
	D Mouth and Pharynx		D Inhalation Anesthetic	D Nitric Oxide
	E Products of Conception		E Stem Cells, Somatic	F Other Gas
	F Respiratory Tract		F Intracirculatory Anesthetic	G Insulin
	G Upper GI		G Other Therapeutic Substance	H Human B-type Natriuretic Peptide
	H Lower GI		H Radioactive Substance	J Other Hormone
	J Biliary and Pancreatic Tract		K Other Diagnostic Substance	K Immunostimulator
	K Genitourinary Tract		L Sperm	L Immunosuppressive
	L Pleural Cavity		M Pigment	M Monoclonal Antibody
	M Peritoneal Cavity		N Analgesics, Hypnotics, Sedatives	N Blood Brain Barrier Disruption
	N Male Reproductive		P Platelet Inhibitor	P Clofarabine
	P Female Reproductive		Q Fertilized Ovum	X Diagnostic
	Q Cranial Cavity and Brain		R Antiarrhythmic	Z No Qualifier
	R Spinal Canal		S Gas	
	S Epidural Space		T Destructive Agent	
	T Peripheral Nerves and Plexi		U Pancreatic Islet Cells	
	U Joints		V Hormone	
	V Bones		W Immunotherapeutic	
	W Lymphatics		X Vasopressor	
	X Cranial Nerves			
	Y Pericardial Cavity			

4: Measurement and Monitoring

A: Physiological Systems

Operation–Character 3	Body System–Character 4	Approach–Character 5	Function/Device–Character 6	Qualifier–Character 7
Ø Measurement	Ø Central Nervous	Ø Open	Ø Acuity	Ø Central
1 Monitoring	1 Peripheral Nervous	3 Percutaneous	1 Capacity	1 Peripheral
	2 Cardiac	4 Percutaneous Endoscopic	2 Conductivity	2 Portal
	3 Arterial	7 Via Natural or Artificial Opening	3 Contractility	3 Pulmonary
	4 Venous	8 Via Natural or Artificial Opening Endoscopic	4 Electrical Activity	4 Stress
	5 Circulatory	X External	5 Flow	5 Ambulatory
	6 Lymphatic		6 Metabolism	6 Right Heart
	7 Visual		7 Mobility	7 Left Heart
	8 Olfactory		8 Motility	8 Bilateral
	9 Respiratory		9 Output	9 Sensory
	B Gastrointestinal		B Pressure	A Guidance
	C Biliary		C Rate	B Motor
	D Urinary		D Resistance	C Coronary
	F Musculoskeletal		F Rhythm	D Intracranial
	H Products of Conception, Cardiac		G Secretion	F Other Thoracic
	J Products of Conception, Nervous		H Sound	G Intraoperative
	Z None		J Pulse	Z No Qualifier
			K Temperature	
			L Volume	
			M Total Activity	
			N Sampling and Pressure	
			P Action Currents	
			Q Sleep	
			R Saturation	

4: Measurement and Monitoring

B: Physiological Devices

Operation–Character 3	Body System–Character 4	Approach–Character 5	Function/Device–Character 6	Qualifier–Character 7
Ø Measurement	Ø Central Nervous	X External	S Pacemaker	Z No Qualifier
	1 Peripheral Nervous		T Defibrillator	
	2 Cardiac		V Stimulator	
	9 Respiratory			
	F Musculoskeletal			

5: Extracorporeal Assistance and Performance

A: Physiological Systems

Operation–Character 3	Body System–Character 4	Duration–Character 5	Function–Character 6	Qualifier–Character 7
Ø Assistance	2 Cardiac	Ø Single	Ø Filtration	Ø Balloon Pump
1 Performance	5 Circulatory	1 Intermittent	1 Output	1 Hyperbaric
2 Restoration	9 Respiratory	2 Continuous	2 Oxygenation	2 Manual
	C Biliary	3 Less than 24 Consecutive Hours	3 Pacing	3 Membrane
	D Urinary	4 24-96 Consecutive Hours	4 Rhythm	4 Nonmechanical
		5 Greater than 96 Consecutive Hours	5 Ventilation	5 Pulsatile Compression
		6 Multiple		6 Other Pump
				7 Continuous Positive Airway Pressure
				8 Intermittent Positive Airway Pressure
				9 Continuous Negative Airway Pressure
				B Intermittent Negative Airway Pressure
				C Supersaturated
				D Impeller Pump
				Z No Qualifier

6: Extracorporeal Therapies

A: Physiological Systems

Operation–Character 3	Body System–Character 4	Duration–Character 5	Qualifier–Character 6	Qualifier–Character 7
Ø Atmospheric Control	Ø Skin	Ø Single	Z No Qualifier	Ø Erythrocytes
1 Decompression	1 Urinary	1 Multiple		1 Leukocytes
2 Electromagnetic Therapy	2 Central Nervous			2 Platelets
3 Hyperthermia	3 Musculoskeletal			3 Plasma
4 Hypothermia	5 Circulatory			4 Head and Neck Vessels
5 Pheresis	Z None			5 Heart
6 Phototherapy				6 Peripheral Vessels
7 Ultrasound Therapy				7 Other Vessels
8 Ultraviolet Light Therapy				T Stem Cells, Cord Blood
9 Shock Wave Therapy				V Stem Cells, Hematopoietic
				Z No Qualifier

7: Osteopathic
W: Anatomical Regions

Operation–Character 3	Body Region–Character 4	Approach–Character 5	Method–Character 6	Qualifier–Character 7
Ø Treatment	Ø Head	X External	Ø Articulatory-Raising	Z None
	1 Cervical		1 Fascial Release	
	2 Thoracic		2 General Mobilization	
	3 Lumbar		3 High Velocity-Low Amplitude	
	4 Sacrum		4 Indirect	
	5 Pelvis		5 Low Velocity-High Amplitude	
	6 Lower Extremities		6 Lymphatic Pump	
	7 Upper Extremities		7 Muscle Energy-Isometric	
	8 Rib Cage		8 Muscle Energy-Isotonic	
	9 Abdomen		9 Other Method	

8: Other Procedures
C: Indwelling Devices

Operation–Character 3	Body Region–Character 4	Approach–Character 5	Method–Character 6	Qualifier–Character 7
Ø Other procedures	1 Nervous System	X External	6 Collection	J Cerebrospinal Fluid
	2 Circulatory System			K Blood
				L Other Fluid

8: Other Procedures
E: Physiological Systems and Anatomical Regions

Operation–Character 3	Body Region–Character 4	Approach–Character 5	Method–Character 6	Qualifier–Character 7
Ø Other Procedures	1 Nervous System	Ø Open	Ø Acupuncture	Ø Anesthesia
	2 Circulatory System	3 Percutaneous	1 Therapeutic Massage	1 In Vitro Fertilization
	9 Head and Neck Region	4 Percutaneous Endoscopic	6 Collection	2 Breast Milk
	H Integumentary System and Breast	7 Via Natural or Artificial Opening	B Computer Assisted Procedure	3 Sperm
	K Musculoskeletal System	8 Via Natural or Artificial Opening Endoscopic	C Robotic Assisted Procedure	4 Yoga Therapy
	U Female Reproductive System	X External	D Near Infrared Spectroscopy	5 Meditation
	V Male Reproductive System		Y Other Method	6 Isolation
	W Trunk Region			7 Examination
	X Upper Extremity			8 Suture Removal
	Y Lower Extremity			9 Piercing
	Z None			C Prostate
				D Rectum
				F With Fluoroscopy
				G With Computerized Tomography
				H With Magnetic Resonance Imaging
				Z No Qualifier

9: Chiropractic

W: Anatomical Regions

Operation–Character 3	Body Region–Character 4	Approach–Character 5	Method–Character 6	Qualifier–Character 7
B Manipulation	0 Head	X External	B Non-Manual	Z None
	1 Cervical		C Indirect Visceral	
	2 Thoracic		D Extra-Articular	
	3 Lumbar		F Direct Visceral	
	4 Sacrum		G Long Lever Specific Contact	
	5 Pelvis		H Short Lever Specific Contact	
	6 Lower Extremities		J Long and Short Lever Specific Contact	
	7 Upper Extremities		K Mechanically Assisted	
	8 Rib Cage		L Other Method	
	9 Abdomen			

B: Imaging

Body System–Character 2	Type–Character 3	Meanings–Character 4	Contrast–Character 5	Qualifier–Character 6	Qualifier–Character 7
0 Central Nervous System	0 Plain Radiography	See next page	0 High Osmolar	0 Unenhanced and Enhanced	0 Intraoperative
2 Heart	1 Fluoroscopy		1 Low Osmolar	1 Laser	1 Densitometry
3 Upper Arteries	2 Computerized Tomography (CT Scan)		Y Other Contrast	2 Intravascular Optical Coherence	3 Intravascular
4 Lower Arteries	3 Magnetic Resonance Imaging (MRI)		Z None	Z None	4 Transesophageal
5 Veins	4 Ultrasonography				A Guidance
7 Lymphatic System					Z None
8 Eye					
9 Ear, Nose, Mouth and Throat					
B Respiratory System					
D Gastrointestinal System					
F Hepatobiliary System and Pancreas					
G Endocrine System					
H Skin, Subcutaneous Tissue and Breast					
L Connective Tissue					
N Skull and Facial Bones					
P Non-Axial Upper Bones					
Q Non-Axial Lower Bones					
R Axial Skeleton, Except Skull and Facial Bones					
T Urinary System					
U Female Reproductive System					
V Male Reproductive System					
W Anatomical Regions					
Y Fetus and Obstetrical					

B: Imaging
Body Part—Character 4 Meanings

Body System–Character 2		Body Part–Character 4
0	Central Nervous System	0 Brain
		7 Cisterna
		8 Cerebral Ventricle(s)
		9 Sella Turcica/Pituitary Gland
		B Spinal Cord
		C Acoustic Nerves
2	Heart	0 Coronary Artery, Single
		1 Coronary Arteries, Multiple
		2 Coronary Artery Bypass Graft, Single
		3 Coronary Artery Bypass Grafts, Multiple
		4 Heart, Right
		5 Heart, Left
		6 Heart, Right and Left
		7 Internal Mammary Bypass Graft, Right
		8 Internal Mammary Bypass Graft, Left
		B Heart with Aorta
		C Pericardium
		D Pediatric Heart
		F Bypass Graft, Other
3	Upper Arteries	0 Thoracic Aorta
		1 Brachiocephalic-Subclavian Artery, Right
		2 Subclavian Artery, Left
		3 Common Carotid Artery, Right
		4 Common Carotid Artery, Left
		5 Common Carotid Arteries, Bilateral
		6 Internal Carotid Artery, Right
		7 Internal Carotid Artery, Left
		8 Internal Carotid Arteries, Bilateral
		9 External Carotid Artery, Right
		B External Carotid Artery, Left
		C External Carotid Arteries, Bilateral
		D Vertebral Artery, Right
		F Vertebral Artery, Left
		G Vertebral Arteries, Bilateral
		H Upper Extremity Arteries, Right
		J Upper Extremity Arteries, Left
		K Upper Extremity Arteries, Bilateral
		L Intercostal and Bronchial Arteries
		M Spinal Arteries
		N Upper Arteries, Other
		P Thoraco-Abdominal Aorta
		Q Cervico-Cerebral Arch
		R Intracranial Arteries
		S Pulmonary Artery, Right
		T Pulmonary Artery, Left
		V Ophthalmic Arteries

Continued on next page

B: Imaging

Body Part—Character 4 Meanings

Continued from previous page

Body System–Character 2	Body Part–Character 4	
4 Lower Arteries	Ø	Abdominal Aorta
	1	Celiac Artery
	2	Hepatic Artery
	3	Splenic Arteries
	4	Superior Mesenteric Artery
	5	Inferior Mesenteric Artery
	6	Renal Artery, Right
	7	Renal Artery, Left
	8	Renal Arteries, Bilateral
	9	Lumbar Arteries
	B	Intra-Abdominal Arteries, Other
	C	Pelvic Arteries
	D	Aorta and Bilateral Lower Extremity Arteries
	F	Lower Extremity Arteries, Right
	G	Lower Extremity Arteries, Left
	H	Lower Extremity Arteries, Bilateral
	J	Lower Arteries, Other
	K	Celiac and Mesenteric Arteries
	L	Femoral Artery
	M	Renal Artery Transplant
	N	Penile Arteries
5 Veins	Ø	Epidural Veins
	1	Cerebral and Cerebellar Veins
	2	Intracranial Sinuses
	3	Jugular Veins, Right
	4	Jugular Veins, Left
	5	Jugular Veins, Bilateral
	6	Subclavian Vein, Right
	7	Subclavian Vein, Left
	8	Superior Vena Cava
	9	Inferior Vena Cava
	B	Lower Extremity Veins, Right
	C	Lower Extremity Veins, Left
	D	Lower Extremity Veins, Bilateral
	F	Pelvic (Iliac) Veins, Right
	G	Pelvic (Iliac) Veins, Left
	H	Pelvic (Iliac) Veins, Bilateral
	J	Renal Vein, Right
	K	Renal Vein, Left
	L	Renal Veins, Bilateral
	M	Upper Extremity Veins, Right
	N	Upper Extremity Veins, Left
	P	Upper Extremity Veins, Bilateral
	Q	Pulmonary Vein, Right
	R	Pulmonary Vein, Left
	S	Pulmonary Veins, Bilateral
	T	Portal and Splanchnic Veins
	V	Veins, Other
	W	Dialysis Shunt/Fistula
7 Lymphatic System	Ø	Abdominal/Retroperitoneal Lymphatics, Unilateral
	1	Abdominal/Retroperitoneal Lymphatics, Bilateral
	4	Lymphatics, Head and Neck
	5	Upper Extremity Lymphatics, Right
	6	Upper Extremity Lymphatics, Left
	7	Upper Extremity Lymphatics, Bilateral
	8	Lower Extremity Lymphatics, Right
	9	Lower Extremity Lymphatics, Left
	B	Lower Extremity Lymphatics, Bilateral
	C	Lymphatics, Pelvic

Continued on next page

B: Imaging

Body Part—Character 4 Meanings

Continued from previous page

Body System–Character 2	Body Part–Character 4	
8	Eye	Ø	Lacrimal Duct, Right
		1	Lacrimal Duct, Left
		2	Lacrimal Ducts, Bilateral
		3	Optic Foramina, Right
		4	Optic Foramina, Left
		5	Eye, Right
		6	Eye, Left
		7	Eyes, Bilateral
9	Ear, Nose, Mouth and Throat	Ø	Ear
		2	Paranasal Sinuses
		4	Parotid Gland, Right
		5	Parotid Gland, Left
		6	Parotid Glands, Bilateral
		7	Submandibular Gland, Right
		8	Submandibular Gland, Left
		9	Submandibular Glands, Bilateral
		B	Salivary Gland, Right
		C	Salivary Gland, Left
		D	Salivary Glands, Bilateral
		F	Nasopharynx/Oropharynx
		G	Pharynx and Epiglottis
		H	Mastoids
		J	Larynx
B	Respiratory System	2	Lung, Right
		3	Lung, Left
		4	Lungs, Bilateral
		6	Diaphragm
		7	Tracheobronchial Tree, Right
		8	Tracheobronchial Tree, Left
		9	Tracheobronchial Trees, Bilateral
		B	Pleura
		C	Mediastinum
		D	Upper Airways
		F	Trachea/Airways
		G	Lung Apices
D	Gastrointestinal System	1	Esophagus
		2	Stomach
		3	Small Bowel
		4	Colon
		5	Upper GI
		6	Upper GI and Small Bowel
		7	Gastrointestinal Tract
		8	Appendix
		9	Duodenum
		B	Mouth/Oropharynx
		C	Rectum
F	Hepatobiliary System and Pancreas	Ø	Bile Ducts
		1	Biliary and Pancreatic Ducts
		2	Gallbladder
		3	Gallbladder and Bile Ducts
		4	Gallbladder, Bile Ducts and Pancreatic Ducts
		5	Liver
		6	Liver and Spleen
		7	Pancreas
		8	Pancreatic Ducts
		C	Hepatobiliary System, All
G	Endocrine System	Ø	Adrenal Gland, Right
		1	Adrenal Gland, Left
		2	Adrenal Glands, Bilateral
		3	Parathyroid Glands
		4	Thyroid Gland

Continued on next page

B: Imaging

Body Part—Character 4 Meanings

Continued from previous page

Body System–Character 2		Body Part–Character 4	
H	Skin, Subcutaneous Tissue and Breast	Ø	Breast, Right
		1	Breast, Left
		2	Breasts, Bilateral
		3	Single Mammary Duct, Right
		4	Single Mammary Duct, Left
		5	Multiple Mammary Ducts, Right
		6	Multiple Mammary Ducts, Left
		7	Extremity, Upper
		8	Extremity, Lower
		9	Abdominal Wall
		B	Chest Wall
		C	Head and Neck
		D	Subcutaneous Tissue, Head/Neck
		F	Subcutaneous Tissue, Upper Extremity
		G	Subcutaneous Tissue, Thorax
		H	Subcutaneous Tissue, Abdomen and Pelvis
		J	Subcutaneous Tissue, Lower Extremity
L	Connective Tissue	Ø	Connective Tissue, Upper Extremity
		1	Connective Tissue, Lower Extremity
		2	Tendons, Upper Extremity
		3	Tendons, Lower Extremity
N	Skull and Facial Bones	Ø	Skull
		1	Orbit, Right
		2	Orbit, Left
		3	Orbits, Bilateral
		4	Nasal Bones
		5	Facial Bones
		6	Mandible
		7	Temporomandibular Joint, Right
		8	Temporomandibular Joint, Left
		9	Temporomandibular Joints, Bilateral
		B	Zygomatic Arch, Right
		C	Zygomatic Arch, Left
		D	Zygomatic Arches, Bilateral
		F	Temporal Bones
		G	Tooth, Single
		H	Teeth, Multiple
		J	Teeth, All
P	Non-Axial Upper Bones	Ø	Sternoclavicular Joint, Right
		1	Sternoclavicular Joint, Left
		2	Sternoclavicular Joints, Bilateral
		3	Acromioclavicular Joints, Bilateral
		4	Clavicle, Right
		5	Clavicle, Left
		6	Scapula, Right
		7	Scapula, Left
		8	Shoulder, Right
		9	Shoulder, Left
		A	Humerus, Right
		B	Humerus, Left
		C	Hand/Finger Joint, Right
		D	Hand/Finger Joint, Left
		E	Upper Arm, Right
		F	Upper Arm, Left
		G	Elbow, Right
		H	Elbow, Left
		J	Forearm, Right
		K	Forearm, Left

Continued on next page

B: Imaging

Body Part—Character 4 Meanings

Continued from previous page

Body System–Character 2		Body Part–Character 4	
P	Non-Axial Upper Bones	L	Wrist, Right
		M	Wrist, Left
		N	Hand, Right
		P	Hand, Left
		Q	Hands and Wrists, Bilateral
		R	Finger(s), Right
		S	Finger(s), Left
		T	Upper Extremity, Right
		U	Upper Extremity, Left
		V	Upper Extremities, Bilateral
		W	Thorax
		X	Ribs, Right
		Y	Ribs, Left
Q	Non-Axial Lower Bones	Ø	Hip, Right
		1	Hip, Left
		2	Hips, Bilateral
		3	Femur, Right
		4	Femur, Left
		7	Knee, Right
		8	Knee, Left
		9	Knees, Bilateral
		B	Tibia/Fibula, Right
		C	Tibia/Fibula, Left
		D	Lower Leg, Right
		F	Lower Leg, Left
		G	Ankle, Right
		H	Ankle, Left
		J	Calcaneus, Right
		K	Calcaneus, Left
		L	Foot, Right
		M	Foot, Left
		P	Toe(s), Right
		Q	Toe(s), Left
		R	Lower Extremity, Right
		S	Lower Extremity, Left
		V	Patella, Right
		W	Patella, Left
		X	Foot/Toe Joint, Right
		Y	Foot/Toe Joint, Left

Continued on next page

B: Imaging

Body Part—Character 4 Meanings

Continued from previous page

Body System–Character 2		Body Part–Character 4	
R	Axial Skeleton, Except Skull and Facial Bones	Ø	Cervical Spine
		1	Cervical Disc(s)
		2	Thoracic Disc(s)
		3	Lumbar Disc(s)
		4	Cervical Facet Joint(s)
		5	Thoracic Facet Joint(s)
		6	Lumbar Facet Joint(s)
		7	Thoracic Spine
		8	Thoracolumbar Joint
		9	Lumbar Spine
		B	Lumbosacral Joint
		C	Pelvis
		D	Sacroiliac Joints
		F	Sacrum and Coccyx
		G	Whole Spine
		H	Sternum
T	Urinary System	Ø	Bladder
		1	Kidney, Right
		2	Kidney, Left
		3	Kidneys, Bilateral
		4	Kidneys, Ureters and Bladder
		5	Urethra
		6	Ureter, Right
		7	Ureter, Left
		8	Ureters, Bilateral
		9	Kidney Transplant
		B	Bladder and Urethra
		C	Ileal Diversion Loop
		D	Kidney, Ureter and Bladder, Right
		F	Kidney, Ureter and Bladder, Left
		G	Ileal Loop, Ureters and Kidneys
		J	Kidneys and Bladder
U	Female Reproductive System	Ø	Fallopian Tube, Right
		1	Fallopian Tube, Left
		2	Fallopian Tubes, Bilateral
		3	Ovary, Right
		4	Ovary, Left
		5	Ovaries, Bilateral
		6	Uterus
		8	Uterus and Fallopian Tubes
		9	Vagina
		B	Pregnant Uterus
		C	Uterus and Ovaries
V	Male Reproductive System	Ø	Corpora Cavernosa
		1	Epididymis, Right
		2	Epididymis, Left
		3	Prostate
		4	Scrotum
		5	Testicle, Right
		6	Testicle, Left
		7	Testicles, Bilateral
		8	Vasa Vasorum
		9	Prostate and Seminal Vesicles
		B	Penis

Continued on next page

B: Imaging
Body Part—Character 4 Meanings

Continued from previous page

Body System–Character 2	Body Part–Character 4
W Anatomical Regions	Ø Abdomen 1 Abdomen and Pelvis 3 Chest 4 Chest and Abdomen 5 Chest, Abdomen and Pelvis 8 Head 9 Head and Neck B Long Bones, All C Lower Extremity F Neck G Pelvic Region H Retroperitoneum J Upper Extremity K Whole Body L Whole Skeleton M Whole Body, Infant P Brachial Plexus
Y Fetus and Obstetrical	Ø Fetal Head 1 Fetal Heart 2 Fetal Thorax 3 Fetal Abdomen 4 Fetal Spine 5 Fetal Extremities 6 Whole Fetus 7 Fetal Umbilical Cord 8 Placenta 9 First Trimester, Single Fetus B First Trimester, Multiple Gestation C Second Trimester, Single Fetus D Second Trimester, Multiple Gestation F Third Trimester, Single Fetus G Third Trimester, Multiple Gestation

C: Nuclear Medicine

Body System–Character 2		Type–Character 3		Meanings–Character 4	Radionuclide–Character 5		Qualifier–Character 6		Qualifier–Character 7	
Ø	Central Nervous System	1	Planar Nuclear Medicine Imaging	See next Page	1	Technetium 99m (Tc-99m)	Z	None	Z	None
2	Heart	2	Tomographic (Tomo) Nuclear Medicine Imaging		7	Cobalt 58 (Co-58)				
5	Veins	3	Positron Emission Tomographic (PET) Imaging		8	Samarium 153 (Sm-153)				
7	Lymphatic and Hematologic System	4	Nonimaging Nuclear Medicine Uptake		9	Krypton (Kr-81m)				
8	Eye	5	Nonimaging Nuclear Medicine Probe		B	Carbon 11 (C-11)				
9	Ear, Nose, Mouth and Throat	6	Nonimaging Nuclear Medicine Assay		C	Cobalt 57 (Co-57)				
B	Respiratory System	7	Systemic Nuclear Medicine Therapy		D	Indium 111 (In-111)				
D	Gastrointestinal System				F	Iodine 123 (I-123)				
F	Hepatobiliary System and Pancreas				G	Iodine 131 (I-131)				
G	Endocrine System				H	Iodine 125 (I-125)				
H	Skin, Subcutaneous Tissue and Breast				K	Fluorine 18 (F-18)				
P	Musculoskeletal System				L	Gallium 67 (Ga-67)				
T	Urinary System				M	Oxygen 15 (O-15)				
V	Male Reproductive System				N	Phosphorus 32 (P-32)				
W	Anatomical Regions				P	Strontium 89 (Sr-89)				
					Q	Rubidium 82 (Rb-82)				
					R	Nitrogen 13 (N-13)				
					S	Thallium 2Ø1 (Tl-2Ø1)				
					T	Xenon 127 (Xe-127)				
					V	Xenon 133 (Xe-133)				
					W	Chromium (Cr-51)				
					Y	Other Radionuclide				
					Z	None				

C: Nuclear Medicine

Body Part—Character 4 Meanings

Body System–Character 2		Body Part–Character 4	
Ø	Central Nervous System	Ø	Brain
		5	Cerebrospinal Fluid
		Y	Central Nervous System
2	Heart	6	Heart, Right and Left
		G	Myocardium
		Y	Heart
5	Veins	B	Lower Extremity Veins, Right
		C	Lower Extremity Veins, Left
		D	Lower Extremity Veins, Bilateral
		N	Upper Extremity Veins, Right
		P	Upper Extremity Veins, Left
		Q	Upper Extremity Veins, Bilateral
		R	Central Veins
		Y	Veins
7	Lymphatic and Hematologic System	Ø	Bone Marrow
		2	Spleen
		3	Blood
		5	Lymphatics, Head and Neck
		D	Lymphatics, Pelvic
		J	Lymphatics, Head
		K	Lymphatics, Neck
		L	Lymphatics, Upper Chest
		M	Lymphatics, Trunk
		N	Lymphatics, Upper Extremity
		P	Lymphatics, Lower Extremity
		Y	Lymphatic and Hematologic System
8	Eye	9	Lacrimal Ducts, Bilateral
		Y	Eye
9	Ear, Nose, Mouth and Throat	B	Salivary Glands, Bilateral
		Y	Ear, Nose, Mouth and Throat
B	Respiratory System	2	Lungs and Bronchi
		Y	Respiratory System
D	Gastrointestinal System	5	Upper Gastrointestinal Tract
		7	Gastrointestinal Tract
		Y	Digestive System
F	Hepatobiliary System and Pancreas	4	Gallbladder
		5	Liver
		6	Liver and Spleen
		C	Hepatobiliary System, All
		Y	Hepatobiliary System and Pancreas
G	Endocrine System	1	Parathyroid Glands
		2	Thyroid Gland
		4	Adrenal Glands, Bilateral
		Y	Endocrine System
H	Skin, Subcutaneous Tissue and Breast	Ø	Breast, Right
		1	Breast, Left
		2	Breasts, Bilateral
		Y	Skin, Subcutaneous Tissue and Breast

Continued on next page

C: Nuclear Medicine

Body Part—Character 4 Meanings

Continued from previous page

Body System–Character 2	Body Part–Character 4	
P	Musculoskeletal System	1	Skull
		2	Cervical Spine
		3	Skull and Cervical Spine
		4	Thorax
		5	Spine
		6	Pelvis
		7	Spine and Pelvis
		8	Upper Extremity, Right
		9	Upper Extremity, Left
		B	Upper Extremities, Bilateral
		C	Lower Extremity, Right
		D	Lower Extremity, Left
		F	Lower Extremities, Bilateral
		G	Thoracic Spine
		H	Lumbar Spine
		J	Thoracolumbar Spine
		N	Upper Extremities
		P	Lower Extremities
		Y	Musculoskeletal System, Other
		Z	Musculoskeletal System, All
T	Urinary System	3	Kidneys, Ureters and Bladder
		H	Bladder and Ureters
		Y	Urinary System
V	Male Reproductive System	9	Testicles, Bilateral
		Y	Male Reproductive System
W	Anatomical Regions	Ø	Abdomen
		1	Abdomen and Pelvis
		3	Chest
		4	Chest and Abdomen
		6	Chest and Neck
		B	Head and Neck
		D	Lower Extremity
		G	Thyroid
		J	Pelvic Region
		M	Upper Extremity
		N	Whole Body
		Y	Anatomical Regions, Multiple
		Z	Anatomical Region, Other

D: Radiation Therapy

Body System–Character 2		Modality–Character 3		Meanings–Character 4	Modality–Qualifier Character 5		Isotope–Character 6		Qualifier–Character 7	
Ø	Central and Peripheral Nervous System	Ø	Beam Radiation	See next Page	Ø	Photons <1 MeV	7	Cesium 137 (Cs-137)	Ø	Intraoperative
7	Lymphatic and Hematologic System	1	Brachytherapy		1	Photons 1 - 1Ø MeV	8	Iridium 192 (Ir-192)	Z	None
8	Eye	2	Stereotactic Radiosurgery		2	Photons >1Ø MeV	9	Iodine 125 (I-125)		
9	Ear, Nose, Mouth and Throat	Y	Other Radiation		3	Electrons	B	Palladium 1Ø3 (Pd-1Ø3)		
B	Respiratory System				4	Heavy Particles (Protons, Ions)	C	Californium 252 (Cf-252)		
D	Gastrointestinal System				5	Neutrons	D	Iodine 131 (I-131)		
F	Hepatobiliary System and Pancreas				6	Neutron Capture	F	Phosphorus 32 (P-32)		
G	Endocrine System				7	Contact Radiation	G	Strontium 89 (Sr-89)		
H	Skin				8	Hyperthermia	H	Strontium 9Ø (Sr-9Ø)		
M	Breast				9	High Dose Rate (HDR)	Y	Other Isotope		
P	Musculoskeletal System				B	Low Dose Rate (LDR)	Z	None		
T	Urinary System				C	Intraoperative Radiation Therapy (IORT)				
U	Female Reproductive System				D	Stereotactic Other Photon Radiosurgery				
V	Male Reproductive System				F	Plaque Radiation				
W	Anatomical Regions				G	Isotope Administration				
					H	Stereotactic Particulate Radiosurgery				
					J	Stereotactic Gamma Beam Radiosurgery				
					K	Laser Interstitial Thermal Therapy				

D. Radiation Therapy

Treatment Site—Character 4 Meanings

Body System–Character 2		Treatment Site–Character 4	
0	Central and Peripheral Nervous System	0	Brain
		1	Brain Stem
		6	Spinal Cord
		7	Peripheral Nerve
7	Lymphatic and Hematologic System	0	Bone Marrow
		1	Thymus
		2	Spleen
		3	Lymphatics, Neck
		4	Lymphatics, Axillary
		5	Lymphatics, Thorax
		6	Lymphatics, Abdomen
		7	Lymphatics, Pelvis
		8	Lymphatics, Inguinal
8	Eye	0	Eye
9	Ear, Nose, Mouth and Throat	0	Ear
		1	Nose
		3	Hypopharynx
		4	Mouth
		5	Tongue
		6	Salivary Glands
		7	Sinuses
		8	Hard Palate
		9	Soft Palate
		B	Larynx
		C	Pharynx
		D	Nasopharynx
		F	Oropharynx
B	Respiratory System	0	Trachea
		1	Bronchus
		2	Lung
		5	Pleura
		6	Mediastinum
		7	Chest Wall
		8	Diaphragm
D	Gastrointestinal System	0	Esophagus
		1	Stomach
		2	Duodenum
		3	Jejunum
		4	Ileum
		5	Colon
		7	Rectum
		8	Anus
F	Hepatobiliary System and Pancreas	0	Liver
		1	Gallbladder
		2	Bile Ducts
		3	Pancreas
G	Endocrine System	0	Pituitary Gland
		1	Pineal Body
		2	Adrenal Glands
		4	Parathyroid Glands
		5	Thyroid

Continued on next page

D. Radiation Therapy

Treatment Site—Character 4 Meanings   *Continued from previous page*

Body System–Character 2		Treatment Site–Character 4	
H	Skin	2	Skin, Face
		3	Skin, Neck
		4	Skin, Arm
		5	Skin, Hand
		6	Skin, Chest
		7	Skin, Back
		8	Skin, Abdomen
		9	Skin, Buttock
		B	Skin, Leg
		C	Skin, Foot
M	Breast	Ø	Breast, Left
		1	Breast, Right
P	Musculoskeletal System	Ø	Skull
		2	Maxilla
		3	Mandible
		4	Sternum
		5	Rib(s)
		6	Humerus
		7	Radius/Ulna
		8	Pelvic Bones
		9	Femur
		B	Tibia/Fibula
		C	Other Bone
T	Urinary System	Ø	Kidney
		1	Ureter
		2	Bladder
		3	Urethra
U	Female Reproductive System	Ø	Ovary
		1	Cervix
		2	Uterus
V	Male Reproductive System	Ø	Prostate
		1	Testis
W	Anatomical Regions	1	Head and Neck
		2	Chest
		3	Abdomen
		4	Hemibody
		5	Whole Body
		6	Pelvic Region

F: Physical Rehabilitation and Diagnostic Audiology
0: Rehabilitation

See next page for Character 5 Meanings

Type–Character 3		Body System–Body Region–Character 4		Equipment – Character 6		Qualifier–Character 7	
0	Speech Assessment	0	Neurological System - Head and Neck	1	Audiometer	Z	None
1	Motor and/or Nerve Function Assessment	1	Neurological System - Upper Back / Upper Extremity	2	Sound Field / Booth		
2	Activities of Daily Living Assessment	2	Neurological System - Lower Back / Lower Extremity	4	Electroacoustic Immitance / Acoustic Reflex		
6	Speech Treatment	3	Neurological System - Whole Body	5	Hearing Aid Selection / Fitting / Test		
7	Motor Treatment	4	Circulatory System - Head and Neck	7	Electrophysiologic		
8	Activities of Daily Living Treatment	5	Circulatory System - Upper Back / Upper Extremity	8	Vestibular / Balance		
9	Hearing Treatment	6	Circulatory System - Lower Back / Lower Extremity	9	Cochlear Implant		
B	Cochlear Implant Treatment	7	Circulatory System - Whole Body	B	Physical Agents		
C	Vestibular Treatment	8	Respiratory System - Head and Neck	C	Mechanical		
D	Device Fitting	9	Respiratory System - Upper Back / Upper Extremity	D	Electrotherapeutic		
F	Caregiver Training	B	Respiratory System - Lower Back / Lower Extremity	E	Orthosis		
		C	Respiratory System - Whole Body	F	Assistive, Adaptive, Supportive or Protective		
		D	Integumentary System - Head and Neck	G	Aerobic Endurance and Conditioning		
		F	Integumentary System - Upper Back / Upper Extremity	H	Mechanical or Electromechanical		
		G	Integumentary System - Lower Back / Lower Extremity	J	Somatosensory		
		H	Integumentary System - Whole Body	K	Audiovisual		
		J	Musculoskeletal System - Head and Neck	L	Assistive Listening		
		K	Musculoskeletal System - Upper Back / Upper Extremity	M	Augmentative / Alternative Communication		
		L	Musculoskeletal System - Lower Back / Lower Extremity	N	Biosensory Feedback		
		M	Musculoskeletal System - Whole Body	P	Computer		
		N	Genitourinary System	Q	Speech Analysis		
		Z	None	S	Voice Analysis		
				T	Aerodynamic Function		
				U	Prosthesis		
				V	Speech Prosthesis		
				W	Swallowing		
				X	Cerumen Management		
				Y	Other Equipment		
				Z	None		

F: Physical Rehabilitation and Diagnostic Audiology
0: Rehabilitation
Type Qualifier—Character 5 Meanings

Type–Character 3	Type Qualifier–Character 5
Ø Speech Assessment	Ø Filtered Speech
	1 Speech Threshold
	2 Speech/Word Recognition
	3 Staggered Spondaic Word
	4 Sensorineural Acuity Level
	5 Synthetic Sentence Identification
	6 Speech and/or Language Screening
	7 Nonspoken Language
	8 Receptive/Expressive Language
	9 Articulation/Phonology
	B Motor Speech
	C Aphasia
	D Fluency
	F Voice
	G Communicative/Cognitive Integration Skills
	H Bedside Swallowing and Oral Function
	J Instrumental Swallowing and Oral Function
	K Orofacial Myofunctional
	L Augmentative/Alternative Communication System
	M Voice Prosthetic
	N Non-invasive Instrumental Status
	P Oral Peripheral Mechanism
	Q Performance Intensity Phonetically Balanced Speech Discrimination
	R Brief Tone Stimuli
	S Distorted Speech
	T Dichotic Stimuli
	V Temporal Ordering of Stimuli
	W Masking Patterns
	X Other Specified Central Auditory Processing
1 Motor and/or Nerve Function Assessment	Ø Muscle Performance
	1 Integumentary Integrity
	2 Visual Motor Integration
	3 Coordination/Dexterity
	4 Motor Function
	5 Range of Motion and Joint Integrity
	6 Sensory Awareness/Processing/Integrity
	7 Facial Nerve Function
	9 Somatosensory Evoked Potentials
	B Bed Mobility
	C Transfer
	D Gait and/or Balance
	F Wheelchair Mobility
	G Reflex Integrity
2 Activities of Daily Living Assessment	Ø Bathing/Showering
	1 Dressing
	2 Feeding/Eating
	3 Grooming/Personal Hygiene
	4 Home Management
	5 Perceptual Processing
	6 Psychosocial Skills
	7 Aerobic Capacity and Endurance
	8 Anthropometric Characteristics
	9 Cranial Nerve Integrity
	B Environmental, Home and Work Barriers
	C Ergonomics and Body Mechanics
	D Neuromotor Development
	F Pain
	G Ventilation, Respiration and Circulation
	H Vocational Activities and Functional Community or Work Reintegration Skills

Continued on next page

F: Physical Rehabilitation and Diagnostic Audiology

0: Rehabilitation

Type Qualifier—Character 5 Meanings

Continued from previous page

Type–Character 3	Type Qualifier–Character 5
6 Speech Treatment	Ø Nonspoken Language 1 Speech-Language Pathology and Related Disorders Counseling 2 Speech-Language Pathology and Related Disorders Prevention 3 Aphasia 4 Articulation/Phonology 5 Aural Rehabilitation 6 Communicative/Cognitive Integration Skills 7 Fluency 8 Motor Speech 9 Orofacial Myofunctional B Receptive/Expressive Language C Voice D Swallowing Dysfunction
7 Motor Treatment	Ø Range of Motion and Joint Mobility 1 Muscle Performance 2 Coordination/Dexterity 3 Motor Function 4 Wheelchair Mobility 5 Bed Mobility 6 Therapeutic Exercise 7 Manual Therapy Techniques 8 Transfer Training 9 Gait Training/Functional Ambulation
8 Activities of Daily Living Treatment	Ø Bathing/Showering Techniques 1 Dressing Techniques 2 Grooming/Personal Hygiene 3 Feeding/Eating 4 Home Management 5 Wound Management 6 Psychosocial Skills 7 Vocational Activities and Functional Community or Work Reintegration Skills
9 Hearing Treatment	Ø Hearing and Related Disorders Counseling 1 Hearing and Related Disorders Prevention 2 Auditory Processing 3 Cerumen Management
B Cochlear Implant Treatment	Ø Cochlear Implant Rehabilitation
C Vestibular Treatment	Ø Vestibular 1 Perceptual Processing 2 Visual Motor Integration 3 Postural Control
D Device Fitting	Ø Tinnitus Masker 1 Monaural Hearing Aid 2 Binaural Hearing Aid 3 Augmentative/Alternative Communication System 4 Voice Prosthetic 5 Assistive Listening Device 6 Dynamic Orthosis 7 Static Orthosis 8 Prosthesis 9 Assistive, Adaptive, Supportive or Protective Devices

Continued on next page

F: Physical Rehabilitation and Diagnostic Audiology

0: Rehabilitation

Type Qualifier—Character 5 Meanings

Continued from previous page

Type–Character 3	Type Qualifier–Character 5
F Caregiver Training	Ø Bathing/Showering Technique
	1 Dressing
	2 Feeding and Eating
	3 Grooming/Personal Hygiene
	4 Bed Mobility
	5 Transfer
	6 Wheelchair Mobility
	7 Therapeutic Exercise
	8 Airway Clearance Techniques
	9 Wound Management
	B Vocational Activities and Functional Community or Work Reintegration Skills
	C Gait Training/Functional Ambulation
	D Application, Proper Use and Care of Assistive, Adaptive, Supportive or Protective Devices
	F Application, Proper Use and Care of Orthoses
	G Application, Proper Use and Care of Prosthesis
	H Home Management
	J Communication Skills

F: Physical Rehabilitation and Diagnostic Audiology

1: Diagnostic Audiology

Type–Character 3	Body System–Body Region–Character 4	Meanings–Character 5	Equipment–Character 6	Qualifer–Character 7
3 Hearing Assessment	Z None	See next page	Ø Occupational Hearing	Z None
4 Hearing Aid Assessment			1 Audiometer	
5 Vestibular Assessment			2 Sound Field / Booth	
			3 Tympanometer	
			4 Electroacoustic Immitance / Acoustic Reflex	
			5 Hearing Aid Selection / Fitting / Test	
			6 Otoacoustic Emission (OAE)	
			7 Electrophysiologic	
			8 Vestibular / Balance	
			9 Cochlear Implant	
			K Audiovisual	
			L Assistive Listening	
			P Computer	
			Y Other Equipment	
			Z None	

F: Physical Rehabilitation and Diagnostic Audiology

1: Diagnostic Audiology

Type Qualifier—Character 5 Meanings

Type–Character 3	Type Qualifier–Character 5	
3 Hearing Assessment	0	Hearing Screening
	1	Pure Tone Audiometry, Air
	2	Pure Tone Audiometry, Air and Bone
	3	Bekesy Audiometry
	4	Conditioned Play Audiometry
	5	Select Picture Audiometry
	6	Visual Reinforcement Audiometry
	7	Alternate Binaural or Monaural Loudness Balance
	8	Tone Decay
	9	Short Increment Sensitivity Index
	B	Stenger
	C	Pure Tone Stenger
	D	Tympanometry
	F	Eustachian Tube Function
	G	Acoustic Reflex Patterns
	H	Acoustic Reflex Threshold
	J	Acoustic Reflex Decay
	K	Electrocochleography
	L	Auditory Evoked Potentials
	M	Evoked Otoacoustic Emissions, Screening
	N	Evoked Otoacoustic Emissions, Diagnostic
	P	Aural Rehabilitation Status
	Q	Auditory Processing
4 Hearing Aid Assessment	0	Cochlear Implant
	1	Ear Canal Probe Microphone
	2	Monaural Hearing Aid
	3	Binaural Hearing Aid
	4	Assistive Listening System/Device Selection
	5	Sensory Aids
	6	Binaural Electroacoustic Hearing Aid Check
	7	Ear Protector Attentuation
	8	Monaural Electroacoustic Hearing Aid Check
5 Vestibular Assessment	0	Bithermal, Bionaural Caloric Irrigation
	1	Bithermal, Monaural Caloric Irrigation
	2	Unithermal Binaural Screen
	3	Oscillating Tracking
	4	Sinusoidal Vertical Axis Rotational
	5	Dix-Hallpike Dynamic
	6	Computerized Dynamic Posturography
	7	Tinnitus Masker

G: Mental Health

Z: Body System—None

Type–Character 3	Type Qualifier –Character 4	Qualifier–Character 5	Qualifier–Character 6	Qualifier–Character 7
1 Psychological Tests	Ø Developmental	Z None	Z None	Z None
	1 Personality and Behavioral			
	2 Intellectual and Psychoeducational			
	3 Neuropsychological			
	4 Neurobehavioral and Cognitive Status			
2 Crisis Intervention	Z None			
3 Medication Management	Z None			
5 Individual Psychotherapy	Ø Interactive			
	1 Behavioral			
	2 Cognitive			
	3 Interpersonal			
	4 Psychoanalysis			
	5 Psychodynamic			
	6 Supportive			
	8 Cognitive-Behavioral			
	9 Psychophysiological			
6 Counseling	Ø Educational			
	1 Vocational			
	3 Other Counseling			
7 Family Psychotherapy	2 Other Family Psychotherapy			
B Electroconvulsive Therapy	Ø Unilateral-Single Seizure			
	1 Unilateral-Multiple Seizure			
	2 Bilateral-Single Seizure			
	3 Bilateral-Multiple Seizure			
	4 Other Electroconvulsive Therapy			
C Biofeedback	9 Other Biofeedback			
F Hypnosis	Z None			
G Narcosynthesis	Z None			
H Group Psychotherapy	Z None			
J Light Therapy	Z None			

H: Substance Abuse Treatment

Z: Body System—None

Type–Character 3	Type Qualifier–Character 4	Qualifier–Character 5	Qualifier–Character 6	Qualifier–Character 7
2 Detoxification Services	Z None	Z None	Z None	Z None
3 Individual Counseling	0 Cognitive 1 Behavioral 2 Cognitive-Behavioral 3 12-Step 4 Interpersonal 5 Vocational 6 Psychoeducation 7 Motivational Enhancement 8 Confrontational 9 Continuing Care B Spiritual C Pre/Post-Test Infectious Disease			
4 Group Counseling	0 Cognitive 1 Behavioral 2 Cognitive-Behavioral 3 12-Step 4 Interpersonal 5 Vocational 6 Psychoeducation 7 Motivational Enhancement 8 Confrontational 9 Continuing Care B Spiritual C Pre/Post-Test Infectious Disease			
5 Individual Psychotherapy	0 Cognitive 1 Behavioral 2 Cognitive-Behavioral 3 12-Step 4 Interpersonal 5 Interactive 6 Psychoeducation 7 Motivational Enhancement 8 Confrontational 9 Supportive B Psychoanalysis C Psychodynamic D Psychophysiological			
6 Family Counseling	3 Other Family Counseling			
8 Medication Management	0 Nicotine Replacement 1 Methadone Maintenance 2 Levo-alpha-acetyl-methadol (LAAM) 3 Antabuse 4 Naltrexone 5 Naloxone 6 Clonidine 7 Bupropion 8 Psychiatric Medication 9 Other Replacement Medication			
9 Pharmacotherapy	0 Nicotine Replacement 1 Methadone Maintenance 2 Levo-alpha-acetyl-methadol (LAAM) 3 Antabuse 4 Naltrexone 5 Naloxone 6 Clonidine 7 Bupropion 8 Psychiatric Medication 9 Other Replacement Medication			

Appendix H: Answers to Coding Exercises

Medical Surgical Section

Procedure	Code
Excision of malignant melanoma from skin of right ear	ØHB2XZZ
Laparoscopy with excision of endometrial implant from left ovary	ØUB14ZZ
Percutaneous needle core biopsy of right kidney	ØTBØ3ZX
EGD with gastric biopsy	ØDB68ZX
Open endarterectomy of left common carotid artery	Ø3CJØZZ
Excision of basal cell carcinoma of lower lip	ØCB1XZZ
Open excision of tail of pancreas	ØFBGØZZ
Percutaneous biopsy of right gastrocnemius muscle	ØKBS3ZX
Sigmoidoscopy with sigmoid polypectomy	ØDBN8ZZ
Open excision of lesion from right Achilles tendon	ØLBNØZZ
Open resection of cecum	ØDTHØZZ
Total excision of pituitary gland, open	ØGTØØZZ
Explantation of left failed kidney, open	ØTT1ØZZ
Open left axillary total lymphadenectomy	Ø7T6ØZZ (RESECTION is coded for cutting out a chain of lymph nodes.)
Laparoscopic-assisted total vaginal hysterectomy	ØUT9FZZ
Right total mastectomy, open	ØHTTØZZ
Open resection of papillary muscle	Ø2TDØZZ (The papillary muscle refers to the heart and is found in the *Heart and Great Vessels* body system.)
Radical retropubic prostatectomy, open	ØVTØØZZ
Laparoscopic cholecystectomy	ØFT44ZZ
Endoscopic bilateral total maxillary sinusectomy	Ø9TQ4ZZ, Ø9TR4ZZ
Amputation at right elbow level	ØX6BØZZ
Right below-knee amputation, proximal tibia/fibula	ØY6HØZ1 (The qualifier *High* here means the portion of the tib/fib closest to the knee.)
Fifth ray carpometacarpal joint amputation, left hand	ØX6KØZ8 (A *complete* ray amputation is through the carpometacarpal joint.)
Right leg and hip amputation through ischium	ØY62ØZZ (The *Hindquarter* body part includes amputation along any part of the hip bone.)

Procedure	Code
DIP joint amputation of right thumb	ØX6LØZ3 (The qualifier *low* here means through the distal interphalangeal joint.)
Right wrist joint amputation	ØX6JØZØ (Amputation at the wrist joint is actually complete amputation of the hand.)
Trans-metatarsal amputation of foot at left big toe	ØY6NØZ9 (A *partial* amputation is through the shaft of the metatarsal bone.)
Mid-shaft amputation, right humerus	ØX68ØZ2
Left fourth toe amputation, mid-proximal phalanx	ØY6WØZ1 (The qualifier *High* here means anywhere along the proximal phalanx.)
Right above-knee amputation, distal femur	ØY6CØZ3
Cryotherapy of wart on left hand	ØH5GXZZ
Percutaneous radiofrequency ablation of right vocal cord lesion	ØC5T3ZZ
Left heart catheterization with laser destruction of arrhythmogenic focus, A-V node	Ø2583ZZ
Cautery of nosebleed	Ø95KXZZ
Transurethral endoscopic laser ablation of prostate	ØV5Ø8ZZ
Cautery of oozing varicose vein, left calf	Ø65Y3ZZ (The approach is coded *Percutaneous* because that is the normal route to a vein. No mention is made of approach, because likely the skin has eroded at that spot.)
Laparoscopy with destruction of endometriosis, bilateral ovaries	ØU524ZZ
Laser coagulation of right retinal vessel hemorrhage, percutaneous	Ø85G3ZZ (The *Retinal Vessel* body-part values are in the *Eye* body system.)
Thoracoscopic pleurodesis, left side	ØB5P4ZZ
Percutaneous insertion of Greenfield IVC filter	Ø6HØ3DZ
Forceps total mouth extraction, upper and lower teeth	ØCDWXZ2, ØCDXXZ2
Removal of left thumbnail	ØHDQXZZ (No separate body-part value is given for thumbnail, so this is coded to *Fingernail*.)
Extraction of right intraocular lens without replacement, percutaneous	Ø8DJ3ZZ

Procedure	Code
Laparoscopy with needle aspiration of ova for in vitro fertilization	0UDN4ZZ
Nonexcisional debridement of skin ulcer, right foot	0HDMXZZ
Open stripping of abdominal fascia, right side	0JD80ZZ
Hysteroscopy with D&C, diagnostic	0UDB8ZX
Liposuction for medical purposes, left upper arm	0JDF3ZZ (The *Percutaneous* approach is inherent in the liposuction technique.)
Removal of tattered right ear drum fragments with tweezers	09D77ZZ
Microincisional phlebectomy of spider veins, right lower leg	06DY3ZZ
Routine Foley catheter placement	0T9B70Z
Incision and drainage of external perianal abscess	0D9QXZZ
Percutaneous drainage of ascites	0W9G3ZZ (This is drainage of the cavity and not the peritoneal membrane itself.)
Laparoscopy with left ovarian cystotomy and drainage	0U914ZZ
Laparotomy and drain placement for liver abscess, right lobe	0F9100Z
Right knee arthrotomy with drain placement	0S9C00Z
Thoracentesis of left pleural effusion	0W9B3ZZ (This is drainage of the pleural cavity)
Phlebotomy of left median cubital vein for polycythemia vera	059F3ZZ (This median cubital vein is a branch of the cephalic vein)
Percutaneous chest tube placement for right pneumothorax	0W9930Z
Endoscopic drainage of left ethmoid sinus	099V4ZZ
External ventricular CSF drainage catheter placement via burr hole	009630Z
Removal of foreign body, right cornea	08C8XZZ
Percutaneous mechanical thrombectomy, left brachial artery	03C83ZZ
Esophagogastroscopy with removal of bezoar from stomach	0DC68ZZ
Foreign body removal, skin of left thumb	0HCGXZZ (There is no specific value for thumb skin, so the procedure is coded to *Hand*.)
Transurethral cystoscopy with removal of bladder stone	0TCB8ZZ
Forceps removal of foreign body in right nostril	09CKXZZ (Nostril is coded to the *Nose* body-part value.)
Laparoscopy with excision of old suture from mesentery	0DCV4ZZ
Incision and removal of right lacrimal duct stone	08CX0ZZ

Procedure	Code
Nonincisional removal of intraluminal foreign body from vagina	0UCG7ZZ (The approach *External* is also a possibility. It is assumed here that since the patient went to the doctor to have the object removed, that it was not in the vaginal orifice.)
Right common carotid endarterectomy, open	03CH0ZZ
Open excision of retained sliver, subcutaneous tissue of left foot	0JCR0ZZ
Extracorporeal shockwave lithotripsy (ESWL), bilateral ureters	0TF6XZZ, 0TF7XZZ (The *Bilateral Ureter* body-part value is not available for the root operation FRAGMENTATION, so the procedures are coded separately.)
Endoscopic retrograde cholangiopancreatography (ERCP) with lithotripsy of common bile duct stone	0FF98ZZ (ERCP is performed through the mouth to the biliary system via the duodenum, so the approach value is *Via Natural or Artificial Opening Endoscopic*.)
Thoracotomy with crushing of pericardial calcifications	02FN0ZZ
Transurethral cystoscopy with fragmentation of bladder calculus	0TFB8ZZ
Hysteroscopy with intraluminal lithotripsy of left fallopian tube calcification	0UF68ZZ
Division of right foot tendon, percutaneous	0L8V3ZZ
Left heart catheterization with division of bundle of HIS	02883ZZ
Open osteotomy of capitate, left hand	0P8N0ZZ (The capitate is one of the carpal bones of the hand.)
EGD with esophagotomy of esophagogastric junction	0D848ZZ
Sacral rhizotomy for pain control, percutaneous	018R3ZZ
Laparotomy with exploration and adhesiolysis of right ureter	0TN60ZZ
Incision of scar contracture, right elbow	0HNDXZZ (The skin of the elbow region is coded to *Lower Arm*.)
Frenulotomy for treatment of tongue-tie syndrome	0CN7XZZ (The frenulum is coded to the body-part value *Tongue*.)
Right shoulder arthroscopy with coracoacromial ligament release	0MN14ZZ
Mitral valvulotomy for release of fused leaflets, open approach	02NG0ZZ
Percutaneous left Achilles tendon release	0LNP3ZZ
Laparoscopy with lysis of peritoneal adhesions	0DNW4ZZ

Procedure	Code
Manual rupture of right shoulder joint adhesions under general anesthesia	ØRNJXZZ
Open posterior tarsal tunnel release	01NGØZZ (The nerve released in the posterior tarsal tunnel is the tibial nerve.)
Laparoscopy with freeing of left ovary and fallopian tube	ØUN14ZZ, ØUN64ZZ
Liver transplant with donor matched liver	ØFYØØZØ
Orthotopic heart transplant using porcine heart	Ø2YAØZ2 (The donor heart comes from an animal [pig], so the qualifier value is *Zooplastic.*)
Right lung transplant, open, using organ donor match	ØBYKØZØ
Transplant of large intestine, organ donor match	ØDYEØZØ
Left kidney/pancreas organ bank transplant	ØFYGØZØ, ØTY1ØZØ
Replantation of avulsed scalp	ØHMØXZZ
Reattachment of severed right ear	Ø9MØXZZ
Reattachment of traumatic left gastrocnemius avulsion, open	ØKMTØZZ
Closed replantation of three avulsed teeth, lower jaw	ØCMXXZ1
Reattachment of severed left hand	ØXMKØZZ
Right hand open palmaris longus tendon transfer	ØLX7ØZZ
Endoscopic radial to median nerve transfer	Ø1X64Z5
Fasciocutaneous flap closure of left thigh, open	ØJXMØZC (The qualifier identifies the body layers in addition to fascia included in the procedure.)
Transfer left index finger to left thumb position, open	ØXXPØZM
Percutaneous fascia transfer to fill defect, anterior neck	ØJX43ZZ
Trigeminal to facial nerve transfer, percutaneous endoscopic	ØØXK4ZM
Endoscopic left leg flexor hallucis longus tendon transfer	ØLXP4ZZ
Right scalp advancement flap to right temple	ØHXØXZZ
Bilateral TRAM pedicle flap reconstruction status post mastectomy, muscle only, open	ØKXKØZ6, ØKXLØZ6 (The transverse rectus abdominus muscle (TRAM) flap is coded for each flap developed.)
Skin transfer flap closure of complex open wound, left lower back	ØHX6XZZ
Open fracture reduction, right tibia	ØQSGØZZ
Laparoscopy with gastropexy for malrotation	ØDS64ZZ
Left knee arthroscopy with reposition of anterior cruciate ligament	ØMSP4ZZ
Open transposition of ulnar nerve	Ø1S4ØZZ
Closed reduction with percutaneous internal fixation of right femoral neck fracture	ØQS634Z

Procedure	Code
Trans-vaginal intraluminal cervical cerclage	ØUVC7DZ
Cervical cerclage using Shirodkar technique	ØUVC7ZZ
Thoracotomy with banding of left pulmonary artery using extraluminal device	Ø2VRØCZ
Restriction of thoracic duct with intraluminal stent, percutaneous	Ø7VK3DZ
Craniotomy with clipping of cerebral aneurysm	Ø3VGØCZ (The clip is placed lengthwise on the outside wall of the widened portion of the vessel.)
Nonincisional, trans-nasal placement of restrictive stent in right lacrimal duct	Ø8VX7DZ
Catheter-based temporary restriction of blood flow in abdominal aorta for treatment of cerebral ischemia	Ø4VØ3DJ
Percutaneous ligation of esophageal vein	Ø6L33ZZ
Percutaneous embolization of left internal carotid-cavernous fistula	Ø3LL3DZ
Laparoscopy with bilateral occlusion of fallopian tubes using Hulka extraluminal clips	ØUL74CZ
Open suture ligation of failed AV graft, left brachial artery	Ø3L8ØZZ
Percutaneous embolization of vascular supply, intracranial meningioma	Ø3LG3DZ
Percutaneous embolization of right uterine artery, using coils	Ø4LE3DT
Open occlusion of left atrial appendage, using extraluminal pressure clips	Ø2L7ØCK
Percutaneous suture exclusion of left atrial appendage, via femoral artery access	Ø2L73ZK
ERCP with balloon dilation of common bile duct	ØF798ZZ
PTCA of two coronary arteries, LAD with stent placement, RCA with no stent	Ø27Ø3DZ, Ø27Ø3ZZ (A separate procedure is coded for each artery dilated, since the device value differs for each artery.)
Cystoscopy with intraluminal dilation of bladder neck stricture	ØT7C8ZZ
Open dilation of old anastomosis, left femoral artery	Ø47LØZZ
Dilation of upper esophageal stricture, direct visualization, with Bougie sound	ØD717ZZ
PTA of right brachial artery stenosis	Ø3773ZZ
Transnasal dilation and stent placement in right lacrimal duct	Ø87X7DZ
Hysteroscopy with balloon dilation of bilateral fallopian tubes	ØU778ZZ
Tracheoscopy with intraluminal dilation of tracheal stenosis	ØB718ZZ
Cystoscopy with dilation of left ureteral stricture, with stent placement	ØT778DZ
Open gastric bypass with Roux-en-Y limb to jejunum	ØD16ØZA
Right temporal artery to intracranial artery bypass using Gore-Tex graft, open	Ø31SØJG

Procedure	Code
Tracheostomy formation with tracheostomy tube placement, percutaneous	0B113F4
PICVA (percutaneous in situ coronary venous arterialization) of single coronary artery	02103D4
Open left femoral-popliteal artery bypass using cadaver vein graft	041L0KL
Shunting of intrathecal cerebrospinal fluid to peritoneal cavity using synthetic shunt	00160J6
Colostomy formation, open, transverse colon to abdominal wall	0D1L0Z4
Open urinary diversion, left ureter, using ileal conduit to skin	0T170ZC
CABG of LAD using left internal mammary artery, open off-bypass	02100Z9
Open pleuroperitoneal shunt, right pleural cavity, using synthetic device	0W190JG
Percutaneous placement of ventriculoperitoneal shunt for treatment of hydrocephalus	00163J6
End-of-life replacement of spinal neurostimulator generator, multiple array, in lower abdomen	0JH80DZ (Taking out of the old generator is coded separately to the root operation *Removal*)
Percutaneous insertion of spinal neurostimulator lead, lumbar spinal cord	00HV3MZ
Percutaneous placement of broken pacemaker lead in left atrium	02H73MZ (Taking out the broken pacemaker lead is coded separately to the root operation *Removal*.)
Open placement of dual chamber pacemaker generator in chest wall	0JH606Z
Percutaneous placement of venous central line in right internal jugular	05HM33Z
Open insertion of multiple channel cochlear implant, left ear	09HE06Z
Percutaneous placement of Swan-Ganz catheter in superior vena cava	02HV32Z (The Swan-Ganz catheter is coded to the device value *Monitoring Device* because it monitors pulmonary artery output.)
Bronchoscopy with insertion of brachytherapy seeds, right main bronchus	0BH081Z
Placement of intrathecal infusion pump for pain management, percutaneous	0JH73VZ (The device resides principally in the subcutaneous tissue of the back, so it is coded to body system *Subcutaneous Tissue and Fascia*.)
Open insertion of interspinous process device into lumbar vertebral joint	0QH004Z
Open placement of bone growth stimulator, left femoral shaft	0QHY0MZ
Cystoscopy with placement of brachytherapy seeds in prostate gland	0VH081Z
Percutaneous insertion of Greenfield IVC filter	06H03DZ

Procedure	Code
Full-thickness skin graft to right lower arm, autograft (do not code graft harvest for this exercise)	0HRDX73
Excision of necrosed left femoral head with bone bank bone graft to fill the defect, open	0QR70KZ
Penetrating keratoplasty of right cornea with donor matched cornea, percutaneous approach	08R83KZ
Bilateral mastectomy with concomitant saline breast implants, open	0HRV0JZ
Excision of abdominal aorta with Gore-Tex graft replacement, open	04R00JZ
Total right knee arthroplasty with insertion of total knee prosthesis	0SRC0JZ
Bilateral mastectomy with free TRAM flap reconstruction	0HRV076
Tenonectomy with graft to right ankle using cadaver graft, open	0LRS0KZ
Mitral valve replacement using porcine valve, open	02RG08Z
Percutaneous phacoemulsification of right eye cataract with prosthetic lens insertion	08RJ3JZ
Transcatheter replacement of pulmonary valve using of bovine jugular vein valve	02RH38Z
Total left hip replacement using ceramic on ceramic prosthesis, without bone cement	0SRB03A
Aortic valve annuloplasty using ring, open	02UF0JZ
Laparoscopic repair of left inguinal hernia with marlex plug	0YU64JZ
Autograft nerve graft to right median nerve, percutaneous endoscopic (do not code graft harvest for this exercise)	01U547Z
Exchange of liner in femoral component of previous left hip replacement, open approach	0SUS09Z (Taking out of the old liner is coded separately to the root operation *Removal*)
Anterior colporrhaphy with polypropylene mesh reinforcement, open approach	0UUG0JZ
Implantation of CorCap cardiac support device, open approach	02UA0JZ
Abdominal wall herniorrhaphy, open, using synthetic mesh	0WUF0JZ
Tendon graft to strengthen injured left shoulder using autograft, open (do not code graft harvest for this exercise)	0LU207Z
Onlay lamellar keratoplasty of left cornea using autograft, external approach	08U9X7Z
Resurfacing procedure on right femoral head, open approach	0SUR0BZ
Exchange of drainage tube from right hip joint	0S2YX0Z
Tracheostomy tube exchange	0B21XFZ
Change chest tube for left pneumothorax	0W2BX0Z
Exchange of cerebral ventriculostomy drainage tube	0020X0Z

Procedure	Code
Foley urinary catheter exchange	ØT2BXØZ (This is coded to *Drainage Device* because urine is being drained.)
Open removal of lumbar sympathetic neurostimulator lead	Ø1PYØMZ
Nonincisional removal of Swan-Ganz catheter from right pulmonary artery	Ø2PYX2Z
Laparotomy with removal of pancreatic drain	ØFPGØØZ
Extubation, endotracheal tube	ØBP1XFZ
Nonincisional PEG tube removal	ØDP6XUZ
Transvaginal removal of brachytherapy seeds	ØUPH71Z
Transvaginal removal of extraluminal cervical cerclage	ØUPD7CZ
Incision with removal of K-wire fixation, right first metatarsal	ØQPNØ4Z
Cystoscopy with retrieval of left ureteral stent	ØTP98DZ
Removal of nasogastric drainage tube for decompression	ØDP6XØZ
Removal of external fixator, left radial fracture	ØPPJX5Z
Reposition of Swan-Ganz catheter insertion in superior vena cava	Ø2WYX2Z
Open revision of right hip replacement, with readjustment of prosthesis	ØSW9ØJZ
Adjustment of position, pacemaker lead in left ventricle, percutaneous	Ø2WA3MZ
External repositioning of Foley catheter to bladder	ØTWBXØZ
Taking out loose screw and putting larger screw in fracture repair plate, left tibia	ØQWHØ4Z
Revision of VAD reservoir placement in chest wall, causing patient discomfort, open	ØJWTØWZ
Thoracotomy with exploration of right pleural cavity	ØWJ9ØZZ
Diagnostic laryngoscopy	ØCJS8ZZ
Exploratory arthrotomy of left knee	ØSJDØZZ
Colposcopy with diagnostic hysteroscopy	ØUJD8ZZ
Digital rectal exam	ØDJD7ZZ
Diagnostic arthroscopy of right shoulder	ØRJJ4ZZ
Endoscopy of maxillary sinus	Ø9JY4ZZ
Laparotomy with palpation of liver	ØFJØØZZ
Transurethral diagnostic cystoscopy	ØTJB8ZZ
Colonoscopy, discontinued at sigmoid colon	ØDJD8ZZ
Percutaneous mapping of basal ganglia	ØØK83ZZ
Heart catheterization with cardiac mapping	Ø2K83ZZ
Intraoperative whole brain mapping via craniotomy	ØØKØØZZ
Mapping of left cerebral hemisphere, percutaneous endoscopic	ØØK74ZZ
Intraoperative cardiac mapping during open heart surgery	Ø2K8ØZZ
Hysteroscopy with cautery of post-hysterectomy oozing and evacuation of clot	ØW3R8ZZ
Open exploration and ligation of post-op arterial bleeder, left forearm	ØX3FØZZ

Procedure	Code
Control of post-operative retroperitoneal bleeding via laparotomy	ØW3HØZZ
Reopening of thoracotomy site with drainage and control of post-op hemopericardium	ØW3CØZZ
Arthroscopy with drainage of hemarthrosis at previous operative site, right knee	ØY3F4ZZ
Radiocarpal fusion of left hand with internal fixation, open	ØRGPØ4Z
Posterior spinal fusion at L1-L3 level with BAK cage interbody fusion device, open	ØSG1ØAJ
Intercarpal fusion of right hand with bone bank bone graft, open	ØRGQØKZ
Sacrococcygeal fusion with bone graft from same operative site, open	ØSG5Ø7Z
Interphalangeal fusion of left great toe, percutaneous pin fixation	ØSGQ34Z
Suture repair of left radial nerve laceration	Ø1Q6ØZZ (The approach value is *Open*, though the surgical exposure may have been created by the wound itself.)
Laparotomy with suture repair of blunt force duodenal laceration	ØDQ9ØZZ
Perineoplasty with repair of old obstetric laceration, open	ØWQNØZZ
Suture repair of right biceps tendon laceration, open	ØLQ3ØZZ
Closure of abdominal wall stab wound	ØWQFØZZ
Cosmetic face lift, open, no other information available	ØWØ2ØZZ
Bilateral breast augmentation with silicone implants, open	ØHØVØJZ
Cosmetic rhinoplasty with septal reduction and tip elevation using local tissue graft, open	Ø9ØKØ7Z
Abdominoplasty (tummy tuck), open	ØWØFØZZ
Liposuction of bilateral thighs	ØJØL3ZZ, ØJØM3ZZ
Creation of penis in female patient using tissue bank donor graft	ØW4NØK1
Creation of vagina in male patient using synthetic material	ØW4MØJØ
Laparoscopic vertical (sleeve) gastrectomy	ØDB64Z3
Left uterine artery embolization with intraluminal biosphere injection	Ø4LF3DU

Obstetrics

Procedure	Code
Abortion by dilation and evacuation following laminaria insertion	10A07ZW
Manually assisted spontaneous abortion	10E0XZZ (Since the pregnancy was not artificially terminated, this is coded to *Delivery* because it captures the procedure objective. The fact that it was an abortion will be identified in the diagnosis code.)
Abortion by abortifacient insertion	10A07ZX
Bimanual pregnancy examination	10J07ZZ
Extraperitoneal C-section, low transverse incision	10D00Z2
Fetal spinal tap, percutaneous	10903ZA
Fetal kidney transplant, laparoscopic	10Y04ZS
Open in utero repair of congenital diaphragmatic hernia	10Q00ZK (Diaphragm is classified to the *Respiratory* body system in the *Medical and Surgical* section.)
Laparoscopy with total excision of tubal pregnancy	10T24ZZ
Transvaginal removal of fetal monitoring electrode	10P073Z

Placement

Procedure	Code
Placement of packing material, right ear	2Y42X5Z
Mechanical traction of entire left leg	2W6MX0Z
Removal of splint, right shoulder	2W5AX1Z
Placement of neck brace	2W32X3Z
Change of vaginal packing	2Y04X5Z
Packing of wound, chest wall	2W44X5Z
Sterile dressing placement to left groin region	2W27X4Z
Removal of packing material from pharynx	2Y50X5Z
Placement of intermittent pneumatic compression device, covering entire right arm	2W18X7Z
Exchange of pressure dressing to left thigh	2W0PX6Z

Administration

Procedure	Code
Peritoneal dialysis via indwelling catheter	3E1M39Z
Transvaginal artificial insemination	3E0P7LZ
Infusion of total parenteral nutrition via central venous catheter	3E0436Z
Esophagogastroscopy with Botox injection into esophageal sphincter	3E0G8GC (Botulinum toxin is a paralyzing agent with temporary effects; it does not sclerose or destroy the nerve.)
Percutaneous irrigation of knee joint	3E1U38Z
Epidural injection of mixed steroid and local anesthetic for pain control	3E0S33Z (This is coded to the substance value *Anti-inflammatory*. The anesthetic is added only to lessen the pain of the injection.)
Transfusion of antihemophilic factor, (nonautologous) via arterial central line	30263V1
Transabdominal in vitro fertilization, implantation of donor ovum	3E0P3Q1
Autologous bone marrow transplant via central venous line	30243G0
Implantation of anti-microbial envelope with cardiac defibrillator placement, open	3E0102A
Sclerotherapy of brachial plexus lesion, alcohol injection	3E0T3TZ
Percutaneous peripheral vein injection, glucarpidase	3E033GQ
Introduction of anti-infective envelope into subcutaneous tissue, open	3E0102A

Measurement and Monitoring

Procedure	Code
Cardiac stress test, single measurement	4A02XM4
EGD with biliary flow measurement	4A0C85Z
Right and left heart cardiac catheterization with bilateral sampling and pressure measurements	4A023N8
Temperature monitoring, rectal	4A1Z7KZ
Peripheral venous pulse, external, single measurement	4A04XJ1
Holter monitoring	4A12X45
Respiratory rate, external, single measurement	4A09XCZ
Fetal heart rate monitoring, transvaginal	4A1H7CZ
Visual mobility test, single measurement	4A07X7Z
Left ventricular cardiac output monitoring from pulmonary artery wedge (Swan-Ganz) catheter	4A1239Z
Olfactory acuity test, single measurement	4A08X0Z

Extracorporeal Assistance and Performance

Procedure	Code
Intermittent mechanical ventilation, 16 hours	5A1935Z
Liver dialysis, single encounter	5A1CØØZ
Cardiac countershock with successful conversion to sinus rhythm	5A22Ø4Z
IPPB (intermittent positive pressure breathing) for mobilization of secretions, 22 hours	5AØ9358
Renal dialysis, series of encounters	5A1D6ØZ
IABP (intra-aortic balloon pump) continuous	5AØ221Ø
Intra-operative cardiac pacing, continuous	5A1223Z
ECMO (extracorporeal membrane oxygenation), continuous	5A15223
Controlled mechanical ventilation (CMV), 45 hours	5A1945Z (The endotracheal tube associated with the mechanical ventilation procedure is considered a component of the equipment used in performing the procedure and is not coded separately.)
Pulsatile compression boot with intermittent inflation	5AØ2115 (This is coded to the function value *Cardiac Output*, because the purpose of such compression devices is to return blood to the heart faster.)

Extracorporeal Therapies

Procedure	Code
Donor thrombocytapheresis, single encounter	6A55ØZ2
Bili-lite UV phototherapy, series treatment	6A8Ø1ZZ
Whole body hypothermia, single treatment	6A4ZØZZ
Circulatory phototherapy, single encounter	6A65ØZZ
Shock wave therapy of plantar fascia, single treatment	6A93ØZZ
Antigen-free air conditioning, series treatment	6AØZ1ZZ
TMS (transcranial magnetic stimulation), series treatment	6A221ZZ
Therapeutic ultrasound of peripheral vessels, single treatment	6A75ØZ6
Plasmapheresis, series treatment	6A551Z3
Extracorporeal electromagnetic stimulation (EMS) for urinary incontinence, single treatment	6A21ØZZ

Osteopathic

Procedures	Code
Isotonic muscle energy treatment of right leg	7WØ6X8Z
Low velocity-high amplitude osteopathic treatment of head	7WØØX5Z
Lymphatic pump osteopathic treatment of left axilla	7WØ7X6Z
Indirect osteopathic treatment of sacrum	7WØ4X4Z
Articulatory osteopathic treatment of cervical region	7WØ1XØZ

Other Procedures

Procedure	Code
Near infrared spectroscopy of leg vessels	8EØ23DZ
CT computer assisted sinus surgery	8EØ9XBG (The primary procedure is coded separately.)
Suture removal, abdominal wall	8EØWXY8
Isolation after infectious disease exposure	8EØZXY6
Robotic assisted open prostatectomy	8EØWØCZ (The primary procedure is coded separately.)
In vitro fertilization	8EØZXY1

Chiropractic

Procedure	Code
Chiropractic treatment of lumbar region using long lever specific contact	9WB3XGZ
Chiropractic manipulation of abdominal region, indirect visceral	9WB9XCZ
Chiropractic extra-articular treatment of hip region	9WB6XDZ
Chiropractic treatment of sacrum using long and short lever specific contact	9WB4XJZ
Mechanically-assisted chiropractic manipulation of head	9WBØXKZ

Imaging

Procedure	Code
Noncontrast CT of abdomen and pelvis	BW21ZZZ
Intravascular ultrasound, left subclavian artery	B342ZZ3
Fluoroscopic guidance for insertion of central venous catheter in SVC, low osmolar contrast	B5181ZA
Chest x-ray, AP/PA and lateral views	BW03ZZZ
Endoluminal ultrasound of gallbladder and bile ducts	BF43ZZZ
MRI of thyroid gland, contrast unspecified	BG34YZZ
Esophageal videofluoroscopy study with oral barium contrast	BD11YZZ
Portable x-ray study of right radius/ulna shaft, standard series	BP0JZZZ
Routine fetal ultrasound, second trimester twin gestation	BY4DZZZ
CT scan of bilateral lungs, high osmolar contrast with densitometry	BB240ZZ
Fluoroscopic guidance for percutaneous transluminal angioplasty (PTA) of left common femoral artery, low osmolar contrast	B41G1ZZ

Nuclear Medicine

Procedure	Code
Tomo scan of right and left heart, unspecified radiopharmaceutical, qualitative gated rest	C226YZZ
Technetium pentetate assay of kidneys, ureters, and bladder	CT631ZZ
Uniplanar scan of spine using technetium oxidronate, with first-pass study	CP151ZZ
Thallous chloride tomographic scan of bilateral breasts	CH22SZZ
PET scan of myocardium using rubidium	C23GQZZ
Gallium citrate scan of head and neck, single plane imaging	CW1BLZZ
Xenon gas nonimaging probe of brain	C050VZZ
Upper GI scan, radiopharmaceutical unspecified, for gastric emptying	CD15YZZ
Carbon 11 PET scan of brain with quantification	C030BZZ
Iodinated albumin nuclear medicine assay, blood plasma volume study	C763HZZ

Radiation Therapy

Procedure	Code
Plaque radiation of left eye, single port	D8Y0FZZ
8 MeV photon beam radiation to brain	D0011ZZ
IORT of colon, 3 ports	DDY5CZZ
HDR brachytherapy of prostate using palladium-103	DV109BZ
Electron radiation treatment of right breast, with custom device	DM013ZZ
Hyperthermia oncology treatment of pelvic region	DWY68ZZ
Contact radiation of tongue	D9Y57ZZ
Heavy particle radiation treatment of pancreas, four risk sites	DF034ZZ
LDR brachytherapy to spinal cord using iodine	D016B9Z
Whole body Phosphorus 32 administration with risk to hematopoetic system	DWY5GFZ

Physical Rehabilitation and Diagnostic Audiology

Procedure	Code
Bekesy assessment using audiometer	F13Z31Z
Individual fitting of left eye prosthesis	F0DZ8UZ
Physical therapy for range of motion and mobility, patient right hip, no special equipment	F07L0ZZ
Bedside swallow assessment using assessment kit	F00ZHYZ
Caregiver training in airway clearance techniques	F0FZ8ZZ
Application of short arm cast in rehabilitation setting	F0DZ7EZ (Inhibitory cast is listed in the equipment reference table under E, *Orthosis*.)
Verbal assessment of patient's pain level	F02ZFZZ
Caregiver training in communication skills using manual communication board	F0FZJMZ (Manual communication board is listed in the equipment reference table under M, *Augmentative/ Alternative Communication*.)
Group musculoskeletal balance training exercises, whole body, no special equipment	F07M6ZZ (Balance training is included in the motor treatment reference table under *Therapeutic Exercise*.)
Individual therapy for auditory processing using tape recorder	F09Z2KZ (Tape recorder is listed in the equipment reference table under *Audiovisual Equipment*.)

Mental Health

Procedure	Code
Cognitive-behavioral psychotherapy, individual	GZ58ZZZ
Narcosynthesis	GZGZZZZ
Light therapy	GZJZZZZ
ECT (electroconvulsive therapy), unilateral, multiple seizure	GZB1ZZZ
Crisis intervention	GZ2ZZZZ
Neuropsychological testing	GZ13ZZZ
Hypnosis	GZFZZZZ
Developmental testing	GZ10ZZZ
Vocational counseling	GZ61ZZZ
Family psychotherapy	GZ72ZZZ

Substance Abuse Treatment

Procedure	Code
Naltrexone treatment for drug dependency	HZ94ZZZ
Substance abuse treatment family counseling	HZ63ZZZ
Medication monitoring of patient on methadone maintenance	HZ81ZZZ
Individual interpersonal psychotherapy for drug abuse	HZ54ZZZ
Patient in for alcohol detoxification treatment	HZ2ZZZZ
Group motivational counseling	HZ47ZZZ
Individual 12-step psychotherapy for substance abuse	HZ53ZZZ
Post-test infectious disease counseling for IV drug abuser	HZ3CZZZ
Psychodynamic psychotherapy for drug dependent patient	HZ5CZZZ
Group cognitive-behavioral counseling for substance abuse	HZ42ZZZ

Appendix I: Illustrations

Peripheral Nervous System

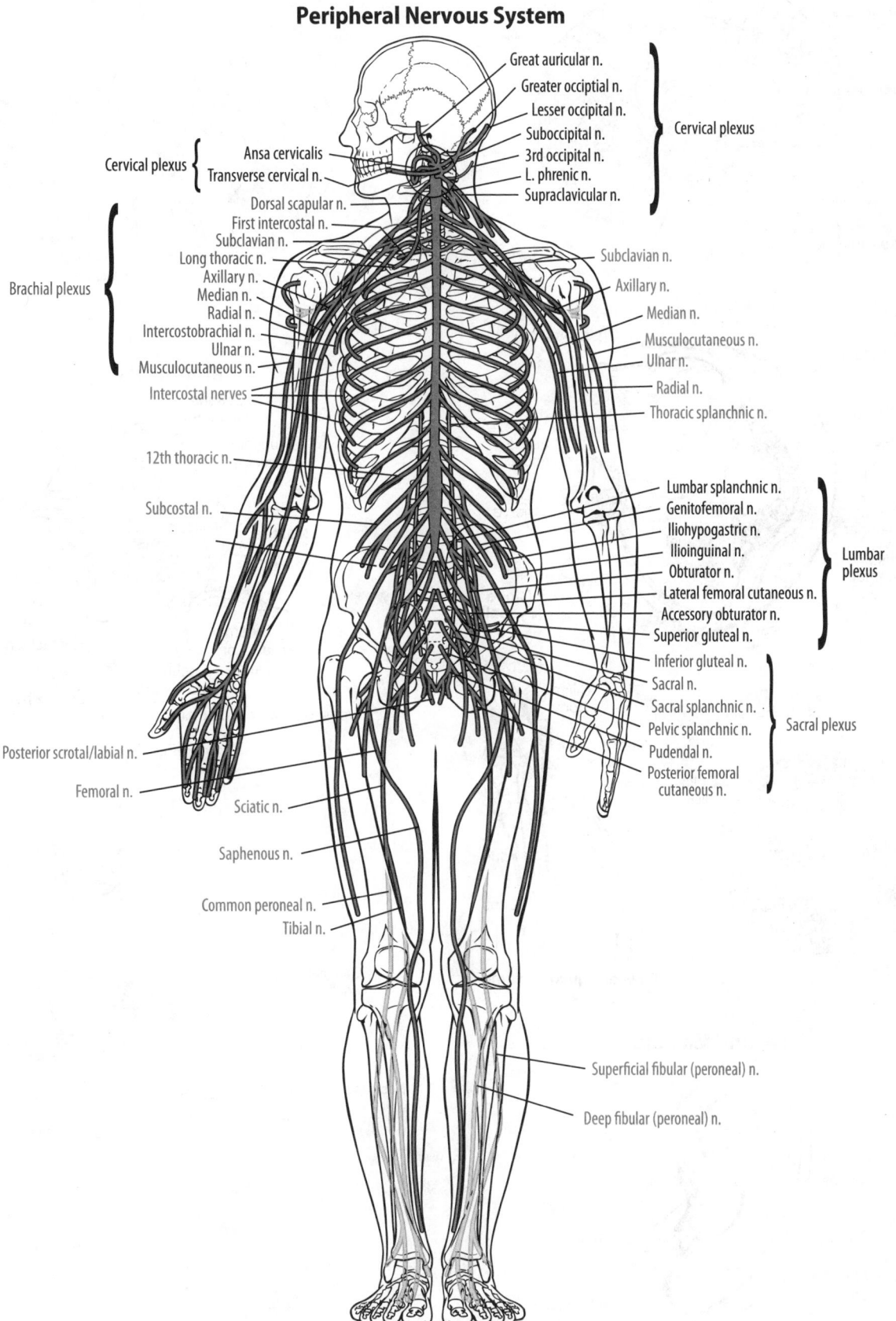

Great auricular n.
Greater occipital n.
Lesser occipital n.
Suboccipital n.
3rd occipital n.
L. phrenic n.
Supraclavicular n.

Cervical plexus

Cervical plexus
Ansa cervicalis
Transverse cervical n.
Dorsal scapular n.
First intercostal n.
Subclavian n.
Long thoracic n.

Brachial plexus
Axillary n.
Median n.
Radial n.
Intercostobrachial n.
Ulnar n.
Musculocutaneous n.
Intercostal nerves

Subclavian n.
Axillary n.
Median n.
Musculocutaneous n.
Ulnar n.
Radial n.
Thoracic splanchnic n.

12th thoracic n.

Subcostal n.

Lumbar splanchnic n.
Genitofemoral n.
Iliohypogastric n.
Ilioinguinal n.
Obturator n.
Lateral femoral cutaneous n.
Accessory obturator n.
Superior gluteal n.

Lumbar plexus

Inferior gluteal n.
Sacral n.
Sacral splanchnic n.
Pelvic splanchnic n.
Pudendal n.
Posterior femoral cutaneous n.

Sacral plexus

Posterior scrotal/labial n.

Femoral n.

Sciatic n.

Saphenous n.

Common peroneal n.
Tibial n.

Superficial fibular (peroneal) n.

Deep fibular (peroneal) n.

Brain

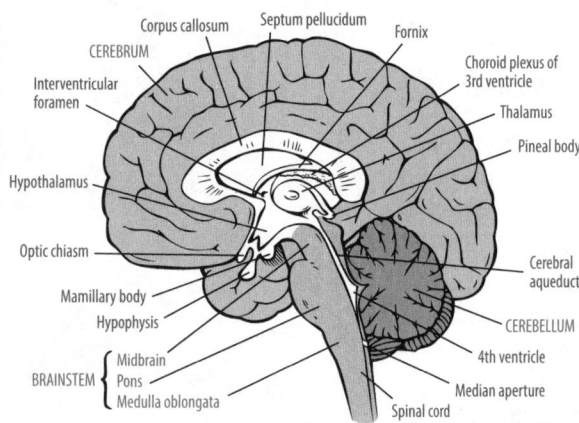

Cranial Nerves

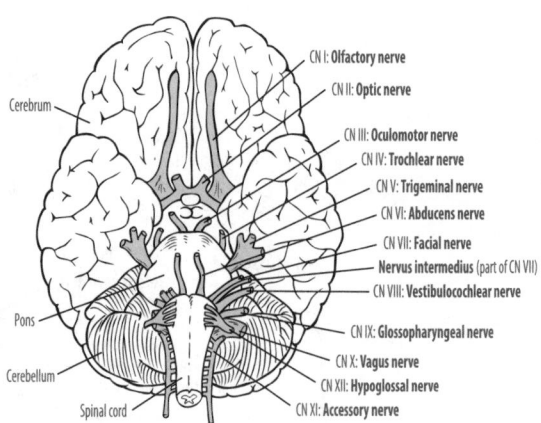

Eye

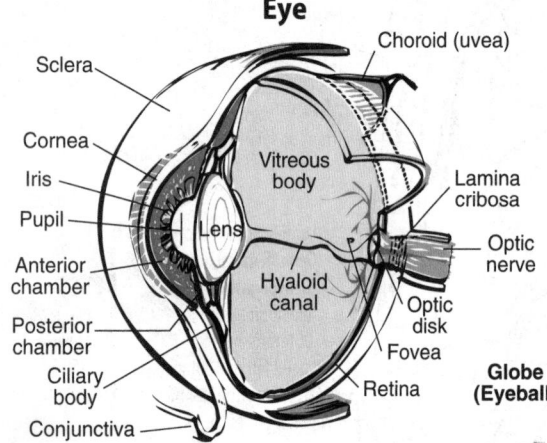

Globe (Eyeball)

Middle Ear

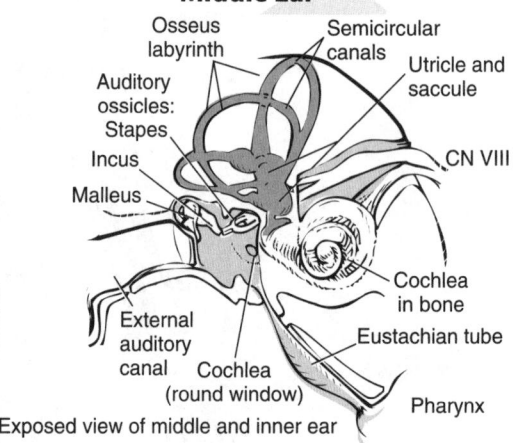

Exposed view of middle and inner ear

Posterior Pole of Globe

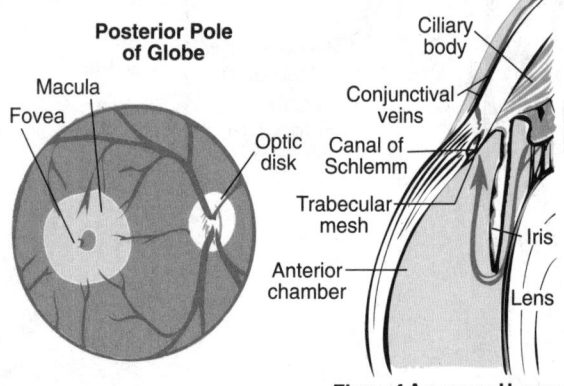

Flow of Aqueous Humor

Lacrimal System

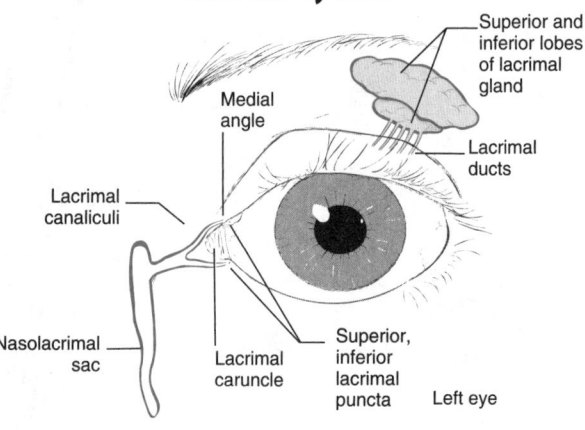

Ear and Mastoid

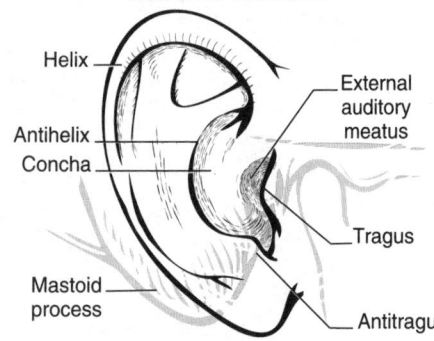

Arteries

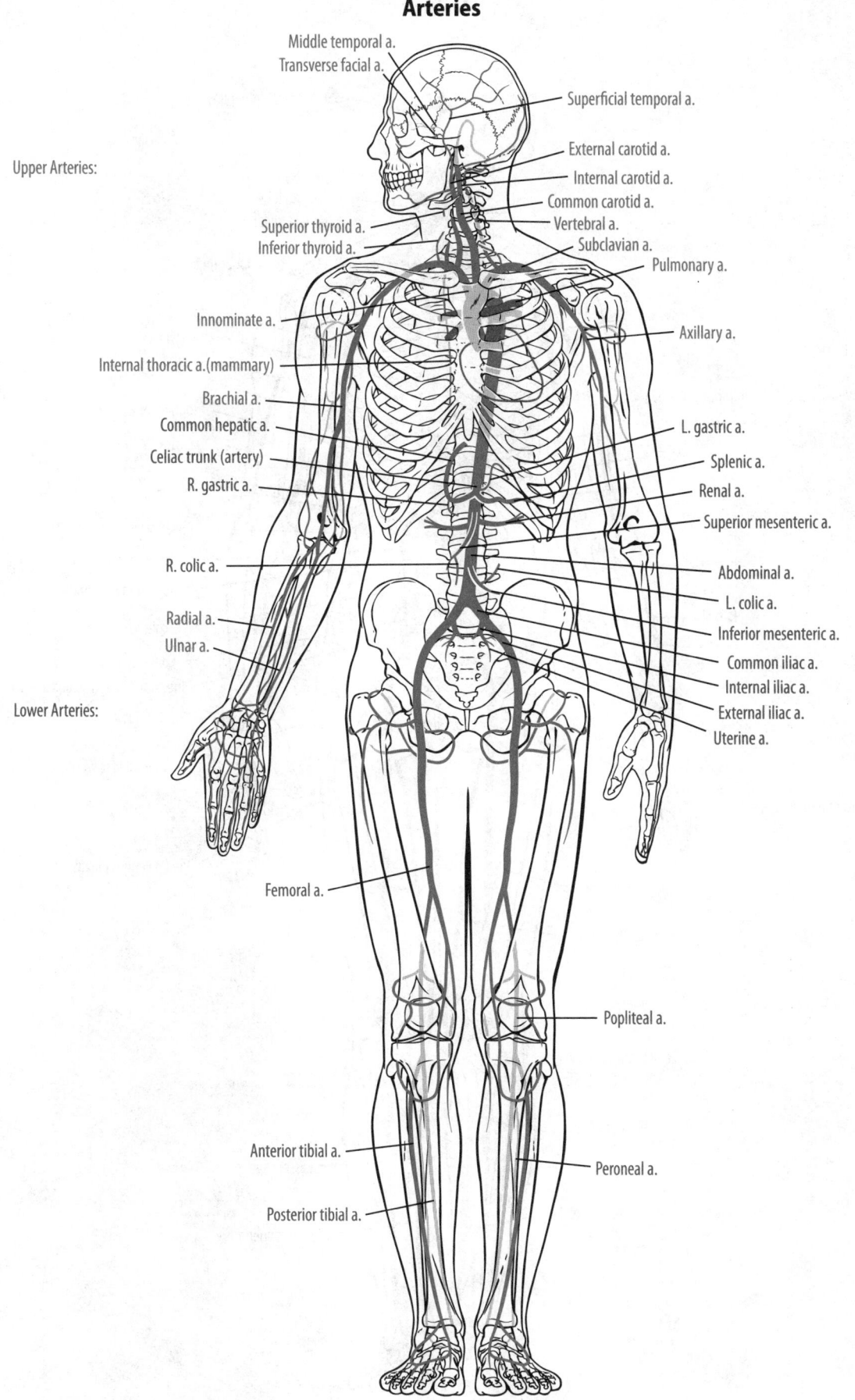

Upper Arteries:

Middle temporal a.
Transverse facial a.
Superficial temporal a.
External carotid a.
Internal carotid a.
Common carotid a.
Vertebral a.
Subclavian a.
Pulmonary a.
Superior thyroid a.
Inferior thyroid a.
Innominate a.
Axillary a.
Internal thoracic a.(mammary)
Brachial a.
Common hepatic a.
L. gastric a.
Celiac trunk (artery)
Splenic a.
R. gastric a.
Renal a.
Superior mesenteric a.
R. colic a.
Abdominal a.
L. colic a.
Radial a.
Inferior mesenteric a.
Ulnar a.
Common iliac a.
Internal iliac a.
External iliac a.
Uterine a.

Lower Arteries:

Femoral a.
Popliteal a.
Anterior tibial a.
Peroneal a.
Posterior tibial a.

Veins

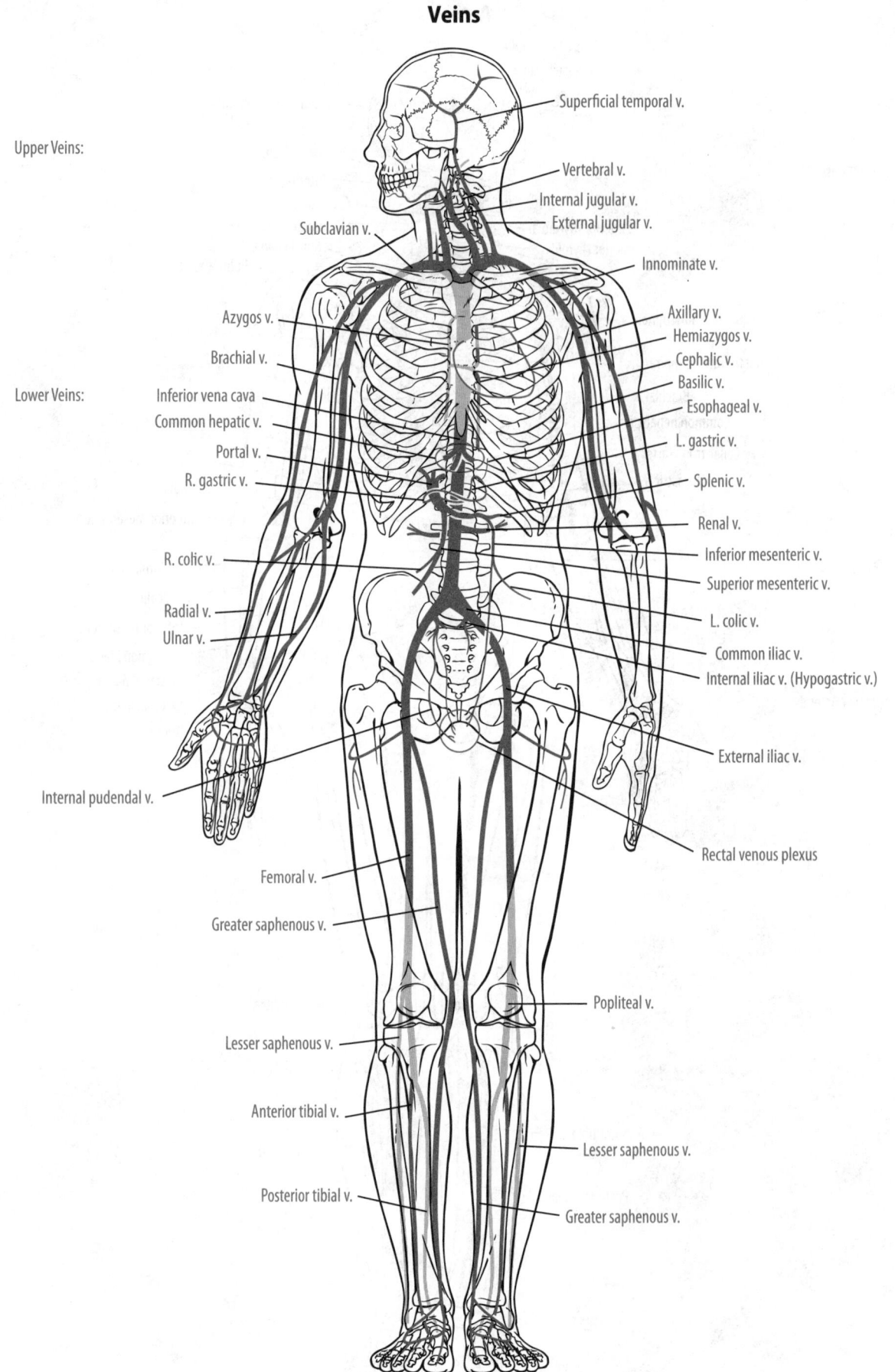

Upper Veins:

Lower Veins:

Superficial temporal v.

Vertebral v.

Internal jugular v.

External jugular v.

Innominate v.

Subclavian v.

Azygos v.

Brachial v.

Inferior vena cava

Common hepatic v.

Portal v.

R. gastric v.

R. colic v.

Radial v.

Ulnar v.

Internal pudendal v.

Femoral v.

Greater saphenous v.

Lesser saphenous v.

Anterior tibial v.

Posterior tibial v.

Axillary v.

Hemiazygos v.

Cephalic v.

Basilic v.

Esophageal v.

L. gastric v.

Splenic v.

Renal v.

Inferior mesenteric v.

Superior mesenteric v.

L. colic v.

Common iliac v.

Internal iliac v. (Hypogastric v.)

External iliac v.

Rectal venous plexus

Popliteal v.

Lesser saphenous v.

Greater saphenous v.

Anatomy of Heart

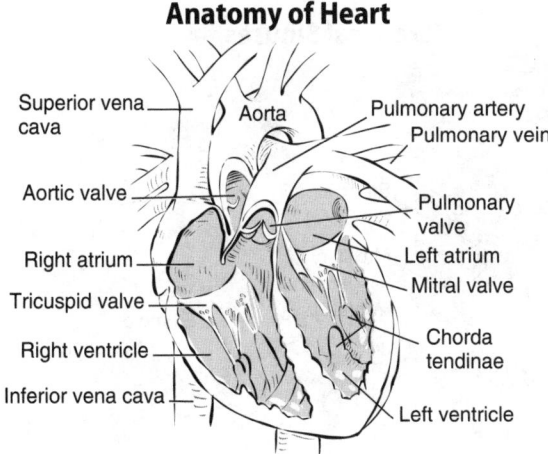

Superior vena cava
Aorta
Pulmonary artery
Pulmonary vein
Aortic valve
Pulmonary valve
Left atrium
Right atrium
Mitral valve
Tricuspid valve
Right ventricle
Chorda tendinae
Inferior vena cava
Left ventricle

Arteries of Heart

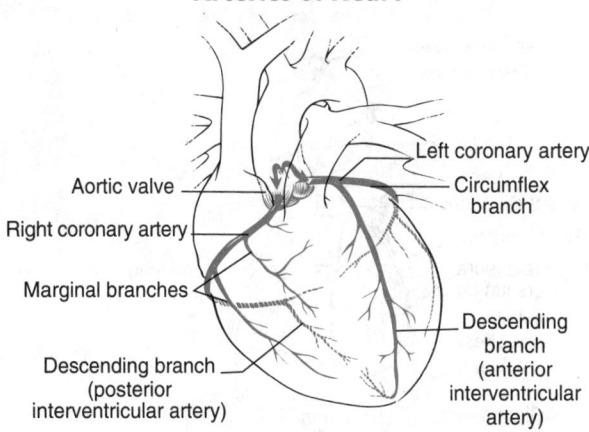

Left coronary artery
Circumflex branch
Aortic valve
Right coronary artery
Marginal branches
Descending branch (anterior interventricular artery)
Descending branch (posterior interventricular artery)

Cerebrovascular Arteries

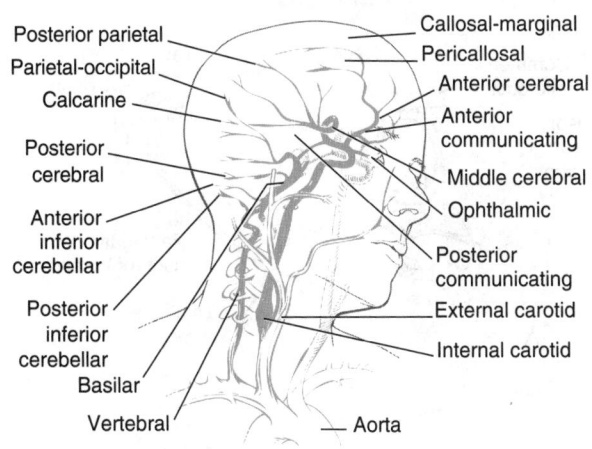

Posterior parietal
Parietal-occipital
Calcarine
Posterior cerebral
Anterior inferior cerebellar
Posterior inferior cerebellar
Basilar
Vertebral
Callosal-marginal
Pericallosal
Anterior cerebral
Anterior communicating
Middle cerebral
Ophthalmic
Posterior communicating
External carotid
Internal carotid
Aorta

Veins of Head and Neck

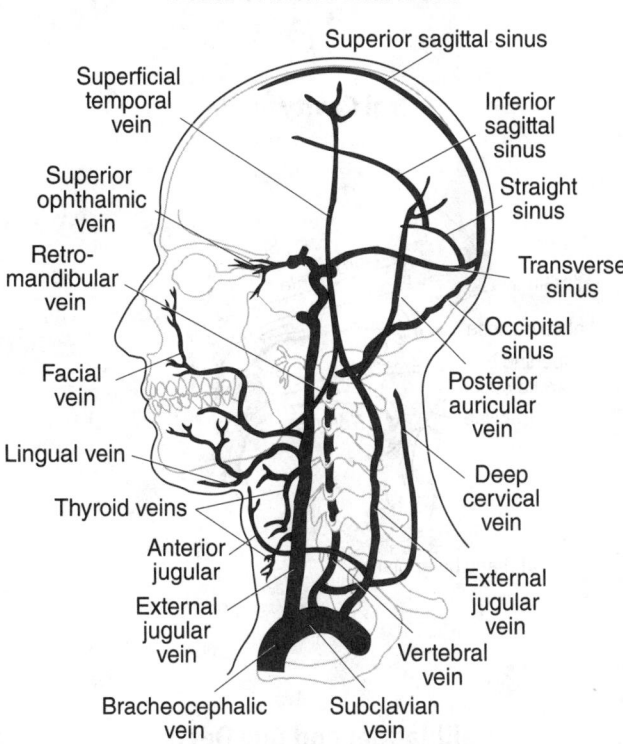

Superior sagittal sinus
Superficial temporal vein
Inferior sagittal sinus
Superior ophthalmic vein
Straight sinus
Retro-mandibular vein
Transverse sinus
Occipital sinus
Facial vein
Posterior auricular vein
Lingual vein
Deep cervical vein
Thyroid veins
Anterior jugular
External jugular vein
External jugular vein
Vertebral vein
Bracheocephalic vein
Subclavian vein

Lymphatic System of Head and Neck

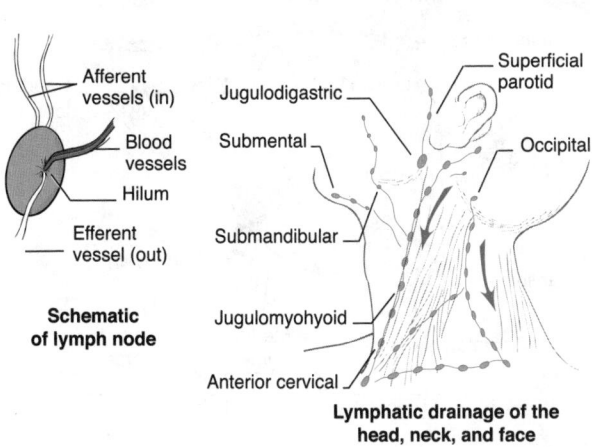

Afferent vessels (in)
Blood vessels
Hilum
Efferent vessel (out)

Schematic of lymph node

Jugulodigastric
Submental
Submandibular
Jugulomyohyoid
Anterior cervical
Superficial parotid
Occipital

Lymphatic drainage of the head, neck, and face

Lymph Nodes

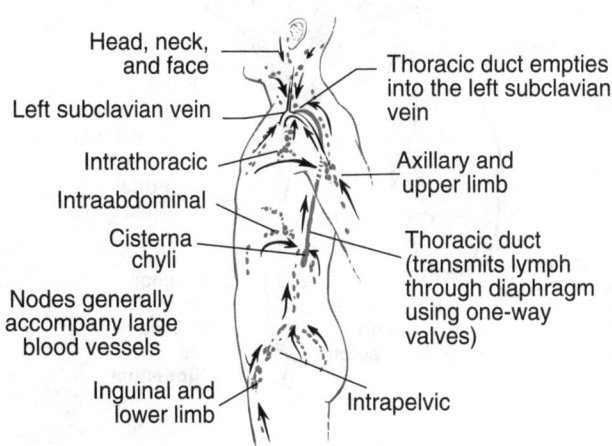

Head, neck, and face
Thoracic duct empties into the left subclavian vein
Left subclavian vein
Intrathoracic
Axillary and upper limb
Intraabdominal
Cisterna chyli
Thoracic duct (transmits lymph through diaphragm using one-way valves)
Nodes generally accompany large blood vessels
Inguinal and lower limb
Intrapelvic

Respiratory System

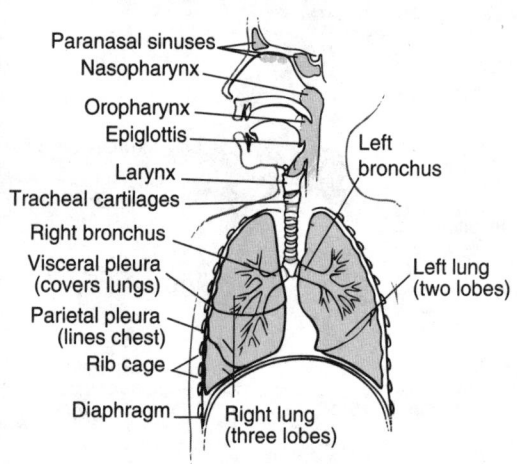

Paranasal sinuses
Nasopharynx
Oropharynx
Epiglottis
Larynx
Tracheal cartilages
Right bronchus
Visceral pleura (covers lungs)
Parietal pleura (lines chest)
Rib cage
Diaphragm
Left bronchus
Left lung (two lobes)
Right lung (three lobes)

Paranasal Sinuses

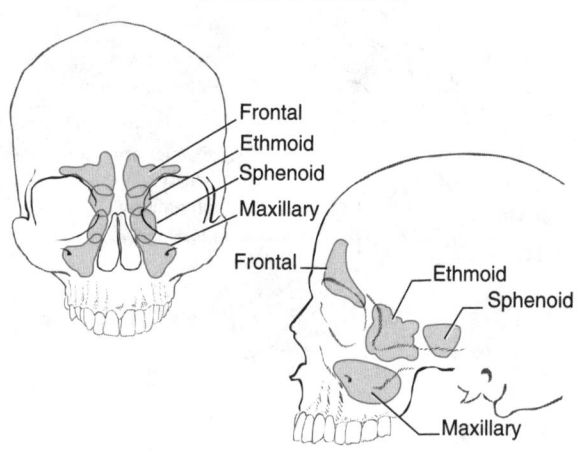

Frontal
Ethmoid
Sphenoid
Maxillary
Frontal
Ethmoid
Sphenoid
Maxillary

Oral Cavity

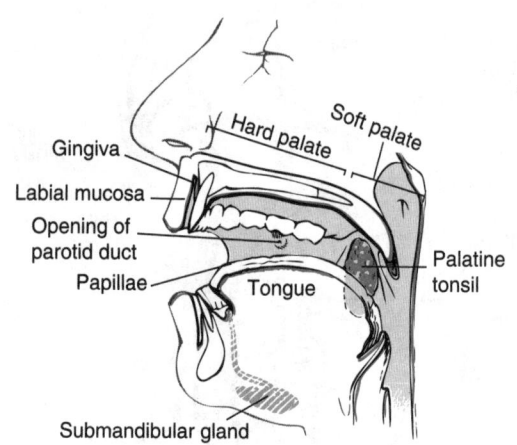

Gingiva
Labial mucosa
Opening of parotid duct
Papillae
Submandibular gland
Hard palate
Soft palate
Tongue
Palatine tonsil

Pancreas

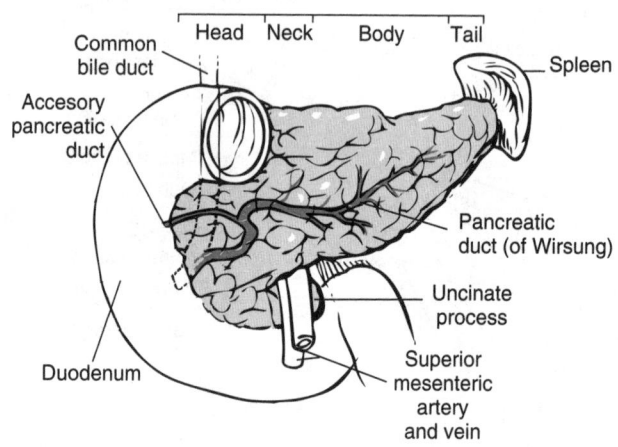

Head Neck Body Tail
Common bile duct
Accesory pancreatic duct
Duodenum
Spleen
Pancreatic duct (of Wirsung)
Uncinate process
Superior mesenteric artery and vein

Gallbladder and Bile Ducts

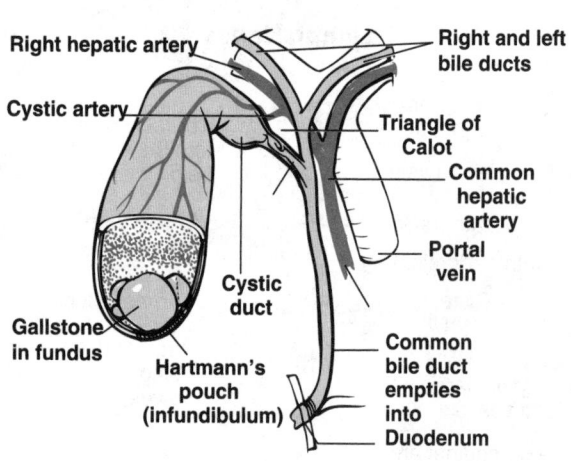

Right hepatic artery
Cystic artery
Gallstone in fundus
Hartmann's pouch (infundibulum)
Cystic duct
Right and left bile ducts
Triangle of Calot
Common hepatic artery
Portal vein
Common bile duct empties into Duodenum

Liver

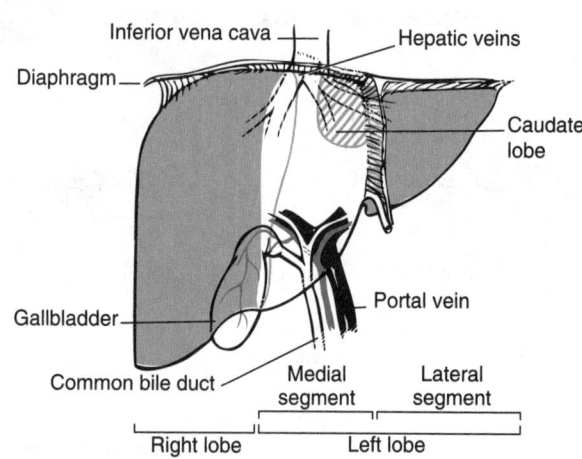

Inferior vena cava
Diaphragm
Gallbladder
Common bile duct
Hepatic veins
Caudate lobe
Portal vein
Medial segment
Lateral segment
Right lobe
Left lobe

Gastrointestinal System

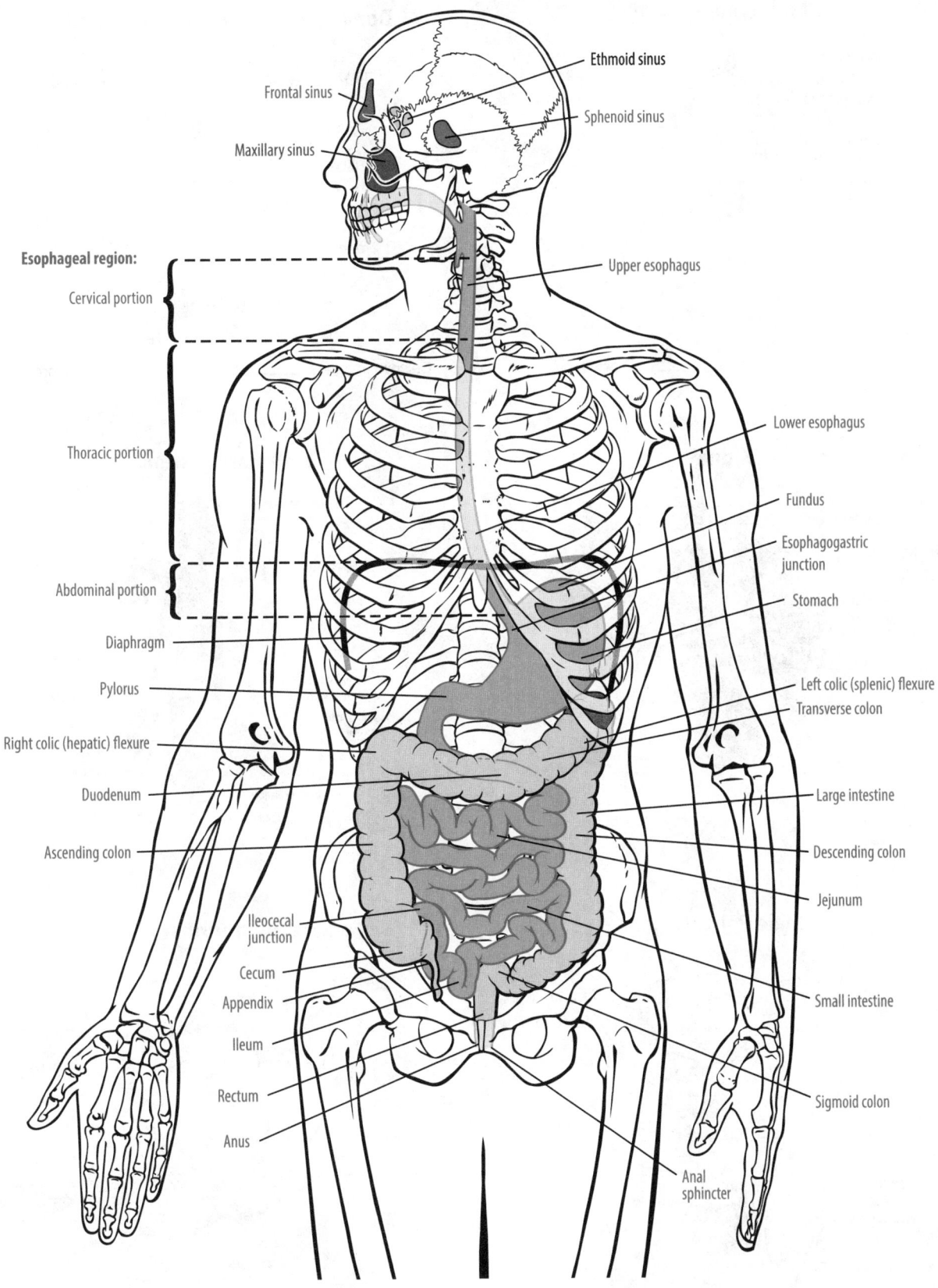

Ethmoid sinus

Frontal sinus

Sphenoid sinus

Maxillary sinus

Esophageal region:

Cervical portion

Upper esophagus

Thoracic portion

Lower esophagus

Fundus

Esophagogastric junction

Abdominal portion

Stomach

Diaphragm

Pylorus

Left colic (splenic) flexure

Transverse colon

Right colic (hepatic) flexure

Duodenum

Large intestine

Ascending colon

Descending colon

Jejunum

Ileocecal junction

Cecum

Appendix

Small intestine

Ileum

Rectum

Sigmoid colon

Anus

Anal sphincter

Endocrine System

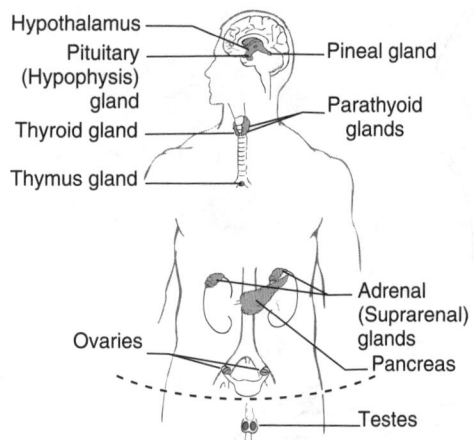

Hypothalamus
Pituitary (Hypophysis) gland
Pineal gland
Thyroid gland
Parathyroid glands
Thymus gland
Ovaries
Adrenal (Suprarenal) glands
Pancreas
Testes

Dorsal View of Parathyroid Gland

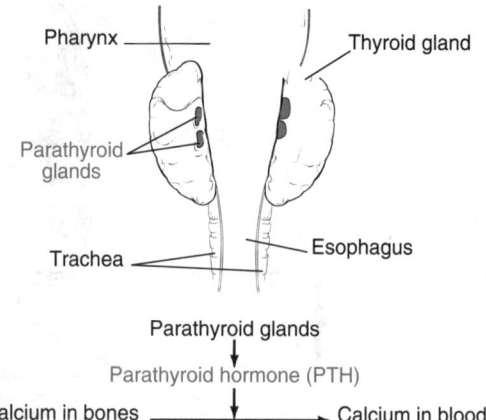

Pharynx
Thyroid gland
Parathyroid glands
Trachea
Esophagus

Parathyroid glands
↓
Parathyroid hormone (PTH)

Calcium in bones ——————→ Calcium in blood

Kidney

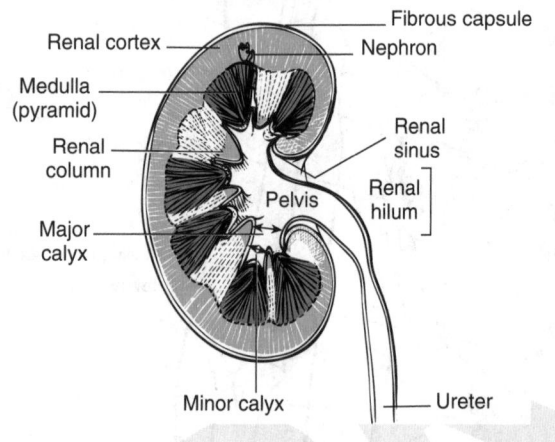

Renal cortex
Fibrous capsule
Nephron
Medulla (pyramid)
Renal sinus
Renal column
Pelvis
Renal hilum
Major calyx
Minor calyx
Ureter

Urinary System

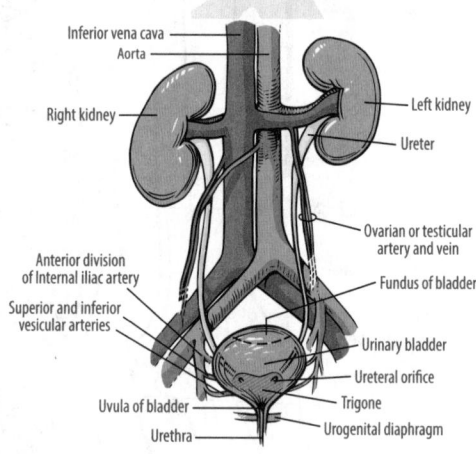

Inferior vena cava
Aorta
Right kidney
Left kidney
Ureter
Ovarian or testicular artery and vein
Anterior division of Internal iliac artery
Fundus of bladder
Superior and inferior vesicular arteries
Urinary bladder
Ureteral orifice
Uvula of bladder
Trigone
Urethra
Urogenital diaphragm

Male Pelvic Organs

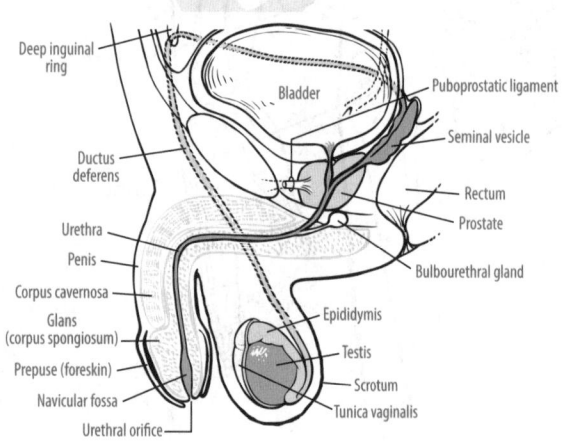

Deep inguinal ring
Bladder
Puboprostatic ligament
Seminal vesicle
Ductus deferens
Rectum
Urethra
Prostate
Penis
Corpus cavernosa
Bulbourethral gland
Glans (corpus spongiosum)
Epididymis
Prepuse (foreskin)
Testis
Navicular fossa
Scrotum
Urethral orifice
Tunica vaginalis

Female Genitourinary System

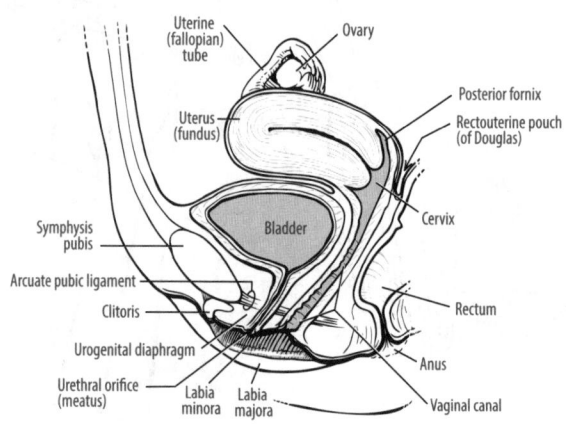

Uterine (fallopian) tube
Ovary
Posterior fornix
Rectouterine pouch (of Douglas)
Uterus (fundus)
Symphysis pubis
Bladder
Cervix
Arcuate pubic ligament
Clitoris
Rectum
Urogenital diaphragm
Anus
Urethral orifice (meatus)
Labia minora
Labia majora
Vaginal canal

Joints

Shoulder (Anterior View)

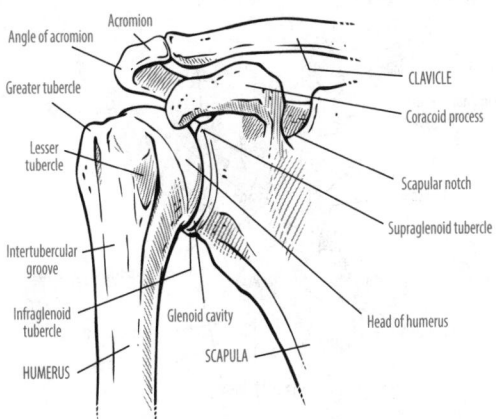

Shoulder (Posterior View)

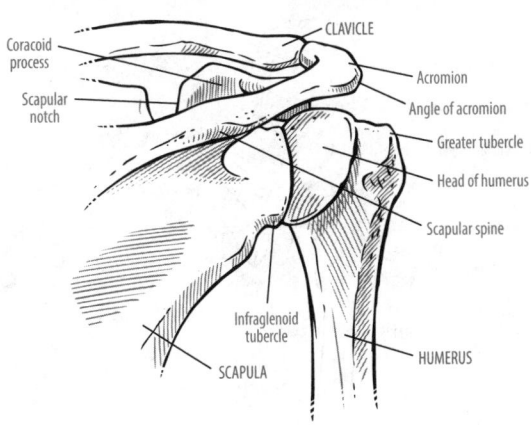

Elbow (Anterior View)

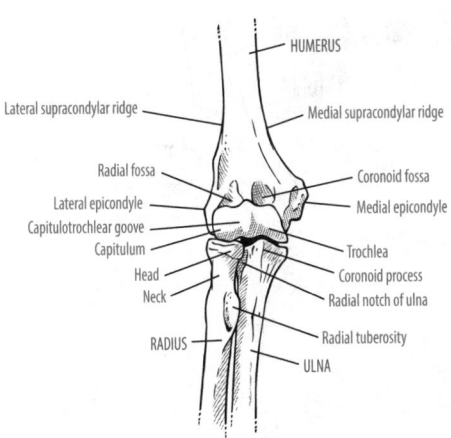

Elbow (Posterior View)

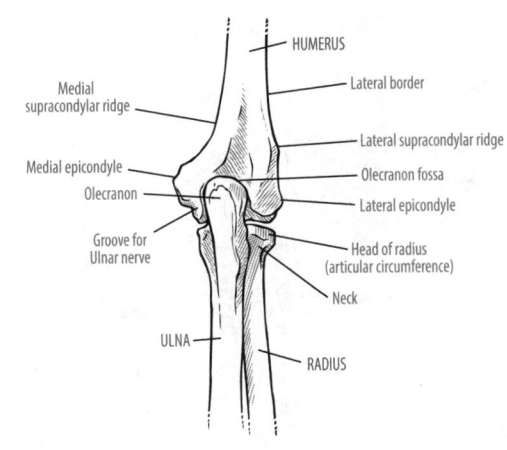

Hand

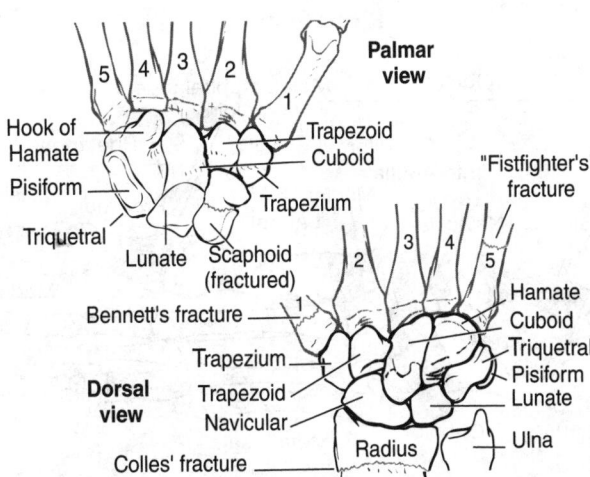

Joints

Hip (Anterior View)

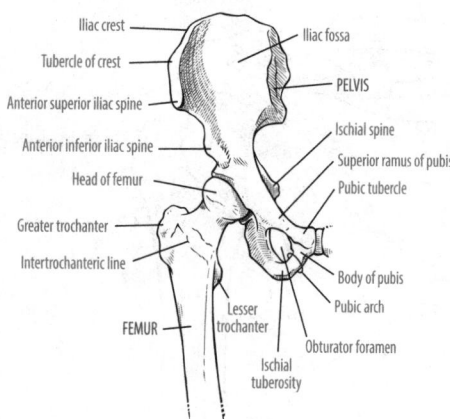

Hip (Posterior View)

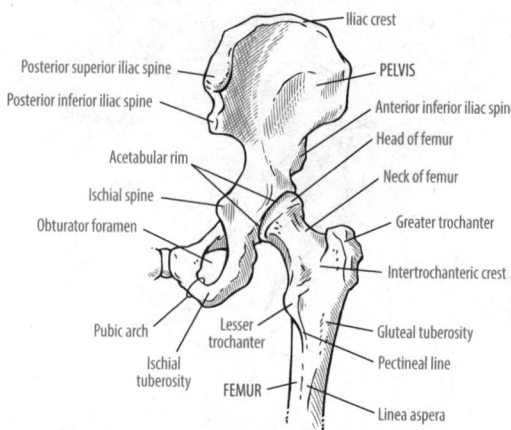

Knee (Anterior View)

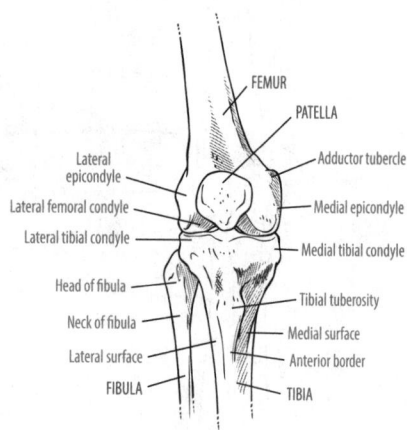

Knee (Posterior View)

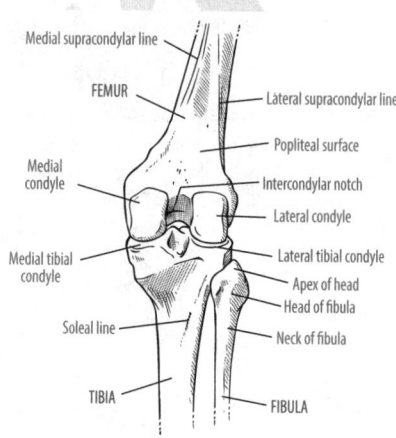

Right Foot

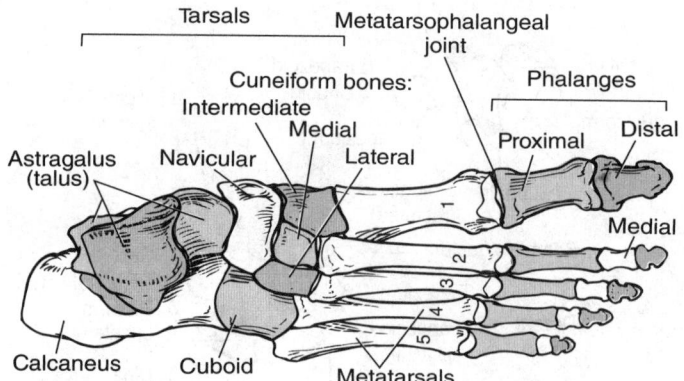

Bones/Joints

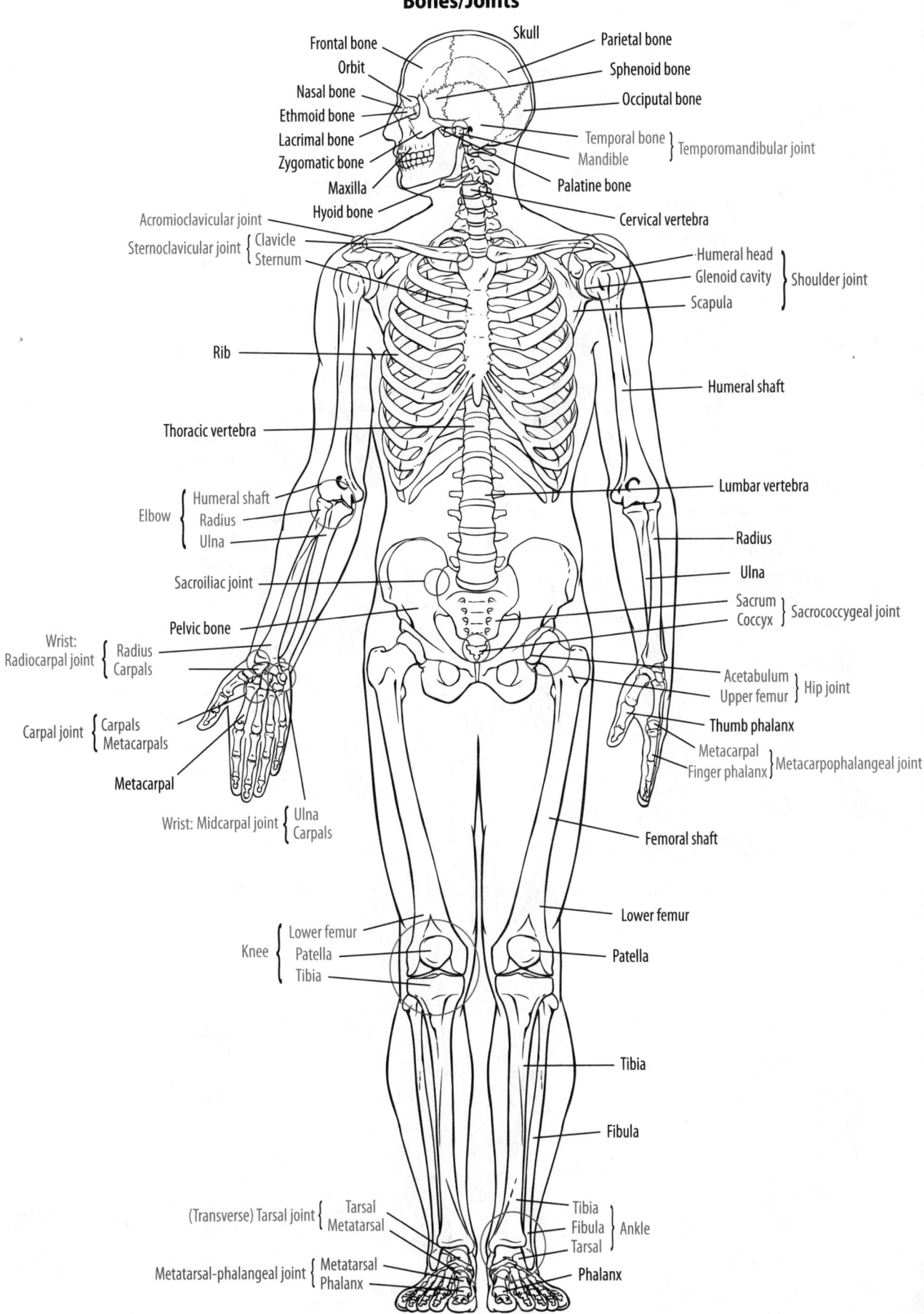

Muscles

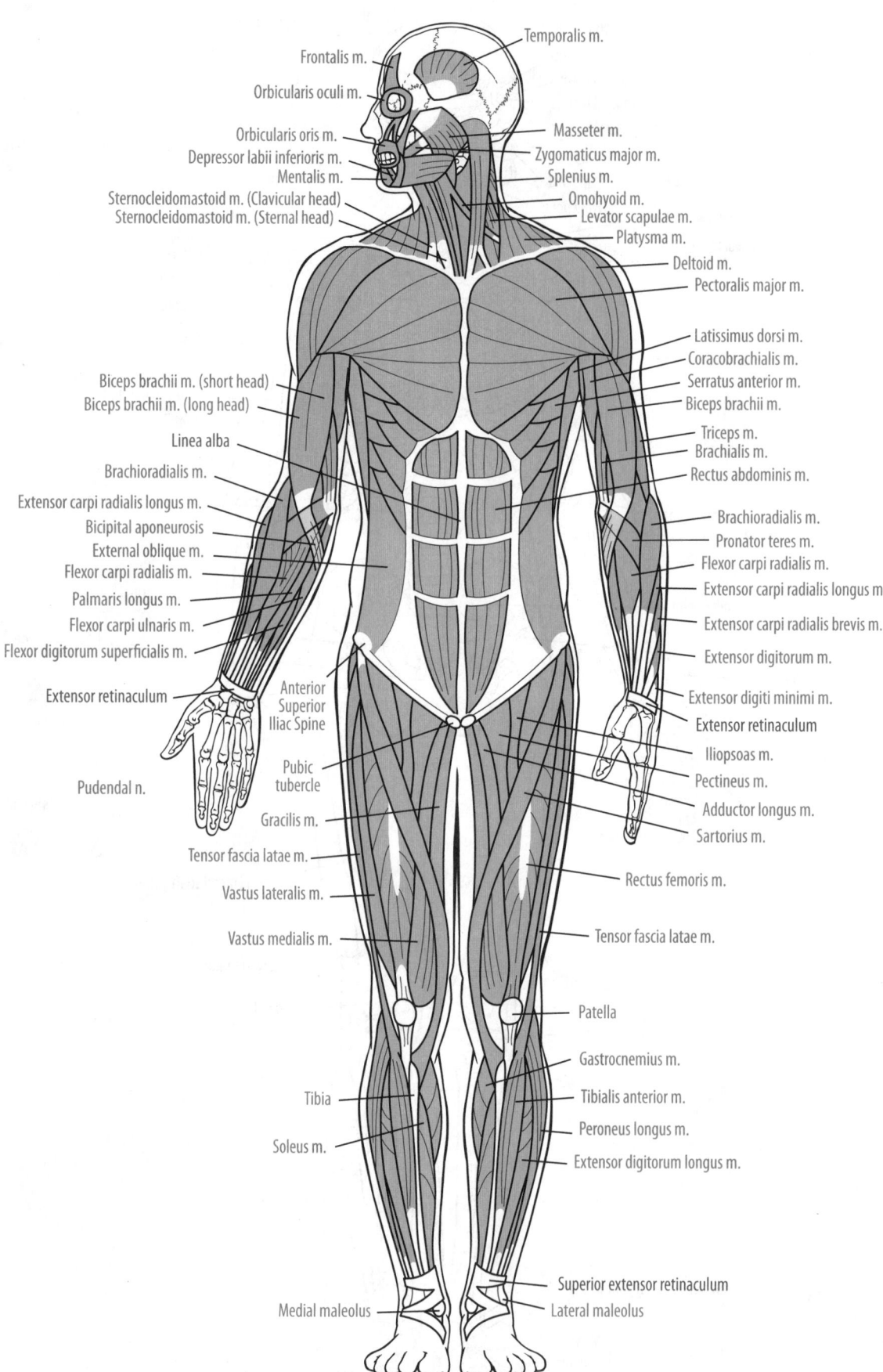

Temporalis m.

Frontalis m.

Orbicularis oculi m.

Orbicularis oris m.

Depressor labii inferioris m.

Mentalis m.

Sternocleidomastoid m. (Clavicular head)

Sternocleidomastoid m. (Sternal head)

Masseter m.

Zygomaticus major m.

Splenius m.

Omohyoid m.

Levator scapulae m.

Platysma m.

Deltoid m.

Pectoralis major m.

Latissimus dorsi m.

Coracobrachialis m.

Serratus anterior m.

Biceps brachii m.

Biceps brachii m. (short head)

Biceps brachii m. (long head)

Linea alba

Brachioradialis m.

Extensor carpi radialis longus m.

Bicipital aponeurosis

External oblique m.

Flexor carpi radialis m.

Palmaris longus m.

Flexor carpi ulnaris m.

Flexor digitorum superficialis m.

Extensor retinaculum

Triceps m.

Brachialis m.

Rectus abdominis m.

Brachioradialis m.

Pronator teres m.

Flexor carpi radialis m.

Extensor carpi radialis longus m.

Extensor carpi radialis brevis m.

Extensor digitorum m.

Extensor digiti minimi m.

Extensor retinaculum

Iliopsoas m.

Pectineus m.

Adductor longus m.

Sartorius m.

Anterior Superior Iliac Spine

Pubic tubercle

Pudendal n.

Gracilis m.

Tensor fascia latae m.

Vastus lateralis m.

Vastus medialis m.

Rectus femoris m.

Tensor fascia latae m.

Patella

Gastrocnemius m.

Tibialis anterior m.

Peroneus longus m.

Extensor digitorum longus m.

Tibia

Soleus m.

Superior extensor retinaculum

Medial maleolus

Lateral maleolus

Notes